a LANGE medical book

Medical Immunology

tenth edition

WITHDRAWN

Edited by

Tristram G. Parslow, MD, PhD
Professor of Pathology and of Microbiology and Immunology
University of California, San Francisco

Daniel P. Stites, MD
Professor of Laboratory Medicine
University of California, San Francisco

Abba I. Terr, MD
Clinical Professor of Medicine
University of California, San Francisco

John B. Imboden, MD
Professor of Medicine
University of California, San Francisco

Lange Medical Books/McGraw-Hill
Medical Publishing Division

Lisbon   London   Madrid   Mexico City   Milan
San Juan   Seoul   Singapore   Sydney   Toronto

McGraw-Hill

*A Division of The **McGraw·Hill** Companies*

Medical Immunology, Tenth Edition

Copyright © 2001 by The **McGraw-Hill Companies,** Inc. All rights reserved. Printed in the United States of America. Except as permitted under the United States Copyright Act of 1976, no part of this publication may be reproduced or distributed in any form or by any means, or stored in a data base or retrieval system, without the prior written permission of the publisher.

Previous editions copyright © 1997, 1993, 1990, by Appleton & Lange

1 2 3 4 5 6 7 8 9 0   DOW/DOW   0 9 8 7 6 5 4 3 2 1

ISBN 0-8385-6300-7
ISSN 0891-2076

This book was set in Times Roman by Rainbow Graphics.
The editors were Janet Foltin, Isabel Nogueira, and Barbara Holton.
The production supervisor was Lisa Mendez.
The cover designer was Mary McKeon.
The illustration manager was Charissa Baker.
The illustrator was Shirley Bortoli.
The index was prepared by Deborah Tourtlotte.

R. R. Donnelley & Sons Company was printer and binder.

This book is printed on acid-free paper.

INTERNATIONAL EDITION ISBN 0-07-112067-X
Copyright © 2001. Exclusive rights by The McGraw-Hill Companies, Inc., for manufacture and export. This book cannot be re-exported from the country to which it is consigned by McGraw-Hill. The International Edition is not available in North America.

Contents

Authors vii

Preface xi

SECTION I. BASIC IMMUNOLOGY _____1

1. Fundamentals of Blood Cell Biology..1
Clifford Lowell, MD, PhD

2. Innate Immunity 19
Tristram G. Parslow, MD, PhD, & Dorothy F. Bainton, MD

3. Lymphocytes & Lymphoid Tissues 40
Tristram G. Parslow, MD, PhD

4. The Immune Response 61
Tristram G. Parslow, MD, PhD

5. Immunogens, Antigens, & Vaccines 72
Tristram G. Parslow, MD, PhD

6. Antigen Presentation & the Major Histocompatibility Complex 82
Frances M. Brodsky, DPhil

7. Immunoglobulins & Immunoglobulin Genes 95
Tristram G. Parslow, MD, PhD

8. B-Cell Development & the Humoral Immune Response 115
Anthony L. DeFranco, PhD

9. T Lymphocytes & Natural Killer Cells 131
John B. Imboden, MD, & William E. Seaman, MD

10. Cytokines 148
Joost J. Oppenheim, MD, & Francis W. Ruscetti, PhD

11. Chemokines 167
Joost J. Oppenheim, MD, & Richard Horuk, PhD

12. Complement & Kinin 175
Kenji M. Cunnion, MD, MPH, Eric Wagner, PhD, & Michael M. Frank, MD

13. Inflammation..189

Abba I. Terr, MD

14. The Mucosal Immune System..204

Warren Strober, MD, & Ivan J. Fuss, MD

SECTION II. IMMUNOLOGIC LABORATORY TESTS   215

15. Clinical Laboratory Methods for Detection of Antigens & Antibodies............................215

Clifford Lowell, MD, PhD

16. Clinical Laboratory Methods for Detection of Cellular Immunity 234

Clifford Lowell, MD, PhD

17. Blood Banking & Immunohematology 250

Maurene Viele, MD, & Elizabeth Donegan, MD

18. Molecular Genetic Techniques for Clinical Analysis of the Immune System 260

Tristram G. Parslow, MD, PhD

19. Histocompatibility Testing 270

Lee Ann Baxter-Lowe, PhD, & Beth W. Colombe, PhD

20. Laboratory Evaluation of Immune Competence.......................................294

Clifford Lowell, MD, PhD

SECTION III. CLINICAL IMMUNOLOGY   299

21. Antibody (B-Cell) Immunodeficiency Disorders 299

Robert L. Roberts, MD, PhD, & E. Richard Stiehm, MD

22. T-Cell Immunodeficiency Disorders 313

Robert L. Roberts, MD, PhD, & E. Richard Stiehm, MD

23. Combined Antibody (B-Cell) & Cellular (T-Cell) Immunodeficiency Disorders 320

E. Richard Stiehm, MD, & Robert L. Roberts, MD, PhD

24. Phagocytic Dysfunction Diseases 333

Robert L. Roberts, MD, PhD, & E. Richard Stiehm, MD

25. Complement Deficiencies 341

Eric Wagner, PhD, & Michael M. Frank, MD

26. The Atopic Diseases 349

Abba I. Terr, MD

27. Anaphylaxis & Urticaria 370

Abba I. Terr, MD

28. Immune-Complex Allergic Diseases 380

Abba I. Terr, MD

29. Cell-Mediated Hypersensitivity Diseases 386

Abba I. Terr, MD

30. Drug Allergy 394

Jeffrey L. Kishiyama, MD, Allyson T. Tevrizian, MD, & Pedro C. Avila, MD

31. Rheumatic Diseases 401

Kenneth E. Sack, MD, & Kenneth H. Fye, MD

32. Endocrine Diseases 422

James R. Baker, Jr., MD

33. Hematologic Diseases 434

J. Vivian Wells, MD, FRACP, FRCPA, & James P. Isbister, FRACP, FRCPA

34. Inflammatory Vasculitides 451

Kenneth H. Fye, MD, FACP, FACR, & Kenneth E. Sack, MD, FACR

35. Gastrointestinal, Hepatobiliary, & Orodental Diseases 460

Warren Strober, MD, Stephen P. James, MD, & John S. Greenspan, BDS, PhD, FRCPath

36. Renal Disease 481

Jean L. Olson, MD

37. Dermatologic Diseases 495

Neil J. Korman, PhD, MD

38. Neurologic Diseases 510

Olaf Stüve, MD, & Scott S. Zamvil, MD, PhD

39. Eye Diseases 527

Mitchell H. Friedlaender, MD, & G. Richard O'Connor, MD

40. Respiratory Diseases 535

John F. Fieselmann, MD, & Hal B. Richerson, MD

41. Reproduction & the Immune System 548

Karen Palmore Beckerman, MD, & Donald J. Dudley, MD

42. Mechanisms of Tumor Immunology 568

Philip D. Greenberg, MD

43. Neoplasms of the Immune System 578

Susan K. Atwater, MD

44. Bacterial Diseases 607

John L. Ryan, MD, PhD, & Steven J. Projan, PhD

45. Viral Infections 617

John Mills, MD

46. AIDS & Other Virus Infections of the Immune System 636

Suzanne Crowe, MD, MBBS, FRACP, & John Mills, MD

47. Fungal Diseases 655

Thomas F. Patterson, MD, & David J. Drutz, MD

48. Parasitic Diseases 673

James H. McKerrow, MD, PhD, & Stephen J. Davies, BVSc, PhD

49. Spirochetal Diseases: Syphilis & Lyme Disease **688**

Linda K. Bockenstedt, MD

SECTION IV. IMMUNOLOGIC THERAPY _____ 699

50. Immunization **699**

Moses Grossman, MD, & Abba I. Terr, MD

51. Allergy Desensitization **714**

Dale T. Umetsu, MD, PhD

52. Clinical Transplantation..**719**

Manikkam Suthanthiran, MD, Peter Stock, MD, Fraser Keith, MD, Charles Linker, MD, & Marvin R. Garovoy, MD

53. Immunosuppressive, Antiinflammatory, & Immunomodulatory Therapy......................................**744**

John B. Imboden, MD, James S. Goodwin, MD, John Davis, Jr. MD, MPH, & David Wofsy, MD

Appendix

The CD Classification of Hematopoietic Cell Surface Markers **761**

Index **763**

Authors

Susan K. Atwater, MD
Staff Pathologist, Kaiser Regional Laboratory, Berkeley, California

Pedro C. Avila, MD
Assistant Clinical Professor, Division of Allergy and Immunology, Departments of Medicine and Pediatrics, University of California, San Francisco

Dorothy F. Bainton, MD
Professor of Pathology, Office of the Vice Chancellor for Academic Affairs, University of California, San Francisco

James R. Baker, Jr., MD
Professor of Medicine; Chief, Division of Allergy; Director, Center for Biologic Nanotechnology, Department of Internal Medicine-Allergy Division, University of Michigan Health System, Ann Arbor

Lee Ann Baxter-Lowe, PhD
Professor in Residence, Department of Surgery, University of California, San Francisco

Karen Palmore Beckerman, MD
Assistant Professor, Department of Obstetrics, Gynecology and Reproductive Sciences, University of California, San Francisco; Director, Bay Area Perinatal AIDS Center, San Francisco

Linda K. Bockenstedt, MD
Harold W. Jockers Associate Professor of Medicine, Yale University School of Medicine, New Haven

Frances M. Brodsky, DPhil
Professor, The G. W. Hooper Foundation, Department of Microbiology and Immunology, School of Medicine; Departments of Biopharmaceutical Sciences and Pharmaceutical Chemistry, School of Pharmacy, University of California, San Francisco

Beth W. Colombe, PhD
Associate Professor, Department of Medicine, Thomas Jefferson University, Philadelphia

Suzanne Crowe, MD, MBBS, FRACP
Professor of Medicine and Infectious Diseases, Monash University; Head, AIDS Pathogenesis Research Unit; Head, Flow Cytometry Laboratory; and Head, Clinical Research Laboratory, Macfarlane Burnet Centre for Medical Research Centre, Victoria, Australia

Kenji M. Cunnion, MD, MPH
Associate Professor, Department of Pediatrics, Duke University Medical Center, Durham, North Carolina

Stephen J. Davies, BVSc, PhD
Postdoctoral Researcher, Tropical Disease Unit, Department of Pathology, University of California, San Francisco

John C. Davis, Jr., MD, MPH, MS
Assistant Professor of Medicine, University of California, San Francisco

Anthony L. DeFranco, PhD
Professor and Chair, Department of Microbiology & Immunology, University of California, San Francisco

Elizabeth Donegan, MD
Assistant Clinical Professor of Anesthesia, Department of Anesthesia, University of California, San Francisco

David J. Drutz, MD
President, Pacific Biopharma Associates, Chapel Hill, North Carolina

Donald J. Dudley, MD
Professor, Department of Obstetrics and Gynecology, University of Texas Health Sciences Center at San Antonio

John F. Fieselmann, MD
Associate Professor, Division of Pulmonary Diseases, Department of Internal Medicine, University of Iowa College of Medicine and University of Iowa Hospitals, Iowa City

Michael M. Frank, MD
Samuel L. Katz Professor and Chairman of Pediatrics; Professor of Immunology and Medicine, Duke University Medical Center, Durham, North Carolina

Mitchell H. Friedlaender, MD
Adjunct Professor, The Scripps Research Institute; Head, Division of Ophthalmology, Scripps Clinic, La Jolla, California

Ivan J. Fuss, MD
Staff Scientist, Mucosal Immunology Section, National Institutes of Health, Bethesda, Maryland

Kenneth H. Fye, MD, FACP, FACR
Clinical Professor of Medicine, Department of Medicine, University of California, San Francisco

Marvin R. Garovoy, MD
Vice President, Clinical and Medical Affairs, XOMA Ltd; Consulting Medical Director, Immunogenetics Transplantation Laboratory, University of California, San Diego; Clinical Consulting Professor of Medicine, Stanford University, Stanford, California

James S. Goodwin, MD
George & Cynthia Mitchell Distinguished Professor; Director, Sealy Center on Aging, The University of Texas Medical Branch, Galveston

Philip D. Greenberg, MD
Professor of Medicine and Immunology, Departments of Medicine and Immunology, University of Washington; Member and Head of Program in Immunology, Fred Hutchinson Cancer Research Center, Seattle

John S. Greenspan, BSc, BDS, PhD, FRCPath
Professor and Chair, Department of Stomatology, University of California, San Francisco

Moses Grossman, MD
Professor Emeritus of Pediatrics, University of California, San Francisco

Richard Horuk, PhD
Principle Scientist, Department of Immunology, Berlex Biosciences, Richmond, Virginia

John B. Imboden, MD
Professor of Medicine, University of California, San Francisco

James P. Isbister, MB, BS, BSc, FRACP, FRCPA
Clinical Professor of Medicine, University of Sydney; Director, Transfusion Medicine, Royal North Shore Hospital of Sydney, Australia

Stephen P. James, MD
Professor of Medicine; Head, Division of Gastroenterology, University of Maryland, Baltimore

Fraser Keith, MD
Associate Clinical Professor, Cardiothoracic Surgery; Director, Cardiopulmonary Transplantation, University of California, San Francisco

Jeffrey L. Kishiyama, MD
Assistant Clinical Professor of Medicine, Department of Medicine, University of California, San Francisco

Neil J. Korman, MD, PhD
Associate Professor of Dermatology, Case Western Reserve University, Cleveland

Charles Linker, MD
Clinical Professor of Medicine; Director, Adult Leukemia and Bone Marrow Transplant Program, University of California, San Francisco

Clifford A. Lowell, MD, PhD
Assistant Professor, Department of Laboratory Medicine, University of California, San Francisco

James H. McKerrow, PhD, MD
Professor, Departments of Pathology and Pharmaceutical Chemistry, University of California, San Francisco

John Mills, MD
Professor, Macfarlane Burnet Centre for Medical Research and the Alfred Hospital, Victoria, Australia

G. Richard O'Connor, MD
Professor Emeritus, Department of Ophthalmology, University of California, San Francisco

Jean L. Olson, MD
Professor of Clinical Pathology, Department of Pathology, University of California, San Francisco

Joost J. Oppenheim, MD
Chief, Laboratory of Immunoregulation, National Cancer Institute, Frederick, Maryland

Tristram G. Parslow, MD, PhD
Professor of Pathology and of Microbiology and Immunology, University of California, San Francisco

Thomas F. Patterson, MD, FACP
Professor of Medicine, Department of Medicine Division of Infectious Diseases, The University of Texas Health Science Center, San Antonio

Steven J. Projan, PhD
Director, Antibacterial Research, Wyeth-Ayerst, Pearl River, New York

Hal B. Richerson, MD
Professor Emeritus, Department of Internal Medicine, University of Iowa, Iowa City

Robert L. Roberts, MD, PhD
Associate Professor, Department of Pediatrics, University of California School of Medicine, Los Angeles

Francis W. Ruscetti, PhD
Chief, Laboratory of Leukocyte Biology, DBS, NCI-FCRDC, Frederick, Maryland

John L. Ryan, MD, PhD
Senior Vice President, Clinical and Research Development, Genetics Institute, Inc., Cambridge, Massachusetts

Kenneth E. Sack, MD
Professor of Clinical Medicine, Department of Medicine, University of California, San Francisco

William E. Seaman, MD
Professor, Department of Medicine, University of California, San Francisco

E. Richard Stiehm, MD
Professor, Department of Pediatrics; Chief, Division of Immunology, Allergy, and Rheumatology, University of California, Los Angeles

Daniel P. Stites, MD
Professor of Laboratory Medicine, University of California, San Francisco

Peter Stock, MD
Associate Professor of Surgery, Division of Transplantation, University of California, San Francisco

Warren Strober, MD
Deputy Chief, LCI, NIAID and Chief, Mucosal Immunity Section, LCI, NIAID, National Institutes of Health, Bethesda, Maryland

Olaf Stüve, MD
Postdoctoral fellow, Department of Neurology, University of California, San Francisco

Manikkam Suthanthiran, MD
Stanton Griffis Distinguished Professor of Medicine, Weill Medical College of Cornell University; Chief, Nephrology and Transplantation Medicine, New York-Presbyterian Hospital, New York Weill Cornell Center; Director, Immunogenetics and Transplantation Center, The Rogosin Institute, New York

Abba I. Terr, MD
Clinical Professor of Medicine, University of California, San Francisco

Allyson T. Tevrizian, MD
Postdoctoral Fellow, Department of Allergy and Immunology, University of California, San Francisco

Dale T. Umetsu, MD, PhD
Professor of Pediatrics; Director, Center for Asthma and Allergic Diseases, Division of Immunology and Allergy, Department of Pediatrics, Stanford University

Maurene K. Viele, MD
Director, Laboratory Medicine Residency Program, Associate Professor of Clinical Lab Medicine and Assistant Director of Blood Bank and Donor Center, University of California, San Francisco

Eric Wagner, PhD
Immunologist, Division of Hematology and Oncology, St. Justine Hospital, Montreal, Canada

J. Vivian Wells, MD, FRACP, FRCPA
Director, Department of Clinical Immunology, Pacific Laboratory Medicine Services, Sydney, Australia

David Wofsy, MD
Professor of Medicine and of Microbiology and Immunology, University of California, San Francisco

Scott S. Zamvil, MD, PhD
Assistant Professor of Neurology, University of California, San Francisco

Preface

With this tenth edition, *Medical Immunology* marks its 25th year as the leading textbook of immunology written specifically for both health care students and practitioners. By combining a state-of-the-art overview of basic immunologic science with a detailed compendium of human immune disorders and their treatments, the book is intended to help busy professionals remain current in this rapidly advancing field. The emphasis is on human immunology throughout, with reference to key experiments or animal models only when they illuminate important aspects of human physiology or pathology. The organization of the book proceeds logically, building from a foundation of cellular and molecular immunology, through clinical laboratory methods, to clinical disorders and their treatment. Every chapter and section emphasizes broad, general principles, but coverage of each specific topic is designed to stand alone for easy reference or review. The authors and editors have made every effort to write in a lucid, readable style without sacrificing important details. As in the past, our goal has been to provide a well-integrated, practical, and accessible survey of basic and clinical immunology.

The book is arranged in four sections that deal, respectively, with Basic Immunology, Immunologic Laboratory Tests, Clinical Immunology, and Immunologic Therapy.

Section I, Basic Immunology, presents a concise but thorough overview of the science of immunology. Designed to be both authoritative and accessible, it can serve as either a textbook for preclinical courses or a timely review and reference book for practicing clinicians, immunologists, and scientists from other fields. The section opens with a chapter that reviews the key molecular processes governing intercellular communication, signal transduction, mitosis, and cell death as they apply to blood cell biology. Chapter 2 then summarizes the humoral and cellular agents of innate immunity, including the vascular inflammatory response and the role of phagocytic cells. This is followed, in Chapters 3 through 9, by progressively sophisticated explorations of acquired immunity, beginning with an introduction to lymphocyte biology and the immune response, followed by discussions of immunogenicity and antigen presentation, and culminating in detailed analyses of B- and T-cell functions. Chapters 10 through 14 then comprehensively review the cytokines, chemokines, inflammatory mediators, and other key aspects of immune function. A list of references is provided at the end of each chapter for readers wishing to explore these subjects further.

Section II, Immunologic Laboratory Tests, serves as a bridge between basic immunology and the clinical sections that follow. The methods used to evaluate various aspects of human immunologic function are described, as are tests that employ immunologic reagents and procedures. Chapter 18 introduces the emerging field of molecular diagnostics in immunology, and other chapters explore the important areas of blood banking, histocompatibility, and immunohematology. A succinct chapter on the evaluation of immune competence in patients brings this section to a close.

Section III, Clinical Immunology, surveys broad categories of human immunologic diseases, organizing them either by organ systems or by common mechanisms of pathogenesis. Chapters 21 through 25 focus on congenital disorders of immunity, highlighting the latest information about their underlying genetic defects. The allergic disorders are reviewed authoritatively in Chapters 26 through 30, followed by detailed coverage of rheumatic disorders in Chapter 31, of major organ system pathologies in Chapters 32 through 41, and of neoplastic diseases in Chapters 42 and 43. The section closes with a series of six chapters on infectious diseases, including a thorough and timely discussion of the acquired immune deficiency syndrome (AIDS).

Section IV, Immunologic Therapy, reviews immunization, allergy desensitization, and treatment modalities currently used in transplantation and immunologic diseases. This section also discusses the available strategies for manipulating immune function, particularly in clinical transplantation or for treating autoimmunity.

New features included in this tenth edition:

- The section on basic immunology has been updated throughout and now includes expanded coverage of innate immunity, apoptosis, dendritic cells, natural killer cells, and other key topics; a new chapter devoted entirely to the chemokines; and the most comprehensive, authoritative review of cytokines available in a textbook of this kind.
- In the section on clinical laboratory methodology, the chapters covering clinical tests for humoral immunity, cell-mediated immunity, histocompatibility, and immunocompetence have each been rewritten by new expert authors, with an emphasis on the molecular diagnostic assays now in widespread clinical use.
- All of the chapters in the section on Clinical Immunology have been revised, streamlined, and updated, many of them under the guidance of a new editor, Dr. John Imboden. The chapters on vasculitis, renal disease, and spirochetal infections have been rewritten by new authors who are experts in these fields.
- Coverage of AIDS, Lyme disease, asthma, reproductive disorders, inflammatory bowel disease, neurologic syndromes, and other important clinical entities have been expanded and updated to reflect the latest research on pathogenesis and treatment.
- Discussions of treatment options incorporate the newest drugs and therapeutic regimens, immunization protocols, immunosuppressive therapies, and approaches to allergy desensitization.
- The Appendix includes a concise table listing the most important hematopoietic cell-surface markers (the CD classification) encountered in clinical medicine or research.

ACKNOWLEDGMENTS

The editors are sincerely grateful to Janet Foltin for her wise counsel and kind indulgence during the preparation of this edition. The book has also benefited immeasurably from the meticulous and painstaking copyediting by Linda Davoli and from the artistry of Charissa Baker. We also thank Dr. Steve Rosen for his expert advice regarding some of the material in Section I.

Recommendations about diagnosis and treatment of disease are based on the best scientific and clinical information currently available. These are intended, however, as guidance to the clinician and not necessarily as recommendations for specific cases. Furthermore, we recognize that we may have overlooked errors despite our best efforts. We would be grateful if our readers would point these out so that they may be corrected in the next edition.

Tristram G. Parslow, MD, PhD
Daniel P. Stites, MD
Abba I. Terr, MD
John B. Imboden, MD

San Francisco
March 2001

Section I.
Basic Immunology

Fundamentals of Blood Cell Biology

1

Clifford Lowell, MD, PhD

Immunology is the study of the ways in which the body defends itself from infectious agents and other foreign substances in its environment. Broadly defined, the field encompasses many layers of defense, including physical barriers like the skin, protective chemical substances in the blood and tissue fluids, and the physiologic reactions of tissues to injury or infection. But by far the most elaborate, dynamic, and effective defense strategies are carried out by cells that have evolved specialized abilities to recognize and eliminate potentially injurious substances. Some of these defensive cells circulate continually through the body in search of foreign invaders; others are stationary sentinels that lie in wait in solid tissues or at body surfaces. Because of their central roles in host defense, these cells are the major focus of contemporary immunology and are the principal subjects of this book.

Virtually all of the specialized defensive cells have two things in common: They all spend at least part of their lives in the bloodstream, and they are all ultimately derived from cells produced in the bone marrow. We therefore begin, in this chapter, by considering the processes involved in cell formation and maturation in the bone marrow—one of the most prolific sites of cell replication in the human body and one that is indispensable for health and even for survival. Investigating these processes provides an opportunity to introduce many of the individual cell types involved in host defense, as well as several regulatory factors that govern their lives. We will also examine the fundamental molecular mechanisms by which cells receive signals from their environments and how these signals control whether cells proliferate, migrate, and carry out specific functions, and even when they die.

HEMATOPOIESIS

Origins of Cells in the Blood & Bone Marrow

The process by which blood cells grow, divide, and differentiate in the bone marrow is called **hematopoiesis.** Three general classes of cells are produced: (1) red blood cells (erythrocytes), responsible for oxygen transport; (2) platelets, responsible for the control of bleeding; and (3) white blood cells **(leukocytes),** the vast majority of which are involved in host defense. All three classes are ultimately derived from a pool of pluripotent **hematopoietic stem cells (HSCs),** which reside in the marrow and have the unique ability to give rise to all of the different mature blood cell types, under the appropriate conditions. The HSCs are **self-renewing** cells: When they proliferate, at least some of their daughter cells remain as HSCs, so that the pool of stem cells does not become depleted.

The other daughters of HSCs, however, can each commit to any of several alternative differentiation pathways that lead to the production of one or more specific types of blood cells (Figure 1–1). A typical pathway involves several cycles of cell division (five or more) and proceeds in stages, with cells at each stage progressively acquiring features of one particular mature cell type while losing the capacity to form any others. Because progression along these pathways is coupled to cell division, the more mature forms greatly outnumber their less differentiated precursors. As the cells differentiate, however, their capacity for replication and self-renewal declines. Indeed, most types of hematopoietic cells lose replicative capacity altogether by the time they are fully mature, and so are said to be **terminally differentiated.** Thus, in general, the less differentiated cells in a given pathway are rare but replicate actively, whereas the mature cells are more numerous but mitotically inert.

The progeny of HSCs initially commit to one of three main alternative differentiation pathways (or **lineages**) that yield erythrocytes, lymphocytes, or myeloid cells, respectively. The most primitive cells in each lineage, called **lineage-committed progenitors,** cannot be identified morphologically; however, their existence and some of their properties can be inferred from their ability to generate particular types of mature cells in biologic assay systems (see later discussion). Erythrocyte development is outside the scope of this book and will not be considered further, but both myeloid cells and lymphocytes are critical to host defense. The mature cells of the myeloid lineage* include neutrophils, monocytes, mast cells, eosinophils, basophils, and megakaryocytes (the cells that produce platelets). All these cells descend from a common myeloid progenitor through a series of intermediate stages, only one of which—the granulocyte–monocyte progenitor, a precursor to both neutrophils and monocytes—is shown in Figure 1–1. Mature cells of the lymphocyte lineage include B lymphocytes, T lymphocytes, and possibly also natural killer (NK) cells; the development and functions of these three cell types is discussed in great detail in later chapters. Altogether, the myeloid and lymphocyte lineages account for roughly 60% and 15%, respectively, of all marrow cells; the remainder are erythroid precursors.

Vast numbers of mature blood cells are produced daily in the marrow, but the rate of production of each cell type is precisely controlled and responsive to physiologic demands. For example, production of leukocytes often increases markedly during systemic infections, whereas red cell production can rise as a reaction to anemia. In addition, many mature leukocytes, particularly neutrophils, are stored in the marrow before being released into the bloodstream. This storage pool, which normally accounts for 10–20% of all marrow cells, provides a reservoir of mature defensive cells that can be mobilized rapidly in times of need. Thus, bone marrow hematopoiesis is precisely controlled at several levels in order to (1) maintain an available pool of HSCs; (2) regulate the commitment, proliferation, and differentiation of cells at all stages of each hematopoietic pathway; and (3) modulate the activity of each pathway in response to physiologic demands. As we shall see, much of this regulation is achieved through physical interactions of the hematopoietic cells with other cells and with soluble factors in the surrounding tissues.

---

* The term *myeloid* means "of the bone marrow." As a group, cells of the myeloid lineage are the most abundant cells in the marrow.

Ontogeny of Hematopoiesis

HSCs arise in the mesoderm of the yolk sac during the first weeks of embryonic life (Figure 1–2). Within 2 months following conception, most HSCs have migrated to the fetal liver, and it is here that the bulk of hematopoiesis occurs during fetal development. Most embryonic and fetal hematopoiesis is devoted to the production of red cells; platelet production first becomes apparent at 3 months of gestation, and leukocytes do not appear until the fifth month. Later in gestation, HSCs begin to colonize the developing bone marrow cavities throughout the skeleton, which contain a network of epithelial cells (called the **bone marrow stroma**) that provide the necessary environment for growth and differentiation of HSC and their progeny. By birth, virtually all of the marrow space is occupied by developing hematopoietic cells, giving the newborn child about the same hematopoietic capacity as his or her adult parents. Hematopoietic activity in the long bones then declines with age, so that after puberty it is largely confined to the axial skeleton—the pelvis, sternum, ribs, vertebrae, and skull. If the bone marrow is injured by infection or malignancy, however, hematopoiesis can resume in the liver and spleen of an adult to maintain the supply of blood cells.

Hematopoietic Cell Growth & Differentiation

Our understanding of hematopoiesis has advanced greatly in recent years with the isolation and characterization of HSCs and the identification of many of the factors that influence the production and differentiation of lineage-committed progenitors (Figure 1–3). HSCs are defined by their abilities to self-renew throughout life and to give rise to committed progenitors that can differentiate along all of the possible hematopoietic lineages. They were first purified from mice as a tiny subpopulation of marrow cells that could completely reconstitute the hematopoietic systems of other mice, whose own marrows had been destroyed by inherited mutations or by radiation. Although similar experiments cannot, of course, be done with human beings, presumptive human HSCs have since been identified that, under certain conditions, are able to repopulate the marrows of mice.

Human HSCs express a characteristic surface protein, **CD34.*** Though CD34 is not unique to HSCs (it

---

* Many of the cell surface proteins important to immunology are referred to by the initials **CD** (which stand for **cluster of differentiation**) followed by a unique identifying number. This CD system of nomenclature was originally developed for membrane proteins or protein complexes that could be identified by their physical properties (eg, molecular weight) or by other means, but whose biologic functions had not yet been determined. Most CD proteins are not related to one another, either structurally or functionally. The CD nomenclature is most often used for proteins expressed on hematopoietic cells, although many are also expressed on one or more nonhematopoietic cell types. A partial listing of CD proteins appears in the Appendix.

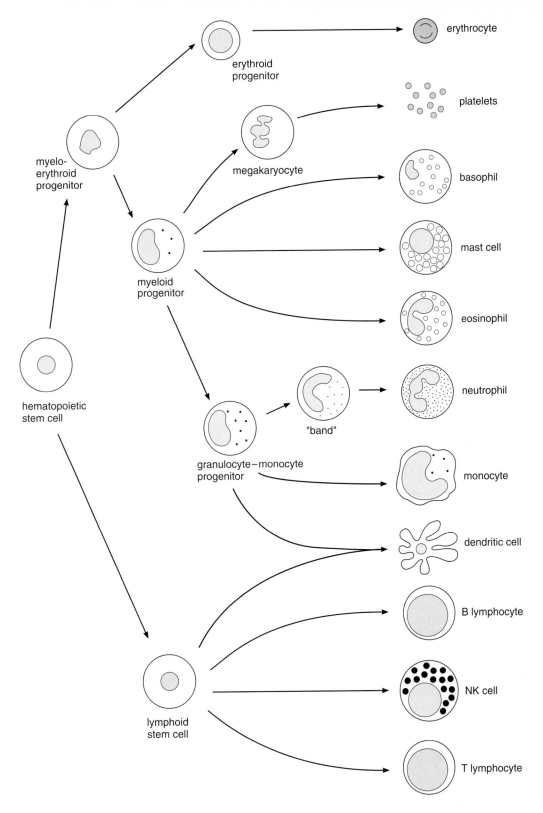

Figure 1–1. Schematic overview of hematopoiesis, emphasizing the erythroid, myeloid, and lymphoid pathways. This highly simplified depiction omits many recognized intermediate cell types in each pathway. All of the cells shown here develop to maturity in the bone marrow, except T lymphocytes, which develop from marrow-derived progenitors that migrate to the thymus (see Chapter 3). A common lymphoid stem cell serves as the progenitor of T and B lymphocytes and of natural killer (NK) cells. Dendritic cells arise from both the myeloid and lymphoid lineages.

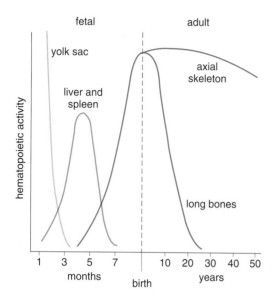

Figure 1–2. Tissue localization of hematopoiesis at various phases of prenatal and postnatal development in humans.

CD34⁺CD38⁻. HSCs make up only 0.01% of total marrow cells in adults but are more abundant in fetal liver and in umbilical cord blood. In adults, HSCs can be induced to leave the bone marrow and enter the peripheral circulation by treatment with certain hormones; these "mobilized" peripheral blood HSCs are being extensively studied for use in clinical bone marrow transplantation.

HSCs are small, morphologically nondescript cells with round nuclei and scant cytoplasm. They vary markedly in their ability to proliferate and differentiate into mature hematopoietic cells (Figure 1–4). At any given moment, about 25% are actively progressing through mitosis, but at varying rates—adult marrow HSCs proliferate slowly, fetal liver HSCs do so rapidly. The entire human HSC pool probably turns over every several months. Since the total number of HSCs in the body normally remains constant, some portion of their daughter cells must undergo differentiation into the various mature cell types. The factors that control this lineage commitment "decision" for any individual HSC are unknown. It is clear, however, that both the self-replication of HSCs and their ability to produce differentiated cells depend on hormonal growth factors called **cytokines.** The cytokines are a diverse group of polypeptides, secreted by both hematopoietic and nonhematopoietic cells. Many cytokines have specific effects on the growth, differentiation, survival, or function of blood cells. There are several different classes of cytokines (see Chapter 10); most of those known to regulate hematopoiesis belong to subgroups called the **colony-**

is also expressed on vascular endothelial cells) and its function is unknown (it is probably involved in cell–cell adhesion), it is useful in recognizing and isolating HSCs. Purified HSCs also generally lack surface proteins, such as CD38, that are found on mature marrow cells; hence HSCs can be said to be

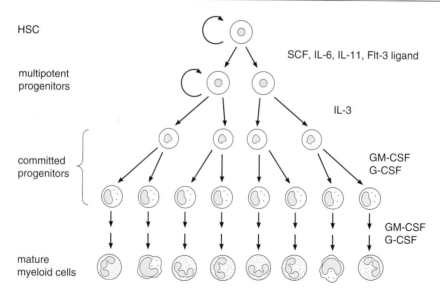

Figure 1–3. Proliferation and differentiation of cells in the myeloid lineage. Early cells are capable of self-renewal and proliferation; later cells are committed to differentiation only. Cytokines required for survival and progression through each stage are indicated at the right. *Abbreviations:* HSC = hematopoietic stem cell; SCF = stem cell factor; IL = interleukin; G-CSF = granulocyte colony-stimulating factor; GM-CSF = granulocyte–monocyte colony-stimulating factor.

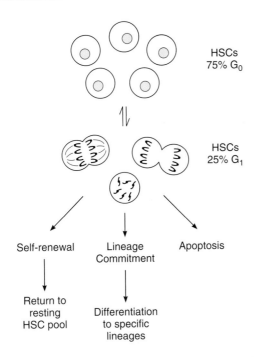

Figure 1–4. Growth and differentiation of hematopoietic stem cells (HSCs). The cells are usually mitotically inactive (ie, they are in the G_0 phase of the cell cycle), but enter mitosis (through the G_1 phase) at some frequency that can be influenced by cytokines or other environmental stimuli. Cycling cells have three potential fates: self-replication, differentiation, or death (apoptosis). In mice, roughly 25% of HSCs are normally in cell cycle at any given moment. Each spends approximately 3–6 days in cycle, so that the entire HSC population goes through the cell cycle every 60 days. The percentages of cycling cells that self-renew, differentiate, or die are not known.

stimulating factors (**CSFs**) or the **interleukins.** Cytokines that can affect HSCs include stem cell growth factor (SCF), Flt3-ligand, interleukin-6 (IL-6), and interleukin-11 (IL-11). These and other cytokines are produced by bone marrow stromal and hematopoietic cells in response to environmental stimuli (eg, anemia or infection) to regulate HSC proliferation and differentiation. Besides self-replication or lineage commitment (differentiation), HSCs have a third option to maintain constant total numbers. This option—cellular suicide, or apoptosis—is available to all types of hematopoietic cells, and will be discussed later on.

A more complete understanding of HSC biology would be extremely valuable in clinical medicine. Many disease states (eg, leukemia or the acquired immune deficiency syndrome) involve injury to the bone marrow and alterations in HSC homeostasis, as do many types of cancer chemotherapy. Moreover, the ability to introduce new genes permanently into HSCs—though not practical at the moment—could

eventually provide a means for curing a host of inherited (genetic) disorders. Indeed, the hope of developing such **gene therapy** is driving much of current research into the biology of HSCs.

Lineage-committed progenitors, the offspring of HSCs, are defined as those cells whose progeny include some, but not all, mature blood cell types. They are often subclassified as either "fully committed progenitors," which give rise to only one particular cell type, or "multipotent progenitors," which can generate two or more. An example of the latter is the granulocyte–monocyte progenitor, which gives rise to both neutrophils and monocytes (see Figure 1–1). Because such progenitors grow readily in tissue culture, they are comparatively easy to study experimentally, and it is from such cultures that most of our knowledge of human progenitor cells has been gained. For example, when a mixed population of bone marrow cells is cultured as a suspension in agar or some other semisolid medium, in the presence of specific cytokines, specific progenitors proliferate and differentiate to produce small multicellular colonies composed of one or more mature cell types. Such experiments are called *colony-forming assays,* and the progenitors themselves are often referred to as **colony-forming units (CFUs).** Using these assays, individual cytokines have been shown to promote the growth of specific types of progenitors: For example, a CSF called erythropoietin (EPO) enhances production of erythrocyte colonies; interleukin-5 (IL-5) favors colonies of eosinophils; and granulocyte–monocyte colony-stimulating factor (GM-CSF) promotes colonies containing both neutrophils and macrophages (from either HSCs or mixed marrow populations).

Progenitors of all types together account for less than 1% of marrow cells, and fully committed progenitors are more abundant than the multipotent forms. Although comparatively rare, these marrow progenitors are the cells that give rise to the various common forms of cancer known as **leukemias**—malignant populations of leukocytes, usually from a particular hematopoietic lineage—that flood the marrow cavities and peripheral blood and that result from excessive proliferation of the progeny from a single founder cell. Most mature cell types in the marrow, despite their greater abundance, cannot give rise to leukemias, in part because they have lost the ability to proliferate.

CELLULAR INTERACTIONS IN THE BONE MARROW

Although it is commonly imagined that hematopoiesis takes place in a liquid environment resembling the blood, with progenitors responding mainly to soluble hormone-like cytokines, this is in fact not the case at all. It is much more accurate to think of the bone marrow as a solid tissue in which different types of hematopoietic cells develop in physically different locations. These microenvironments are visible in histologic sections of bone marrow, which reveal a patchwork of microscopic foci, each devoted to the production of a particular cell type (Figure 1–5). The bone marrow microenvironment is set up and maintained by bone marrow stromal cells. Within each microenvironment, contact of cells with one another or with proteins and other substances that make up the **extracellular matrix (ECM)** greatly facilitates cell division and differentiation.

The physiology of these marrow microenvironments can be studied in artificial systems, called long-term bone marrow cultures (LTBMCs), in which hematopoietic progenitor cells are grown in combination with marrow stromal cells, ECM components, and other factors. The conditions of these cultures can be optimized to support sustained growth and differentiation of either myeloid or lymphoid cells. Studies of such cultures have demonstrated that hematopoiesis depends not only on specific cytokines but also on a group of cell surface macromolecules, known as **adhesion molecules,** that allow different cell types to adhere stably to one another or to the ECM. Among the primary types of adhesive molecules on hematopoietic progenitor cells are the integrins, the selectins, and various forms of CD44. Each of these classes recognizes and binds specific ligands that are present either on the bone marrow stromal cells or in the ECM (Table 1–1).

The **integrins** are a group of heterodimeric proteins, each composed of α-chain and β-chain polypeptides. At least 17 different integrin α chains and eight β chains exist, and these can associate in various combinations to produce dimers with distinct binding properties that are expressed on different cell types. For example, hematopoietic progenitors express primarily α4β1 and α5β1 dimers. The integrins bind a variety of ECM proteins, as well as nonintegrin adhesion molecules, such as vascular cell adhesion molecule 1 (**VCAM-1**) found on the stromal cell surface. These interactions allow progenitors to bind tightly to the marrow stroma and are responsible for sequestering progenitor cells in the appropriate marrow microenvironments. When baboons are injected with reagents that interfere with binding by the integrin β1 chain, for example, large numbers of hematopoietic progenitors are released from the marrow into the peripheral circulation. Contact of an integrin with its ligand also transmits a signal into the integrin-expressing cell, and this signal can directly stimulate its growth or other activities. Consequently, reagents that block ligand binding by integrin α4 or β1 chains in vitro cause progenitors not only to dissociate from the stroma but also to cease proliferation. Beta1 integrins have also been implicated in directing migration of HSCs from the yolk sac

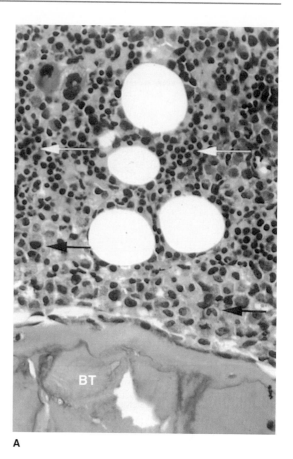

A

Figure 1–5. Bone marrow microenvironments. **A:** Regional variations in hematopoietic activity as demonstrated by histology. This section through a portion of a marrow cavity, stained with hematoxylin and eosin, shows a zone of predominantly myeloid cells *(black arrows)* that is flanked on one side by a bone trabeculum (BT), and on the other by a zone of predominantly erythroid cells *(white arrows).* (Contributed by Susan Atwater.) *(Continued)*

mesenchyme into the fetal liver during embryogenesis and, subsequently, of HSCs from the fetal liver to the bone marrow. The **selectins** are a class of adhesion proteins that recognize specific oligosaccharide residues displayed on cell surface glycoproteins called mucins. The term **mucin** refers to any heavily glycosylated protein composed of an elongated polypeptide backbone containing many serine and threonine residues that serve as attachment sites for carbohydrate sidechains. Selectins derive their name from the term **lectin,** which refers to any protein that binds specific sugar groups; hence, the selectins are only one of many different types of lectin proteins. The selectins bind primarily to sugar residues in the mucin sidechains, though features of the polypeptide backbone may also contribute to recognition. One ex-

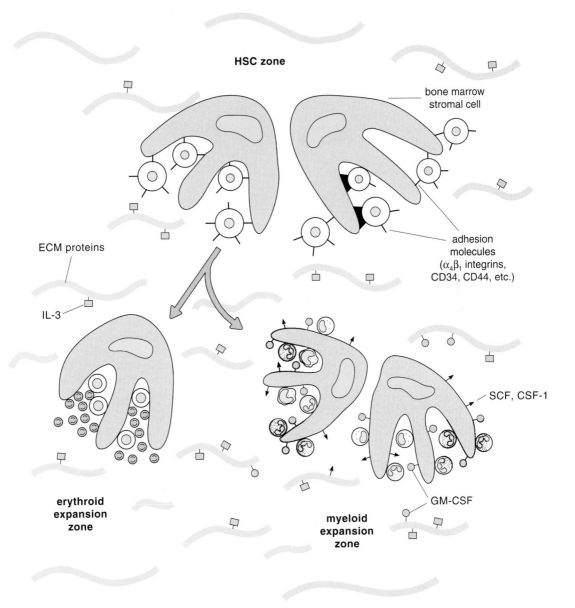

HSC zone

bone marrow
stromal cell

ECM proteins

IL-3

adhesion
molecules
($\alpha_4\beta_1$ integrins,
CD34, CD44, etc.)

SCF, CSF-1

GM-CSF

**erythroid
expansion
zone**

**myeloid
expansion
zone**

Figure 1–5 *(Continued).* **B:** Model for the establishment of marrow microenvironments. Self-renewing pluripotent hematopoietic stem cells (HSC), as well as lineage-committed progenitors, are localized to marrow niches based on the expression of specific surface adhesion molecules, such as integrins, CD34, and CD44. Different regions of the marrow serve as niches for myeloid or erythroid cell expansion based on expression of cell surface-bound cytokines (eg, colony-stimulating factor 1 [CSF-1] or stem cell factor 1 [SCF-1]) on stromal cells or because of localized deposition of such cytokines in the extracellular matrix (ECM).

ample of a mucin is the HSC surface marker CD34, which serves as a major ligand for L-selectin, a selectin found on all mature leukocytes. (As previously mentioned, CD34 is found on certain nonhematopoietic cells, including stroma and vascular endothelium, as well as on HSCs.) Marrow progenitor cells and stroma express various combinations of selectins and mucins, which mediate cell–cell interactions between them. The importance of these carbohydrate-mediated interactions is illustrated by the finding that addition of synthetic oligosaccharides (which would competitively interfere with binding) to LTBMCs strongly inhibits hematopoietic cell division and differentiation.

Table 1–1. Selected adhesion proteins and their ligands.

Adhesion Protein	Principal Ligands
Integrins	ECM and cell surface proteins.
β1 family	
α1β1, α2β1, α6β1	Collagens, laminin.
α4β1, α5β1	Fibronectin, collagen, laminin, VCAM-1.
β2 family	
αLβ2	Fibrinogen, ICAM-1, ICAM-2.
αMβ2	Fibrinogen, ICAM-1, complement protein C3b.
αXβ2	Fibrinogen.
β3 family	
αvβ3	Vitronectin, thrombospondin, osteopontin.
Selectins[a]	Carbohydrate residues found on various cell surface mucins and other macromolecules.
L-selectin	CD34, GlyCAM-1, MAdCAM-1, and others.
E-selectin	CLA[b]
P-selectin	PSGL-1.
CD44[c]	Hyaluronic acid, collagen, fibronectin.

Abbreviations: ECM = extracellular matrix; VCAM-1 = vascular cell adhesion molecule 1; ICAM-1, -2 = intracellular adhesion molecules 1 and 2; GlyCAM-1 = glycosylated cell adhesion molecule 1; PSGL-1 = P-selectin glycoprotein ligand 1.
[a] The selectin ligands listed here are the major mucins and other macromolecules that carry the specific carbohydrate modifications recognized by each selectin and that serve as its main physiologic ligands in vivo.
[b] CLA denotes an incompletely characterized family of surface proteins on cutaneous lymphocytes.
[c] Multiple isoforms of CD44, with varying affinities for different ligands, are produced by alternative mRNA splicing.

The cell surface protein **CD44** can exist in a variety of alternative forms that differ in their extracellular ligand-binding regions (and hence in their binding specificities) as a result of alternative RNA splicing.

Hematopoietic progenitor cells express the most truncated form of CD44, which binds hyaluronic acid, an abundant glycosaminoglycan found in the ECM. Compounds that interfere with this binding block hematopoietic cell proliferation in LTBMCs.

Thus, a wide variety of adhesive interactions, both of the cell-cell and cell-ECM variety, are critical for hematopoiesis. Abnormal interactions between hematopoietic progenitors and ECM components or stromal cells can be observed in many diseases that involve abnormal hematopoiesis. For example, the malignant cells in certain types of leukemias, particularly those arising from myeloid cells, often show significantly reduced adhesion to ECM proteins and stromal cells. Conversely, stromal cells from patients with leukemia often produce abnormal cytokines and ECM protein components.

As will be discussed in Chapters 2 and 3, all of these adhesions molecules—selectins, integrins, and CD44—also help guide the migration of mature hematopoietic cells through the body.

Besides providing the appropriate adhesive and ECM molecules for progenitor cells, bone marrow stromal cells also synthesize and express a host of cytokines needed for hematopoietic proliferation (Table 1–2). Some of these are not only secreted but also expressed as membrane-bound proteins that remain attached to the surface of the stromal cell. Much evidence suggests that these membrane-bound cytokines may have much greater biologic activity on hematopoietic progenitors than the secreted forms, presumably because the effective concentration of the cytokine is much higher on the stromal cell surface. In addition, the strong adhesive contacts between the two cell types prolong the much weaker interaction between a membrane-bound cytokine and its receptor on the hematopoietic cell. In a similar fashion, IL-3, GM-CSF, and several other cytokines

Table 1–2. Major lineage-specific effects of the hematopoietic cytokines.[a]

Progenitors Affected	Cytokine	Principal Source
Multilineage		
Erythroid, myeloid, megakaryocyte	IL-3	Activated T lymphocytes.
Myeloid, megakaryocyte	GM-CSF	Stromal cells, activated macrophages.
Lineage-Restricted		
Granulocyte	G-CSF	Stromal cells, activated macrophages.
Monocyte	M-CSF (= CSF-1)	Stromal cells, endothelial cells, activated macrophages.
Eosinophils	IL-5	Activated T lymphocytes, mast cells.
Erythroid	EPO	Kidney epithelium.
Megakaryocyte	TPO	Stromal cells, liver
Lymphoid	IL-2	Activated T lymphocytes.
Synergistic		
All lineages	SCF	Stromal cells, endothelial cells, hepatocytes.
	IL-6	Fibroblasts, endothelial cells, stromal cells, activated macrophages.
	IL-1	Virtually all cell types.
	Flt-3 ligand	Stromal cells.

Abbreviations: IL = interleukin; GM-CSF = granulocyte–macrophage colony-stimulating factor; G-CSF = granulocyte colony-stimulating factor; M-CSF = monocyte colony-stimulating factor; EPO = erythropoietin; TPO = thrombopoietin; SCF = stem cell factor.
[a] Properties of most of these cytokines are considered in detail in Chapter 10.

bind tightly to glycosaminoglycans and other components of the ECM, which immobilizes them, increases their local concentrations, and maximizes their availability to hematopoietic cells. Localized secretion of cytokines from stromal cells into the ECM may have a role in delineating specific microenvironments within the bone marrow.

HEMATOPOIETIC CYTOKINES & THEIR RECEPTORS

Cytokine Effects on Hematopoiesis

Hematopoietic progenitors depend on a variety of cytokines to control their growth and differentiation. These include several different types of CSFs and interleukins that each act on specific cell types to promote or inhibit particular types of responses. Detailed discussions of individual cytokines are presented in Chapter 10; for the present, we focus on general principles of cytokine action as illustrated in their effects on hematopoiesis.

In general terms, cytokines that influence hematopoiesis can be divided into three categories (see Table 1–2): (1) those that act on multipotent progenitors, (2) those that act on lineage-committed progenitors, and (3) those that have little effect by themselves but dramatically augment or inhibit the effects of the preceding cytokines. These divisions are not absolute, however, and many cytokines could appropriately be assigned to more than one category. For example, GM-CSF supports proliferation of both multipotential progenitors and precursors committed to monocyte formation. Similarly, thrombopoietin (TPO) supports growth and survival of HSCs but also promotes platelet formation. Certain cytokines can also substitute for one another: For example, large doses of either IL-3 or GM-CSF can sustain HSC proliferation in vitro. Thus, it is important to recognize that the effects of cytokines often are redundant or overlap one another. In addition, many cytokines that influence hematopoiesis also can affect the functions of fully differentiated blood cells. GM-CSF, for example, is an important regulator of the defensive activities of mature neutrophils (see Chapter 2). Similarly, interleukin-2 (IL-2) promotes not only the development of lymphocytes but also many of their protective functions (see Chapters 3 and 4).

In light of these complexities, it is best to view the cytokines as acting in a cooperative, interactive network. This makes it difficult (and sometimes misleading) to assign unique roles to any individual cytokine, particularly in the intact host. Nevertheless, hints to the predominant effects of cytokines have been obtained from experiments in which animals are genetically altered to lack a particular cytokine. In most cases, these studies show that the absence of one or several cytokines has minimal effect on blood cell development but often a more pronounced effect on mature leukocyte function. For example, mice deficient in GM-CSF show only minor decreases in myeloid cell production, but the neutrophils they produce are dysfunctional.

Although it was long believed that specific cytokines acted by inducing HSCs and progenitors to differentiate along a certain pathway, the weight of evidence currently favors another view. It now appears instead that each cell is intrinsically predisposed toward one lineage or another (apparently choosing among them at random) but is unable to proliferate, or even survive, unless the cytokines appropriate to that lineage are present. In other words, cytokines do not direct cells into a particular pathway but instead act as lineage-specific growth and survival factors. Thus, when progenitor cells are deprived of an essential cytokine, they not only cease growing but often die—actively committing suicide through a process called apoptosis (see later discussion). On the other hand, progenitors that have been genetically manipulated so that they cannot undergo apoptosis continue growing and differentiating along a particular lineage even when the cytokine is withdrawn, implying that the differentiative fate of each cell is intrinsically programmed. The concept that lineage commitment is a stochastic (ie, random) process and that one major function of cytokines is to promote survival, rather than induce differentiation, explains why so many cytokines seem to use so few signal transduction pathways, as will be described in the following section.

Cytokine Receptors & Signal Transduction

The overlapping functions of cytokines largely reflect the properties of the cell surface receptors to which they bind. All cytokine receptors function as multiprotein complexes made up of two or more integral membrane polypeptides, called subunits (Figure 1–6). A typical subunit polypeptide has an extracellular domain that participates in cytokine binding, a transmembrane region, and an intracellular domain (also called a cytoplasmic tail) involved in **signal transduction**—the molecular events that transmit signals to the cell interior and induce specific cellular responses when the receptor binds its appropriate cytokine ligand. Some receptors (eg, EPO-R) function as homodimers of a single type of subunit; others (eg, GM-CSFR) function as heterodimers, and still others (eg, IL-2R) as heterotrimers. In general, although the preformed subunits are present on the cell surface at all times, they do not assemble into a complete receptor complex until the appropriate cytokine is bound. It is this ligand-dependent assembly of the receptor complex that initiates the intracellular events in signal transduction.

Most cytokine receptors belong to a family of proteins called the **hematopoietin receptor family.** Members of this family all have a number of features in common, including extracellular domains that share common amino acid residues at key positions

receptor tyrosine kinase family   **hematopoietin receptor family**

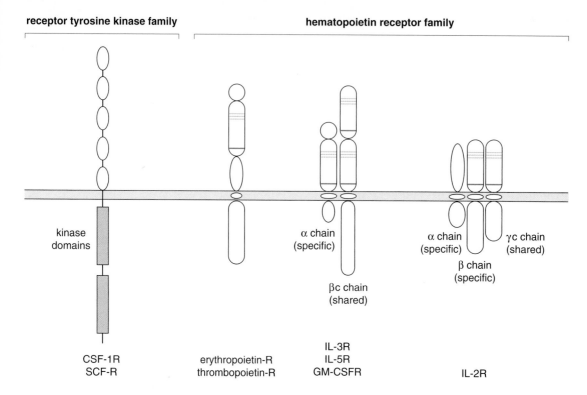

Figure 1–6. Cytokine receptor families. The receptor tyrosine kinase family is characterized by the presence of tyrosine kinase domains *(shaded boxes)* within the intracellular portion of the receptor protein. Hematopoietin receptors lack tyrosine kinase domains, but their extracellular regions share conserved cysteine residues *(thick lines)* and the sequence motif TrpSerXTrpSer *(narrow lines),* where X is any amino acid. Hematopoietin receptors can be composed of one, two, or three polypeptide chains. Examples of each receptor type are listed at bottom of the figure. *Abbreviations:* CSF = colony-stimulating factor; SCF = stem cell factor; IL = interleukin; GM-CSFR = granulocyte-macrophage colony-stimulating factor R.

and that fold into a similar three-dimensional structure composed of 14 antiparallel β strands. Each receptor consists of an α chain and a β chain; the α chain determines the specificity of cytokine binding, but the β chain is also required for maximal binding affinity. Trimeric receptors, such as IL-2R, may also include a γ subunit. As shown in Figure 1–6, many of these receptors share subunits; for example, IL-3R, IL-5R, and GM-CSFR all use a common β chain. These shared subunits are in part responsible for the overlapping functions of many cytokines because they allow receptors with different ligand specificities to trigger identical signaling events inside a cell.

Attached noncovalently to the cytoplasmic tail of most hematopoietin receptor subunits is a cytoplasmic enzyme with **protein tyrosine kinase (PTK)** activity—that is, a protein with the ability to catalyze phosphorylation of tyrosine residues in other proteins. Phosphorylation, either at tyrosine or at serines and threonines, is a common mechanism of regulating protein function; indeed, many of the PTKs must themselves be phosphorylated before they can become active. When a cytokine binds, the component

subunits of its receptor are brought into physical proximity with one another, along with their associated PTKs in the cytoplasm. Clustering of the PTKs allows these enzymes to phosphorylate and activate one another as well as other proteins in the cytoplasm. This PTK activation is the first step in cytoplasmic signal transduction by all known cytokine receptors. Interestingly, the few cytokine receptors (CSF-1R and SCF-R) that do not belong to the hematopoietin receptor family use a slightly different strategy to achieve the same result: The subunits of these receptors have intrinsic PTK enzymatic activity in their cytoplasmic domains, and these **receptor PTKs** become activated in a similar manner when the subunits are brought together. In each case, ligand binding causes the cytokine receptor subunits to associate with one another, which triggers PTK activity in the cytoplasm and initiates signal transduction. As we will see in later chapters, this same principle also applies to many other types of cell surface receptors.

The sequences of events that occur following PTK activation and that lead to specific cellular responses vary among different cytokines, receptors, and cell types. Perhaps the best characterized signaling pathways are those that affect cell proliferation or modulate the transcription of particular genes. Following the onset of PTK activity, many such signals are commonly transmitted to the nucleus through three primary pathways, called the Ras-dependent pathway, the Jak-Stat pathway, and the nuclear factor κB(NF-κB) pathway (Figure 1–7).

The Ras-Dependent Signaling Pathway

The Ras-dependent pathway can be triggered by a variety of cytokine receptors, as well as by certain adhesion molecules and by many other surface receptors when they contact appropriate ligands. Signaling in this pathway can be initiated by cytosolic proteins called **Src-family kinases,** so named because they bear regions of sequence homology to the oncoprotein Src. These Src-like kinases contain specialized protein domains, termed **SH2 domains** (for Src-homology region 2), that enable them to bind other proteins containing phosphorylated tyrosine residues. When a cytokine receptor binds ligand, subunits of the receptor become phosphorylated and can immediately be bound by a Src-family kinase. This interaction leads to the binding of other cytoplasmic proteins, so that a multicomponent signaling complex forms on the inner aspect of the cell membrane. This complex then activates proteins of the **Ras** family, each of which has intrinsic guanosine triphosphatase (GTPase) activity. The cleavage of GTP to guanosine diphosphate (GDP) by Ras-family proteins induces a structural change that triggers activation of the Raf kinase (via a direct interaction of GTP–Ras with Raf). This, in turn, activates protein kinases called Mek and mitosis-associated protein kinase (**MAPK),** which phosphorylate and activate each other in sequence. Once activated, MAPK migrates into the nucleus, where it phosphorylates transcriptional regulatory proteins that control specific genes. Among the effects of MAPK activation are enhanced cell proliferation (see later discussion), gene activation, and changes in cytoskeletal organization that promote migration and function of hematopoietic cells.

The Ras pathway is actually much more complicated than the foregoing explanation would suggest. For example, at least three different forms of MAPK are expressed by various tissues. The activities of individual Ras-pathway components can also be either enhanced or inhibited by other signaling factors in the cells. In addition, signaling through the Ras pathway also can affect cell functions independently of MAPK. How all these intricacies result in specific cellular responses is the subject of intense research.

The Jak/Stat Signaling Pathway

Perhaps the most exciting recent advance in the cytokine signaling field has been the elucidation of the Jak/Stat pathway. The Janus kinase (**Jak**) family consists of four known enzymes (Jak1, Jak2, Jak3,

and Tyk2), each of which associates specifically with the cytoplasmic tails of one or more cytokine receptor subunits. For example, IL-2R associates with both Jak1 and Jak3, which bind its α and γ subunits, respectively. Cytokine binding brings the receptor subunits together and allows the associated Jak proteins to phosphorylate and activate one another. The primary substrates of the activated Jaks are a family of transcription factors called the **Stat** (for signal transducers and activators of transcription) proteins. The Stat proteins contain SH2 domains and so are recruited to the vicinity of an activated receptor when its kinases become active. As a consequence, the Stat factors become phosphorylated, which causes them to dimerize and then translocate into the nucleus, where they act directly to promote expression of specific genes. At least seven Stat proteins (called Stat1-Stat7) are known, each of which acts on different genes. There is no evidence that any individual Jak acts preferentially on a particular Stat. Therefore, the genes activated in response to a given cytokine are determined mainly by the combination of receptor subunits and Stat factors expressed by the responding cell.

Recent work has unearthed another layer of complexity in Jak/Stat signaling. A class of proteins known as suppressors of cytokine signaling, or SOCS, has been found to block this pathway by directly binding and inhibiting Jak kinases. There are as many as eight SOCS proteins, some of which (such as SOCS1) seem to inhibit all Jak-family members, whereas others have more limited effects. Animals that genetically lack SOCS1 respond excessively to cytokines, leading to inflammatory diseases and early death. The possibility that mutations inactivating SOCS proteins in marrow progenitors might lead to hematopoietic cancer is an area of intense interest.

It is tempting to envision that one of the earliest events in lineage commitment by a hematopoietic progenitor may be expression of receptor subunits and Stat proteins that enable it to respond to lineage-specific cytokines. The redundancy of cytokine function therefore reflects the fact that different cytokines bind to structurally similar receptors that activate the same types of signaling molecules. This explains why absence of one or a few cytokines has minimal effect on hematopoiesis in vivo. Moreover, if the stochastic model for lineage commitment is correct, then relatively few signaling pathways are needed, since individual cytokines all produce the same effect, thus supporting survival of the developing progenitors. By contrast, because many cytokines signal through common receptor subunits and signaling pathways, one might predict that loss of a particular subunit or signaling kinase would have a much more profound effect. This is indeed the case: In mice that carry mutations in Jak3 and in both humans and mice with mutations in the IL-2R γ chain, these genetic defects impair signaling by many cytokines simultane-

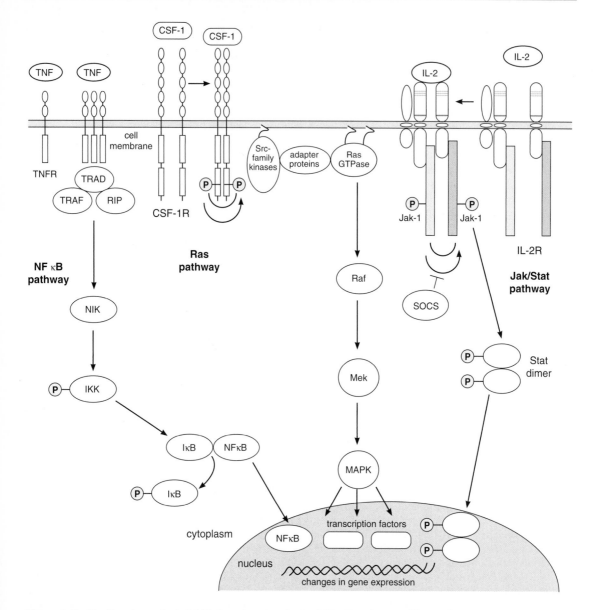

Figure 1–7. The Ras-dependent, Jak/Stat, and nuclear factor (NF)-κB pathways of intracellular signal transduction. In each case, ligand binding to cell surface receptors causes oligomerization and activation of the associated tyrosine kinases *(arrows)*. In the Ras pathway, signals communicated through Src-family kinases and a variety of adapter proteins (such as Grb-2) serve to activate the guanosine triphosphatase protein Ras, which is anchored to the inner aspect of the plasma membrane by fatty acyl groups *(wavy lines)*. Ras signaling then proceeds through sequential activation of several other kinases (including Raf, Mek, and mitosis-associated protein kinase [MAPK]), and ultimately leads to phosphorylation of transcription factors in the nucleus. Jak/Stat signaling is initiated by phosphorylation of cytoplasmic Stat proteins, which causes these proteins to dimerize, translocate to the nucleus, and regulate gene expression by binding to DNA. Jak kinase activation is inhibited by suppressors of cytokine signaling (SOCS)-family proteins. NF-κB activation is shown here as a consequence of tumor necrosis factor (TNF)α stimulation. Treatment of cells with TNFα leads to trimerization of the TNFα receptor and association with a variety of adapter proteins (including TRAD, TRAF, and RIP). This complex activates a pathway leading to phosphorylation and degradation of I-κB, allowing NF-κB to migrate into the nucleus. The NF-κB pathway is also activated by many other stimuli, all of which function similarly through I-κB.

ously and result in profound deficits in hematopoiesis and in cellular defense functions.

The NF-κB Signaling Pathway

A third major signaling pathway involves proteins related to **NF-κB,** which was first identified as a nuclear transcription factor required for expression of specific genes in B lymphocytes. We now know that the NF-κB family includes five related transcription factors that control a plethora of cellular responses to cytokines and other environmental stimuli. NF-κB proteins exist as dimers (either heterodimers between different NF-κB proteins or homodimers) and are normally held in an inactive state within the cytoplasm through association with inhibitory proteins termed the **I-κB** family. Many types of stimuli initiate signaling cascades that lead to phosphorylation of the I-κB proteins, which then are rapidly degraded. The NF-κB dimers are thus liberated and move into the nucleus, where they bind and activate specific genes, which, depending on the cell type involved and other factors, can lead to cell proliferation, activation of particular functions, or cellular suicide (apoptosis). A remarkably large number of the body's defenses are controlled through the NF-κB pathway, making it an important target for drug therapy of immune and inflammatory disorders. Indeed, the classic antiinflammatory drugs, the **corticosteroids,** act in part by increasing the synthesis of I-κB proteins, which in turn suppress activity of NF-κB.

CONTROL OF CELL PROLIFERATION & SURVIVAL

The Cell Cycle

One ultimate effect of many cytokines, ECM proteins, and cell–cell interactions is to influence the rate at which hematopoietic cells divide. The sequence of events that occurs in a cell during each round of mitosis is called the **cell cycle** and is traditionally divided into four phases (Figure 1–8), designated G_1, S (when DNA synthesis occurs), G_2, and M (mitosis, when the cell actually divides). Cells that have ceased dividing (temporarily or permanently) are said to be in a resting phase called G_0. The ordered progression from one phase to the next is coordinated by a complex set of proteins, and the cellular signals that control cell division do so by modulating the activities of those proteins.

Cell cycle regulation takes place mainly at the transition points, or boundaries, between the different phases. Each of these boundaries serves as a **checkpoint:** Specific requirements (eg, completion of DNA synthesis or DNA repair) must be met before a cell can move through the checkpoint from one phase to the next. In mammals, most variation in cell cycle timing is due to variation in the length of G_1, and the G_1/S checkpoint is tightly regulated. Three main classes of proteins are directly involved in checkpoint regulation: (1) the **cyclins,** whose levels rise and fall in specific phases of the cycle; (2) the cyclin-

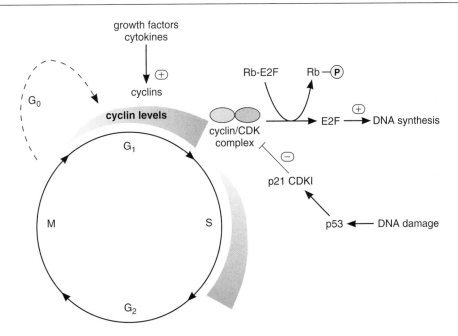

Figure 1–8. The cell cycle. This simplified depiction illustrates a few of the molecular factors that influence the G_1/S transition. *Abbreviations:* CDK = cyclin-dependent kinase; CDKI = CDK inhibitor; sharp arrowheads = activation; blunt arrowheads = inhibition.

dependent kinases **(CDKs),** a class of serine–threonine kinases that regulate cyclin activity by phosphorylation; and (3) the CDK inhibitors **(CDKIs),** which inactivate the CDKs.

There are at least seven different cyclins and CDKs, each operative at different phases of the cycle. The intracellular levels of specific cyclins are in part responsive to external stimuli: For example, CSF-1 acts on cells of the monocyte lineage to increase expression of cyclins required for progression through the G_1/S checkpoint. The expression levels of particular cyclins can be used to determine which stage of the cell cycle a population of cells has reached. As cyclin levels increase during a given phase, they form a complex with the corresponding CDKs; this activates the CDKs, which then phosphorylate other substrates that allow checkpoint progression. In hematopoietic cells, for example, one of the predominant species that accumulates during G_1 is the cyclinD/CDK6 complex, whose primary substrate is the nuclear retinoblastoma (Rb) protein. Rb ordinarily exists as a complex with transcription factors of the E2F family. When the cyclinD/CDK6 complex hyperphosphorylates Rb, the E2F proteins dissociate from it and instead bind and activate specific genes, such as those encoding DNA polymerase and thymidine synthetase, which are required for DNA synthesis and, hence, for entry into the S phase.

Other signals can inhibit cell cycle progression by inducing CDKIs. The CDKIs are small molecules, numbered according to their molecular weights, which bind and inhibit specific cyclin/CDK complexes. In hematopoietic cells, for example, the cytokine called transforming growth factor beta (TGFβ) induces expression of CDKIs called p15 and p18, which inactivate the cyclinD/CDK6 complex and prevent entry into the S phase.

Progression through G_1 is also marked by the accumulation of other transcription factors, including the proteins Fos, Jun, and **c-Myc,** which presumably act on other genes required for DNA replication. Like the E2F proteins, several of these factors are regulated by association with other proteins. For example, c-Myc must dimerize with another protein, called Max, in order to bind DNA and promote gene expression; however, Max can instead form dimers with other proteins that antagonize Myc/Max activity and slow cell cycle progression. Thus, a critical balance of cyclin/CDK and transcription factor activities is required for progression from G_1 to S. If this balance is not achieved, the cell stops dividing and either enters the G_0 resting state or dies through apoptosis (see later discussion). In some circumstances, the G_0 state is maintained by high-level expression of CDKIs.

A number of other factors can also inhibit progression through the G_1/S boundary. One of the most important is DNA damage, which occurs to some degree under normal conditions but is greatly enhanced by ultraviolet or gamma irradiation and by many of the chemotherapeutic agents used to treat cancer. The integrity of chromosomal DNA is continually monitored through an unknown mechanism that involves a protein called **p53.** When DNA damage is present, p53 directly induces a CDKI called p21, which blocks G_1/S progression until the damage is repaired. This process helps ensure that mutations caused by the damage are not replicated and passed on to daughter cells. Cells with mutations in p53 manifest extreme genomic instability (ie, they accumulate numerous mutations) and are highly prone to becoming malignant. Indeed, p53 mutations are an important factor in the development of a wide variety of human cancers.

Programmed Cell Death

Under some circumstances, cells respond to environmental or internal signals by committing suicide—a phenomenon known as programmed (or physiologic) cell death, or **apoptosis.** Such programmed deaths are extremely common in many cell types and, in fact, are essential for maintaining stable cell populations by ensuring that the rate of new cell production is balanced by an equal rate of cell death. This is particularly true in the hematopoietic system, where vast numbers of new cells are generated each day. Programmed deaths are also critical for shaping and maintaining other tissues, such as in resorption of the tail bud and finger webs during embryogenesis, in selecting neural connections of the developing brain, and in regression of the mammary epithelium after lactation. Apoptosis also has a defensive function: Cells that are infected by a virus or other intracellular pathogen may kill themselves—often after having been instructed to do so by other host cells—to help limit the spread of the infection.

In all of these settings, a cell undergoing apoptosis shows characteristic morphologic changes. Over the course of several hours, it shrinks overall as its nucleus and cytoplasm contract; surface features such as microvilli disappear; fragments of cytoplasm pinch off from the surface (a phenomenon called blebbing); the nuclear chromatin condenses; and cellular endonucleases cleave the chromosomal DNA into segments. Ultimately, the cell disintegrates into small fragments (called apoptotic bodies) that are quickly engulfed and digested by adjacent cells. All of this occurs so efficiently that very few dead cells can be seen microscopically, even in tissues in which the rate of apoptosis is extremely high. These tidy, inconspicuous suicides are very different from the uncontrolled, accidental form of cell death called **necrosis,** in which the dying cell often swells and then bursts, producing further damage by spewing its contents onto its neighbors.

The biochemical processes that occur during the final ("execution") phase of apoptosis are thought to be similar in all cell types. Perhaps most important is the activation of cytoplasmic proteases called

caspases, which are distinguished from other proteases by having an essential cysteine in their active sites and by their preference for cleaving target proteins at particular aspartate residues. Caspases are normally expressed in the cytoplasm as larger, inactive precursors, called procaspases, but become activated when they are cleaved proteolytically, usually by other caspases. This allows the caspases to activate one another in a self-amplifying, proteolytic cascade. More than ten different human caspases have been identified, at least five of which become activated during apoptosis. Some (including caspases-8 and -9) have large prodomains that can interact with specific regulatory proteins; these are often the first caspases to become active during an apoptotic response, whereas those with shorter prodomains (such as caspases-3, -6, and -7) generally become active later in the cascade.

In addition to cleaving one another, the activated caspases directly attack other cellular proteins, producing many of the hallmarks of apoptotic death. For example, caspases break down structural proteins of the nuclear matrix and cytoskeleton, leading to collapse of the nucleus and cytoplasm. Proteins required for cell–cell adhesion are also broken down, causing the cell to detach from its neighbors, round up, and become easier to engulf. Caspases proteolytically activate a cellular endonuclease that then attacks and degrades chromosomal DNA, and they simultaneously destroy DNA repair enzymes that might otherwise limit the damage. Numerous signaling molecules, cell cycle regulators, and transcription factors are also degraded, crippling the cell's vital functions. The importance of caspases as cellular executioners is confirmed by the finding that drugs that inhibit these enzymes can completely prevent apoptosis in laboratory studies. Perhaps for this reason, human cells encode at least four related proteins, called inhibitors of apoptosis (IAPs), that can directly bind and inhibit caspases; their physiologic role is not yet clear. The same strategy is used by some poxviruses and herpesviruses, which encode caspase-inhibitor proteins that prevent infected cells from committing apoptosis.

The procaspases needed for suicide are always ready and can be activated by various signals from inside or outside the cell. One important receptor for death signals is a surface protein called **Fas** (or **CD95**). Many cells express Fas when they are suicide-prone because it allows them to be killed by other cells expressing a surface protein called **Fas ligand (FasL).** Contact with a FasL-bearing cell causes clustering of Fas receptors, whose cytoplasmic tails then associate with specific adapter proteins in the cytoplasm (Figure 1–9). These adapters then bind and activate procaspase-8 which, in turn, triggers the rest of the caspase cascade and leads quickly to apoptosis. (In some cases, stressed cells express both Fas and FasL on their surfaces, and so trigger their own death!) Binding of TNFα by the TNF receptor can likewise lead to caspase activation, as well as activating the NF-κB pathway, as previously described. An even more direct approach can be used by specialized lymphocytes to kill virally infected cells. These lymphocytes bind the target cell, create minute openings in its surface, and secrete into its cytoplasm a protease called **granzyme B,** which cleaves and activates multiple caspases, causing apoptosis (see Chapter 9).

Mitochondria play a key role in many apoptotic responses, including those induced by cytokine withdrawal or gamma irradiation. Abnormalities in mitochondrial function occur early, including the release of specific proteins from within these organelles to the cytoplasm. The mechanism of this release is uncertain, but it does not require rupture of the mitochondrial membranes. One of the released proteins is **cytochrome** *c,* a component of the electron-transport chain which, when it enters the cytoplasm, potently activates the caspase cascade. Cytochrome *c* produces this effect by associating with a cytosolic protein to form a complex that activates caspase-9. A second released protein, called **apoptosis-inducing factor (AIF),** is able to induce nuclear collapse, chromosome breakage, and other signs of apoptosis through unknown pathways that do not require caspase activity. AIF also causes the lipid **phosphatidylserine,** normally found on the inner leaflet of the plasma membrane, to become exposed on the cell's surface. This change in surface lipids promotes engulfment of the dying cell and is one of the earliest signs of apoptosis. Some apoptotic cells also show evidence of injury caused by **reactive oxygen species,** which are toxic byproducts of mitochondrial aerobic metabolism; however, it is unclear whether such injury is essential to the apoptotic process.

The mitochondrial pathways of apoptosis are tightly controlled by a family of cytoplasmic proteins related to the human oncoprotein **Bcl2** (see Chapter 7). Members of the Bcl2 family have been identified in mammalian cells, viruses, and other organisms (Table 1–3). Most are integral membrane proteins that associate with organelles throughout the cytoplasm, including the endoplasmic reticulum, outer nuclear envelope, and inner plasma membrane, as well as with mitochondria. All Bcl2 family members share conserved amino acid sequences and tend to dimerize with themselves or with one another. Remarkably, however, they fall into two classes with opposite biologic effects: When expressed individually within cells, some of these proteins (eg, Bax) actively induce or promote apoptosis, whereas others (eg, Bcl2) inhibit apoptosis, making cells resistant to an assortment of stimuli that would otherwise trigger cell death. These two classes of protein antagonize each other (perhaps by forming mixed heterodimers), so that the overall tendency of a cell to undergo apoptosis partly reflects the relative levels at which it expresses proteins of each class.

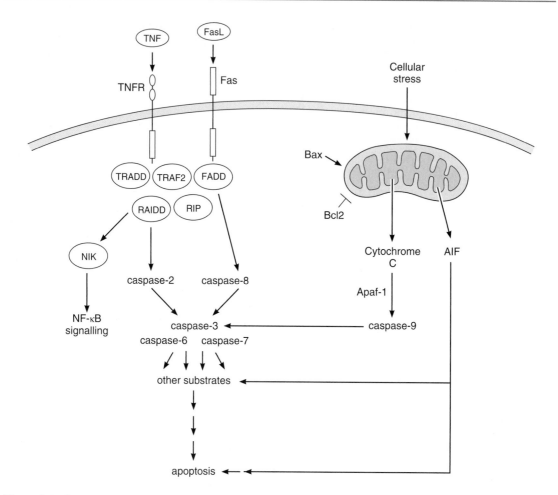

Figure 1–9. Apoptosis-signaling pathways. Contact of responsive cells with either TNFα or FasL results in trimerization of the respective receptors and association of cytoplasmic adapter proteins to form a signaling complex at the membrane, which leads to caspase activation. Note that many of the same adapter proteins are implicated in TNFα signaling whether it leads to activation of NF-κB or of caspases. However, some of these adapter proteins (eg, RAIDD) have specific protein recognition domains (called CARD domains, or caspase activation/recognition domains) that allow them to bind and activate certain caspases. Activation of the distal caspases is also accomplished by release of cytochrome *c* from mitochondria; these organelles are also targets of the Bcl2 family of apoptotic regulatory proteins.

Table 1–3. Proteins of the Bcl2 family.[a]

Inhibit Apoptosis	Promote Apoptosis
Bcl2	Bax
BclX$_L$	BclX$_S$
Mcl-1	Bak
A-1	Bik
Bhrf-I (Epstein–Barr virus)	Bad
p35 (Baculovirus)	
Ced-9 (Nematode)	

[a] Each of these proteins is expressed by mammalian cells unless otherwise indicated. BclX$_L$ and BclX$_S$ are alternatively spliced products from a single gene.

The mechanisms by which Bcl2 and related proteins regulate apoptosis are not fully known. Their structures resemble those of certain bacterial pore-forming proteins, and Bax and Bcl2 have each been shown to form ion channels with somewhat different properties in artificial membranes. Bax and Bid normally reside in the cytosol but move to mitochondria after apoptotic stimulation, when they trigger the release of cytochrome *c* into the cytoplasm. By contrast, Bcl2 antagonizes this release, and BclX$_L$ may interfere with cytochrome *c*-mediated activation of caspase-9. It also appears that some cytokines regulate the expression of Bcl2 family members. For example, withdrawing a particular cytokine may lead to reduced Bcl2 expression in some hematopoietic progenitors, leaving these cells vulnerable to the unopposed effects of Bax. Certain viruses also manipulate expression of these proteins: For example, the Epstein-Barr virus not only encodes a Bcl2-like protein of its own, but also specifically activates expression of cellular Bcl2, thereby preventing the infected cell from committing apoptosis.

In addition, apoptosis in hematopoietic cells is closely tied to the cell cycle. Many cytokine-dependent hematopoietic cells must pass through the G_1 phase of the cell cycle before commencing apoptosis following cytokine withdrawal. In the process, these cells accumulate G_1-specific proteins such as c-Myc, which may, paradoxically, have a role in initiating cell death under these conditions. Another critical cell cycle regulator, p53, is also directly linked to apoptosis: If the DNA damage that triggers p53-dependent cell cycle arrest (see earlier discussion) cannot be repaired in a timely manner, p53 acts to initiate apoptosis (possibly by inducing Bax) and in that way eliminates the damaged cell for the benefit of the host.

CONCLUSION

The regulation of hematopoiesis reflects the individual and combined effects of soluble factors and direct cell–cell interactions in the marrow. By activating specific signal transduction pathways inside the developing cells, these external stimuli modulate the activities of transcription factors, cell cycle regulatory factors, and other intracellular proteins that determine whether a cell will proliferate, differentiate, or die. These mechanisms are essential for controlling not only blood cell production but also the defensive functions carried out by mature blood cells. Indeed, many of these same signaling responses control aspects of cell division and differentiation in nonhematopoietic cells as well. Hence, many of the themes that have been outlined here will be encountered again in subsequent chapters.

REFERENCES

HEMATOPOIESIS AND HEMATOPOIETIC STEM CELLS
Akashi K et al: Lymphoid development from hematopoietic stem cells. Int J Hematol 1999;69:217.

Eaves C et al: Introduction to stem cell biology in vitro. Threshold to the future. Ann N Y Acad Sci 1999;872:1.

Cheshier SH et al: In vivo proliferation and cell cycle kinetics of long-term self-renewing hematopoietic stem cells. Proc Natl Acad Sci U S A 1999;96:3120.

Glimm H, Eaves CJ: Direct evidence for multiple self-renewal divisions of human in vivo repopulating hematopoietic cells in short-term culture. Blood 1999;94:2161.

Osawa M et al: Long-term lymphohematopoietic reconstitution by a single CD34-low/negative hematopoietic stem cell. Science 1996;273:242.

CYTOKINES AND SIGNAL TRANSDUCTION
Starr R, Hilton DJ: Negative regulation of the JAK/STAT pathway. Bioessays 1999;21:47.

Wallach D et al: Tumor necrosis factor receptor and Fas signaling mechanisms. Ann Rev Immunol 1999;17:331.

Ghosh S et al: NF-κB and Rel proteins: Evolutionarily conserved mediators of immune responses. Ann Rev Immunol 1998;16:225.

Ihle JN et al: Signaling by the cytokine receptor superfamily. Ann N Y Acad Sci 1998;865:1.

Liu KD et al: JAK/STAT signaling by cytokine receptors. Curr Opin Immunol 1988;10:271.

Socolovsky M et al: Control of hematopoietic differentiation: lack of specificity in signaling by cytokine receptors. Proc Natl Acad Sci U S A 1998;95:6573.

Darnell JE: STATs and gene regulation. Science 1997;277:1630.

BONE MARROW STROMA
Torok-Storb B et al: Dissecting the marrow microenvironment. Ann N Y Acad Sci 1999;872:164.

Papayannopoulou T: Hematopoietic stem/progenitor cell mobilization. A continuing quest for etiologic mechanisms. Ann N Y Acad Sci 1999;872:187.

Verfaillie CM: Adhesion receptors as regulators of the hematopoietic process. Blood 1998;92:2609.

Oostendorp RA, Dormer P: VLA-4-mediated interactions between normal human hematopoietic progenitors and stromal cells. Leukemia Lymphoma 1997;24:423.

CELL CYCLE CONTROL
Sherr CJ, Roberts JM: CDK inhibitors: Positive and negative regulators of G1-phase progression. Genes Dev 1999;13:1501.

Obaya AJ et al: Mysterious liaisons: The relationship between c-Myc and the cell cycle. Oncogene 1999;18:2934.

Tsihlias J et al: The prognostic significance of altered cyclin-dependent kinase inhibitors in human cancer. Ann Rev Med 1999;50:401.

Pavletich NP: Mechanisms of cyclin-dependent kinase regulation: Structures of Cdks, their cyclin activators, and Cip and INK4 inhibitors. J Mol Bio 1999;287:821.

Furukawa Y: Cell cycle regulation of hematopoietic stem cells. Hum Cell 1998;11:81.

APOPTOSIS

Wickremasinghe RG, Hoffbrand AV: Biochemical and genetic control of apoptosis: Relevance to normal hematopoiesis and hematological malignancies. Blood 1999;93:3587.

Lundberg AS, Weinberg RA: Control of the cell cycle and apoptosis. Eur J Cancer 1999;35:531.

Gross A et al: BCL-2 family members and the mitochondria in apoptosis. Genes Dev 1999;13:1899.

Scaffidi C et al: Apoptosis signaling in lymphocytes. Curr Opin Immunol 1999;11:277.

Tschopp J et al: Apoptosis: Silencing the death receptors. Curr Biol 1999;9:381.

Raff M: Cell suicide for beginners. Nature 1998;396:19.

Chao DT, Korsmeyer SJ: Bcl-2 family: Regulators of cell death. Ann Rev Immunol 1998;16:395.

Innate Immunity

2

Tristram G. Parslow, MD, PhD, & Dorothy F. Bainton, MD

The human body protects itself in many ways. The first line of defense is provided by physical barriers, such as the skin, which cover body surfaces and prevent microorganisms and other potentially injurious agents from entering the tissues beneath. In addition to being structurally impervious, these barriers often have specialized features that help them repel foreign invaders. For example, lactic acid and other substances in sweat maintain the surface of the epidermis at an acidic pH, which helps prevent colonization by bacteria and other organisms. Similarly, the more delicate epithelia lining the respiratory and digestive tracts are bathed in a protective, flowing layer of mucus, which can trap, dissolve, and sweep away foreign substances. Although these physical barriers are relatively static, they often can be enhanced to some degree in times of need: A chronically irritated epidermis may thicken to form a callus, and the respiratory tract's efforts to cleanse itself by copious mucus production are familiar to anyone who has suffered from a cold or "hay fever" allergy. The importance of these physical defenses becomes most obvious in people who lack them: For example, burn patients are at greatly increased risk for many types of infections, owing to loss of the cutaneous barrier.

Whenever a **pathogen** (ie, any microorganism with the potential to cause tissue injury or disease) succeeds in breaching the surface barriers and entering the body, it encounters a panoply of other factors that guard the inner tissues. Traditionally, these inner defenses have been grouped into two more-or-less distinct functional systems, based on whether the resistance (immunity) they confer against a particular pathogen is present from the outset or instead develops only after contact with the pathogen. **Innate (or natural) immunity** refers to any inborn resistance that is already present the first time a pathogen is encountered; it does not require prior exposure and is not modified significantly by repeated exposures to the pathogen over the life of an individual. **Acquired immunity** refers to resistance that is weak or absent on first exposure, but that increases dramatically with subsequent exposures to the same specific pathogen.

The innate and acquired immune systems are each made up of numerous components that can carry out particular types of protective functions. Some are specialized cells that have the ability to recognize, sequester, and eliminate various types of organisms or harmful substances; the defenses provided by such cells are collectively known as **cell-mediated immunity.** The remainder are soluble macromolecules (usually proteins) that circulate in the blood and extracellular fluid, making these liquids (which were once called the body's humors) inhospitable to foreign invaders even when all cells have been removed; cell-free defenses of this type are called **humoral immunity.**

The innate and acquired immune systems each play critical roles in host defense. Both systems are essential for health; they usually act in concert and often depend on each other to produce their maximum effects. Nor are they entirely separate. The actions of one system frequently influence the other, and certain individual cell types or humoral proteins are pivotal to the workings of both systems. Of the two, the acquired immune system has received much more attention in recent years, and indeed most contemporary usage of such terms as "immunology," "immune response," and so on, refers primarily to the acquired immune system. That same emphasis will be apparent in this book, as most of the following chapters focus on the cells and proteins that mediate acquired immunity. Nevertheless, there is a growing recognition that the innate immune system is critical for human health, not only in its own right but also in activating and regulating acquired immunity. We will therefore begin by describing the capabilities and limitations of the innate immune system, to understand how it functions as a guardian of the body, and to consider why this system alone cannot provide a sufficient defense against many types of pathogens.

HUMORAL PROTEINS OF INNATE IMMUNITY

The body's innate resistance to many pathogens is provided by enzymes and other proteins in the blood and tissue fluids. These proteins are the **effectors** (ie, the active agents) of humoral innate immunity, and they have features in common with one another that are also characteristics of the innate immune system as a whole. First, these proteins are continually expressed throughout life, regardless of whether or not their protective effects are needed at a given moment. Second, although many of these proteins can be produced in higher quantities in times of need, their intrinsic properties (eg, substrate specificity and binding affinity) never change: The characteristics of these proteins have been shaped by evolution, are genetically determined, and are fixed at birth, so that they do not vary during an individual's lifetime. Third, although these proteins carry out highly specific functions at the molecular level, they generally recognize targets or substrates that are found on a wide range of different microorganisms but that are not normally present in the human body. Some examples of these pathogen-specific macromolecules are listed in Table 2–1. Many are chemically distinctive carbohydrates or lipids that are displayed in spatially repetitive arrays on an organism's surface. Because they occur repeatedly both among different pathogen groups and on each individual pathogen, these targets of innate immunity are sometimes called **pathogen-specific molecular patterns,** and the host proteins that recognize them can be thought of as pattern recognition molecules. By recognizing these common patterns, the host proteins are able to provide relatively nonspecific protection against a broad array of pathogens. This strategy is highly efficient, enabling the innate system to immediately recognize many pathogens as chemically foreign even if they have never been encountered before. It also helps minimize the risk that these proteins might inadvertently attack host tissues. The ability to recognize and respond to distinctive carbohydrates, lipids, or nucleic acids is also a key feature that distinguishes the innate from the acquired immune system, because, as we shall see in later chapters, the acquired immune system recognizes pathogens mainly by the specific proteins they express.

Antimicrobial Enzymes & Binding Proteins

A few of the best known humoral effectors of innate immunity are listed in Table 2–2, along with the

Table 2–1. Pathogen-specific macromolecules.[a]

Macromolecules	Sources
Peptidoglycan	Bacterial cell walls
Lipopolysaccharide (LPS)	Gram-negative bacterial cell walls
Lipoteichoic acid	Gram-positive bacterial cell walls
N-Formylmethionyl peptides	Bacteria
Distinctive glycolipids	Mycobacteria
Mannans	Yeast, mycobacteria
DNA with unmethylated CpG[b]	Bacteria
Double-stranded RNA	Certain viruses

[a] Only selected representative examples are listed.
[b] Denotes the dinucleotide base sequence cytosine–guanosine in DNA; in this context, the cytosine base is usually methylated in eukaryotes but not in bacteria.

types of target molecules they recognize. Some are enzymes that can directly injure or kill microbial pathogens. An example is **lysozyme,** an endoglycosidase found in human saliva, mucus, tears, and other secretions, which attacks the protective cell wall encasing every bacterial cell. Lysozyme acts by digesting the **peptidoglycan**—a meshwork formed by long carbohydrate chains of alternating N-acetylmuramic acid and N-acetylglucosamine residues, crosslinked covalently by short oligopeptide sidechains—which is a major constituent of all bacterial cell walls but is not found in mammalian tissues. By cleaving the linkages between carbohydrate residues in the peptidoglycan, lysozyme weakens the cell wall and leaves bacteria vulnerable to killing by osmotic lysis.

Other humoral factors bind to pathogens but produce little or no effect on their own; instead, they mark the pathogen for destruction by other humoral or cell-mediated processes. One very important example is the liver-derived serum protein known as **mannan-binding lectin (MBL),** which binds residues of the sugars mannose, glucose, fucose, or N-acetylglucosamine, found commonly at the exposed ends of carbohydrate sidechains on microbial glycoproteins or glycolipids. MBL (which is sometimes called mannose-binding lectin or mannose-

Table 2–2. Major humoral effector proteins of the innate immune system.

Protein	Major Microbial Targets	Effects
Lysozyme	Peptidoglycan of bacterial cell walls	Digestion of cell wall
Mannan-binding lectin (MBL)	High-mannose glycoproteins and glycolipids	Opsonization; complement activation
C-Reactive protein	Polysaccharides and phosphorylcholine on microbial surfaces	Opsonization; complement activation
Serum amyloid protein P	Carbohydrates in cell walls	Opsonization
LPS-binding protein[a] (LBP)	LPS	Promotes LPS binding to CD14
Soluble CD14	LPS	Promotes LPS binding by host cells
Defensins	Microbial membranes	Membrane lysis
Complement protein C3	Covalent binding to carbohydrates and proteins on microbial surfaces	Opsonization; complement activation; many other effects

[a] LPS, bacterial lipopolysaccharide.

binding protein) is composed of three identical polypeptide chains that can each bind one sugar residue independently, but optimal binding occurs when all three chains are bound by sugars spaced about 45 Å apart, as occurs on the surfaces of bacteria, yeast, mycobacteria, parasites, and some viruses. Although mammalian glycoproteins also contain the target sugars, these usually are present in smaller amounts, are masked by other carbohydrates such as galactose or sialic acid at the sidechain termini, and do not form repetitive arrays, so that they do not bind MBL efficiently. Binding of MBL has little direct effect on a pathogen, but greatly increases the efficiency with which pathogens are captured and destroyed by certain host cells, through a phenomenon called opsonization, and it also triggers pathogen destruction by humoral factors known as the complement cascade (see later sections). Other effectors that function similarly include **serum amyloid protein P, C-reactive protein** in the blood, and **lung surfactant protein A,** each of which binds a subset of carbohydrate or lipid determinants found on many different types of bacteria.

Peptide Antibiotics

Other humoral effectors have the ability to lyse microorganisms directly. The best studied of these are a class of small peptide antibiotics known as **defensins,** which in their active forms are all roughly 30 amino acids long (3–5 kilodaltons), positively charged, and protease-resistant. Each also has three internal disulfide bonds. They are classified as either α or β defensins based on the arrangement of the disulfides, but both classes have nearly the same compact, folded structure consisting of three strands of antiparallel β-pleated sheets. Their mechanism of action is not fully understood, but they appear to kill by forming voltage-dependent ion channels in microbial membranes, allowing solutes to leak out. Defensins are active against a broad spectrum of bacteria, fungi, and enveloped viruses, but not against mammalian cells; it has been suggested that they act preferentially on membranes that lack cholesterols.

Numerous α defensins are produced and stored within human granulocytes and specialized intestinal epithelial cells, called Paneth cells, and can be discharged from these cells in response to infections. Only two human β defensins have been identified. One (hDB-1) is continually made and secreted by epithelial cells lining the airways and urogenital tract and can be found in mucus bathing these epithelia as well as in the blood. It has been proposed that the high salt concentrations in airway secretions of people with cystic fibrosis inactivate hDB-1, accounting for the increased susceptibility of these patients to chronic airway colonization by *Pseudomonas, Staphylococcus,* and other bacteria. The other human β defensin (hDB-2) is secreted by skin, lung, and tracheal epithelial cells in response to the cytokine tumor necrosis factor α (TNFα) or on contact with bacteria or fungi.

Humoral Factors That Recognize Bacterial Lipopolysaccharide

One especially favored target for immune recognition is bacterial **lipopolysaccharide (LPS)**. This macromolecule is found only in the outer lipid bilayer that surrounds the cell walls of gram-negative bacteria, such as *Neisseria, Salmonella,* and *Escherichia coli.* Each molecule of LPS consists of a core carbohydrate linked on one side to a phospholipid (called lipid A) that is anchored in the bilayer and on the other side to a long polysaccharide chain (called the O sidechain) that extends outward from the bacterial surface (Figure 2–1). The sequence of sugars making up the O sidechain is species-specific and highly variable, even within a single bacterial genus: For example, more than 1000 variants in *Salmonella* are known. The core carbohydrate and lipid A, by contrast, are essentially invariant and serve as the target for binding by several different human serum proteins.

Two important humoral proteins that recognize LPS are **LPS-binding protein (LBP)** and **soluble CD14.** These proteins can each form complexes with LPS on a bacterial surface, and these complexes are, in turn, very efficiently recognized by specialized surface receptors on endothelial cells, neutrophils, monocytes, and many other human cell types. Because they form complexes that bind to these receptors at even minute concentrations of LPS ($<10^{-12}$ M), LBP and soluble CD14 greatly enhance recognition and destruction of gram-negative bacteria by cells. At the same time, the interaction of these LPS complexes with at least one class of receptors, called Toll-like receptors (see later section) transmits signals into the cell, which can lead to powerful physiologic changes in the host. For example, LPS binding induces many types of cells to secrete various cytokines, which, in turn, trigger a wide array of other innate and acquired immune phenomena that we will encounter later in this book.

Soluble CD14 (and its cell surface counterpart, a protein called membrane CD14) can bind not only LPS but also other lipid-containing ligands, including gram-positive bacterial and mycobacterial cell walls. LBP also binds LPS directly, and the resulting complex binds more efficiently to soluble or membrane CD14. Another LPS-binding humoral effector with a different mechanism of action is **bactericidal permeability-increasing protein (BPI),** a 55-kilodalton serum protein that, when it binds, opsonizes a bacterium and can also lyse it directly through an unknown mechanism.

The Complement Cascade

An especially elaborate and important type of innate antimicrobial defense is provided by a group of

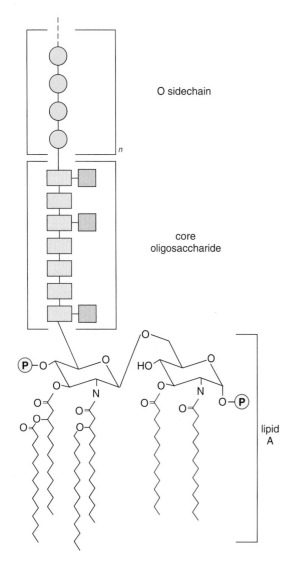

Figure 2–1. Structure of lipopolysaccharide (LPS) from gram-negative bacteria. Lipid A contains two residues of phosphorylated glucosamine bearing six O- and N-linked saturated fatty acids and accounts for half the lipids in the outer lipid bilayer. The core oligosaccharide is composed of ten sugar residues. The O antigen comprises 25–50 repeating tetrasaccharide units, and its sequence varies widely among bacterial strains. Total mass of the LPS unit is about 10,000 daltons.

serum proteins that together make up the **complement** pathway. This group comprises more than two dozen different liver- and macrophage-derived proteins, called complement factors or components, most of which normally circulate in the form of proenzymes that have latent protease activity. As a rule, each of the proteases becomes active when proteolytically cleaved and will then catalyze cleavage

and activation of a different complement component. These cleavages occur in a defined sequence, with each activated protein subsequently activating many copies of the next component, so that the reactions proceed in a self-amplifying cascade. When complement becomes activated on the surface of a pathogen, it leads to four distinct types of protective effects: (1) Some of the complement components assemble into pores that create holes in the microbial surface membrane; (2) others coat the organism and enhance its killing by host cells through opsonization; (3) others acts as chemoattractants for various leukocytes; and (4) still others bind to receptors on nearby host cells and trigger different types of defensive reactions that will be described later. Because it plays a key role in many aspects of immunity, the complement cascade is considered in great detail in Chapter 12. In the present discussion, we consider only a very simplified outline of its contributions to the innate defense against pathogens.

Complement can become activated through three distinct routes, all of which involve activation of a complement protein called C3, a fairly abundant protein with a normal serum concentration of 1 g/L or more. The **classical pathway** uses proteins from the acquired immune system to activate C3 (see Chapter 12), but the alternative and lectin pathways (Figure 2–2) are examples of innate immunity.

The **alternative pathway** depends on the fact that, under normal conditions, a small proportion of C3 molecules in the serum are continually becoming activated due to spontaneous hydrolysis. These activated C3 proteins can interact with two other serum complement components (factors B and D) to form a highly reactive, extremely short-lived species capable of bonding covalently to virtually any protein or carbohydrate molecule in its vicinity. With a half-life of only 0.1 ms, this active C3 derivative cannot diffuse far from its site of formation before decaying to an inactive form. If during this time it encounters an appropriate molecule on a cell surface, however, the C3 derivative binds and is stabilized and can then act on other complement proteins in the surrounding serum to trigger the entire complement cascade. Human cells express on their surfaces a number of complement-inhibitory proteins whose function is to inactivate immediately any molecule of this C3 species that attaches itself to the cell; in this way, human cells protect themselves from the effects of spontaneously activated C3. Many pathogens, however, lack such protection. When such organisms enter the bloodstream, their surfaces quickly become coated with the active C3 species, triggering localized complement activation.

The same result can be achieved through the **lectin pathway** (see Figure 2–2), which is initiated by specific binding of MBL to a pathogen surface; this triggers activation of two MBL-associated serum proteases, called MASP1 and MASP2, which in turn

alternative pathway

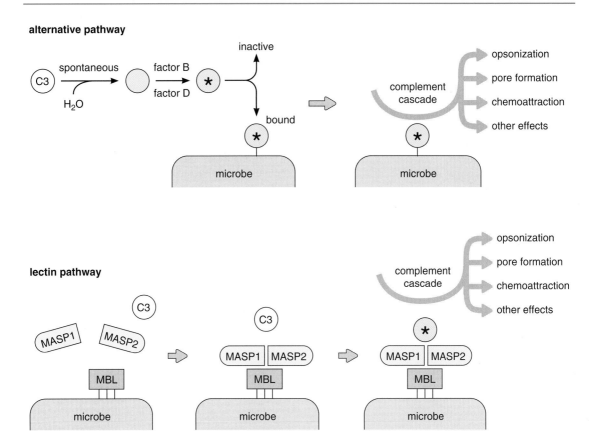

Figure 2–2. Complement activation through the alternative pathway. For details, see Chapter 12. Abbreviations: MBL = mannan-binding lectin; MASP = MBL-associated serum protein.

activate C3. Regardless of the pathway involved, complement activation at the pathogen surface results in membrane perforation, enhanced killing by host defensive cells, leukocyte chemoattraction, and the activation of many other types of defensive reactions in the surrounding tissues.

The Acute-Phase Response

With the exception of C3, most soluble mediators of innate immunity are found in relatively small amounts in the serum under normal conditions. The concentrations of several of these proteins, however, can increase as much as 1000-fold during serious infections or other crises, as part of a coordinated protective reaction called the **acute-phase response.** In this response, the liver temporarily increases its synthesis of more than 30 different serum proteins, often called **acute-phase proteins** (Table 2–3). Many of these, such as complement factors C3 and B, MBL, LBP, C-reactive protein, and serum amyloid protein P, participate in antimicrobial defense. Others include coagulation factors, such as fibrinogen; granulocyte colony-stimulating factor; antioxidants; and serum

metal-binding proteins that sequester iron, zinc, and copper, making these essential nutrients unavailable to invading organisms.

The acute-phase response occurs when hepatocytes are exposed to particular cytokines—chiefly interleukin-6 (IL-6), as well as IL-1 or TNFα—released locally or into the bloodstream by other host cells (see Chapter 10). Significantly, one of the most potent inducers of these cytokines, and hence of the acute-phase response, is bacterial LPS. These same cytokines, in concert with poorly defined neural mechanisms, give rise to the fever, somnolence, and loss of appetite that commonly occur as part of the acute-phase response. If the response is prolonged, they can also produce the anemia and generalized loss of body mass (called wasting, or **cachexia**) that accompany many chronic illnesses.

The acute-phase response can thus be viewed as a primitive, nonspecific defense reaction, mediated by the liver, that intensifies some aspects of innate immunity and other protective functions in times of distress. It can be triggered not only by infections, but also by trauma, burns, tissue necrosis, advanced can-

Table 2–3. The acute-phase response.[a]

Proteins whose plasma concentrations increase
  Antimicrobial protein
    C-reactive protein
    LPS-binding protein
    Mannan-binding lectin
    Serum amyloid protein A
    Complement proteins C3, C4, C9, and factor B
  Coagulation and fibrinolytic proteins
    Fibrinogen
    Protein S
    Plasminogen
    Tissue plasminogen activator
    Urokinase
    Vitronectin
  Protease inhibitors
    α_1-Protease inhibitor
    α_1-Antichymotrypsin
  Transport and metal-binding proteins
    Ceruloplasmin
    Haptoglobin
    Hemopexin
    Ferritin
  Other proteins
    Granulocyte colony-stimulating factor
    IL-1 receptor antagonist
    Fibronectin
    Angiotensinogen
    Secreted phospholipase A
Proteins whose plasma concentrations decrease
  Albumin
  Transferrin
  Transthyretin
  α-Fetoprotein
  Thyroxine-binding globulin
  Insulin-like growth factor I
  Coagulation factor XII
Other acute-phase phenomena
  Fever
  Somnolence
  Anorexia
  Anemia
  Leukocytosis
  Thrombocytosis
  Cachexia (loss of muscle mass, fat, and bone)

Abbreviations: LPS = bacterial lipopolysaccharide, IL-1 = interleukin-1.
[a] A more complete listing and discussion can be found in Gabay C, Kushner I: Acute-phase proteins and other systemic responses to inflammation, *N Engl J Med* 1999; **340**:448.

cer, or a variety of immunologically mediated diseases, either localized or systemic. Measurement of this response is very useful in clinical practice as a general indicator of ill health, or for assessing severity and prognosis in chronic disorders such as rheumatoid arthritis. One traditional assay is the **erythrocyte sedimentation rate,** a measure of the rate at which red cells fall through plasma, which increases as the fibrinogen concentration rises during an acute-phase response. This assay is gradually being supplanted, however, by direct quantitation of serum fibrinogen or C-reactive protein, both of which are more sensitive and precise measures of the acute-phase response.

INFLAMMATION: VASCULAR RESPONSES TO INJURY OR INFECTION

Some of the immediate sequelae of injury are uncomfortably familiar: Soon after an injury occurs, the affected site and its surrounding tissues become **reddened, warm, swollen, and painful.** These four signs—which are probably the most useful and ubiquitous diagnostic clues in all of clinical medicine—are hallmarks of acute **inflammation,** the body's initial physiologic reaction to tissue distress. In its simplest form, inflammation is a response carried out by blood vessels and by the endothelial cells that line them. It serves an important protective function by setting in motion the processes of defense, healing, and repair. Inflammation is not considered an immune reaction, because it can be triggered not only by microbial infection but also by blunt trauma, thermal or chemical burns, lacerations, radiation injury (eg, sunburn), vascular obstruction, or myriad other causes. Nevertheless, immune and inflammatory reactions are closely linked, and they often promote and enhance one another. In particular, many types of innate or acquired immune reactions (eg, those that lead to complement activation) trigger inflammation in nearby blood vessels, so that the involved tissues become red, warm, swollen, and painful. On the other hand, as we shall see, the changes that take place in inflamed blood vessels are key to attracting cells of the immune system into an injured or infected tissue. Before discussing the cells of innate immunity, we begin with a brief overview of the vascular events of inflammation that set the stage for their arrival.

Mediators of Inflammation

The spectrum of events that occur during inflammation varies according to the tissue and type of injury involved. The most fundamental are changes in the diameter and permeability of local blood vessels, and in the surface molecules expressed on their lining endothelial cells. But a given response may also involve an influx of particular types of leukocytes from the bloodstream, activation of the clotting or coagulation systems, fever, or a host of other phenomena. Individual aspects of the response are controlled by diffusible signaling molecules known as **inflammatory mediators,** a class that encompasses many unrelated proteins, peptides, and small organic compounds, each with unique biologic effects. Some, called **vasoactive mediators,** act principally on the vasculature, whereas others mediate pain, fever, coagulation, or leukocyte chemotaxis. Table 2–4 lists the mediators believed to be most important for certain key aspects of inflammation. In general, these mediators come from three main sources. Some are secreted by injured or distressed host cells; others are byproducts either of tissue injury per se (eg, fragments of colla-

Table 2–4. Inflammatory mediators.[a]

	Vasodilatation	Vascular Permeability	Endothelial Activation	Leukocyte Chemotaxis	Pain	Fever
Secreted by Host Cells						
Histamine	***	***	***			
Prostaglandins[b]	***				***	
Leukotrienes[c]		***		***		***
PAF		***				
Nitric Oxide	***d				***	
Chemokines				***		***
Cytokines (eg, IL-6, TNFα)		***	***	***	***	
Byproducts of tissue injury and host reactions						
Complement byproducts (eg, C5a)		***	***	***		
Coagulation factors (eg, fibrin, thrombin)			***	***		
Collagen fragments					***	
Bradykinin		***				
Unique Microbial Macromolecules						
LPS			***			
N-Formylated oligopeptides				***		

Abbreviations: PAF = platelet-activating factor; IL-6 = interleukin-6; TNFα = tumor necrosis factor α; LPS = bacterial lipopolysaccharide.
[a] For detailed discussions of individual mediators, see Chapters 11 and 12.
[b] Especially PGD_2 and PGE_2.
[c] Especially LTC_4, LTD_4, and LTE_4.
[d] Nitric oxide directly dilates large, but not small, blood vessels; however, it also dilates small vessels indirectly by stimulating the release of histamine and other mediators.

gen) or of the host's reaction to it (eg, activation of the clotting or complement cascades); and still others are unique microbial macromolecules (eg, LPS) that may also serve as targets for innate immunity. Thus, as a rule, the inflammatory response is triggered by molecules that broadly signify tissue damage, infection, or distress, regardless of its specific cause.

Dilatation & Increased Permeability of Microscopic Blood Vessels

The response to injury usually begins with dilatation of small blood vessels in and around the injured site (Figure 2–3). This response (called **vasodilatation**) results from relaxation of smooth muscle in the vascular walls. It can begin within seconds after an

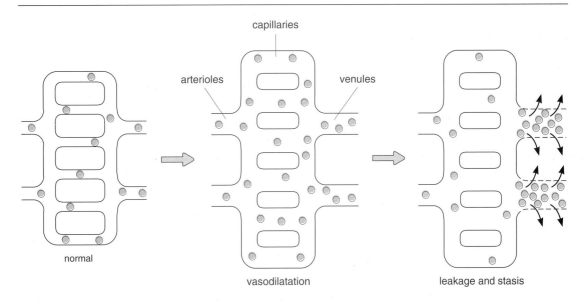

Figure 2–3. Vasodilatation and vascular leakage. Vasodilatation affects arterioles, capillaries, and venules. Leakage results from endothelial retraction that occurs only in postcapillary venules.

acute injury or develop over hours or days of low-grade irritation or infection. Vasodilatation initially results in increased blood flow through arterioles, capillaries, and venules of the affected region, leading to redness (**erythema**) and warmth. As the vessels dilate, endothelial cells lining some of the vessels actively retract away from one another to create temporary, microscopic gaps in the endothelial lining. Endothelial retraction occurs only in the smallest venules (often called **postcapillary venules**), which are thin-walled vessels with lumenal diameters of 20–60 μm (Table 2–5). Retraction results in **increased permeability** of the venule wall, which allows protein-rich fluid from the blood to leak out through the gaps, percolate through the endothelial basement membrane, and flow into the extracellular space of the surrounding tissue. The leakage of fluid, in turn, produces swelling of the injured tissue. It also creates a condition called stasis (or sludging) within the venules, as densely packed blood cells accumulate inside the distended lumens and the rate at which they travel along the length of the vessels decreases.

The dilatation and increased permeability of vessels near injured tissue result in part from a spinal reflex. Pain receptors stimulated by the injury transmit signals along sensory nerves to the spinal cord, where they act on autonomic motor neurons to cause relaxation of arteriolar smooth muscles at the injured site. Even if the neurons are cut, however, vasodilatation and vascular leakage still occur, though to a somewhat lesser degree. This neural-independent component of the vascular response is triggered by vasoactive mediators that are produced at the injured site and act directly on the local vessels. Among the best studied is **histamine,** an amino acid metabolite stored in large amounts by cells called **mast cells,** which reside in connective tissues throughout the body, particularly near blood vessels. Within seconds after various physical or chemical stimuli, mast cells can discharge histamine into the surrounding tissues, where it acts as a potent vasodilator and increases venular permeability. Similar effects are produced by certain **prostaglandins** and **leukotrienes**—members of a class of mediators derived from cell membrane lipids, which can be secreted by mast cells and many other cell types after trauma or other stimuli.

Vasodilatation and increased vascular permeability are protective responses that benefit the host in several ways. For example, the enhanced local blood supply helps improve delivery of oxygen, platelets, and clotting factors to the injured site, which in turn helps stabilize damaged tissues and facilitates wound healing and repair. Moreover, the vascular fluid that leaks into the tissues can immediately dilute or dissolve harmful substances in the tissues and carries with it many of the antimicrobial proteins from the serum, thereby helping to deliver innate, nonspecific defensive factors rapidly to the site where they are needed.

Even more importantly, vasodilatation alters the pattern of blood flow within the venules in such a way as to promote random collisions between blood leukocytes and the endothelium. In any normal vessel, circulating blood cells tend to be drawn toward the center of a lumen, where frictional resistance with the wall is minimized and the flow rate is highest. When a vessel dilates and its average flow rate diminishes, however, the cells within it distribute more uniformly throughout the lumen and, as a result, collide more frequently and at lower velocities against the endothelial lining. In an inflamed tissue, these collisions are especially significant because the surfaces of the venular endothelial cells have become "sticky," allowing them to bind tightly to passing leukocytes on contact. The stickiness of these vessels results from the process called endothelial activation, which is another key aspect of the inflammatory response.

Endothelial Activation

The properties of endothelial cells normally vary among organs and among different types and sizes of blood vessels. The cells lining postcapillary venules, in particular, have the unique ability to express high levels of certain surface adhesion molecules when the surrounding tissue is distressed. Endothelial cells express these proteins as part of a process called **endothelial cell activation,** which occurs when they are exposed to particular inflammatory mediators, including histamine, LPS, byproducts of the coagulation or complement cascades, or cytokines such as IL-1 or TNFα (Tables 2–4 and 2–6). Among the mol-

Table 2–5. Physical and hydrodynamic properties of human blood vessels.

Vessel Type	Wall Thickness (μm)	Lumen Diameter (μm)	Total Cross-Sectional Area (cm²)	Mean Flow Velocity (mm/s)
Aorta	2000	25,000	5	185
Artery	1000	4,000	20	42
Arteriole	20	30	400	2
Capillary	1	5	4500	0.2
Venule[a]	2	20	4000	0.2
Vein	500	5,000	40	21
Vena cava	1500	30,000	18	46

Source: Modified, with permission, from data in Ganong WF: *Review of Medical Physiology,* 17th ed. Appleton & Lange, 1995, for a resting, supine person with cardiac output of 5.0 L/min.

[a] All venules have a thin wall and low flow rate. The smallest venules (called postcapillary venules, with lumen diameters of 20–60 μm) also have endothelium specialized to retract and express leukocyte adhesion proteins when activated (see text).

Table 2–6. Major adhesion proteins induced on activated endothelial cells.

Adhesion Protein	Kinetics[a]	Major Inducers
P-selectin	Rapid (min)	Thrombin Histamine Complement derivatives Peroxide
E-selectin	Slow (h)	Interleukin-1 Tumor necrosis factor LPS
ICAM-1, VCAM-1	Slow (h)	Interleukin-1 Tumor necrosis factor Interferon gamma LPS

Abbreviations: ICAM = intercellular adhesion molecule; VCAM = vascular cell adhesion molecule; LPS = lipopolysaccharide.
[a] Kinetics of appearance of binding activity after activating stimulus.

Table 2–7. Properties of three major human cell lineages involved in host defense.[a]

	Neutrophils	Monocyte–Macrophages	Lymphocytes[b]
Primary effector function	Phagocytosis	Phagocytosis	Varies
Cytoplasmic granules	Many	Moderate	Few
Can synthesize new membrane or secretory proteins	Very limited	Yes	Yes
Terminally differentiated	Yes	Usually	No
Principal normal location	Blood and marrow	All tissues	Lymphoid tissues
Immunoregulatory cytokine production	No[c]	Yes	Yes
Antigen presentation[d]	No	Yes	Yes

[a] The properties as listed apply to the mature cells of each lineage.
[b] Several distinct subtypes of lymphocytes have been described, and their functional properties differ widely (see Chapter 3). Properties shown are those of B and α/β T lymphocytes.
[c] Except certain chemokines (see Chapter 10).
[d] To helper T lymphocytes (see Chapter 4).

ecules that are expressed on activated endothelium are intercellular adhesion molecule 1 (**ICAM-1**) and vascular cell adhesion molecule 1 (**VCAM-1**), each of which can bind specific integrins on other cells (see Chapter 1), as well as two members of the selectin family of carbohydrate-binding proteins, called **E-selectin** and **P-selectin.** Some of these adhesion molecules appear only after the endothelium has been activated for several hours, so as to allow time for synthesis of the appropriate mRNAs and protein, but others can be induced within minutes. For example, endothelial cells normally store P-selectin on the membranes of intracytoplasmic secretory granules called Weibel-Palade bodies; when the cell is stimulated appropriately, these organelles quickly fuse with the plasma membrane, transferring P-selectin onto the cell surface. Each endothelial adhesion protein has an affinity for surface molecules expressed by one or more types of leukocytes. Thus, the postcapillary venules in inflamed tissue not only are dilated and leaky, but also are lined by activated endothelial cells that have markedly increased affinity for leukocytes. As we shall see in the following section, binding of blood leukocytes onto the endothelium is the first, essential step in attracting these defensive cells to the site of an injury or infection.

THE PHAGOCYTES

Although virtually all types of leukocytes contribute to host defense, three types play especially preeminent roles (Table 2–7). Two of these (the **neutrophils** and the **monocyte–macrophage** series) are phagocytic cells, which act primarily by engulfing and digesting bacteria, cellular debris, and other particulate matter. The third group, made up of the **lymphocytes** and their relatives, has little phagocytic capacity but instead carries out a host of other protective reactions known collectively as immune responses. Lymphocytes are the main agents of acquired immunity, and their properties will be considered at length in later chapters. The phagocytes, on the other hand, can act in cooperation with lymphocytes, but also are able to recognize and kill many pathogens directly and so constitute the most important cellular effectors of the innate immune system.

Neutrophils

Neutrophils make up an army of more-or-less identical circulating phagocytes that are poised to respond quickly and in vast numbers wherever tissue injury has occurred. The mature cells, which are also known as segmented neutrophils (segs) or polymorphonuclear leukocytes (polys, or PMNs), can easily be identified by their characteristic multilobed nucleus and by the abundant storage granules in their cytoplasm (Figure 2–4). These granules store bactericidal agents and lysosomal enzymes until they are needed to kill and digest an ingested microorganism. Synthesis of the granule proteins, and their incorporation into granules, occurs as immature neutrophil precursors develop in the bone marrow. The mature neutrophil contains three chemically distinct granule types, which appear at different stages of maturation (Table 2–8). The azurophilic (or primary) granules are formed early, during the promyelocyte stage, and

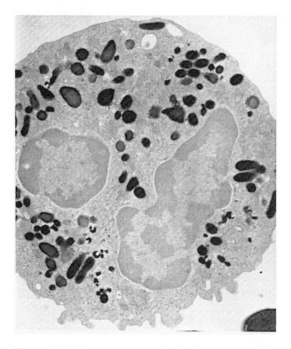

Figure 2–4. Electron micrograph of a human neutrophil. The single elongated nucleus is constricted at multiple sites to form segments, only two of which appear in this section. The cytoplasm contains numerous storage granules that differ in appearance and enzyme content; the myeloperoxidase-containing (azurophilic) granules are stained darkly in this preparation. Note the absence of rough endoplasmic reticulum.

contain an antibacterial enzyme called myeloperoxidase, as well as defensins, lysozyme, numerous lysosomal enzymes, and other proteins. The specific (or secondary) granules are formed later, during the myelocyte stage, and contain lysozyme, the iron-binding protein lactoferrin, and several important membrane receptors but lack myeloperoxidase. Gelatinase-containing granules are formed last, at the metamyelocyte stage. Thus, each neutrophil contains a diverse armamentarium of preformed antimicrobial proteins. Immature neutrophil precursors have a well-developed rough endoplasmic reticulum and Golgi apparatus that are used to synthesize the granules, but those organelles become greatly diminished as the cells mature, leaving the fully developed neutrophil with very limited ability to produce new secretory or membrane proteins. The mature neutrophil is also terminally differentiated—that is, it lacks the ability to replicate by cell division.

Neutrophils grow to full maturity in the bone marrow and are usually retained in the marrow for an additional 5 days as part of a large reserve pool. They are then released into the bloodstream, where they normally constitute one half to two thirds of all circulating white blood cells. An adult has approximately 50 billion neutrophils in the circulation at all times, each of which is programmed to die by apoptosis less than 12 hours, on average, after entering the bloodstream. Thus, the marrow must produce vast numbers of neutrophils each day to maintain a stable circulating population. To meet this demand, roughly 60% of all marrow hematopoietic activity is devoted to neu-

Table 2–8. Representative contents of human neutrophil granules.

	Azurophilic Granules	Specific Granules	Gelatinase Granules
Soluble Proteins			
Microbicidal proteins	Myeloperoxidase Lysozyme Defensins	Lysozyme	
Other enzymes	Lysosomal acid hydrolases Elastase Cathepsin G Proteinase 3 Azurocidin	Collagenase Gelatinase	Gelatinase
Other proteins		Lactoferrin β_2-microglobulin Vitamin B$_{12}$-binding protein	
Membrane Proteins			
Receptors for:		Complement proteins (CR3) Chemokines *N*-Formyl peptides Laminin Vitronectin	Immunoglobulin (FcγRIII)
Other proteins	CD63	Mac-1 (CD11b/CD18)	Mac-1 (CD11b/CD18)

Abbreviations: FcγRIII = type-3 Fc receptor specific for immunoglobulin G (see Chapter 7). Mac-1 is an integrin composed of the CD11b and CD18 chains.

trophil production, as compared with only 20–30% devoted to erythrocyte formation.

Once released from the marrow, neutrophils normally circulate continuously in the blood throughout their brief lives. If their journey carries them into an inflamed tissue, however, the cells rapidly adhere to the activated endothelium of local postcapillary venules, migrate through the vessel walls, and invade the affected tissues, where they may accumulate in vast numbers. As is true for all leukocytes, the process by which neutrophils adhere to a vessel wall is called **margination** and occurs in three phases (Figure 2–5). The first, **selectin-mediated phase** begins when a passing neutrophil or other leukocyte collides with the vessel wall, allowing P-selectin and E-selectin molecules on the activated endothelium to bind leukocyte surface mucins that bear the appropriate carbohydrate sidechains. The selectins and their mucin ligands are elongated molecules often located at the tips of microvilli, which enhances their accessibility for binding. In contrast to other types of adhesion molecules, selectins bond tightly to their ligands in less than a millisecond, so that even momentary contact can tether a moving leukocyte firmly to the wall. Because this tethering involves only a few bonds at a time, however, and because the individual bonds dissociate after no more than a second, the leukocyte may, under the force of the flowing blood, continue to roll or skip intermittently along the vessel wall during this phase.

Once it is tethered onto the venule wall, the neutrophil or other leukocyte comes into contact with a wide variety of inflammatory mediators (see Table 2–4) that may either be expressed by the activated endothelium or simply diffuse into the blood from the injured tissue. Among these mediators are a diverse subset of intermediaries known as **leukocyte chemotactic factors** which bind to receptors on the leukocyte surface and trigger the second, **activation phase** of margination. The most important leukocyte chemotactic factors are the **chemokines,** a structurally diverse group of protein cytokines that can be secreted by activated endothelial cells and by many other cell types in response to tissue distress, and which each selectively attract particular types of leukocytes that bear the corresponding surface receptors (see Chapter 11). Although they are soluble proteins, the chemokines tend to adhere to the surfaces of endothelial cells and also to the extracellular matrix, forming an immobilized gradient of chemokine concentration that begins at the venular endothelium, rises through the tissues, and peaks at the site of injury. A number of other inflammatory mediators also are leukocyte chemoattractants: These include fragments of fibrin or collagen (as might be generated in a wound), factors released by activated platelets or mast cells, and certain byproducts of the complement cascade. Another notable example are peptides containing **N-formylmethionine** residues, a modified amino acid that is present at the amino termini of proteins from most types of bacteria but is not found in proteins of human origin and that therefore serves as a telltale sign that bacteria are present in a host tissue.

Each leukocyte chemotactic factor is recognized by a specific receptor on the leukocyte surface. Despite the diversity of their ligands, all of these receptors belong to the **7-transmembrane** receptor family, a very large group of receptors that each consists of a single polypeptide threaded across the plasma membrane seven times (see Figure 2–5B). Every neutrophil carries a host of receptors for different chemotactic factors. Contact with even minuscule amounts of such a factor, either dissolved in the blood or bound to the endothelial surface, triggers dramatic changes in the surface adhesion properties of the neutrophil. One such change is that a surface protein called **L-selectin,** which is ordinarily present on neutrophils and all other leukocytes, is shed from the cells, so it can no longer contribute to selectin-mediated interactions. At the same time, activation by chemotactic factors changes the conformations of **integrins** on the leukocyte surface, enabling them to bind to specific glycoproteins on the endothelium. For example, exposure of a neutrophil to either N-formylmethionyl peptides or certain chemokines unmasks the binding activities of integrins called **Mac-1** and leukocyte functional antigen 1 **(LFA-1),** which can each then bind to ICAM-1 on an activated endothelial cell. These latter changes usher in the final, **integrin-mediated phase** of margination (see Figure 2–5). Integrin-mediated interactions develop relatively slowly, but lead to stable, long-lasting molecular contacts that prevent further movement of the neutrophil, so that it stops rolling along the vessel wall within seconds and then flattens out against the endothelium over the course of a few minutes.

Once attached, neutrophils actively insinuate themselves between endothelial cells to migrate out of the venule and into the adjacent tissue in a process termed **emigration.** The neutrophils then travel by ameboid motion up the concentration gradient of chemotactic factors until they arrive at the focus of injury or infection. Emigration and chemotaxis are facilitated in part by binding of neutrophil surface integrins to fibronectin and other components of the extracellular matrix.

On arrival at an injured site, neutrophils immediately begin the process of engulfing any bacteria, cellular debris, or foreign particulate matter in the area. The mechanisms by which these cells are able to recognize such a wide range of target particles are not fully understood. Some types of targets, such as unencapsulated bacteria, carbon particles, or polystyrene beads, are probably recognized by virtue of nonspecific surface properties such as hydrophobicity. Others may carry particular oligosaccharides or other chemical features that are recognized by recep-

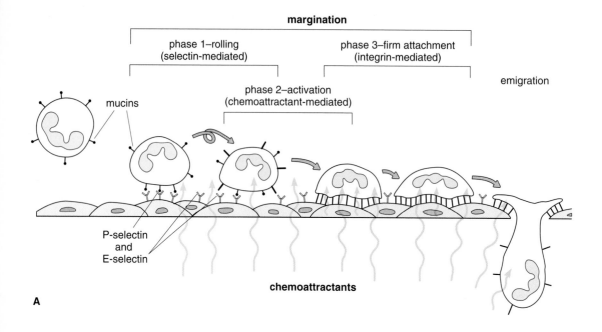

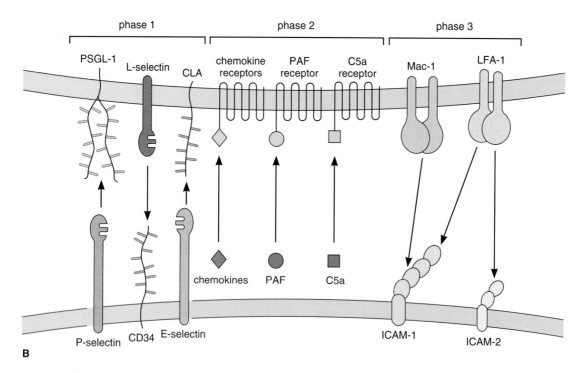

Figure 2–5. Neutrophil margination and emigration. **A:** Leukocyte adhesion to activated endothelium occurs in three overlapping phases, each mediated by a particular class of molecules. **B:** Molecular interactions in the three phases of neutrophil adhesion. Representative surface molecules on the neutrophil (*above*) and endothelial cell (*below*) are shown with their corresponding ligands. Similar interactions also mediate endothelial binding by other leukocytes, though the specific molecules involved may vary. *Abbreviations:* PSGL-1 = P-selectin glycoprotein ligand; CLA = cutaneous lymphocyte antigen; PAF = platelet-activating factor; ICAM = intercellular adhesion molecule; LFA = leukocyte function-associated antigen; C5a = complement derivative 5a (see Chapter 12). (Modified and redrawn, with permission, from Springer TA, *Ann Rev Physiol* 1995;**57**:827.)

tors on the neutrophil surface. Individual macromolecules or submicroscopic particles such as viruses that bind an individual receptor may be taken into the cell through **receptor-mediated endocytosis,** but larger (>100-nm diameter), multivalent particles, such as bacteria, undergo **phagocytosis,** which is thought to occur through a progressive "zippering" process in which increasing numbers of receptors on the cell surface membrane come into contact with the particle surface until it is completely engulfed (Figure 2–6).

Many types of particles, including most species of encapsulated bacteria, do not interact effectively with any cellular receptor and hence cannot be phagocytized directly. Phagocytosis of such particles can occur, however, when their surfaces are coated with certain host-derived proteins. Proteins that have this ability to enhance phagocytosis are known as **opsonins.** Many different human proteins function as

opsonins (eg, see Table 2–1), but by far the most important are the complement derivatives and a group of proteins called **immunoglobulins** that are secreted by some cells of the lymphocyte lineage (see Chapters 3 and 7). Opsonization occurs because the phagocyte carries surface receptors for the opsonin protein: When such a protein coats a target particle, it allows efficient receptor-mediated engulfment (Figure 2–7). The opsonizing effect of immunoglobulins, for example, is mediated through immunoglobulin receptors, called **Fc receptors,** on the phagocyte surface. Similarly, some components of the complement pathway act as very potent opsonins because the phagocytes express surface **complement receptors.**

Particles that have been engulfed by a neutrophil are initially contained within membrane-bounded vacuoles called **phagosomes.** Seconds after engulfment, storage granules in the neutrophil cytoplasm

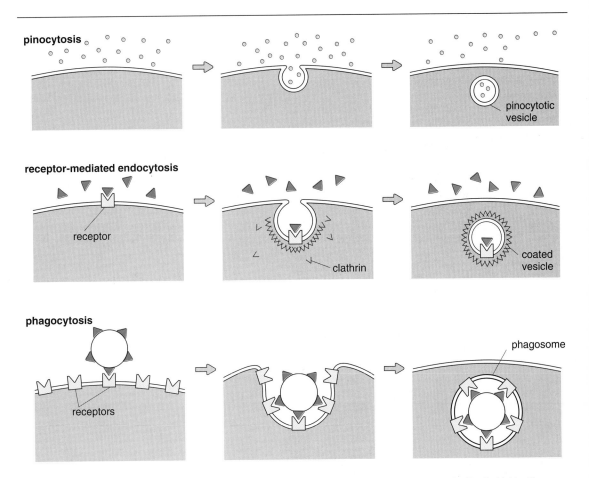

Figure 2–6. Three major pathways for bringing extracellular materials into a cell. Pinocytosis ("cell drinking") occurs through formation of minute surface vesicles filled with unmodified extracellular fluid. Receptor-mediated endocytosis is triggered by the binding of a soluble ligand to one or more specific surface receptors; the resulting polymerization of clathrin protein on the cytoplasmic aspect of the plasma membrane leads to invagination of the receptor and formation of a coated pit. Phagocytosis occurs when multiple surface receptors sequentially engage the surface of a target particle, usually >100 nm in diameter. Pinocytotic and coated vesicles, like phagosomes, are lined by a single lipid bilayer derived from the plasma membrane.

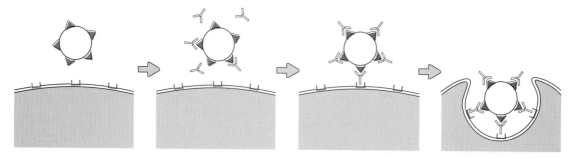

Figure 2–7. Opsonization. The opsonin protein (in this case, an immunoglobulin) binds to the surface of a particle, enabling the particle to be recognized by opsonin-specific receptors on the phagocyte surface.

begin to fuse with each phagosome, emptying their contents into its lumen (Figure 2–8). This process is known as **degranulation.** The neutrophil granules contain an extensive array of enzymes and other substances that can kill and degrade bacteria or dissolve other phagocytized materials (see Table 2–8). Among the most abundant are the α-**defensins,** which kill by making microbial membranes permeable and which constitute 30–50% of total granule protein. Other granule contents, including lysozyme, lactoferrin, and numerous proteases, also have powerful antimicrobial effects. The cell also acidifies the phagosome by actively pumping hydrogen ions into its interior; this not only promotes hydrolysis of the target directly, but also enhances the activities of many granular enzymes.

The contents of the phagosome are also subjected to powerful oxidizing agents generated by a multiprotein complex called reduced nicotinamide adenine dinucleotide phosphate **(NADPH)-dependent oxidase.** This complex is assembled from at least five different protein subunits, three of which normally reside in the cytosol and the remaining two of which are located in the membranes of secretory vesicles and specific granules. During degranulation, the cytosolic and membrane components rapidly come together at the membrane to assemble an active oxidase, which projects into the lumen of the phagosome. The oxidase acts to convert molecular oxygen into highly reactive singlet oxygen, which spontaneously dismutates to form hydrogen peroxide (Figure 2–9). In the presence of **myeloperoxidase** (which accounts for 5% of the dry weight of a neutrophil), this hydrogen peroxide combines with chloride ions to form hypochlorous acid (HOCl)—a potent oxidizing agent that is the active ingredient of household bleach. The hypochlorous acid is consumed almost instantaneously as it oxidizes amines, thiols, nucleic acids, proteins, and other biomolecules in the target particle, but a substantial portion reacts to form organic chloramines (R-NCl)—a less powerful but much longer lived class of oxidizing agents.

Oxidative killing also occurs through a second pathway involving production of **nitric oxide (NO)** a soluble, highly labile free-radical gas. When activated, neutrophils express an enzyme called inducible nitric oxide synthase, which can generate NO from the amino acid arginine and molecular oxygen (see Figure 2–9). In the presence of other reactive oxygen species within the phagocytic vacuole, NO is

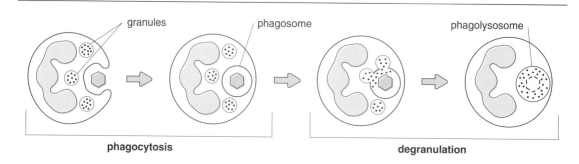

Figure 2–8. Engulfment and digestion of a target by a neutrophil. In the process of degranulation, multiple types of cytoplasmic granules may fuse with the phagosome, disgorging their contents into its lumen to inactivate and degrade the target particle.

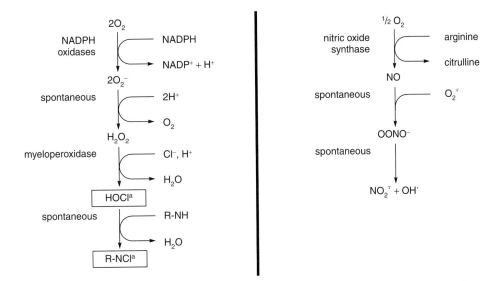

Figure 2–9. The major oxidative microbial pathways in neutrophils.
[a] Hypochlorous acid (HOCl) and organic chloramines (R-NCl) probably account for most of the target oxidation that takes place in vivo. The superoxide (O_2^-) and hydrogen peroxide (H_2O_2) intermediates in this pathway are also strong oxidizing agents but probably proceed along the pathway too quickly to play a major direct role in attacking target particles. "R-NH" denotes any organic primary or secondary amine.

converted to other products, such as peroxynitrite, which are highly toxic to bacteria, yeast, viruses, and other pathogens.

Together, these oxidative pathways provide some of the neutrophil's most important antimicrobial effects. Their vigorous action is manifested by a pronounced, transient increase in overall oxygen consumption by the neutrophil (called a **respiratory burst,** or **metabolic burst**) that occurs immediately after phagocytosis and can persist for as long as 3 hours.

The types of injuries that attract neutrophils into a tissue are nearly always accompanied by the local release of inflammatory mediators that produce swelling, redness, heat, and pain at the involved site (see Chapter 13). Inflammation associated with an infiltration of neutrophils is known as **acute inflammation.** The first wave of invading neutrophils can be detected as early as 30 minutes after an acute injury; the cells generally accumulate to significant levels within 8–12 hours and continue to arrive in increasing numbers until the production of chemotactic signals subsides. Because neutrophils cannot replicate and because they survive for only a few hours within tissues, many die at the site of inflammation and must be replaced by new cells from the circulation. In severe acute infections or other periods of high demand, the rate at which neutrophils are produced and released from storage in the bone marrow often increases dramatically, so that the blood neutrophil concentration rises several fold. This greatly

increases the number of cells available for delivery to the injured site. If marrow output is especially great, immature neutrophils that have unsegmented, rod-shaped nuclei (and hence are called **bands**) may also be released to the bloodstream. When the demand eventually wanes, the peripheral neutrophil concentration gradually returns to normal over a period of days or weeks.

If a localized response is prolonged or intense, enzymes released from dying neutrophils may liquefy nearby host cells and foreign material alike to form a viscous semifluid residue called **pus**—another hallmark of acute inflammation. Granule contents can also escape accidentally from living neutrophils during the course of phagocytosis because degranulation often begins before a target particle has been completely engulfed (Figure 2–10). An extreme example of this occurs when neutrophils confront a target (eg, a splinter) that is too large to engulf: In such a case, the cells attach themselves to the target and discharge granule contents onto its surface in a process called **extracellular degranulation.** Although beneficial in some cases, extracellular release of granule contents carries the risk of serious damage to host tissues and plays a prominent role in the pathogenesis of several human diseases, including gout, some forms of glomerulonephritis, and autoimmune arthritis.

The neutrophilic phagocyte system has many advantageous properties as an agent of innate immunity. First, neutrophils are attracted by a limited number of stimuli that generally signal the presence of

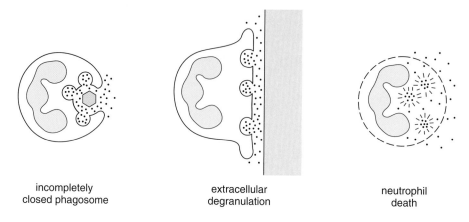

incompletely
closed phagosome

extracellular
degranulation

neutrophil
death

Figure 2–10. Some means by which the contents of neutrophil granules may be released into the extracellular milieu. Extracellular degranulation (also called "frustrated phagocytosis") occurs when the cell encounters a target that is too large to engulf. Neutrophil death and the inadvertent release of granule contents from incompletely closed phagosomes are common during intense or prolonged neutrophil reactions.

tissue injury regardless of cause. This ensures that the cells can respond to many different types of injuries, including those that the host has never encountered before. Thus, acute trauma, foreign bodies, burns, bacterial infections, and many other types of injuries each can provoke an intense neutrophil response. In addition, because large numbers of neutrophils are continually present in the blood and because nearly all of them respond to the same set of chemotactic factors, vast numbers of the cells can be mobilized without delay. Moreover, neutrophils are highly effective at killing certain bacteria, and their ability to digest cellular debris and exogenous particulate matter provides an important first step in the healing process.

Nevertheless, a defense system based solely on neutrophils would have some very significant limitations. In particular, these cells are completely unable to recognize many types of potentially injurious agents and so do not respond to them until tissue damage has occurred. For example, neutrophils cannot detect or eradicate most types of proteinaceous toxins or individual viral particles circulating in the blood because these generally do not bind to any neutrophil surface receptor. When neutrophils are called into action, they have only a limited repertoire of possible responses, consisting mainly of phagocytosis and the intracellular or extracellular discharge of their granule contents. Finally, the neutrophil system by itself has almost no ability to modify its responses on the basis of past exposure. Left on its own, this system of phagocytes would respond (or fail to respond) in the same stereotypical manner to a given pathogen no matter how many times it had encountered that same pathogen before.

Mononuclear Phagocytes: The Monocyte–Macrophage System

Nearly all tissues, organs, and serosal cavities harbor a population of resident phagocytes. Most contain only a diffuse scattering of individual phagocytic cells that remain inconspicuous under normal conditions and are very similar to one another in appearance and function. In some tissues, however, phagocytes are especially abundant or have distinctive morphologic features and are known by specific names. Examples include the Kupffer cells that line sinusoids of the liver (and account for nearly 10% of total liver mass), osteoclasts in bone, or microglial cells of the brain (Table 2–9). Regardless of their location or appearance, all of these tissue-associated phagocytes belong to a single lineage known as the **mononuclear phagocyte system** and are derived from a circulating white blood cell called the monocyte.

Monocytes are relatively large (12–20 μm in diameter) cells with kidney-shaped nuclei, loose nuclear chromatin, and fairly abundant cytoplasm that is well stocked with the types of organelles needed to synthesize secretory and membrane proteins (Figure 2–11). They also contain a substantial supply of cytoplasmic **lysosomes,** which contain most of the same enzymatic constitutents found in neutrophil azurophilic granules; however, these are less numerous than the granules in neutrophils and are not readily seen under the light microscope. Monocytes are not very abundant in the peripheral circulation, accounting for only 1–6% of all nucleated blood cells. They are produced in the bone marrow and are then released into the blood, where they circulate for only about a day before settling into a permanent site of residence in a

Table 2–9. Cells of the monocyte–macrophage lineage.

Tissue	Cell Type Designation
Blood	Monocytes
Bone marrow	Monocytes and monocyte precursors (monoblasts, promonocytes)
Any solid tissue	Resident macrophages (histiocytes) and myeloid dendritic cells
Skin	Langerhans' cells
Liver	Kupffer cells
Lung	Alveolar macrophages
Bone	Osteoclasts
Synovium	Type A synovial cells
Central nervous system	Microglia
Pleural cavity	Pleural macrophages
Peritoneal cavity	Peritoneal macrophages
Chronic inflammatory exudate	Exudate macrophages
Granuloma	Epithelioid cells, multinucleated giant cells

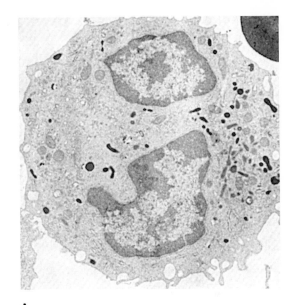

A

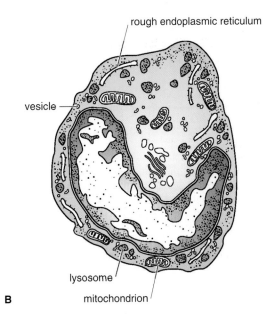

B

Figure 2–11. A: Electron micrograph and **B:** diagram of a human monocyte. Cytoplasmic granules (lysosomes) are present but are much less numerous than in neutrophils. However, the cell retains the abundant Golgi apparatus and rough endoplasmic reticulum needed to synthesize additional granules or secretory proteins as needed.

tissue. Once settled in this manner, the cells are called tissue **macrophages,** or **histiocytes.** The criteria by which the cells select their tissue residence is presently unknown. Like other leukocytes, blood monocytes can be attracted into a site of injury or infection through a three-phase process of endothelial attachment that is essentially identical to that described for neutrophils and uses many of the same adhesion proteins and chemotactic factors (see earlier section). The specific chemokines recognized by monocytes and neutrophils differ, however, because the cells express different chemokine receptors; as a result, the particular combination of chemokines produced in a distressed tissue determines whether monocytes, neutrophils, or other leukocytes will be attracted. It appears likely that chemokines or similar factors also govern the entry and distribution of monocytes into normal tissues. Monocytes that colonize some tissues (eg, liver or brain) subsequently undergo changes in morphology or function, presumably in response to factors in the local microenvironment.

A tissue macrophage lives for approximately 2–4 months. During this time, some macrophages remain immobile, whereas others wander incessantly by ameboid motion. In either case, the cell continually samples its surrounding environment by pinocytosis (see Figure 2–6) and through an extensive array of receptors on its surface (Table 2–10). Whenever it encounters certain inflammatory mediators or other signals of tissue distress, the cell undergoes a process known as **macrophage activation,** in which it rapidly increases its metabolic rate, motility, and phagocytic activity. Activated macrophages are somewhat larger than their inactive counterparts, owing mainly to an increase in cytoplasmic volume, and are much more efficient at killing bacteria and other pathogens. Many new proteins are synthesized on ac-

tivation, including the inducible nitric oxide synthase, whose product (NO) has a major role in macrophage bactericidal function. The range of stimuli that can activate macrophages is very large: Direct surface contact with certain microorganisms or inert

Table 2–10. Ligands bound by macrophage surface receptors.

Opsonins
Complement components (C3 and C4 products)
Immunoglobulins (especially IgG; via Fc receptors)
Carbohydrates and carbohydrate-binding proteins (mannose-, fucose-, galactose-, and *N*-acetylglucosamine-containing oligosaccharides)
Chemotactic factors
N-Formyl oligopeptides
Complement components (C5a)
Thrombin
Fibrin
Growth factors and cytokines
Colony-stimulating factors (GM-CSF, M-CSF)
Interleukins (IL-1, IL-3, IL-6, IL-10)
Interferons (IFNα, IFNβ, IFNγ)
Tumor necrosis factors (TNF)
Transforming growth factor β (TGFβ)
Hormones and other mediators
Insulin
Histamine
Epinephrine
Calcitonin
Parathyroid hormone
Somatomedins
Miscellaneous
Transferrin
Lactoferrin
Modified low-density lipoproteins
Fibronectin

Source: Modified and reproduced, with permission, from Klein J: *Immunology,* Blackwell Scientific, 1990.

particles, with bacterial LPS or host tissue breakdown products, or with protein components of the complement or blood coagulation systems can each lead to activation. Another potent activator is bacterial DNA, which is characterized by its high content of cytosine-phosphate-guanosine (CpG) dinucleotides that lack the cytosine methylation found in vertebrate DNA. These **unmethylated CpG dinucleotides** are thought to be recognized by specific intracellular receptors, presumably after a bacterium has been phagocytosed and digested. Activation can also be induced by certain cytokines (notably one known as interferon-γ, or **IFNγ**) that may be secreted by nearby lymphocytes (see Chapter 10).

Activated macrophages are avid phagocytes that engulf whatever foreign particles or cellular debris they encounter. They move somewhat less rapidly than neutrophils, but have the advantage of being much longer lived. They also are larger and hence can engulf larger targets, including entire apoptotic, senescent, or damaged host cells. Like neutrophils, macrophages recognize some target particles directly by their surface properties. Some macrophage surface receptors have target specificities resembling those of the humoral proteins of innate immunity (see Table 2–1). For example, macrophages express a specific **mannose receptor,** an LPS receptor called

membrane **CD14** that is a membrane-bound version of soluble CD14, and a family of very broad-specificity receptors, called **scavenger receptors,** that recognize diverse, usually negatively charged ligands, such as the phosphatidylserine on the surfaces of apoptotic host cells and certain carbohydrates or lipids in bacterial and yeast cell walls.

Receptors belonging to the newly discovered **Toll-like receptor (TLR)** family are especially important for activating macrophages. At least ten different TLRs are known in humans. Among these is TLR-4, which is expressed selectively on macrophages and other immune cells and serves as a signal-transducing partner for CD14. Although the soluble and membrane forms of CD14 can each bind LPS, neither can directly signal to cells that binding has occurred. Instead, these LPS/CD14 complexes must first associate with the extracellular part of TLR-4, whose cytoplasmic domain then transmits signals that activate the macrophage (Figure 2–12). The importance of this signaling is indicated by the finding that mice that congenitally lack TLR-4 have increased susceptibility to fatal gram-negative infection. Other TLRs are expressed on a wide range of cell types and can directly bind LPS, mycobacterial lipoproteins, and other lipid-rich foreign molecules. TLRs, which derive their name from a related protein (called Toll) that functions similarly in the innate immune system of fruit flies, are evolutionarily very ancient. They probably play a critical role in allowing all cells to recognize microbial pathogens and initiate protective responses.

Macrophages also have receptors for complement components, immunoglobulins, and other opsonins, and a coating of such opsonins is essential for phagocytosis of many types of particles. Engulfment occurs through the zippering process described earlier (see Figure 2–6) and encloses the target particle in a phagosome. Cytoplasmic lysosomes then fuse with the phagosome, disgorging their contents into its lumen. Interestingly, the events that occur during and after phagocytosis depend in part on the receptors involved. For example, particles opsonized by immunoglobulins are engulfed by pseudopods, whereas complement-opsonized particles sink into the surface of the macrophage. Moreover, phagocytosis involving Toll-like or Fc receptors promotes oxidative killing, whereas complement-mediated phagocytosis does not.

In comparison with the action of neutrophils, macrophage phagocytosis tends to be a slower, less dramatic process: The metabolic burst that occurs after engulfment is less pronounced, and engulfed matter tends to be broken down gradually and relentlessly over time. This is partly due to the limited number of lysosomes that are available in the macrophage at a given moment. Unlike neutrophils, however, macrophages retain all of the organelles needed to synthesize secretory proteins and so can

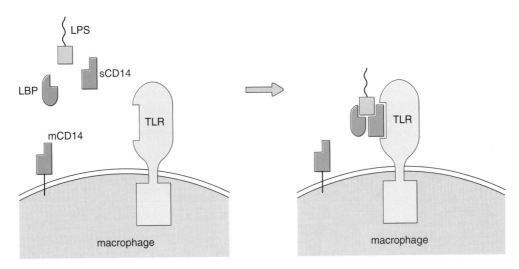

Figure 2–12. Role of a Toll-like receptor (TLR) in cellular signaling by lipopolysaccharide (LPS). The humoral proteins soluble CD14 (sCD14) and LPS-binding protein (LBP) can bind LPS but are not cell-associated. Membrane CD14 (mCD14) is attached to the cell surface via a glycolipid anchor but cannot transmit a signal. A TLR may bind LPS directly, as a complex with sCD14 or mCD14 alone, or as a complex with LPS and sCD14 (as depicted here), and can then transmit signals to the cell through the NFκB pathway.

produce new lysosomes as needed. Ultimately, the offending particles are usually completely annihilated. For example, red blood cells that leak from a damaged vessel to form a bruise, as well as any host cells that die by apoptosis (see Chapter 1), are soon engulfed by tissue macrophages and broken down into their component molecules. Most engulfed bacteria meet the same fate, but some, such as mycobacteria, can survive and even replicate inside these defensive cells. Other materials may resist degradation, but still remain sequestered within the macrophage and so are prevented from contacting the surrounding tissue. For example, inhaled carbon particles often persist for years within macrophages in the lungs of cigarette smokers.

Activated macrophages not only function as phagocytes, but also specifically secrete an enormous variety of biologically active substances into the surrounding tissues. Over 100 macrophage secretory products have been identified so far, a partial list of which is presented in Table 2–11. Some of these can be secreted individually in response to specific stimuli, whereas others are released in combination with one another as part of a more generalized response. Certain products, such as lysozyme, complement components, and hydrogen peroxide, have antimicrobial activity. Others, such as elastases and collagenases, act to liquefy and remodel the extracellular matrix. This process facilitates cellular migration and helps clear the way for the healing process. Macrophages also secrete numerous **cytokines** that influence the growth and activities of other cell types

(Chapter 10). These include colony-stimulating factors (eg, granulocyte–macrophage colony-stimulating factor [GM-CSF], which prolongs neutrophil survival in tissues by suppressing apoptosis), IL-6 (which induces the acute-phase response), fibroblast growth factors, prostaglandins, and chemokines that draw lymphocytes and other leukocytes into the vicinity. Interestingly, the NO secreted by activated macrophages not only has broad-spectrum antimicrobial activity but also acts as a messenger to regulate functions of other nearby cells. For example, NO triggers release of histamine and other vasoactive mediators from mast cells and platelets and so promotes the local vascular response of inflammation.

Most macrophages are thought to be terminally differentiated although some appear capable of limited replication within tissues. Some of the factors secreted by activated macrophages attract other nearby macrophages and blood monocytes, but the relatively slow movement and small numbers of such cells limit the speed of their response. In most cases, little or no accompanying increase occurs in marrow production or blood concentration of these cells. Generally, 7–10 days must pass before significant numbers of macrophages arrive at an injury site. Their presence (usually accompanied by an influx of lymphocytes) defines a pattern of host response known as **chronic inflammation** or **delayed-type hypersensitivity** (see Chapter 14).

Eventually, large numbers of macrophages may congregate around targets that are large, numerous, or resistant to digestion. Such macrophage aggregates

Table 2–11. Secretory products of macrophages.

Enzymes
  Lysozyme
  Acid hydrolases (proteases, nucleases, glycosidases,
    phosphatases, lipases, etc)
  Elastase
  Collagenase
  Plasminogen activator
  Angiotensin-converting enzyme

Mediators
  Interferons (IFNα, IFNβ)
  Colony-stimulating factors (GM-CSF, M-CSF, G-CSF, and
    others)
  Interleukins (IL-1, IL-6, IL-8, IL-10, IL-12)
  Chemokines
  Tumor necrosis factor α (TNFα)
  Platelet-derived growth factor
  Platelet-activating factor (PAF)
  Transforming growth factor β (TGFβ)
  Angiogenesis factors
  Nitric oxide (NO)
  Arachidonate metabolites (prostaglandins, leukotrienes)

Complement components
  C1–C9
  Properdin
  Factors B, D, I, and H

Coagulation factors
  Factors V, VII, IX, and X
  Prothrombin
  Thromboplastin

Reactive oxygen species
  Hydrogen peroxide
  Superoxide anion
  Nitric oxide (NO)
  Singlet oxygen
  Hydroxyl radicals

Miscellaneous
  Glutathione
  Nucleotides (adenosine, thymidine, guanosine, etc)

Abbreviations: GM-CSF = granulocyte–macrophage colony-stimulating factor; M-CSF = monocyte colony-stimulating factor; G-CSF = granulocyte colony-stimulating factor.

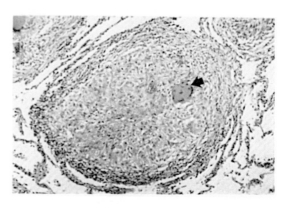

Figure 2–13. A granuloma—a distinctive pattern of macrophage reaction against foreign material. This photomicrograph shows a single roughly spherical granuloma, 1–2 mm in diameter, in the lung. It is composed almost entirely of epithelioid macrophages, with a thin, surrounding rim of fibroblasts and normal lung tissue. At one site, several individual macrophages have fused to form a multinucleated giant cell (*arrow*). In addition to macrophages, granulomas often contain other types of defensive cells (especially lymphocytes), fibroblasts, and collagen. (Courtesy of Martha Warnock)

are called **granulomas** (Figure 2–13) and usually contain subpopulations of lymphocytes, fibroblasts, and other cell types. Macrophages in such lesions are often called **epithelioid cells** because they tend to interdigitate closely with one another through complex surface folds and microvilli and so form a continuous sheet of cells that resembles an epithelium. This interdigitation serves to entrap material within the granuloma. Newly arrived monocytes entering the lesion may also fuse to form large, **multinucleate giant cells,** which are able to engulf correspondingly larger targets, such as splinters, multicellular parasites, or surgical suture material.

Viewed in isolation, macrophages are major effectors of innate immunity, but suffer from many of the same limitations described earlier for neutrophils. They are a fairly homogeneous group of phagocytic cells that recognize a fixed number of potential targets. They are, moreover, less numerous, slower to respond, and less effective than neutrophils at killing most bacteria. However, an additional facet of their biology places macrophages among the most important components of the immune system. Unlike neutrophils, macrophages are able to control the actions of lymphocytes—a far more abundant and versatile population of defensive cells—and the principal cells of acquired immunity. Macrophages affect lymphocyte responses in at least major two ways. First, activated macrophages secrete cytokines, such as TNFα and IL-12, that control lymphocyte proliferation, differentiation, and effector function. Secondly, activated macrophages are also among the most important types of **antigen-presenting cells**—cells that process and display foreign substances in a form that can be recognized and responded to by lymphocytes. Through these two types of regulatory interactions with lymphocytes, macrophages have the ability to initiate and coordinate acquired immune responses. We will explore the mechanisms and consequences of these interactions in detail in subsequent chapters.

REFERENCES

INNATE IMMUNITY

Fearon DT, Locksley RM: The instructive role of innate immunity in the acquired immune response. *Science* 1996;272:50.

Hoffmann JA et al: Phylogenetic perspectives in innate immunity. *Science* 1999;284:1313.

INNATE HUMORAL EFFECTORS

Boman HG: Peptide antibiotics and their role in innate immunity. *Ann Rev Immunol* 1995;13:61.

Gabay C, Kushner I: Acute-phase proteins and other systemic responses to inflammation. *N Engl J Med* 1999; 340:448.

Krieg AM: The role of CpG motifs in innate immunity. *Curr Opin Immunol* 2000;12:35.

Turner MW: Mannose-binding lectin (MBL) in health and disease. *Immunobiology* 1998;199:327.

INFLAMMATION

Gallin JI, Snyderman R (editors): *Inflammation: Basic Principles and Clinical Correlates,* 3rd ed. Lippincott Williams & Wilkins, 1999.

PHAGOCYTOSIS & ENDOCYTOSIS

Aderem A, Underhill DM: Mechanisms of phagocytosis in macrophages. *Ann Rev Immunol* 1999;17:593.

Allen L-A, Aderem A: Molecular definition of distinct cytoskeletal structures involved in complement- and Fc receptor-mediated phagocytosis in macrophages. *J Exp Med* 1996;184:627.

Kornfeld S: The biogenesis of lysosomes. *Ann Rev Cell Biol* 1989;5:483.

Platt N et al: Recognizing death: The phagocytosis of apoptotic cells. *Trends Cell Biol* 1998;8:365.

PHAGOCYTE EFFECTOR MECHANISMS

Babior BM: NADPH oxidase: An update. *Blood* 1999;93: 1464.

Ganz T: Oxygen-independent microbicidal mechanisms of phagocytes. *Proc Assoc Am Phys* 1999;111:390.

Hampton MB et al: Inside the neutrophil phagosome: Oxidants, myeloperoxidase, and bacterial killing. *Blood* 1998;92:3007.

MacMicking J et al: Nitric oxide and macrophage function. *Ann Rev Immunol* 1997;15:323.

Weiss SJ: Tissue destruction by neutrophils. *N Engl J Med* 1989;320:365.

NEUTROPHILS & MONOCYTE–MACROPHAGES

Borregaard N, Cowland JB: Granules of the human neutrophilic polymorphonuclear leukocyte. *Blood* 1997;89: 3503.

Cotter TG et al: Cell death in the myeloid lineage. *Immunol Rev* 1994;142:93.

Fais S et al.: The biological relevance of polykaryons in the immune response. *Immunol Today* 1997;18:522.

ADHESION PROTEINS & LEUKOCYTE–ENDOTHELIAL INTERACTIONS

Baggiolini M: Chemokines and leukocyte traffic. *Nature* 1998;392:565.

Bokoch GM: Chemoattractant signaling and leukocyte activation. *Blood* 1995;86:1649.

Luster AD: Chemokines—Chemotactic cytokines that mediate inflammation. *N Engl J Med* 1998;338:436.

Ruoslahti E: Integrins. *J Clin Invest* 1991;87:1.

Springer TA: Traffic signals on endothelium for lymphocyte recirculation and leukocyte emigration. *Ann Rev Physiol* 1995;57:827.

Vestweber D, Blanks JE: Mechanisms that regulate the function of the selectins and their ligands. *Physiol Rev* 1999;79:181.

3 Lymphocytes & Lymphoid Tissues

Tristram G. Parslow, MD, PhD

The normal adult human body contains on the order of a trillion (10^{12}) lymphocytes, most of which appear virtually identical to one another when examined by conventional histologic techniques. The typical lymphocyte is a small, round, or club-shaped cell, 5–12 μm in diameter, with a spherical nucleus, densely compacted nuclear chromatin, and cytoplasm so scanty as to be scarcely detectable under the light microscope. The cytoplasm contains scattered mitochondria and free ribosomes but lacks any distinctive organelles (Figure 3–1). Despite this uniform appearance, several very different types of lymphocytes can be distinguished on the basis of their functional properties and by the specific proteins they express. The most fundamental distinction is the division of these cells into two major lineages known as T (thymus-derived) cells and B (bone-marrow-derived) cells.

The relative proportions of T and B cells vary among tissues (Table 3–1); in peripheral blood, they account for about 75% and 10% of all lymphocytes, respectively. The remaining 15% of peripheral blood lymphocytes belong to a separate and rather enigmatic lineage known as natural killer (NK) cells, which differ from other lymphocytes in many significant respects and have some unusual properties that will be described later in this book (see Chapter 9). The present chapter focuses exclusively on T and B cells, which are the cells involved in most types of immune responses.

T- and B-lineage cells both arise from a subset of hematopoietic stem cells in the bone marrow or fetal liver that become committed to the lymphoid* pathway of development (Figure 3–2). They are descendants of a committed marrow progenitor, called the **lymphoid stem cell,** that serves as a common precursor for both T and B cells, as well as for NK cells and some dendritic cells. The progeny of these putative stem cells follow divergent pathways to mature into either B or T lymphocytes. Human B-lymphocyte development takes place entirely within the bone marrow. T cells, on the other hand, develop from immature precursors that leave the marrow and travel through the bloodstream to the thymus, where they proliferate and differentiate into mature T lymphocytes.

The thymus and bone marrow are sometimes referred to as **primary lymphoid organs** because they provide unique microenvironments that are essential for **lymphopoiesis**—the initial production of lymphocytes from uncommitted progenitor cells. Together, the thymus and marrow produce approximately 10^9 mature lymphocytes each day, which are

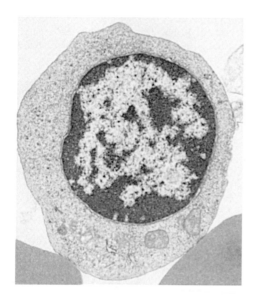

Figure 3–1. Electron micrograph of a normal human lymphocyte. This slightly tangential section exaggerates the amount of cytoplasm present: In most resting lymphocytes, the nucleus accounts for 90% of total cell volume. Note the dense nuclear chromatin and the bland cytoplasm, which lacks any obvious secretory organelles. (Courtesy of Imok Cha and Noel Weidner.)

---

* The word *lymphocyte* refers to cells at a specific stage in the T- or B-cell lineage. The term *lymphoid* is used to denote the entire lineages (encompassing cells at all developmental stages) or tissues in which cells from these lineages normally predominate.

Table 3–1. Proportions of lymphoid cell types in normal human tissues.

Tissue	Approximate % of [a]		
	T Cells	B Cells	NK Cells
Peripheral blood	70–80	10–15	10–15
Bone marrow	5–10	80–90	5–10
Thymus	99	<1	<1
Lymph node	70–80	20–30	<1
Spleen	30–40	50–60	1–5

[a] Includes cells at all recognizable stages of development in each lineage.

then released into the circulation. Lymphopoietic activity is controlled in part by soluble factors elaborated within these organs. For example, growth of early lymphoid progenitors requires at least two cytokines, called interleukin-7 (**IL-7**) and stem cell factor (**SCF**), found in both the thymic and marrow microenvironments. In addition, the thymus produces a number of hormones that selectively promote later stages of T-cell development. Lymphopoiesis also depends on direct contact of the lymphoid precursor cells with marrow and thymic stromal elements, with the extracellular matrix, and with one another. In general, lymphocytes are produced and released by the marrow and thymus at a more or less constant rate, irrespective of whether the cells are needed for an immune response at the moment. T lymphopoiesis in the thymus continues until about the time of puberty, at which time the organ normally involutes, but B cells continue to be produced by the marrow throughout life.

Mature lymphocytes that emerge from the thymus or bone marrow are in a quiescent, or **"resting,"** state: They are mitotically inactive (ie, they are in the G_0 phase of the cell cycle), and, although they are potentially capable of undergoing cell division and of carrying out immunologic functions, they have not yet been stimulated to do either. When dispersed into the bloodstream, these so-called **naive,** or "virgin," lymphocytes migrate efficiently into various **secondary** (or **peripheral**) **lymphoid organs,** such as the spleen, lymph nodes, or tonsils. The function of the secondary lymphoid organs is to maximize encounters between lymphocytes and foreign substances, and it is from these sites that most immune responses are launched.

Most naive lymphocytes have an inherently short life span and are programmed to die within a few days after leaving the marrow or thymus. If such a cell receives signals that indicate the presence of a specific foreign substance or pathogen, however, it may respond through a phenomenon known as **activation,** in the course of which it may undergo several successive rounds of cell division over a period of several days (Figure 3–3). Some of the resulting

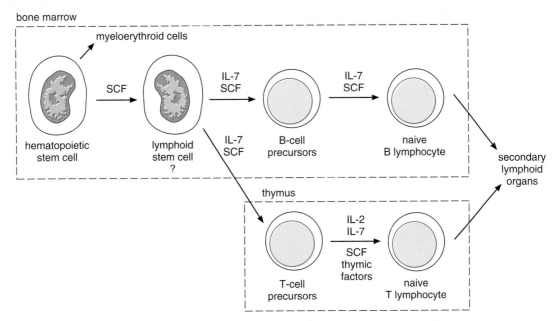

Figure 3–2. Schematic overview of lymphocyte development (lymphopoiesis). In this simplified diagram, most intermediate stages are omitted. The characteristics of cells that migrate to the thymus are unknown. A few of the regulatory molecules needed for proliferation at particular stages of development are indicated. *Abbreviations:* SCF = stem cell factor; IL = interleukin.

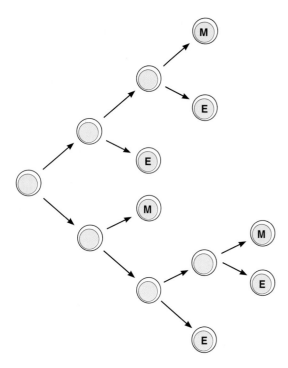

Figure 3–3. Lymphocyte activation leads to both cell division and differentiation. At each cell division, individual cells can cease dividing and differentiate into memory (M) or effector (E) cells. In this example, a single activated lymphocyte gives rise to four effector and three memory cells after four cycles of division.

progeny cells then revert to the resting state to become **memory lymphocytes**—cells that resemble the naive T or B lymphocyte from which they are derived but which can survive for many years. Such memory lymphocytes make up a large proportion of the cells in the immune system of an adult, and, like naive lymphocytes, are constantly poised to undergo further cycles of activation and cell division. Thus, one consequence of activating a naive lymphocyte is that some of its progeny become long-term constituents of the host immune system. The other progeny of an activated naive lymphocyte differentiate into **effector cells,** which survive for only a few days but, during that time, carry out specific defensive activities against the foreign invader.

Lymphocyte proliferation can thus take place in two very different contexts. The first (primary lymphopoiesis) is confined to the thymus and marrow and results in the de novo production of short-lived, quiescent naive lymphocytes that are then released into the periphery. This occurs autonomously at a rate dictated by the marrow and thymus themselves. The second form of replication takes place in peripheral tissues and occurs only when lymphocytes become activated as part of an immune response. This stimulus-dependent proliferation gives rise to long-

lived memory cells and also to short-lived effector cells that actively carry out specific immune functions. The nature of these latter functions depends on the lymphocyte lineage from which the effector cells arose.

B CELLS

The defining feature of cells in the B-cell lineage is their ability to synthesize proteins called **immunoglobulins** (Figure 3–4). No other cell expresses these proteins. The immunoglobulins are an extremely diverse family of proteins, each made up of two related types of polypeptides called **heavy chains** and **light chains.** Each immunoglobulin binds specifically and with high affinity to its own particular small molecular ligand, which may be any of a vast number of chemical determinants found in proteins, carbohydrates, lipids, or other macromolecules. The molecular determinants bound by various immunoglobulin proteins can be referred to collectively as **antigens**—an important term that is considered more thoroughly in Chapter 5.

Mature B cells can express immunoglobulin in two different forms that each serve unique functions (Figure 3–5). In resting (naive or memory) B lymphocytes, immunoglobulins are expressed only on the cell surface, where they serve as membrane-bound receptors for specific antigens. Each resting lympho-

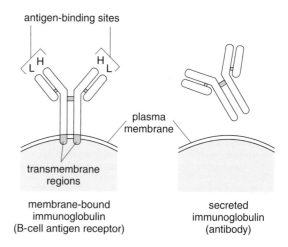

Figure 3–4. Membrane-bound and secreted forms of an immunoglobulin protein. This diagram depicts one of the many types of immunoglobulins, each of which is composed of paired light-chain (L) and heavy-chain (H) polypeptides. The amino termini of the L and H chains are juxtaposed to form the binding site for an antigen. A hydrophobic region (shaded) at the carboxy termini of the heavy chains anchors the membrane-bound protein onto the cell surface. When this region is absent, the immunoglobulin is secreted from the cell.

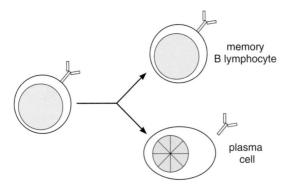

Figure 3–5. The progeny of an activated B lymphocyte can differentiate into either memory B lymphocytes or antibody-secreting plasma cells.

cyte may express tens of thousands of membrane immunoglobulins on its surface. By contrast, the effector cells of the B lineage (called **plasma cells**) are uniquely specialized to secrete large amounts of immunoglobulin proteins into their surrounding milieu. Secreted immunoglobulins retain the ability to recognize and bind their specific ligands and are often referred to as **antibodies;** they normally circulate at a serum concentration of 7–26 g/L in an adult and so account for about 25% of total serum protein. Binding of an antibody to its target antigen can have a variety of effects that are beneficial to the host. For example, antibody binding may sequester and inactivate a toxic protein in the blood or may block receptors on a viral particle that would otherwise enable the virus to adhere to host cells. Many secreted immunoglobulins also are potent opsonins, in that they promote phagocytosis of bacteria or other targets to which they bind. The properties of immunoglobulins are discussed in much more detail in Chapter 7. For the present, it is enough to say that these binding proteins not only serve as surface receptors for foreign substances but also can be released to search out and bind their targets at a considerable distance from the cell.

When an activated B lymphocyte divides, some of its progeny become memory B cells, and the remainder differentiate into plasma cells. Plasma cells are oval or egg-shaped and have abundant cytoplasm and eccentrically placed round nuclei (Figure 3–6). Clumps of dark-staining chromatin are often distributed around the inner aspect of the nuclear membrane in plasma cells, giving the nuclei a characteristic "pinwheel" or "clock face" appearance under the light microscope. The protein-secretory organelles are well represented, including a large paranuclear Golgi apparatus and abundant rough endoplasmic reticulum. Immunoglobulins usually are not present on the surface of a plasma cell but are produced in copious amounts in the cytoplasm and are then se-

creted into the extracellular space. Plasma cells have a relatively short life span (on the order of days to a few weeks) and are terminally differentiated. Unless new plasma cells are continually produced, the existing ones soon die out and immunoglobulins are no longer secreted. Thus, activation of B cells typically results in a transient wave of proliferation, followed by a burst of antibody secretion that increases and then subsides over several days or a few weeks.

The main function of B-lineage cells is to secrete antibodies into the blood and other body fluids and hence to make these fluids inhospitable to foreign invaders. They are the principal cell type involved in **humoral acquired immunity**—that is, in protective effects that are mediated through tissue fluids. B cells also play two additional roles in the immune system. First, they can function as **antigen-presenting cells,** by processing and displaying foreign substances in a manner that can be recognized by T lymphocytes. Second, activated B cells can secrete certain **lymphokines** and other factors that influence the growth and activities of other immunologically important cells. These last two functions are discussed in more detail in later chapters.

T CELLS

T lymphocytes do not express immunoglobulins but, instead, detect the presence of foreign substances by way of surface proteins called **T-cell receptors.** These receptors form a heterogeneous class of membrane proteins, which, on most T cells, are made up of a pair of transmembrane polypeptides known as the α and β chains. T-cell receptors are closely related to immunoglobulins in evolution and share with them a number of structural and functional properties (see Chapters 7 and 9), including the ability to detect specific small molecular ligands called **antigens.** Unlike immunoglobulins, however, T-cell receptor proteins are never secreted, and, as a result, T cells lack the ability to strike their targets at long distance. Instead, they exert their protective effects either through direct contact with a target or by influencing the activity of other immune cells. Together with macrophages, T cells are the primary cell type involved in the category of immune responses called **cell-mediated acquired immunity.**

Unlike B cells, T cells can detect foreign substances only in specific contexts. In particular, T lymphocytes recognize a foreign protein only if it is first cleaved into small peptides, which are then displayed on the surface of a second host cell, called an **antigen-presenting cell.** Virtually all types of host cells can present antigens under some conditions, but certain cell types are specially adapted for this purpose and are particularly important in controlling T-cell activity. This specialized group, sometimes called the "professional" antigen-presenting cells, includes macrophages,

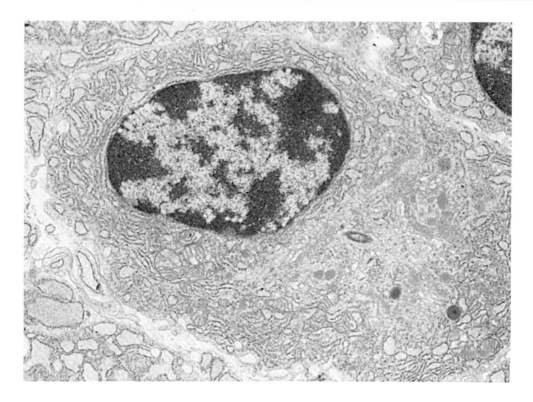

A

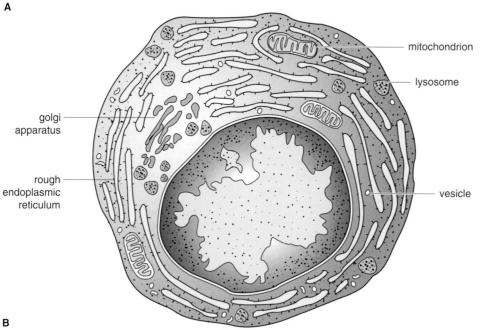

golgi
apparatus

rough
endoplasmic
reticulum

mitochondrion

lysosome

vesicle

B

Figure 3–6. A: Electron micrograph and **B:** diagram of a plasma cell, the effector cell of the B-lymphoid lineage. The abundant rough endoplasmic reticulum and Golgi complex in the cytoplasm allow these cells to synthesize large amounts of immunoglobulin in a form that is then secreted from the cell. (Courtesy of DF Bainton.)

B lymphocytes, and a family of bone-marrow-derived cells known as **dendritic cells.** Dendritic cells are found in nearly all tissues and have a distinctive stellate shape due to the many long, spidery cytoplasmic projections, called dendrites, that extend outward from their surfaces. These and other properties of dendritic cells make them extremely adept at antigen presentation and T-cell activation; in fact, they appear to be the only cell type that can efficiently activate naive T cells. As a result, dendritic cells are probably the most important class of antigen-presenting cells in the body. We will encounter some of these cells later in this chapter and will consider them in detail in Chapters 4 and 6.

Antigen presentation depends in part on specific proteins, called **major histocompatibility complex (MHC)** proteins, on the surface of the presenting cells. Foreign peptides are attached noncovalently onto the MHC proteins for display, and it is the combination of peptide and MHC protein that can be recognized by a T-cell receptor. Thus, T lymphocytes must directly touch the surfaces of other cells to detect antigens as well as to produce most of their immunologic effects.

Mature, functional T lymphocytes express a number of characteristic surface proteins in addition to T-cell receptors (Table 3–2). For example, surface T-cell receptors are always expressed in conjunction with five other transmembrane surface polypeptides that are known collectively as the **CD3 complex.** These CD3 proteins are physically associated with the T-cell receptors through noncovalent attachments; they serve to transmit signals from the receptors into the cytoplasm and must be present for the receptors to be transported onto the cell surface. Because the CD3 proteins are expressed almost exclusively by T-lineage cells and are easier to detect and much less structurally diverse than the receptors themselves, their presence is commonly used to identify T lymphocytes. Surface expression of the receptor–CD3 complex, however, occurs relatively late in T-cell ontogeny. A different protein, called **CD2,** appears at an earlier stage of T-cell development in the thymus, continues to be displayed on the surfaces of virtually all T-lineage cells, and is almost never found on other cell types. CD2 therefore serves as a very useful general marker for recognizing all cells in this lineage.

Nearly all mature T lymphocytes that are found in peripheral blood and secondary lymphoid organs are CD2$^+$CD3$^+$—that is, they each express CD2 and CD3 on their surface. The class of CD2$^+$CD3$^+$ T lymphocytes as a whole, however, is actually made up of distinct subpopulations that have very different immunologic functions and express their own distinctive surface markers. These subpopulations are often referred to as **T-cell subsets** (Table 3–3). The two most important T-cell subsets can be distinguished by two additional surface proteins known as CD4 and CD8. Mature, functional T lymphocytes almost always ex-

Table 3–2. Some important surface molecules on T lymphocytes.

Marker	Major Function or Significance
T-cell receptor	Antigen binding
CD3 complex	Signal transduction from T-cell receptor; lineage-specific marker
CD2, CD5, CD7	Lineage-specific markers
CD4	Subset-specific marker (mainly on helper cells); interaction with class II MHC proteins
CD8	Subset-specific marker (mainly on cytotoxic cells); interaction with class I MHC proteins
CD28	Activation-specific marker; receives B7-mediated costimulation from APC
CD40 ligand (CD40L)	Activation-specific marker; delivers contact-mediated help to B cells
IL-2 receptor Class II MHC proteins Transferrin receptor CD25, CD29, CD54, CD69	Other activation-specific markers
IL-1 receptor IL-6 receptor TNFα receptor	Other cytokine receptors
Fc receptors	Immunoglobulin binding
LFA-1, ICAM-1	Cell–cell adhesion molecules

Abbreviations: APC = antigen-presenting cell; IL = interleukin; TNF = tumor necrosis factor; LFA = leukocyte functional antigen; ICAM = intercellular adhesion molecule.

press only one of these two proteins, and this correlates with important differences in cell function (Figure 3–7). Most T lymphocytes that express surface **CD8** protein have **cytotoxic** activity—the ability to kill cells that have foreign macromolecules on their surfaces. Cytotoxic T lymphocytes (**T$_c$ cells,** or **CTLs**) are extremely important in the defense against viral infections: For example, host cells that are infected by a virus can often be identified by the presence of viral peptides on their surfaces, and killing

Table 3–3. Major T-cell subsets found in blood and peripheral tissues.

Surface Phenotype	Predominant Function	Proportion of Total Blood T Lympho-cytes	T-Cell Receptor Type
CD4$^+$CD8$^-$	Helper	70%	α/β
CD4$^-$CD8$^+$	Cytotoxic	25%	α/β, rarely γδ
CD4$^-$CD8$^-$	Cytotoxic	4%	γ/δ
CD4$^+$CD8$^+$	?	1%	α/β

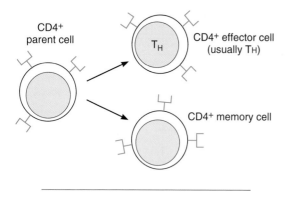

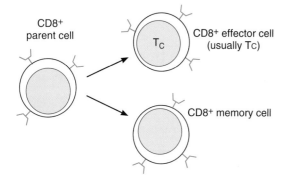

Figure 3–7. The progeny of activated T lymphocytes retain the surface phenotype (CD4⁺ or CD8⁺) of their parents.

cells are cytotoxic. Expression of CD4 or CD8 actually correlates most closely with the type of MHC protein that a T cell can recognize, as will be described in Chapters 4 and 6. Nor are these the only functionally important ways in which T cells can differ from one another. Within the T_H-cell population, for example, additional subsets of cells can be distinguished that each secrete a characteristic group of cytokines when activated and so promote particular types of defensive reactions. This heterogeneity among T_H cells will be discussed in Chapter 9.

Naive and memory T lymphocytes ordinarily remain in the resting state, and in this state they do not exhibit significant helper or cytotoxic activity. When activated, however, these cells can undergo several rounds of mitotic division to produce multiple daughter cells. Some of these daughter cells return directly to the resting state as memory cells, but others become effector cells that actively express helper or cytotoxic activity. The daughter cells resemble their parents: Activated CD4⁺ cells can produce only CD4⁺ daughter cells, whereas activated CD8⁺ cells yield only CD8⁺ progeny. The effector cells of the T lineage tend to have slightly more cytoplasm and looser chromatin than their resting counterparts but cannot reliably be distinguished from them under the light microscope. The effector cells, however, display several types of surface proteins (eg, CD25, CD28, CD29, CD40L, transferrin receptors, and a group of MHC proteins known as class II MHC proteins) that are not found on resting T cells, and they also express increased amounts of some constitutive T-cell markers (eg, CD2). When the activating stimuli are withdrawn, cytotoxic or helper activity gradually subsides over a period of several days as the effector cells either die or revert to the resting state.

AN OVERVIEW OF LYMPHOCYTE ACTIVATION

The term **lymphocyte activation** denotes an ordered series of events through which a resting lymphocyte is stimulated to divide and produce progeny, some of which become effector cells (Figure 3–8). The full response thus includes both the induction of cell proliferation (**mitogenesis**) and the expression of immunologic functions. Lymphocytes become activated when specific ligands bind to receptors on their surfaces. The ligands required are different for T cells and B cells (see the following discussion), but the response itself is similar in many respects for all types of lymphocytes.

The earliest event known to take place when a T or B cell binds ligands that cause activation is a marked increase in activity of cytoplasmic **protein tyrosine kinases (PTKs)**—proteins that have the ability to catalyze the phosphorylation of tyrosine residues in other proteins. This increase occurs within seconds

these cells is essential to eradicating the disease. In contrast, T lymphocytes that express **CD4** protein generally are not cytotoxic but instead function as **helper T cells (T_H cells),** which promote proliferation, maturation, and immunologic function of other cell types. For example, specific lymphokines secreted by helper T cells are very important in controlling the activities of B cells, macrophages, and cytotoxic T cells.

Altogether, roughly 70% of T cells in human blood or secondary lymphoid tissues are CD4⁺CD8⁻ (also called CD4 cells), whereas 25% are CD4⁻CD8⁺ (or simply CD8 cells). Cells with either of these phenotypes are often referred to as **single-positive** lymphocytes and are the cells most commonly involved in immune responses. Approximately 4% of T cells outside the thymus are CD4⁻CD8⁻ **double-negative** lymphocytes; nearly all of these express an alternative form of T-cell receptor composed of polypeptides called γ and δ (see Chapter 9). The remaining 1% of extrathymic T cells are **double-positive** CD4⁺CD8⁺ cells, whose function is unknown.

The correlation of CD4 or CD8 with T_H and T_C cell function, respectively, is strong but not absolute: A few CD8 cells have helper activity, and a few CD4

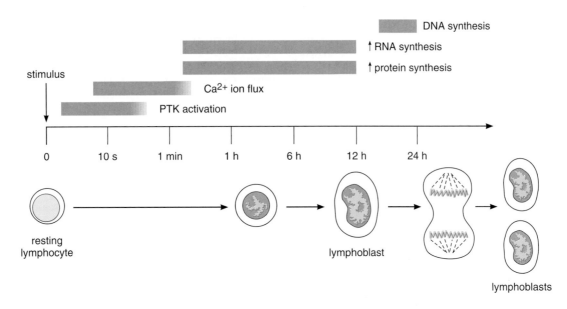

Figure 3–8. Major biochemical and morphologic events in lymphocyte activation. *Abbreviation:* PTK = protein tyrosine kinase.

and reflects the functional activation of numerous different PTKs. Several important types of lymphocyte surface receptors (including membrane immunoglobulin and T-cell receptor proteins) are physically linked to specific cytoplasmic PTK proteins, which become active when the receptor binds its target ligand. As in many other receptor systems (see Chapter 1), the ligand-induced clustering of receptors on the B- or T-lymphocyte surface appears to be a key event in triggering PTK activation. The receptor-associated PTKs, in turn, may then activate other types of PTKs through phosphorylation, so that almost immediately a host of different PTKs are recruited into the response. By phosphorylating still other types of substrates, such as proteins that control cytoskeletal organization, expression of specific genes, and entry into the cell cycle, these newly activated PTKs appear to be either directly or indirectly responsible for triggering all subsequent events in lymphocyte activation. At present, however, the functions of most individual PTKs are uncertain.

One almost immediate effect of the PTK cascade is to activate the cytosolic enzyme **phospholipase C-γ1,** which then acts to hydrolyze a specific class of phospholipids, called phosphatidylinositides, that are found in cellular membranes. The products of this hydrolysis include two small organic molecules, **diacylglycerol (DAG)** and **inositol 1,4,5-trisphosphate (IP$_3$)**, which serve as second messengers to trigger additional changes in cellular physiology. DAG remains within the membrane of origin, where it binds and allosterically activates **protein kinase C**—a family of cytosolic enzymes that can phosphorylate other

proteins at serine and threonine residues. IP$_3$ is released into the cytoplasm; binds to specific membrane receptors; and triggers a rapid, marked increase in the concentrations of **intracellular free calcium ions,** which flood into the cytosol from organellar storage pools, reaching maximal concentrations within 1 minute after contact with the activating stimulus. Like the PTK cascade, protein kinase C activation and these rapid calcium fluxes are thought to be critical for initiating the subsequent events in activation, though how they accomplish this is not yet known.

Within the first hour after stimulation, the rates of oxidative metabolism and of overall protein and RNA synthesis in the lymphocyte rise. The chromatin becomes less dense as previously silent genes are transcribed and the cell prepares to undergo mitosis. After 2–4 hours, specific proteins that are thought to regulate cell proliferation, such as the product of the protooncogene **c-*myc*,** become detectable in the nucleus. In parallel with these biochemical events, the morphology of the cell changes in a process known as **blast transformation:** its overall diameter increases to 15–30 μm as both its nucleus and cytoplasm enlarge; the nuclear chromatin becomes loose and pale-staining; and the cell acquires a prominent nucleolus (reflecting a high rate of RNA synthesis). Within 8–12 hours, the changes are sufficiently marked that the cell can be recognized under the light microscope as a **lymphoblast**—a lymphocyte poised to begin mitosis. DNA synthesis takes place at around 18–24 hours after stimulation. The first cell division occurs 2–4 hours later and, depending on the conditions, can be repeated five or more times in succession, at intervals as brief as 6 hours. The effector cells produced as a result of each division mature completely within a few days and express the immune functions typical of their lineage for several days thereafter.

REQUIREMENTS FOR ACTIVATION OF B OR T LYMPHOCYTES

What are the stimuli that can lead to lymphocyte activation in vivo? Certainly, the most important are the innumerable foreign **antigens** that are recognized and bound by membrane immunoglobulins or T-cell receptor proteins. A few types of antigens are in themselves sufficient to activate B cells—these are usually highly polymeric proteins or polysaccharides that are able to interact simultaneously with many immunoglobulin proteins on the surface of a single cell. Such multivalent antigens act to **cross-link** the immunoglobulins to one another, so that eventually a great many immunoglobulins are gathered at one pole of the cell surface at the point of contact with antigen—a phenomenon known as **capping** (Figure 3–9A). This dense local aggregation of immunoglobulins, each of which is bound to antigen, transmits a very effective signal and is enough to trigger B-cell activation.

Activation can also be induced under artificial conditions by cross-linking other types of surface molecules (Table 3–4). Among the agents used for this purpose are certain lectins (sometimes called **mitogens**), which can activate T or B cells (or both) by cross-linking surface glycoproteins. Similar results can be obtained by using multivalent antibody complexes to cross-link some T-cell surface proteins (such as CD3) that are able to transmit signals to the cytoplasm. Alternatively, lymphocytes can be activated pharmacologically by treating them with agents that directly induce calcium fluxes and other important signaling events, thereby bypassing the surface receptors entirely. Such potent artificial activators are often used in clinical testing to study lymphocyte responses in vitro.

The majority of antigens encountered in nature, however, are not polymeric and so do not cross-link large numbers of receptors. Even when many copies of such an antigen bind individual immunoglobulins on a B cell, they generate only an incomplete signal, which fails to activate the cell. B cells can be activated by these more common antigens only if they are simultaneously stimulated by a nearby activated helper T lymphocyte. This stimulation, which will be referred to in this book as **help,** can be delivered by lymphokines secreted from the T_H cell, but it occurs most effectively when the cells contact each other directly. This contact allows a surface protein called

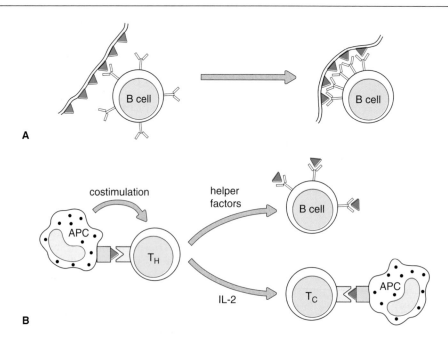

Figure 3–9. General requirements for lymphocyte activation. **A:** Some highly polymeric antigens that cross-link multiple antigen receptors are sufficient to activate B cells. **B:** Activation by a monomeric antigen requires additional stimuli supplied by another cell type. Costimulators from the antigen-presenting cell (APC) are necessary to activate a helper T cell (T_H), which in turn provides helper factors for B cells or interleukin-2 (IL-2) for T_C cells.

Table 3–4. Mitogens and conditions used
to activate lymphocytes in vitro.

Mitogen or Condition	Specificity
Lectins	
Concanavalin A	T cells
Helix pomatia lectin	T cells
Phytohemagglutinin	T cells; few B cells
Pokeweed mitogen	T and B cells
Wheat germ agglutinin	T cells
Artificial cross-linking of specific surface proteins	
Immunoglobulins	B cells
T-cell surface markers (eg, CD3)	T cells
Pharmacologic agents	
Phorbol myristyl acetate plus calcium ionophore (eg, ionomycin)	T and B cells

CD40 ligand (CD40L) on the activated T_H cell to bind a nonimmunoglobulin surface receptor called **CD40** on the B cell. Binding of CD40L by CD40 transmits a second signal into the B cell, and the combined effects of this help signal together with the bound antigen then act synergistically to cause B-cell activation.

In a similar manner, T-lymphocyte responses to most antigens also require two types of stimuli simultaneously. The first is provided by the antigen, which, if appropriately displayed by MHC proteins on an antigen-presenting cell, can be recognized and bound by T-cell receptors. When it binds an antigen–MHC complex, the T-cell receptor sends a signal to the cell interior, but this signal alone is usually not enough to cause activation. For helper T cells, full activation also requires contact with other specific ligands, known as **costimulators,*** that are expressed on the surface of the antigen-presenting cell. The best characterized costimulators are the **B7** proteins, called B7.1 and B7.2, which bind a surface receptor called **CD28** on the T_H cell surface. Activation of a cytotoxic T cell, on the other hand, generally requires **IL-2,** a cytokine secreted by activated helper T cells.

In summary, it is important to recognize that activation of a lymphocyte is controlled not only by antigen binding but also by interactions with other cells (Figure 3–9B): All T cells must cooperate with antigen-presenting cells, whereas B cells and cytotoxic

cells depend on helper T lymphocytes. These interactions either require direct surface-to-surface contact or are mediated by cytokines that act only over extremely short distances. Owing to this interdependence among cell types, lymphocyte activation occurs most commonly and efficiently in the secondary lymphoid organs, where lymphocytes, antigens, and antigen-presenting cells encounter one another at close quarters.

LYMPHOID ORGANS

Lymphocytes are normally present in the blood at a concentration of approximately 2500 cells/mm³ and so account for roughly one third of all peripheral white blood cells. Each individual lymphocyte, however, spends most of its life within solid tissues, entering the circulation only periodically to migrate from one resting place to another. Indeed, at any given moment, no more than 1% of the total lymphocyte population can be found in the blood. Most of the remaining cells are contained in specialized lymphoid organs, such as the lymph nodes, thymus, white pulp of the spleen, or mucosal regions of the respiratory and digestive tracts, where they carry out most of their functions.

Lymph Nodes & Lymphatic Circulation

Driven by the hydrostatic pressure within capillary lumens, water and low-molecular-weight solutes from the blood plasma continually leach out through blood vessel walls and into the lower pressure interstitial space. This slow leakage occurs in all solid organs and is the source of the nutrient-rich **interstitial fluid** that permeates every available niche in the tissues and bathes each individual cell. Most of this fluid returns directly to the bloodstream through the walls of nearby venules, but a substantial amount (totaling approximately 120 mL/h in an adult at rest) does not. Instead, this portion of the interstitial fluid flows through the tissues at an almost imperceptible rate and is eventually collected in a branching network of flaccid, thin-walled channels known as primary lymphatic vessels. These vessels ramify throughout almost all organs of the body (except the brain, eyeballs, marrow cavities, cartilage, and placenta) but are often difficult to discern in tissue sections, since they collapse easily and are delimited only by a single delicate layer of lymphatic endothelial cells. Once the fluid enters these vessels, it is known as **lymph.** Flowing slowly along the primary lymphatics, the lymph empties into progressively larger caliber lymphatic vessels, which ultimately converge and drain their contents into the right and left subclavian veins in the thorax (Figure 3–10). Thus, the lymphatic vasculature serves as a slow-flowing, low-pressure drainage system that collects a small proportion of the interstitial fluid from

---

* Immunologists commonly use the prefix "co-" to indicate that a molecule intensifies or contributes to a particular function (and may even be essential for it) but cannot carry out that function by itself. Thus, any molecule that can activate T cells in the presence of antigen, but cannot do so alone, is a costimulator of T-cell activation. Examples of similar usage include the terms *coreceptor, comitogen,* and *coactivator.*

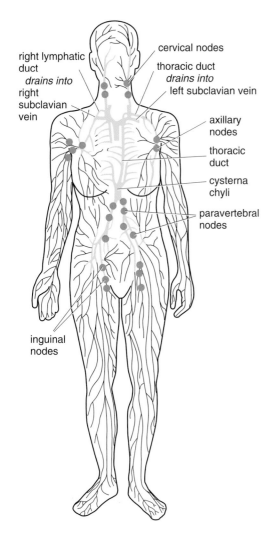

right lymphatic duct *drains into* right subclavian vein

cervical nodes

thoracic duct *drains into* left subclavian vein

axillary nodes

thoracic duct

cysterna chyli

paravertebral nodes

inguinal nodes

Figure 3–10. Lymphatic vascular system. Lymphatic vessels draining the right arm and right side of the head and neck converge to form the right lymphatic duct; the thoracic duct receives lymph from the remainder of the body. Only a few major collections of lymph nodes are depicted.

throughout the body and returns it to the bloodstream.

During its passage along the lymphatic vessels, the lymph flows through a series of bean-shaped organs called **lymph nodes,** which range from as little as 1 mm to about 25 mm in diameter. Nodes are distributed along the entire length of the lymphatic vasculature, tend to increase in size toward the venous end of the system, and often occur in chains or clusters that receive flow exclusively from a particular organ or region of the body (see Figure 3–10). Especially prominent clusters of lymph nodes can be found in the neck and axillae (draining the head and arms), in

the inguinal and paravertebral regions (draining the legs and pelvis), and in the root of the mesentery (draining the gut).

In its simplest form, a lymph node can be viewed as a localized dilatation of the lymphatic vessel, filled with dense aggregates of lymphocytes and macrophages that cling to a loose meshwork of connective tissue fibers called **reticulin** fibers. The reticulin mesh is produced by specialized fibroblasts known as **reticular cells,** small numbers of which are also present in the node. The node functions as a physical and biologic filter: As lymph fluid percolates through its internal lattice of cells, the macrophages and lymphocytes survey the fluid for any bacteria, viruses, or foreign macromolecules that may have been carried along with it from the tissues.

Larger nodes show an organized internal structure, which is schematized in Figure 3–11. The entire node is surrounded by a fibrous capsule. Lymph flows into the node along several **afferent lymphatic vessels** on one surface of the node and enters a narrow **subcapsular sinus** that is lined primarily by macrophages. The lymph then percolates sequentially through two more or less distinct regions of predominantly lymphoid tissue, called the **cortex** and the **medulla,** and finally exits through an **efferent lymphatic vessel** on the opposite side, at a region known as the hilus. Each node also receives a rich supply of blood that enters via an arteriole at the hilus, flows through a dense bed of capillaries and venules in the cortex and medulla, and then returns to the hilus to drain out through small veins.

The lymph node cortex usually contains several discrete spherical or ovoid cellular aggregates called **lymphoid follicles** (see Figure 3–11). These follicles are composed mainly of memory B lymphocytes, a smaller number of T cells (virtually all of which are helper cells), and a specialized type of supporting cell called the **follicular dendritic cell.** The latter cells are so named because they are found only in lymphoid follicles and exhibit many long, delicate cytoplasmic processes that radiate out like tentacles to encircle each follicular lymphocyte. The origin and function of follicular dendritic cells are poorly understood: Despite their name and morphology, they are not related to the marrow-derived dendritic cells and are not antigen-presenting cells, but instead appear to be responsible for assembling memory B cells into follicles and regulating their subsequent activities.

Lymphoid follicles are labile structures that can disappear and re-form at different sites over time and can enlarge in response to infections or other immune challenges. They are of two types (Figure 3–12). **Primary follicles** contain predominantly mature, resting B cells; since these have dense nuclei and little cytoplasm, a primary follicle appears as a relatively dark-staining mass on conventional histologic preparations. **Secondary follicles,** on the other hand, appear

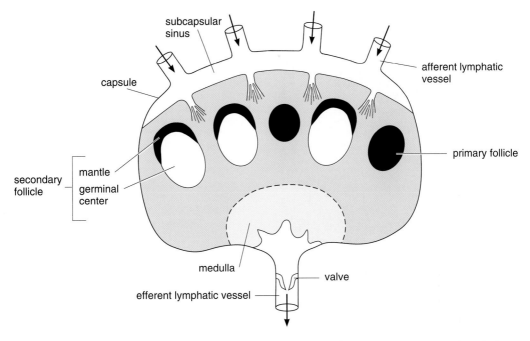

Figure 3–11. Idealized structure of a lymph node. Lymph enters via afferent vessels, passes through the cortex (shaded) and medulla, and exits via a single efferent vessel. Large lymphatic vessels often contain valves that prevent backward flow of the lymph.

as a pale-staining sphere known as the **germinal center,** with a cap (or **mantle**) of more darkly staining mature B lymphocytes overlying it on the afferent side of the node. The pale staining of the germinal center reflects the fact that, in this portion of the follicle, most of the lymphocytes are in various stages of activation and blast transformation and hence have more cytoplasm and looser chromatin than do resting lymphocytes. Numerous individual macrophages are also present in the germinal center, and occasional plasma cells may be seen.

Secondary follicles are not present at birth, and they form only after repeated exposure to substances that provoke an immune response. The presence of secondary follicles clearly denotes an ongoing B-cell immune response. Secondary follicles are thought to arise when a few B cells become activated in response to an antigen, migrate into a primary follicle, undergo blast transformation, and begin to proliferate rapidly. Some of their progeny differentiate into plasma cells, which migrate from the follicle toward the medulla of the node; the antibodies that these cells secrete are carried away by the lymph flow into the bloodstream. Proliferating B cells in a germinal center also undergo a process called **affinity maturation,** in which the B cells that respond most vigorously to the antigen are allowed to proliferate while others selectively die (see Chapter 8). The phagocytosed remains of B cells that have died in this process

can be seen within the macrophages of a germinal center.

The regions of lymph node cortex lying outside the follicles are populated primarily by T cells, about two thirds of which are helper cells. T cells are especially abundant in the poorly demarcated region of cortex known as the **paracortex,** which lies between the lymphoid follicles and the medulla. Here, as in the T-cell-rich zones of all secondary lymphoid organs, the T cells are accompanied by a smaller population of specialized dendritic cells, called **interdigitating dendritic cells,** that have antigen-presenting activity. The **medulla** usually is less densely cellular than the cortex and often contains a scattering of plasma cells along with mature B and T lymphocytes and macrophages.

The lymph that flows into a node may carry with it microorganisms or other foreign matter from the tissues. When such a substance enters a lymph node, some of the lymphocytes and macrophages in the node may respond by activation. As a result, some of the resident lymphocytes begin to proliferate, inflammatory mediators are released locally, blood flow to the node increases markedly, and the normal, continual lymphocyte emigration from the node ceases entirely. If these responses are sufficiently pronounced, the node may become noticeably enlarged—a condition known as **lymphadenopathy.** Rapid enlargement of a lymph node can occur, for example, when

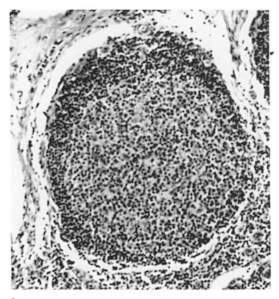

Figure 3–12. Structures of lymphoid follicles. **A:** A secondary follicle in the cortex of a lymph node, from a hematoxylin–eosin-stained section. Note the round, pale-staining germinal center and darker, overlying cap (mantle). Because follicles are often cut tangentially in standard tissue sections, the mantle is sometimes erroneously thought to completely encircle the germinal center. (Contributed by Brian Herndier.) **B:** At the top are photomicrographs of a primary *(left)* and a secondary *(right)* follicle from a hematoxylin–eosin-stained section of a lymph node. (Contributed by Roger Warnke.) **C:** The diagrams schematically depict the relationship between a follicular dendritic cell (white with shaded nucleus) and the surrounding lymphoid cells in a primary follicle *(left)*) and a germinal center *(right)*. The relatively pale-staining properties of the germinal center result mainly from the abundant cytoplasm and large, pale-staining nuclei of the B-cell blasts it contains.

A

primary

secondary

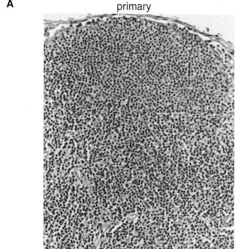

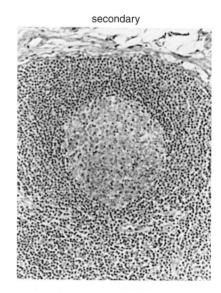

B

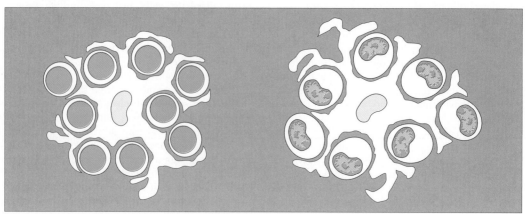

primary follicle

germinal center
of secondary follicle

C

an infection develops in the region it drains. Swelling usually decreases when the infection ends, although repeated bouts of swelling can lead to permanent enlargement and induration by scarring the interior of a node.

Spleen

The spleen (Figure 3–13) filters blood much as the lymph nodes filter lymph. Located just below the diaphragm on the left side of the abdomen, the spleen weighs approximately 150 g in an adult and is enclosed in a thin and rather fragile connective tissue capsule. Blood enters by way of the splenic artery at the hilum and passes into a branching network of progressively smaller arterioles that radiate throughout the organ. Each arteriole is encased in a cylindrical cuff of lymphoid tissue that consists mainly of mature T cells and is called the **periarteriolar lymphoid sheath.** Primary and secondary lymphoid follicles protrude at intervals from the sheath; these are identical to the follicles found in other lymphoid tissues and are composed mainly of B cells. Surrounding the follicles and sheaths together is a region called the **marginal zone,** composed mainly of B cells and macrophages. The arterioles, sheaths, follicles, marginal zones, and a small amount of associated connective tissue are together called the splenic

white pulp, which is visible as a delicate latticework on the cut surface of the organ. Blood flows from the arterioles into the **red pulp**—a spongy, blood-filled network of reticular cells and macrophage-lined vascular sinusoids that makes up the bulk of the spleen—and then exits by way of the splenic vein.

During the course of each day, approximately half the total blood volume passes through the spleen, where lymphocytes, dendritic cells, and macrophages survey it continually for evidence of infectious agents or other contaminants. The spleen thus serves as a critical line of defense against blood-borne pathogens. Splenic macrophages also have the important function of recognizing and eliminating any abnormal, damaged, or senescent red or white cells from the blood. Surgical removal of the spleen (most often performed because it has been lacerated by trauma) is usually well tolerated in an adult but causes a persistent rise in the percentage of malformed circulating erythrocytes and a modestly increased risk of sepsis due to diplococci or other pyogenic bacteria.

Tonsils, Peyer's Patches, & Other Subepithelial Lymphoid Organs

Vast numbers of individual T and B lymphocytes, macrophages, and plasma cells lie just below the mu-

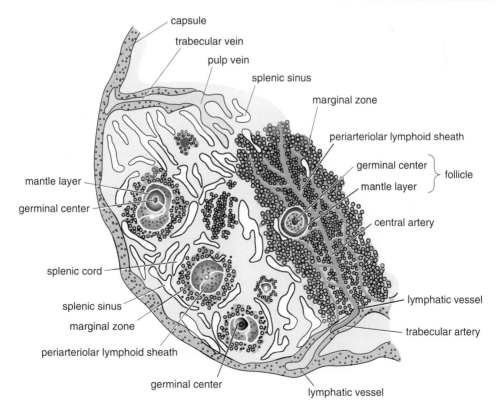

Figure 3–13. Microscopic anatomy of the spleen.

cosal epithelia in many regions of the alimentary, genitourinary, and respiratory tracts. Especially dense populations of such cells can normally be found around bronchial lumens or in the lamina propria and submucosa of the large and small intestines, where they are well situated to detect any foreign substances that contact these body surfaces. In most areas, the cells form a diffuse, disorganized mass, punctuated only occasionally by isolated lymphoid follicles.

At other sites, the cells are organized into discrete, stable anatomic structures. For example, **tonsils** are nodular aggregates of macrophages and lymphoid cells located immediately beneath the stratified squamous epithelium of the nasopharynx and soft palate. Tonsils lack a capsule and afferent lymphatic vessels but have many of the other constituents of a lymph node, including lymphoid follicles; their function is to detect and respond to pathogens in the respiratory and alimentary secretions. The overlying epithelium plunges downward into the substance of a tonsil to form deep crypts whose contents are continually monitored by the tonsillar cells. Similar unencapsulated lymphoid nodules, called **Peyer's patches,** are present in the ileal submucosa of the small bowel, where they serve to detect substances that diffuse across the intestinal epithelium (Figure 3–14). Together, all of the organized and diffuse lymphoid tissues found in submucosal regions of the body can be viewed as a single functional unit, called the **mucosa-associated lymphoid tissue (MALT),** which is the largest lymphoid organ, containing roughly half the lymphoid cells in the body. MALT will be discussed in detail in Chapter 14. One important function of these tissues is to secrete antibodies across the mucosal surface as a defense against external pathogens.

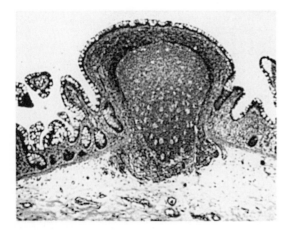

Figure 3–14. Microscopic anatomy of a Peyer's patch, a secondary lymphoid follicle beneath the mucosal epithelium of the small intestine. (Contributed by Linda Ferrell.)

The skin, too, is an important site of immune surveillance. Small populations of lymphocytes are constantly present in the dermis and epidermis, although they usually are inconspicuous and do not normally form lymphoid follicles. In addition, the epidermis contains a resident subpopulation of antigen-presenting dendritic cells, called **Langerhans' cells,** each of which sends out a network of cytoplasmic processes that intertwine between epidermal epithelial cells over a relatively large area. These Langerhans' cells account for about 5% of all epidermal cells. When it encounters foreign substances, a Langerhans' cell secretes cytokines that attract additional lymphocytes from the nearby circulation and it also captures and presents the foreign substances on its surface to help initiate an immune response. Macrophages in the dermis play a similar role as antigen-presenting sentinels.

Thymus

Unlike the other lymphoid organs described earlier, the thymus is involved in lymphocyte production and maturation rather than in immune surveillance per se. It is the primary site at which T lymphocytes differentiate and become functionally competent. The organ itself arises during embryogenesis as two endodermal buds from the third pharyngeal pouches; these invade downward into the superior mediastinum and then fuse to form a solid, V-shaped epithelial mass. During the third month of gestation, this mass becomes colonized by primitive, marrow-derived lymphoid stem cells that are carried to it by way of the blood. It is not yet clear whether these migrating stem cells are already committed to T-cell differentiation or become committed only after entering the thymus. The epithelial component of the thymus is made up of sheets and islands of squamous cells that make and secrete factors that attract T-cell precursors from the blood and also promote subsequent maturation within the thymus. These factors include a chemokine called thymus-expressed cytokine (TECK), and a number of small, incompletely characterized peptide hormones known as thymulin, thymopoietin, thymic humoral factor, and thymosin. Once inside the organ, T cells pack themselves densely into the interstices between epithelial cells, stretching them apart until the epithelium comes to resemble a loose network of stellate cells that cling to one another via desmosomes. In this microenvironment, T cells proliferate briskly, giving the thymus one of the highest rates of cell division in the body.

The fully developed thymus is composed of two lobes, each comprising multiple lobules (Figure 3–15). Lymphocytes are packed more densely toward the periphery of each lobule than near its center, which gives rise to the appearance of an outer cortex and inner medulla, although there is no sharp anatomic border between these two zones. In some areas of the medulla, the epithelium forms small ker-

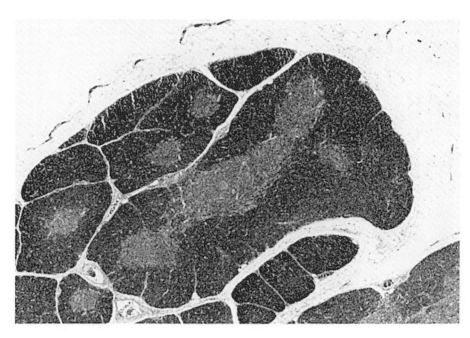

Figure 3–15. Microscopic anatomy of the thymus. This photomicrograph shows a portion of a thymic lobule from a hematoxylin–eosin-stained section, illustrating the dense outer cortex and pale inner medulla. (Contributed by Gordon Honda.)

atinized whorls, called **Hassall's corpuscles,** whose significance is unknown. Apart from the epithelial cells and a few macrophages and other supporting elements, virtually all cells in the thymus are T cells. T lymphocytes residing in the thymus are often called **thymocytes.** Of these, a minor proportion (approximately 10%) are CD4-CD8- cells. Unlike the rare double-negative T cells found outside the thymus, these are somewhat enlarged, have a high rate of mitotic activity, and are presumed to be primitive T-cell precursors. A second subpopulation (15% of thymic T cells) consists of single-positive thymocytes that express only CD4 or CD8 alone and are nearly indistinguishable from the mature T lymphocytes found elsewhere throughout the body. Such single-positive cells are most abundant in the thymic medulla and are thought to be fully mature naive T lymphocytes that are preparing to leave the organ.

The vast majority of lymphoid cells in the thymus, however, are small T cells that express both CD4 and CD8 proteins together on their surfaces. These double-positive thymocytes account for roughly 75% of all thymic T cells. They are not immunologically functional and are thought to represent a transient intermediate stage in T-cell development. Amazingly, nearly all of these double-positive thymocytes (at least 99%) die without ever leaving the thymus: The thymic cortex is studded with individual dying thymocytes, and phagocytosed debris from the dead thy-

mocytes can be seen within cortical macrophages and epithelial cells. Thus, the thymus is a site for both prolific replication and wholesale slaughter of T cells. As discussed in later chapters, the T-cell deaths that occur in the thymus are part of a rigorous **selection** process that is essential for creating a functioning immune system.

The developmental relationships among the various classes of thymocytes are outlined in Figure 3–16. Blood-borne lymphocyte progenitors enter the thymus and form a pool of replicating cells located mainly near the periphery of the cortex; it is not known whether this replicating pool is stable or must continually be replenished with new marrow precursors. The progeny of the replicating cells appear first as double-negative thymocytes and then progress to the double-positive stage in which they express T-cell receptors along with both CD4 and CD8 on their surfaces. Each individual thymocyte then selectively and permanently shuts off expression of either CD4 or CD8 (apparently choosing between these two markers at random), and so becomes a single-positive thymocyte. This differentiation process is plainly arduous, since fewer than 1% of the cells produced in the thymus are able to complete it. Although the factors that determine which thymocytes will survive are not entirely known, the selection process depends in part on specific interactions with thymic macrophages or epithelial cells, at least some of which are mediated

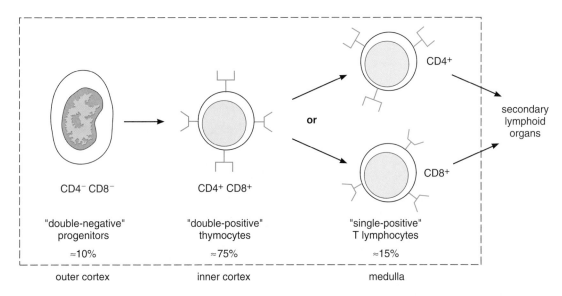

outer cortex   inner cortex   medulla

Figure 3–16. Model for intrathymic T-cell maturation. Developing thymocytes pass through three successive stages of differentiation as they migrate from the outer cortex to the medulla and then exit the thymus. Some identifiable intermediate stages have been omitted. The sequence depicted applies to most T cells that express α/β T-cell receptors. For details, see Chapter 9.

through the T-cell receptor (see Chapter 9). The small percentage of single-positive cells that survive ultimately leave the thymus as mature T lymphocytes. The general tendency is for the cells to migrate from the cortex toward the medulla as they differentiate, although this may not be true of all thymocytes.

The thymus is relatively large and highly active at birth, weighing an average of 22 g. It continues to enlarge for several years, although at a lower rate than the rest of the body, and reaches its peak weight (around 35 g) at puberty. Thereafter, it begins to involute as the lymphoid components recede and are replaced by fatty connective tissue. Little more than 6 g of thymic tissue (most of it epithelial) persists into adulthood. In the past, this involution was believed to signify that the thymus becomes inactive and irrelevant after puberty. Consistent with that view, congenital absence of the thymus results in the absence of T lymphocytes and produces profound, life-threatening immunodeficiency, but the organ can be surgically removed at any time after birth without causing significant immunologic problems. Surprisingly, however, recent studies have shown that T-lymphopoiesis normally continues into old age, though at a much reduced rate that parallels the declining lymphoid cell mass in the thymus. Thymic T-cell production at age 35 averages only 20%, and at age 65 only 2%, of the rates in newborns, but even these low rates raise hope that measures to maintain or restore thymic function could be developed to treat immunodeficiencies in adults.

Growing evidence also suggests that some naive T cells are produced outside the thymus, particularly in diffuse lymphoid tissue contacting the gut epithelium. Although thymic hormones may contribute, a significant proportion of these cells develop fully independently of the thymus. The functional importance of this extrathymic T-lymphopoiesis is unknown.

LYMPHOCYTE CIRCULATION & HOMING

Lymphocytes are migratory cells; their distribution in the body reflects the rates at which they enter and depart particular sites, as well as their local replication. Individual lymphocytes in a lymph node, for example, linger there for an average of only 12 hours before detaching from the reticulin matrix and exiting through efferent lymphatics, swept along by the flowing lymph. These emigrating cells eventually are carried into the bloodstream, which disperses them throughout the body, but they generally remain in circulation for only a few minutes or hours before again taking up residence temporarily in another lymphoid organ (Figure 3–17). In a similar fashion, mature lymphocytes continually migrate in and out of all other secondary lymphoid tissues as well, changing locations on average once or twice each day, with roughly 1–2% of the total population in transit at any given moment. In most types of lymphoid organs, lymphocytes enter via blood vessels and exit through lymphatics, but in the spleen they enter and exit directly from the blood.

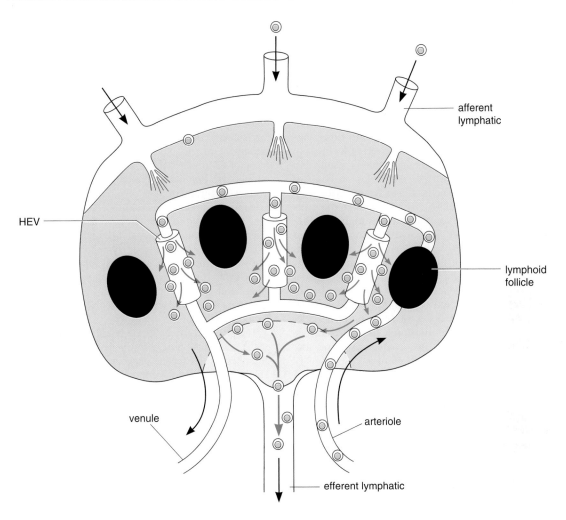

Figure 3–17. Schematic view of lymphocyte traffic through a lymph node. Some lymphocytes arrive from other nodes through the afferent lymphatic channels, but most enter from the blood by way of a high endothelial venule (HEV), migrate through the substance of the node and exit through efferent lymphatics. Average residence time in the node is approximately 12 hours. Note that the HEVs are located predominantly in the paracortex between lymphoid follicles.

These restless migrations serve several functions. First, as lymphocytes travel from organ to organ, they can survey the entire body for foci of infection or foreign antigens. This is especially important because, as we shall see in Chapter 4, only a small percentage of lymphocytes are able to respond to any given antigen—continually dispersing and reshuffling the population helps ensure that these rare, responsive lymphocytes will be present wherever in the body that antigen might appear. Second, such movements help maintain a balanced overall distribution of lymphocytes among tissues. In addition, because the microenvironments found in different tissues tend to favor specific aspects of lymphocyte development, migration through various sites can sequentially modulate and optimize a cell's growth and function. Finally, like a game of musical chairs, the shuttling

process also places strong darwinian pressure on the population, as the migrating lymphocytes are forced to compete with one another for the limited space available in each tissue. Lymphocytes confront this competition from the earliest stages of their lives; for example, the bone marrow exports more new naive B cells each day than can be accommodated in the periphery. Cells that compete least effectively for entry to the most favorable microenvironments tend to be weeded out over time, while the best adapted cells thrive.

Lymphocyte traffic among organs is not random. Resting, naive lymphocytes shuttle almost exclusively among the lymph nodes, Peyer's patches, tonsils, and spleen and have a roughly equal tendency to migrate into any of these tissues. In comparison, memory and effector cells can invade not only those sites but also the diffuse submucosal lymphoid tissues of the gut and lung, the pulmonary interstitium, and inflamed or infected sites in virtually any other organ. Moreover, once activated, individual effector and memory cells often show a very strong preference to return to the same type of tissue in which activation originally occurred. A memory cell originally activated in a lymphoid organ of the gut, for example, will tend to home preferentially to other gut-associated lymphoid tissues for the rest of its life.

These tissue-selective homing patterns result from interactions between surface molecules on lymphocytes and endothelial cells. Blood lymphocytes most commonly enter tissues by passing through the walls of specialized blood vessels known as **high endothelial venules (HEVs).** These vessels are a modified form of postcapillary venules, are found in all lymphoid organs except the spleen, and can be recognized under the light microscope by the cuboidal shape of the endothelial cells that line them (Figure 3–18). High endothelial cells in different target organs, such as lymph nodes or Peyer's patches, express particular surface glycoproteins, called **vascular addressins,** which are characteristic of that organ. Each type of addressin, in turn, is specifically recognized by one or more surface proteins, called **homing receptors,** on lymphocytes that home to that organ. Thus, when a circulating lymphocyte expresses a particular homing receptor, it will tend to bind HEV addressins found in the corresponding tissue or organ. Different types of lymphocytes are predisposed to express particular homing receptors, but the level of expression may increase or decrease markedly depending on whether the cell is activated, the nature of the activating antigen, and the microenvironment where activation occurred. Several of the receptor-addressin pairs that are known to mediate lymphocyte homing to lymph nodes, skin, the gastrointestinal tract, or sites of inflammation are listed in Table 3–5; addressins and receptors for other tissues are believed to exist but have not yet been identified. In particular, homing to lymph nodes can be initiated by contact between lymphocyte **L-selectin** and various endothelial surface glycoproteins, including **CD34.** Homing to gastrointestinal sites, on the other hand, depends on contact between a specific integrin on the lymphocyte and a glycoprotein ligand on the endothelium.

The process of lymphocyte binding and penetration of the vessel wall progresses in phases similar to those described earlier for the phagocytes (see Figure 2–5). The initial interaction of most nonintegrin-homing re-

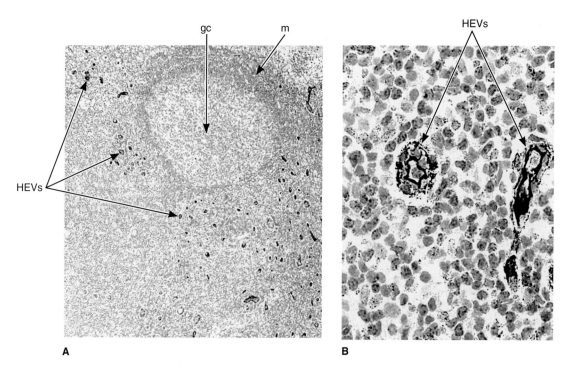

Figure 3–18. High endothelial venules (HEVs). **A:** Histologic section of a human lymph node, showing the distribution of HEVs, which are primarily found in the paracortex. The germinal center (gc) and mantle (m) of a single lymphoid follicle are also visible. **B:** High-power view showing the distinctive cuboidal shape of the high endothelial cells. The tissue in both photographs has been treated with reagents specific for the L-selectin ligand, which stain the high endothelial cell surfaces black. (Contributed by Michael Bell.)

Table 3–5. Receptor–addressin interactions involved in lymphocyte homing.[a]

Lymphocyte Homing Receptor	Vascular Addressin	Homing Specificity Conferred
L-selectin	CD34, glyCAM-1, others[b]	Naive lymphocytes to lymph nodes
L-selectin	MAdCAM	Naive lymphocytes to Peyer's patches
$\alpha_4\beta_7$ integrin	MAdCAM, VCAM-1	Naive lymphocytes to Peyer's patches; memory–effector cells to lamina propria of GI tract
CLA	E-selectin	Memory–effector cells to skin
VLA-4	VCAM-1	Activated lymphoblasts and memory–effector cells to sites of inflammation
CD44	Hyaluronate	Activated lymphoblasts to sites of inflammation
PSGL-1	P-selectin	Unknown

Abbreviations: CLA = cutaneous lymphocyte antigen; glyCAM = glycosylated cell adhesion molecule; MAdCAM = mucosal addressin cell adhesion molecule; VCAM = vascular cell adhesion molecule; VLA = very late antigen; PSGL = P-selectin glycoprotein ligand.
[a] Interactions involving the $\alpha_4\beta_7$ and VLA-4 integrins can support both the primary and secondary phases of adhesion (see Fig. 2–5). All other molecular interactions listed here are sufficient for primary adhesion only. In most instances, secondary adhesion requires activation of surface integrins, particularly lymphocyte LFA-1, which binds ICAM-1 and ICAM-2 on the endothelial surface.
[b] L-selectin is thought to recognize a sulfated carbohydrate determinant based on sialyl Lewis-X, which is found on several distinct endothelial surface glycoproteins.

ceptors with a vascular addressin is relatively weak and short-lived, so that the cell often continues to roll along the HEV wall under the force of the flowing blood. During this **primary adhesion** phase, which lasts only a few seconds, the lymphocyte must receive signals that induce it to progress into the **secondary adhesion** phase, in which it rapidly translocates presynthesized integrin proteins (especially leukocyte function-associated antigen **[LFA]-1**) onto its surface, stops rolling, and becomes firmly anchored to the endothelium. Among the signals that trigger this progression in lymphocytes is a chemokine called secondary lymphoid-tissue chemokine (SLC), which is displayed on HEV surfaces and recognized by receptors on naive T cells.

After adhering to the HEV wall, a lymphocyte can then pass between high endothelial cells to enter the surrounding tissue. This process, called **diapedesis,** is usually completed within 10 minutes and depends on the continued expression of surface integrins that provide attachment to adjacent cells and to the extracellular matrix. The efficiency of lymphocyte recruitment can be very high; for example, about 25% of blood lymphocytes that enter a lymph node's vascular bed will invade across the HEVs. After exiting the bloodstream, each lymphocyte must then continue its migration within the lymphoid organ until it reaches an appropriate resting place, such as the paracortical region (for most T cells) or lymphoid follicles (for most B cells) of a lymph node. Each cell's migration into and localization within a lymphoid organ is guided by specific chemokines. For example, SLC

and another chemokine called ELC are expressed in the T-cell zones of lymphoid organs, and are responsible for attracting naive T cells to these areas, whereas a chemokine called BLC serves to attract B lymphocytes into follicles. Individual lymphocytes may also migrate from one location to another within an organ as they become activated, and this migration, too, is controlled by chemokines. For example, soon after binding an antigen through its surface immunoglobulins, a B cell may begin to express surface receptors for ELC, and so be attracted out of a follicle and into the ELC-rich T-cell zones; this increases its likelihood of contacting an activated T_H cell that can provide the help signal needed for B-cell activation.

High endothelial venules are a constant feature of all secondary lymphoid organs (except the spleen) but may also appear transiently at any site in the body where an immune response is occurring. They arise by differentiation of preexisting capillaries in response to factors elaborated locally by activated immune cells. These vessels then serve as a portal through which blood lymphocytes and other defensive cells can enter tissues to join in a response wherever they are needed. If the response is sufficiently intense and prolonged, the assembled lymphocytes, plasma cells, and antigen-presenting cells may arrange themselves spatially in a manner that resembles a permanent lymphoid organ, complete with secondary follicles. Such reactive, and usually temporary, encampments are sometimes referred to as **tertiary lymphoid organs.**

REFERENCES

ONTOGENY AND SUBTYPES
OF T AND B LYMPHOID CELLS

Ahmed R, Gray D: Immunological memory and protective immunity: Understanding their relation. *Science* 1996; 272:54.

Akashi K et al: Lymphoid development from hematopoietic stem cells. *Int J Hematol* 1999;69:217.

Fischer A, Malissen B: Natural and engineered disorders of lymphocyte development. *Science* 1998;280:237.

Opferman JT et al: Linear differentiation of cytotoxic effectors into memory T lymphocytes. *Science* 1999;283:1745.

Shortman K, Wu L: Early T lymphocyte progenitors. *Annu Rev Immunol* 1996;14:29.

Sprent J, Tough DF: Lymphocyte life-span and memory. *Science* 1994;265:1395.

Weissman IL: Developmental switches in the immune system. *Cell* 1994;76:207.

LYMPHOID ORGANS

Bohnsack JF, Brown EJ: The role of the spleen in resistance to infection. *Annu Rev Medicine* 1986;37:49.

Fu Y-X, Chaplin DD: Development and maturation of secondary lymphoid tissues. *Annu Rev Immunol* 1999;17:399.

Gretz JE et al: Cords, channels, corridors and conduits: Critical architectural elements facilitating cell interactions in the lymph node cortex. *Immunol Rev* 1997;156: 11.

Imai Y, Yamakawa M: Morphology, function and pathology of follicular dendritic cells. *Pathol Int* 1996;46:807.

Jamieson BD et al: Generation of functional thymocytes in the human adult. *Immunity* 1999;10:569.

Kuper CF et al: The role of nasopharyngeal lymphoid tissue. *Immunol Today* 1992;13:219.

Liu YJ, Arping C: Germinal center development. *Immunol Rev* 1997;156:111.

MacLennan ICM: Germinal centers. *Annu Rev Immunol* 1994;12:117.

Rodewald H-R: The thymus in the age of retirement. *Nature* 1998;396:630.

Sminia T et al: Structure and function of bronchus-associated lymphoid tissue (BALT). *Crit Rev Immunol* 1989;9:119.

Steinman RM et al: Dendritic cells in the T-cell areas of lymphoid organs. *Immunol Rev* 1997;156:25.

LYMPHOCYTE ACTIVATION

Janeway CA, Bottomly K: Signals and signs for lymphocyte responses. *Cell* 1994;76:275.

Weiss A, Littman DR: Signal transduction by lymphocyte antigen receptors. *Cell* 1994;76:263.

LYMPHOCYTE RECIRCULATION AND HOMING

Butcher EC, Picker LJ: Lymphocyte homing and homeostasis. *Science* 1996;272:60.

Cyster JG et al: Chemokines and B-cell homing to follicles. *Curr Topics Microbiol Immunol* 1999;246:87.

Goodnow CC, Cyster JF: Lymphocyte homing: The scent of a follicle. *Curr Biol* 1997;7:219.

Gunn MD et al: A chemokine expressed in lymphoid high endothelial venules promotes the adhesion and chemotaxis of naive T lymphocytes. *Proc Natl Acad Sci USA* 1998;95:258.

Rosen SD, Bertozzi CR: The selectins and their ligands. *Curr Opin Cell Biol* 1994;6:663.

Springer TA: Traffic signals for lymphocyte recirculation and leukocyte emigration: The multistep paradigm. *Cell* 1994;76,301.

The Immune Response

4

Tristram G. Parslow, MD, PhD

We now turn our attention to the protective reactions underlying acquired immunity, which are called immune responses. The acquired immune system differs profoundly from the innate system in its interactions with pathogens. Innate immunity mainly recognizes substances such as distinctive carbohydrates, lipids, and *N*-formylated peptides, that are foreign per se, but acquired immune responses are most commonly directed against proteins—a class of molecules found both in pathogens and in the host. Nevertheless, the acquired immune system **discriminates between self and nonself,** so that it normally coexists peacefully with all of the proteins and other organic materials that make up the host but responds vigorously against foreign organisms, and even against cells or tissues from other people. It does so with extreme **specificity,** detecting subtle differences among vast numbers of proteins and responding (or not responding) to each of these individually. It is not unusual for the immune system to discriminate between proteins based on a single amino acid or a minor difference in conformation. Most remarkably, acquired immunity has **memory,** that is, the ability to be molded by its experience so that subsequent contacts with a particular foreign organism provoke a much more rapid and vigorous response than occurred at the initial encounter. These properties of the immune system seemed impenetrable mysteries only a few decades ago, but in recent years they have yielded rapidly to research. A great deal is now understood about the mechanisms that give rise to immunologic specificity and memory, and the processes underlying self–nonself discrimination are beginning to be unraveled as well. What has emerged is the realization that the lymphocyte population in each person constitutes an extraordinarily interactive network of mobile cells that are almost as diverse as the foreign substances they respond to and that their diversity is the result of molecular genetic processes that may well be unique to these cells. Moreover, it is now recognized that each person's immune system is continually evolving in response to its environment and experience as the individual cells communicate and cooperate with one another to control their own proliferation, differentiation, and immunologic functions.

The interplay of molecular and cellular events that takes place during even the simplest immune response is dauntingly complex, and many aspects of immune system function are still incompletely understood. As a result, the subject can be especially bewildering and intimidating on first encounter. The goal of this chapter is therefore to present an introduction to the subject by describing the organization of lymphocyte populations and the essential elements of an immune response in a stepwise and simplified fashion. Each of these topics will then be addressed more rigorously and in much greater detail in subsequent chapters of this book.

CLONAL ORGANIZATION & DYNAMICS OF LYMPHOCYTE POPULATIONS

Naive lymphocytes are continually released from the primary lymphoid organs into the periphery, each carrying surface receptors that enable it to bind substances called **antigens.** Antigen binding in B cells is mediated by surface immunoglobulin proteins, whereas in T cells it is mediated by T-cell receptors. The sequences of these two types of proteins are extremely diverse, so that as a group they can bind an enormous variety of antigens (see Chapters 7 and 9). Antigen binding, when accompanied by other stimuli, can lead to activation of a T or B cell. Naive lymphocytes that fail to become activated die within a few days after entering the periphery, but those that become activated survive and proliferate, yielding daughter cells that may then undergo further cycles of activation and proliferation.

All of the progeny cells derived from any single naive lymphocyte constitute a lymphocyte **clone.** Some members of each clone differentiate into effector cells, whereas the remainder are memory cells; apart from this, however, all cells within a clone are identical to one another in nearly all respects, reflecting their common ancestry. For example, B-cell clones contain only B cells, and each T-cell clone is made up entirely of either CD4 or CD8 cells.

A fundamental property of lymphocytes is that all of the immunoglobulin or T-cell receptor proteins expressed by cells in a given clone are identical. Although each individual lymphocyte typically has thousands of such proteins on its surface, all of these have precisely the same amino acid sequence and are identical to those expressed by all other cells in the same clone. Since the sequence of an immunoglobulin or T-cell receptor protein determines which antigens it will bind, it follows that any single lymphocyte can recognize and respond to only a very small subset of the total universe of possible antigens. This same antigen specificity, moreover, is shared by all other cells in the clone (with the exception of occasional somatic mutants, discussed in Chapter 8). Thus, each lymphocyte or clone of lymphocytes has a uniquely restricted specificity for antigens—a phenomenon known as **clonal restriction.** The immune system as a whole is able to recognize many different antigens because it is made up of a vast number of different lymphocyte clones, each of which has very limited antigen specificity.

The antigen specificity of each naive lymphocyte is determined through an essentially random genetic process during the early stages of its development and is permanently fixed by the time the cell enters the periphery (see Chapter 7). It has been estimated that the lymphopoietic system is able to produce lymphocytes with approximately 10^8 alternative antigen specificities. This range of possible specificities is known collectively as the **primary lymphocyte repertoire.** Roughly 10^9 naive lymphocytes enter the periphery each day, so that at least a few with any given specificity are likely to be present at all times. Whenever any one of these encounters its specific antigen under conditions that favor activation, it can give rise to multiple daughter cells, some of which are long-lived memory cells. With each successive exposure to the same antigen, the antigen-specific clone expands further and so comes to represent an increasing proportion of the total lymphocyte population (Figure 4–1). In this manner, exposure to an antigen selectively promotes the growth of any clones that recognize it without affecting other cells in the population—a phenomenon known as **clonal selection.** On the other hand, if no further contact with that antigen occurs, the specific memory cells tend to die out, though this usually takes place over a period of years or decades. Thus, the lymphocyte population is continually evolving over time as individual clones expand or subside, depending on the specific antigens to which the host is exposed.

The antigen specificity of a given clone applies not only to its ability to recognize antigens but also to its effector functions. For example, cytotoxic effector T cells generally attack a target cell only if it bears the particular surface antigen recognized by their T-cell receptors; hence, the sequence of the T-cell receptor defines not only the antigen that can activate the T-cell clone but also the targets it will attack. Similarly, the antibodies secreted by a B-cell clone have exactly the same binding specificity as the surface immunoglobulins expressed on that clone. Clonal restriction thus ensures that the immune response

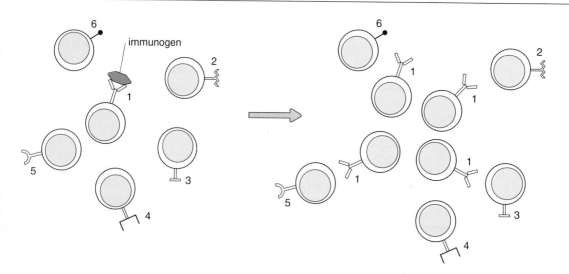

Figure 4–1. Clonal selection of lymphocytes by a specific immunogen. **Left:** The unimmunized lymphocyte population is composed of cells from many different clones, each with its own antigen specificity, indicated here by the distinctive shapes of the surface antigen receptors. **Right:** Contact with an immunogen leads to selective proliferation (positive selection) of any clone or clones that can recognize that specific immunogen.

mounted by a lymphocyte clone is directed with a high degree of specificity against the antigen that induced its activation. The speed and intensity of response to a given antigen is determined largely by clonal selection: The larger the specific clone, the more lymphocytes are available that can recognize the antigen and can participate in the immune response.

The principles of clonal restriction and clonal selection were first postulated by Burnet, Jerne, Talmadge, and others in the 1950s and still rank among the most important conceptual insights in the history of immunology. Clonal restriction is the primary basis for the extreme specificity of immune responses: Each clone of lymphocytes can respond only to the limited set of antigens recognized by its unique immunoglobulin or T-cell receptor proteins and, when activated, carries out effector functions that are specifically directed against that same antigen. Clonal selection, on the other hand, is principally responsible for the phenomenon of immunologic memory: Exposure to an antigen sculpts and hones the lymphocyte population so that it can respond more quickly and more vigorously the next time the same antigen is encountered.

THE IMMUNE RESPONSE

Every **immune response** is a complex and intricately regulated sequence of events involving several cell types. It is triggered when an antigen enters the body and encounters a specialized class of cells called antigen-presenting cells (APCs). These APCs capture a minute amount of the antigen and display it in a form that can be recognized by antigen-specific helper T lymphocytes. The helper T cells become activated and, in turn, promote the activation of other classes of lymphocytes, such as B cells or cytotoxic T cells. The activated lymphocytes then proliferate and carry out their specific effector functions, which, in most cases, successfully inactivate or eliminate the antigen. At each stage in this process, the lymphocytes and APCs communicate with one another through direct contact or by secreting regulatory cytokines. They also may interact simultaneously with other cell types or with components of the complement, kinin, or fibrinolytic systems, resulting in phagocyte activation, blood clotting, or the initiation of wound healing. Immune responses may be either localized or systemic but are nearly always highly specific, focusing their full force against the antigen while causing little or no damage to normal host tissues. The responses are also precisely controlled and normally terminate soon after the inciting antigen is eliminated.

Figure 4–2 provides a schematic overview of the sequence of events that take place during a prototypical immune response. The following sections describe each step of this response in turn.

Immunogens & Antigens

Immunologists commonly use the term **antigen** when referring to the agent that triggers an immune response. Strictly speaking, however, this term actually refers to the ability of a molecule to be recognized by an immunoglobulin or T-cell receptor and hence to serve as the target of a response. For reasons that will be explained in Chapter 5, not all antigens are capable of inducing immune responses. Instead, a molecule or collection of molecules that can induce an immune response in a particular host is most properly referred to as an **immunogen.** Typical immunogens include pathogenic microorganisms (eg, viruses, bacteria, or parasites), foreign tissue grafts, or otherwise innocuous environmental substances, such as the proteins in pollen, grasses, or food.

Proteins are, in general, the most potent immunogens. Other classes of molecules, such as lipids, carbohydrates, or nucleic acids, most commonly become the targets of immune responses when they are linked to an immunogenic protein (as in lipoproteins, glycoproteins, or nucleoprotein complexes). Many of the immunogens encountered in nature are actually composites of several different immunogenic substances. A single bacterium, for example, is made up of a multitude of proteins and other molecules that may each elicit a specific immune response. In the prototypic immune response depicted in Figure 4–2, the immunogen is a virus that, like most viruses, contains several immunogenic proteins.

ANTIGEN PROCESSING & PRESENTATION

Responses to most proteinaceous immunogens can begin only after the immunogen has been captured, processed, and presented by an APC (see Figure 4–2). The reason for this is that T cells only recognize immunogens that are bound to **major histocompatibility complex (MHC)** proteins on the surfaces of other cells (see Chapter 6). There are two different classes of MHC proteins, each of which is recognized by one of the two major subsets of T lymphocytes. **Class I MHC** proteins are expressed by virtually all somatic cell types and are used to present substances to **CD8** T cells, most of which are cytotoxic. Almost any cell can therefore present antigens to cytotoxic T cells and thus serve as the target of a cytotoxic response. **Class II MHC** proteins, on the other hand, are expressed only by macrophages and a few other cell types and are necessary for antigen presentation to **CD4** T cells—the subset that includes most helper cells. Since helper cell activation is necessary for virtually all immune responses, the class II-bearing APCs play a pivotal role in controlling such responses. In fact, unless otherwise stated, the term *antigen-presenting cell* usually refers only to these specialized cells that bear class II MHC pro-

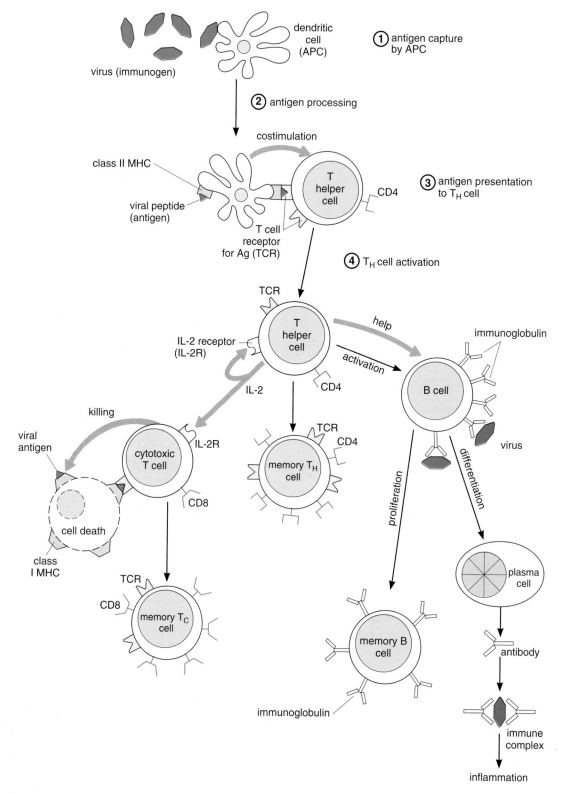

Figure 4–2. Sequence of events in a prototypical immune response (see text for details). *Abbreviations:* MHC = major histocompatibility class; APC = antigen-presenting cell; TCR = T-cell receptor.

teins. These cells, sometimes called "professional" APCs, include dendritic cells, macrophages, and B lymphocytes.

The APC depicted in Figure 4–2 is a **dendritic cell** and so represents the class of APCs that initiates most immune responses (see Chapter 6). Dendritic cells are present in nearly all tissues, including surface epithelia and the T-cell-rich zones of lymphoid organs, which allows them to monitor the skin, gastrointestinal and respiratory tracts, blood, and lymph continually for foreign invaders. The cytoplasm of dendritic cells extends outward in sheet-like structures called veils, and in long, narrow tendrils called dendrites, which provides a large surface area for contacting immunogens. They also express numerous surface receptors—such as receptors for mannose or for bacterial lipopolysaccharide (LPS), similar to those found on macrophages—that can recognize and bind pathogens. Dendritic cells readily capture particulate immunogens through phagocytosis and can also capture smaller immunogens through pinocytosis or receptor-mediated endocytosis (see Figure 2–6). All three of these pathways are also used by macrophages. B lymphocytes are poor phagocytes, but can efficiently endocytose antigens that bind to their surface immunoglobulins or other receptors (see Chapter 8). As a group, the APCs are able to capture a very broad range of immunogens, which helps to ensure that potential immunogens will not escape detection.

Immunogens that are captured and engulfed by an APC become enclosed within membrane-lined vesicles in its cytoplasm and, within these vesicles, undergo a series of alterations called **antigen processing** (Figure 4–3). For proteinaceous immunogens, this involves denaturation (unfolding) and partial proteolytic digestion, so that the immunogen is cleaved into short peptides. A limited number of the resulting peptides then associate noncovalently with class II MHC proteins and are transported to the APC surface, where they can be detected by helper T cells. This process is called **antigen presentation.** A CD4 helper T lymphocyte that comes into direct contact with an APC may become activated, but only if it expresses a T-cell receptor that is able to recognize and bind the particular peptide-MHC complex presented by that APC.

Statistically, the odds that any given T cell will respond to a given antigen are very poor: Even for highly potent immunogens, fewer than one in 100,000 naive T cells have the necessary specificity. Moreover, T cells are normally quite scarce at most locations in the body. Fortunately, dendritic cells have the ability to transport antigens from the site where they were captured into lymph nodes or other lymphoid tissues, where T cells are abundant. Within minutes after an immunogen contacts the skin, for example, the resident dendritic cells (Langerhans' cells) migrate out of the epidermis and into the underlying lymphatic vessels, which carry them and their cargo of antigens into the regional lymph nodes in search of a responsive T cell. This ability to transport antigens rapidly to lymphoid tissues is one of the features responsible for the extreme efficiency of dendritic cells as APCs and for their central role in launching immune responses.

Activation of Helper T Lymphocytes

Helper T (T_H) cells are the principal orchestrators of the immune response because they are needed for activation of the two other lymphoid effector cell types: cytotoxic T (T_C) cells and antibody-secreting plasma cells. T_H cell activation occurs early in an immune response (see Figure 4–2) and requires at least two signals. One signal is provided by binding of the T-cell antigen receptor to the antigenic peptide–MHC

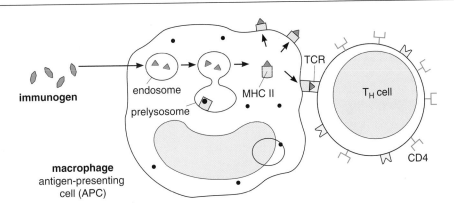

Figure 4–3. Capture, processing, and presentation of antigen by an antigen-presenting cell (APC). The immunogen is captured by phagocytosis, receptor-mediated endocytosis, or pinocytosis and is broken down into fragments. Some fragments (antigens) become associated with major histocompatibility (MHC) class II proteins and are transported to the cell surface, where they can be recognized by CD4 T cells. *Abbreviation:* TCR = T-cell receptor.

complex on the APC surface and is transmitted through the CD3 protein complex (see Chapter 9). The second, **costimulatory** signal also requires close contact between the APC and T_H cell surfaces and is usually delivered by the T_H-cell protein called **CD28** when it binds to either one of a pair of **B7** proteins on the APC surface (Figure 4–4).

Together, the two signals induce the helper T cell to begin secreting a cytokine known as interleukin-2 (**IL-2**) and also to begin expressing specific high-affinity **IL-2 receptors** on its surface (see Figure 4–4). IL-2 is a highly potent mitogenic factor for T lymphocytes and is essential for the proliferative response of activated T cells. The IL-2 protein has a very short half-life outside the cell and so acts only over extremely short distances. In fact, IL-2 is thought to exert its greatest effects on the cell from which it is secreted—a phenomenon known as an **autocrine effect.** Even if a T cell has received both activation signals from contact with an APC, it will not begin to proliferate in the absence of IL-2 activity or if its own surface IL-2 receptors are blocked. The IL-2 secreted by an activated T_H cell can also act on cells in the immediate vicinity, in a so-called **paracrine effect;** this is especially important for activating T_C cells, which generally do not produce enough IL-2 to stimulate their own proliferation (see later discussion). In addition to IL-2, activated T_H cells secrete other cytokines that promote the growth, differentiation, and functions of B cells, macrophages, and other cell types (see Chapter 9).

Activation of B Cells & Cytotoxic T Cells

While the T_H cells are being activated as described earlier, some B cells may also have been engaging the immunogen through their antigen receptors, which are membrane-bound forms of the antibodies they will later secrete (see Chapters 7 and 8). Unlike T cells, B cells recognize an immunogen in its free, unprocessed form (see Figure 4–2). Specific antigen binding provides one of the two signals needed for B-cell activation. The second is provided by activated T_H cells, which express proteins that help activate the B cell by binding to nonimmunoglobulin receptors on its surface. This second type of signal, called **T-cell help,** can act on any B cell regardless of its antigen specificity. The most effective form of help occurs when a protein called CD40 ligand (**CD40L**), which is expressed on T_H cells only after they become activated, binds to a protein called **CD40** on B cells (Figure 4–5). In fact, direct contact with an activated T_H cell may be sufficient to activate a resting B cell even though its surface immunoglobulins have not engaged an antigen; this is known as **bystander** B-cell activation. The combination of antigen binding and helper factors, however, yields the strongest mitogenic signals, so that over time antigen-specific clones quickly outgrow any activated bystanders. Some cells in each activated clone differentiate into plasma cells that secrete antibodies specific for the immunogen.

T_C lymphocytes function to eradicate cells that express foreign antigens on their surfaces, such as virus-infected host cells (Figure 4–6). Most T_C cells express CD8 rather than CD4 and hence recognize antigens in association with class I rather than class II MHC proteins. When a somatic cell is infected by a virus, some immunogenic viral proteins may undergo processing within the cell, and the resulting peptides may then appear as surface complexes with class I MHC molecules. These peptide–MHC com-

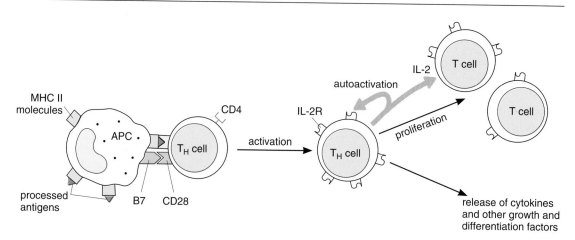

Figure 4–4. T_H-cell activation. The antigen-presenting cell (APC) presents an antigenic peptide, bound to major histocompatibility class (MHC) II, to the T_H cell and also provides a costimulatory signal when a B7 protein on its surface binds CD28 on the T_H cell. The two signals lead to activation of the T_H cell. Activation leads to interleukin (IL)-2 receptor expression and IL-2 secretion by the T_H cell, resulting in autocrine growth stimulation.

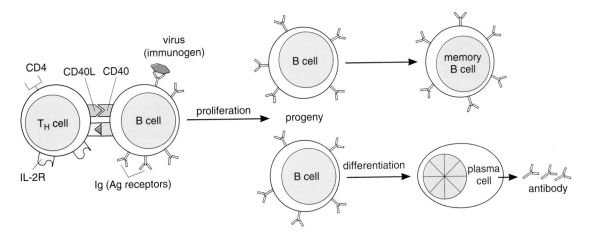

Figure 4–5. B-cell activation. Antigen binding to the surface immunoglobulins, coupled with soluble or contact-mediated helper factors from an activated T_H cell, lead to proliferation and differentiation. Cytokines involved in T_H-cell help include interleukin (IL)-2, IL-4, and IL-6. Contact-mediated help generally involves binding of CD40 on the B-cell surface to CD40 ligand (CD40L) on the activated T_H cell.

plexes may then be recognized by the T-cell receptor of an antigen-specific clone, providing one of two signals necessary for T_C-cell activation. This first signal alone induces high-affinity IL-2 receptors on the T_C cell. The second signal is furnished by IL-2 secreted from a nearby activated T_H lymphocyte. On receiving both signals, the activated T_C cell acquires cytotoxic activity, enabling it to kill the cell to which it is bound, as well as any other cells bearing the same peptide-MHC class I complexes. In some cases, killing occurs because the T_C releases cytolytic toxins onto the target cell; in others, the T_C induces the target cell to commit suicide by apoptosis (see later discussion). The activated T_C cell also proliferates, giving rise to additional T_C cells with the same antigen specificity.

MECHANISMS OF ANTIGEN ELIMINATION

The ultimate function of the immune system is to seek out and destroy foreign substances in the body. Depending in part on the nature of the foreign substance, this can be accomplished in several ways. One, described in the preceding section, is the direct **cytotoxic** killing of antigen-bearing target cells by activated T_C cells (see Figure 4–6). Most other immunologic effector mechanisms require antibodies; the most important of these will now be described.

Toxin Neutralization

Antibodies specific for bacterial toxins or for the venom of insects or snakes bind these antigenic pro-

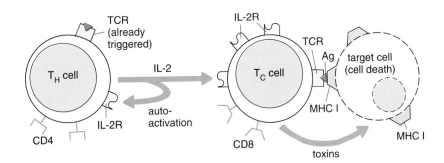

Figure 4–6. T_C-cell activation requires contact with a specific antigen complexed with a major histocompatibility class (MHC) I molecule on the surface of a target cell. It also requires interleukin(IL)-2 from a nearby activated T_H cell. The activated T_C cell kills the target cell either by secreting cytotoxins (as shown) or by inducing it to commit suicide. *Abbreviation:* TCR = T-cell receptor.

teins and, in many cases, directly inactivate them by steric effects. In addition, formation of an antigen-antibody complex promotes the capture and phagocytosis of these toxins by macrophages and other phagocytes (see the section on opsonization). Because of their effectiveness, preformed antibodies against toxins or venom are often injected prophylactically or therapeutically as a means of protecting unimmunized individuals who have recently been, or are at risk of being, exposed to specific toxins.

Virus Neutralization

Antibodies specific for proteins on the surface of a virus may block the attachment of the virus to target cells, particularly if the antibodies bind at or close to the site of cell binding on the virus. This provides a means by which preexisting antibodies can protect against new viral infections. Once viral infection has become established, however, neutralization is often less important than the cytotoxic action of T_C cells for eradicating the infection.

Opsonization & Phagocyte Activation

Antibodies that coat bacteria or other particulate antigens can function as **opsonins** to promote phagocytosis. This occurs because macrophages and other phagocytes carry surface **Fc receptors** that facilitate engulfment of antibody-coated particles (see Chapters 2 and 7). Thus, just as macrophages control lymphocyte function through their role as APCs, B lymphocytes regulate macrophage function by directing these phagocytes to specific antigenic targets through the process of opsonization.

Immune responses also affect phagocyte functions in other ways. For example, some activated T_H cells release interferon gamma (**IFNγ**) and other cytokines that are potent macrophage activators. The resulting activation increases the phagocytic activity of the macrophage and may cause it to secrete numerous other cytokines and mediators (see Chapter 2). Activated lymphocytes also produce IL-2, IL-3, and IL-4, as well as colony-stimulating factors (see Chapter 10), which regulate macrophage growth and function.

Activation of Complement

Certain types of antibodies can activate the **complement pathway** when they are complexed with an antigen (see Chapters 7 and 12). If the antibody is bound to the surface of a cell, such as a bacterium, the cascade of complement enzyme reactions may lead to lysis of the cell, providing an important means of killing these pathogens. Some products of the complement cascade also act as opsonins when bound to an antigen–antibody complex, whereas others are chemoattractive for neutrophils. Still others cause the release of inflammatory mediators such as histamine from mast cells and basophils (see Chapter 13).

Antibody-Dependent Cell-Mediated Cytotoxicity

One major class of antibodies, called IgG (see Chapter 7), binds to Fc receptors on the surfaces of natural killer (NK) cells and certain other cell types and enables them to carry out a form of antigen-specific cell killing called **antibody-dependent cell-mediated cytotoxicity (ADCC).** The IgG antibodies bound on its surface enable the cell to bind specifically to antigen-bearing target cells, which might be bacteria or multicellular parasites, and to kill the target cells with cytotoxins. The antibodies are said to "arm" the cells to perform ADCC, and they are absolutely required for such killing; this fact distinguishes ADCC from T_C-mediated cytotoxicity, which occurs independently of antibodies.

INFLAMMATION

Although lymphocytes and APCs are the key cells in all immune responses, other types of cells may be recruited into the response. For example, cytokines, chemokines, or other products released by activated lymphocytes and macrophages may chemoattract neutrophils or eosinophils, stimulate proliferation of fibroblasts and endothelial cells, or cause mast cells and basophils to discharge other bioactive substances into the local tissues (see Chapter 13). These agents, as well as products of the complement cascade, may lead directly or indirectly to increased blood flow, increased vascular permeability, leakage of fluid into the extravascular space, and pain. Those four responses are, of course, the cardinal signs of acute inflammation, which often accompanies immune responses. In some instances, other enzymatic pathways such as the kinin, clotting, and fibrinolytic systems may also become activated (see Chapters 12 and 13). Different features of inflammation predominate in different settings, giving rise to several distinct categories of inflammatory reactions that will be described in Chapter 13.

LOCALIZATION OF IMMUNE RESPONSES

The initial response to an immunogen depends partially on its route of entry into the body. Most immunogens enter via one of three routes. Those that enter through the bloodstream are most likely to be detected by dendritic cells and macrophages in the spleen, which then becomes the principal site of the immune response. By contrast, immunogens that enter the skin and subcutaneous connective tissues are usually detected by resident APCs, such as epidermal Langerhans' cells or dermal macrophages, and, in addition, may be carried via the lymphatic circulation into regional lymph nodes; the immune response then begins both at the site of contact and in the affected nodes. Alternatively, an immunogen may enter the body by traversing mucosal surfaces of the respiratory or gastrointestinal tract; in this case, it immediately encounters the submucosal lymphoid tissues, which launch a response that is directed both locally and into the adjacent lumen from which the immunogen came (see Chapters 3 and 14).

Regardless of the site at which a response begins, some trafficking of dendritic cells and lymphocytes to other sites via the blood and lymphatic vessels always takes place, so that the entire immune system can eventually be recruited into the response if the immunogen is especially abundant, widely disseminated, or resistant to immune elimination.

QUANTITATIVE & KINETIC ASPECTS OF IMMUNE RESPONSES

The quantitative aspects of immune function have been studied most extensively for B cells, since B-cell activity can easily be monitored by the concentrations of specific antibodies in the serum—an area of investigation known as **serology.** The general conclusions of such studies, however, are thought to be applicable to T-cell responses as well.

At any given moment, active T- and B-effector cells account for roughly 1% of the total lymphoid population in a normal host. These belong to many different clones (the exact number is unknown and no doubt varies widely), most of which are probably involved in ongoing, low-level immune responses against the many antigens encountered in everyday life. As a result, the serum of a normal, healthy adult contains innumerable different types of antibody molecules. Each is present in only minute amounts, but altogether they account for roughly 20% of total serum protein. Each of these circulating antibodies provides a low level of protection against its specific antigen.

When a person or animal is exposed to significant amounts of an antigen and mounts a B-cell response, the concentration of serum antibodies against that antigen generally rises. Serum from such an immunized individual is often called a **specific antiserum.** It is important to remember, however, that even in the serum of highly immunized individuals, antibodies against a given antigen make up only a small fraction of the total and antibodies with many other specificities are also present.

An individual's first encounter with a particular immunogen is called a **priming** event and leads to a relatively weak, short-lived response designated the **primary immune response.** This is divisible into several phases (Figure 4–7). The **lag,** or **latent, phase** is the time between the initial exposure to an immunogen and the detection of antibodies in the circulation, which averages about 1 week in humans. During this period, activation of T_H and B cells is taking place. The **exponential phase** is marked by a rapid increase in the quantity of circulating antibodies and reflects the increasing numbers of secretory plasma cells. After an interval during which the antibody level remains relatively constant because secretion and degradation are occurring at approximately equal rates (the **steady-state,** or **plateau, phase**), the antibody level gradually declines (**declining phase**) as synthesis of new antibody wanes. The decline indicates that new plasma cells are no longer being produced and that existing plasma cells are dying or

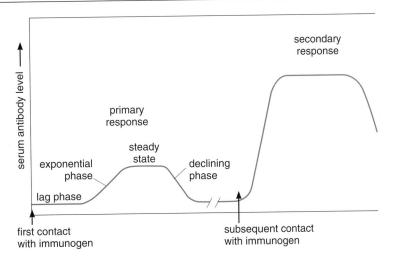

Figure 4–7. Primary and secondary immune responses (see text for details).

ceasing antibody production; this generally signifies that the immunogen has been eradicated. Thus, the duration of a humoral immune response is limited primarily by the duration of the antigenic stimulus and by the relatively short life spans of the plasma cells involved in the response.

Subsequent encounters with the same immunogen lead to responses that are qualitatively similar to the primary response but manifest marked quantitative differences (see Figure 4–7). In such a **secondary, or anamnestic, immune response,** the lag period is short and antibody levels rise more rapidly to a much higher steady-state level, thereafter remaining in the serum at detectable levels for much longer periods. The large numbers of antigen-specific memory T and B cells generated during the primary response are responsible for the rapid kinetics and the greater intensity and duration of secondary responses.

PROGRAMMED CELL DEATH IN THE IMMUNE SYSTEM

Antigen-dependent proliferation of a lymphocyte clone is an example of **positive selection;** that is, the antigen promotes growth of the cells on which it acts. Under some conditions, however, contact with antigens or other stimuli results in **negative selection** of a responsive clone, meaning that cells in the clone selectively die. Negative selection of lymphocytes is a common event and is essential to the ability of the immune system to discriminate self from nonself. In particular, most naive T or B cells whose antigen receptors recognize components found in normal host tissues are thought to be selectively killed before they leave the bone marrow or thymus, as a means of protecting the host against attack by these potentially **autoreactive** (ie, self-reactive) cells. This may account for the observation that at least 99% of developing thymocytes die within the thymus (see Chapter 3). Thus, the clonal composition of the immune system is shaped not only by positive clonal selection but also by the active elimination of potentially deleterious clones.

Lymphocytes frequently die after being instructed to commit suicide by signals in their environment. These signals often include events such as antigen binding to surface immunoglobulins or TCRs which, under other circumstances, would lead to clonal proliferation. When delivered in particular combinations or at certain vulnerable stages in a cell's life, however, these signals instead induce death by **apoptosis** (see Chapter 1). In particular, repeated or intense activation of a T or B cell commonly leads to apoptosis, a phenomenon termed **activation-induced cell death (AICD).** AICD triggered by contact with self-antigens is an important mechanism for eliminating au-

toreactive B- and T-lymphoid cells (see Chapters 8 and 9) and occurs commonly among normal thymocytes, bone marrow progenitors, and germinal center B cells.

Another signaling pathway that is especially important for killing of and by lymphocytes involves the surface transmembrane protein called **Fas** (also called APO-1 or **CD95**), which is expressed constitutively by many normal or neoplastic cell types as well as on activated B and T lymphocytes. The extracellular portion of Fas serves as a receptor for a different surface protein—a homotrimer of polypeptides called Fas ligand **(FasL),** found on many activated T cells and certain other cell types. When cells expressing these two proteins contact one another, binding of FasL causes Fas to trimerize and this, in turn, induces apoptosis in the Fas-bearing cell (see Chapter 1). Cytotoxic T lymphocytes exploit this as one mechanism for killing: Activated T_C cells express FasL, which enables them to induce apoptosis in target cells that express Fas. But lymphocytes themselves can also be killed in this way. For example, after prolonged or repeated activation, helper T cells express both Fas and FasL and so may kill either themselves or one another; this is a major pathway of AICD and is thought to be one mechanism for limiting the intensity of an immune response. The same mechanism might also act to eradicate autoreactive T_H cells that encounter abundant self-antigens in peripheral tissues—and indeed, mutations in Fas are responsible for certain rare autoimmune diseases. Fas-mediated killing may also account in part for the phenomenon of **immune privilege**—the observation that foreign tissues transplanted to certain sites in the body are much less prone to immunologic attack than they would be at other sites. Cells in two of the best studied privileged sites (the testes and anterior chamber of the eye) have been found to express FasL constitutively; this tends to induce apoptosis of any lymphocytes that become activated (and hence express Fas) within these tissues and so suppresses any local immune responses.

The importance of negative selection is also illustrated by **follicular lymphoma,** the most common form of B-cell cancer in humans (see Chapters 7 and 43). A major factor in the genesis of this disease is **Bcl-2**—a normal cellular protein that acts to inhibit apoptosis in some lymphocytes and other cell types (see Chapter 1). Follicular lymphoma arises when a clone of B cells expresses abnormally high levels of Bcl-2 protein and so becomes resistant to killing; as a result, these cells accumulate in abnormally large numbers and eventually evolve into a cancer. This implies that a high, controlled rate of programmed lymphocyte death normally benefits the host by restricting the growth of individual clones and of the lymphoid population as a whole, providing a counterforce against the stimuli that might otherwise drive excessive lymphocyte proliferation.

REFERENCES

Abbas AK: Die and let live: Eliminating dangerous lymphocytes. *Cell* 1996;84:655.

Banchereau J, Steinman RM: Dendritic cells and the control of immunity. *Nature* 1998;392:245.

Cory S: Regulation of lymphocyte survival by the BCL-2 gene. *Annu Rev Immunol* 1995;13:513.

Mellman I et al: Antigen processing for amateurs and professionals. *Trends Cell Biol* 1998;8:231.

Streilein JW: Unraveling immune privilege. *Science* 1995; 270:1158.

Watts C: Capture and processing of exogenous antigens for presentation on MHC molecules. *Annu Rev Immunol* 1997;15:821.

5 Immunogens, Antigens, & Vaccines

Tristram G. Parslow, MD, PhD

Any substance capable of inducing an immune response is called an **immunogen** and is said to be **immunogenic.** Some immunogens activate either the humoral or the cellular limb of the immune system exclusively, but most activate both. As a rule, immune responses are carried out only by those B- and T-cell clones whose surface immunoglobulin or T-cell receptor (TCR) proteins recognize the immunogen. Substances that are recognized by a particular immunoglobulin or TCR, and so can serve as the target of an immune response, are called **antigens** and are said to be **antigenic.** Thus, all immunogens are also antigens (Figure 5–1).

Most of the immunogens encountered in nature, including essentially all microbial pathogens, are complex assemblages made up of several different types of molecules, not all of which are antigenic. For example, the response to an enveloped virus is directed against proteins of the viral particle but not against the lipids that make up much of the viral envelope. Even when a single pure protein serves as an immunogen, the response is usually directed against only a few discrete clusters of amino acid residues within the larger polypeptide. The specific set of chemical features that is recognized by a given antibody or TCR is called an **epitope** (or, in older terminology, an **antigenic determinant**). In other words, an epitope is the specific site to which a particular immunoglobulin or TCR binds. It follows that every immunogen must contain one or more epitopes that enable it to serve as an antigen. Not all antigens or epitopes are immunogenic, however; in other words, not every chemical substance that can be bound by an immunoglobulin or TCR is, by itself, capable of inducing an immune response. This chapter explores the properties that enable a substance to serve as the stimulus for, or the target of, an immunologic attack.

IMMUNOGENS

The ability to evoke an immune response, and the nature and intensity of this response, depend not only on the physicochemical properties of the immunogen itself but also on other factors, such as the characteristics of the organism being immunized, the route of contact, and the sensitivity of the methods used to detect the response. The factors that influence immunogenicity are complex, but several important generalizations can be made.

Properties of the Immunogen

Proteins are, as a rule, the most effective immunogens. Polysaccharides, short polypeptides, and some synthetic organic polymers (eg, polyvinyl pyrrolidone) can also be immunogenic under certain circumstances. Nucleic acids and lipids from mammalian cells are not immunogenic, but antibodies that react with them can be elicited by immunization with nucleoprotein or lipoprotein complexes; this is probably the mechanism of origin of the anti-DNA antibodies found in the serum of many patients with autoimmune diseases (see Chapter 31). Thus, nucleic acids and most lipids are examples of molecules that are antigenic but not immunogenic.

Immunogenicity is influenced by molecular size

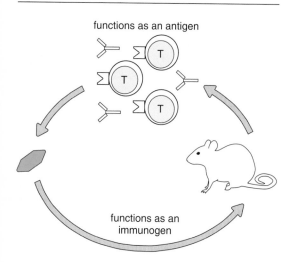

functions as an antigen

functions as an immunogen

Figure 5–1. Immunogens and antigens. An immunogen induces an immune response; antigens serve as the target of the response.

and complexity. The most effective immunogens are proteins with molecular weights greater than 100,000. Extremely small molecules, such as amino acids, monosaccharides, and most other species smaller than MW 10,000, usually are not immunogenic. Homopolymers of a single amino acid may be poor immunogens regardless of size, whereas copolymers of two or more are often quite active, with aromatic amino acids such as tyrosine contributing more to immunogenicity than do nonaromatic residues. A few substances with molecular weights below 1000 can induce immune responses but in most cases will do so only when bound to a larger, host-derived macromolecule such as a protein; this is the mechanism by which many people become allergic to metals (such as nickel) or to certain drugs.

Most important, however, is foreignness: The immune system normally discriminates between self and nonself, so that only molecules that are foreign to the host are immunogenic. Thus, albumin isolated from the serum of a rabbit and injected back into the same or another rabbit will not yield an immune response—every rabbit is **tolerant** to this endogenous protein. Yet the same protein, if injected into other vertebrate species, is likely to evoke substantial antibody responses, depending on the dose of antigen and the route and frequency of injection. The mechanisms of tolerance are beginning to be understood and will be considered in later chapters.

Genetic Constitution of the Host Animal

The ability to respond to a particular immunogen is genetically predetermined. For example, pure polysaccharides are immunogenic when injected into mice or human adults but not when injected into guinea pigs or rabbits. Much information about the genetics of immune responsiveness has accrued from studies using inbred strains of animals. For example, some strains of guinea pig produce a vigorous antibody response against the simple polypeptide poly-L-lysine, whereas other strains give no detectable response; crossbreeding studies among these strains indicate that the ability to respond to poly-L-lysine is inherited as an autosomal-dominant trait. Many analogous phenomena have been described in humans. Selective responsiveness of this type reflects a number of hereditary factors, the best understood of which include the particular collection (**repertoire**) of different immunoglobulins and TCR proteins that an individual is able to produce (Chapters 7–9) and the ability of antigen-presenting cells (APCs) to present specific types of molecules to T lymphocytes (Chapter 6). Individuals whose APCs cannot present a substance or whose lymphocytes cannot recognize it will not respond to this substance as an immunogen.

Mode of Contact

Whether a substance will evoke an immune response also depends on the dosage and the route by which it enters the body. A quantity of substance that has no effect when injected intravenously may evoke a copious antibody response when injected subcutaneously. Route of contact also can influence the qualitative nature of a response; for example, an immunogen that contacts the intestinal mucosa typically evokes the production of a different type of antibody than would be produced if it entered through the bloodstream, and this can affect subsequent events in the immune response (see Chapters 7 and 14). The threshold dose required for a response under particular conditions varies among immunogens. In general, once the threshold dose is exceeded, increasing doses lead to increasing, though less than proportionate, responses. Excessive doses, however, may not only fail to induce a response but may instead establish a state of specific unresponsiveness, or tolerance, to subsequent exposures to that substance—a phenomenon that is sometimes referred to as **high-zone tolerance.**

Both the intensity and the character of the response to an immunogen can be altered if it is administered in combination with other immunogens. This is because an ongoing response to one substance can affect local cytokine concentrations as well as the type and activation state of local immune cells, and these may, in turn, favor or disfavor particular types of responses to other immunogens. Certain substances, called **adjuvants** and **immunomodulators,** are especially effective at enhancing or modifying the responses to many different immunogens when administered along with them and have been exploited therapeutically for this purpose in the development of vaccines (see later section).

B-CELL ANTIGENS & B-CELL EPITOPES

Large molecules are the strongest immunogens and usually are correspondingly strong antigens. Any given antibody or TCR, however, will recognize and bind to only a limited portion of such a molecule, and this binding site is called an epitope. A single antigenic molecule may contain several distinct epitopes, and most large antigens do (Figure 5–2). For any given antigen in a particular individual, the regions that are recognized by immunoglobulins (called **B-cell epitopes**) are usually different from those recognized by TCRs (called **T-cell epitopes**). The concept of T-cell epitopes is somewhat complicated in that T cells only recognize their epitopes in association with major histocompatability class (MHC) molecules on cell surfaces. In contrast, epitope recognition by an antibody is a relatively straightforward bimolecular interaction that occurs in solution and so is easier to study experimentally and to understand. We therefore begin by focusing on B-cell antigens and epitopes.

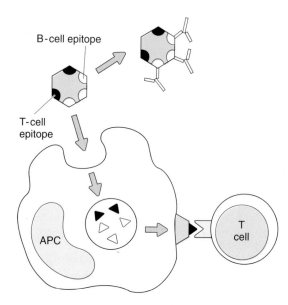

Figure 5–2. Most large antigens contain multiple epitopes. B-cell epitopes (white) are regions that can be bound by immunoglobulin proteins. T-cell epitopes (black) are recognized by T lymphocytes only after being processed and presented in association with a major histocompatibility complex (MHC) protein on the surface of an antigen-presenting cell (APC).

Size and Locations of B-Cell Epitopes

Antibody responses against native, folded proteins are almost always directed against residues on the protein surface because these residues are exposed and accessible for binding. X-ray crystallographic studies have revealed the precise, three-dimensional structures of several protein antigens with individual antibodies bound to them, so that we now understand the interactions involved in great detail.

Globular proteins tend to fold into compact masses with the majority of their constituent amino acids (particularly those with hydrophobic sidechains) buried in the interior, leaving a minority of residues (including most of those that have polar sidechains) on the surface, exposed to the surrounding environment. Because the overall folding pattern is fairly rigid, the exposed residues occupy more-or-less fixed locations with respect to one another, which together define the contoured, water-accessible surface of the protein. A given antibody typically binds to a specific subset of residues that are clustered together on this surface. The epitope for such an antibody, then, is best thought of as a particular array of chemical features arranged in a specific spatial contour on the accessible surface of the antigen.

Studies of antibody binding to very short, synthetic polypeptides indicate that an epitope can be formed by as few as three to six amino acids. On the other hand, the antigen–antibody complexes that

have been analyzed by x-ray crystallography generally show the antibody contacting as many as 20 amino acid residues on the antigen simultaneously. Thus, a reasonable rule of thumb might be that B-cell epitopes generally comprise 6–20 amino acid residues on the antigen surface. The antigen-binding site on any single immunoglobulin molecule has a fixed size (Chapter 7), and this, in turn, dictates the maximum spatial dimensions of its epitope. A typical epitope extends over a total area of up to about 700 $Å^2$ on the antigen surface, which means that a single epitope might occupy roughly 10% of the total surface of a small protein such as human lysozyme (130 amino acids; MW 14,700).

The number of separate epitopes on an antigenic molecule generally is proportional to its size and chemical complexity. One way to estimate how many B-cell epitopes are present on a given antigen is to determine the number of antibody molecules that can bind to each molecule of antigen under saturating conditions. Using this approach, it has been estimated, for example, that hen egg albumin (MW 42,000) has about five distinct B-cell epitopes, whereas thyroglobulin (MW 700,000) has about 40. This approach provides only minimal estimates, however, because epitopes can overlap one another, so that not all possible epitopes on a molecule can be occupied by bound antibodies simultaneously. Moreover, these numbers are somewhat misleading, since different regions of an antigen can be used preferentially as epitopes by different individuals or different animal species, or even by a single individual at different times. In fact, the weight of evidence currently suggests that virtually any region on the exposed surface of a folded protein has the potential to serve as a B-cell epitope.

These observations can be of use in predicting the locations of B-cell epitopes on a folded protein whose sequence is known but whose precise structure is not: Because polar residues are situated on the surface much more frequently than nonpolar residues, the regions of highest average polarity within a polypeptide sequence have the highest likelihood of being targets for antibody binding.

Conformational & Linear Epitopes

In many instances, all of the amino acid or sugar residues that form a given epitope are positioned sequentially in the linear sequence of a protein or polysaccharide antigen. Because these residues are covalently linked to one another and cannot move far apart, epitopes of this type are not affected by heat denaturation or other treatments that alter the three-dimensional structure of a protein. Such epitopes are called **linear** (or **sequential**) **epitopes** (Figure 5–3).

Other B-cell epitopes, by contrast, form only when the critical residues are brought together in space through folding of the polypeptide or polysaccharide chain into its normal three-dimensional conforma-

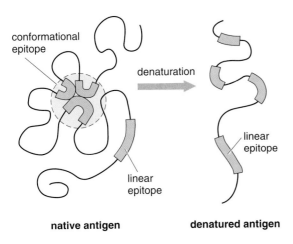

native antigen   **denatured antigen**

Figure 5–3. Conformational and linear epitopes in a polypeptide antigen. After denaturation, the conformational epitope can no longer be recognized by antibodies, but the linear epitope is unaffected.

tion. Epitopes of this type are called **conformational epitopes,** and, by definition, are lost if the antigen is denatured and fails to refold properly. Many conformational epitopes are made up of residues located at two or more discontinuous sites along the linear sequence of an antigen, as depicted in Figure 5–3. This is not always the case, however. For example, antibodies raised against a short, α-helical peptide may not recognize the same peptide in denatured form; thus, even a contiguous sequence of amino acids can function as a conformational epitope.

Antibodies that recognize conformational epitopes are often used to study changes that occur in the three-dimensional structures of proteins during physiologic processes such as ligand binding. Such conformational shifts may eliminate certain epitopes on a protein while causing new ones to form. For example, antibodies have been described that can discriminate between the oxygenated and nonoxygenated

forms of hemoglobin by detecting small differences in alignment of the globin subunits. There are many other examples of such conformation-specific antibody binding.

THE PHYSICOCHEMICAL BASIS OF ANTIGEN–ANTIBODY BINDING

As is the case in other types of protein–protein interactions, antibodies bind to their antigens because the areas of contact between the two molecules are **complementary** to each other: The antigen-binding residues on an antibody form a contoured surface that closely mirrors that of its epitope, so that epitope and antibody can mold smoothly against each other (Figure 5–4A). This complementarity refers not only to the shapes of the two binding surfaces (with peaks in one fitting into valleys in the other) but also to their chemical features: Individual amino acids from the antigen and antibody are positioned so as to allow the formation of salt bridges (ie, bonding between positively and negatively charged residues), hydrogen bonds, van der Waals contacts, and localized hydrophobic interactions between the two surfaces. These multiple, discrete, noncovalent linkages are the basis for bonding between an antibody and its epitope, and the aggregate of the individual strengths of these linkages determines the overall bonding energy. The more perfectly an epitope matches the chemical and spatial contours of an antibody, the more tightly it is bound. Understanding the nature of the complementarity between immunoglobulins and their epitopes is extremely important because it is the mechanism by which the humoral immune system recognizes and distinguishes among antigenic molecules.

Changes in chemical structure of an epitope tend to distort its complementarity with the antibody, weakening or eliminating individual chemical contacts and so weakening the interaction overall. Systematic study of this phenomenon shows that not all chemical linkages contribute equally; in general, salt

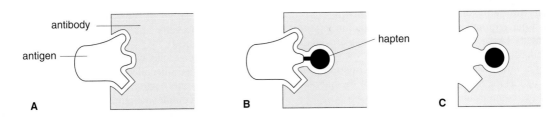

Figure 5–4. Schematic illustration of the complementarity between a B-cell epitope and the antigen-binding site on an antibody protein. Antibodies raised against **A:** an antigen or **B:** a hapten–carrier complex are fully complementary to their cognate epitopes. **C:** An antibody whose epitope includes a hapten will also bind the isolated hapten, although it usually has lower affinity for the free hapten than for the hapten–carrier complex. Note that binding of the hapten interferes with binding of the hapten–carrier complex; this fact is often used as a basis for demonstrating low-affinity hapten binding by hapten-specific antibodies.

bridges and hydrogen bonds are individually more critical than van der Waals or hydrophobic interactions, and in some cases the loss of even one salt bridge or hydrogen bond can abolish antigen–antibody binding. As a result, mutation of an amino acid residue within an epitope may reduce or eliminate binding, depending on how much that residue contributed quantitatively to the binding and to what extent the new amino acid can substitute for it.

Quantitative Aspects of Antigen-Antibody Interactions

Humoral immune responses to most antigens involve many structurally different antibody molecules, which may each recognize separate or overlapping epitopes. Because each makes a different set of chemical contacts, some antibodies bind very strongly, and others more weakly, to the same antigen. By the same token, any given antibody can bind not only its original (or **cognate**) antigen, but also other molecules containing regions that happen to resemble its epitope. The binding of an antibody to an antigen other than the one that induced its formation is called a **cross-reaction.** Cross-reacting antigens generally have some, but not all, of the features responsible for the strong binding of the cognate epitope, and generally bind more weakly, though this is not always the case. Indeed, although we generally think of antibodies as highly specific, it is important to remember that every antibody can bind very weakly to a vast number of different antigens, though it binds very strongly to only a few.

The term **affinity** is used to describe the strength of interaction between two molecules that interact reversibly in a simple one-to-one fashion. It reflects the relative rates at which such molecules tend to associate and disassociate from each other, which can be depicted as:

$$[AB] \underset{k_2}{\overset{k_1}{\rightleftharpoons}} [A] + [B]$$

where k_1 and k_2 are the rate constants for dissociation and association, respectively. Affinity can be described in terms of the **dissociation half-life** $(t_{1/2})$—the time required for half of a population of preformed [AB] complexes to come apart under standard conditions. A more common measure is a single value, called the **dissociation constant** (K_d), defined as the ratio of concentrations of the unbound and bound molecules at equilibrium:

$$K_d = \frac{[A]\ [B]}{[AB]}$$

so that small K_d values indicate strong, high-affinity interactions. In the case of antigen-antibody binding, K_d values in the range of 10^{-7} to 10^{-10} molar (M) are typical for high-affinity interactions with cognate antigens. Cross-reactions and low-affinity cognate interactions may be characterized by K_d values as high as 10^{-4} to 10^{-6} M; weaker interactions often are not detectable and may not be physiologically significant.

The situation is very different, however, for **multivalent** antigens and antibody molecules—that is, those that can bind each other at multiple sites. As we shall see in Chapter 7, every antibody molecule has at least two identical antigen-binding sites, each of which can bind independently to its epitope. Conversely, some large antigens, including many viruses, bacteria, and parasites, have repeating arrays of molecules on their surfaces (see Chapter 2) that offer many identical epitopes to an appropriate antibody. When antigen and antibody are both multivalent, $t_{1/2}$ for the complex is much longer than for the individual contacts because even if one contact dissociates the others remain. The effect can be striking: The apparent "affinity" of divalent or trivalent interactions can be 10^3 or 10^6-fold higher, respectively, than for monovalent binding of a particular antibody-epitope pair.* Increased valency can thus make a low-affinity antibody functionally equal to a high-affinity one—a fact which the immune system exploits by producing antibodies with up to ten antigen-binding sites per molecule. As a result, even low-affinity antibodies can protect against infection provided they are present in sufficient concentration. Experiments based on inoculation of a rabies-like virus indicate that 200–500 bound antibody molecules are needed to neutralize each viral particle and that protection requires a serum concentration of at least 10^{-8} M virus-specific antibodies; this corresponds to about 0.01% of the total antibody concentration in normal serum.

Haptens

Many small molecules that are not immunogenic can nevertheless serve as B-cell epitopes—that is, they can be bound by antibodies that have the appropriate specificity (Figure 5–5). Antibodies against such molecules are commonly prepared by attaching them covalently onto an immunogenic protein; when this complex is then injected into animals, the resulting immune response often includes antibodies capable of binding the small molecule alone. Molecules that have this property are called **haptens,** from the Greek word *haptien* ("to fasten"), and the proteins or other immunogens onto which they are fastened for such experiments are called **carriers.** As a rule, a hapten forms only part of an epitope on the hapten–carrier complex (Figure 5–4B), but is also able to bind independently, though at lower affinity, to antibodies that recognize this epitope (Figure 5–4C). This provides a useful way to obtain antibod-

---

* The term **avidity** is often used to refer to the higher apparent affinity of multivalent interactions.

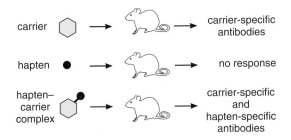

Figure 5–5. Haptens are substances that are antigenic but not immunogenic.

ies directed against peptides, drugs, or virtually any other small molecule, regardless of its inherent immunogenicity. Even antibodies that are specific for particular metal ions have been prepared in this manner.

T-CELL ANTIGENS & T-CELL EPITOPES

The antigen-binding site of a TCR has a structure much like that of an immunoglobulin, and it recognizes epitopes through complementary interactions like those described earlier. But there are important differences. Unlike an antibody, a TCR does not bind free antigens. Instead, proteinaceous antigens must first undergo processing, in the course of which they are degraded into peptides, some of which then associate with an MHC protein and are presented on the APC surface. Although the peptide is considered to be the epitope, a TCR that recognizes it does so by binding to a surface created by both the peptide and MHC molecule. In fact, the MHC protein provides the majority of chemical contacts with the TCR. Most of the peptide in a peptide–MHC complex is buried and inaccessible, with only a few of its amino acid sidechains exposed on the surface, but these are critical for T-cell recognition, and changing them can reduce or eliminate binding of a cognate TCR.

In comparison to antigen–antibody interactions, TCR binding is remarkably weak and short-lived. All TCRs are monovalent (ie, they have only a single binding site for an antigen-MHC complex), and epitopes that activate T cells typically bind with K_d around 10^{-6} M or less and $t_{1/2}$ of 10–50 seconds. The short duration of binding is especially problematic because the initial activation, proliferation, and differentiation of T cells requires an hour or more of prolonged, sustained contact with an APC. Moreover, although most APCs express 10^4–10^6 MHC proteins on their surfaces, the vast majority of these are occupied by peptides derived from normal host proteins that do not provoke immune responses (see Chapter 6). Even during an infection, only about 10^2–10^4

MHC molecules on any single APC present peptides derived from the pathogen.

To become activated, then, a T cell must use a very low affinity receptor to detect an epitope that is present on as few as 0.01% of the surface MHC molecules on an APC. This is possible only because of a specialized intercellular junction that forms between an APC and an antigen-specific T cell (Figure 5–6). As T cells and APCs migrate through tissues, they frequently collide and bind briefly to one another by means of surface adhesion proteins such as ICAM-1, CD2, and LFA-1 (see Chapter 1). During their brief encounters, TCRs on the T cell scan the APC surface for peptide–MHC complexes to which they can bind. If none are found, the cells soon detach and continue on their separate ways. If, on the other hand, the TCR detects its specific epitope, it transmits signals that immediately cause the T cell to stop moving and adhere more tightly to the APC. The APC, in turn, responds by increasing its expression of adhesion and MHC proteins, so that within about 30 seconds a disk-shaped zone of adhesion molecules collects at the point of contact between the cells. Around the periphery of this zone, where membranes of the two cells are in close contact, TCRs continue to search for the rare epitope–MHC complexes to which they can bind. Whenever one is found, it is translocated toward the center of the contact zone, and adhesion molecules shift toward the periphery. Over the course of 5–20 minutes, the specific epitope-MHC complexes are corralled into a small cluster on the cell-cell interface, where they are confined by a surrounding ring of adhesion molecules. Within this specialized junction, called the **immunologic synapse,** the high local concentration of specific epitope-MHC complexes allows many TCRs to bind and dissociate repeatedly over the course of an hour or more. The T cell appears to "count" these binding events and, provided it also receives costimulatory signals from the APC, becomes fully activated after about 1500 have occurred.

Like an antibody, every TCR can recognize some cross-reacting epitopes when appropriately presented, though peptide-MHC complexes that are bound extremely weakly may inhibit, rather than activate, the T cell. A specialized pathway is also available for presenting certain unusual **lipids** and **glycolipids,** such as those found in mycobacterial cell walls, which can then serve as epitopes for cytotoxic T cells (see Chapter 6); TCRs discriminate the structures of sugars, phosphates, and other polar groups in these antigens, rather than the lipids themselves.

T-Cell Epitopes & Immunogenicity

Because they recognize only processed antigens, T cells show no preference for epitopes that lie on the surfaces (as opposed to the interior) of globular proteins and rarely recognize specific conformational features of the native antigen. Moreover, APCs often

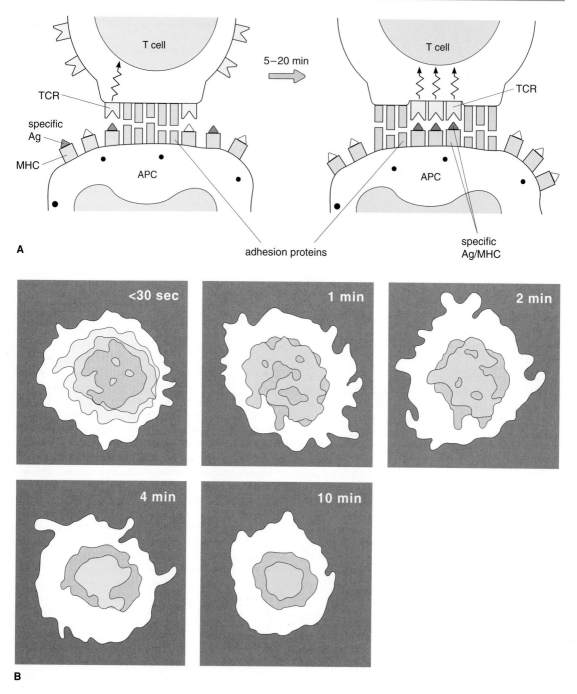

Figure 5–6. The immunological synapse. **A:** Initial binding (depicted at the *left*) of a T cell to an antigen-presenting cell (APC) is mediated by adhesion molecules such as LFA-1 and ICAM-1, which accumulate in a disk at the zone of contact. T-cell receptors (TCRs) then scan the many peptide/MHC complexes on the adjacent APC surface to identify the few that contain a specific epitope (black triangles). These specific complexes are translocated (possibly by an active process) to the center of the contact zone, while adhesion molecules move to the periphery. The mature synapse (at *right*) consists of a central cluster of 100–10,000 specific epitope–MHC complexes with a surrounding ring of adhesion proteins. It forms within 5–20 minutes after contact and may persist for hours, allowing repeated TCR binding events that eventually activate the T cell. **B:** Synapse formation viewed from the perspective of the APC. In this experimental model, a single T cell binds to an artificial planar lipid membrane containing fluorescently tagged ICAM-1 (blue) and specific peptide-MHC complexes (blue). The zone of contact is photographed at the indicated times after binding. Peptide-MHC complexes are initially distributed around the periphery of the synapse, but are translocated to its center as the synapse matures. (Photomicrographs courtesy of M. Dustin, from studies described by Grakoui et al, *Science* 1999;258: 221.)

present only a few of the many possible peptides that can be obtained from an antigen (see Chapter 6), which strictly limits the number that can function as T-cell epitopes. Nevertheless, some large proteins have been found to contain as many as 50 separate T-cell epitopes.

Studies with small, well-defined antigens have shown that humoral and cell-mediated immune responses can be directed against different regions of a single molecule. For example, the human hormone glucagon, which is only 29 amino acids long, contains separate B-cell and T-cell epitopic regions: When mice are immunized with human glucagon, they produce antibodies only against the amino-terminal part of the molecule, whereas their T cells respond only to the carboxy-terminal portion.

T-cell epitopes not only serve as the targets for cytotoxic T-cell responses but are also essential for nearly all B-cell responses. This is because T-cell epitopes are needed to activate helper T lymphocytes, which, in turn, are required for B-cell responses against nearly all antigens. Thus, as a rule, a molecule must contain at least one T-cell epitope to be immunogenic. Molecules that contain only B-cell epitopes (eg, haptens or the amino-terminal portion of human glucagon) may serve very well as targets for antibody responses but are unable to induce such responses themselves.

Immunodominance

Individual residues within a single epitope that contribute disproportionately to interactions with an antibody or TCR are said to be **immunodominant** residues. This might be said, for example, of a residue that forms a salt bridge with the antibody or TCR. When an antibody recognizes a sequence at the end of a polymer, the terminal residue of this polymer is almost invariably the most critical for binding and, hence, is immunodominant, whereas the other residues generally exhibit decreasing degrees of immunodominance with increasing distance from the terminus. The same term can also be applied to a particular epitope within a large antigen that contains multiple epitopes; in a given individual, and under a given set of circumstances, only one or a few of these may serve as the primary target of an immune response. In a B-cell response, for example, one epitope might evoke antibodies in larger quantities and with higher binding affinities than do the other available epitopes and so would be said to be the immunodominant epitope.

VACCINES

A **vaccine** is a nonpathogenic immunogen that, when inoculated into a host, induces protective immunity against a specific pathogen. Vaccines rank among the most important contributions of science to human health, and the development of the first vaccines against smallpox (by Edward Jenner, in 1798) and rabies (by Louis Pasteur, in 1880) are landmarks in the history of immunology. Effective vaccination programs have drastically reduced the incidence of many infectious diseases that once were common, and in the case of smallpox eradicated the disease. To be effective, a vaccine must induce long-standing immunity that acts at the appropriate body sites and against the appropriate microbial antigens to prevent disease in all persons at risk; to be practical, it must also be safe, inexpensive, and easy to store and administer. Vaccines currently in use, some of which are listed in Table 5–1, generally satisfy these criteria. But useful vaccines have yet to be developed against many major infectious diseases, including malaria and AIDS, and for this reason, as well as the need to improve existing preparations, vaccinology remains a very active area of research.

Some useful vaccines consist of live, naturally occurring microbes that share important antigens with a pathogen but are not pathogenic themselves. For example, **vaccinia** (cowpox) virus, a relative of the smallpox virus, causes an inapparent, self-limiting infection in normal people while inducing immunity against smallpox as well as against itself. Similarly, the nonpathogenic mycobacterium called **bacille Calmette-Guérin (BCG)** can be used as a live vaccine against *Mycobacterium tuberculosis*. An advantage of these agents is that, being infectious, they can be transmitted from vaccinees to others in the population; a drawback is that they may cause serious disease in persons with defective immune systems (see Chapter 21–23).

Table 5–1. Representative vaccines for human use.[a]

Vaccine	Type	Administration
Smallpox	Nonpathogen (vaccinia virus)	Subcutaneous
Polio—Salk	Killed	subcutaneous
Polio—Sabin	Live, attenuated	Oral
MMR: Measles Mumps Rubella	Live, attenuated Live, attenuated Live, attenuated	Subcutaneous Subcutaneous Subcutaneous
DTP: Diphtheria Tetanus Pertussis	Toxoid Toxoid Killed	Intramuscular Intramuscular Intramuscular
Haemophilus influenzae B	Glycoconjugate	Intramuscular
Hepatitis A virus	Killed	Intramuscular
Hepatitis B virus	Subunit	Intramuscular

[a] Properties of some vaccine preparations as approved for use in the United States; alternative forms of some are also available. Smallpox vaccine is no longer in general use, as the disease has been eradicated worldwide. MMR and DTP are combination vaccines, each directed against three pathogens as shown.

Other vaccines are prepared from potentially pathogenic bacteria or viruses that have either been **killed** (with heat or chemical treatments) or are **attenuated** (ie, have lost the ability to produce disease in humans). Because of the way in which their antigens are presented to T cells (see Chapter 6), killed vaccines induce humoral but not cell-mediated immunity, whereas attenuated vaccines induce both types of immunity and are generally much more potent and efficacious than killed vaccines. Efficacy is one reason why the original, killed-virus polio vaccine developed by Jonas Salk was quickly superseded by the Sabin vaccine, which uses live, attenuated poliovirus. The usual method of attenuating a virus is to grow it for prolonged periods in cells from a species other than its usual host; over time, the virus accumulates mutations that favor growth under the new conditions but which often reduce its growth and virulence in the original host. This approach was first developed by Pasteur, who attenuated the canine rabies virus by adapting it to growth in rabbits. In many cases, the exact mutations responsible for attenuation are unknown. One problem with attenuated vaccines is that, very rarely, further mutations allow the virus to revert to a pathogenic form. For example, approximately one case of polio occurs among every million vaccinees receiving the Sabin virus. A newer approach to attenuation is to employ recombinant DNA techniques to introduce large gene deletions and other mutations that may be less prone to reversion.

Certain vaccines are made of purified macromolecules rather than entire microorganisms. For example, the tetanus and diphtheria vaccines contain only inactive forms of the soluble bacterial toxins responsible for these diseases; these **toxoid** vaccines induce antitoxin antibodies but no immunity against the bacteria themselves. **Subunit vaccines,** such as the hepatitis B vaccine, consist of only a single immunogenic protein from the pathogen of interest, usually produced in laboratory bacteria, yeast, or cultured cells using recombinant DNA techniques. Several effective **glycoconjugate vaccines** against *Haemophilus influenzae* type B have been produced by linking polysaccharide B-cell epitopes from the capsule of this organism onto immunogenic carriers such as tetanus toxoid; similar vaccines against pneumococci and some meningococci are also under development. A related approach is to attach short, chemically synthesized peptides (usually < 20 amino acids) that correspond to known epitopes from an infectious organism onto a carrier to create **peptide vaccines.** These strategies are based on the concept that isolated carbohydrate or polypeptide epitopes can act as haptens to induce antibodies, which may then recognize the same epitopes in the native pathogen, though usually with lower affinity. For this approach to succeed, however, the vaccine must incorporate both B- and T-cell epitopes, since B-cell epitopes alone induce little or no immunologic memory. Moreover, T-cell epitopes must be carefully

chosen to ensure that they can be recognized, presented, and responded to by all members of the populations at risk.

One very new strategy for immunization is the use of **DNA vaccines.** These are based on the discovery that when DNA encoding a chosen microbial protein is injected intramuscularly or intradermally, host cells can take up these artificial genes and express the foreign protein for several weeks. Depending on the protein expressed, this can induce specific humoral or cellular immunity, or both. DNA vaccines appear to offer many advantages of safety and convenience and have yielded promising results in animals, but their clinical usefulness has not yet been proven.

Adjuvants

The response to an immunogen can often be enhanced if it is administered as a mixture with substances called **adjuvants.** Adjuvants function in one or more of the following ways: (1) by prolonging retention of the immunogen, (2) by increasing the effective size of the immunogen, and so promoting phagocytosis and presentation by macrophages, (3) by stimulating the influx of macrophages or other immune cell types to the injection site, or (4) by promoting local cytokine production and other immunologic activities of such immune cells.

A number of adjuvants have been used in experimental animals, the most potent being **complete Freund's adjuvant (CFA),** a water-in-oil emulsion containing killed mycobacteria. CFA appears to work by providing a depot for the immunogen and by stimulating macrophages and certain lymphocytes, but its very strong inflammatory effects preclude its use in humans. The only adjuvants approved for clinical use in the United States are **aluminum salts**—fine particles of aluminum phosphate or hydroxide onto which the immunogen is adsorbed. These widely used adjuvants increase the stability and effective particle size of an immunogen and also promote release of certain cytokines, such as interleukin-1. Unfortunately, aluminum adjuvants only stimulate humoral immunity, do not work with all antigens, and cannot be frozen or freeze-dried. Several other types of adjuvants are being explored for human use, most of which contain either mycobacterial cell walls or specific glycosylated protein fragments, called **muramyl di-** or **tripeptides,** derived from such walls, usually emulsified with oils, phospholipids, or other surfactants as a complex mixture. Another promising approach may be to incorporate specific **immunomodulators** into vaccines in order to promote particular types of immune responses. For example, **interleukin-12** influences helper T-cell development so as to promote cell-mediated, as opposed to humoral, immune reactions (see Chapter 9); its inclusion in a vaccine preparation might selectively promote a protective cytotoxic response against the target pathogen.

REFERENCES

Bachmann MF et al: The role of antibody concentration and avidity in antiviral protection. *Science* 1997;276: 2024.

Davies DR, Cohen GH: Interactions of protein antigens with antibodies. *Proc Natl Acad Sci USA* 1996;93:7.

Donnelly JJ et al: DNA vaccines. *Annu Rev Immunol* 1997;15:617.

Germain RN, Stefanova I: The dynamics of T cell receptor signaling: Complex orchestration and the key role of tempo and cooperation. *Annu Rev Immunol* 1999;17: 467.

Grakoui A et al: The immunologic synapse: A molecular machine controlling T cell activation. *Science* 1999;285: 221.

Moody DB et al: Structural requirements for glycolipid antigen recognition by CD1b-restricted T cells. *Science* 1997;278:283.

Rabinovich NR et al: Vaccine technologies: View to the future. *Science* 1994; 265:1401.

Robinson HL, Torres CA: DNA vaccines. *Semin Immunol* 1997;9:271.

6 Antigen Presentation & the Major Histocompatibility Complex

Frances M. Brodsky, DPhil

The cells and humoral factors of the innate immune system have, for the most part, evolved to recognize distinctive carbohydrate or lipid markers found on many types of pathogens but not in the normal host (see Chapter 2). The acquired immune system, by contrast, mainly targets peptide antigens derived from foreign proteins. This focus on peptides reflects the antigen specificity of T lymphocytes, whose antigen receptors (TCRs) only recognize the complexes formed by peptides bound to **major histocompatibility complex (MHC) proteins** on the surfaces of host cells. The use of a peptide-based recognition system has important advantages: since the structural diversity of peptides is much greater than that of carbohydrates or lipids, the acquired immune system is able to detect and discriminate among a much broader range of immunogens, which allows for much greater specificity in its responses. In addition, peptide-specific responses can be directed against virally encoded proteins that are synthesized by infected host cells even though they lack any unusual carbohydrate or lipid modifications.

As part of this focus on peptide antigens, the immune systems of humans and other mammals have evolved mechanisms for sampling the many proteins in their environments and cleaving them into peptides (a sequence of events called **antigen processing**) and then making those peptides accessible for recognition by T cells **(antigen presentation).** These are early,

indispensible steps in nearly all acquired immune responses, and so are critical to the immune system's ability to detect and respond to antigenic challenges. In this chapter, we examine in detail the cellular and molecular basis of antigen processing and presentation, emphasizing the ways in which these processes influence whether and how lymphocytes react to a potential immunogen. Against this backdrop, we also explore the important role these processes play in determining resistance or susceptibility to disease and their unique importance in the context of organ transplantation.

ORIGINS OF ANTIGENIC PEPTIDES

To function as T-cell antigens, proteins must first be processed into peptides that can associate with host cell MHC molecules. Depending on the source of the antigen, processing can occur through either of two major pathways, and the pathway that is used has decisive consequences for any subsequent immune response (Table 6–1).

The Endocytic (Class II) Pathway

Many antigenic peptides are derived from proteins that have been captured and taken into a cell from its external environment. These include proteins that were part of a microorganism or other

Table 6–1. The antigen-processing pathways.

	Endocytic Pathway	Cytosolic Pathway
Major antigen sources	Endocytosed extracellular proteins (host and foreign) Membrane proteins (host and foreign)	Cytosolic proteins of host or intracellular pathogens (viral, bacterial, parasitic) Signal peptides (host and foreign)
Processing machinery	Lysosomal enzymes	Proteasomes (including LMPs)
Cell types where active	Professional APCs	All nucleated cells
Site of antigen–MHC binding	Endocytic vesicles, prelysosomes	Rough endoplasmic reticulum
MHC utilized	Class II	Class I
Presents to	CD4 (helper) T cells	CD8 (cytotoxic) T cells

Abbreviations: MHC = major histocompatability complex; APC = antigen-presenting cell; LMP = low-molecular-weight protein.

large particle engulfed through phagocytosis; smaller particles or individual proteins that were bound to the cell surface and then captured through receptor-mediated endocytosis; or free, soluble proteins in the extracellular fluid that were imbibed nonspecifically during pinocytosis (Figure 2–6). Proteins captured through any of these routes are taken into the cell in membranous endosomal vesicles, where they are then gradually broken down by exposure to an acidic pH and to cellular proteolytic enzymes. Although the bulk of each protein is ultimately destroyed, many short peptides are produced as intermediates in this process, their lengths and sequences varying in accordance with the sequence of the original protein, the cleavage specificities of the proteinases acting on it, its folded conformation and accessibility to cleavage, and many other factors. Through a mechanism that will be described later, some of these peptides are spared from further degradation and are instead transported back to the cell surface for presentation to T cells. This is sometimes termed the "exogenous" pathway of antigen processing because it acts mainly on proteins from outside the presenting cell.

Peptides generated by the endocytic pathway vary widely in sequence and in length. Importantly, this pathway delivers peptides to **MHC class II** molecules, which are expressed by macrophages and other "professional" antigen-presenting cells (APCs) that present antigens to CD4 T lymphocytes, most of which are helper cells. The endocytic pathway therefore supplies the antigenic peptides used by specialized APCs to activate helper T cells.

The Cytosolic (Class I) Pathway

Antigenic proteins can also be derived from pathogens that live inside infected host cells. This category includes not only viruses, which rely on the protein synthetic machinery of the host, but also some intracellular bacteria (such as *Chlamydia, Shigella, Rickettsia,* and *Listeria*) and intracellular parasites (eg, *Toxoplasma*), which synthesize their own proteins. Antigens from such intracellular pathogens are processed through a sequence of events involved in normal protein turnover. In this case, protein cleavage occurs in the cytosol within large, multisubunit enzyme assemblages called **proteasomes,** which ordinarily carry out the routine function of degrading host cytosolic proteins that have been damaged, improperly folded, or otherwise targeted for destruction or rapid turnover. Two distinct size classes of proteosomes (20S and 26S) have been described, and both are implicated in antigen processing. Each proteasome is made up of 15–20 different proteolytic subunits and has multiple substrate specificities. As a result, they can degrade a broad range of cytosolic proteins, including not only normal cellular constituents but also proteins from intracellular pathogens.

In the process of cleaving these substrates, the proteasomes liberate a myriad of short peptides into the cytosol. Selected peptides from this pool are then actively pumped into the lumen of the rough endoplasmic reticulum (RER) through channels created by a pair of proteins called the transporters of antigenic peptides: **TAP-1** and **TAP-2.** Each of the TAP subunits is an integral RER membrane protein that has seven transmembrane regions and an adenosine triphosphate (ATP)-hydrolyzing domain on its cytoplasmic surface; the TAPs therefore belong to the family of structurally related membrane channel proteins called ATP-binding cassette (ABC) transporters—a family that also includes P-glycoprotein (which pumps drugs and other small molecules out of cells, conferring drug resistance in some human cancers) and the cystic fibrosis transmembrane conductance regulator (an ion channel whose mutation causes cystic fibrosis). TAP-1 and TAP-2 together form a heterodimeric channel that selectively pumps a wide assortment of peptides of 8–12 residues (or occasionally longer) from the cytosol into the RER lumen in an ATP-dependent manner. As described later on, some of these peptides then associate with **MHC class I** proteins and are delivered to the cell surface for presentation to CD8 T lymphocytes. All components of this cytosolic pathway, including class I MHC proteins, are expressed by nearly every nucleated human cell type, ensuring that any cell that becomes infected can present antigens to cytotoxic T cells. This, in turn, leads to killing of the infected cell, which helps to limit spread of the pathogen it contained.

Though the endocytic and cytosolic degradative pathways are largely separate, some pathogens are processed through both. For example, the contents of endocytic vesicles are occasionally released into the cytosol (perhaps by lysis of the vesicle membrane) in a phenomenon called **macropinocytosis,** which transfers potential antigens from the endocytic to the cytosolic pathway. Conversely, virally encoded proteins that integrate into cellular membranes (eg, the surface glycoproteins of enveloped viruses) are targeted to endocytic vesicle membranes and consigned to the endocytic pathway, as are membrane proteins of the host cells. Interestingly, the signal peptides that target membrane proteins to the RER, and which are proteolytically removed during protein synthesis, often survive in the RER lumen and bind class I MHC proteins, whereas the remainder of the same polypeptide enters the endocytic pathway and is presented by class II MHC. Despite these exceptions, however, most immunogenic proteins primarily follow one pathway or the other. That is why, for example, live virus vaccines (which are processed through the cytosolic pathway) stimulate cytotoxic immune responses much more effectively than killed virus or subunit vaccines (which must be processed through the endocytic pathway).

STRUCTURE, FUNCTION, & GENETICS OF MHC PROTEINS

Before describing how antigenic peptides become bound to MHC proteins, we must first consider the proteins themselves. The human MHC proteins were first discovered in the 1950s, when it was recognized that many people, especially those who had received multiple blood transfusions or had been pregnant several times, had antibodies in their serum that reacted against a new class of surface glycoproteins on leukocytes from other members of the population. The membrane proteins recognized by these antibodies were termed **human leukocyte antigens (HLA)**— a term that is still used as a synonym for the human MHC proteins. It was soon realized that these same HLA molecules could also be targets of cellular immunity: When leukocytes from two unrelated individuals are incubated together, T cells from each nearly always react strongly (by activation and proliferation) against HLA proteins expressed by the other. Similarly, HLA proteins are usually the main targets of the cellular immune reactions that cause rejection of solid tissues transplanted between unrelated individuals. In these artificial settings, the HLA proteins behave as immunogenic markers that distinguish each person's cells from most others in the population and are the major barrier to **histocompatibility**—the ability of tissue transplants from one person to be accepted by another, rather than rejected immunologically. Despite their clinical importance, however, these properties of the MHC proteins are simply byproducts of their normal function of presenting antigenic peptides to T cells.

The Structures of Classical MHC Proteins & Their Peptide-Binding Sites

Most peptide antigens are presented as complexes with the **"classical"** MHC proteins: class I, which presents antigens to CD8 (usually cytotoxic) T cells, and class II, which presents to CD4 (usually helper) T cells. Class I and class II proteins are encoded by separate genes but are closely related in evolution and structurally similar in many respects. Each is expressed on the cell surface as a heterodimer composed of two noncovalently linked polypeptide chains (Figure 6–1). A class II molecule is formed by polypeptides called α and β, which are similar in size and are both anchored in the surface membrane at their carboxy termini. The extracellular regions of the class II α and β chains each fold to form a pair of globular domains, designated α_1 and α_2, or β_1 and β_2, respectively. Each class I molecule, by contrast, consists of a structurally distinct α chain associated with a second, shorter polypeptide called β_2**-microglobulin.** The class I α chain is organized in three folded domains (α_1, α_2, and α_3) and has a carboxy-terminal membrane anchor. The smaller β_2-microglobulin, with one folded domain, is linked to the membrane

only indirectly through its association with the α chain; this association is critical for stabilizing the class I molecule and for facilitating its transport to the cell surface.

Each MHC molecule can bind one antigenic peptide. Binding occurs at a site formed by the two domains that are situated farthest from the cell surface and, hence, are most accessible to other cells. The **peptide-binding site** in a class I protein is formed by the α_1 and α_2 domains; the corresponding site in a class II protein is formed by the α_1 and β_1 domains. In either case, sequences from the two adjacent domains combine to create an eight-stranded β-pleated sheet that serves as the floor of the binding site, above which are positioned two α helices, oriented adjacent and roughly parallel to each other, so that they form two walls with a groove between them (Figure 6–2).

Peptides bind inside the groove of an MHC protein in an extended conformation. The structure of the groove determines the types of peptides that can bind (Figure 6–3). For example, the groove in a class I molecule is constricted at both ends, and so can only accommodate peptides that are eight to ten amino acids long. The ends of the class II binding cleft are more open, which enables these proteins to bind the somewhat longer and irregular peptides (9–20 amino acids) generated by the endocytic processing pathway.

The specificity of binding in both class I and class II proteins is further determined by the amino acid residues that make up the β-sheet floor and α-helical walls of the peptide-binding groove: These create minute pockets with unique spatial and chemical features that can bind complementary features in a peptide, such as a particular amino acid sidechain at a particular position. The characteristics of these pockets, which reflect the sequence of the MHC protein, determine whether a given peptide can be bound. The constraints are fairly liberal, however, so that any single MHC protein can accommodate peptides with a wide variety of different sequences. The important point is that peptide binding by a given MHC protein is somewhat selective but much less specific than antigen binding by a TCR or an immunoglobulin protein. Because a single cell may express on the order of 10^6 class I proteins on its surface, each cell has the potential to present many alternative peptides simultaneously.

MHC Polymorphism

The MHC genes have evolved by successive duplications so that each person inherits multiple class I and class II genes (Figure 6–4). There are three separate genes, designated **HLA-A, -B,** and **-C,** that each code for classical MHC class I α chains. Similarly, there are three classical MHC class II gene loci, known as **HLA-DP, -DQ,** and **-DR,** each of which includes genes for one α and at least one β polypep-

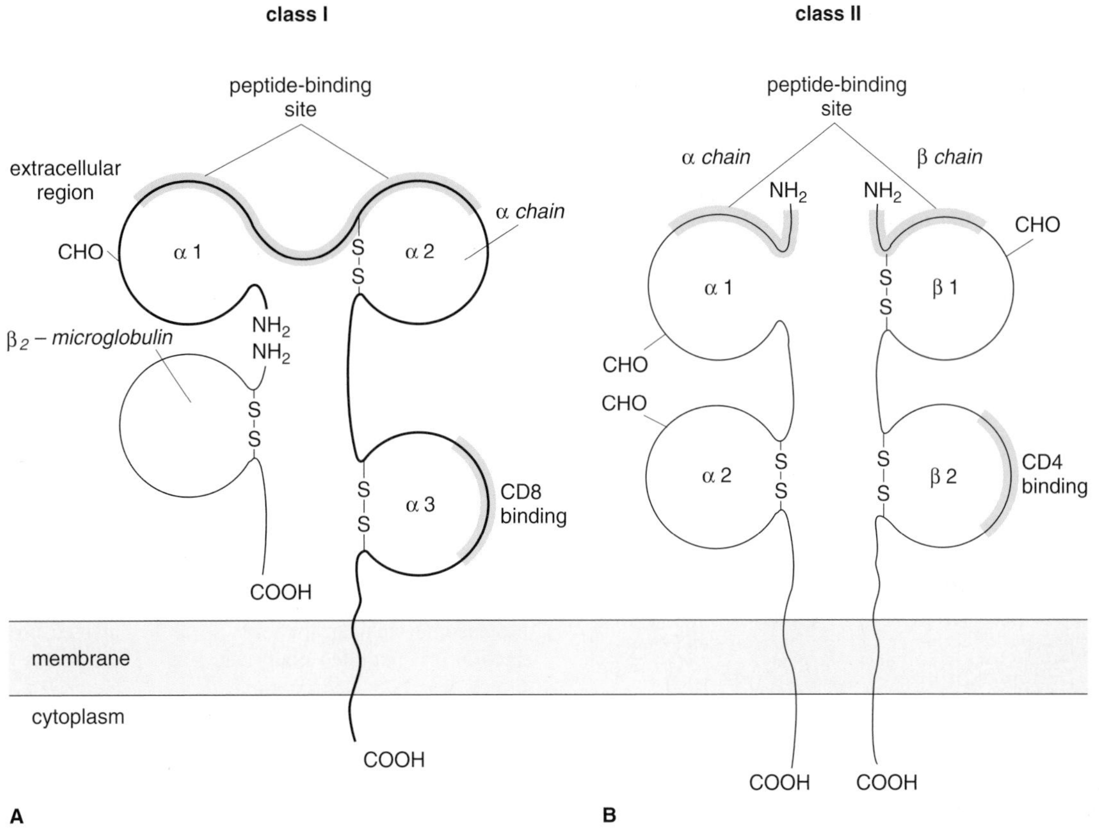

Figure 6–1. Schematic representations of MHC class I and class II proteins. **A:** The class I molecule consists of a MW 44,000 polymorphic transmembrane polypeptide (α chain) noncovalently associated with a MW 12,000 nonpolymorphic polypeptide (β$_2$-microglobulin) that is not anchored in the membrane. The three extracellular domains of the α chain are designated α$_1$, α$_2$, and α$_3$. The binding site for antigenic peptides is formed by the cleft between the α$_1$ and α$_2$ domains; CD8 contacts a portion of the α$_3$ domain. **B:** The class II molecule consists of a MW 34,000 α chain noncovalently associated with a MW 29,000 β chain, both of which are polymorphic. Antigenic peptides bind a cleft formed by the α$_1$ and β$_2$ domains; CD4 contacts sequences in the β$_2$ domain. Locations shown for the peptide-, CD4-, and CD8-binding sites are approximations only.

tide. A person normally inherits two copies of each gene locus (one from each parent), and so carries a total of six class I and six class II loci. Moreover, multiple different **alleles** of each locus exist in the human population—that is, there are many alternative versions of each MHC gene that yield proteins with slightly distinct sequences (Table 6–2). For example, there are at least 151 known HLA-A alleles, 301 HLA-B alleles, and 282 HLA-DR-β alleles. Diversity of this type is called allelic **polymorphism,** and the MHC genes are the most polymorphic genetic system known.

Almost all of the polymorphism among MHC alleles involves amino acid residues located in and around the peptide-binding groove. As a result, each allelic form has its own unique peptide-binding properties. Because many allelic forms are common in the population, a typical person is likely to inherit two

different alleles of many of the MHC loci. This is advantageous to the individual because it increases the range of different antigenic peptides that can be presented to T cells. MHC polymorphism also benefits humanity at large because it increases the likelihood that at least some individuals will be able to present antigens from any new pathogen that might be encountered, thus helping to ensure survival of the population as a whole.

The HLA Gene Complex

All of the classical MHC gene loci previously described reside together in the HLA gene complex (see Figure 6–4), which spans 3.6 million basepairs on the short arm of chromosome 6. The three class I α loci (HLA-A, -B, and -C) are together on one side of this region, and the three class II loci (HLA-DP, -DQ, and -DR, each with its α and β genes) occupy

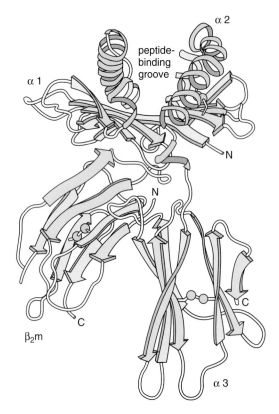

Figure 6–2. Diagrammatic structure of a class I MHC molecule (side view). In this ribbon diagram of the polypeptide backbone, the protein is oriented as in Figure 6–1, but only the extracellular region is depicted. The peptide-binding site is a groove (or cleft) formed by eight strands of β-pleated sheet and a pair of α helices from the α_1 and α_2 domains. The β sheet forms the floor and the two α helices form the walls of the cleft. Beta strands are depicted as broad arrows and α helices as narrow coils. (Modified and reproduced, with permission, from Bjorkman PJ et al: Structure of the human class I histocompatibility antigen HLA-A2. *Nature* 1987;329:506.)

the other. The particular combination of alleles found at these six loci on any single chromosome (and which are therefore inherited together) is called a **haplotype.**

MHC genes are expressed **codominantly,** which means, for example, that all six class I alleles (three on each copy of chromosome 6) are expressed together on the surface of every nucleated cell. HLA-C, however, is generally expressed at a lower level than HLA-A and HLA-B. All of these class I α chains pair with β_2-microglobulin, which is the product of a single, nonpolymorphic gene located on chromosome 15. The class II loci are also expressed codominantly but are only active in the subset of cells that express class II (as well as class I). HLA-DR tends to be expressed at higher levels than HLA-DP or HLA-DQ.

The α and β genes of each class II locus pair preferentially with each other, so that cross-locus pairings do not contribute significantly to HLA diversity.

Also encoded in the HLA complex are several other proteins that contribute to antigen processing or presentation. These include the genes for **TAP-1** and **TAP-2,** which transport peptides into the RER as part of the endogenous pathway and are encoded in the class II region. Although some allelic variability of the human TAP proteins has been observed (see Table 6–2), this is thought to have little effect on their peptide-transporting function; by contrast, TAP genes in rats are more polymorphic and strongly influence the repertoire of endogenous peptides that can be processed. The class II region also includes the gene for **tapasin** (also called TAP-binding protein, or TAPBP), a protein that mediates interaction between class I MHC molecules and the TAP transporter. Two other genes in the class II region encode low-molecular-weight proteins **(LMPs)** that also participate in the endogenous pathway. The LMPs are subunits of proteasomes and appear to modify proteasome cleavage patterns so as to enhance production of peptides that can bind MHC class I molecules.

The HLA locus also includes genes for certain **nonclassical MHC proteins,** which are structurally similar to class I or class II but have different roles in immunity. One of these, **HLA-G,** is encoded in the class I region and forms a dimer with β_2-microglobulin that acts to control immune responses at the fetal–maternal interface. Another nonclassical class I molecule encoded in the class I region is **HLA-E.** This molecule binds peptides derived from the signal sequences of the classical HLA-A, -B, and -C molecules, creating complexes that are recognized by receptors on natural killer (NK) cells (see Chapter 9). Recognition of these HLA-E complexes inhibits NK cells from attacking normal cells, so that they only kill cells that fail to express class I proteins—something that often occurs when cells become infected by viruses or undergo malignant transformation. (Some other nonclassical class I MHC proteins are encoded outside the MHC locus, such as the CD1 family of molecules, which will be discussed later.) Nonclassical class II MHC molecules are encoded in the class II region and include **HLA-DM** and **HLA-DO,** both of which are heterodimers that localize to endocytic vesicles. HLA-DM helps promote loading of peptides processed through the endocytic pathway onto MHC class II proteins, whereas HLA-DO modulates the function of HLA-DM, as described later on.

The HLA complex can thus be regarded as a cluster of tightly linked genes, many of which are evolutionarily related and contribute to antigen processing or presentation. Altogether, about 40% of the genes in the MHC locus encode proteins with an immunologic function; these include the genes for the cy-

class I

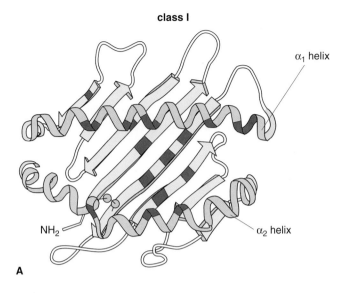

A

class II

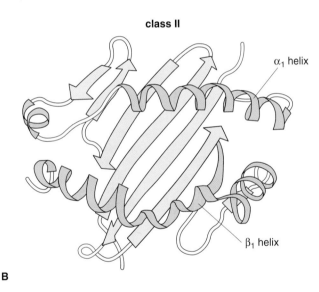

B

Figure 6–3. Peptide-binding sites of MHC class I and class II molecules. Each binding site has a floor composed of eight β strands and two α-helical walls. **A:** In the class I molecules, β sheets appear as broad arrows, α helices as narrow coils, and residues that are highly polymorphic among alleles are shown in black. The helices at either end of the class I binding site are closely apposed, so that peptides of only eight to nine residues can be bound. **B:** The class II groove, by comparison, has relatively open ends, which enable it to accommodate somewhat longer peptides. (Modified and reproduced, with permission, from Bjorkman PJ et al: Structure of the human class I histocompatibility antigen HLA-A2. *Nature* 1987;329:506, with additional data supplied by Peter Parham; and from Brown JH et al: Three-dimensional structure of the human class II histocompatibility antigen HLA-DR1. *Nature* 1993;364:33.)

tokines tumor necrosis factor α and β (see Chapter 10), and for complement factors C2, C4, B, and F (see Chapter 12). The MHC also contains many other genes that have no known role in immunology, such as those encoding two heat shock proteins or the steroidogenic enzyme 21-β-hydroxylase. The functional significance of the latter associations, if any, is unknown.

ASSEMBLY & PRESENTATION OF PEPTIDE-MHC COMPLEXES

Like other integral membrane proteins, class I and class II MHC proteins are synthesized in association with the RER. The individual chains translocate across the RER membrane as they are produced, so that when synthesis is complete the majority of each protein pro-

HLA Complex

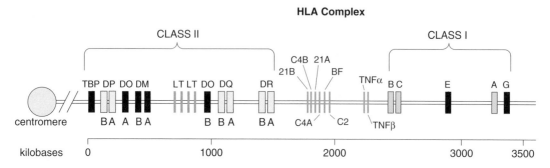

Figure 6–4. Organization of the HLA gene complex on the short arm of human chromosome 6. Regions encoding the class I and class II MHC proteins are indicated by braces. This map is simplified in that one to three tandem copies of genes encoding the subunits of each classical class II gene (HLA-DP, -DQ, and -DR) may be present on a single chromosome. Genes designated A, encode α chains and those designated B, encode β chains. A cluster of four genes within the class II region encodes TAP (T) and LMP (L) proteins, which are peptide-transport proteins and proteasome components, respectively, required for processing cytosolic antigens (see text). The TAPBP gene encodes the tapasin protein involved in TAP function. Of the several genes for nonclassical MHC molecules encoded in the HLA locus, only those for HLA-E (E), HLA-G (G), HLA-DM (DM), and HLA-DO (DO) are shown. The region between the class I and class II loci (sometimes called the class III locus) contains genes for tumor necrosis factors α and β (TNFα and TNFβ), steroid 21-β-hydroxylase (21A and 21B), and complement factors C2, C4, B, and F. Based on the complete sequence and gene map of the human MHC, reported by the MHC Sequencing Consortium, *Nature* 1999;401:921. Scale is approximate. *Abbreviations:* TAP = transporter of antigenic peptide; LMP = low-molecular-weight proteins; HLA = human leukocyte antigen; MHC = major histocompatibility complex.

Table 6–2. Number of alleles in the human MHC (HLA region).[a]

Locus	Known Alleles
Class I	
Classical	
HLA-A	151
HLA-B	301
HLA-C	83
Nonclassical	
HLA-G	14
Class II	
Classical	
HLA-DRA[b]	2
HLA-DRB	282
HLA-DQA	20
HLA-DQB	43
HLA-DPA	18
HLA-DPB	87
Accessory Molecules[c]	
HLA-DMA	4
HLA-DMB	6
HLA-DOA	8
HLA-DOB	3
TAP-1	6
TAP-2	4

Abbreviations: HLA = human leukocyte antigen; TAP = transporter of antigenic peptides; LMP = low-molecular-weight protein.
[a] These are the number of alleles officially assigned by the WHO Nomenclature Committee for Factors of the HLA System, as of October 1999. Provided by Steven G. E. Marsh.
[b] The class II genes designated A or B encode the α or β subunits, respectively.
[c] Allelic variation of the LMP genes in humans has not yet been fully characterized.

jects into the RER lumen, with its carboxy terminus remaining embedded in the membrane (see Figure 6–1). The class I and class II biosynthetic pathways then diverge immediately, as the subunits begin to assemble in the lumen of the RER (Figure 6–5).

MHC Class I. Each newly formed class I α chain associates with β_2-microglobulin and binds antigenic peptide during its assembly in the RER. The chaperone proteins calnexin and calreticulin help to mediate the initial folding and association of the α-chain/β_2-microglobulin heterodimer, which then physically associates with TAP transporter complexes in the membrane through interaction with the MHC-encoded chaperone, tapasin (TAPBP). The TAP proteins deliver cytosolically processed peptides to the peptide-binding site, inducing an additional conformational change that stabilizes the peptide-MHC complex. Although the TAP proteins preferentially import peptides 8–12 residues long, most peptides bound to class I proteins are only 8–9 residues long, suggesting that some exopeptidase trimming may occur within the RER. The peptide-MHC complex is then transported through the cytoplasm along the usual route of vesicular transport, passing sequentially through the Golgi apparatus and *trans*-Golgi network (where the single carbohydrate sidechain is attached to the α chain in the RER and modified to a complex carbohydrate) before emerging on the cell surface (see Figure 6–5). Class I proteins that fail to bind peptides are unstable and are degraded within the cell.

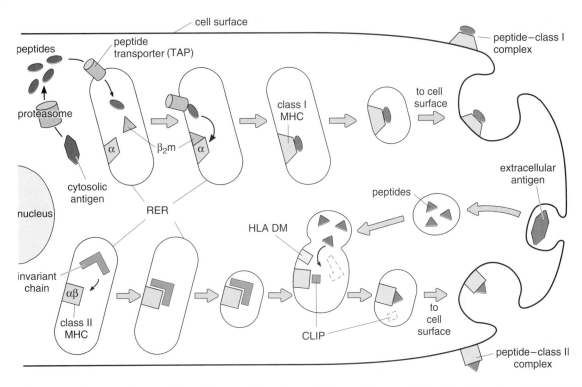

Figure 6–5. Pathways of assembly and transport for antigen–MHC complexes containing **(top)** class I and **(bottom)** class II HLA molecules. MHC polypeptides of both classes are initially expressed in the RER lumen. Peptides from cytosolic antigens processed by proteasomes are actively pumped into the RER by TAP transporters; they bind class I α chain and β_2-microglobulin in the RER lumen and are then transported to the cell surface. Class II proteins associate with the invariant chain in the RER and so are prevented from binding cytosolically processed peptides. Class II proteins are instead translocated to an endosomal compartment (either directly or by way of the cell surface), where the invariant chain is degraded to the CLIP peptide and then removed entirely to be replaced by peptides from the endocytic pathway. Peptide loading onto class II is assisted by the nonclassical MHC molecule HLA-DM. *Abbreviations:* RER = rough endoplasmic reticulum; TAP = transporter of antigenic peptides; HLA = human leukocyte antigen; MHC = major histocompatibility complex; CLIP = corticotropin-like intermediate lobe peptide.

MHC Class II. Class II α and β chains associate with each other soon after synthesis in the RER, where they, like class I proteins, are exposed to the pool of cytosolically processed peptides. The class II molecules, however, do not bind these peptides, because they associate instead with a third polypeptide, called the **invariant chain,** which blocks the class II peptide-binding site (see Figure 6–5). The invariant chain received its name because it has no polymorphic variants in the human population, though it is expressed in four different forms as a result of alternative splicing and alternative translational initiation sites. The major form of the invariant chain polypeptide spans the RER membrane and has an amino-terminal domain that projects into the cytoplasm; it assembles to form a trimer that can bind three class II α/β heterodimers simultaneously. In addition to blocking peptide binding, the bound invariant chain functions as a chaperone that promotes stable folding of the class II proteins. It also alters the intracellular

trafficking so that, after passing through the *trans*-Golgi network (where carbohydrate sidechains on the α, β, and invariant chains are modified) vesicles containing the class II protein complex are routed into the endocytic pathway. The signals that trigger this change in trafficking are provided mainly by the cytoplasmic portion of the invariant chain, though lumenal sequences may also play a role. It is unclear whether the class II-containing vesicles enter the endocytic pathway directly from the *trans*-Golgi network or instead are first delivered to the cell surface for endocytosis, or both. Whatever the route, this is a critical event because it directs the class II proteins toward an encounter with endocytosed peptides from the extracellular environment.

As vesicles bearing the class II/invariant chain complexes mature into **prelysosomes,** cellular proteinases (including cathepsins B, D, and S) in the vesicle lumen progressively cleave the invariant chain to produce a shorter, residual peptide called corticotropin-like intermediate lobe peptide **(CLIP).** The CLIP peptide is then catalytically removed by the **HLA-DM** molecule, which is exclusively localized to the class II-rich prelysosomal compartment. This process is modulated in APCs by interaction with another nonclassical class II molecule, **HLA-DO.** Removal of CLIP exposes the peptide-binding groove and allows endocytically processed peptides to bind the class II molecule. Peptide binding stabilizes the MHC proteins and allows the peptide/class II complex to be transported to the cell surface (see Figure 6–5).

Thus, class I and class II MHC molecules travel different routes within the cell and acquire antigenic peptides in different cellular compartments. The effect is to segregate these two groups of molecules, so that class I proteins selectively present peptides derived from proteins synthesized within the cell, whereas class II proteins present peptides from the extracellular environment. MHC proteins of both classes that fail to bind peptides are unstable and are rapidly degraded within the cell, ensuring that most MHC molecules are displayed on the cell surface as peptide–MHC complexes.

Control of the Antigen-Processing & Presentation Pathways

Though antigen processing and presentation occur constitutively, their efficiencies can be enhanced in times of need. For example, levels of expression of class I molecules, TAP transporters, and LMP subunits all increase in response to interferon-gamma (IFNγ), a cytokine produced by macrophages, helper T lymphocytes, and other cell types during immune responses. IFNγ also can induce the expression of class II molecules on a variety of cell types (including endothelial cells, fibroblasts, and epithelial cells) that normally do not express them, temporarily enabling these cells to present antigens to helper T cells. On the other hand, some infectious pathogens actively subvert these processes: for example, herpes simplex viruses have been found to produce proteins that bind and inactivate the TAP transporters, enabling these viruses to block the endogenous pathway in an infected cell and so evade detection by the immune system. Many other viruses (including adenoviruses and cytomegalovirus) encode proteins that achieve the same result by inhibiting expression of class I molecules on infected cells.

PEPTIDE-MHC RECOGNITION BY T CELLS

TCRs recognize peptide-MHC complexes by binding simultaneously to specific residues both in the peptide and in the highly polymorphic region of the MHC molecule in and around the peptide-binding groove. As a result, individual TCRs are capable of discriminating not only among peptides but also among different allelic forms of a given MHC protein.

A T cell's ability to distinguish among peptide-MHC complexes is further enhanced by the CD4 or CD8 proteins on its surface. These two coreceptor molecules each specifically recognize one of the nonpolymorphic, immunoglobulin-like domains found in MHC proteins: CD4 binds the β_2 domain in all MHC class II polypeptides, whereas CD8 binds the α_3 domain of MHC class I. Recognition by CD4 or CD8 increases the overall avidity of the interaction and delivers a strong activation signal to the T cell (see Chapter 9). As a consequence, CD8 T cells generally recognize peptides bound to class I MHC proteins and are said to be **class I-restricted,** whereas CD4 T cells recognize peptides complexed with MHC class II and are said to be **class II-restricted.** This is an important factor in determining the type of immune response induced by a particular antigen. Cytosolic (class I-associated) antigens are mainly recognized by CD8 cytotoxic T cells, which can kill the infected cells that present them. On the other hand, peptides from the endocytic pathway, associated with class II molecules, are mainly presented to CD4 helper T cells, and these, in turn, may help to initiate a B-cell antibody response against the extracellular antigen.

Positive & Negative T-Cell Selection

The antigen-processing machinery operates continually within all normal cells, even in the absence of infection. Malfolded or otherwise unstable cellular proteins from the cytosol are constantly being cleaved into peptides that are then processed through the cytosolic pathway. Consequently, every nucleated human cell normally presents a great many host-derived ("self") peptides as MHC class I complexes on its surface. Similarly, class II-bearing cells routinely endocytose and present self-peptides from proteins in the extracellular fluid and from their own surface membranes. When an infection occurs, peptides from the pathogen commingle with those from the host in the endogenous or exogenous pools (or both) and are presented along with them on the cell surface. Even during an intense infection, foreign peptides rarely account for more than a small fraction of all surface complexes. In short, the antigen presentation pathways do not distinguish between foreign and self-peptides.

If self-antigens are processed and presented at all times, why do they not trigger immune reactions? The answer lies mainly in an important, but incompletely understood, process of **negative selection** that operates on T cells as they develop in the thymus. Through negative selection, any T cells whose TCRs can bind to a self-peptide/MHC complex are either killed or functionally inactivated before they are released to the periphery. This thymic censorship functions to eliminate **autoreactive** (ie, self-reactive) T cells that might otherwise attack normal host tissues.

A different selective process in the thymus, called **positive selection,** acts to ensure that mature T cells recognize peptides in the context of MHC proteins. This process selectively favors the growth of T cells whose TCRs recognize epitopes that include at least some residues from the MHC molecule—particularly those that flank the peptide-binding groove. Because this region of the MHC is highly polymorphic in the population, one consequence of this selection is that any individual's T cells respond primarily to pathogen peptides bound to a specific MHC allele expressed by that individual, that is, to "self" MHC. This limited recognition that develops in an individual immune response against pathogen is known as **MHC restriction.** T cells that are not positively selected in this way fail to survive in the thymus.

The mechanisms of positive and negative selection during thymic T-cell development are considered in more detail in Chapter 9. For the present, it is enough to say that they are critical to the adaptive immune system's ability to discriminate self from nonself. Positive selection ensures that an individual's T cells respond primarily to peptides complexed with self-MHC proteins. Negative selection ensures that any T cells capable of recognizing MHC complexes that contain a self-peptide are eliminated or inactivated before they can attack host tissues.

Alloreactivity & Transplant Rejection

When cells or tissues are transplanted between individuals who express different alleles at one or more MHC loci, the recipient's T cells encounter the donor's MHC molecules, which carry different polymorphic residues and also present a very different set of self-peptides derived from the donor's proteins. Responding to highly diverse features in both the foreign MHC and the foreign peptides as mimicking foreign peptide plus self-MHC, a high proportion of the recipient's T cells (as much as 30%) are strongly activated. This so-called **alloreaction** (*allo-* means "other") is a major cause of transplant rejection. Avoiding it requires finding donors whose MHC alleles match those of the recipient as closely as possible, but the extensive polymorphism of these alleles makes matching difficult except between related individuals. Determining an individual's MHC alleles is called **HLA typing,** or histocompatibility typing. Ideally, if data from several family members are available to provide information about heredity, complete haplotypes can be determined. Although HLA typing has in the past relied on the use of antibodies to detect specific alleles, this has now been almost entirely supplanted by methods based on DNA sequence analysis of the HLA genes, which are far more accurate in determining allelic variation (see Chapter 19).

ANTIGEN-PRESENTING CELLS

Unless otherwise stated, the term *antigen-presenting cell* (APC) refers to cells that constitutively express class II MHC molecules and so can present antigens to helper T cells. (These are sometimes also called "professional" APCs.) Three major classes of cells function as APCs (dendritic cells, macrophages, and B cells), and each has unique properties that make it important for particular aspects of the immune response.

Dendritic Cells

Dendritic cells have numerous specialized features that make them extremely efficient at capturing and presenting antigens and at activating T cells. They are responsible for launching most acquired immune responses, and particularly for primary responses (ie, to pathogens that have not been encountered before). Dendritic cells arise from both the myeloid and lymphoid lineages of the bone marrow, but it is not yet clear whether this correlates with any functional differences, and they are currently regarded as a single cell type. They are found as a diffuse, minor resident population in all surface epithelia and most other solid tissues, and also as rare migratory cells in the blood and lymph. They have historically been given a variety of names depending on their locations in the body, including epidermal **Langerhans' cells,** the "veiled" cells of lymph, **blood dendritic cells** (which make up less than 0.1% of nucleated blood cells), and the **interdigitating cells** that are scattered throughout the T-cell zones of lymphoid organs. All have in common an unusual, spidery shape imparted by their many cytoplasmic projections—long, narrow dendrites, and sheet-like structures called veils—which can extend or retract and tend to insinuate between and encircle adjacent cells. (Follicular dendritic cells, discussed in Chapters 3 and 8, are not included in this group, though they have a similar morphology.) The cells themselves are also motile, and can migrate as rapidly as neutrophils into sites of viral or bacterial infection, attracted by particular chemokines or defensins.

Under normal conditions, tissue dendritic cells are said to be **immature** because, although they store large amounts of class II MHC protein in late-endosomal vesicles in the cytoplasm, they express very little class II protein on their surfaces and are unable to activate T cells. However, their large surface area and the numerous receptors they express—including receptors for bacterial lipopolysaccharide (LPS), microbial mannans, and the Fc portions of IgG and IgE—enable them to capture a broad array of potential pathogens and antigen–antibody complexes. These can then be taken into the cell through phagocytosis, receptor-mediated endocytosis, or macropinocytosis. Antigen uptake alone generally has no effect, however, unless the cell also receives signals that indicate infection or tissue distress. Such signals may be delivered directly to the dendritic cell if, for example, LPS or other bacterial macromolecules contact the Toll-like receptors on its surface. Alternatively, an infection or injury may stimulate other nearby cells to express CD40 ligand (CD40L) on their surfaces, to secrete certain defensins, or to release cytokines such as tumor necrosis factor α, interleukin-1, or granulocyte-macrophage colony-stimulating factor (GM-CSF), any of which may bind receptors on the immature dendritic cell and transmit signals to it through the NFκB pathway.

These signals trigger **maturation** of the dendritic cell into a highly effective APC. During the initial stage of maturation, processed peptides from any captured immunogen are loaded onto preformed class II MHC proteins in the cytoplasm and are rapidly transported to the cell surface. Through macropinocytosis, peptides from the same immunogens can also be diverted into the endocytic pathway, and so be presented in the context of class I MHC molecules. Antigen uptake and MHC protein synthesis cease within minutes, but by that time very large numbers of antigen–MHC complexes have accumulated on the cell surface (up to 100 times as many as are found on other types of APCs), and these can remain stable for several days. Laden with these antigen complexes, the maturing dendritic cell then crawls rapidly into nearby lymphatic vessels and is transported to the T-cell-rich zones of lymphoid tissues, guided by many of the same types of homing signals used by lymphocytes (see Chapter 3).

Once in the T-cell zone, the fully mature dendritic cell begins to secrete substances that attract and stimulate T cells specific for the antigen. Among these are the chemokines ELC and MDC, which preferentially attract naive and activated T cells, respectively, as well as IL-12, which potentiates T-cell activation and differentiation (see Chapters 10 and 11). Mature dendritic cells also strongly express the T-cell costimulatory molecules B7.1 and B7.2, along with cell adhesion molecules such as ICAM-1 and LFA-3. As a result, T cells migrate toward the dendritic cells and are enveloped in the folds of their cytoplasm, where they encounter high densities of antigen–MHC complexes and costimulatory proteins. For T cells with the appropriate antigen specificity, this creates a powerful environment for activation.

Their unique efficiency at capturing, transporting, and presenting antigen, and at attracting and activating specific T cells, make mature dendritic cells the most potent APCs known. Under some conditions, a single dendritic cell can activate up to 3000 T cells. They are prime targets of alloreactions during transplant rejection and also appear to be critical for establishing T-cell tolerance to self-antigens, both during intrathymic development (negative selection) and in the peripheral circulation, as will be described in

Chapter 9. Certain factors they secrete regulate other immune cells as well: for example, IL-12 potentiates NK-cell function, and the chemokine ELC is thought to attract antigen-specific B cells into the T-cell zones of lymphoid organs, where they receive help and become activated. Dendritic cells are also an important source of interferon α, a cytokine that activates innate antiviral mechanisms in other cells (see Chapter 10). For this reason, and because they respond to many stimuli (eg, LPS and defensins) that regulate innate defenses, dendritic cells have a key role in integrating innate and acquired immunity.

Macrophages

Most types of macrophages express class II MHC proteins, and their levels of class II, B7.1, and B7.2 protein expression increase when they become activated (see Chapter 2). Macrophages are widely distributed in lymphoid and nonlymphoid tissues and, because of their prodigious phagocytic capacity, are especially important for presenting antigens from particulate immunogens such as bacteria. Their many broad-specificity receptors enable macrophages to capture a wide range of pathogens, but their affinity for most ligands is low, so that most unopsonized immunogens must accumulate to relatively high local concentrations (micromolar, as opposed to nanomolar or picomolar for dendritic cells) to be presented efficiently by macrophages. They lack the ability to transport antigens to distant lymphoid organs, and so mainly function at sites of antigen deposition. Macrophages are highly efficient at capturing antibody-coated antigens using their surface Fc receptors, however, and so can play an important role in processing antigens during secondary immune responses.

B Lymphocytes

Although B cells lack significant phagocytic activity, they are able to capture, process, and present some antigens to helper T cells. They are especially effective in presenting the antigens that bind specifically to their surface immunoglobulins. B cells with appropriate specificity are usually very scarce the first time an antigen is encountered but become increasingly significant as APCs with each subsequent exposure. Antigen presentation by B cells and its importance for humoral immunity are considered in detail in Chapter 8.

Specialized Forms of Antigen Presentation

As noted earlier, cytokines (especially IFNγ) released at sites of ongoing immune reactions can induce class II MHC expression in epithelial and mesenchymal cells, enabling these cells to function temporarily as APCs. In addition, certain cells are able to present nonpeptide antigens to T cells by means of a small family of nonclassical class I MHC molecules called the **CD1** proteins. Cells that express the CD1 proteins include immature thymocytes, dendritic cells, and a variety of hematopoietic cells. The antigens presented by CD1 are generally **lipids** and **glycolipids,** including various forms of the mycobacterial cell wall lipid, mycolic acid. Four different CD1 proteins are present in humans, each comprising an α chain (encoded outside the MHC locus, on chromosome 1) associated with β_2-microglobulin; two of these are known to present nonpeptide antigens. The structure of the antigen-binding groove of the mouse CD1 molecule has been determined; it is narrower and deeper than the peptide-binding groove of a classical class I molecule and contains two highly hydrophobic cavities, consistent with its lipid-binding function. Although the CD1 molecule resembles a class I MHC protein, it behaves intracellularly like a class II protein in that it localizes primarily to the endocytic pathway in the cells in which it is expressed. Furthermore, the antigen that it presents is generated through the endocytic pathway, though its mechanism of loading into the CD1 molecule has yet to be characterized. Presentation of antigen by CD1 molecules stimulates a variety of defensive responses needed for elimination of intracellular bacteria and parasites, depending on the particular CD1 family member presenting the antigen.

MHC & DISEASE

The allelic forms of class I and class II MHC molecules that are expressed by any one individual dictate the repertoire of peptides that can be presented. Due to the relatively small number of proteins in a typical pathogen and the peptide-binding constraints imposed by a given set of MHC alleles, usually only a few epitopes from any one pathogen can be presented effectively to an individual's T cells. These few epitopes therefore dominate the cellular response to that pathogen and are called the dominant T-cell epitopes with respect to that individual (see Chapter 5). This genetically determined capacity to react immunologically against a particular immunogen is called **immune responsiveness.** Historically, the phenomenon was first observed in mice, where it became evident that inbred strains differed in their ability to mount an antibody response against particular synthetic peptide antigens; this was attributed to "immune response" genes, which were ultimately shown to be class II MHC alleles.

Because immune responses directed against some features of a pathogen are likely to be more effective than others at preventing or limiting infection, it might be expected that different individuals would show differences in their ability to resist infectious diseases and that these differences would be genetically correlated with the presence of particular MHC

alleles. This expectation has been confirmed repeatedly in animals but has been harder to demonstrate in humans, in part because the population is highly outbred, and in part because disease development is influenced by numerous other genetic and environmental factors in addition to the MHC. Nevertheless, a few recent studies in humans indicate a role for MHC alleles in susceptibility to infectious diseases. For example, in Gambia, where malaria is highly prevalent, it has been observed that three specific HLA alleles are statistically less common among children dying of this disease than in the Gambian population at large. Those alleles are, conversely, more frequent among children who develop a low-level, less virulent infection, suggesting that these alleles may confer the ability to mount a more effective immune response.

Studies on MHC-binding epitopes from human immunodeficiency virus (HIV) proteins have also revealed the importance of the interplay between host and pathogen in modulating immune responsiveness. The HLA-B8 allele is known to present a peptide derived from a region of the HIV Gag protein where mutations do not interfere with Gag function; therefore, the virus easily escapes a T-cell response directed against this epitope. The antigenic peptide presented by the HLA-B27 allele, however, is derived from a region of HIV Gag that is less tolerant of mutation; as a result, the cytotoxic T-cell responses generated by individuals expressing HLA-B27 have a more sustained antiviral effect in vitro. It has not yet been determined whether this particular difference in immune responsiveness is associated with a more effective antiviral immune response or a better clinical outcome overall. Nevertheless, such observations support a role for HLA alleles in natural disease resistance in humans and suggest their importance for designing effective vaccination strategies.

Another statistical link between MHC alleles and human disease has been observed in the case of **autoimmune disorders**—that is, disorders that are thought to involve an inappropriate immune attack against self-tissues (see Chapter 31). As indicated in Table 6–3, several autoimmune disorders have been found to occur significantly more frequently among persons who carry particular HLA alleles than among those who do not. For example, in the US white population, inheritance of the HLA-B27 allele is associated with an 80-fold increased risk of developing ankylosing spondylitis, a degenerative inflammatory disease of the spine whose cause is unknown. One possible interpretation of this finding is that the HLA-B27 allele confers susceptibility to an as-yet-unidentified infectious agent that is directly responsible for the disease. Another possibility is that HLA-B27 presents peptides derived from a normal component of vertebral tissue, which resemble peptides from such an agent and so become the target of

Table 6–3. Some MHC-associated disorders
in the US white population.

Disorder	HLA Allele	Relative Risk[a]
Ankylosing spondylitis	B27	87
Juvenile rheumatoid arthritis	DR4	4
Reiter's syndrome	B27	40
Insulin-dependent diabetes mellitus	DR3 and DR4	3
Acute anterior uveitis	B27	8
Sjögren's syndrome	DR3	6
Graves' disease	DR3	4
Systemic lupus erythematosus	DR2	3

Abbreviations: MHC = major histocompatibility complex; HLA = human leukocyte antigen.
[a] Chance that a person who is heterozygous for the indicated allele will develop the disease, expressed as a multiple of risk in the population that does not carry this allele.

an immunologic cross reaction in infected individuals. Still another hypothesis is that no external agent is required, but that HLA-B27 inappropriately presents self-antigens from vertebral tissues in such a way that it becomes the target of an immune attack, due to a failure of T-cell negative selection. Although investigations of these and other possible causes are continuing, it is important to emphasize that no HLA allele is associated with disease in 100% of cases. Hence, the effect of MHC proteins is likely to be only one among several genetic and environmental factors that determine susceptibility to autoimmune disease.

REFERENCES

Alfonso C et al: The role of H2-O and HLA-DO in major histocompatibility complex class II-restricted antigen processing and presentation. *Immunol Rev* 1999;172:255.

Banchereau J, Steinman RM: Dendritic cells and the control of immunity. *Nature* 1998;392:245.

Borrego F et al: Recognition of human histocompatibility leukocyte antigen (HLA)-E complexed with HLA class I signal sequence-derived peptides by CD94/NKG2 confers protection from natural killer cell-mediated lysis. *J Exp Med* 1998;187:813.

Brodsky FM et al: Human pathogen subversion of antigen presentation. *Immunol Rev* 1999;168:199.

Chapman HA: Endosomal proteolysis and MHC class II function. *Curr Opin Immunol* 1999;10:93.

Geraghty D et al: Complete sequence and gene map of a human major histocompatibility complex: The MHC sequencing consortium. *Nature* 1999;401:921.

Hill AVS: The immunogenetics of human infectious diseases. *Annu Rev Immunol* 1998;16:593.

Jones EY: MHC class I and class II structures. *Curr Opin Immunol* 1997;9:75.

Lopez de Castro JA: The pathogenetic role of HLA-B27 in chronic arthritis. *Curr Opin Immunol* 1998;10:59.

Mellman I et al: Antigen processing for amateurs and professionals. *Trends Cell Biol* 1998;8:231.

Pamer E, Cresswell P: Mechanisms of MHC class I-restricted antigen processing. *Annu Rev Immunol* 1998;16:323.

Pieters J: MHC class II restricted antigen presentation. *Curr Opin Immunol* 1997;9:89.

Ploegh HL: Viral strategies of immune evasion. *Science* 1998;280:248.

Porcelli SA, Modlin RL: The CD1 system: Antigen-presenting molecules for T cell recognition of lipids and glycolipids. *Annu Rev Immunol* 1999;17:297.

Rock KL, Goldberg AL: Degradation of cell proteins and the generation of MHC class I-presented peptides *Annu Rev Immunol* 1999;17:739.

Tang HL, Cyster JG: Chemokine up-regulation and activated T cell attraction by maturing dendritic cells. *Science* 1999;284:819.

Wilson IA, Bjorkman PJ: Unusual MHC-like molecules: CD1, Fc receptor, the hemochromatosis gene product, and viral homologs. *Curr Opin Immunol* 1998;10:67.

Immunoglobulins & Immunoglobulin Genes

7

Tristram G. Parslow, MD, PhD

Immunoglobulin proteins are the critical ingredients at every stage of a humoral acquired immune response. When expressed on the surfaces of resting B lymphocytes, they serve as receptors that can detect and distinguish among the vast array of potential antigens present in the environment. On binding their cognate antigens, surface immunoglobulins can initiate a cascade of molecular signaling events that may culminate in B-cell activation, clonal proliferation, and the generation of plasma cells. The immunoglobulins that are secreted as a result then function as **antibodies,** traveling through the tissue fluids to seek out and bind to the specific antigens that triggered their production.

The two hallmarks of immunoglobulins as antigen-binding proteins are the **specificity** of each for a particular epitope target and their **diversity** as a group. In addition to antigen binding, however, immunoglobulins also possess **secondary biologic activities** that are critical for host defense. These include, for example, the ability to function as opsonins, to activate the complement cascade, or to cross the placental barrier. Immunoglobulin proteins are heterogeneous with respect to these latter activities, which are determined by structural features independent of those that dictate antigen specificity. In this chapter, we first consider how the structures of immunoglobulins account for their specificity, diversity, and secondary biologic activities. We then examine the remarkable genetic mechanisms that give rise to these proteins.

IMMUNOGLOBULIN PROTEINS

Organization & Diversity of Immunoglobulin Proteins

The immunoglobulins are an enormous family of related, but nonidentical glycoproteins. It has been estimated that each person is capable of producing at least 10^8 different antibody molecules, each with its own distinct properties. Though carbohydrate may account for up to one fifth of an antibody's mass, almost all of its significant biologic attributes are deter-

mined by its polypeptide components. Antibodies are bifunctional molecules in that they bind specifically to antigens and also initiate a variety of secondary phenomena—such as complement activation, opsonization, or signal transduction—that are unrelated to their antigen-binding specificity. As we shall see, these two independent aspects of immunoglobulin function reside in separate regions of each protein.

The sheer diversity of immunoglobulins was for a long time a major barrier to understanding their structures. A serum specimen from any normal person contains a tremendous number of different antibody molecules, each of which is present in only minute amounts and (owing to its unique structure) has its own distinctive set of physical properties, such as molecular weight and isoelectric point. When a serum specimen is fractionated by electrophoresis, for example, most immunoglobulins are found to migrate as a broad band (called the **gamma-globulin** fraction) that reflects the presence of innumerable different proteins, each with slightly different electrophoretic properties. This extreme diversity made it virtually impossible to isolate sufficient amounts of any single antibody protein from a normal donor to permit a thorough biochemical analysis.

A series of key discoveries beginning in the 1950s finally opened up the field of immunoglobulin protein chemistry. The first was the finding that enzymes and reducing agents could be used to digest or dissociate immunoglobulins into smaller components. This revealed that diversity was largely confined to specific regions of the immunoglobulin molecules; other regions were much more uniform and could be isolated in pure form that made them accessible for structural analysis. A second breakthrough came with the realization that patients who had certain types of B-lymphoid cancers (eg, **multiple myeloma**) contained in their blood and urine large amounts of a single, homogeneous type of immunoglobulin protein secreted by a single malignant B-cell clone. Purification of such **myeloma proteins** made it possible to study individual antibodies and permitted (by 1969) the determination of the first complete amino acid sequence of an immunoglobulin. The development, in 1975, of laboratory methods for immortalizing individual clones of antibody-secreting cells gave birth to **monoclonal antibody** technology (see later section) and made it possible to obtain homogeneous antibodies of virtually any specificity in unlimited quantities. At about the same time, the isolation and analysis of immunoglobulin genes revolutionized the study of this protein family by making it relatively easy to isolate, modify, and even design immunoglobulin proteins of all types. Information gleaned from all these approaches forms the basis for our current, detailed understanding of immunoglobulin protein structure.

The Four-Chain Basic Unit. Every immunoglobulin molecule is made up of two different types of polypeptides. The larger, **heavy (H) chains** are roughly twice as large as the smaller, **light (L) chains.** Every immunoglobulin contains equal numbers of heavy- and light-chain polypeptides and can be represented by the general formula $(H_2L_2)n$. The chains are held together by noncovalent forces and also by covalent interchain disulfide bridges to form a bilaterally symmetrical structure as depicted in Figure 7–1. All

normal immunoglobulins conform to this basic structure, although some, as we shall see, are composed of more than one of these four-chain units.

The heavy and light polypeptide chains are both composed of folded globular **domains,** each of which is 100–110 amino acids long and contains a single intrachain disulfide bond (see Figure 7–1). Although the amino acid sequences of the individual domains vary, they fold into very similar three-dimensional conformations (a roughly cylindrical assembly of β strands known as the **immunoglobulin barrel**), owing in part to the fairly constant location of the intrachain disulfide. Light chains always contain two of these domains, whereas heavy chains contain either four or five.

All of the light chains and all of the heavy chains in any single immunoglobulin protein are identical. When compared among different immunoglobulins, however, the sequences of these chains vary widely. In both heavy and light chains, this variability is most pronounced in the N-terminal domain, whereas the sequences of the other domains remain relatively constant. For this reason, the N-terminal domain in a

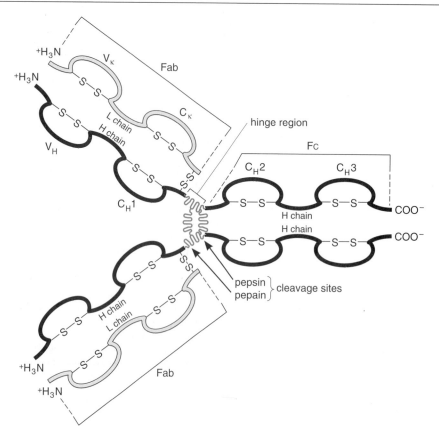

Figure 7–1. Schematic model of an IgG1 (κ) human antibody molecule showing the basic four-chain structure and domains (V_H, C_H1, etc). Sites of enzymatic cleavage by pepsin and papain are shown.

heavy- or light-chain polypeptide is called the **variable region,** abbreviated V_H or V_L, respectively. The other domains are collectively termed the **constant region,** abbreviated C_H or C_L. Light-chain polypeptides contain only a single C_L domain, but heavy chain C_H regions comprise three or more domains that are numbered sequentially (C_H1, C_H2, etc) beginning with the domain closest to V_H.

Within an immunoglobulin unit, the heavy and light chains are aligned in parallel as shown in Figure 7–1. Each V_H domain is always positioned directly beside a V_L domain, and this pair of domains together forms a single **antigen-binding site.** Each basic four-chain unit thus contains two separate but identical antigen-binding sites and so is said to be **divalent** with respect to antigen binding. The antigen specificity of a given protein is determined by the combined sequences of its V_H and V_L domains and for this reason varies widely among immunoglobulins. Each C_H1 domain interacts closely with the C_L domain, and in most types of immunoglobulins the two are linked covalently by one or more disulfide bridges. Each of the remaining C_H domains is aligned with its counterpart on the opposite heavy chain and may be linked to it by disulfide bonds. Overall, the protein has a T- or Y-shaped configuration when viewed schematically. The region at the base of each arm in the T or Y, located between the C_H1 and C_H2 domains, is called the **hinge region;** in most immunoglobulins, it has a loose secondary structure that makes it flexible, enabling the two arms to move relatively freely with respect to each other.

Enzymatic Digestion Products of Immunoglobulins. Immunoglobulins are rather resistant to proteolytic digestion but are most susceptible to cleavage near the hinge region (see Figure 7–1), which usually lies adjacent to the site of interchain disulfides linking the two heavy chains together. The enzyme **papain** happens to cleave this region on the N-terminal side of the inter-heavy-chain disulfides, and so splits an immunoglobulin into three fragments of roughly similar size. Two of these are identical to each other, consisting of an entire light chain along with the V_H and C_H1 domains of one heavy chain; these fragments thus contain the antigen-binding sites of the protein, and so are called **Fab fragments** (ie, antigen-binding fragments). Each Fab fragment is **monovalent** with respect to antigen-binding activity. The third fragment comprises the carboxy-terminal portions of both heavy chains held together by disulfides. The structure of this third fragment is identical for many different immunoglobulin molecules, so that fragments of this type can often be crystallized even if they are derived from a heterogeneous antibody population. Hence, this third fragment is designated the crystallizable, or **Fc, fragment.** Most of the secondary biologic properties of immunoglobulins (eg, the ability to activate complement) are determined by sequences in the Fc region of the protein.

This is also the region that is recognized by the **Fc receptors** found on many types of cells.

A somewhat different pattern of cleavage occurs with the enzyme pepsin, which cleaves on the carboxy-terminal side of the inter-heavy-chain disulfides. This yields a single large fragment called an **F(ab)′2** fragment, which roughly corresponds to two disulfide-linked Fab fragments and has divalent antigen-binding activity. The Fc region, on the other hand, is extensively degraded by pepsin, and usually does not survive as an intact fragment.

Characterization of these proteolytic fragments in the 1960s was an important step toward understanding antibody structure because it provided the first evidence that the antigen-binding and secondary functions of antibodies reside in separate regions of the protein. Such fragments are still used today when it is necessary to dissociate different aspects of antibody function for diagnostic or research purposes.

Classification of Immunoglobulins & Their Constituent Chains

Immunoglobulins are composed of heavy and light chains. The N-terminal domain (V region) in both types of chains is highly variable and mediates antigen binding. The remaining portion (C region) of each chain, by comparison, is far less variable. Nevertheless, every normal person produces several alternative forms of heavy and light chains that each have distinctly different C-region amino acid sequences (Table 7–1). These alternative forms of the immunoglobulin chains can be distinguished from one another by their physical properties (eg, molecular weight) or serologically by using antibodies (usually obtained from animals that have been immunized with human Fc fragments) that recognize specific features in the various human C regions. Although these normal variations in sequence of the C_L region have no effect on immunoglobulin function, those in the C_H region significantly affect the secondary biologic properties of immunoglobulins.

Light-Chain Types and Subtypes. All light chains have protein molecular weights of approximately 23,000 but can be classified into two distinct **types,** called **kappa (κ)** and **lambda (λ),** on the basis of their C_L-region sequences. No known functional differences exist between these two types, and each can associate with any of the various classes of heavy chains. Nevertheless, expression of two distinct light-chain types is common among mammals. Indeed, the amino acid sequence similarities between human and mouse kappa chains are much greater than those between the kappa and lambda chains within each species—indicating that the primordial kappa and lambda genes separated from one another during evolution prior to the divergence of these mammalian species.

The C regions of all κ light chains produced by an individual are essentially identical. In contrast, a single person may express as many as six slightly differ-

Table 7–1. Properties of human immunoglobulin chains and related polypeptides.

Chain	H Chains					L Chains		Secretory Component	J Chain
	γ	α	μ	δ	ε	κ	λ	SC	J
Classes in which chain occurs	IgG	IgA	IgM	IgD	IgE	All classes	All classes	IgA	IgA, IgM
Subclasses or subtypes	1,2,3,4	1,2	—	—	—	—	1,2,3,4,5,6	—	—
Molecular weight (approximate)	50,000[a]	55,000	70,000	62,000	70,000	23,000	23,000	70,000	15,000
V region subgroups	V_{HI}–V_{HIV}					$V_{\kappa I}$–$V_{\kappa IV}$	$V_{\lambda I}$–$V_{\lambda IV}$		
Carbohydrate (average percentage)	4	10	15	18	18	0	0	16	8
Number of oligosaccharides (average)	1	2 or 3	5	?	5	0	0	?	1

[a] 60,000 for γ3.

ent forms of the λ C region. These various **subtypes** of λ differ from one another only slightly in C-region amino acid sequences and are functionally identical, though each is encoded by a separate chromosomal locus.

A given immunoglobulin molecule always contains exclusively κ or one of the λ chains, never a mixture. Similarly, any given B-lineage cell produces only one type of light chain. When the entire population of serum immunoglobulins (or of B-lineage cells) in an individual is considered, the proportion of kappa to lambda chains produced varies from species to species; in humans, the ratio is about 2:1.

Heavy-Chain Classes and Subclasses. Humans express five different classes (or isotypes) of immunoglobulin heavy chains, which differ considerably in their C_H-region sequences and in their physical and biologic properties. All of the heavy chains in any given immunoglobulin are identical. The five classes of heavy chains are designated μ, δ, γ, α, and ε, and immunoglobulins that contain these heavy chains are designated the IgM, IgD, IgG, IgA, and IgE classes, respectively. The γ and α classes are further divided into subclasses (γ1, γ2, γ3, γ4, α1, and α2) based on relatively minor differences in C_H sequence and function; the corresponding immunoglobulin subclasses are denoted IgG1, IgG2, and so on. Heavy chains representing the various subclasses within a class are much more similar to one another than to the other classes. Normal individuals express all nine classes and subclasses, because each is encoded by a separate genetic locus and is inherited independently.

The heavy-chain polypeptides range in molecular weight from about 50,000 to 70,000. The μ and ε chains are made up of five globular domains apiece (one V_H and four C_H), whereas γ, α, and δ chains each contain only four (one V_H and three C_H). The δ chain has an intermediate molecular weight attributable to an enlarged hinge region. The γ3 chain also

has a large hinge that consists of about 60 amino acid residues; of these, 14 are cysteines, which accounts for the large number of inter-heavy-chain disulfide bonds in IgG3 (see the section on IgG). In some mammalian species, the charge characteristics of the various IgG subclasses differ sufficiently to permit their separation by electrophoretic techniques, but this is not true of humans.

Composition of Immunoglobulin Classes and Subclasses. The class of the H chain determines the class of the immunoglobulin. Thus, there are five classes of immunoglobulins: IgG, IgA, IgM, IgD, and IgE. A given molecule in any of these classes may contain either κ or λ light chains. For example, two γ chains (of any of the four subclasses), combined with either two κ or two λ L chains, constitute an IgG molecule—the most abundant class of immunoglobulins in sera from adults. Similarly, two μ chains together with two L chains form an IgM monomer unit of the type found on the surfaces of many B cells. The secreted form of IgM, however, is a pentameric macroglobulin, which consists of five of these basic four-chain units along with an additional polypeptide called J chain (Figure 7–2). Each IgM pentamer contains ten identical antigen-binding sites and so has polyvalent binding activity. IgA accounts for only about 10–15% of serum immunoglobulin but is the predominant class of antibody found in body secretions. The membrane-bound or circulating form of IgA is a single four-chain unit, but the secreted form can polymerize to form assemblages comprising two to five of these basic units along with J chain and (in secreted IgA) yet another polypeptide called secretory component (see Figure 7–2). The properties of the individual chains are summarized in Table 7–1, and those of the immunoglobulin classes are compared in Table 7–2.

One noteworthy structural difference among the immunoglobulin classes or subclasses lies in the number and arrangement of interchain disulfide

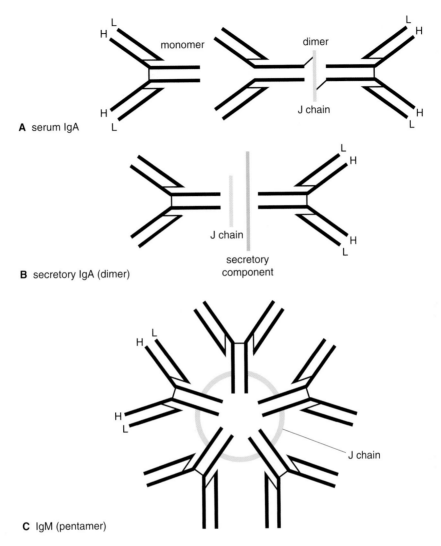

Figure 7–2. Highly schematic illustration of polymeric human immunoglobulins. Polypeptide chains are represented by thick lines; disulfide bonds linking different polypeptide chains are represented by thin lines.

bridges within each four-chain unit (Figure 7–3). In IgA2, for example, the L chains are covalently linked to each other rather than to the H chains, so that L–H binding is entirely due to noncovalent forces. In other subclasses, the L–H bond may be situated either close to the junction of the V_H and C_H1 domains (as in IgG2 or IgA1) or, alternatively, near the junction between C_H1 and C_H2 (as in IgG1).

Membrane and Secreted Immunoglobulins. Immunoglobulins of all classes can exist in either membrane-bound or secreted forms. The membrane forms always exist as individual four-chain units and have on their heavy chains an additional carboxy-terminal sequence of approximately 40 amino acid residues. This sequence consists of a highly acidic region of 12–14 residues, followed by a strikingly hy-drophobic sequence of about 26 residues. The hy-drophobic portion is the transmembrane component, which anchors the heavy chain (and, hence, the entire four-chain unit) into the cell membrane. It is similar in hydrophobicity and length to known transmem-brane segments of other proteins and probably forms a single membrane-spanning α helix. The acidic por-tion of the membrane segment shows little amino acid sequence conservation among heavy-chain classes, but the hydrophobic sequences tend to be quite similar. This reflects the requirement that mem-brane-bound heavy chains of all classes must associ-ate with the same pair of integral membrane proteins, called Ig-α and Ig-β, in order to transduce signals into the cell (see Chapter 8). The direct anchoring of immunoglobulins into surface membranes occurs

Table 7–2. Properties of human immunoglobulins.

	IgG	IgA	IgM	IgD	IgE
H-chain class	γ	α	μ	δ	ϵ
H-chain subclasses	$\gamma1, \gamma2, \gamma3, \gamma4$	$\alpha1, \alpha2$			
L-chain type	κ and λ	κ and λ	κ and λ	κ and λ	κ and λ
Molecular formula	γ_2L_2	$\alpha_2L_2{}^a$ or $(\alpha_2L_2)_2SC^bJ^c$	$(\alpha_2L_2)_5J^c$	δ_2L_2	ϵ_2L_2
Sedimentation coefficient (S)	6–7	7	19	7–8	8
Molecular weight (approximate)	150,000	160,000[a] or 400,000[d]	900,000	180,000	190,000
Electrophoretic mobility (average)	γ	Fast γ to β	Fast γ to β	Fast γ	Fast γ
Complement fixation (classic)	+	0	++++	0	0
Serum concentration (approximate; mg/dL)	1000	200	120	3	0.05
Serum half-life (days)	23	6	5	3	2
Placental transfer	+	0	0	0	0
Mast cell or basophil degranulation	?	0	0	0	++++
Bacterial lysis	+	+	+++	?	?
Antiviral activity	+	+++	+	?	?

[a] For monomeric serum IgA.
[b] Secretory component.
[c] J chain.
[d] For secretory IgA.

only in B-lineage cells and should not be confused with the indirect association that results when soluble antibodies bind to Fc receptors found on many cell types.

Secreted immunoglobulins lack the terminal transmembrane segment as a result of alternative RNA splicing (see later discussion). In its place, the secreted forms of μ and α (but not of the other classes) contain a short terminal sequence, called the **tail segment,** that mediates polymerization of four-chain units and also serves as contact site for the J chain.

Allotypic (Allelic) Forms of Heavy and Light Chains. The heavy-chain classes and subclasses and the light-chain types and subtypes are each encoded by separate genetic loci, so that all are normally present in a single haploid genome. Some of these individual loci, however, exist in more than one form within the population; the alternative forms (alleles) generally differ from one another by only one or, at most, a few amino acid substitutions. Such minor alternative forms at a given immunoglobulin locus are called allotypes. In humans, allotypes have been found for γ, α, and ϵ H chains and for κ L chains. Thus far, allotypic forms of λ L chains or of μ and δ H chains have not been observed.

Allotypic variation has no effect on immunoglobulin function and is primarily of interest because the variant C-region sequences can be immunogenic in some circumstances. For example, mothers may become immunized during the course of pregnancy against paternal allotypic determinants expressed on fetal immunoglobulins. Alternatively, immunization may result from blood transfusions. In addition, patients with rheumatoid arthritis can develop **rheumatoid factors**—antibodies that are directed against normal IgG—which occasionally recognize allotypic determinants.

J Chain and Secretory Component. As noted earlier, the secreted forms of IgM and IgA generally exist as polymers of the basic four-chain unit that include a single additional polypeptide called the J chain. The J chain is a small (MW 15,000) acidic protein that is structurally unrelated to heavy and light chains but is synthesized by all plasma cells that secrete polymeric immunoglobulins. In these polymeric assemblies, the J chain is disulfide-bonded to the penultimate cysteine residue in the tail segment of the α or μ chains. Its function seems to be to facilitate proper polymerization.

Secretory component is a single glycopeptide with a peptide molecular weight of approximately 70,000 and a high carbohydrate content. It is associated only with IgA and is found almost exclusively in body secretions. Its amino acid sequence is invariant and shows no resemblance to the J chain or to any of the immunoglobulin polypeptides. Secretory component can exist either in free form or bound to dimeric or polymeric (but not monomeric) IgA molecules; the latter interaction is usually noncovalent, but disulfide bonds have been implicated in a small proportion of human IgA. Free secretory component can even be observed in secretions from individuals who lack measurable IgA in their serum or secretions.

Secretory component is not synthesized by lym-

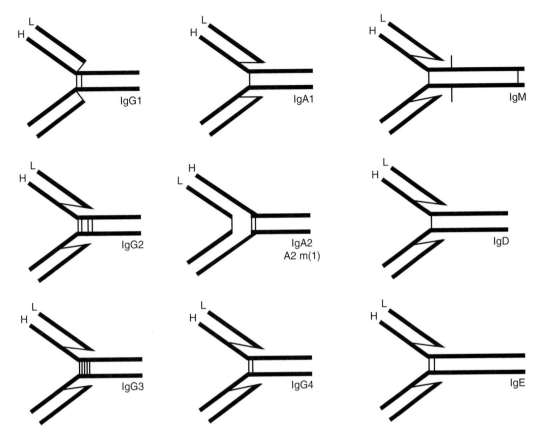

Figure 7–3. Distribution of interchain disulfide bonds in various human immunoglobulin classes and subclasses. H chains are represented by long thick lines and L chains by short thick lines. Disulfide bonds are represented by thin lines. The number of inter-heavy-chain disulfide bonds in IgG3 may be as large as 14.

phocytes but rather by mucosal epithelial cells that overlie Peyer's patches and other submucosal lymphoid tissues (see Chapter 14). Such epithelial cells take up IgA that is secreted from the lymphoid cells beneath them, link it with secretory component, and transport the resulting complex across the epithelial barrier into secretions. Linkage with secretory component is presumed to facilitate the transepithelial passage of IgA.

Biologic Activities of Immunoglobulins

As previously noted, immunoglobulins are bifunctional molecules that bind antigens and, in addition, initiate other biologic processes that are independent of antibody specificity. These two kinds of activities are each localized to a particular part of the protein: antigen binding to the combined V_H and V_L domains, and the other activities to the C_H domains (particularly those of the Fc segment). The latter activities, some of which are summarized in Table 7–2, are considered in this section.

Immunoglobulin G. Immunoglobulin G (IgG) ac-

counts for approximately 75% of the total serum immunoglobulin in normal adults and is the most abundant antibody produced during secondary humoral immune responses in the blood. Within the IgG class, the relative concentrations of the four subclasses are approximately as follows: IgG1, 60–70%; IgG2, 14–20%; IgG3, 4–8%; and IgG4, 2–6% (Table 7–3). These values vary somewhat among individuals; it appears that the propensity to produce IgG antibodies of one subclass or another is at least partly an inherited trait.

Table 7–3. Properties of human IgG subclasses.

	IgG1	IgG2	IgG3	IgG4
Abundance (% of total IgG)	70	20	6	4
Half-life in serum (days)	23	23	7	23
Placental passage	+++	+	+++	+++
Complement fixation	+	+	+++	—
Binding to Fc receptors	+++	−	+++	+

Semiquantitative values are indicated for some properties, ranging from − = none, to +++ = highest.

IgG is the only class of immunoglobulin that can cross the placenta in humans, and it is responsible for protection of the newborn during the first months of life (see Chapter 41). The subclasses are not equivalent in this respect, IgG2 being transferred less efficiently than the others, but the biologic significance of this inequality, if any, is unknown.

Antigen-bound IgG is also capable of fixing (ie, binding and activating) serum complement, and once again the subclasses do so with unequal efficiency (IgG3 > IgG1 > IgG2). IgG4 is completely unable to fix complement by the classical pathway, which requires binding of a protein called C1q, but it may be active in the alternative pathway (see Chapter 12). The C1q binding site on the other IgG proteins appears to reside in the C_H2 domain.

Macrophages and certain other cell types express surface receptors that bind the Fc regions of IgG molecules. These interact principally with C_H2 domains and bind IgG1 and IgG3 with much higher affinity than the other subclasses. The properties of these receptors are considered in a later section.

Immunoglobulin A. Immunoglobulin A (IgA) is the predominant immunoglobulin produced by B cells in Peyer's patches, tonsils, and other submucosal lymphoid tissues. Thus, although it accounts for only 10–15% of serum immunoglobulin, it is by far the most abundant antibody class found in saliva, tears, intestinal mucus, bronchial secretions, milk, prostatic fluid, and other secretions. On B-cell surfaces or in the blood, IgA exists as a monomer (MW 160,000) comprising only one four-chain unit. In secretions, it multimerizes to form disulfide-linked polymers of up to five such units that are associated with one molecule each of J chain and (in secretions) secretory component. The predominant secreted forms of IgA are dimers and trimers (see Figure 7–2). The two subclasses, IgA1 and IgA2, are expressed at a 5:1 ratio in the blood and have similar properties. High-affinity Fc receptors specific for IgA have been identified.

Immunoglobulin M. Immunoglobulin M (IgM) constitutes approximately 10% of normal serum immunoglobulins and is normally secreted as a J-chain-containing pentamer with a molecular mass of approximately 900 kilodaltons. IgM antibody predominates in early primary immune responses to most antigens, although it tends to become less abundant subsequently. IgM (often accompanied by IgD) is the most common immunoglobulin expressed on the surfaces of B cells, particularly naive B lymphocytes. IgM is also the most efficient complement-fixing immunoglobulin: A single molecule of antigen-bound IgM suffices to initiate the complement cascade. Fc receptors specific for IgM have been characterized.

Immunoglobulin D. The immunoglobulin D (IgD) molecule is a monomeric four-chain unit with a molecular mass of approximately 180 kilodaltons. Although IgD is commonly found on the surfaces of B lymphocytes that also bear surface IgM, it is rarely secreted in significant amounts, and only traces of it are normally found in the blood. In cells that coexpress IgD and IgM, both classes of heavy chains are produced by alternative splicing of a single RNA (see later discussion) and have identical antigen specificity. The IgD on these cells can bind antigen and transmit signals to the cell interior, with consequences that appear identical to those produced by IgM. When such B cells become activated, surface IgD expression ceases.

The physiologic function of IgD is unknown. It is relatively labile to degradation by heat or proteolytic enzymes. There are isolated reports of IgD with antibody activity toward insulin, penicillin, milk proteins, diphtheria toxoid, nuclear components, or thyroid antigens. Its presence on many mature naive lymphocytes has suggested an as-yet-unproven role in B-cell differentiation or tolerance.

Immunoglobulin E. Although it normally represents only a minute fraction (0.004%) of all serum antibodies, immunoglobulin E (IgE) is extremely important from the clinical standpoint because of its central involvement in allergic disorders. Two specialized types of inflammatory cells involved in allergic responses—the mast cell and the basophil—carry a unique, high-affinity Fc receptor that is specific for IgE antibodies. Thus, despite the very low concentration of IgE (roughly 10^{-7} M) in blood and tissue fluids, the surfaces of these cells are constantly decorated with IgE antibodies, adsorbed from the blood, that serve as antigen receptors. When its passively bound IgE molecules contact an antigen, the mast cell or basophil releases inflammatory mediator substances that produce many of the acute manifestations of allergic disease (see Chapters 13 and 27). Elevated levels of serum IgE may also signify infection by helminths or certain other types of multicellular parasites (Chapter 48). Like IgG and IgD, IgE exists only in monomeric form. Fc receptors appear to recognize primarily the C_H3 domain of the ε chain.

Immunoglobulin Variable Regions

The V regions, which coincide with the N-terminal domains of light and heavy chains, mediate antigen binding and are by far the most heterogeneous portions of these proteins. Indeed, no two human myeloma proteins from different patients have ever been found to have identical V-region sequences. Some clear patterns can be discerned, however. V_H regions show significantly more resemblance to one another than to V_L regions, whereas V_κ and V_λ sequences each have characteristic features that distinguish them from each other and from V_H. Thus, V_H, V_κ, and V_λ sequences can be recognized as separate groups that each associate with their own characteristic constant regions. There is never any mixing: a given V_H sequence, for example, may be found on heavy chains of any class (μ, δ, γ, α, or ε), but is never found on a light chain.

Framework and Hypervariable Regions. Variable regions within any single group are not uniformly variable across their entire 110-amino-acid spans. Instead, they consist of relatively invariant stretches (called framework regions) of 15–30 amino acids, separated by shorter regions of extreme variability (called hypervariable regions) that are each 9–12 amino acids long. V_H and V_L regions each contain three hypervariable regions, whose approximate locations are depicted in Figure 7–4. Antigen binding is mediated by noncovalent interactions that primarily involve amino acids in the hypervariable regions of each chain; hence, the sequences of these regions are the primary determinants of antigen specificity. Hypervariable regions are also called complementarity-determining regions (CDRs), and within each chain are designated CDR1, CDR2, and CDR3, beginning with the one nearest the amino terminus. CDR3 is usually the longest and most variable of the three, as specialized genetic mechanisms act to increase sequence diversity in this region (see later section).

V-Region Subgroups. When sequences of many variable regions from any one type of chain (V_H, $V_κ$, or $V_λ$) are compared, they are found to form subgroups that are more similar to one another than to the remaining V regions in the group. For example, human $V_κ$ regions have been classified into four subgroups, and similar subgroups exist for the V_H and $V_λ$ regions. The subgroups differ from one another principally in the length and position of amino acid insertions and deletions within their framework regions.

Idiotypes. The term *idiotype* refers to the unique V-region amino acid sequences of the homogeneous immunoglobulin molecules produced by a single B-cell clone. Thus, there are as many idiotypes as there are B-cell clones (perhaps about 10^8 in an adult).

The concept of idiotype (which means "self-type") was first derived from experiments in which inbred animals were inoculated with purified antibody proteins that had been raised against a particular antigen in genetically identical animals. The inoculated animals mounted an antibody response against the injected immunoglobulin, implying that some sequences within it were recognized as foreign, but these antibodies would not react with other immunoglobulins from the same strain of animal. The antiserum produced in such a response was called an **antiidiotype** antiserum. It was soon observed that the reaction between an antihapten antibody and its corresponding antiidiotypic antiserum could, in some cases, be inhibited by the hapten, indicating that the idiotypic determinants were close to or within the antigen-binding site. It is now known that antiidiotype antibodies specifically recognize sequences in the hypervariable regions of the target antibody, which are unique to that antibody and determine its antigen specificity. Thus, in current usage, the term *idiotype* refers to the global characteristics of the antigen-binding site in a given immunoglobulin, which are determined by the hypervariable sequences of its particular V_H and V_L domains.

The Three-Dimensional Structure of Immunoglobulins

The complete three-dimensional structures of many immunoglobulin molecules have been deduced from x-ray crystallographic studies. Such studies provided conclusive evidence that all of the individual globular domains in heavy and light chains share a common folded structure, despite the considerable differences in their amino acid sequences. Each domain is folded into a rigid, roughly cylindrical scaffold made up of seven to nine strands of antiparallel β sheets that are aligned like the staves of a barrel (Figure 7–5). In V_H and V_L domains, the three hypervariable sequences each occupy a position between individual β strands and form relatively flexible

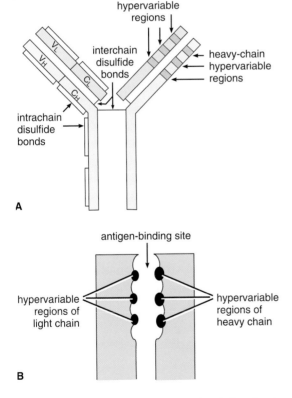

Figure 7–4. A: Schematic depiction of an IgG molecule showing the approximate locations of the hypervariable regions (also called complementarity-determining regions [CDRs]) in the heavy and light chains. Each CDR is roughly 9–12 residues long and is centered on residues 30–33, 56, or 94–98 of the polypeptide chain. **B:** Schematic depiction of how the three CDRs in each heavy- and light-chain pair form an antigen-binding site.

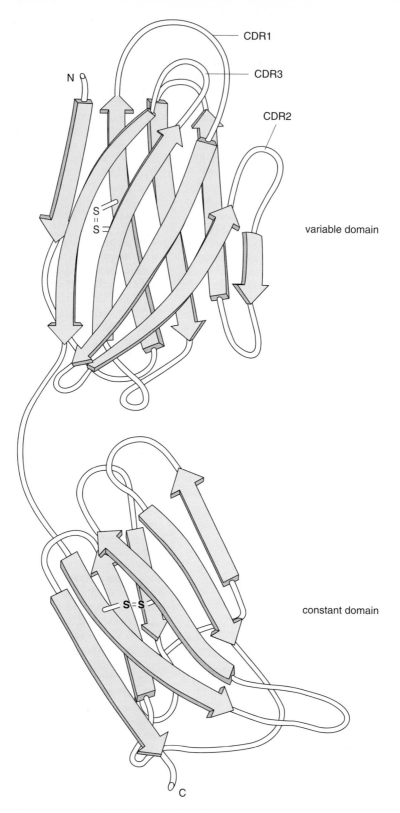

Figure 7–5. Three-dimensional structure of a light chain. In this ribbon diagram tracing the polypeptide backbone, β strands are shown as wide ribbons, other regions as narrow strings. Each of the two globular domains consists of a barrel-shaped assembly of seven to nine antiparallel β strands. The three hypervariable regions (CDR1, CDR2, and CDR3) are flexible loops that project outward from the amino-terminal end of the V_L domain.

loops that project outward from one "rim" of the barrel to participate in antigen binding. A single antigen-binding site is formed by the apposition of six hypervariable loops: three from V_H and three from V_L.

Complete crystallographic structures have also been obtained for antibodies or Fab fragments complexed with their target antigens or with haptens. These structures confirm the expectation that antigen binding is mainly carried out by residues in the hypervariable regions (especially CDR3) but demonstrate that nearby residues in the framework regions can also participate in binding. In general, haptens tend to bind by nestling into small (10–15 Å) crevices in the antigen-binding site, whereas macromolecular antigens interact over larger regions on the surface of the site. For example, 16 separate residues in lysozyme were found to interact with nearly 20 residues spread over a 20 × 30 Å surface formed by the six CDR loops of one antilysozyme Fab fragment.

Structural studies also reveal the strong tendency of immunoglobulin domains to adhere to one another laterally through noncovalent (especially hydrophobic) interactions (Figure 7–6). Thus, pairs of heavy and light chains are held together side by side not only by disulfide bonds but also by extensive noncovalent interactions between the C_H1 and C_L domains. Similarly, the heavy chains within each four-chain unit adhere to one another in part through strong hydrophobic contacts between C_H3 domains. These interdomain interactions are mediated by hydrophobic residues that occupy one lateral face of the barrel and that tend to be relatively conserved among all immunoglobulin domains.

The Immunoglobulin Supergene Family

The repetitive domain structure of immunoglobulin polypeptides reflects the manner in which their genes evolved. It is thought that the common ancestor of all immunoglobulin proteins was a small primordial gene that encoded a single copy of the barrel-like polypeptide domain. In light of the tendency of modern immunoglobulin domains to adhere to one another noncovalently, it could be speculated that the protein product of this gene originally served to mediate some useful protein–protein interaction in—or, perhaps, cell-cell interactions among—the ancestral cells that expressed it. Over evolutionary time, this single progenitor gene appears to have been reduplicated many times at the DNA level, so that additional copies were produced at both nearby and distant chromosomal locations. The sequences of individual copies then diverged as a result of random mutations and natural selection. Every modern immunoglobulin light chain can thus be viewed as a tandemly duplicated descendant of the primordial domain, whereas heavy chains each represent four or five tandem variants of this domain.

The descendants of this hypothetical primordial domain can be found not only in immunoglobulins but also in many other types of proteins (Table 7–4). Although their sequences have diverged greatly, the single or multiple immunoglobulin-like domains in each of these proteins can be recognized by their size and three-dimensional shape, by the characteristic position of the intrachain disulfide bond, and by a

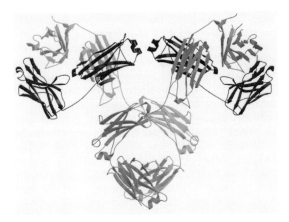

Figure 7–6. Three-dimensional structure of an immunoglobulin molecule. (Redrawn by L. Brinen, with permission, from Silverton EW et al: Three-dimensional structure of an intact human immunoglobulin. *Proc Natl Acad Sci U S A* 1977;74:5140.)

Table 7–4. The immunoglobulin gene superfamily.

Immunoglobulin heavy and light chains
T-cell receptor α, β, γ, and δ chains
CD3 complex γ, δ, and ε chains
MHC proteins: class I α and $β_2$-microglobulin, and class II α and β
T-cell differentiation antigens CD2, CD4, CD7, and CD8
B-cell signal transducers Ig-α and Ig-β
Costimulatory surface proteins (B7.1 and B7.2) and their receptor (CD28)
Fc receptor α chains: FcαRI, FcεRI, FcεRII (CD23), FcγRI (CD64), FcγRII (CD32), and FcγRIII (CD16)
Killer inhibitory receptors (KIRs) on natural killer cells
Complement receptors: CR1 (CD35) and CR2 (CD21)
Adhesion proteins: VCAM-1 (CD106), ICAM-1 (CD54), ICAM-2 (CD102), LFA-3 (CD58), and NCAM
Other CD proteins: eg, CD1, CD5, CD19, CD22, CD31, CD33, CD48, and CD56
Cytokine receptors for IL-1, IL-6 family, M-CSF, G-CSF, stem cell factor (SCF), and platelet-derived growth factor (PDGF)
Poly-Ig receptor
Thy-1
Carcinoembryonic antigen
Myelin protein Po

Abbreviations: VCAM-1 = vascular cell adhesion molecule type 1; ICAM-1 and -2 = intercellular adhesion molecule types 1 and 2; LFA-3 = leukocyte functional antigen type 3; NCAM = neural cell adhesion molecule; M-CSF = monocyte colony-stimulating factor; IL = interleukin.

few other conserved features. In recognition of their common ancestry, these proteins (or their corresponding genes) are known collectively as the **immunoglobulin gene superfamily.** Most, but not all, are integral membrane proteins. In any given member of this family, the immunoglobulin-like domains may be found in association with other unrelated types of domains that confer specialized activities, such as transmembrane signaling. Superfamily members are found at widely scattered chromosomal locations, are expressed in diverse cell types, and subserve many different functions, but in each case the immunoglobulin-like sequences appear to retain their ancestral function of interacting with other immunoglobulin-like domains in the same or other proteins.

ANTIBODY TECHNOLOGIES

The diversity and specificity of antibodies make them potentially invaluable reagents for diagnostics and research. Early serologists discovered, for example, that **antiserum** from an animal immunized against a particular microbe could be used to detect that microbe in blood or tissue specimens to diagnose infections. Even today, antisera raised in this way against snake venom proteins are widely used to treat snake bites, and antisera against human T cells have been used to suppress rejection of transplanted tissues. But this approach has serious limitations: Even when a well-defined immunogen is used, the antiserum obtained is a complex mixture of structurally diverse antibodies recognizing multiple epitopes on the immunogen, and its composition fluctuates unpredictably over the life of the animal. Moreover, the supply of antiserum from any single animal is limited, and there is no way of ensuring that antiserum obtained from a different animal would have identical properties.

To harness the full potential of antibodies, it was necessary to devise a way of obtaining abundant, pure preparations of homogeneous immunoglobulin directed against any desired antigen. This was first accomplished in 1975 by Kohler and Milstein, who discovered that fusing a normal B cell with an immortal, malignant plasma cell could give rise to a hybrid cell line that proliferated indefinitely while secreting the immunoglobulin encoded by the parental B cell. An immortal, antibody-producing clone of hybrids obtained in this way is called a **hybridoma,** and the antibody it produces is termed a **monoclonal antibody.** The production of hybridomas (Figure 7–7) is now routine and typically uses one of several mouse plasma cell lines developed for this purpose that do not express immunoglobulins of their own, so that any hybrids they form secrete only antibodies derived from the B-cell parent. First, a mouse is immunized with the target antigen in order to maximize the number of cognate B cells, and a single-cell suspension of its splenic cells is then combined with plasma cells in the presence of an agent that induces cell fusion. The mixture is next treated with a combination of antibiotics that selectively kill the parental plasma cells but not B cells or hybrids. Because any unfused B cells have a short life span in culture, the only proliferating cells that remain after a few weeks are hybrids, whose nuclei contain a mixture of chromosomes from both parents in varying proportions. These can then be grown as individual clones and screened to identify those that secrete antibody with the desired properties, which can then be produced in large quantities by propagating the hybridoma in culture or in animals.

Monoclonal antibodies have revolutionized the study of immunology and cell biology and have found numerous applications in diagnosis (see Chapter 15). They are also being explored as tools for clinical imaging and therapy, especially in cancer. For example, certain radioactively labeled monoclonal antibodies that recognize tumor surface antigens can, if injected into the bloodstream, home to the tumor and reveal its location by radioactive emission. Similarly, monoclonal antibodies coupled to toxins such as ricin or diphtheria toxin (forming a so-called **immunotoxin**) have shown some promise as antitumor chemotherapeutic agents capable of targeting toxin activity specifically to tumor cells. Unfortunately, the use of mouse monoclonal antibodies in humans is often limited by their immunogenicity, and it can be technically difficult to obtain the immunized human B cells needed to produce useful human hybridomas. One possible solution is to isolate the heavy- and light-chain genes encoding a murine antibody of interest, use recombinant DNA techniques to alter their C-region sequences to encode proteins that more closely resemble a human antibody, and then reintroduce this **humanized** antibody gene into a plasma cell for expression. Even more elegant approaches have been developed using new techniques for manipulating the genes of living mice. For example, strains of mice have been created whose own immunoglobulin genes are inactivated but which instead carry genes encoding a large assortment of human H and L chains. When immunized, these mice can produce authentic human antibodies directed against the antigen and can be used to make hybridomas secreting antigen-specific human monoclonal antibodies.

Antibody diversity can also be exploited for less obvious purposes. For example, certain V regions have been found to have enzymatic activity, in that they can catalyze specific organic chemical reactions. As is true of other enzymes, such **catalytic antibodies** generally have affinity for a transition state intermediate along the reaction pathway, and deliberate immunization with a transition-state analog offers one approach to obtaining monoclonal antibodies that promote a particular reaction. But catalytic antibodies also occur spontaneously; among the anti-

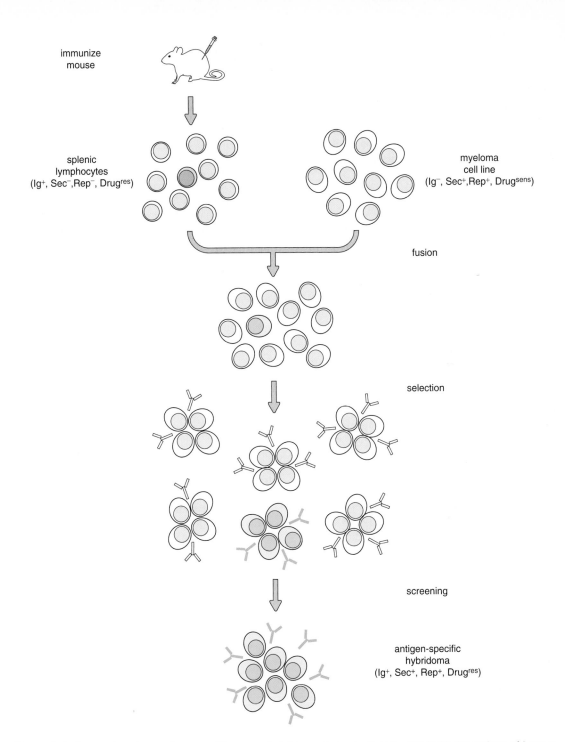

Figure 7–7. Preparation of an antigen-specific mouse hybridoma. A mouse is immunized with the antigen of interest, and its splenocytes are isolated as a source of B cells, a few of which *(dark blue)* express surface immunoglobulin (Ig) specific for the antigen. The B cells express Ig but do not secrete it and cannot replicate in cell culture (ie, they are Ig^+, Sec^-, Rep^-). The splenocytes are fused with a myeloma cell line that replicates actively in culture and has an intact secretory apparatus but does not express endogenous Ig (ie, it is Ig^-, Sec^+, Rep^+). The myeloma cells also carry a mutation ($Drug^{sens}$) that makes them vulnerable to killing by a drug or other conditions to which the normal B cells are resistant ($Drug^{res}$). The B cells and myeloma cells are fused in vitro to produce hybrid cells carrying chromosomes from both parental cells together in a single nucleus. The mixed population that results from this fusion also includes a few unfused parental cells of each type. The population is exposed to the drug for 2 weeks or more, which kills any unfused myeloma cells ($Drug^{sens}$). Unfused B cells (Rep^-) also die during this time, so that the only proliferating cells that remain are hybrids with features of both parents (Rep^+, $Drug^{res}$). These are then grown as individual clones and screened to identify those that secrete antibody with the desired specificity. The antigen-specific hybridomas identified in this way can be grown indefinitely in culture or as ascites tumors and produce a limitless supply of the desired monoclonal antibody.

DNA antibodies produced by patients with autoimmune disorders, for example, one can identify rare antibodies that catalyze cleavage of the DNA strand! The study of catalytic antibodies is in its infancy, but the range of reactions they can catalyze is already surprisingly broad, and it appears likely they will find many industrial and research applications.

FC RECEPTORS

Many cell types are able to bind circulating antibodies or antigen–antibody complexes using surface **Fc receptors.** The physiologic function of these receptors varies among cell types. Receptors have been identified for each of the heavy-chain classes, but the best studied are those for γ and ε. Three types of Fcγ receptors and two types of Fcε receptors can be distinguished based on their binding affinities, which differ from one another by one or two orders of magnitude (Table 7–5). Moreover, humans express up to three structurally different forms of a given Fcγ receptor, each encoded by a separate gene on chromosome 1, and each with a characteristic tissue distribution and biologic activity. Some of these receptors consist only of a single ligand-binding (α) polypeptide, but others are complexes containing an α subunit along with the CD3-γ or -ζ chains (or both). These are the same CD3-γ and -ζ polypeptides that form part of the antigen-receptor complex in T cells (see Chapters 3 and 9), and they serve an identical function in transducing signals from the Fc receptors into the cell interior. FcεRI also includes CD3-γ, as well as a unique signal-transducing β chain.

Only the high-affinity receptors of each type (FcγRI and FcεRI) are able to bind monomeric immunoglobulins to a significant degree at the concentrations normally found in the blood. Cells that express these high-affinity Fc receptors can therefore adsorb circulating antibodies onto their surfaces, where they may function as antigen receptors. For example, binding of unliganded IgG molecules onto FcγRI receptors on macrophages or natural killer cells serves to "arm" these cells to carry out **antibody-dependent cell-mediated cytotoxicity (ADCC)** (Chapter 4). On the other hand, antigen binding to FcεRI-associated IgE on the surface of a basophil or mast cell can stimulate these cells to degranulate, producing symptoms of **allergy** (see Chapter 13).

Cells that carry only the low-affinity Fc receptors (FcγRII, FcγRIII, and FcεRII) cannot adsorb appreciable amounts of free antibody but instead bind their cognate immunoglobulin only in antigen–antibody complexes, where its effective concentration is increased. Binding of such multivalent complexes also serves to cross-link the Fc receptors and transmit signals into the cell. Interactions of this type are responsible for facilitating phagocytosis through the phenomenon of **opsonization** (Chapter 2) and are also important for triggering chemotaxis and degranulation in neutrophils and other phagocytes. In addition, low-affinity Fc receptors on B-lymphoid cells enable these cells to sense the presence of antigen–antibody complexes, providing an important feedback-signaling pathway that limits further antibody production in the late stages of an immune response (see Chapter 8).

IMMUNOGLOBULIN GENES

Immunoglobulin Genes Are Formed Through DNA Rearrangement in B Cells

To contend with the almost unlimited variety of antigens that it may encounter, the human immune system is able to produce antibody molecules with an estimated 10^8 different unique specificities for antigen. How can so many different antibody proteins be encoded in the genes of every human being? The antigen specificity of an antibody is determined by amino acid sequences within its paired heavy- and light-chain variable domains, which together form the antigen-binding site. To produce antibodies with many different specificities, the immune system must

Table 7–5. Properties of human Fc receptors.

	Associated Markers[a]	Affinity (Kd)	Relative Subclass Preference	Cell Type Distribution
IgG receptors				
FcγRI	CD64	10^{-8}M	IgG1 = IgG3 > IgG4	Monocytes, macrophages.
FcγRII	CD32	10^{-7}M	IgG1 = IgG3 > IgG2	Monocytes, macrophages, neutrophils, eosinophils, B lymphocytes.
FcγRIII	CD16	10^{-6}M	IgG1 = IgG3	Macrophages, neutrophils, eosinophils, NK cells.
IgE receptors				
FcεRI	—	10^{-9}M	—	Mast cells, basophils.
FcεRII	CD23	10^{-7}M	—	Eosinophils, monocytes, macrophages, platelets, some T and B cells.

Abbreviation: NK = natural killer (see Chapter 9).
[a] CD designations generally apply only to the ligand-binding (α) chains of these receptors.

have the genetic capability to produce a very large number of different variable domain sequences. The sequence of the constant region, on the other hand, is generally the same for all heavy or light chains of a given immunoglobulin class and has no effect on antigen specificity. In fact, the entire family of immunoglobulin proteins consists of a relatively small number of different constant region domains linked in various combinations with an almost unlimited assortment of variable region sequences. In 1965, Dreyer and Bennett first recognized that these interchangeable combinations of protein domains must be the result of an active reshuffling of gene fragments that took place within the B-cell chromosomes. This was a revolutionary insight, because it implied that a cell could efficiently manipulate its chromosomes to change the structure of genes that it had inherited. And yet this proved to be only a part of the story: Nearly a decade later, Tonegawa made the astonishing discovery that the inherited chromosomes contain no immunoglobulin genes at all, but only the building blocks from which these genes can be assembled. Since that time, studies by many investigators have revealed in detail the extraordinary process through which a B-cell precursor assembles an immunoglobulin gene.

As with most human genes, the information that codes for an immunoglobulin protein is dispersed along the DNA strand in multiple coding segments **(exons)** that are separated by regions of noncoding DNA **(introns)**; after the gene is transcribed into RNA, introns are removed from the transcript and the exons are joined together by RNA splicing. Unlike nearly all other genes, however, the immunoglobulin DNA sequences that are found in germ cells or other nonlymphoid cell types do not exist as intact, functional genes. This is because the exons that code for variable domains are normally broken up along the chromosome into still smaller gene segments; these segments each lack some of the features needed for proper RNA splicing and so cannot function individually as exons. Before a developing B cell can begin to synthesize immunoglobulin, it must first fuse two or three of these gene segments together to assemble a complete variable region exon. This fusion of gene segments is achieved through a highly specialized process that requires cutting, rearrangement, and rejoining of the chromosomal DNA strands. Only developing lymphocytes possess the enzymatic machinery needed to carry out this process of immunoglobulin gene rearrangement.

Light-Chain Genes. The kappa light-chain genes are simplest and are therefore considered first. All of the genetic information needed to produce kappa chains lies within a single locus on chromosome 2 (Figure 7–8). The constant domain of the protein (amino acid residues 109–214) is encoded by an exon called C_κ, and only one copy of this exon is found on the chromosome. The sequence encoding

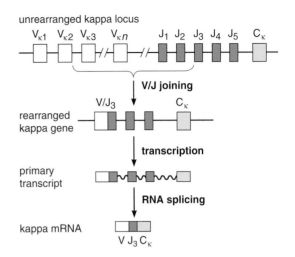

Figure 7–8. Assembly and expression of the κ light-chain locus. A DNA rearrangement event fuses one V segment (in this example, $V_{\kappa2}$) to one J segment ($J_{\kappa3}$) to form a single exon. The V/J exon is then transcribed together with the unique C_κ exon, and the transcript is spliced to form mature κ mRNA. Note that any unrearranged J segments on the primary transcript are removed as part of the intron during RNA splicing.

any given variable domain, however, is contained in two separate gene segments called the variable (V_κ) and joining (J_κ) segments. The V_κ segment encodes approximately the first 95 amino acids of the variable domain; the shorter J_κ segment codes for the remaining 13 (amino acids 96–108). In contrast to the single C_κ exon, multiple V_κ and J_κ segments are present, each with a somewhat different DNA sequence. The five J_κ segments are clustered together near the C_κ exon, whereas approximately 30–35 different V_κ segments lie scattered over a region that spans roughly 1 million base pairs (bp) of DNA (less than 1% of the length of chromosome 2). This wide separation between V_κ and J_κ segments is found in the DNA of all nonlymphoid cells. When an immature hematopoietic cell becomes committed to the B-lymphocyte lineage, however, it selects one V_κ and one J_κ segment and fuses these together. This process of V/J joining is accomplished by highly precise enzymatic manipulation of specific sites in the chromosomal DNA. In some instances, this involves precise deletion of all the DNA that normally separates the V_κ and J_κ segments; in others, the two segments are brought together by inverting a portion of the chromosomal strand with no overall loss of DNA (Figure 7–9). The result in either case is that the V_κ and J_κ segments become permanently and covalently joined to one another, side by side on the rearranged chromosome, to form a single continuous exon. Transcription can then begin at one end of the V_κ segment, and pass through both the fused V_κ/J_κ exon and the nearby C_κ

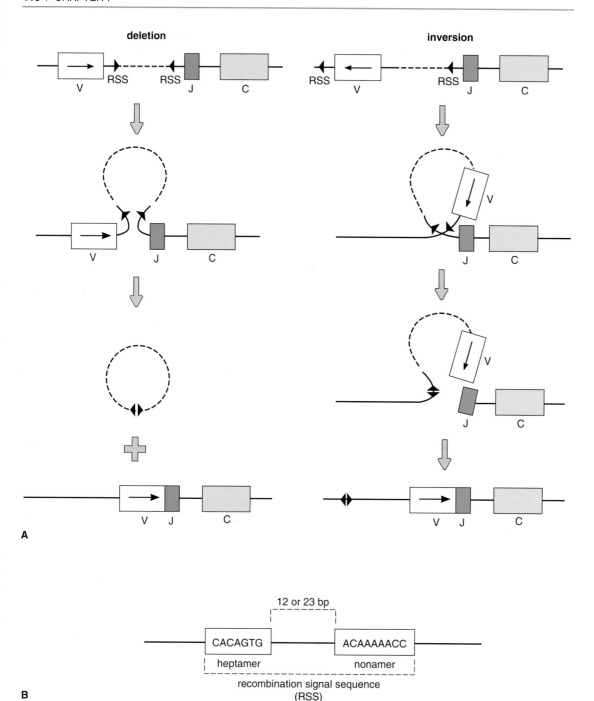

Figure 7–9. Mechanism of immunoglobulin κ gene rearrangement. **A:** Site-specific cleavage and religation of the chromosomal DNA is guided by a pair of recombination signal sequences (RSS) flanking V and J gene segments. The chromosome segment undergoes either deletion (*left*) or inversion (*right*), depending on the original orientation of the V segment with respect to the J and C segments. If deletion occurs, the DNA that originally separated V and J is released as a covalently closed circle and subsequently is degraded. **B:** The RSS, consisting of a pair of short DNA sequences (heptamer and nonamer) separated by either 12 or 23 bp of DNA, marks all sites of recombinase action in both heavy- and light-chain genes.

exon. When transcribed together, these two exons contain all of the information needed to synthesize a particular kappa protein.

The organization of the kappa genes thus accounts for the unusual properties of this light-chain protein family. As there is only one C_κ exon, all kappa proteins must have identical constant region sequences. On the other hand, because the cell can choose from among many alternative V_κ and J_κ segments, and can join these together in various combinations, a large number of different variable domain sequences can result. For example, 30 V_κ and 5 J_κ segments could in theory give rise to (30 × 5 =) 150 different variable domains. This reshuffling process, known as **combinatorial joining,** is the most important source of light-chain protein diversity.

Lambda light chains arise from a similar gene complex on chromosome 22. Joining of V_λ and J_λ segments occurs in a manner identical to that of the kappa segments. A given chromosome 22, however, may contain up to six slightly different copies of the C_λ exon (corresponding to various subtypes of lambda protein), each with a nearby J_λ segment. A V_λ segment (of which there are approximately 100) may fuse to any of these alternative J_λ segments, and the resulting V_λ/J_λ exon can then be transcribed together with the adjacent C_λ exon. The B cell selects only one of the available J_λ segments for V/J joining, and in so doing determines which C_λ subtype will be expressed (Figure 7–10).

Heavy-Chain Genes. All immunoglobulin heavy chains are derived from a single region spanning 685,000 bp on chromosome 14 (Figure 7–11). Each heavy-chain constant region is encoded by a cluster of several short exons. The μ constant region, for example, is divided among five exons known collectively as the C_μ sequence. Constant region (C_H) sequences for each of the nine heavy-chain isotypes are arrayed in tandem along the chromosome in the following order: C_μ, C_δ, $C_\gamma3$, $C_\gamma1$, $C_\alpha1$, $C_\gamma2$, $C_\gamma4$, C_ε, $C_\alpha2$; only a single copy of each is present. The six J_H segments and approximately 65 V_H segments are arranged in a manner analogous to those of the kappa

gene. In contrast to the light-chain genes, however, a third type of gene segment, called the diversity (D_H) segment, must also be used in forming a heavy-chain variable region. Several of these D_H segments (the exact number is unknown), each coding for two or three amino acids, lie between the J_H and V_H segments on the unrearranged chromosome. In assembling the heavy-chain gene, a B cell must complete two DNA rearrangement events, first bringing together one D_H and one J_H segment and subsequently linking these to a V_H segment—a sequence termed V/D/J joining.

Use of the D_H segment greatly increases the amount of heavy-chain diversity that can be produced. For example, 65 V_H, 10 D_H, and 6 J_H segments could give rise to (65 × 10 × 6 =) 3900 different heavy-chain variable domains, and these, when combined with 150 kappa-chain variable domains, could form (150 × 3900 =) nearly *600,000* different antigen-binding sites! Even using a relatively small number of gene segments, then, the immune system can generate enormous antibody diversity through combinational joining.

Additional diversity of immunoglobulin variable regions arises because the V/(D)/J (ie, either V/J or V/D/J) rearrangement process is somewhat imprecise, so that the site at which one segment fuses with another can vary by a few nucleotides. As a result, the DNA coding sequence that remains at the junction between any two segments can also vary. Moreover, during assembly of a heavy-chain gene (but not of light-chain genes), a few nucleotides of random sequence (called **N regions**) are often inserted at the points of joining between the V, D, and J segments; these insertions are carried out by **terminal deoxynucleotidyl transferase (TdT),** a nuclear enzyme that is expressed in immature lymphocytes. The variations in gene sequence that result from **imprecise joining** or from the insertion of N regions contribute substantially to overall antibody diversity. Moreover, these processes affect the sequences within each V/(D)/J exon that code for the **third hypervariable region (CDR3)** of the heavy- or light-

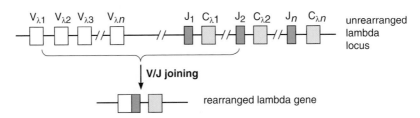

Figure 7–10. Assembly of a λ light-chain gene. An individual λ locus contains up to six alternative C_λ exons, each with a nearby Jλ segment. In this example, DNA rearrangement fuses $V_{\lambda1}$ with $J_{\lambda2}$; the resulting gene produces light chains that contain $C_{\lambda2}$.

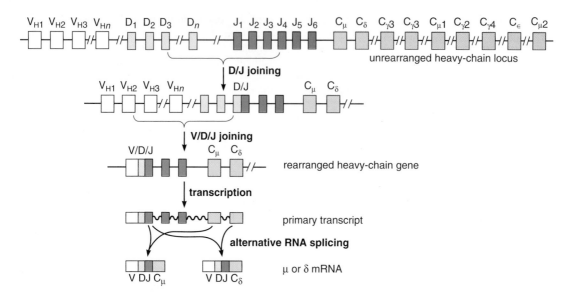

Figure 7–11. Rearrangement and expression of the heavy-chain locus. Unlike the light-chain genes, assembly of a heavy-chain V region exon requires two sequential DNA rearrangement events involving three different types of gene segments. The D_H and J_H segments are joined first and are then fused to a V_H segment. Nine alternative C-region sequences are present; of these, however, only C_μ and C_δ are initially transcribed. The primary transcript can be spliced in either of two ways to generate mRNAs that encode μ or δ heavy chains with identical V domains. This diagram is highly schematic: Each C_H sequence is actually composed of multiple exons whose aggregate length is more than three times longer than that of the V/D/J exon.

chain variable domain; hence, the diversity they engender has a disproportionately strong effect on antigen specificity. At the same time, however, these processes greatly increase the risk that two segments may be joined in an improper translational reading frame, resulting in a nonfunctional gene. In practice, such unsuccessful rearrangements occur frequently and generally cannot be reversed or repaired; they represent a cost paid by the immune system in exchange for greater potential gene diversity.

In general, only the C_H region located immediately downstream of the V/D/J exon can be expressed. Because the V/D/J exon is originally assembled at a site adjacent to the C_μ locus, the gene always produces μ heavy chains when it is first rearranged. For this reason, naive B lymphocytes always express IgM on their surfaces. Expression of one of the other C_H regions can occur only after a cell becomes activated in the periphery, as is described in Chapter 8. One important exception to this rule is the C_δ sequence, which lies very near the C_μ region and is often transcribed along with the V/D/J and C_μ exons. This produces RNA that can be spliced to yield either μ or δ mRNA (see Figure 7–11) and so enables the cell simultaneously to express IgM and IgD antibodies that have identical variable domain sequences. Such coexpression of IgM and IgD on the surface membrane is a common phenotype of mature B lymphocytes.

The Molecular Basis of V/(D)/J Rearrangement

Active gene rearrangements of the type that produce V/(D)/J joining were first thought to be a unique property of the immunoglobulin genes. Subsequently, however, it was found that the genes encoding T-cell antigen receptors (TCRs) also are assembled from germline V, D, J, and C segments through a virtually identical series of DNA rearrangements (see Chapter 9). Among the similarities, for example, the rearrangement sites in both immunoglobulin and TCR genes always coincide with so-called **recombination signal sequences** (see Figure 7–9B)—a pair of short DNA sequences (7 and 9 bp long, respectively) that are located immediately adjacent to each unrearranged V, D, or J segment. It is now thought that rearrangement of both the immunoglobulin and TCR gene families is carried out by the same molecular machinery: a system of enzymes and other proteins known collectively as the **V/(D)/J recombinase.** The most important components of the recombinase are two nuclear proteins called **RAG-1** and **RAG-2** (the products of recombination activating genes 1 and 2, respectively), which are expressed in immature B- and T-lineage cells. Acting together, RAG-1 and RAG-2 have the ability to recognize and cleave DNA specifically at a recombination signal sequence, making them the critical ingredients in these early steps of recombination. By contrast, later steps of recombination, such as religating the various gene segments together, are carried out by cellular enzymes that are also involved in more common forms of DNA repair that occur in all cell types.

Because RAG-1 and RAG-2 (and possibly unknown accessory factors) are expressed only in lymphoid cells, V/(D)/J recombination appears to be absolutely confined to this lineage: no nonlymphoid cell type has yet been proven to manipulate its chromosomes in this way. Until recently, it was also thought that recombinase was expressed only in the early phases of lymphoid development that take place within the lymphopoietic organs. It is true that, by the time a naive B cell emerges from the marrow, it has rearranged both its heavy- and light-chain genes, and has ceased to express recombinase activity, so that it is unable to perform further V/(D)/J rearrangements. We now know, however, that under some circumstances recombinase can become active again in mature lymphocytes, which use it to modify their rearranged genes further in a process called **receptor editing** (see Chapter 8). The orderly manner in which recombinase is expressed and carries out its tasks thus defines specific stages of lymphocyte ontogeny, as will be discussed in the following chapters.

Natural Antibiotics

In both humans and animals, a high proportion of circulating antibodies normally are able to bind pathogen-specific molecules such as bacterial lipopolysaccharide (LPS), phosphatidylcholine, or mannans. Because these antibodies are continually expressed even without specific immunization, can activate complement, and presumably have a role in innate (ie, natural) immunity against pathogens, they are called natural antibodies. Other natural antibodies react with endogenous antigens that are expressed by injured or distressed host cells. For example, when a tissue is deprived of oxygen, preexisting antibodies may bind the injured cells, activate complement, and immediately trigger an inflammatory response. The origins and function of natural antibodies are controversial. In mice, most are IgM antibodies produced by a subset of B lymphocytes called B-1 B cells (see Chapter 8), using a very limited number of V_H and V_L gene segments. This may indicate that part of the immunoglobulin gene repertoire has evolved to provide rapid, innate recognition of pathogens and distressed tissues.

Immunoglobulin Gene Rearrangements & B-Cell Malignancy

Apart from their role in generating antibody diversity, immunoglobulin gene rearrangements are gaining increasing importance in clinical diagnosis and research. Rearrangement of these genes can be detected in biopsies or blood specimens by using a technique known as the Southern blot, and their pres-

ence provides a highly sensitive and specific means of diagnosing lymphoid cancers (see Chapter 18). Perhaps more importantly, errors in immunoglobulin gene rearrangement are now thought to contribute to the genesis of several major types of leukemia and lymphoma. For example, the cells of **Burkitt's lymphoma,** a B-lymphocytic malignancy, usually contain a specific chromosomal abnormality called **t(8,14),** in which a portion of chromosome 8 has been translocated onto chromosome 14 (Figure 7–12). In this translocation, breakage of chromosome 14 occurs within the immunoglobulin heavy-chain locus, whereas the breakpoint on chromosome 8 coincides with a cellular protooncogene known as **c-myc,** which encodes the transcription factor c-Myc (see Chapter 1). As a result, the c-*myc* gene is moved to a position directly adjacent to the heavy-chain gene. It is thought that this proximity to the transcriptionally active heavy-chain locus alters the expression of the protooncogene, and that this, along with other damage to c-*myc* that can occur during translocation, contributes to malignant transformation. Less commonly, Burkitt's lymphoma may lack t(8,14) and instead exhibit a closely related anomaly in which the c-*myc* locus is translocated into the kappa or lambda light-chain gene on chromosomes 2 or 22, producing the same effects.

A similar type of chromosomal anomaly, designated **t(14,18),** is observed in at least 90% of cases of **follicular lymphoma**—the most common human B-

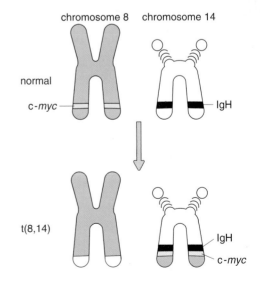

Figure 7–12. The t(8,14) chromosomal anomaly of Burkitt's lymphoma. A reciprocal translocation of genetic material exchanges the distal ends of the long arms of chromosomes 8 and 14. This transposes the c-*myc* protooncogene from chromosome 8 into the active immunoglobulin heavy-chain locus on chromosome 14 and contributes to the development of a malignancy.

cell malignancy. In this translocation, the gene on chromosome 18 that encodes the cytoplasmic membrane protein **Bcl-2** is moved to a position immediately adjacent to the heavy-chain locus on chromosome 14. B-cells carrying the t(14,18) anomaly express unusually high levels of structurally normal Bcl-2 protein and hence are resistant to being killed by many of the physiologic processes that normally induce apoptosis (Chapter 1). As a result, they tend to accumulate in great numbers and evolve into a malignancy (Chapter 43). In both t(14,18) and the Burkitt's anomalies, the chromosomal breakpoint in affected immunoglobulin loci occurs directly beside a J segment, which strongly implies that each of these translocations results in part from an error in immunoglobulin gene rearrangement.

REFERENCES

Agrawal A et al: Transposition mediated by RAG1 and RAG2 and its implications for the evolution of the immune system. *Nature* 1998;394:744.

Alzari PN et al: Three-dimensional structures of antibodies. *Annu Rev Immunol* 1988;6:555.

Daëron M: Fc receptor biology. *Annu Rev Immunol* 1997; 15:203.

Davies DR, Cohen GH: Interactions of protein antigens with antibodies. *Proc Natl Acad Sci U S A* 1996;93:7.

Davies DR, Padlan EA: Antibody-antigen complexes. *Annu Rev Biochem* 1990;59:439.

Dreyer WJ, Bennett JC: The molecular basis of antibody formations: A paradox. *Proc Natl Acad Sci U S A* 1965;54:864.

French DL et al: The role of somatic hypermutation in the generation of antibody diversity. *Science* 1989;244:1152.

Garman SC et al: Crystal structure of the human high-affinity IgE receptor. *Cell* 1998;95:951.

Gellert M: Recent advances in understanding V(D)J recombination. *Adv Immunol* 1997;64:39.

Honjo T et al (editors): *Immunoglobulin Genes.* Academic Press, 1989.

Kohler G, Milstein C: Continuous cultures of fused cells secreting antibody of predefined specificity. *Nature* 1975; 256:659.

Korsmeyer SJ: Chromosomal translocations in lymphoid malignancies reveal novel protooncogenes. *Annu Rev Immunol* 1992;10:785.

Lerner RA et al: At the crossroads of chemistry and immunology: Catalytic antibodies. *Science* 1991;252:659.

Lonberg N, Huszar D: Human antibodies from transgenic mice. *Int Rev Immunol* 1995;13:65.

Lorenz M, Radbruch A: Developmental and molecular regulation of immunoglobulin class switch recombination. *Curr Topics Microbiol Immunol* 1996;217:151.

Morrison SL: In vitro antibodies: Strategies for production and application. *Annu Rev Immunol* 1992;10:239.

Ravetch JV, Kinet J-P: Fc receptors. *Annu Rev Immunol* 1991;9:457.

Ravetch JV: Fc receptors: Rubor redux. *Cell* 1994;78:553.

Rowen L et al: The complete 685-kilobase DNA sequence of the human B T cell receptor locus. *Science* 1996;272:1755.

Schatz D et al: V(D)J recombination: Molecular biology and regulation. *Annu Rev Immunol* 1992;10:359.

Schultz PG, Lerner RA: From molecular diversity to catalysis: Lessons from the immune system. *Science* 1995;269:1835.

Spiegelberg HL: Biological activities of immunoglobulins of different classes and subclasses. *Adv Immunol* 1974;19:259.

Tonegawa S: Somatic generation of antibody diversity. *Nature* 1983;302:575.

Williams AF, Barclay N: The immunoglobulin superfamily—domains for cell surface recognition. *Annu Rev Immunol* 1988;6:381.

B-Cell Development & the Humoral Immune Response

8

Anthony L. DeFranco, PhD

The clonal selection theory, formulated by Burnet in the 1950s to explain the specificity of immune responses, postulates that each of the cells that make antibodies—the B lymphocytes—makes only antibodies of a single specificity and, moreover, that each antigen selectively induces the expansion of those cells that can make antibody against it. This theory was soon expanded to account for the fact that the immune system normally makes antibodies to foreign entities but not to self-components. In subsequent years, a great deal has been learned about B lymphocytes and how they participate in immune responses. The tenets of the clonal selection theory have been upheld, and the molecular mechanisms by which it occurs are now largely understood. In this chapter, we consider the mechanisms by which B lymphocytes develop from precursors and how these mechanisms ensure that each B cell makes a unique antibody molecule. This, in turn, forms the basis for clonal selection. We then consider how antigen induces an immune response from the appropriate B cells and the role of helper T cells in this process, as well as the mechanisms by which B-cell responses are diversified to give different classes of immunoglobulin (IgM, IgG, etc) and to maximize the affinities of the antibodies produced. Finally, we review what is known about the mechanisms that act to prevent B-cell immune responses directed against self.

B-LYMPHOCYTE ONTOGENY

THE GENERATION OF B LYMPHOCYTES

Development of B cells from hematopoietic stem cells occurs in the bone marrow. In humans, approximately 10^9 B cells are generated each day. Their development proceeds through a series of distinct stages that are accompanied and, in many cases defined, by the DNA rearrangements that assemble their immunoglobulin genes. These rearrangements occur in a strict developmental sequence (Figure 8–1). The first rearrangements take place in a population of mitotically active bone marrow cells, sometimes referred to as **pro-B cells,** which are the most primitive recognizable cells in the B lineage. These cells express the surface proteins CD10 and CD19, as well as the nuclear proteins terminal deoxynucleotidyl transferase (TdT) and recombination-activating gene products RAG-1 and RAG-2 (Figure 8–2). These latter proteins play important roles in V/D/J recombination as described in Chapter 7.

The first rearrangement that occurs in a pro-B cell is the joining of D_H and J_H segments in the heavy-chain genes. This occurs on both copies of chromosome 14 in virtually all developing B cells. The cell then joins a V_H segment to the fused D_H/J_H segment on one of its two chromosomes. If this first attempt yields a functional gene in which the V and J regions are linked in such a way that they can be translated in the same reading frame of the genetic code and hence produce a functional protein, the cell (for reasons that will be discussed presently) carries out no further rearrangements of its other heavy-chain locus. If, on the other hand, the first rearrangement fails, a second attempt at V/D/J assembly is made using the other chromosome 14. Because of the error-prone nature of V/D/J joining, about 50% of pro-B cells fail at both tries to produce a functional heavy-chain gene; unable to proceed further through the maturation pathway, these cells simply die in the marrow.

Successful V/D/J rearrangement on either chromosome allows the cell immediately to begin synthesizing heavy-chain proteins. The heavy chains produced at this stage are all of the μ isotype and have a short hydrophobic region at their carboxy termini that causes them to integrate into cellular membranes. This membrane-associated form of μ protein is called $μ_m$. Heavy chains ordinarily cannot be transported to the cell surface unless they are complexed with light chains. Pro-B cells express two proteins, known as **surrogate light chains,** that can bind to heavy chains, take the place of light chains, and be displayed transiently on the surface membranes of these

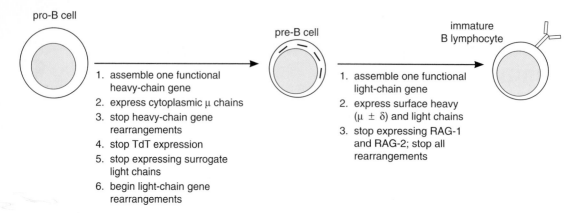

Figure 8–1. Major genetic events in early B-cell ontogeny. Listed are the sequences of events that occur in progressing from each stage of development to the next. Note that the ability to perform V/(D)/J rearrangements is lost by the time the cell becomes an immature B lymphocyte.

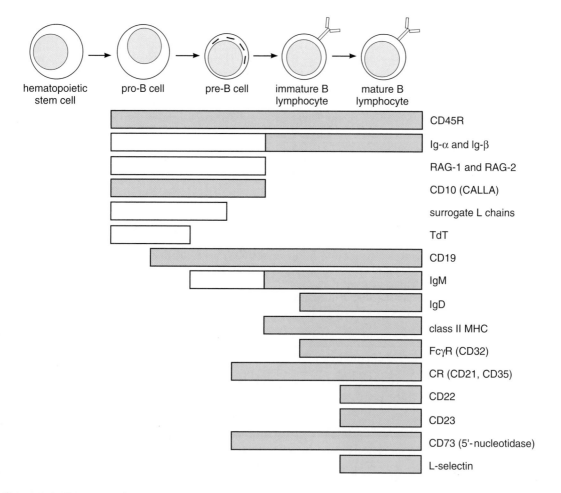

Figure 8–2. Expression of selected marker proteins at various stages of B-cell development. Open bars indicate that a protein is expressed only within the cytoplasm of a cell; filled bars indicate surface expression. *Abbreviations:* RAG = recombination-activating gene; CR = complement receptors; TdT = terminal deoxynucleotidyl transferase; MHC = major histocompatibility complex.

immature cells. The surrogate light chains are not true immunoglobulin proteins; they are expressed only in primitive B-cell precursors, are derived from genes that do not undergo somatic rearrangement, and have no role in immune responses per se. Nevertheless, they are essential for regulating early B-cell development. When the μ_m and surrogate light-chain proteins reach the cell surface, they are believed to transmit a signal back into the cell, perhaps after contacting some unknown ligand. In effect, this signal notifies the cell that it has produced a functional heavy-chain protein. In response, the cell permanently halts any further rearrangements of its heavy-chain genes and stops expressing TdT. At about the same time, the cell gains the ability to rearrange its light-chain genes. This shift from heavy-chain to light-chain rearrangements does not appear to be due to changes in the recombinase machinery itself, but rather to changes in accessibility of the various immunoglobulin loci on the chromosomes, and is probably mediated by many of the same proteins that control transcription of these genes. Once the developing B cell expresses μ_m, it also ceases to synthesize new surrogate light chains, so that the temporary signaling complex soon disappears from the cell surface. The μ_m chain, now lacking a light-chain partner, is trapped in the endoplasmic reticulum at this stage. These events mark the transition into the next phase of ontogeny, known as the pre-B cell stage (see Figure 8–1).

Pre-B cells are defined as cells that do not yet express immunoglobulin light chains but contain μ_m heavy chains intracellularly (Figs 8–1 and 8–2). They are found almost exclusively in the bone marrow and represent a transient phase in B-cell development that lasts for about 2 days. Interestingly, generation of pre-B cells is deficient in a fairly common hereditary immunodeficiency disease known as **X-linked agammaglobulinemia,** or Bruton's agammaglobulinemia. The defect in this disorder is in the gene encoding an intracellular protein tyrosine kinase, called **Btk.** Although the exact role of Btk in B-cell development is not understood, its absence leads to decreased maturation of pro-B cells to pre-B cells and also to a reduction in subsequent steps in B-cell development. As a result, the affected patients have very few B cells, and they make little or no antibody.

On entering the pre-B-cell phase, the B-cell precursors divide several times in response to interleukin 7 (IL-7) produced locally by bone marrow stromal cells. Pre-B cells then cease dividing and do not resume mitosis until they have become fully mature B cells and encounter antigen in the periphery. The most important event taking place in pre-B cells is the rearrangement of light-chain genes, which begins only after heavy-chain rearrangements have ceased. Because TdT is no longer expressed, no N-region nucleotides are inserted as the light-chain genes rearrange. V/J joining is attempted on each chromo-

some 2 or 22 in succession, until a functional κ or λ gene is produced. As soon as either type of light-chain protein appears, it associates with the existing μ_m heavy chains, and the resulting four-chain units are transported to the cell surface as membrane IgM. At that moment, the cell enters the B-lymphocyte stage of development and ordinarily loses the ability to perform additional V/J rearrangements because RAG-1 and RAG-2 expression ceases. It seems likely that the signal to shut off the recombinase is sent by the IgM molecules themselves when they first reach the cell surface.

The successful assembly of a single heavy- or light-chain gene prevents all other genes of that type from undergoing rearrangement in the same cell. Consequently, only one heavy-chain and one light-chain gene can give rise to protein in any individual B lymphocyte—a phenomenon termed **allelic and isotypic exclusion.** If the lymphocyte subsequently divides in the periphery, chromosomes bearing the active rearranged genes are passed on to its progeny, and the daughter cells continue to express these genes without performing further V/J or V/D/J rearrangements. For this reason, all of the immunoglobulin molecules produced by a given B lymphocyte and its progeny have identical antigen specificity and light-chain type (κ or λ). This is the molecular basis of the phenomenon known as **clonal restriction** (Chapter 4). The diversity of antibody molecules produced by the immune system as a whole reflects the fact that innumerable B-cell precursors each rearrange their genes independently and in different combinations, resulting in a large assortment of clones that each possess a unique specificity for antigen.

MATURATION & RELEASE OF NAIVE B LYMPHOCYTES

The moment it begins to express surface IgM, a cell is considered to have become a B lymphocyte. Nevertheless, it is not yet ready to participate in immune responses. Instead, such **immature B lymphocytes** remain in the marrow for another 1–3 days before exiting to the periphery, where they continue their maturation. During this process, the cells acquire additional surface molecules that distinguish them as **mature B lymphocytes** (see Figure 8–2). One such marker is surface **IgD,** which, as noted in Chapter 7, is produced by alternative splicing of some of the RNA transcripts arising from the rearranged heavy-chain gene. The IgM and IgD on any individual lymphocyte both incorporate the same light chains and have identical antigen specificity. Other surface markers that appear on mature B lymphocytes include complement receptors (CR1 and CR2, the latter also known as CD21); a membrane-anchored enzyme called **5′-nucleotidase (CD73),** whose function is unknown; the lectin-like oligosaccharide-binding protein **CD23;** and the adhesion proteins **leukocyte function-associated antigen-1 (LFA-1), intercellular adhesion molecule-1 (ICAM-1),** and **CD22.** Individual cells also begin to express surface-homing receptors, such as **L-selectin,** which target them to lymph nodes or other peripheral sites. At about the same time, the cells acquire **class II major histocompatibility complex (MHC)** proteins, which enable them to present antigens to helper T cells, and they also begin surface expression of **CD40**—a protein involved in receiving T-cell help (see later discussion). With the acquisition of these various accessory molecules, the mature B lymphocytes become competent for immunologic function.

Mature B cells have a long life span, with a half-life of more than 3 weeks. Most immature B cells that exit the bone marrow, however, never mature fully and instead die with a half-life of less than 1 week. Maturation of these cells occurs only if they receive some low level of signaling through the B-cell antigen receptor (BCR), and even mature B cells rapidly die if they are deprived of such signals. (This phenomenon, called **"death by neglect,"** also applies to T-cell development, as will be described in Chapter 9). Thus, there is a darwinian competition among peripheral B cells to remain in the circulating pool. This is presumably advantageous to the host because signaling implies that a cell must have a functional BCR and may be more likely to respond to foreign antigens.

The developmental pathway outlined earlier is typical of the B-cell population as a whole but does not apply strictly to all of its cells. Individual B-lineage cells may differ significantly in the types and amounts of surface markers they express or the sequence in which these markers are acquired. This may reflect the existence of functionally distinct subsets of B cells. Indeed, there is considerable circumstantial evidence for the existence of distinct subsets. At present, however, only two types of B cells are clearly recognizable: the "conventional" B cells and a small, enigmatic subpopulation of B cells that express on their surface CD5—a protein of unknown function that is also expressed on most T lymphocytes. These **CD5 B cells** are long-lived cells that are found principally in the peritoneal cavity and that appear to be derived from precursor cells present in infant but not adult bone marrow. As these B cells arise soon after birth, they are the major source of antibody production in young individuals. The heavy-chain gene rearrangements of these B cells principally involve a few V_H genes near the D_H and J_H gene segments and often lack N regions. Thus, these cells have a less diverse antibody repertoire than do the B cells that dominate mature individuals. No unique immunologic function has yet been assigned to CD5 B cells, although they may be especially important for T-cell-independent antibody responses such as those directed at antigens

of bacterial cell walls (see next section). Curiously, CD5 B cells are disproportionately more likely than other B cells to produce autoreactive immunoglobulins (ie, antibodies that recognize determinants in host tissues). Remarkably, the malignant cells in nearly all cases of human B-cell **chronic lymphocytic leukemia** carry the CD5 marker, suggesting that this malignancy arises from the CD5 B cell subpopulation.

THE HUMORAL IMMUNE RESPONSE

THE B-CELL ANTIGEN RECEPTOR

The production of large amounts of specific antibody in response to antigenic challenge depends on the ability of the immune system to activate only those rare B cells capable of producing antibody that can react with the antigen. These cells are induced to proliferate rapidly to expand their numbers. Subsequently, they either differentiate into antibody-secreting plasma cells or become memory B cells, which are long-lived cells that produce an antibody response later on reexposure to the antigen. This process is referred to as **clonal selection,** because a small number of B cells are selected, based on their antigen specificity, and then divide and give rise to a clone of progeny, all of which produce the same or nearly the same antibody as the founder cell.

Clonal selection requires each B cell to recognize the antigen that binds to the antibody secreted by that cell. This is accomplished by differential RNA splicing, yielding the expression of two forms of immunoglobulin heavy chains—a secreted form and a membrane form, the latter containing a hydrophobic transmembrane domain and a very short cytoplasmic tail. All heavy-chain isotypes can give rise to both secreted and membrane forms. The membrane form combines with immunoglobulin light chains to make membrane immunoglobulin. Interestingly, membrane immunoglobulin is retained in the endoplasmic reticulum unless it can associate with two additional proteins expressed exclusively in cells of the B-cell lineage. These proteins, called **Ig-α and** Ig-β, associate with membrane immunoglobulin to form the **B-cell antigen receptor (BCR),** which can transit to the cell surface (Figure 8–3A). Ig-α and Ig-β are transmembrane glycoproteins, each of which has a moderately large cytoplasmic domain. These cytoplasmic domains each include a short region important for transmitting into the cell a signal indicating that antigen has bound. This region is called an **immunoreceptor tyrosine-based activation motif (ITAM),** and its key features are two precisely spaced tyrosine residues within a partially conserved surrounding sequence. ITAM sequences are found not only in components of the BCR, but also in the T-cell antigen receptor complexes, in various Fc receptors, and in the activating receptors of natural killer cells. In each case, ITAM sequences are thought to induce transmembrane signaling in a fundamentally similar way. In B cells, cross-linking of two or more BCRs by a bivalent or multivalent antigen brings together several Ig-α and Ig-β cytoplasmic domains with their ITAMs. This clustering leads to phosphorylation of the ITAM tyrosines by protein tyrosine kinases belonging to the Src-family (see Chapter 1). The phosphorylated ITAM, in turn, becomes a binding site for a second type of tyrosine kinase, called **Syk,** which binds and becomes activated to phosphorylate other cytoplasmic proteins that activate various signaling pathways leading, for example to hydrolysis of phosphatidylinositol 4,5-bis-phosphate (PIP$_2$) and to activation of Ras (see Figure 8–3). The subsequent events are poorly understood at this time, although a number of transcription factors ultimately become activated, which leads to the expression of specific genes that contribute to cellular activation. In any case, it is the ability of bivalent or multivalent antigen to bring together multiple antigen receptors and their attached ITAMs that initiates the signaling events that inform a B cell it has encountered antigen.

T-CELL-INDEPENDENT ANTIGENS

The consequences of antigen contact with the BCR depend on the nature of the antigen and on other signals received by the B cell at that time. Generally, antigen contact alone is insufficient to activate B cells because most protein antigens require antigen-specific T-cell help to generate an antibody response. Some antigens do not require the presence of helper T cells, however, and are called **T-independent antigens.** These antigens typically fall into either of two categories, with different mechanistic properties (Figure 8–4). The first group, called **TI-1 antigens,** can, at high concentrations, induce activation of many B cells, both specific and nonspecific. Because many B cells are activated, these antigens are called **polyclonal B-cell activators.** Many polyclonal B-cell activators also potently stimulate macrophages to produce cytokines such as interleukin-1 (IL-1) and tumor necrosis factor alpha (TNFα), which augment immune responses. Typical TI-1 antigens are bacterial cell wall components, and their recognition by cells of the immune system appears to be an evolved feature of innate immunity. For example, the TI-1 antigen **lipopolysaccharide (LPS),** from gram-negative bacterial cell walls, can induce immunologic defense reactions in a number of invertebrate as well as vertebrate organisms. Mammalian cells recognize LPS with **Toll-like receptor 4 (TLR4)** and several other bacterial cell wall components with the closely related TLR2 (See Chapter 2). Interestingly, at low concentrations TI-1 antigens often do elicit an antigen-specific antibody response. It has been postulated that this occurs because BCRs that specifically recognize the TI-1 antigen can concentrate it onto the surfaces of specific B cells, where it can then stimulate Toll-like receptors more efficiently and trigger activation.

In contrast, **TI-2 antigens** do not have polyclonal B-cell activator properties, nor do they activate macrophages. These antigens are generally highly repetitive polymeric antigens such as polysaccharides from bacterial cell walls, or polymeric protein structures such as bacterial flagella. It has been postulated that their B-cell-activating properties derive from their ability to cross-link numerous BCR molecules and induce either intense, or especially prolonged, intracellular-signaling reactions (see Figure 8–4). Antibody responses to TI-2 antigens, although they do not require helper T cells, do appear to require low levels of cytokines, such as might be generated by a nearby immune response.

T-CELL HELP & ACCESSORY SIGNALS

Most protein antigens only induce antibody production in the presence of CD4 helper T cells. Typically, T-cell help can be provided in two forms: by soluble cytokines (especially IL-4 and IL-5) or by a cell–cell contact-dependent signal (Figure 8–5). Contact-mediated help results from specific interactions between membrane proteins on the T$_H$- and B-cell surfaces. The most important interaction of this type occurs between the B-cell protein **CD40** and a protein called **CD40 ligand** (or **CD40L**), which appears on T$_H$ cells only after they become activated. In some circumstances, the CD40L signal in combination with the cytokines IL-4 and IL-5 can fully activate B cells even in the absence of antigen. In other circumstances, however, CD40L stimulation in the absence of antigen contact leads to death of the B cell via apoptosis. In general, however, the combination of antigen binding and CD40L acts synergistically to trigger B-cell activation. Binding of CD40 to CD40L is an extremely important mechanism of delivering T-cell help in vivo. An inherited defect in CD40L causes a form of congenital immunodeficiency known as **hyper-IgM syndrome,** in which humoral immunity is impaired due to a deficiency of T-cell help. In these patients, the antibody response to many antigens is markedly abnormal, and no IgG, IgA, or IgE is produced. IgM levels, on the other hand, are abnormally high, possibly as a secondary effect of recurrent infections. This IgM response may be due to T-independent antigen stimulation or possibly to residual T-cell-dependent antibody responses in the absence of CD40L.

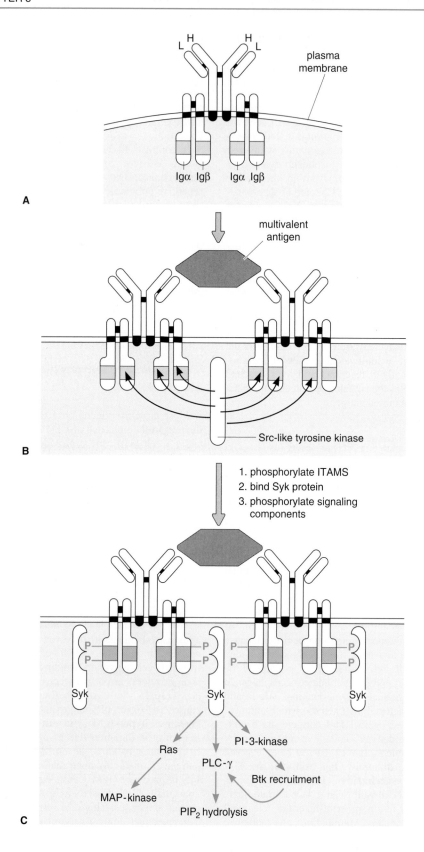

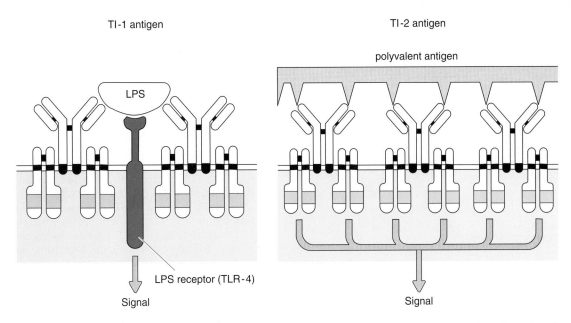

TI-1 antigen

TI-2 antigen

polyvalent antigen

LPS

LPS receptor (TLR-4)

Signal

Signal

Figure 8–4. B-cell activation by T-independent antigens. **(Left)** TI-1 antigens activate B cells by signaling primarily through nonimmunoglobulin receptors, most likely members of the Toll-like receptor (TLR) family, although specific surface antibodies can enhance signaling by concentrating the antigen on the cell surface. **(Right)** TI-2 antigens are highly repetitive structures and therefore can activate B cells by specifically binding and cross-linking numerous surface immunoglobulins.

In B cells that coexpress surface IgM and IgD, both are capable of antigen binding and signal transduction, and they produce identical effects. Certain accessory molecules on the B cell (eg, CD22, complement receptors, and class II MHC proteins) can also send signals that augment activation when they bind their cognate ligands. Antigens that have complement fragments bound to them can simultaneously bind the BCR and CR2 complement receptor, bringing them together in the plasma membrane; this bridging greatly promotes B-cell activation (Figure 8–6B). In contrast, activation is suppressed by the binding of antigen–antibody complexes (especially those containing IgG) to B-cell surface **Fc receptors**—this provides a negative feedback mechanism that may be important for terminating B-cell responses once saturating amounts of antibody have been produced. The mechanism of this suppression involves the clustering of the Fc receptors together with the engaged BCRs, leading to the engagement of molecules that inactivate Ras and counter PIP_2 signaling (see Figure 8–6C). Thus, the B cell can recognize complex antigenic ligands in which the antigen has either complement components or antibodies

Figure 8–3. Signaling through the B-cell antigen receptor (BCR). **A:** Antigen receptor transmembrane-signaling complex on mature B cells. Ig-α and Ig-β are disulfide-linked to each other but associate with membrane immunoglobulins noncovalently through their transmembrane and extracellular domains. The number of Ig-α/Ig-β heterodimers per membrane immunoglobulin unit is unknown but is believed to be two, as shown, for reasons of symmetry. Both Ig-α and Ig-β cytoplasmic domains contain copies of the immunoreceptor tyrosine-based activation motif (ITAM). The consensus sequence for the ITAM is YxxL/I$xxxxxxx$YxxL/I, where Y = tyrosine; L/I = leucine or isoleucine; and x = any amino acid. In the resting state, the ITAM tyrosines (Y) of Ig-α and Ig-β are largely unphosphorylated. **B:** On cross-linking with multivalent antigen, an Src-family tyrosine kinase phosphorylates ITAM tyrosines. **C:** Doubly phosphorylated ITAMS serve as binding sites for a second type of tyrosine kinase, called Syk. Once bound, Syk becomes phosphorylated on tyrosines and its activity is increased. Syk is thought to be largely responsible for phosphorylating downstream signaling targets, such as activators of Ras and phosphatidylinositol 3-kinase (PI 3-kinase). The latter enzyme synthesizes PIP_3 which, in turn, attracts to the membrane a third type of tyrosine kinase, called Btk, which then participates in BCR signaling. Btk and Syk are both needed to phosphorylate and activate phospholipase Cγ (PLC-γ), which hydrolyzes inositol-containing phospholipids (eg, PIP_2), leading to elevation of intracellular free calcium and activation of protein kinase C.

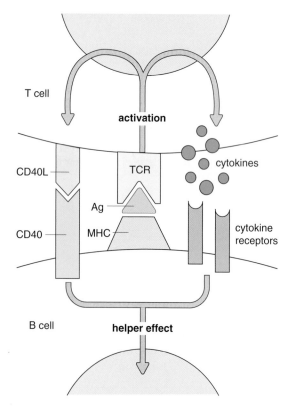

Figure 8–5. B-cell activation by a helper T cell. Antigen-specific B cells are stimulated by antigen contact with the B-cell receptor (BCR). They also take up the antigen (Ag) for digestion into peptides that combine with class II major histocompatibility complex (MHC) molecules and then go to the cell surface to be presented to antigen-specific helper T cells. T-cell-receptor (TCR)-based recognition of the antigen leads to T-cell activation, which stabilizes the association between the T and B cells and induces T-cell synthesis of CD40L and cytokines, which provide coactivating signals for the B cell.

bound to it, as distinct from simple antigens, and can modulate its response appropriately.

Another surface protein that may modulate lymphocyte activation is **CD45,** a membrane-spanning glycoprotein whose cytoplasmic domain has **protein tyrosine phosphatase** activity (ie, the ability to dephosphorylate phosphotyrosines of other proteins). CD45 is found on all hematopoietic cells, but its molecular mass varies considerably among cell types owing to differences in the size of the extracellular domain that result from alternative mRNA splicing. B lymphocytes express the largest (220 kd) isoform of CD45, designated **CD45R.** Although its precise role is unknown, CD45 paradoxically stimulates BCR or TCR signaling. It appears to do this by removing an inhibitory tyrosine phosphorylation of the Src-family tyrosine kinases, which initiate signal

transduction by phosphorylating ITAMs in clustered antigen receptors.

B LYMPHOCYTES AS ANTIGEN-PRESENTING CELLS

The activation of B cells in response to T-cell-dependent antigens usually requires direct contact between the antigen-stimulated B cell and an antigen-activated T_H cell. T cells are constantly binding to other cells to determine whether they have ligands (specific antigenic peptide bound to an MHC molecule) for the TCR of that T cell. This interaction is short-lived if the T cell fails to detect the appropriate ligand. On the other hand, if a T cell encounters antigen presented by the bound cell, the interaction between the two cells is greatly strengthened. In the case of T_H cells, the resulting interaction can last for many hours and allow for efficient delivery of cytokines and contact-dependent signals involving CD40L. For efficient activation of B cells to occur, the B cell must present antigen to T_H cells to induce such a stable interaction. B cells are inefficient at taking up antigens by phagocytosis or pinocytosis but are extremely efficient at taking up antigen via the BCR. This is because the immunoglobulin acts as a high-affinity receptor, enabling the B cell to capture its cognate antigen at concentrations several orders of magnitude lower than those needed to engage the low-affinity, broad-specificity receptors on other types of antigen-presenting cells. The bound antigen is taken into the B cell by receptor-mediated (in this case, immunoglobulin-mediated) endocytosis. It is then processed by proteases in late endosomes or lysosomes. The resulting antigenic peptides can combine with newly synthesized class II MHC molecules, which are specially routed to endocytic compartments. Class II MHC molecules are constitutively synthesized by B cells, but their synthesis is upregulated by various activation stimuli, including specific antigen, IL-4, and polyclonal B-cell activators. The resulting class II MHC–peptide complexes are then displayed on the B-cell surface, where they may be recognized by T cells that have the appropriate antigen- and MHC-specificities (Figure 8–7). Note that, if the antigen is a complex protein, the B cell may produce and display from it many different processed peptides that can serve as T-cell epitopes; these may or may not correspond to the B-cell epitope originally recognized by the immunoglobulin. If this sequence of events leads to helper T-cell activation, the presenting B cell is also likely to become activated because it not only receives signals from the bound antigen but is also already in direct contact with the helper cell (see Figure 8–6). Activated B cells express surface **B7.1** and **B7.2** proteins, which are T-cell costimulators that are important for activating naive T cells. In the absence of costimulation, B-cell

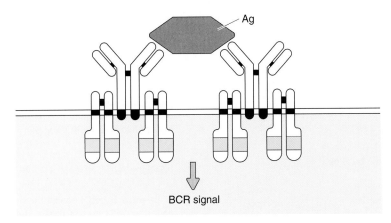

A   antigen alone

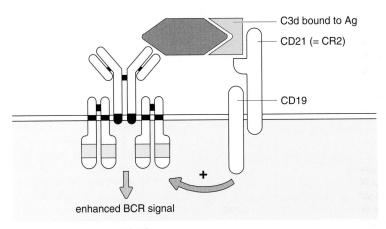

B   antigen + complement (C3d)

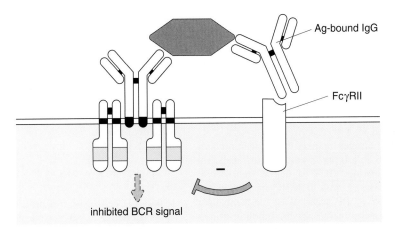

C   antigen – antibody complex

Figure 8–6. Recognition of complex ligands by B cells. **A:** Immunoglobulin cross-linking by antigen can transmit a signal through the B-cell antigen receptor (BCR) alone. **B:** Signaling is enhanced when the antigen is complexed with other immunologically relevant ligands such as the C3d fragment of complement (see Chapter 12), which engages a separate receptor called complement receptor 2 (CR2) that synergizes with the BCR. **C:** Signaling may be inhibited if the antigen is complexed with an antibody (ie, the antigen exists as an antigen–antibody complex) because the antibody engages a surface Fc receptor (in this case, FcγRII), which antagonizes signaling by the BCR by recruiting signaling molecules that inactivate Ras and oppose PI 3-kinase.

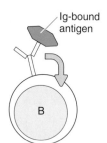

1. internalize
2. process to peptides
3. bind peptides to
   class II MHC
4. Express peptide–MHC II
   complex on cell surface

A   antigen uptake by B cell

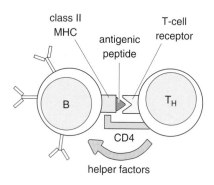

B   antigen presentation to T$_H$ cell

Figure 8–7. Antigen presentation by a B lymphocyte to a CD4 T lymphocyte. **A:** The antigen-specific B cell can bind antigen via membrane immunoglobulin (Ig) and **B:** internalize the antigen and present it to helper T cells. Presentation does not require, but is likely to result in, activation of the B cell.

presentation of antigen to naive T cells leads to their inactivation. In contrast, a T$_H$ cell that has recently been activated by antigen presented by other cells expressing B7.1 or B7.2 can provide help to a B cell even if it does not express the costimulatory molecules. Activated B cells may also secrete IL-6 and TNFα, which (like IL-1) increase the efficiency of T$_H$-cell activation.

In addition to antigen uptake, the BCR stimulates the ability of a B cell to present antigen to T cells via its signaling function. BCR signaling induces increased expression of class II MHC molecules, induces expression of B7.1 and B7.2, and enhances cell–cell adhesion by increasing the binding affinity of the adhesion molecule LFA-1. These features of BCR function serve to promote antigen-specific antibody responses by favoring interactions between antigen-specific T$_H$ cells and antigen-stimulated B cells.

Although they offer unique advantages, B cells also have important limitations as antigen-presenting cells. They are not present in large numbers at most sites in the body, and, because they have little phago-

cytic capacity, they are unable to process many types of particulate antigens. Most importantly, in an unimmunized person, B cells specific for any given antigen are exceedingly rare. Consequently, other types of antigen-presenting cells, particularly dendritic cells, usually play the dominant role in initiating primary humoral responses. B cells then become increasingly important in this capacity at each subsequent encounter with antigen.

IMMUNOGLOBULIN SECRETION

When a B cell becomes activated and divides, its daughter cells do not regain the capacity for V/(D)/J rearrangement, but rather continue to express the rearranged genes they inherited from their clonal forebears. Some undergo further differentiation to become **plasma cells,** which secrete large amounts of immunoglobulin derived from the same genes (up to thousands of antibody molecules per second). Some of the cells that commit to becoming plasma cells migrate to the bone marrow in order to do so. Whereas plasma cells that remain in lymphoid tissue produce antibody for about a week and then die, plasma cells in the bone marrow have a much longer life span. As a result, the marrow contains the great majority of the body's plasma cells and is the main source of circulating antibodies.

The shift from producing membrane-bound to secreted immunoglobulin that occurs in plasma cells reflects a subtle change in the structure of the heavy-chain mRNA. The short hydrophobic tail that anchors a heavy-chain protein onto the cell membrane is encoded by the final two exons of every C$_H$ region; when a B cell differentiates into a plasma cell, it produces an alternative form of heavy-chain mRNA that lacks these final exons and so encodes a heavy-chain protein that can be secreted from the cell (see Figure 3–4). In the case of μ heavy chains, this slightly truncated mRNA is designated μ$_s$. B cells that coexpress surface IgM and IgD almost always secrete only IgM (in pentameric form, complexed with J chains); IgD is rarely secreted.

MEMORY B LYMPHOCYTES

Most B cells within a proliferating clone that do not differentiate into plasma cells instead revert to the resting state to become memory B lymphocytes. Many of these memory cells ultimately take up residence within lymphoid follicles, where they survive for years; if subsequently activated, they undergo further cycles of replication to produce still more memory and plasma cells. In general, the progeny at each stage continue to express the same immunoglobulin genes as their parents. Two specialized types of genetic processes, however, occur at high frequency whenever memory B cells proliferate in the periphery. These processes—known as class switching and somatic hypermutation—further diversify the immunoglobulin genes expressed by some of the replicating cells and can permanently alter the characteristics of the B-cell clone. In the following sections, we consider each of these phenomena in turn.

THE HEAVY-CHAIN CLASS SWITCH

As a B-cell clone proliferates, individual daughter cells often appear that express a heavy-chain class (such as γ or α) that differs from that of the founder (Figure 8–8A). This phenomenon is called **class switching,** or isotype switching. It results from a specialized type of DNA rearrangement in the expressed heavy-chain gene, whereby a new C_H region is moved to a position adjacent to the existing V/D/J exon by deleting all intervening C_H sequences on the chromosome (see Figure 8–8B). Although class switching bears some resemblance to V/(D)/J joining, the two processes are believed to occur through entirely different enzymatic pathways. In particular, switching occurs in mature B cells that no longer express RAG-1 and RAG-2 and hence cannot carry out V/(D)/J joining. In addition, switching takes place at distinct chromosomal sites (called **switch regions**)

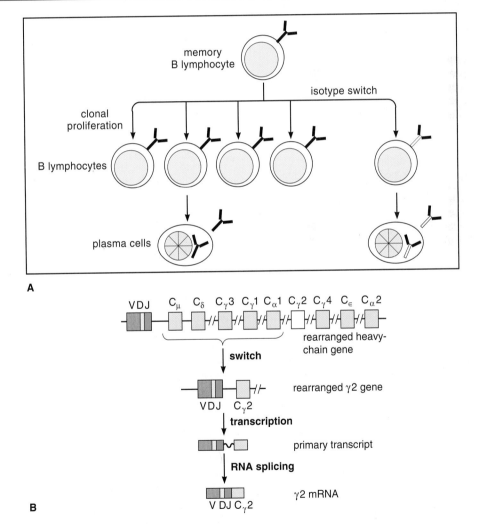

Figure 8–8. Heavy-chain class switch. **A:** During clonal proliferation of an activated memory B cell, some daughter cells may arise that express a different heavy-chain isotype and pass this trait on to their progeny. **B:** Class switching takes place when a fully assembled heavy-chain locus undergoes an additional DNA rearrangement event that places a new C_H sequence adjacent to the V/D/J exon. This occurs by deletion of the intervening C_H exons and is carried out by an enzymatic pathway distinct from that of V/D/J rearrangement. In the example shown, the gene switches to the $C_{\gamma2}$ isotype.

that are located within the introns upstream of the first C_H exon of each heavy-chain gene. As switching occurs within introns, it does not change the structure of the V/D/J exon and therefore does not affect antigen specificity. Because class switching occurs by deleting one or more heavy-chain isotype genes, it is normally irreversible.

Through the process of class switching, a pre-assembled V/D/J exon that was originally linked to C_μ can become associated with any of the other heavy-chain constant-region sequences. By this means, the effector function of an antibody can be changed without altering its specificity for antigen. The choice of a new C_H isotype is strongly influenced by cytokines and other factors acting on the B cell. For example, the microenvironment found in Peyer's patches favors switching to $C_{\alpha 1}$, resulting in the production of IgA. This appears to be due to the action of a cytokine called transforming growth factor beta (TGFβ). Similarly, exposure of the activated B cell to IL-4 promotes switching to C_ε. In the mouse, IL-4, TGFβ, and interferon gamma (IFNγ) each promote class switching to different IgG subtypes. In the human, less is known about the control of switching, although IFNγ and IL-4 are known to promote switching to IgG1 and IgG4, respectively. If a cell that has switched continues to divide, its progeny (both memory and plasma cells) also express the new heavy-chain isotype. As a rule, subclones expressing non-μ isotypes become increasingly prevalent during a T-cell-dependent antibody response, and their isotype distribution increasingly reflects the peripheral tissue in which the proliferation has occurred: Memory cells in subepithelial regions most commonly express IgA, whereas IgM- and IgG-expressing memory cells are predominant elsewhere.

SOMATIC HYPERMUTATION

Fully assembled V/J and V/D/J exons in B cells undergo point mutation at an unusually high rate during the course of an immune response. The mechanism of this phenomenon, termed **somatic hypermutation,** is unknown but appears quite specific in that adjacent regions on the chromosome (including the C_H exon) are not affected. As the mutations are introduced into the variable region exon at random, they can have the effect of either increasing or decreasing affinity of the resulting immunoglobulin for its target antigen. Individual cells that express higher affinity mutants are selected from this pool of cells by virtue of their high affinity for antigen. This occurs by a complicated process in the germinal center, which is described later. This selection process is thought to account for a phenomenon known as **affinity maturation:** the observation that antibodies produced later in an immune response tend to have higher affinity for the target antigen than those produced earlier.

LYMPHOID FOLLICLES & GERMINAL CENTERS

The initial encounter between B cells and antigen most commonly occurs within a lymphoid organ, such as a lymph node or submucosal lymphoid tissue because that is where most B cells normally reside. An antigen may be transported into the lymphoid organ by a dendritic cell (see Chapter 6), which can then present it directly to cognate T_H cells. Alternatively, free antigen may enter by way of lymphatic channels to be captured and presented to the antigen-specific B cell by resident macrophages or may be captured directly by the specific B cell itself. In each case, antigen stimulates the B cell to alter its responsiveness to chemokines that direct traffic of lymphocytes within the lymph node. As a result, the antigen-activated B cell migrates toward the T-cell zone, where it may encounter antigen-specific helper T cells that have been activated by dendritic cells and that can recognize the complexes of antigen with class II MHC molecules on the B-cell surface. Recognition of this antigen by the activated T cell leads to a stable interaction between the two antigen-specific lymphocytes within the T-cell zone. This interaction promotes the proliferation of both cells. Some B cells soon terminally differentiate into plasma cells in the lymph node, whereas others migrate, along with some of the antigen-specific T_H cells, from the T-cell zone into a nearby lymphoid follicle, where they proliferate and differentiate (Figure 8–9A).

In the absence of an ongoing immune response, a lymphoid follicle consists mainly of a polyclonal collection of resting B lymphocytes, each enveloped within the spidery cytoplasmic processes of specialized supportive cells called **follicular dendritic cells (FDCs).** The FDCs, which are unrelated to other types of dendritic cells despite the unfortunate similarities in name and morphology, appear to be responsible for organizing the follicle and controlling many of its activities. Unlike dendritic cells, FDCs are not derived from a bone marrow precursor cell, and they do not ordinarily present antigens to T cells. FDCs express abundant surface Fc receptors, however, and are therefore very efficient at capturing antigen–antibody complexes; in the presence of preformed antibodies, this enables FDCs to trap unprocessed antigens within follicles, where they may persist for weeks or even months on the FDC surface.

Activated B cells that enter the follicle then begin to proliferate very rapidly, with a generation time as short as 6 hours. The clonal progeny of the founder B cells become visible within 3 days to a week as a **germinal center**—a roughly spherical group of blast cells that tend to push aside the surrounding FDCs and resting lymphocytes of the original follicle (see Figure 8–9B). Each germinal center results from the

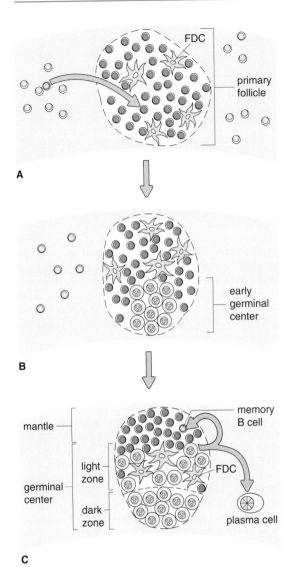

A

B

C

Figure 8–9. Dynamics of a lymphoid follicle during a humoral response. **A:** An antigen-specific B cell *(in dark blue)* contacts antigen and receives help from an activated T_H cell in the T-cell-rich zone of a lymphoid organ (in this case, the paracortex of a lymph node). It migrates into an adjacent primary lymphoid follicle and undergoes blast transformation. *Abbreviation:* FDC = follicular dendritic cell. **B:** After 3–7 days, clonal progeny of the B cell *(in dark blue)* appear as an early germinal center, which displaces the FDCs and resting polyclonal B cells of the original follicle toward the afferent surface of the node. **C:** After 1–4 weeks, the germinal center has matured to form a dark zone, populated mainly by proliferating blasts, and an apical light zone, where nonproliferating progeny of these blasts contact FDCs. Cells that survive selection in the light zone emerge as memory cells or plasma cells. The newly formed memory B cells, as well as those from the original primary follicle, make up the follicular mantle overlying the germinal center. Photographs of germinal centers exhibiting these features can be seen in Figures 3–12 and 3–14.

clonal expansion of only one or a few activated B-cell founders. Over time, the germinal center enlarges and becomes polarized into two morphologically distinct zones (see Figure 8–9C). The **dark zone** (which, in a lymph node, tends to be located near the efferent side of the follicle, ie, near the medulla) is composed of rapidly proliferating B cells called **centroblasts.** It is during the proliferation of centroblasts in the dark zone that hypermutation takes place within the V/D/J and V/J exons of the rearranged immunoglobulin genes.

As individual centroblasts cease dividing, they move into the adjacent **light zone,** where they acquire the name **centrocytes** and come into contact with FDCs that bear unprocessed antigens. The light zone is believed to be a region of intense selective pressure where numerous centrocytes compete to bind a limited amount of cognate antigen on the surface of the FDCs. Centrocytes whose BCR binds antigen survive, whereas those that fail to bind die by apoptosis. This is thought to be the basis for selecting cells that produce high-affinity immunoglobulins: In a competitive situation, surface immunoglobulins of higher affinity are thought to compete for antigen more effectively than those of lower affinity. Cells with higher affinity immunoglobulins not only are stimulated more strongly through their BCRs, but also compete more effectively in internalizing antigen and presenting it to local T_H cells, and hence receive more effective help, as described earlier. Together, these selective processes likely account for the antibody affinity maturation that occurs as a humoral response proceeds.

Centrocytes that survive the selection process emerge from the germinal center as either plasma cells or memory B cells. The plasma cells generally exit the follicle, either remaining in the lymphoid organ or migrating to the bone marrow. Memory cells often move into the follicular mantle, joining the original polyclonal population of memory B cells that remain in the follicle after the immune response subsides and the germinal center regresses. The T_H-cell surface molecule CD40L appears to play a role in inducing centrocytes to develop into memory cells rather than into plasma cells. Interestingly, patients with the X-linked hyper-IgM syndrome, in which CD40L is defective, fail to develop germinal centers at all.

PRIMARY & SECONDARY HUMORAL RESPONSES

Of necessity, the properties of a primary humoral immune response (ie, the antibody response that occurs the first time an individual encounters a given antigen) reflect the properties of naive lymphocytes. Because B cells with the appropriate specificity are rare in unimmunized hosts, most of the antigen must be processed by dendritic cells and presented to antigen-specific helper T cells, which are also correspondingly rare. These antigen-activated T_H cells multiply and then must contact and promote the activation of antigen-specific B cells, which must in turn proliferate and differentiate into plasma cells in sufficient numbers to be effective. The initially low frequencies of antigen-specific T cells and B cells and the necessity of their expansion account for the lag time (typically 5–10 days) required to reach peak serum antibody concentrations in a primary response, and for the relatively low concentrations achieved (Table 8–1). The antibodies initially produced are predominantly IgM—the type secreted by most direct progeny of naive B cells—and have, on average, low antigen affinities. The pentameric structure of IgM helps compensate for this low intrinsic affinity by providing multiple binding sites so that antigens with multiple copies of individual epitopes can be bound with a higher avidity.

Subsequent responses, by contrast, are increasingly dominated by antigen-specific memory cells, whose sheer numbers enhance both the speed and intensity of the response (see Table 8–1). In a highly immunized lymph node, as many as one in a few hundred B cells may be specific for the target antigen. Memory B cells may serve as the principal antigen-presenting cells in secondary responses, and so enable helper T cells to become activated at very low concentrations of antigen. In the process, the B cells themselves are ideally positioned for activation because they are stimulated strongly both by antigen induction of BCR signaling and by direct contact with the helper cells (see Figure 8–7). The responding B cells are more likely to express high-affinity antibodies, following selection in the germinal center during either the initial response or the secondary response. Although some plasma cells still produce IgM in a secondary response, a substantial number of plasma cells arise from class-switched B-cell subclones and instead secrete IgG, IgA, or IgE. These latter isotypes therefore tend to predominate in secondary responses, depending on the site at which the response occurs: Secondary responses in the peripheral lymph nodes are predominantly IgG, whereas those at mucosal surfaces are mainly IgA.

B-CELL TOLERANCE

The random assembly of V, D, and J segments during lymphopoiesis inevitably produces some B-cell clones whose immunoglobulins recognize self-determinants on normal host cells or tissues. Because such autoreactive immunoglobulins are potentially deleterious to the host, stringent measures are needed to ensure that they are not secreted. In most cases, these measures operate successfully; the immune system remains specifically **tolerant** toward the many self-determinants to which it is continually exposed. In contrast, in some people antibodies to certain self-components are made and lead to tissue or organ damage. These diseases are referred to as **autoimmune diseases** because the immune system has lost tolerance to certain self-components.

The B cells that make autoreactive immunoglobulins are normally silenced in two main ways. The first applies to the situation in which an immature B cell contacts antigen in the bone marrow shortly after it begins expressing surface immunoglobulins. This results in maturational arrest; the cell fails to mature further and does not exit the marrow. Instead, the cell reactivates expression of the RAG-1 and RAG-2 recombinase proteins, so that it is able to resume rearranging its light-chain genes. Like 60–70% of all human B lymphocytes, many autoreactive B cells initially express κ light chains; in those cells, the reactivated recombinase is able to carry out a special type of DNA rearrangement in which a V_κ or J_κ segment in the active κ-gene locus becomes fused to a site downstream of the C_κ segment, which is called the κ-**deleting element** (Figure 8–10). As a result of this rearrangement, the C_κ segment and other important regions are deleted, the gene is permanently inactivated, and the cell can then attempt to assemble a new κ or λ gene on one of its other chromosomes. This process has been called **receptor editing.** If the

Table 8–1. Comparison of primary and secondary humoral immune responses.

	Primary response	Secondary response
Antigen presentation	Mainly by non-B cells	B lymphocytes increasingly important
Antigen concentration needed to induce response	Relatively high	Relatively low

Antibody response
  Lag phase
  Peak concentration
  Class(es)
	5–10 days
	Relatively low
	Mostly IgM
		2–5 days
		Relatively high
		Other classes (IgG, IgA, etc) often predominate, in tissue-specific manner

Average antigen affinity	Relatively low	Relatively high

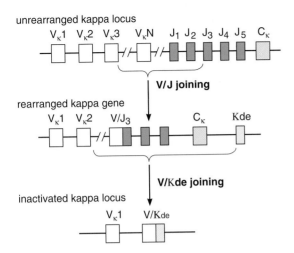

unrearranged kappa locus

Figure 8–10. Rearrangements that remove a functionally rearranged κ light-chain gene. In immature B cells that contact self-antigen, maturation is arrested and the recombination-activating genes RAG-1 and RAG-2 are reexpressed. Among the reactions that can be performed by the V/D/J recombinase is a rearrangement between either an unrearranged V_κ gene (as shown) or a sequence in the intron between J_κ and C_κ with a sequence 24 kb downstream of the C_κ gene called the κ-deleting element (Kde). This deletes the intervening DNA, including C_κ, and results in a nonfunctional gene. This reaction may occur as part of receptor editing, whereby a self-reactive immature B cell attempts to change light chain and thereby its antigen specificity.

original κ chain contributed to recognition of self-antigen, then replacing it with a new light chain may eliminate autoreactivity. In that case, the cell can resume maturation, shut off its recombinase activity,

and be released from the marrow. If receptor editing fails, then the autoreactive B cell remains arrested in the undifferentiated state and eventually dies.

The receptor-editing mechanism applies only to immature B cells, and so would be effective only for eliminating cells that recognize self-antigens found in the bone marrow, such as serum proteins and ubiquitous cell surface or extracellular matrix proteins. Many other self-antigens, however, are found only outside the marrow, and for these antigens a different mechanism is needed to ensure B-cell tolerance. This mechanism acts only on B cells in peripheral tissues and relies on the fact that B-cell activation by most protein antigens requires the participation of helper T cells. When a mature B cell contacts antigen in the absence of appropriate T-cell help, the B cell either dies or loses its ability to carry out an immune response. The fate of the B cell depends on the physical nature of the antigen involved. In the case of membrane-bound or particulate antigens, the self-reactive B cell generally dies—a phenomenon referred to as **clonal deletion.** Soluble protein antigens, which presumably generate weaker signals through the BCR of a self-reactive B cell, do not cause cell death but instead make the cell unresponsive to activating stimuli—a phenomenon called **clonal anergy.** Anergic B cells can become activated under some circumstances, so clonal anergy is thought to be a less absolute mechanism for enforcing tolerance to self. Anergic B cells, however, cannot compete effectively with nonanergic B cells for survival and proliferation in the body; as a result, the anergic cells probably die within a few days, so that clonal anergy and clonal deletion differ only in the short term. It remains to be determined precisely how clonal anergy and clonal deletion are circumvented in people who develop autoimmune disease.

REFERENCES

B-CELL DEVELOPMENT

Burnet FM: A modification of Jerne's theory of antibody production using the concept of clonal selection. *Aust J Sci* 1957;20:67.

Kantor AB, Herzenberg LA: Origin of murine B cell lineages. *Annu Rev Immunol* 1993;11:501.

Kincade PW et al: Cells and molecules that regulate B lymphopoiesis in bone marrow. *Annu Rev Immunol* 1989;7:111.

Kitamura D et al: A B cell-deficient mouse by targeted disruption of the membrane exon of the immunoglobulin μ chain gene. *Nature* 1991;350:423.

Li Y-S et al: The regulated expression of B lineage associated genes during B cell differentiation in bone marrow and fetal liver. *J Exp Med* 1993;178:951.

Nussenzweig MC: Immune receptor editing: Revise and select. *Cell* 1998;95:875.

Rolink A, Melchers F: Molecular and cellular origins of B lymphocyte diversity. *Cell* 1991;66:1081.

Vetrie D et al: The gene involved in X-linked agammaglobulinemia is a member of the Src-family of protein-tyrosine kinases. *Nature* 1993;361:226.

B-CELL SURFACE RECEPTORS & SIGNALING

DeFranco AL: Transmembrane signaling by antigen receptors of B and T lymphocytes. *Curr Opin Cell Biol* 1995;7:163.

Kurosaki T: Genetic analysis of B cell antigen receptor signaling. *Annu Rev Immunol* 1999;17:555.

Lam KP et al: In vivo ablation of surface immunoglobulin on mature B cells by inducible gene targeting results in rapid cell death. *Cell* 1997;90:1073.

Reth M: Antigen receptors on B lymphocytes. *Annu Rev Immunol* 1992;10:97.

Scharenberg AM, Kinet JP: The emerging field of receptor-mediated inhibitory signaling: SHP or SHIP? *Cell* 1996; 87:961.

Zola H: The surface antigens of human B lymphocytes. *Immunol Today* 1987;8:308.

B-CELL ACTIVATION

Arpin C et al: Generation of memory B cells and plasma cells in vitro. *Science* 1995;268:720.

Aruffo A et al: The CD40 ligand, gp39, is defective in activated T cells from patients with X-linked hyper-IgM syndrome. *Cell* 1993;72:291.

Banchereau J et al: The CD40 antigen and its ligand. *Annu Rev Immunol* 1994;12:881.

Clark EA, Lane PJL: Regulation of human B-cell activation and adhesion. *Annu Rev Immunol* 1991;9:97.

Clark EA, Ledbetter JA: How B and T cells talk to each other. *Nature* 1994;367:425.

Cyster JG: Chemokines and cell migration in secondary lymphoid organs. *Science* 1999:286:2098.

MacLennan ICM: Germinal centers. *Annu Rev Immunol* 1994;12:117.

Mond JJ et al: T cell-independent antigens type 2. *Annu Rev Immunol* 1995;13:655.

Parker DC: T cell-dependent B-cell activation. *Annu Rev Immunol* 1993;11:331.

Rajewsky K: Clonal selection and learning in the antibody system. *Nature* 1996;381:751.

Slifka MK, Ahmed R: Long-lived plasma cells: A mechanism for maintaining persistent antibody production. *Curr Opinion Immunol* 1998;10:252.

Vitetta ES et al: Cellular interactions in the humoral immune response. *Adv Immunol* 1989;45:1.

HEAVY-CHAIN CLASS SWITCHING & IMMU-NOGLOBULIN SECRETION

Early P et al: Two mRNAs can be produced from a single immunoglobulin μ gene by alternative RNA processing pathways. *Cell* 1979;20:313.

Finkelman FD et al: Lymphokine control of in vivo immunoglobulin isotype selection. *Annu Rev Immunol* 1990; 8:303.

Harriman W et al: Immunoglobulin class-switch recombinations. *Annu Rev Immunol* 1993;11:385.

Wagner SD, Neuberger MS: Somatic hypermutation of immunoglobulin genes. *Annu Rev Immunol* 1996;14:441.

B-CELL TOLERANCE

Cyster JG et al: Competition for follicular niches excludes self-reactive cells from the recirculating B-cell repertoire. *Nature* 1994;371:389.

Goodnow CC et al: The need for central and peripheral tolerance in the B repertoire. *Science* 1990;248:1373.

Goodnow CC: Transgenic mice and analysis of B cell tolerance. *Annu Rev Immunol* 1992;10:489.

Schwartz RH: Acquisition of immunological self-tolerance. *Cell* 1989;57:1073.

Tiegs SL et al: Receptor editing in self-reactive bone marrow B cells. *J Exp Med* 1993;177:1009.

T Lymphocytes & Natural Killer Cells

9

John B. Imboden, MD, & William E. Seaman, MD

The acquired immune response relies heavily on the ability of thymus-derived (T) lymphocytes to recognize and discriminate among a wide range of different foreign antigens. As is the case with B lymphocytes, the enormous diversity of the T-cell repertoire stems from the ability of developing T cells to rearrange and modify the genes that encode their antigen receptors. An appreciation of the structure and function of the T-cell antigen receptor (TCR) is essential for understanding T-cell development and the complexities of the responses of mature T cells to antigen.

T-CELL ANTIGEN RECEPTOR

T lymphocytes do not "see" soluble antigens, but rather recognize antigen bound to specialized molecules on the surfaces of other cells. Although some T cells recognize glycolipids and other nonprotein antigens, most T cells respond to protein antigens and recognize these antigens in the form of peptide fragments associated with class I or class II molecules of the major histocompatibility (MHC) locus. Mature T cells express one of two types of TCR: a heterodimer composed either of α and β chains or of γ and δ chains. Because T cells expressing $\alpha\beta$ receptors account for T-cell helper function and cytotoxic activity, the major focus of this chapter will be on this type of TCR. $\gamma\delta$ T cells, whose physiologic role is still unclear, will be reviewed later on.

The $\alpha\beta$ TCR dimer recognizes peptides bound to MHC molecules. The amino-terminal regions of the α and β chains are polymorphic, so that within the entire T-cell population a large number of different TCR $\alpha\beta$ dimers occur, each capable of recognizing a particular combination of antigenic peptide and MHC. The TCRs on individual T cells generally contain only a single type of $\alpha\beta$ dimer and, therefore, individual T cells respond only to a specific combination of antigen and MHC.

The $\alpha\beta$ dimer is associated with a complex of proteins designated CD3 (Figure 9–1). The CD3 chains are not polymorphic and range in size from 16 to 28 kd. They are involved in signal transduction and thus allow the TCR to convert the recognition of antigen–MHC into intracellular signals for activation. Compared with TCR α and β, whose intracellular regions are only several amino acids in length, the CD3 chains have large cytoplasmic domains, ranging from 45 to 55 amino acids for CD3 ε, δ, and γ to 113 amino acids for CD3ζ.

TCR α & β GENES & THE GENERATION OF TCR DIVERSITY

To generate the diversity of TCRs required to recognize a wide spectrum of antigenic determinants, the TCR α and β genes use a strategy of recombination similar to that of the immunoglobulin genes (see Chapter 7). The germline TCR β-gene locus contains 20–30 V (variable), 2 D (diversity), and 13 J (joining) gene segments (Figure 9–2). When the TCR β gene rearranges early in T-cell ontogeny, one of the V_β segments is linked to one of the D_β regions and to one of the J_β segments to form a complete exon. After transcription, RNA processing combines the V/D/J exon with a C_β (constant) region to form a TCR β-messenger RNA that encodes a functional protein. The potential diversity generated by this combinatorial joining is equal to the product of the number of possible V segments $\times$ the number of D segments $\times$ the number of J segments. Similarly, in the TCR α locus, there are approximately 100 V segments and 50 J segments (but no D segments). To form a functional TCR α-chain gene, a V_α segment joins to a J_α segment. As in immunoglobulin genes, diversity is further enhanced by imprecise joining and by the insertion of nongermline-encoded nucleotides (N regions) between segments during the rearrangement process. These mechanisms each enhance the diversity of sequences at the junctions between V_α and J_α and between the V_β, D_β, and J_β segments (junctional diversity). N-region insertion is carried out by the enzyme terminal deoxynucleotidyltransferase (TdT), which is

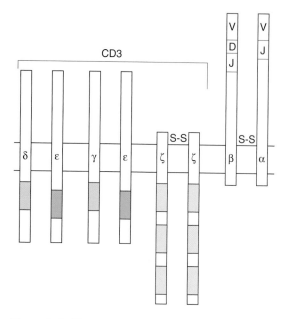

Figure 9–1. The T-cell antigen receptor (TCR). The TCR is a complex of eight transmembrane proteins. The α and β chains form a disulfide-linked (S–S) dimer that is responsible for the recognition of antigenic peptides bound to class I and class II major histocompatability class (MHC) molecules. The amino-terminal regions of the α and β chains, which are formed through rearrangements of V, D, and J segments, are highly polymorphic. The αβ dimer is noncovalently associated with the CD3 complex, which converts the recognition of antigen into transmembrane signals. The CD3 polypeptides are not polymorphic and have larger cytoplasmic domains than TCR α and β. The CD3 complex consists of three sets of dimers. There are two CD3ε chains, one paired with CD3γ and the other with CD3δ. The ζ chain exists either as a disulfide-linked ζ/ζ homodimer (as shown here) or as a heterodimer with either η (an alternatively spliced form of ζ) or the γ chain. The functional importance of this variation in the ζ dimer is not understood. The cytoplasmic domains of CD3 chains contain one or more immune receptor tyrosine-based activation motifs (ITAMs), depicted here as shaded boxes.

expressed in the nuclei of immature T cells at the stage when V/(D)/J recombination occurs. Unlike immunoglobulin genes, TCR genes do not undergo somatic hypermutation.

αβ TCR STRUCTURE & RECOGNITION OF ANTIGEN

αβ TCRs recognize antigen in the form of peptides bound in the groove on the "top" of class I or class II MHC molecules. The TCR αβ dimer resembles an immunoglobulin Fab fragment in its overall structure, with the hypervariable regions (or complementarity-determining regions, CDRs) forming loops that ex-

tend from the end of a barrel-like variable-region domain. X-ray crystallographic studies of αβ TCR proteins bound to peptide-class I MHC complexes reveal that the TCR interacts directly with both the peptide and the MHC protein. The TCR binds so that the loops with greatest sequence diversity (ie, the CDR3 loop of each antigen-binding site) lie directly over the center of the peptide. The TCR interacts with the MHC molecule along the exposed surfaces of the two α helices that form the sides of the peptide-binding groove. Most contacts with the MHC molecule are formed with amino acids that are conserved in each MHC allele. Interactions with polymorphic MHC residues, however, are also critical and form the structural basis for the long-standing observation that the T-cell system is heavily biased toward recognizing peptides bound to self–MHC molecules. This "MHC restriction" results from a process of positive selection in the thymus that selectively favors the growth and survival of developing T cells whose TCRs have the potential to recognize peptides presented by self-MHC, as will be described later on.

INTERACTION OF THE TCR WITH SUPERANTIGENS

Superantigens are a class of bacterial toxins and retroviral proteins that have the ability to bind both MHC class II molecules and the TCR β chain. In so doing, they act as a "clamp" between the TCR and class II molecule, providing signals to the T cells. It is important to grasp the differences between classical antigenic peptides and superantigens. Superantigens are not processed and interact with the MHC molecule outside of the peptide-binding groove. On the T-cell side, superantigens bind to V_β segments only, without regard to the D_β and J_β regions or to any part of the TCR α chain (Figure 9–3). Superantigens differ in the V_β sequences they can bind, with any given superantigen binding only those encoded by one or a few V_β gene segments. Activation of T cells by individual superantigens, therefore, is selective for T cells whose TCRs express particular V_β segments.

Because superantigens only recognize the V_β segment and not the other components of the TCR αβ dimer, a superantigen has the capability of activating 1–10% of peripheral T cells (this is orders of magnitude more than a conventional antigen). Exposure to a superantigen, therefore, can lead to massive T-cell activation, and the ensuing release of large amounts of lymphokines accounts for many of the manifestations of acute exposure to bacterial toxins that have superantigen capabilities. This likely explains the clinical features of **toxic shock syndrome,** which can be induced by *Staphylococcus aureus* toxin TSST-1, a superantigen that activates human T cells expressing $V_{\beta 2}$. In the acute phase of toxic shock syndrome there is a marked, and selective, expansion of T cells

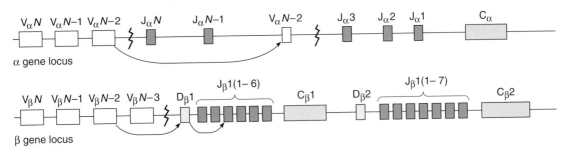

Figure 9–2. Rearrangement of the TCR α and β genes. The TCR α-gene locus contains multiple V and J segments, only several of which are shown here. Similarly, the TCR β-gene locus contains multiple V, D, and J segments. During T-cell ontogeny, the TCR genes rearrange *(arrows)*, so that one of the V_α segments pairs with the J_α segment and a V_β segment pairs with a D_β and J_β segment. The two C (constant) segments in the β gene are very similar, and differential use of $C_{\beta 1}$ and $C_{\beta 2}$ does not contribute to TCR diversity.

that bear $V_{\beta 2}$: in one case, 70% of peripheral T cells were $V_{\beta 2}{}^+$ in the acute phase of the disease. Under other conditions, however, the activation induced by a superantigen leads to apoptosis of the activated cells, so that eventually T cells expressing the cognate V_β segment are selectively depleted from the population.

CD4 & CD8 CORECEPTORS

The expression of CD4 and CD8 divides mature T cells into two mutually exclusive subsets: those that recognize antigen in the context of class II MHC molecules (CD4 cells) and those that recognize antigen bound to class I molecules (CD8 cells). CD4 binds to a membrane-proximal region of MHC class II molecules that is not directly involved in peptide binding; CD8, on the other hand, binds to a corresponding region on MHC class I molecules (see Figure 6–1). It is possible, therefore, that CD4 or CD8 interacts with the same MHC molecule as the TCR

during T-cell activation (Figure 9–4). There is considerable evidence to support this notion and to suggest that CD4 and CD8 are in close proximity to the TCR, functioning as coreceptors.

T-CELL ONTOGENY

STAGES OF THYMOCYTE DEVELOPMENT

T cells develop from bone-marrow-derived progenitor cells that undergo maturation in the thymus (Figure 9–5). Early in development, thymocytes ex-

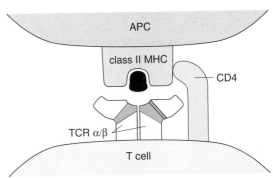

Figure 9–4. CD4 coreceptor. CD4 binds class II MHC molecules at a membrane-proximal region not directly involved in peptide binding. In the model depicted here, the coreceptor binds the same MHC molecule that engages the TCR. CD8 plays a similar coreceptor role on T cells that recognize antigen in association with class I MHC molecules. CD8 binds a nonpolymorphic region on MHC class I molecules. Because the cytoplasmic domains of CD4 and CD8 interact with Lck, the coreceptors can bring this Src-like protein tyrosine kinase into proximity with the TCR.

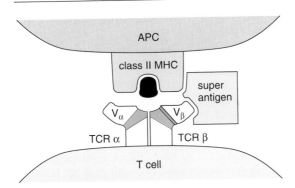

Figure 9–3. Model of the interactions between the TCR, class II MHC molecule, and a superantigen. The superantigen interacts with the MHC molecule outside the peptide groove and binds only to the V_β segment of the TCR.

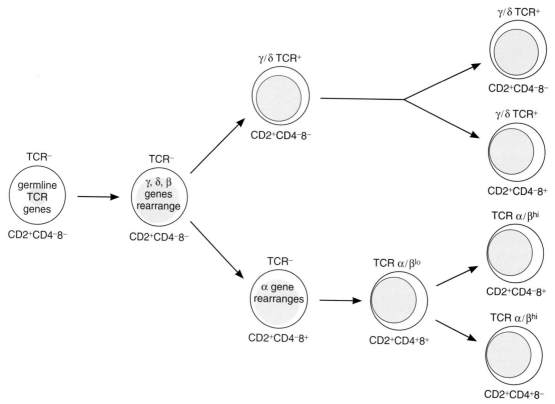

Figure 9–5. Stages in thymocyte development. Progenitor cells migrate from the bone marrow to the thymus. At the earliest stages of development, thymocytes express several T-cell surface molecules, such as CD2, but still have germline configurations of their TCR genes. Thymocytes destined to become αβ T cells pass through a critical CD4$^+$CD8$^+$ phase during which positive and negative selection occur.

press several cell surface molecules, such as CD2, that are characteristic of the T-cell lineage, but they lack many others, including CD4 and CD8, and thus are known as **double-negative thymocytes.** Rearrangement of the TCR genes begins in the double-negative stage. Cells that are destined to become αβ T cells rearrange the β gene first. If rearrangement at the TCR β locus is successful, the resulting β-chain polypeptide pairs with an invariant polypeptide called pTα. The pTα-TCRβ dimer then associates with CD3 chains and is expressed on the cell surface as a pre-TCR. Expression of the pre-TCR serves to terminate further rearrangements at the TCR β gene locus and is required for efficient transition to the next major stage in development, when thymocytes express both CD4 and CD8 and are called **double-positive** cells. Rearrangement of the TCR α gene occurs during the double-positive stage and, if successful, leads to low-level expression of an αβ TCR. As thymocytes mature into T cells, the level of TCR expression increases and the cells lose expression of either CD4 or CD8, becoming **single-positive.** At this stage, thymocytes have acquired

the phenotype of mature peripheral T cells and soon exit the thymus.

POSITIVE & NEGATIVE SELECTION OF THYMOCYTES

The generation of TCRs is a largely stochastic process and can produce T cells with undesirable antigen specificities. For this reason, enormous selective pressures are exerted within the thymus to allow survival of only those mature T cells whose TCRs are restricted by self–MHC molecules and are not autoreactive. The great majority of thymocytes fail this process: At least 99% of developing T cells die within the thymus. Two distinct types of selection have been observed, both of which occur at the stage when thymocytes are CD4$^+$CD8$^+$ (double-positive) and express low levels of TCR on the cell surface. **Positive selection** promotes the survival of thymocytes whose TCRs have the capability of recognizing antigens bound to self–MHC molecules.

Negative selection leads to the deletion of thymocytes whose TCRs recognize peptides derived from self-proteins.

Thymocytes are programmed to die by apoptosis unless they are rescued on the basis of the ability of their TCRs to recognize antigen in association with self–MHC molecules. A remarkable feature of this positive selection is that it leads to the selection of TCRs with specificity for foreign antigens bound to self–MHC yet occurs in the absence of the foreign antigen. Positive selection takes place in the thymic cortex, where developing thymocytes encounter epithelial cells that express both class I and class II MHC molecules loaded with self-peptides (Figure 9–6). The molecular basis for positive selection remains uncertain, but clearly involves signaling through the TCR. It appears that TCR binding to self-peptide–MHC complexes in the thymic cortex transmits a survival signal to the thymocyte, resulting in its positive selection. Thymocytes whose TCRs are completely unable to recognize self-peptide–MHC do not receive a survival signal, fail positive selec-

tion, and die. Failure of positive selection accounts for the great majority of intrathymic death.

Negative selection, which eliminates potentially autoreactive T cells, appears to occur primarily in the thymic medulla, where double-positive thymocytes migrate from the cortex. There, thymocytes encounter self-peptides presented in association with class I and class II MHC molecules on bone-marrow-derived dendritic cells and macrophages (see Figure 9–6). If a thymocyte recognizes these self-peptides with high affinity, it undergoes apoptosis. Thus, at this stage in T-cell development and in this context, recognition of antigen delivers signals that result in cell death rather than activation. Cells that do not receive this cell death signal mature and are exported from the thymus.

One recent hypothesis, called the **avidity model** of T-cell selection, proposes that, to a large extent, positive and negative selection represent qualitatively different responses to different intensities of signaling through the TCR. The overall strength of signaling in a T cell is proportional to TCR occupancy, which in

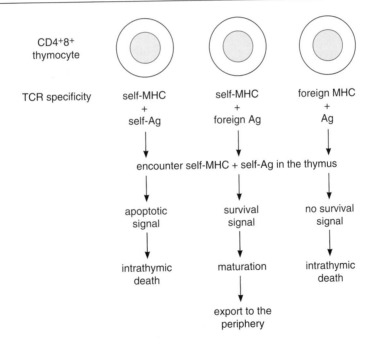

Figure 9–6. Positive and negative selection of thymocytes. CD4+CD8+TCR+ thymocytes encounter self-antigens bound to class I and class II major histocompatibility complex (MHC) molecules on epithelial cells in the thymic cortex and on macrophages and dendritic cells in the thymic medulla. In the resulting interactions, thymocytes whose T-cell receptors (TCRs) recognize self-MHC plus self-antigen will receive an apoptotic signal and undergo apoptosis in the thymus (negative selection). In contrast, thymocytes whose TCRs have specificity for self-MHC plus foreign antigens receive a survival signal that results in their positive selection. Thymocytes whose TCRs are unable to recognize antigens in association with self-MHC die of neglect (failure of positive selection). Differences in the binding affinities of TCRs for self-MHC plus self-antigen may explain these outcomes. Excessive signaling from high-affinity interactions leads to cell death, but intermediate levels of signaling from lower affinity interactions promote cell survival and rescue cells from death by neglect. The net result of thymic selections is the survival of T cells whose TCRs are restricted by self-MHC but that are not autoreactive.

turn reflects both the number of TCRs engaged and their affinity for binding the antigen–MHC complex. Below a certain level of TCR occupancy, no effective signal is transmitted. According to the avidity model, a moderate level of occupancy provides a positive signal that allows thymocyte growth and maturation, whereas excessive occupancy (above a certain, undefined threshold) causes cell death by apoptosis. Thymocytes whose receptors bind strongly to self-peptide–MHC complexes in the medulla would thus be eliminated (negative selection), whereas those that give weak but perceptible binding to the same complexes in the cortex would be positively selected. We do not yet know, in biochemical terms, exactly what constitutes the critical difference between the survival signal delivered by low-avidity TCR binding and the apoptotic signal triggered by high-avidity interactions. Nevertheless, the avidity model offers a plausible schema by which TCR–MHC interactions could guide both positive and negative thymic selection, and considerable evidence is accruing to support it.

For negative selection to eliminate all potentially autoreactive T cells, one might imagine that thymic medullary dendritic cells and macrophages would need to present all potential antigenic self-peptides, including those derived from proteins expressed in a highly tissue-specific fashion. To what extent this occurs is not yet clear; the array of peptides presented in the thymus is an area of ongoing investigation. It is known, however, that negative selection is not 100% effective and that some potentially autoreactive T cells do escape. Normally, these autoreactive cells are then either deleted in peripheral tissues or are rendered anergic (unresponsive to antigen). Alternatively, such cells may never encounter antigen simply because their cognate antigens are normally sequestered from the immune system. In certain pathologic states, however, one or more of these mechanisms for **peripheral tolerance** fails, leading to autoimmunity.

T-CELL ACTIVATION

When a T cell encounters an antigen-presenting cell (APC), the specificity of its TCR determines the outcome. Only if the TCR recognizes its particular antigen–MHC combination does activation occur. The recognition of appropriately presented antigen activates T cells to proliferate, differentiate, and perform their effector functions. Activation of helper T cells leads to the production of lymphokines that promote cellular and humoral immune responses, whereas activation of cytotoxic T cells results in killing of the antigen-bearing cells. Each of these T-cell responses depends on the ability of the TCR to generate intracellular signals for activation.

SIGNAL TRANSDUCTION BY THE TCR

Key to the ability of the TCR to deliver intracellular signals is its interactions with protein tyrosine kinases (PTKs). In unstimulated T cells, **Fyn,** a member of the Src family of PTKs, associates with the cytoplasmic domains of CD3 chains (Figure 9–7). A second Src-like PTK, called **Lck,** binds to the cytoplasmic domains of CD4 and CD8 and thus can be brought into proximity with the TCR through the interactions of these coreceptors with the MHC. Stimulation of the TCR by antigen-MHC triggers the phosphorylation of tyrosine residues in the cytoplasmic domains of the CD3 chains of the receptor complex. According to a widely accepted model of TCR signaling, Lck and Fyn are responsible for these initial phosphorylation events.

The antigen-induced tyrosine phosphorylation sites lie within particular amino acid sequences, designated immune receptor tyrosine-based activation motifs **(ITAMs),** found in the cytoplasmic domains of CD3 molecules. ITAMs are also present in the signaling chains of the B-cell antigen receptor and of certain Fc receptors. When tyrosine-phosphorylated, the CD3 ITAMs form a recognition unit for another PTK, called **ZAP-70,** and thus recruit ZAP-70 to the TCR complex. ZAP-70, either alone or together with the Src-like PTKs, appears largely responsible for the phosphorylation of a number of intracellular proteins. Mutations in ZAP-70 result in immunodeficiency in humans, underscoring the importance of ZAP-70 in TCR signaling.

Key signaling molecules activated by TCR stimulation include Ras and phospholipase C (PLC)γ-1 (see Chapter 1). The coupling of the TCR to the Ras and PLCγ-1 pathways involves complex linker molecules such as LAT (Figure 9–8). TCR stimulation triggers the tyrosine phosphorylation of LAT, a transmembrane protein. This phosphorylation induces LAT to associate with Grb2-Sos (an initiator of Ras activation) and PLCγ-1. The recruitment of these molecules to LAT is required for TCR-mediated activation of Ras and PLCγ-1. Activated Ras, in turn, stimulates the MAP kinase cascade of serine–threonine kinases (see Chapter 1). PLCγ-1 hydrolyzes the membrane phospholipid called phosphatidylinositol-(4,5)-bisphosphate (PIP_2). The ensuing breakdown of PIP_2 generates two second messengers: diacylglycerol and inositol-1,4,5-tris-phosphate (IP_3). Diacylglycerol activates the protein kinase C family of serine-threonine protein kinases. IP_3 releases Ca^{2+} from internal stores into the cytoplasm, causing an increase in the concentration of cytoplasmic free calcium ($[Ca^{2+}]_i$). Elevations in $[Ca^{2+}]_i$, activated protein kinase C, and the Ras pathway appear to be important mediators for many of the T-cell responses, including the induction of lymphokine gene transcription and the trig-

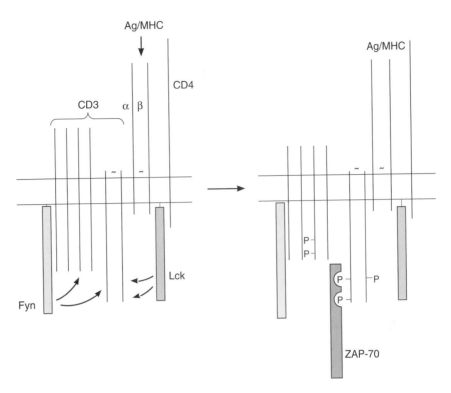

Figure 9–7. Model for the interactions of the T-cell antigen receptor with protein tyrosine kinases. In resting T cells, the CD3 components of the T-cell receptor (TCR) are associated with the protein tyrosine kinase Fyn, and the CD4 coreceptor is associated with Lck. On stimulation of the TCR, the CD3 chains are tyrosine phosphorylated on immunoreceptor tyrosine-based activation motifs (ITAMs), probably through the action of Fyn or Lck. The tyrosine-phosphorylated ITAMs in turn recruit a third protein tyrosine kinase, ZAP-70, to the receptor.

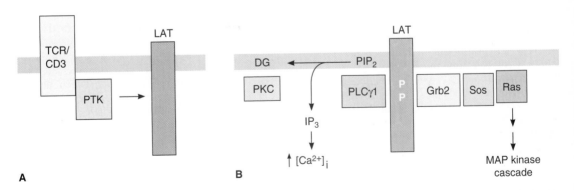

Figure 9–8. Activation of the phospholipase C (PLC) and Ras pathways by the T-cell receptor (TCR). **A:** Following TCR stimulation, protein tyrosine kinases (PTK) phosphorylate the linker protein LAT. **B:** Tyrosine-phosphorylated LAT then associates with phospholipase C γ-1 (PLCγ-1) and with Grb2-Sos. PLCγ-1 hydrolyzes phosphatidylinositol-(4,5)-bisphosphate (PIP_2), producing two second messengers: diacylglycerol (DG), which activates the protein kinase C (PKC) family of serine–threonine kinases, and inositol trisphosphate (IP_3), which triggers an increase in the concentration of cytosolic free calcium ions ($[Ca^{2+}]_i$). Grb2-Sos recruits and activates Ras, leading to activation of the MAP kinase cascade (see Chapter 1).

gering of cytolytic activity. One consequence of the increase in $[Ca^{2+}]_i$ is the activation of calcineurin, a Ca^{2+}-dependent serine phosphatase that plays a key role in activating the interleukin-2 (IL-2) gene. Calcineurin is the target of **cyclosporin** and FK506, two immunosuppressive drugs that block TCR-mediated production of IL-2. These drugs are widely used after clinical transplantation to prevent graft rejection.

CD45: A TYROSINE PHOSPHATASE REQUIRED FOR TCR SIGNALING

CD45 is a large (180–220 kd) transmembrane cell surface molecule that is expressed by all leukocytes, including all T lymphocytes. The cytoplasmic domain of CD45 has tyrosine phosphatase activity. Variants and mutants of T-cell lines that lack CD45 have been isolated in vitro. Remarkably, these CD45-negative T cells cannot respond to antigen, even though they express normal levels of the TCR. The block is at the very early steps of TCR signaling, indicating that CD45 is required for the functional coupling of the TCR and its PTKs. At first glance a positive role for a tyrosine phosphatase in TCR signaling seems counterintuitive. It appears, however, that the CD45 phosphatase removes tyrosine phosphorylations that inhibit the activation of Src-like PTKs. Phosphorylation of a tyrosine residue found in the carboxy-terminal tails of Src-like PTKs inactivates these kinases (Figure 9–9). By removing this inhibitory phosphorylation, CD45 allows these PTKs to be activated during antigen recognition.

COSTIMULATION BY CD28

Despite their complexity, the signals delivered by the TCR are insufficient to fully activate T cells. Rather, T-cell activation requires the delivery of both the TCR signals and a second set of signals generated by costimulatory molecules. In the absence of the proper costimulus, stimulation of the TCR alone can induce a T cell to enter a state in which it remains viable but is refractory to stimulation by antigen. This state, which is known as **anergy,** can be long-lived, persisting for weeks to months in vitro.

The best characterized (and probably the most important) costimulatory molecule is **CD28,** a 44-kd glycoprotein that is expressed as a homodimer on the surfaces of virtually all CD4 T cells and approximately 50% of CD8 T cells. CD28 binds two distinct cell surface molecules, **B7.1** and **B7.2,** found on dendritic cells, macrophages, and activated B cells. The combination of TCR stimulation and the interaction

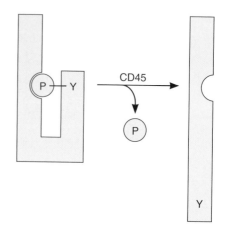

Figure 9–9. Regulation of Src-like protein tyrosine kinases by CD45. Src-like protein kinases, such as Lck and Fyn, can be phosphorylated (P) on a carboxy-terminal tyrosine (Y) by a kinase designated Csk. Phosphorylation at this site induces a conformational change in Src kinases that renders them catalytically inactive. The CD45 phosphatase removes the phosphate from this regulatory tyrosine and restores activity. An inability to activate Lck and Fyn likely explains the impaired TCR signaling observed in T cells that lack CD45.

of CD28 with its B7 ligands fully activates T cells and results in substantially greater lymphokine production than can be induced by TCR signals alone (Figure 9–10). This enhanced lymphokine production reflects the ability of CD28 signals to promote lymphokine gene transcription and to increase the stability of lymphokine messenger RNAs. The signaling pathways involved in costimulation by CD28 have not been defined.

Because T-cell activation requires both the TCR signals and a costimulus, costimulatory molecules such as CD28 may provide a means of manipulating the immune response to specific antigens. Indeed, in vivo blockade of B7.1 and B7.2 (which prevents CD28 from binding) results in prolongation of allograft survival in experimental animals and reverses autoimmunity in mouse models, raising the possibility that disrupting the CD28/B7 interaction may prove to be a powerful means of suppressing undesirable immune responses. The CD28 costimulus can also be exploited to enhance responses. For example, the immune response to many types of tumors, which generally lack B7.1 and B7.2, is inadequate to prevent tumor growth following implantation in mice. In certain experimental models, however, an effective antitumor immune response is initiated in animals immunized with tumor cells that have been genetically altered so that they express B7.1.

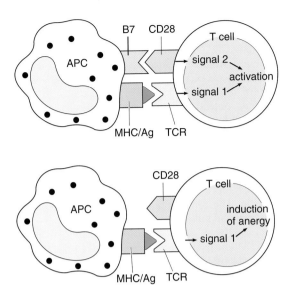

Figure 9–10. The role of CD28 in T-cell activation. Activation of T cells is thought to require T-cell receptor (TCR)-derived signals (signal 1) and a costimulus (signal 2). The major costimulatory molecule, CD28, binds to two cell surface molecules, B7.1 and B7.2, on antigen-presenting cells (APC). The combination of TCR signals and CD28 signals results in a substantial increase in lymphokine production over that seen with TCR stimulation alone. In the absence of the costimulus, the unopposed TCR signals can cause the T cell to enter a state of unresponsiveness known as anergy. *Abbreviations:* MHC = major histocompatibility complex; Ag = antigen.

T-CELL-MEDIATED IMMUNE RESPONSES

Naive T cells circulate through the bloodstream and lymphatics to the spleen, lymph nodes, and Peyer's patches, where they encounter antigens trapped by resident antigen presenting cells (APCs) or imported by dendritic cells that have migrated from their sentinel positions in other tissues. In nonimmunized individuals, the frequency of T cells specific for any particular antigen is very low—on the order of 1 in 10,000 or less. An important component of T-cell immune responses is a rapid expansion in the numbers of antigen-specific T cells. Studies of viral infections in mice, for example, have documented increases from several hundred antigen-specific cytotoxic T lymphocytes (CTLs) at the time of inoculation to nearly 10^8 cells by day 8 of the infection—at which time antigen-specific CTLs account for 50% of T cells in the spleen. At the peak of expansion the antigen-specific CTL population doubles every 6–8 hours. During the expansion period, antigen-specific T cells differentiate into potent effector cells. The ef-

fector function of naive T cells is limited but evolves rapidly following initial activation. The immune response, therefore, entails qualitative as well as quantitative changes in the responding cells.

The number of antigen-specific T cells falls dramatically when an immune response terminates. Following successful clearance of virus, the number of virus-specific CTLs in a mouse can drop from 10^8 to 10^6—a decrease of 99%. The decline reflects apoptosis, perhaps triggered by cytokine withdrawal or by engagement of Fas or other members of the tumor necrosis factor (TNF) receptor family. One important negative regulator of T-cell activation is CTLA-4, a T-cell surface molecule induced on activation and not found on resting cells. CTLA-4 shares considerable sequence homology with CD28 and, like CD28, binds B7.1 and B7.2 on the APC. Unlike CD28, however, CTLA-4 delivers inhibitory signals to T cells, so that engagement of CTLA-4 tends to strongly diminish T-cell responses. CTLA-4 is also critical for maintaining T-cell homeostasis: Mice genetically engineered to lack CTLA-4 die with massive polyclonal expansion of T lymphoblasts.

The T-cell population is heterogeneous with respect to both functional capabilities and cell surface phenotypes. Broadly speaking, T cells are divided into helper cells, which promote cell-mediated and antibody responses, and cytotoxic cells, which kill antigen-bearing target cells. Helper T cells usually express CD4, and cytotoxic T cells generally express CD8. It should be emphasized, however, that expression of CD4 and CD8 primarily correlates with MHC restriction. Thus, some CD4 T cells have cytolytic activity, and certain CD8 T cells function as helper cells. In addition to the classic helper T cells and CTLs, the peripheral T-cell population contains several less well-characterized subsets, including those that express the γδ TCR and cells that share certain phenotypic features with natural killer cells (called NKT cells; see later section).

HELPER T CELLS: THE T_H1 & T_H2 SUBSETS

Helper T cells provide signals that augment cell-mediated immune responses and that are necessary for B cells to differentiate into antibody-producing cells. When activated, helper T cells produce soluble lymphokines that can regulate the activities of T cells, B cells, monocyte–macrophages, and other cells of the immune system. T-cell help for B-cell differentiation also involves direct contact between the two cell types, which exposes the B cell to high local concentrations of T_H-derived lymphokines and which also results in direct stimulation of B-cell surface receptors, most notably CD40. T-cell activation induces T cells to express a ligand for CD40 (called CD40L), and the interaction of CD40 with CD40L provides critical signals for B-cell differentiation. Inherited defects in the expression of CD40L lead to a state of immunodeficiency characterized by low levels of circulating IgG and IgA with increased levels of IgM.

The lymphokine repertoire of naive helper T cells is very limited; on their initial encounter with antigen, helper T cells produce IL-2 but little in the way of other lymphokines. When activated, however, naive T_H cells give rise to effector T cells that can produce a considerable array of different lymphokines. Most of these mature T_H effector cells belong to one of two distinct subsets, designated T_H1 and T_H2 cells, that are distinguished by the particular lymphokines they produce (Table 9–1). Their divergent patterns of lymphokine expression, in turn, allow each of these T_H subsets to promote distinct types of immune reactions that are best suited to eliminating particular types of microorganisms.

Table 9–1. Lymphokine expression by T_H1 and T_H2 cells.

TH Subtype	Cytokines Secreted	Major Immunologic Effects[a]
T_H1	IFNγ	Activate macrophages
		Promote B-cell proliferation and class switching to IgG1
	IL-2	Promotion activation of antigen-specific T_H and T_C cells
	TNFβ	Activate macrophages and neutrophils
		Promote B-cell growth and immunoglobulin production
T_H2	IL-4	Chemoattract lymphocytes, mast cells, and basophils
		Enhance growth of mast cells and eosinophils
		Promote B-cell proliferation and class switching to IgE and IgG4
		Inhibit T_H1-cell differentiation.
		Inhibit cytokine production by macrophages
	IL-5	Enhance growth and development of eosinophils
	IL-6	Promote B-cell growth and immunoglobulin production
	IL-10	Inhibit production of cytokines (including IFNγ) by T_H1 cells, macrophages, and other APCs
		Inhibit T_H1-cell differentiation
		Promote B-cell growth and immunoglobulin production
	IL-13	Same as IL-4

Abbreviations: IFNγ = interferon gamma, IL = interleukin, TNFβ = tumor necrosis factor beta, APC = antigen-presenting cell.

[a] Only a few pertinent effects of these cytokines are listed here; a more complete discussion can be found in Chapter 10. Each of the processes listed is enhanced by the cytokine unless otherwise stated.

T_H1 **cells** produce IL-2, interferon-gamma (IFNγ), and tumor necrosis factor beta (TNFβ, also called lymphotoxin alpha). Broadly speaking, these lymphokines promote defensive reactions that are mediated by macrophages and other phagocytes, and so involve intracellular killing of pathogens. IFNγ, for example, potently activates macrophages by inducing nitric oxide synthase and other metabolic enzymes that increase microbicidal activity. At the same time, IFNγ acts on activated B cells to induce immunoglobulin class switching to IgG1—an isotype that binds strongly to all three classes of macrophage Fcγ receptors and so functions as an extremely potent opsonin. The overall effect is to potentiate both engulfment and killing by phagocytes.

T_H2 **cells,** by contrast, do not make IL-2, IFNγ, or TNFβ but instead secrete IL-4, IL-5, IL-6, IL-10, and IL-13. These T_H2-derived cytokines act together to chemoattract B cells, mast cells, basophils, and eosinophils and then to promote the growth and differentiation of those cell types at the site of an immune response. In addition, IL-4 promotes B-cell class switching to IgE—the isotype bound uniquely by Fcε receptors on mast cells and eosinophils, and which enables those cells to recognize and respond to antigens. By these means, T_H2 cells cause an influx of mast cells and eosinophils and help focus their attack on an antigen. This type of defense reaction is particularly effective against large, multicellular parasites such as helminths, which can often be killed extracellularly by eosinophils but are too large to be engulfed by macrophages. Indeed, macrophages play little role in T_H2-mediated immune reactions, in part, because IL-10 acts to inhibit IFNγ production and because IL-4 selectively favors production of two immunoglobulin isotypes (IgE and IgG4) that are not recognized by macrophage Fc receptors.

T_H1 and T_H2 cells derive from common precursor cells that have the capacity to differentiate into either T_H type (Figure 9–11). Cytokines are the most important determinants of T_H differentiation. IL-12, produced by activated macrophages, causes antigen-primed naive T cells to differentiate into T_H1 cells which, in turn, amplify the macrophage response. In contrast, the presence of IL-4 during an immune response promotes differentiation of naive T cells into T_H2 cells. The source of IL-4 at the initiation of an immune response (ie, before the appearance of T_H2 cells) is uncertain; possibilities include memory T cells, NKT cells, mast cells, eosinophils, and basophils. Differentiation from naive cells to either T_H1 or T_H2 may involve an intermediary cell, designated T_H0, which is defined by its ability to secrete both IFNγ and IL-4.

The cytokines produced by each of the two T_H subsets reciprocally inhibit the development of the other. Thus, T_H1-derived IFNγ inhibits the development of T_H2 cells, and the IL-4 produced by T_H2 cells prevents development of T_H1 cells. Unchecked cytokine-

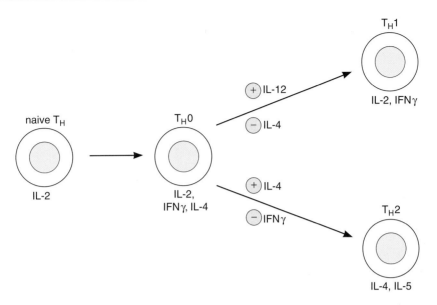

Figure 9–11. Differentiation of helper T cells into T_H1 and T_H2 cells. Naive T_H cells produce IL-2 and little in the way of other cytokines on initial activation. Repeated stimulation in the presence of IL-12, a macrophage-derived cytokine, causes T_H cells to differentiate into T_H1 cells, which produce IL-2 and IFNγ and are particularly effective in enhancing immune responses that involve macrophages and other phagocytes. Stimulation in the presence of IL-4, on the other hand, promotes the development of T_H2 cells, which produce IL-4 and other cytokines that promote mast cell- and eosinophil-mediated responses. The differentiation into either T_H subtype probably involves a common intermediary, designated T_H0, which produces IL-2, IFNγ, and IL-4. T_H1 and T_H2 cells have the ability to mutually down-regulate the development of the other: the T_H1 product IFNγ impairs the generation of T_H2 cells, and the T_H2 cytokine IL-4 inhibits the development of T_H1 cells.

mediated immune responses can cause considerable damage. Transforming growth factor beta (TGFβ) inhibits the development of both T_H1 and T_H2 cells, and regulatory T cells that produce TGFβ (sometimes designated T_H3 cells) may play a role in the suppression of T_H1- and T_H2-mediated immune responses (eg, see the discussion of oral tolerance in Chapter 14).

An immune response can become strongly polarized toward either T_H1 or T_H2 production over time, so that one subtype or the other comes to dominate. Immune responses that are chronic, such as those to parasitic infections, are especially prone to such polarization. This can be highly advantageous if it yields the optimal response against a pathogen. A well-characterized example of a T_H1-dominated response is the brisk cell-mediated reaction of most mouse strains against the protozoan *Leishmania major*. This intracellular pathogen invades macrophages, stimulating them to produce IL-12 and thus promoting T_H1 development. The T_H1 lymphokines, in turn, activate the macrophages to kill the parasites and clear the infection. For reasons that are not well understood, certain mouse strains develop a T_H2-dominated response to *L major;* this leads to a vigorous antibody response but no macrophage response. In these strains, the parasite evades killing, disseminates widely, and eventually kills the host.

The divergent effects of T_H1 and T_H2 cells are also seen in their association with deleterious immune reactions in humans. In particular, **autoimmune disorders** associated with the destruction of host tissues, as occurs in diabetes mellitus, multiple sclerosis, or inflammatory bowel disease, predominantly involve T_H1 responses. By contrast, **allergic disorders** (eg, seasonal rhinitis, asthma, and contact dermatitis) in which IgE, mast cells, and eosinophils play a prominent role are dominated by T_H2 cells. It is not yet clear to what extent the development of such disorders might reflect an inborn predisposition toward T_H1 or T_H2 responses. Nevertheless, it may someday be possible to treat or prevent these disorders by selectively influencing the development or functions of individual T_H subtypes. Similar approaches might also be used to promote desirable immune responses. For example, IL-12 administered at the time of vaccination has been found to enhance protective T_H1 reactions against certain pathogens in animals.

CYTOLYTIC T CELLS

Cytolytic T lymphocytes (CTLs) respond to antigen recognition by killing the antigen-bearing cell. These cells are usually CD8 and recognize antigen in the context of MHC class I molecules. CTLs play a prominent role in the host defense against viral infections. Proteins from viral pathogens enter the endogenous pathway for antigen presentation, resulting in the expression of MHC class I molecules bearing viral peptides. CTLs also are involved in the response to certain intracellular bacterial pathogens, including *Listeria* and mycobacteria. CTLs are important in allograft rejection and may play a role in immune surveillance against malignancy.

Killing by Cytotoxic Granules

CTLs arise from naive T precursors that have limited killing capability. Differentiation into cytolytic cells results from the combination of antigen recognition and exposure to IL-2. In addition to triggering proliferation, IL-2 increases the expression of cytoplasmic granules involved in the killing of target cells (Figure 9–12). The CTL granules contain **perforin** (also known as cytolysin) and **granzymes,** a family of related serine proteases. During target cell recognition, the contents of these granules are directionally released toward the target. The perforin molecules, which are evolutionarily related to complement component C9, form 10- to 20-nm pores in the plasma membrane of the target. These perforin pores are not sufficient to kill nucleated target cells, which have the ability to repair membranes and thereby avoid osmotic lysis. Rather, the pores appear to function as a means of delivering granzymes into the target, and it is the granzymes that induce death of the target by triggering apoptosis. One important step in this process is carried out by granzyme B, which proteolytically cleaves and activates caspases in the target cell, which are components of the apoptotic pathway (see Chapter 1).

Killing by the Fas Ligand–Fas Pathway

The release of cytolytic granules is not the only means by which CTLs can kill antigen-bearing cells. Antigen recognition stimulates CTLs to express Fas ligand, a member of the tumor necrosis factor (TNF) family. The interaction of Fas ligand with Fas (a cell surface molecule related to TNF receptors) induces apoptosis in the Fas-expressing cell (see Chapter 4). The Fas death pathway is also used by CD4 T_H1 cells, which do not express cytolytic granules.

T cells can be activated to express Fas, and activated T cells can become susceptible to Fas-induced apoptosis. Fas-mediated death of T cells, triggered by

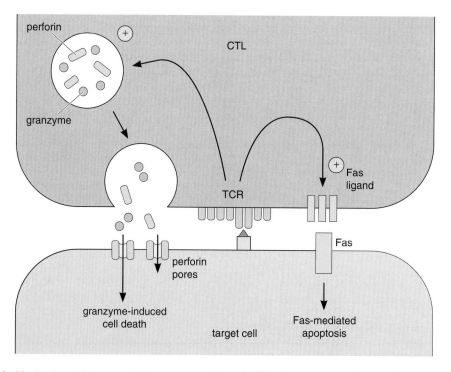

Figure 9–12. Mechanisms of target cell killing by cytolytic T cells (CTL). Antigen recognition by CTLs triggers the exocytosis of granules, leading to the release of perforins, which form pores in the target cell membrane and permit the entry of granzymes into the target cell. Granzymes trigger target cell death through apoptosis. CTLs also can kill targets through the Fas ligand-Fas pathway. T-cell receptor (TCR) stimulation induces the expression of Fas ligand on the cytolytic T cell. If the target cell expresses Fas, its engagement by Fas ligand transduces a signal that triggers apoptosis in the target cell.

Fas ligand-expressing T cells, is important for immune regulation. Humans and mice with mutations that interfere with Fas expression or function develop a clinical disorder characterized by massive accumulation of T cells and by autoimmunity.

MEMORY T CELLS

A remarkable feature of the adaptive immune system is its memory; a second challenge with an antigen results in a prompter and more effective immune response than does the initial exposure to the same antigen. T-cell memory reflects antigen-induced differentiation of naive T cells into memory cells and can involve T_H cells and CTLs.

One important aspect of T-cell memory is quantitative; exposure to an antigen results in a prolonged increase in the numbers of T cells whose TCRs have specificity for that antigen. Unlike the short-lived naive T cells, which exist for a matter of weeks, memory T cells are either long-lived or capable of self-renewal and persist for years. Indeed, antigen-specific memory CTLs have been detected in humans as long as 30 years after vaccination. On rechallenge, therefore, up to 100 times more T cells can be available to respond to the antigen in question.

Important qualitative distinctions also exist between memory T cells and naive T cells. Memory T_H cells, for example, proliferate sooner and express a broader array of lymphokines after contact with an antigen and are more effective helpers. Memory and naive T cells also differ in their surface phenotypes, most notably in their expression of CD45 isoforms. Alternative splicing of CD45 mRNA gives rise to a number of different isoforms of CD45 that differ in the size and composition of their extracellular domains. Naive T cells express 205- to 220-kd isoforms designated CD45RA, whereas memory T cells express a 180-kd isoform called CD45RO. Memory T cells also express higher levels of adhesion molecules on their surfaces; this enables them to adhere more tightly to APCs and may account for their ability to respond to lower concentrations of antigens. In addition, memory and naive T lymphocytes express different types of surface homing receptors and so follow different patterns of trafficking to and within tissues (see Chapter 3).

γδ T CELLS

A small subset (<5%) of mature T cells does not express a TCR αβ dimer. These cells have a second form of the TCR, composed of a CD3 complex together with a dimer of polypeptides designated γ and δ. The TCRγ and δ genes are highly homologous to the TCRα and β genes and, as is the case with α and β, functional gene products are formed by the re-

arrangements of germline V and J segments (in the case of γ) or V, D, and J segments (TCRδ). Indeed, the TCRδ gene lies within the TCRα locus.

Interestingly, the first T cells to mature during fetal development are γδ T cells. The development of these early γδ T cells is highly regulated. They appear in successive waves, with each wave characterized by the use of particular Vγ segments. Remarkably, the initial wave of γδ T cells in the mouse expresses an invariant TCR and, therefore, is composed of T cells that all have identical specificity for antigen. These γδ T cells populate the epidermis, where they assume a dendritic morphology. The γδ T cells that mature in the postnatal thymus, by contrast, use a variety of different Vγ segments and therefore express diverse TCRs.

Relatively little is known about how γδ T cells recognize antigen. In terms of length, the CDR3 loops of γδ TCRs resemble those of immunoglobulins more than of αβ TCRs, suggesting a mode of antigen recognition quite different from that used by αβ T cells. Indeed, with few exceptions, γδ T cells do not recognize antigen in an MHC-restricted fashion. The relatively few antigens for γδ T cells that have been identified fall into three categories: unprocessed proteins, small organic compounds containing alkylphosphate, and alkylamines.

The physiologic roles of γδ T cells are also uncertain. Mature γδ T cells are either double-negative or CD8 and constitute a major component of the T-cell populations in the epidermis and the mucosal epithelia of the tongue, intestine, female reproductive tract, and lung. Roughly 5% of peripheral blood T cells are γδ cells. The invariant T-cell population in the epidermis responds to signals expressed by damaged keratinocytes and, when activated, produces cytokines, such as keratinocyte growth factor, that may facilitate wound healing. Thus, one function of γδ T cells may be to protect the integrity of epithelial tissues. γδ T cells likely have regulatory and effector functions in the response to infection, but it has been difficult to define those roles precisely. γδ T cells have cytolytic capabilities and can produce IFNγ and other immunoregulatory cytokines. Substantial increases in the numbers of peripheral blood γδ T cells can occur in certain bacterial infections, including tuberculosis, brucellosis, and listeriosis, and in several parasitic diseases, such as leishmaniasis and malaria. The ability of γδ T cells to recognize and proliferate in response to alkylphosphates and alkylamines produced by pathogens may explain these responses.

NATURAL KILLER CELLS

Natural killer (NK) cells are large granular lymphocytes that, like CTLs, use cytoplasmic granules containing perforins to kill target cells. NK cells were defined initially by their ability to lyse certain tumor cell lines and virally infected cells in vitro. In contrast to T cells, NK cells can lyse these cells without prior immunization, and so mediate a form of innate (or natural) immunity that is termed "natural killing."

Unlike T cells, NK cells do not productively rearrange their TCR genes, and they do not express a cell surface TCR/CD3 complex. They also lack CD4, the marker for T helper cells. About half of human NK cells express CD8, the marker for cytolytic T cells, but only one form of CD8 is expressed (a homodimer of two α chains), and it does not appear to be required for natural killing. (It is not found on mouse NK cells.) Most NK cells express CD16 (a receptor for the Fc portion of IgG) and CD56 (a variant of neural cell adhesion molecule, NCAM). Neither of these is required for natural killing, and they are expressed at different levels in different tissues. They nonetheless serve to identify NK cells, which are generally CD16+, CD56+, CD3−, whereas T cells are CD3+, CD16−, CD56−.

DEVELOPMENT & TISSUE DISTRIBUTION OF NK CELLS

Like T and B lymphocytes, NK cells derive from a bone marrow precursor. Unlike T cells, they do not require the thymus for development, and they develop fully in mice lacking the recombinase enzymes required for rearranging the TCR or immunoglobulin genes. Similarly, patients with combined T- and B-cell immunodeficiency may have normally functional NK cells. NK cells do not, however, develop in mice lacking either IL-15 or the IL-15 receptor.

NK cells account for about 10–15% of blood lymphocytes. They are rare in lymph nodes and do not circulate through the lymph. Interestingly, NK cells are abundant in the pregnant uterine decidua, where they constitute most of the hematopoietic cells. The function of these uterine NK cells, however, is unknown.

NK EFFECTOR FUNCTIONS

The cell surface molecules that NK cells use to selectively recognize targets for **natural killing** have not been well defined. All NK cells express a surface receptor called NKp46, and blockade of this receptor impairs natural killing. Almost all NK cells also express and are activated by 2B4, a receptor that binds to CD48, which is expressed on most hematopoietic cells. These receptors may be important in natural killing, but their role is not yet fully defined.

When NK cells are stimulated by IL-2, their cytotoxic capacity is enhanced, and the range of target cells they can kill is greatly broadened. These **lymphokine-activated killer (LAK) cells** have been used clinically to treat tumors. Treatment, however, requires the administration of IL-2 in toxic doses, and success has been limited, so this therapy has not gained wide use. Activation by IL-2 induces NK cells to express NKp44, an activating cell surface receptor that is not expressed by resting NK cells and that may help to enhance killing.

The CD16 Fc receptor on NK cells permits them to bind and lyse cells that are coated with antibody. This **antibody-dependent cell-mediated cytotoxicity (ADCC)** provides a bridge between the innate and acquired immune systems. Natural killing, by contrast, occurs independently of antibodies.

NK cells also kill hematopoietic blasts, and so present a barrier against bone marrow transplantation. As discussed later on, inhibitory receptors on NK cells that recognize class I MHC antigens influence graft rejection. The preferential activation of NK cells by hematopoietic cells may account for the reduction in formed blood elements, including white cells, red cells, and platelets, that has been found in patients with abnormal proliferation of NK-like cells.

Activated NK cells produce cytokines such as IFNγ, TNFα, granulocyte-monocyte colony-stimulating factor, and colony-stimulating factor-1. The production of IFNγ by NK cells may serve to bias a T-cell response toward T_H1 differentiation. NK cells are not, however, required for all T_H1 responses because these can also be generated through the production of IFNγ by T cells.

INHIBITORY RECEPTORS ON NK CELLS RECOGNIZE CLASS I MHC ANTIGENS

Unlike T cells, NK cells do not require the expression of MHC molecules on target cells for activation. Instead, NK cells are generally inhibited by the expression of class I MHC proteins on target cells. This inhibition is mediated by receptors on NK cells that specifically recognize class I antigens and deliver inhibitory signals. NK cells express inhibitory receptors that identify both self and nonself class I MHC antigens. All NK cells, however, express at least one inhibitory receptor for a self class I MHC antigen. By this means, NK cells are prevented from killing cells from their host.

The inhibitory receptors on NK cells are of two structural types: immunoglobulin-like (Ig-like) and lectin-like. The Ig-like receptors are members of the immunoglobulin gene superfamily (see Chapter 7) and are called **killer inhibitory receptors (KIRs).** The KIRs are encoded by a gene family on chromosome 19, and different members of the family interact with different sets of class I MHC proteins. Different KIRs recognize features that are common to large groups of class I MHC molecules, so that two KIRs, for example, identify mutually exclusive subsets that together make up all of the HLA-C proteins. Class I recognition by KIRs is relatively unaffected by the particular peptides bound in the peptide-binding groove of the MHC protein.

Other families of KIR-like receptors are encoded on chromosome 19. These are variably expressed on different subsets of hematopoietic cells, sometimes including NK cells. For most of these, the ligands are not yet identified, although at least some of them also interact with class I MHC.

The **lectin-like receptors,** like the KIRs, include inhibitory receptors on NK cells, and they are also encoded in gene families, although on a different chromosome. In mice, these include the Ly-49 receptor family. Mice lack KIRs, and they instead use Ly-49 receptors to recognize class I MHC. Humans, on the other hand, lack Ly-49 receptors. Both humans and mice, however, share the expression of some lectin-like receptors. One is a receptor formed by the joining of two different lectin-like chains, called CD94 and NKG2A. The CD94/NKG2A receptor inhibits NK cells when it binds to HLA-E, a nonclassical class I MHC molecule. HLA-E has the unusual property that it is only expressed when certain classical class I proteins (HLA-A, -B, or -C) are expressed on the same cell. Most classical class I MHC proteins support the expression of HLA-E; thus, HLA-E indirectly and nonspecifically identifies cells as expressing a classical class I protein. The recognition of HLA-E by the CD94/NKG2A receptor may thus provide a "backup" to prevent NK cells from lysing targets for which they do not have an inhibitory receptor.

The finding that NK cell function is inhibited by class I MHC has given rise to the "**missing self" hypothesis.** This model proposes that unlike cytotoxic T lymphocytes, which must be activated from a resting state by contact with an appropriately presented foreign antigen, NK cells are always predisposed to kill any cell they encounter, but are prevented from killing host cells because they recognize the host class I proteins. Thus, they only attack cells whose class I MHC proteins are lost or altered (missing self), as occurs frequently in malignancy or viral infection.

Our understanding of MHC-specific inhibitory receptors has been complicated by the recent discovery that the gene families encoding both KIRs and lectin-like receptors encode activating receptors for class I MHC as well as inhibitory receptors. The activating receptors are not required for natural killing because NK cells kill targets that lack class I expression. The role of these receptors is thus unclear.

ROLE OF NK CELLS IN HOST DEFENSE

The ability of NK cells to kill tumor cells has been a focus of research interest and of therapeutic trials, but there is little evidence that NK cells normally protect against the development of tumors. Instead the most important role for NK cells appears to be in host defense against infection by intracellular agents, including certain viruses, bacteria, and parasites. Selective deficiency of NK cells in humans has been associated with recurrent viral infections, particularly with DNA viruses. Similarly, in mice, NK cells have been shown to help defend against infection by cytomegalovirus. NK cells alone are insufficient protection, but they provide an early innate barrier to infection by eliminating infected host cells, and they also help activate T cells in the acquired antiviral response.

NKT CELLS

In certain strains of mice, all NK cells express the NKR-P1C (NK1.1) surface receptor. This activating receptor is also found on a small subset of T cells (<5%), and these "NKT" cells have distinct properties. Similar NKT cells are found in humans, where they also express a member of the NKR-P1 receptor family, called NKR-P1A (CD161), an antigen that is also found frequently on T cells as well as on NK cells. The majority of NKT cells use the same TCR α chain. They differ from conventional T cells in that they do not respond to peptide antigens complexed with classical class I or class II MHC molecules, but instead respond to **glycolipid** antigens bound to a nonclassical class I protein called **CD1d.** These glycolipids include glycosylphosphatidylinositol (GPI), a glycolipid that is abundant in the cell membrane and is used to anchor a variety of proteins onto the cell surface. Although the structure of GPI is known to vary among organisms, it is not known whether NKT cells recognize pathogens by distinguishing particular forms of GPI. The most potent known stimulus to NKT cells, however, is the glycolipid α-galactosylceramide (α-GalCer). This glycolipid is derived from sponges and is not found in mammals, which instead express β-GalCer. Thus, it has no natural role in regulating NKT cells, but is nevertheless a very useful agent for activating them in vitro and in vivo. Activation of NKT cells through this mechanism secondarily activates NK cells as well.

NKT cells require the expression of CD1d for their development. CD1d is expressed in the thymus, and NKT development is impaired in athymic mice but it is not absent, indicating that NKT cells may develop in response to CD1 outside the thymus.

NKT cells, like NK cells, demonstrate spontaneous cytotoxicity. Of greater importance, however, may be their capacity to produce cytokines, notably IFNγ and IL-4. These cytokines have opposing effects in shaping the immune response, and their production by NKT cells is currently the subject of intense investigation. NKT cells are the major source of IL-4 in mice stimulated with antibody to CD3, but their capacity to produce IFNγ appears to be of particular importance in shaping the immune response.

NKT cells are deficient in both numbers and function in patients with insulin-dependent diabetes or with scleroderma, as well as in certain mouse models of diabetes. IL-12 can induce the rejection of tumor cells by mice through a mechanism that involves NKT cells, and rejection of tumors can also be induced in mice by treatment with α-GalCer.

REFERENCES

THE TCR, T-CELL ONTOGENY, & T-CELL ACTIVATION

Bevan MJ: In thymic selection, peptide diversity gives and takes away. *Immunity* 1997;7:175.

Bluestone JA: New perspectives of CD28-B7-mediated T cell costimulation. *Immunity* 1995;2:555.

Chan AC et al: ZAP-70: A 70 kd protein tyrosine kinase that associates with the TCR ζ chain. *Cell* 1992;71:649.

Clements JL, Koretsky GA: Recent developments in lymphocyte activation: Linking kinases to downstream signaling events. *J Clin Invest* 1999;103:925.

Garboczi DN, Biddison WE: Shapes of MHC restriction. *Immunity* 1999;10:1.

Harding FA et al: CD28-mediated signalling co-stimulates murine T cells and prevents induction of anergy in T-cell clones. *Nature* 1992:356:607.

Janeway CA: The T cell receptor as a multicomponent signaling machine: CD4/CD8 coreceptors and CD45 in T cell activation. *Annu Rev Immunol* 1992;10:645.

Janeway CA: Thymic selection: Two pathways to life and two to death. *Immunity* 1994;1:3.

Jenkins MK et al: CD28 delivers a costimulatory signal involved in antigen-specific IL-2 production by human T cells. *J Immunol* 1991;147:2461.

Kappler JW et al: T cell tolerance by clonal deletion in the thymus. *Cell* 1987;49:273.

Killeen N et al.: Signaling checkpoints during the development of T lymphocytes. *Curr Opin Immunol* 1998;10:360.

Marrack P, Kappler J: The staphylococcal enterotoxins and their relatives. *Science* 1990;248:705.

Murali-Krishna K et al.: Counting antigen-specific CD8 T cells: A reevaluation of bystander activation during viral infection. *Immunity* 1998;8:177.

Rudd CE et al: The CD4 receptor is complexed in detergent lysates to a protein tyroine kinase (pp58) from human T lymphocytes. *Proc Natl Acad Sci U S A* 1988;85:5190.

Schreiber SL, Crabtree GR: The mechanism of action of cyclosporin and FK506. *Immunol Today* 1992;13:136.

Van Leeuwen JEM, Samelson LE: T-cell antigen-receptor signal transduction. *Curr Opin Immunol* 1999;11:242.

Veillette A et al: The CD4 and CD8 T cell surface molecules are associated with the internal membrane tyrosine protein kinase p56*lck*. *Cell* 1988;55:301.

Von Boehmer H et al.: Pleiotropic changes controlled by the pre-T-cell receptor. *Curr Opin Immunol* 1999;11:135.

T-CELL SUBSETS & EFFECTOR FUNCTION

Boismenu R, Havran WL: Modulation of epithelial cell growth by intraepithelial gamma delta T cells. *Science* 1994;266:1253.

Born W et al.: Immunoregulatory functions of γδ T cells. *Adv Immunol* 1999;71:77.

Bukowski JF et al: Human γδ T cells recognize alkylamines derived from microbes, edible plants, and teas: Implications for innate immunity. *Immunity* 1999;11:57.

Henkart PA: Lymphocyte-mediated cytotoxicity: Two pathways and multiple effector molecules. *Immunity* 1994;1:343.

Kojima H et al: Two distinct pathways of specific killing revealed by perforin mutant cytotoxic T lymphocytes. *Immunity* 1994;1:357.

O'Garra A: Cytokines induce the development of functionally heterogeneous T helper cell subsets. *Immunity* 1998;8:275.

Paul WE, Seder RA: Lymphocyte responses and cytokines. *Cell* 1994;76:241.

Sprent J: T and B memory cells. *Cell* 1994;76:315.

Watanabe-Fukunaga R et al: Lymphoproliferation disorder in mice explained by defects in Fas antigen that mediates apoptosis. *Nature* 1992;356:314.

NK CELLS

Biron CA et al: Natural killer cells in antiviral defense: Function and regulation by innate cytokines. *Annu Rev Immunol* 1999;17:189.

Cantoni C et al: NKp44, a triggering receptor involved in tumor cell lysis by activated human natural killer cells, is a novel member of the immunoglobulin superfamily. *J Exp Med* 1998;189:787.

George T et al: Allorecognition by murine natural killer cells: Lysis of T-lymphoblasts and rejection of bone-marrow grafts. *Immunol Rev* 1997;155:29.

Lanier LL: NK cell receptors. *Annu Rev Immunol* 1998;16:359.

Long EO: Regulation of immune responses through inhibitory receptors. *Annu Rev Immunol* 1999;17:875.

Yokoyama WM: Natural killer cell receptors. *Curr Opin Immunol* 1998;10:298.

NK T CELLS

Bendelac A et al: Mouse CD1-specific NK1 T cells: Development, specificity, and function. *Annu Rev Immunol* 1997;15:535.

Falcone M et al: A Defect in Interleukin 12-induced activation and interferon gamma secretion of peripheral natural killer T cells in nonobese diabetic mice suggests new pathogenic mechanisms for insulin-dependent diabetes mellitus. *J Exp Med* 1999;190:963.

Kronenberg M et al: Conserved lipid and peptide presentation functions of nonclassical class I molecules. *Immunol Today* 1999;20:515.

Schofield L at al: CD1d-restricted immunoglobulin G formation to GPI-anchored antigens mediated by NKT cells. *Science* 1999;283:225.

10

Cytokines

Joost J. Oppenheim, MD, & Francis W. Ruscetti, PhD

Many critical interactions among cells of the immune system are controlled by soluble mediators called **cytokines.** These cytokines are a diverse group of intercellular signaling peptides and glycoproteins with molecular weights (MW) between 6000 and 60,000, and most of them are genetically and structurally unrelated to one another. Several hundred have been identified to date. Each is secreted by particular cell types in response to a variety of stimuli and produces characteristic effects on the growth, mobility, differentiation, or function of target cells. Collectively, they regulate not only immune and inflammatory responses but also wound healing, hematopoiesis, angiogenesis, and many other biologic processes. They are extremely potent compounds that act at concentrations of 10^{-9}–10^{-15} M by binding to specific surface receptors on target cells. Unlike endocrine hormones, they are not produced by specialized glands and secreted into the circulation, but rather are produced locally by a variety of tissues and cells. Only a few cytokines, such as transforming growth factor β (TGFβ), erythropoietin (EPO), stem cell factor (SCF), and monocyte colony-stimulating factor (M-CSF), are normally present in detectable amounts in the blood and are able to influence distant target cells. Most other cytokines, unless produced in excess, act only locally over short distances, in either a **paracrine** manner (ie, on adjacent cells) or an **autocrine** manner (ie, on the producing cell itself).

Cytokine nomenclature has little to do with structural relationships among molecules; some of them have been termed interleukins (IL) and been assigned a number (Table 10–1), but many others retain their descriptive and frequently misleading historical names (Table 10–2). Some can be classified into families based on their use of receptors that share a common chain or exhibit other sequence homologies. Cytokines produced by lymphocytes are also called **lymphokines,** whereas those produced by monocytes or macrophages are called **monokines.** A given cytokine may be secreted individually or as part of a coordinated response along with other, unrelated cytokines. Many have activities that overlap extensively, and others may be antagonistic. Furthermore, one cytokine may induce expression of other cytokines or mediators, thus producing a cascade of biologic effects.

This chapter will focus primarily on the role of cytokines and their receptors in immune and inflammatory responses. We will consider the interleukins, TNFα, transforming growth factor β (TGFβ), colony-stimulating factors (CSFs), and interferons (IFNs), emphasizing their effects on growth, differentiation, and function of leukocytes. Cytokines that act primarily on other tissue types will not be covered. Because it can be quite perilous to extrapolate from in vitro studies, much of what we know about cytokine functions in vivo has come from studying humans or animals with mutations that inactivate a particular cytokine or cytokine-receptor gene. Some of these mutations occur naturally, and others have been introduced deliberately into the chromosomes of laboratory mice to create so-called **knockout mouse** strains with defects in specific genes. In addition, the ability to produce cytokines in large quantities using recombinant DNA techniques has allowed them to be tested as potential therapeutic agents. We will briefly summarize the information available to date; readers may consult the accompanying references for additional details.

INTERLEUKIN-1 & TUMOR NECROSIS FACTOR

IL-1 and TNFα are structurally unrelated and use different receptors, yet their spectra of biologic effects overlap considerably (Table 10–3). For example, each can directly promote growth and differentiation of B cells, activate neutrophils and macrophages, stimulate hematopoiesis, and produce a broad range of effects on nonhematopoietic cell types. They also induce expression of many other cytokines and mediators that promote inflammation and are therefore known as proinflammatory cytokines. Their main importance for immunity, however, lies in their ability to enhance the activation of T helper (T_H) lymphocytes by antigen-presenting cells (APCs). IL-1 and

Table 10–1. Major properties of human interleukins.

Interleukin	Principal Cell Source	Principal Effects[a]
IL-1α and β	Macrophages, other APCs, other somatic cells	Costimulation of APCs and T cells B-cell growth and Ig production Acute-phase response Phagocyte activation Inflammation and fever Promotes hematopoiesis
IL-2	Activated T_H2 cells, CTLs, NK cells	Proliferation of activated T cells Apoptosis of T cells after prolonged or repeated activation NK-cell and CTL functions B cell proliferation and IgG2 expression
IL-3	T lymphocytes	Growth of early hematopoietic progenitors
IL-4	T_H2 cells, mast cells	B-cell proliferation, IgE expression, and class II MHC expression T_H2-cell and CTL proliferation and functions Eosinophil and mast cell growth and function Inhibits monokine production
IL-5	T_H2 cells, mast cells	Eosinophil growth and function
IL-6	Activated T_H2 cells, APCs, other somatic cells	Synergistic effects with IL-1 or TNFα Fever Acute-phase response B-cell growth and Ig production Hematopoiesis
IL-7	Thymic and marrow stromal cells	T and B lymphopoiesis CTL functions
IL-8	Macrophages, other somatic cells	Chemoattracts neutrophils and T cells Angiogenic
IL-9	T cells	Some hematopoietic and thymopoietic effects
IL-10	Activated T_H2, CD8 T, and B lymphocytes; macrophages	Inhibits cytokine production by T_H1 cells, NK cells, and APCs Promotes B-cell proliferation and antibody responses Suppresses cell-mediated immunity
IL-11	Stromal cells	Synergistic effects on hematopoiesis and thrombopoiesis
IL-12	B cells, macrophages	Proliferation and function of activated CTLs and NK cells IFNγ production Promotes T_H1-cell induction; suppresses T_H2-cell functions Promotes cell-mediated immunity
IL-13	T_H2 cells	Similar, but additive, to IL-4 effects
IL-15	Epithelial cells and monocytes, nonlymphocytic cells	Mimics IL-2 T-cell effects Mast-cell and NK activation
IL-16	CD8 and some CD4 T lymphocytes	Chemoattracts CD4 T cells, eosinophils, and monocytes Comitogenic for CD4 T cells
IL-17	Activated memory T cells	Promotes T-cell proliferation, neutrophil development
IL-18	Macrophages, keratinocytes	Coinduces IFNγ production Coactivates T_H1- and NK-cell development

Abbreviations: APC = antigen-presenting cell; NK = natural killer cell; IL = interleukin; CTL = cytotoxic T lymphocyte; MHC = major histocompatibility complex; TNF = tumor necrosis factor; IFN = interferon.
[a] All of the indicated processes are increased or enhanced unless otherwise indicated.

TNFα are each secreted by APCs on contact with a T_H cell that has the appropriate antigen and major histocompatibility complex (MHC) specificity. They then act in an autocrine manner to induce or increase expression of various adhesion molecules, IFNγ receptors, and class II MHC proteins on the APC surface and so increase the efficiency with which the APC can bind and activate T_H cells. They also act in a paracrine fashion on the T_H cell, augmenting secretion of IL-2, expression of surface receptors for IL-2 and IFNγ, and other events leading to clonal T-cell proliferation. As a result, IL-1 and TNFα help to initiate both humoral and cellular immune responses. Although each can function independently, they also synergize with one another, or with IL-6, to produce markedly augmented effects.

Table 10–2. Major properties of human noninterleukin cytokines.

Cytokine	Principal Cell Source	Principal Effects[a]
TNFα	Activated macrophages, other somatic cells	IL-1-like effects Vascular thrombosis and tumor necrosis
LTα	Activated T_H1 cells	IL-1-like and TNFα-like effects
LTα-LTβ complex	Activated T_H1 cells	Development of peripheral (secondary) lymphoid organs
IFNα and β	Macrophages, neutrophils, other somatic cells	Antiviral effects Induction of class I MHC on all somatic cells Activation of macrophages and NK cells
IFNγ	Activated T_H1 and NK cells	Induction of class I MHC on all somatic cells Induction of class II MHC on APCs and somatic cells Activation of macrophages, neutrophils, and NK cells Promotion of cell-mediated immunity (inhibits T_H2 cells) Antiviral effects
TGFβ	Activated T lymphocytes, platelets, macrophages, other somatic cells	Antiinflammatory (suppression of cytokine production and class II MHC expression) Antiproliferative for stem cells, monomyelocytic cells and lymphocytes Promotion of fibroblast proliferation and wound healing

Abbreviations: TNF = tumor necrosis factor; LT = lymphotoxin; IFN = interferon; TGF = transforming growth factor; NK = natural killer; IL = interleukin; MHC = major histocompatibility complex.
[a] All of the listed processes are enhanced unless otherwise indicated.

IL-1 Proteins & Their Receptors

Like all species examined to date, humans express two distinct molecular forms of IL-1, called IL1α and IL-1β. These are peptides, 159 and 153 amino acids long, respectively, that are encoded by separate genes and share only 26% amino acid sequence similarity, but have virtually identical potency and biologic activities and bind with about the same affinity to the same cell surface receptors. Virtually all nucleated cells can produce IL-1, and although many cell types express both forms, their relative levels of expression vary widely. For example, human monocytes produce predominantly IL-1β, whereas keratinocytes produce mainly IL-1α. The biologic significance of this disparity is unknown. IL-1α and IL-1β are initially synthesized as propeptides, which are then processed enzymatically to mature form, either at or beyond the outer cell membrane. IL-1β is processed by **caspase-1** (also called IL-1β-converting enzyme, or ICE) and is then released in soluble form. By contrast, IL-1α most often remains on the cell surface and may thus participate in interactions that require cell-to-cell contact. A number of cell types can also express a third gene that codes for a protein called **IL-1 receptor antagonist (IL-1RA),** which has no intrinsic activity but competes for binding of IL-1 receptors and so is a competitive inhibitor of IL-1α and IL-1β.

A few tissues express IL-1, constitutively; for example, the skin, sweat, urine, and amniotic fluid contain significant amounts. In contrast, macrophages and most other cell types produce IL-1 only in response to external stimuli, such as bacterial lipopolysaccharide **(LPS);** urate or silicate particles; or adjuvants such as aluminum hydroxide (see Chap-

ter 5). It is thought that, during the process of antigen presentation, IL-1 production by the APC is initially triggered by contact with a specific T_H cell and may then increase further in response to TNFα or IL-2 released from the T cell when it becomes activated. Prostaglandins, a class of lipid-derived inflammatory mediators, can also regulate IL-1 expression; for example, IL-1 production by macrophages is enhanced by leukotrienes, but is suppressed by products of the cyclooxygenase pathway, such as prostaglandin E_2 (see Chapter 13). Increased circulating levels of IL-1 are also observed during the luteal phase of the menstrual cycle and during strenuous exercise.

IL-1α and IL-1β bind to high-affinity receptors ($K_d = 10^{-10}$ M) present on most nucleated cell types. A fibroblast may carry several thousand IL-1 receptors; resting T cells express as few as 50, but this number increases after activation. Binding leads to endocytosis of IL-1 together with its receptor. Two distinct IL-1 receptors have been characterized, both of which are membrane glycoproteins that share only 28% sequence similarity but have comparable three-dimensional structures and bind IL-1α and IL-1β equally. The type-I receptor **(IL-1RI)** has a large cytoplasmic domain and transmits signals when it binds IL-1; the signaling pathway is not fully known, but shares some components with those used by the IL-18 and Toll-like receptor families. Binding to as few as five copies of IL-1RI on a cell can be sufficient to produce a response. The type-II receptor **(IL-1RII),** by contrast, has a small cytoplasmic domain and cannot transduce signals. The extracellular domain of IL-1RII is released in soluble form at sites of local inflammation and into the serum during times of systemic inflammation. This soluble IL-1RII is pro-

Table 10–3. Target cells and actions of IL-1α or -β and of TNFα.

Target Cells or Tissues	Effects	IL-1	TNF
T lymphocytes	Costimulate T-cell activation	+	+
	Induce IL-2 and IFNγ receptors	+	+
	Induce lymphokine production	+	+
B lymphocytes	Promote proliferation	+	+
	Enhance immunoglobulin expression	+	+
Monocytes and macrophages	Chemoattract	–	±
	Activate cytotoxic state	+	+
	Induce production of prostaglandins, IL-1, IL-6, GM-CSF, and chemokines	+	+
Neutrophils	Activate to produce cytokines	+	+
Endothelial and vascular smooth muscle cells	Increase adhesiveness for leukocytes (ICAM-1)	+	+
	Induce procoagulant activity, cytokine production, and class I MHC	+	+
	Induce mitogenesis and angiogenesis	+	+
Hematopoietic cells	Inhibit some precursor growth and differentiation	–	+
	Stimulate precursor cells	+	–
Hepatocytes	Induce some acute-phase proteins	+	+
	Decrease cytochrome P-450	+	+
	Increase plasma Cu; decrease plasma Fe and Zn	+	+
Neuroendocrine cells	Stimulate glucocorticoid secretion	+	+
	Induce fever	+	+
	Induce somnolence and anorexia	+	+
Osteoblasts	Decrease alkaline phosphatase	+	+
Osteoclasts	Increase bone resorption and collagenase	+	+
Chondrocytes	Increase cartilage turnover	+	+
Fibroblasts and synovial cells	Induce collagenase, chemokines, other cytokines	+	+
Adipocytes	Decrease lipoprotein lipase	+	+
	Increase lipolysis	+	+
Epithelial cells	Induce proliferation	+	ND[a]
	Increase type IV collagen secretion	+	ND
Pancreatic β cells	Modulate insulin secretion	+	–
Dendritic cells	Enhance ability to activate T cells	+	ND
Tumor cells	Cytostatic and cytolytic effects	+	+

Abbreviations: IFN = interferon; IL = interleukin; GM-CSF = granulocyte–monocyte colony-stimulating factor; ICAM = intercellular adhesion molecule; MHC = major histocompatibility complex; TNF = tumor necrosis factor.
[a] ND, no data available.

duced in relatively large amounts, binds IL-1β much more strongly than it binds IL-1α or IL-1RA, and functions as an endogenous inhibitor of IL-1β. Both the soluble and cell-associated forms of IL-1RII have therefore been called IL-1 **decoy receptors.**

TNFα & Its Receptors

TNFα was first described as an activity in the serum of LPS-treated animals that could induce hemorrhagic necrosis of certain tumors, and it was later discovered independently as **cachectin,** a circulating mediator of the wasting syndrome (cachexia) associated with certain chronic diseases. It is part of a large superfamily comprising at least 15 proteins that have diverse functions (Table 10–4) and that associate with at least 24 different receptors. Every member of the TNF superfamily has some effect on the immune system (see Table 10–4), and several (notably, **FasL**

and **CD40**) have been highlighted in previous chapters. We will focus initially on TNFα itself, many of whose properties also apply to other members of the family.

TNFα is synthesized as a propeptide and then processed intracellularly by an enzyme called TNFα-converting enzyme (TACE) to its mature, secreted form, which is 157 amino acids long. An active membrane-bound form of TNFα has also been described. Like other members of its family, TNFα binds as a trimer to its receptor, with each trimer binding to two or three copies of the receptor simultaneously. This results in ligand-mediated cross-linking of the receptors, which then transmit signals into the cell.

Two different TNFα receptors have been identified. The type-II receptor (**TNFRII**) binds TNFα with about tenfold higher affinity ($K_d = 5 \times 10^{-11}$ M)

Table 10–4. TNF superfamily ligands.

Ligand	Receptor	Major Effects
TNFα and LTα	TNFRI TNFRII	Cytotoxicity and lymphocyte proliferation Apoptosis and septic shock
LTα/β complex	LTβR	Development of lymph nodes and Peyer's patches
Nerve growth factor (NGF)	NGFR (low-affinity)	Promotes neuronal survival and differentiation Autocrine growth factor for memory B cells
Fas ligand (FasL)	Fas	Apoptosis Target-cell killing by CTL
CD40 ligand (CD40L)	CD40	Promotes B-cell growth, survival, differentiation, and Ig class-switching Costimulates T cells
CD27 ligand (CD27L; CD70)	CD27	Costimulates T-cell activation and CTL development Promotes B-cell development and IgE production
CD30 ligand (CD30L)	CD30	Costimulates T-cell activation, especially of T_H2 cells
Ox40 ligand	Ox40	Costimulates CD4 T cells
TRAIL	DR4, DR5, DCR1, DCR2	Selectively apoptotic for tumor cells
TRANCE (RANK-ligand; osteoprotegerin ligand)		Prevents osteopetrosis by promoting osteoclast differentiation Stimulates dendritic cell/cytokine production and antigen presentation to T cells Supports normal thymic and B-cell development

Abbreviations: TNF = tumor necrosis factor; TNFR = TNFα receptor; Ig = immunoglobulin; TRAIL = TNF-related apoptosis-inducing ligand; DR = death receptor; LT = lymphotoxin; CTL = cytotoxic T lymphocyte; Ig = immunoglobulin; DC = dendritic cell.

than does the type-I receptor **(TNFRI).** Each has a large cytoplasmic domain and can transmit signals through the NFκB pathway (see Chapter 1) that give rise to most of the immunologic effects of TNFα. In most respects, TNFRI is the principal mediator of TNFα activity, with TNFRII serving an auxiliary role. Moreover, unlike TNFRII, the cytoplasmic portion of TNFRI includes an 80-amino-acid sequence known as the **death domain,** which is also found in the Fas protein (the receptor for FasL). The death domains of TNFRI and Fas allow these proteins to trigger **apoptosis** when they bind their respective ligands; they do so by activating caspase-8, which in turn activates the downstream caspase cascade. Like the IL-1 receptors, TNFα receptors are internalized (endocytosed) after ligand binding. IL-2 increases expression of both types of TNFα receptors, whereas IFNγ selectively induces TNFRII. Activated cells shed their TNFα receptors, which can bind TNFα and may antagonize its activity during inflammatory responses. An inherited inability to shed TNFRI results in a syndrome of recurrent localized inflammatory episodes and fevers.

Nonimmunologic Inflammatory Effects of IL-1 & TNFα

TNFα is primarily responsible for a laboratory phenomenon known as the localized **hemorrhagic Shwartzman reaction,** in which repeated injection of LPS into a solid tissue leads to hemorrhagic infarction. This occurs because LPS-induced TNFα secretion by macrophages can stimulate endothelial cells to release prostaglandins, IL-6, and other mediators that cause coagulation, clotting, and obstruction of the local blood supply. A similar mechanism probably accounts for the ability of TNFα to cause infarcts and hemorrhagic necrosis of tumors—the property that led to its discovery. There is also a systemic form of the Shwartzman reaction in which intravenous LPS induces **disseminated intravascular coagulation (DIC)**—widespread thrombosis that blocks capillaries and may lead to hemorrhages, shock, and death. This systemic reaction resembles the effects of overwhelming bacterial sepsis and is mediated, at least in part, by TNFα. Repeated injections of IL-1 can also yield localized Shwartzman reactions, and low doses of IL-1 act synergistically with TNFα to mimic the fatal systemic effects of **septic shock.**

TNFα and IL-1 are important inducers of the **acute-phase response** (see Chapter 2), although they are exceeded in this regard by IL-6. Acting alone or synergistically, they can induce a number of effects that are mediated through the hypothalamus: they are **endogenous pyrogens** (ie, they induce **fever**) and stimulate the secretion of corticotropin-releasing factor, which stimulates the release of adrenocorticotropic hormone (ACTH) from the pituitary and in turn induces the production of **glucocorticoids** by the adrenals. Both IL-1 and TNFα have effects on bones and synovia and are present at increased concentration in inflammatory joint fluids, suggesting that they may contribute to the fibrosis and thickening of arthritic joints.

Other effects of IL-1 and TNFα are listed in Table 10–3. Overall, the functional overlap between these cytokines is probably beneficial because it provides parallel pathways for mobilizing host defenses. IL-1 and TNFα induce each other as well as IL-6, and their ability to synergize enables them to achieve maximal effects at suboptimal concentrations. Despite this redundancy, however, the disparate phenotypes of various IL-1 and TNFα ligand- and receptor-knockout mice indicate that each of these cytokines does have unique pathophysiologic roles (Table 10–5).

Table 10–5. Phenotypes of proinflammatory cytokine knockout mice.

Targeted Gene	Phenotypic Abnormalities
IL-1β	Reduced IL-6 production and acute-phase response Resistance to collagen-induced arthritis
IL-1RI	Same as IL-1β knockout, but more susceptible to *Listeria monocytogenes*
Caspase-1 (ICE)	Reduced production of IL-1β and partially of IL-1α Resistance to LPS lethality
IL-1RA	Decreased body mass Greater LPS susceptibility More resistant to *L monocytogenes* Develop arthritis
TNF-RI	Lower LPS lethality and decreased serum IL-6 levels Lower resistance to intracellular bacteria Decreased germinal centers
TNF-RII	Lower LPS lethality More susceptible to *L monocytogenes* Decreased induction of cutaneous hypersensitivity
TNFα	Lower LPS lethality and reduced resistance to intracellular bacteria Lack germinal centers and abnormal IgG synthesis
LTα	Failure of lymph node development, absent Peyer's patches, and splenic hypoplasia Defective isotype switching
LTβ or LTβR	Failure of lymph node development (except mesenteric and cervical) Absent Peyer's patches; splenic hypoplasia
CD30	Impaired negative selection in the thymus
CD40 Ligand	No immunoglobulin response to T-cell-dependent antigens Human gene defect results in hyper-IgM syndrome with neutropenia and intracellular bacterial infections
Fas Ligand	Failure of apoptosis in T cells and CTL target cells Mice with gld gene defect develop lymphoid hyperplasia and autoimmunity
Fas	Mice (lpr/lpr) develop lymphoid hyperplasia and autoimmunity due to failure to delete lymphocytes Humans with gene defect develop ALPS
TRANCE	Impaired thymic development and osteopetrosis due to osteoclast deficiency
Osteoprotegerin	Decreased bone density and bone size
IL-6	LPS increases serum TNFα, but fever response reduced. Diminished local inflammation Reduced acute-phase response Reduced plasma cell tumorigenesis Defective IgG and IgA responses Impaired hematopoiesis
IL-6Rβ	Embryonic lethal with cardiac hypoplasia, reduced hematopoietic progenitor cells, impaired placental development
LIF	Failure of blastocyst implantation
LIF-R	Embryonic lethal with disrupted placental architecture, increased osteoclasts and osteopenia, reduced glial cells and decreased neural cell survival
CNTF	Loss of motor neurons and muscle atrophy
TGFβ-1	Neonatal death from wasting and polyinflammatory state
TGFβ-2 or 3	Embryonic lethal

Abbreviations: IL = interleukin; TNF = tumor necrosis factor; LT = lymphotoxin; LIF = leukemia inhibitory factor; TGF = transforming growth factor; CNTF = ciliary neurotrophic factor; LPS = lipopolysaccharide; Ig = immunoglobulin; CTL = cytotoxic T lymphocyte; ALPS = autoimmune lymphoproliferative syndrome

IL-1 & TNFα as Therapeutic Agents

Both IL-1 and TNF have been investigated as possible therapeutic agents, with emphasis on their immunostimulatory and antineoplastic activities, but neither has proven useful in practice, largely because of their numerous side effects. Antagonists of IL-1 and TNFα, on the other hand, are also of interest as a means of ameliorating chronic inflammatory diseases such as rheumatoid arthritis. Potent nonspecific antagonism to both these cytokines is exhibited by TGFβ and by corticosteroids. In addition to reducing IL-1 production, TGFβ inhibits IL-1RI expression and induces production of IL-1RA—it is a "triple threat!" Corticosteroids not only reduce the production of IL-1 and TNFα, but also increase expression of IL-1RII, which can further inhibit IL-1 effects. Inhibitors of the lipoxygenase pathway likewise reduce IL-1 secretion, whereas leukotrienes appear to increase it (see Chapter 13).

Other TNF & TNF-Receptor Superfamily Proteins

Proteins of the TNF receptor superfamily (see Table 10–4) differ from most other receptors in that they bind trimeric ligands and contain one or more copies of a cysteine-rich 40-amino-acid sequence in their extracellular domains. Nearly all members of this family characterized to date are involved in regulating immune functions, though they may do so through divergent signaling pathways. Indeed, the cytoplasmic signaling domains of these proteins resemble one another very little, except that a few of them (eg, TNFRI, Fas, and NGFR) contain death domains.

One prominent member is **CD40,** the principal receptor on B cells for contact-mediated help provided by T cells that express the CD40L protein (see Chapter 9). CD40 is also expressed on APCs and participates in T-cell costimulation. Another member is **Fas,** which, in conjunction with its ligand (FasL), transmits signals that trigger apoptosis in various settings, including target-cell killing by cytotoxic T lymphocytes (CTLs; see Chapters 4 and 9). Resting human B lymphocytes express the nerve growth factor (**NGF**) receptor and secrete NGF, which functions as an autocrine growth factor that is essential for survival of memory (ie, class-switched), but not naive, B cells. **CD27** is expressed on activated T cells, B cells, and natural killer (NK) cells. The CD27 ligand (also known as CD70) is expressed on monocytes and some T and B cells and is thought to participate in IL-2-independent T-cell stimulation and CTL development. CD27–CD70 interactions augment IgE secretion by promoting B-cell maturation. **CD30** is a T-cell costimulatory receptor that is reported to act preferentially on T_H2 cells and is also found on the Reed–Sternberg cells of Hodgkin's disease. Interaction of Ox-40 with Ox-40L likewise provides costimulatory signals that sustain primary T_H-cell responses, and interference with these signals has been reported to suppress inflammatory bowel disease and autoimmune encephalomyelitis in animal models. **TRAIL** and its receptors are of interest because of their ability to induce apoptosis in cancer cells but, unlike TNFα or Fas, not in most normal cells. **TRANCE** is expressed on mature dendritic cells and serves both to induce cytokine production from these cells and to costimulate T_H cells that express its ligand.

Lymphotoxin α (LTα, also known as TNFβ) is only 28% similar to TNFα but binds both TNFα receptors and has many of the same biologic effects. Unlike TNFα, however, LTα appears to be required for normal formation of lymph nodes and Peyer's patches during development, at least in mice. This reflects the fact that LTα also binds to a cell-surface protein known as LTβ, which is found on T and B lymphocytes and, to a limited degree, on myelomonocytic cells. The LTα/LTβ complex binds and stimulates a receptor, called LTβR, which mediates the unique effects of LTα. The TNFα, LTα, and LTβ genes lie adjacent to one another within the MHC gene cluster.

INTERLEUKIN-2

IL-2 is an autocrine and paracrine growth factor secreted by activated T lymphocytes and is essential for clonal T-cell proliferation. The discovery of IL-2 (then called T-cell growth factor) represented a major advance in immunology, because it made it possible to propagate and study individual clones of normal T cells that maintained their immunologic properties in cell culture. Its role in promoting T-cell proliferation, cytokine production, and the functional properties of B cells, macrophages, and NK cells, make IL-2 critical for activating all types of acquired immune responses. Paradoxically, however, this cytokine appears equally important in limiting such responses and eliminating autoreactive T cells: prolonged or repeated activation in the presence of IL-2 causes T-cell apoptosis, and mutations that inactivate IL-2 or its receptor lead to excessive T-cell proliferation and autoimmunity in both humans and animal models (Table 10–6). IL-2 is thus a two-edged sword that initiates immune responses but also limits their intensity and duration.

IL-2 is 133 amino acids long and is encoded by a single gene on human chromosome 4. Although it bears little obvious sequence similarity to other known cytokines, its three-dimensional structure—consisting of two α helices forming planar faces around a very hydrophobic core—is similar to those of IL-4 and granulocyte–monocyte CSF (GM-CSF). This configuration is maintained in part by the single intrachain disulfide bond, which is essential for biologic activity.

Resting T lymphocytes neither synthesize nor se-

Table 10–6. Phenotypes of immunoregulatory cytokine knockout mice.

Targeted Gene	Phenotypic Abnormalities
IL-2	Lethal gastrointestinal ulcerations, inflammatory bowel disease Lymphoid hypertrophy in survivors
IL-2Rα	Older mice develop massive enlargement of lymphoid organs, with autoimmunity
IL-2Rβ	Hyperactivation of T-cells, with autoimmunity
IL-2Rγ	Greatly reduced lymphoid numbers, including NK cells (humans develop severe combined immune deficiency)
IL-7	Failure of thymic and peripheral lymphocyte development
IL-7R	Greatly underdeveloped thymic and lymphoid tissues
IFNγ	Susceptible to bacterial and viral infections No deficiency in T_H1 responses Deactivated macrophages
IFNαβR	Reduced antiviral resistance
IFNγR	Reduced LPS lethality and cytokine production Lower resistance to bacterial infection
IL-4	Reduced IgG_1 and IgE levels Reduced T_H2 cytokine production
IL-4 + IL-13	Absence of IgG_1 and IgE Absence of T_H2 cytokine production
IL-10 or IL-10R	Chronic enterocolitis secondary to elevated levels of proinflammatory cytokines; growth defects

Abbreviations: IL = interleukin; IFN = interferon; NK = natural killer; LPS = lipopolysaccharide.

crete IL-2, but can be induced to do both by the appropriate combinations of antigen and costimulatory factors or by exposure to polyclonal mitogens (Chapters 4 and 9). Although CD4 T_H cells are the main source of IL-2, CD8 T cells and NK cells also can be induced to secrete it under certain conditions. Several signaling pathways, including the NFκB pathway, regulate the IL-2 gene, and immunosuppressive drugs that interfere with NFκB signaling (eg, cyclosporin A) produce their effects in part by inhibiting IL-2 production. When human lymphocytes are exposed to a T-cell mitogen, IL-2 mRNA expression becomes detectable after 4 hours, reaches peak concentration at 12 hours, and thereafter declines rapidly. The abrupt disappearance of IL-2 mRNA reflects not only cessation of IL-2 gene transcription but also the instability of IL-2 mRNA, which has a half-life of less than 30 minutes. Synthesis and release of IL-2 protein follow a similar time course, resulting in a transient burst of secretion that quickly subsides. Because IL-2 has very short half-life in the circulation, it primarily acts as an autocrine or paracrine mediator.

IL-2 Receptors & Signal Transduction

The high-affinity IL-2 receptor (IL-2R) is composed of three subunits, designated α, β, and γ, each of which is an integral membrane protein. This heterotrimer binds IL-2 with a K_d of 1.3×10^{-11} M and a dissociation half-life of 50 minutes. The α chain alone (also called Tac or CD25) binds IL-2 with intermediate affinity (K_d 1.4×10^{-8} M), but cannot sig-

nal. The β and γ subunits alone can each transmit signals, but the β chain binds IL-2 with only low affinity (K_d 1.2×10^{-7} M), and the γ does not bind it detectably. Receptors composed of α/γ or β/γ heterodimers bind with K_d of about 10^{-9} M and, like the heterotrimer, can mediate IL-2 signaling. The IL-2R γ chain is also a functional component of the IL-4, IL-7, IL-9 and IL-15 receptor complexes (Figure 10–1), enabling all of these cytokines to act as T-cell growth factors.

Several distinct cytoplasmic regions of the IL-2R β chain contribute to signaling: A serine-rich region is required for induction of c-Myc protein; an acidic region mediates interaction with Lck and other Src-like protein tyrosine kinases and activation of the Ras pathway; and phosphorylation of this chain activates phosphatidylinositol 3-kinase (see Chapters 1 and 9). In addition, both the β and γ chains can interact with components of the Jak/Stat pathway (Chapter 1), and mutations either in the γ chain or in Jak-3-kinase can lead to severe immune deficiency in humans.

Resting T cells express the β/γ receptor dimer, but not the α subunit. Activation of T-cells by antigens or polyclonal mitogens leads to α-chain expression and assembly of high-affinity receptor trimers, which reach maximal levels within 2–3 days, coinciding with the peak of the T-cell proliferative response. Interference with either IL-2 or its receptor (eg, by treatment with specific antibodies) blocks proliferation. Unless the cell is repeatedly stimulated, receptor expression then declines to undetectable levels by 6–10 days after activation. This decline occurs re-

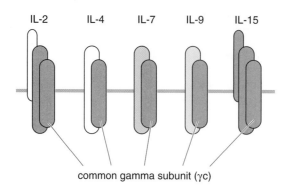

Figure 10–1. Receptors that use the common IL-2R γ chain (γ_c).

gardless of whether IL-2 is present and ensures that, within a few days after activation, T cells become refractory to IL-2 and clonal proliferation ceases. The transient nature of IL-2R expression helps to maintain the cyclical, self-limiting pattern of normal T-cell growth in vivo. CD8 T cells are generally unable to produce adequate amounts of IL-2 and so require exogenous IL-2 from T_H cells in order to proliferate. In contrast, T cells that have been transformed by **human T-cell lymphotropic virus type I (HTLV-I),** the etiologic agent of **adult T-cell leukemia,** constitutively express the IL-2R α chain, giving these cells a growth advantage. Some HTLV-1-infected cells also constitutively produce IL-15, suggesting that autocrine growth stimulation can play a role in T-cell transformation.

IL-2 Effects on Non-T Cells

NK cells constitutively express IL-2R β/γ dimers and thus are IL-2-responsive even in a resting state, although they respond only to relatively high IL-2 concentrations. Once stimulated by IL-2, however, NK cells begin to express the IL-1-2R α chain and assemble high-affinity receptors. IL-2-stimulated NK cells have enhanced cytolytic activity and secrete numerous chemokines and cytokines, including several (IFNγ, GM-CSF, and TNFα) that potently activate macrophages. IL-2 also induces lymphokine-activated killer (LAK) activity, which is predominantly due to NK cells (see Chapter 9).

Activated or transformed B lymphocytes express high-affinity IL-2R at approximately 30% the density found on activated T cells. IL-2 enhances proliferation and antibody secretion by normal B cells, although at concentrations two- to threefold higher than are required to obtain T-cell responses. Human monocytes and macrophages constitutively express low levels of IL-2R β chain, but inducibly express high-affinity receptors containing all three chains on exposure to IL-2, IFNγ, or other activating agents. Continued exposure of an activated macrophage to higher concentrations of IL-2 enhances its microbici-

dal and cytotoxic activities and promotes secretion of hydrogen peroxide, TNFα, and IL-6. High concentrations of IL-2 can activate neutrophils as well.

IL-2 as a Therapeutic Agent

Administration of IL-2 to normal or immunodeficient mice has been shown to enhance immune responses, particularly those mediated by CTLs or NK cells. Its potential use in humans, unfortunately, is limited by the severe toxic side effects of pharmacologic IL-2 dosages. One of the most important of these is the "vascular leak syndrome," characterized by the accumulation of edema fluid in the pleural cavities, peritoneum, and other extravascular spaces; this may result from the ability of IL-2 to induce other cytokines that activate endothelial cells and increase vascular permeability. IL-2 treatment can also increase serum cortisol levels, with consequent immunosuppressive effects. High-dose IL-2 has been tested as an immunostimulatory agent in the treatment of various cancers and has produced partial remissions in some cases, most notably in some renal cell cancers. IL-2 has been tested at low doses as a treatment for the T-cell anergy that occurs in patients with lepromatous leprosy; although some clinical benefit was observed, the anergy persisted, and the beneficial effects have been attributable to activation of macrophages and NK cells. Low doses of IL-2 have also been shown to improve T-cell production and function in patients with the acquired immune deficiency syndrome (**AIDS**) or with idiopathic CD4 T-cell deficiency.

INTERLEUKIN-4 & INTERLEUKIN-13

IL-4 is a glycoprotein cytokine secreted by activated T_H cells, mast cells, and a subset of NK cells. IL-4 is now best known for the role it plays in **allergic diseases** by promoting IgE production, expression of low-affinity Fcε receptors, and the growth and function of mast cells and eosinophils. Secretion of IL-4 is a hallmark, as well as an inducer, of T_H2 differentiation in T cells.

IL-4 and the closely related cytokine IL-13 are produced in the same cell types and are regulated in similar ways. They also produce many of the same biologic effects, in part because their receptors share at least one common chain called IL-4Rα. Two IL-4 receptors have been described: One is a heterodimer of IL-4R α and IL-2R γ chains; the second consists of IL-4Rα and IL-13Rα1 and can transduce both IL-4 and IL-13 signals. Specific IL-13 receptors are either IL-4Rα/IL-13Rα2 heterodimers or are homodimers of IL-13Rα chains. All of these receptors appear to use similar signaling pathways.

Both IL-4 and IL-13 favor T_H2-cell development while suppressing development and function of T_H1 cells. They promote CTL activity, growth of mast cells and other hematopoietic cells, and expression of vascular cell adhesion molecule 1 (VCAM)-1 on endothelial cells. They also have multiple effects on macrophages, activating cytocidal functions and increasing expression of class II MHC proteins, but suppressing the synthesis of proinflammatory cytokines, such as IL-1, IL-6, IL-8, and TNFα. Studies in knockout mice indicate that, despite their overlapping functions, IL-4 and IL-13 have additive effects in T_H2-mediated immune responses: Pulmonary granuloma formation, eosinophil infiltration, and levels of serum IgE and IL-5 were all reduced in schistosome-infected mice that lacked either one of these cytokines, but were completely eliminated in mice that lacked both (see Table 10–6).

INTERLEUKIN-5

IL-5 is a disulfide-linked homodimeric glycoprotein that was originally described as a B-cell growth factor in mice, but functions mainly as an **eosinophil** growth and differentiation factor in humans. T_H2 cells are the major source of IL-5. The human IL-5 receptor shares a common β chain with the IL-3 and GM-CSF receptors, and an α chain expressed only in eosinophils and basophils. IL-5 may have an important role in the pathogenesis of certain allergic diseases and asthma, as well as in helminth infections. Human IL-5 also enhances the activities of basophils by priming them to release mediators such as histamine and leukotrienes in response to other signals (Chapter 13).

INTERLEUKIN-6 & RELATED CYTOKINES

Major activities of IL-6 include synergizing with IL-1 and TNFα to promote T-cell activation by APCs; inducing the **acute-phase response** (Chapter 2); enhancing B-cell replication, differentiation and immunoglobulin production; and promoting hematopoiesis and thrombopoiesis (Table 10–7). It does not induce production of any other cytokines and has relatively little direct effect on immune cells at physiologic concentrations, suggesting that its main immunologic function is to potentiate the effects of other cytokines. IL-6 is a single polypeptide, but can be glycosylated and phosphorylated to various degrees. It is produced by many cell types, including activated B and T cells, monocytes, and endothelial cells. Stimuli that induce its expression include TNFα, IL-1, and agents that activate lymphocytes or macrophages. The malignant plasma cells of multiple myeloma both secrete and respond to IL-6, suggesting it may be an autocrine growth factor for these cells.

IL-6-responsive cells typically express 10^2–10^4 high-affinity IL-6 receptors with an apparent K_d of 10^{-10}–10^{-12} M. The receptor consists of two glycoprotein chains. IL-6 first binds with low affinity to the IL-6R α chain, which has a short cytoplasmic domain and does not signal; the resulting complex then associates with the IL-6R β chain, which increases the affinity of IL-6 binding and transmits a signal into the cell.

The IL-6R β chain also forms part of the receptors for five other cytokines that are structurally unrelated to IL-6 (see Table 10–7). Each has it own specific receptor made up of one or more unique ligand-binding chains together with the IL-6R β chain, which functions as a common signal-transducing subunit. As a result, these cytokines have both unique and overlapping activities, as summarized in Table 10–7. Three members of the family (IL-6, IL-11, and leukemia inhibitory factor [LIF]) promote multilineage hematopoiesis.

INTERLEUKIN-7

IL-7 is a glycoprotein secreted by thymus, spleen, and bone marrow stromal cells. It provides critical signals for the development of both T- and B-cell precursors. The receptor for IL-7, composed of a ligand-binding IL-7R α chain and the common IL-2R γ signal transducer, is expressed on lymphoid progenitors, mature T cell, monocytes, and macrophages. IL-7 provides an essential survival signal to thymocytes and pre-B cells; when IL-7 is withdrawn, these cells rapidly die through apoptosis. IL-7 is also thought to provide a signal that initiates T-cell receptor gene rearrangement during thymocyte development, and it enhances β integrin-mediated adhesion of thymocytes onto extracellular matrix proteins.

Mature human peripheral blood T cells do not respond significantly to IL-7 unless activated, but after activation this cytokine enhances cytotoxic activity and other effector functions of mature cells. It can also induce lymphokine-activated killer (LAK) activ-

Table 10–7. The human IL-6 family of cytokines.

	IL-6	IL-11	LIF	OSM	CNTF	CT-1
Prominent cell sources	Activated T$_H$2 cells, Macrophages, Endothelial, Fibroblasts	Stromal cells	T cells, Macrophages, Fibroblasts	Macrophages, T cells	Glial cells	Embryonic stem cells, heart and skeletal muscle, Fibroblasts
Unique effects	T-cell costimulator, Coinduces cachexia, Induces glucocorticoids, Increases bone resorption, Promotes keratinocyte growth		Inhibits leukemic cell growth	Promotes smooth muscle and fibroblast growth	Enhances survival of ciliary neurons	Cardiac myocyte hypertrophy
Shared effects[a]						
Acute-phase response	+		+	+	+	+
B-cell and plasma-cell growth, Ig production	+		–	–	–	–
Hematopoiesis	+		+	+	–	?
Leukemic cell growth	?		↓	↓	–	↓
Neurotrophic activity	?		+	+	+	+
Endothelial cell growth	?		+	+	–	?

Abbreviations: IL = interleukin; LIF = leukemia inhibitory factor; OSM = oncostatin M; CNTF = ciliary neurotrophic factor; CT-1 = cardiotrophin.
[a] Ability to induce or enhance the indicated processes.

ity, although much less potently than IL-2. At higher dosages, IL-7 increases macrophage cytotoxic activity and induces cytokine secretion by monocytes. Pharmacologic doses of IL-7 produce marked leukocytosis in normal mice and hasten recovery of bone marrow leukocytopoiesis in mice exposed to sublethal irradiation or cytotoxic agents. At these dosages, it produces greater effects on B-lineage than T-lineage cells.

INTERLEUKIN-9

IL-9 is a heavily glycosylated polypeptide lymphokine secreted by activated T cells and has growth-promoting effects on T cells and mast cells. The IL-9 receptor is a heterodimer composed of IL-9R α and IL2R γ chains. Mice that express high levels of IL-9 systemically develop mucosal mastocytosis and allergic eosinophilia in the lungs, as well as enhanced T-cell transformation. IL-9 can synergize with IL-2 or IL-4 in T-cell costimulation and may also stimulate hematopoietic progenitors. Its physiologic role has not been firmly established.

INTERLEUKIN-10

IL-10 is a potent inhibitor of inflammatory and immune responses, in part because it inhibits APC function by suppressing class II MHC expression on dendritic cells and macrophages. It is a product of activated T$_H$2 and CD8 T cells, B cells, monocytes, and keratinocytes and was originally identified because of its ability to inhibit cytokine production by activated T cells, often acting synergistically with TGFβ. For example, IL-10 inhibits the production of IL-2 and IFNγ by T$_H$1 cells, thereby favoring T$_H$2-dependent responses. It inhibits production of cytokines by NK cells, and of cytokines, reactive oxygen species, nitric oxide, and adhesion proteins by macrophages. It is also thought to promote immune tolerance to ingested antigens in the gut (Chapter 14) and may have a more general role in anergy. Mice lacking IL-10R develop severe gastrointestinal inflammatory disease due to overexpression of proinflammatory cytokines. High-level endogenous expression of IL-10 correlates with graft survival in skin, cardiac, and islet-cell transplantation. On the other hand, IL-10 is not entirely immunosuppressive because it has direct comitogenic effects on T cells, B cells, and mast cells and promotes B-cell antibody production.

INTERLEUKIN-12

IL-12 is a critical regulator of both innate and acquired immunity. By selectively promoting differentiation of T_H1 lymphocytes, it potentiates cell-mediated immunity while suppressing T_H2-dependent functions such as the production of IL-4, IL-10, and IgE antibodies. It enhances proliferation of activated T and NK cells, enhances lytic activity of NK and LAK cells, and is the most potent inducer of IFNγ production by resting or activated T and NK cells. In addition, IL-12 induces the production of GM-CSF, TNFα, IL-6, and, to a small extent, IL-2, and it synergizes with IL-2 in promoting CTL and NK-cell responses. It is being explored for potential clinical usefulness as an immunomodulator.

IL-12 is produced by "professional" APCs (macrophages, dendritic cells, and activated B cells) and also by astrocytes. It is a heterodimer composed of a smaller protein subunit expressed by many cell types that is disulfide-linked to a larger subunit expressed preferentially by APCs. The IL-12 receptor is composed of two chains, called β1 and β2. IL-12 synthesis is controlled in part through a feedback mechanism: the T_H2-cell products IL-4 and IL-10 suppress it, whereas IFNγ (a T_H1 cytokine) is required for sustained IL-12 production.

INTERLEUKIN-15

IL-15 shares many of the biologic properties of IL-2 in that it enhances proliferation of activated T cells, generation of CTLs, and activation of LAK cells. It is also essential for NK-cell survival, development, and activation. Unlike IL-2, IL-15 is expressed most abundantly by epithelial cells and monocytes, as well as by numerous other cell types, including placenta, skeletal muscle, kidney, lung, liver, heart and bone marrow stroma, but not by T lymphocytes. It is thought to provide a means by which diverse non-lymphoid cells can potentiate T-cell-mediated immune responses. It has been reported to promote T_H1 responses preferentially. IL-15 generally binds to a receptor composed of the IL-2R β and γ chains and a unique IL-15R α chain, but on mast cell it uses a distinct receptor that does not incorporate any IL-2R subunits.

INTERLEUKIN-16

IL-16 is a product of CD8 T cells and acts as a chemoattractant for CD4 T cells through direct inter-

action with CD4 molecules on their surfaces. Binding of IL-16 inhibits IL-2 production by CD4 T cells and inhibits mixed lymphocyte reactions, suggesting a possible role in T-cell anergy. IL-16 binds to the region in CD4 that mediates CD4 dimerization. Although it does not interfere with CD4 binding or cell entry by the human immunodeficiency virus (HIV), IL-16 does inhibit HIV replication, reportedly by blocking viral mRNA expression.

INTERLEUKIN-17

IL-17 is a homodimeric cytokine that is produced by activated memory T cells and binds to receptors on a wide variety of cells, particularly resting T lymphocytes and cells of the spleen and kidney. It was first identified as the cellular homologue of a protein encoded by the T-cell-tropic virus *Herpesvirus saimiri*. Il-17 induces target cells to express IL-6, IL-8, G-CSF, and the chemokine MCP-1. It stimulates T-cell proliferation and the growth and differentiation of neutrophil precursors and may have a role in organ transplant rejection.

INTERLEUKIN-18

IL-18 was originally discovered by its ability to induce release of IFNγ and other proinflammatory mediators from macrophages and has since been shown to influence expression of other cytokines as well. In synergy with IL-12, for example, it potentiates IFNγ and GM-CSF production by T, B, and NK cells, and promotes T_H1 differentiation. It also synergizes with IL-2 to induce IL-13 production by T and NK cells. IL-18 is constitutively produced by keratinocytes and macrophages. It is structurally related to IL-1 and, like IL-1, is synthesized as a precursor that is then processed by caspase-1 to yield the mature cytokine. The IL-18 receptor is likewise remarkably similar to IL-1R and signals through the same pathways. IL-12 can induce IL-18R expression on T and NK cells. An IL-18 decoy receptor also exists.

INTERFERONS

In 1957, it was discovered that cells exposed to inactivated viruses produce at least one soluble factor that can "interfere" with viral replication when applied to newly infected cells. The factor was named interferon (IFN). It has since been shown that the interferons consist of a large family of secretory proteins that not only share antiviral activity, but also have the ability to inhibit proliferation of vertebrate cells and to modulate immune responses. Interferons do not exert their antiviral effects by acting on viral particles, but rather by inducing an antiviral state within the host cell that makes it inhospitable to viral replication. This, as well as the antiproliferative and immunomodulatory effects of interferons, reflects their ability to regulate specific gene expression and metabolic activity in their target cells. Several types of proteins can induce an antiviral state in vertebrate cells and therefore are, by definition, interferons. The molecular and immunoregulatory properties of IFNγ are so different from those of the other interferons, however, that it must be considered separately.

The Antiviral IFNs

IFNs with relatively high antiviral potency are called antiviral, or **type I,** IFNs. They are not normally found in tissues or serum, but can be synthesized and released rapidly by most cell types in response to infection by viruses, bacteria, or protozoa, or on exposure to certain cytokines (Figure 10–2). These IFNs can also be induced artificially by treating cells with double-stranded RNA molecules, which presumably mimic the genomes of certain RNA viruses. One commonly used inducer of type I IFN is poly(I:C)—a heteroduplex of polyinosine and polycytidine RNA chains.

There are three major forms of type I IFN: IFNα, IFNβ, and IFNω. **IFNα** is the primary IFN produced by leukocytes and consists of at least 14 glycoproteins encoded by a closely related family of genes. The amino acid sequences of these various IFNα proteins are approximately 73% identical to one another. Fibroblasts and most other nonleukocytes primarily express **IFNβ,** a protein that is only about 30% identical to IFNα. Small amounts of IFNβ are also expressed by leukocytes. **IFNω** has only a single functional gene, which resembles the **IFNγ** gene and is primarily expressed by leukocytes.

All type I IFNs bind to a single multichain receptor, which is expressed on nearly all cell types and is structurally related to the IL-10 receptor. Binding of type I IFN to this receptor leads to increased expression of at least 30 different proteins in the target cell. Among these are the **class I MHC** proteins, which enable an infected cell to present viral antigens and so to be killed by CTLs. The type I IFNs also stimulate IL-12-independent production of **IFNγ,** which promotes T-cell and macrophage function. Other IFN-inducible proteins include an RNA-dependent protein kinase (**PKR**) and **2′-5′ oligoadenylate (2-5A) synthetase,** each of which requires the presence of double-stranded RNA for activity. When activated, PKR phosphorylates a component of the cellular translational machinery (called eukaryotic initiation factor 2, or eIF2), thereby inhibiting protein synthesis. The 2-5A synthetase produces short chains of adenylate residues joined by 2′-5′ phosphodiester bonds; these bind and activate a cellular endoribonuclease that specifically degrades single-stranded RNA. These enzymes, together with other IFN-inducible proteins, combine to confer a relatively nonspecific but potent intracellular defense against viruses.

In addition to inhibiting viral replication, type I IFNs can modulate specific cellular functions. They

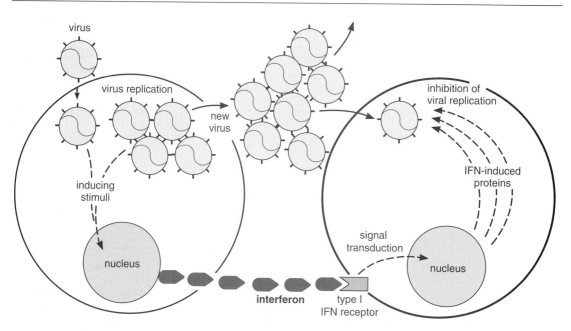

Figure 10–2. Schematic representation of the induction and activity of a type I interferon.

arrest the growth of (but generally do not kill) many types of cells in culture, including transformed cell lines. They also may either inhibit or promote cellular differentiation, depending on the cell type, timing, and dosage of treatment.

Clinically, type I interferons have proven most useful in treating hematologic disorders. Recombinant IFNα, either alone or in combination with chemotherapy, is used to treat hairy cell leukemia, chronic lymphocytic leukemia (CLL), cutaneous T cell lymphoma, and certain other non-Hodgkin's lymphomas. Both IFNα and IFNβ have been effective in subsets of patients with acute and chronic hepatitis B and C infections, and in patients with relapsing remitting multiple sclerosis.

Immune IFN

IFNγ (also called **type II** IFN or **immune IFN**) arises from a single gene and differs in virtually all respects from the type I IFNs. There is only a single active form of IFNγ protein—a homodimer of polypeptides that can be glycosylated to various degrees. The receptor to which it binds is likewise unrelated to the receptor for type I IFN. Although IFNγ has some antiviral activity (which led to its discovery and is the source of its name), it is much less active in this regard than the type I IFNs. Moreover, IFNγ expression is not directly inducible by infection or by double-stranded RNA. It is involved in the regulation of nearly all phases of the immune and inflammatory responses, including the activation and differentiation of T cells, B cells, NK cells, macrophages, and others. It is therefore best regarded as a distinct **immunoregulatory** cytokine and has found clinical application as an immunostimulator in chronic granulomatous disease and other disorders.

IFNγ secretion is a hallmark of T_H1 lymphocytes. It is also secreted by nearly all CD8 T cells, by some T_H0 cells, and by NK cells. Each of these cell types secretes IFNγ only when activated, usually as part of an immune response and especially in response to IL-2 and IL-12. IFNγ production is inhibited by IL-4, IL-10, TGFβ, glucocorticoids, cyclosporin A and FK506. Nearly all cell types express the heterodimeric receptor for IFNγ and respond to this cytokine by increasing the surface expression of class I MHC proteins. As a result, virtually any cell in the vicinity of an IFNγ-secreting cell becomes more efficient at presenting endogenous antigens and hence a better target for cytotoxic killing if it harbors an intracellular pathogen. Unlike the type I IFNs, IFNγ also increases the expression of **class II MHC** proteins on professional APCs, and so promotes antigen presentation to helper T cells as well. It also induces de novo expression of class II MHC proteins on venular endothelial cells and on some other epithelial and connective tissue cells that do not otherwise express them, thus enabling these cell types to function as temporary APCs at sites of intense immune reactions.

IFNγ is also a potent activator of **macrophages.** Exposure to IFNγ greatly enhances the microbicidal (and, to a lesser degree, cytotoxic) activity of macrophages and induces them to secrete nitric oxide and monokines such as IL-1, IL-6, IL-8, and TNFα. It also activates neutrophils, NK cells, and vascular endothelial cells. IFNγ synergistically enhances the cytotoxic effects of TNFα. Although IFNγ tends to promote the differentiation of B cells and CD8 T cells into immunologically active effectors, it does not promote lymphocyte proliferation. It enhances the activity of T_H1 cells, but inhibits the production of T_H2 cells. IFNγ not only decreases the production of IL-4 by T_H2 cells but also potently blocks the effects of IL-4 on B cells, promoting IgG1 production at the expense of IgE production.

TRANSFORMING GROWTH FACTOR β

TGFβ was initially discovered as a growth factor for fibroblasts that promoted wound healing. It also has considerable antiproliferative activity, however, and acts as a negative regulator of immunity and hematopoiesis. TGFβ is produced by many cell types, including activated macrophages and T lymphocytes. Humans express at least three forms of TGFβ: TGFβ-1, -2, and -3. These are the products of separate genes, but they all bind to five types of high-affinity cell surface receptors. Type I and II receptors transduce signals, whereas the function of type III, IV, and V receptors is not yet clear. TGFβ receptors are expressed in widely different numbers by many cell types. Studies in mice suggest that TGFβ-1 is the most important immunoregulator in this group; mice that lack it die of fulminant inflammatory and autoimmune disease.

TGFβ has antiproliferative effects on a wide variety of cell types, including macrophages, endothelial cells, and T and B lymphocytes (Figure 10-3). It also suppresses the production of most lymphokines and monokines and reduces the cellular expression of class II MHC proteins and of IL-1 receptors. At 10^{-10}–10^{-12} M, it blocks the proliferative effects of IL-2 on T and B cells, as well as of IL-1 on thymocytes. In addition, TGFβ inhibits T-cell-dependent antibody production by B cells, mixed-leukocyte reactions, and the generation of CTLs. It also inhibits induction of NK-cell activities and of LAK cells by IL-2. Thus, TGFβ is unique in that it can act as a negative-feedback regulator that dampens immunologically mediated reactions. Recently, a new subset of helper T cells (dubbed **T_H3 cells**) has been identified that mainly produces TGFβ; these cells appear important in maintaining tolerance to orally administered antigens in the gut (see Chapter 14), further demonstrating the role of TGFβ as a major immunosuppressive cytokine.

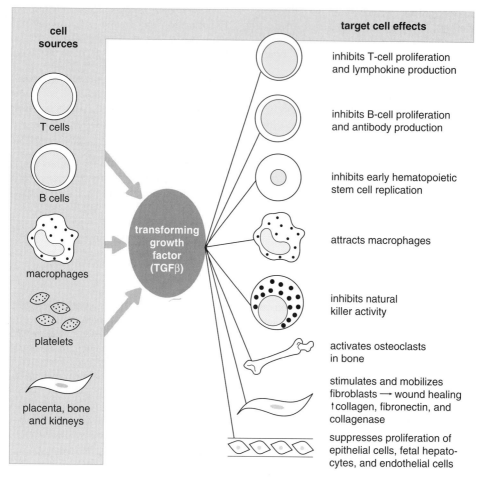

Figure 10–3. Cell sources and effects of TGFβ.

TGFβ also has some proinflammatory activities. It is a chemoattractant for neutrophils and monocytes, and it increases expression of adhesion proteins on monocytes. These effects may account for the observation that injecting TGFβ directly into inflamed joints exacerbates the inflammation. On the other hand, systemic administration of TGFβ-1 has antiinflammatory effects.

HEMATOPOIETIC COLONY-STIMULATING FACTORS

CSFs are cytokines that support the production of particular mature blood cell types from pluripotent stem cells or committed progenitors in the bone marrow. Examples include G-CSF, GM-CSF, EPO, thrombopoietin (TPO), SCF, and IL-3 (also known as multi-CSF because it promotes formation of all hematopoietic cell types). The biologic properties of

the CSFs and their receptors have been summarized in Chapter 1; only a few points will be highlighted here.

The various CSFs are unrelated to one another structurally and bind to distinct receptors. Nevertheless, many have overlapping functions and induce quite similar biologic effects. This is particularly true of CSFs that influence granulocyte and macrophage production. The biologic significance of this redundancy is unclear. Some CSFs have unique functions that become apparent in knockout mice that lack them (Table 10–8), although these are not always relevant to hematopoiesis. Certain cytokines (eg, IL-1, IL-6, and IL-11) that have little or no independent effect on hematopoiesis act synergistically with CSFs. SCF is the most potent synergistic CSF; it interacts with many other cytokines to promote growth of myeloerythroid and lymphoid stem cells, and hence increases the production of all blood cells. Nevertheless, hematopoietic stem cells will not proliferate in

Table 10–8. Phenotypes of hematopoietic cytokine knockout mice.

Targeted Gene	Phenotypic Abnormalities
G-CSF	Defective myelopoiesis Neutropenia Susceptible to *Listeria* infections
GM-CSF	Accumulation of pulmonary surfactant; pulmonary fibrosis No hematopoietic defects
cMPL (thrombopoietin receptor)	Thrombocytopenia
SCF(c-kit ligand)	*Steel* locus mutation in mice results in altered coat color, anemia, and defective gonadal development
SCF-receptor (c-kit)	Maldevelopment of melanocyte, germ cell, and hematopoietic lineages Piebaldism: dominant hypopigmented spotting
M-CSF	Reduced bone resorption, osteopetrosis in mice Hypoactive macrophages
Flt-3	Defective hematopoiesis

Abbreviations: G-CSF = granulocyte colony-stimulating factor; GM-CSF = granulocyte–monocyte colony-stimulating factor; SCF = stem cell factor; M-CSF = monocyte colony-stimulating factor; cMPL = cellular counterpart of viral myeloproliferative leukemia gene.

response to any single cytokine; instead, their growth is promoted by combinations of cytokines that include one from each of the following three groups: (1) SCF or Flt-3 ligand; (2) IL-1, IL-6, IL-11, IL-12, TPO, or G-CSF; and (3) IL-3, IL-4, or GM-CSF. These synergistic effects are direct and can be observed in single-cell assays.

The production of some CSFs is selectively increased during immune or inflammatory responses. For example, activated T cells can secrete IL-3, IL-5, and GM-CSF, and activated macrophages produce a host of CSFs and other cytokines. Similarly, fibroblasts and endothelial cells secrete G-CSF and GM-CSF only when stimulated by IL-1, TNFα, or other products of activated macrophages.

Several of the CSFs profoundly affect immune and inflammatory cells. Those that act on granulocytes, for example, help prolong the survival and function of neutrophils and eosinophils at an infected site by suppressing apoptosis. Macrophages produced in the presence of GM-CSF alone have more potent APC function and, when activated, have greater cytotoxic activity than those produced with M-CSF, in part because M-CSF reduces MHC protein expression and stimulates production of IL-1RA. GM-CSF also is essential for the generation of **dendritic cells** from their marrow-derived precursor cells, and the local release of this cytokine by activated macrophages, T cells, and keratinocytes in the course of an immune response is thought to trigger dendritic cell maturation into functional APCs.

Many CSFs are currently being tested for possible clinical use. GM-CSF and G-CSF may prove to be of value in preventing the therapy-induced granulocytopenia that is the major cause of death among cancer patients undergoing chemotherapy or radiation therapy. Both of these cytokines may also help protect against bacterial septicemia. In contrast to many of the other cytokines, G-CSF, EPO, and TPO, which act on more limited cell populations, produce relatively few toxic side effects and are in clinical use to increase the production of neutrophils, red cells, and platelets, respectively. In addition, G-CSF is the agent of choice for mobilizing hematopoietic stem cells into the peripheral blood for harvest and use in autologous bone marrow transplantation.

CYTOKINE RECEPTOR FAMILIES

The characterization of many cytokine receptors and their corresponding genes has revealed that most belong to larger multigene families (Table 10–9). The members of each family share distinctive structural features and are thought to be evolutionarily related. The divisions among families are not mutually exclusive, however, and some receptors (eg, IL-6R) can be assigned to multiple families. The receptors for IL-1, IL-6, M-CSF, G-CSF, and SCF each contain an immunoglobulin-like domain in their extracellular regions and thus belong to the **immunoglobulin gene superfamily** (see Chapter 7). Many of the remaining cytokines belong to the **hematopoietin receptor family,** whose members can be recognized by a distinctive set of four spaced cysteines in their extracellular domains as well as by a conserved sequence motif (Trp-Ser-X-Trp-Ser, where X is any amino acid) located near the external membrane surface. It has been proposed that receptor dimerization is required for signal transduction by hematopoietin receptors; the dimers can be either homodimers, as in IL-4R, or more complex heterodimers, as in IL-6R and some others.

Table 10–9. Cytokine receptor families.

	Distinguishing Features	Ligands of Member Receptors
Hematopoietin superfamily	Trp-Ser-X-Trp-Ser motif; 4 extracellular Cys residues	IL-2, IL-3, IL-4, IL-5, IL-6 family, IL-7, IL-9, GM-CSF, G-CSF, Epo, growth hormone, prolactin
Immunoglobulin superfamily	Ig-like extracellular domain	IL-1, IL-6, M-CSF, G-CSF, SCF
TNF family	4 Cys-rich extracellular regions	TNFα, CD27, CD30, CD40, Fas, LTα & α/β complex, NGF
IL-3 family	Common β subunit	IL-3, IL-5, GM-CSF
IL-6 family	Common β subunit	IL-6, IL-11, LIF, OSM, CNTF, CT-1
IL-8 family	7 transmembrane domains	Chemokines
Tyrosine kinase family	Intrinsic Tyr kinase activity in cytoplasmic domain	M-CSF, SCF, platelet-derived growth factor, fibroblast growth factor
TGFβ family	Intrinsic Thr/Ser kinase activity in cytoplasmic domain	TGFβ, inhibins, activins, Mullerian inhibiting substance, bone morphogenetic protein
IFN family	Type I (for IFNα, β, and ϖ), type II (for IFNγ)	IFNα, β, ϖ, and γ, IL-10

Abbreviations: TNF = tumor necrosis factor; IL = interleukin; TGF = transforming growth factor; IFN = interferon; GM-CSF = granulocyte–monocyte colony-stimulating factor, G-CSF = granulocyte colony-stimulating factor; M-CSF = macrophage colony-stimulating factor; SCF = stem cell factor; LIF = leukemia inhibitory factor; OSM = oncostatin M; CNTF = ciliary neurotrophic factor; CT-1 = cardiotrophin-1.

VIROKINES & VIRORECEPTORS

Many viruses encode proteins that resemble specific cytokines or cytokine receptors. These probably play an important role in the viral life cycles, particularly in immune evasion. It has been proposed that these so-called virokines or viroreceptors are descended from cellular proteins whose genes were usurped by the viruses. For example, **Epstein–Barr virus,** which infects and immortalizes B lymphoid cells, encodes an IL-10-like protein which, like IL-10 itself, stimulates B-cell proliferation and differentiation (and so enhances viral replication) while suppressing cellular immune responses. Similarly, the T-cell-tropic virus *Herpes saimiri* encodes a protein resembling IL-17, which promotes T-cell proliferation. Other viruses, such as the **poxviruses,** encode proteins that resemble cellular receptors (eg, those for IL-1, TNFα, IFNγ, or certain chemokines) and that appear to suppress immune reactions by binding and inhibiting these cytokines in vivo. Interestingly, the cowpox virus also encodes an intracellular inhibitor of caspase-1; this inhibitor not only blocks processing and secretion of IL-1β, but also helps suppress apoptosis of the infected cell.

OVERVIEW & PROSPECTS

The cytokines as a group serve as crucial intercellular signaling molecules that are responsible for the multidirectional communication among cells engaged in host defense, tissue repair, and other essential functions. Cytokines regulate one another's production and activities through competition, synergism, and mutual induction, resulting in a complex network of cytokine cascades and regulatory circuits with positive and negative feedback effects. In addition, other types of biologic mediators, such as corticosteroids and prostaglandins, can enhance or antagonize cytokine activities. The biologic responses to cytokines can also be regulated through effects on the specific cytokine receptors expressed by responsive cells, and these receptors may provide a useful therapeutic target for modulating cytokine activity. Owing to the complexity of cytokine interactions, the therapeutic use of these agents is still in its infancy. Nevertheless, the potential of this approach has already been demonstrated in some clinical settings. Specific agonists and antagonists of the cytokines and their receptors can be expected to play an important role in future therapy of inflammatory, infectious, autoimmune, and neoplastic diseases.

REFERENCES

GENERAL

Durum SK, Muegge K. (editors): *Cytokine Knockouts.* Humana Press, 1998.

Krakauer T et al: Proinflammatory cytokines: TNF and IL1 families, chemokines and others. In: *Fundamental Immunology,* 4th ed. Paul WE (editor). Lippincott-Raven Pub. 1999.

Leonard WJ. Type I cytokines and interferons and their receptors. In: *Fundamental Immunology,* 4th ed. Paul WE (editor). Lippincott-Raven Pub., 1999.

Mire-Sluis A. Thorpe R: *Cytokines.* Academic Press, 1998.

Nicola NA (editor): *Guidebook to Cytokines and Their Receptors.* Oxford Univ Press, 1994.

Oppenheim JJ et al (editors): *Cytokine Reference: A Compendium of Cytokines and Other Mediators of Host Defense.* Academic Press, Ltd. Inc., 2000.

Thompson AW (editor): *The Cytokine Handbook,* 3rd ed. Academic Press, 1998.

INTERLEUKIN-1

Alcami A, Smith GL: A mechanism for the inhibition of fever by a virus. *Proc Natl Acad Sci U S A* 1996;93: 11029.

Bresnihan B et al: Treatment of rheumatoid arthritis withrecombinant human interleukin-1 receptor antagonist. *Arthritis Rheum* 1998;41:2196.

Colotta F et al: The type II decoy receptors: a novel regulatory pathway for IL-1. *Immunol Today* 1994;15:562.

Dinarello CA: Biologic basis for interleukin-1 in disease. *Blood* 1996;87:2095.

Dinarello CA: IL-1, IL-1R and IL-1RA. *Int Rev Immunol* 1998;16:457.

Fantuzzi G, Dinarello CA: The inflammatory response in IL-1β-deficient mice: Comparison with other cytokine-related knockout mice. *J Leuk Biol* 1996;59:489.

TUMOR NECROSIS FACTOR FAMILY

Beutler B, Can Huffel C: Unraveling function in the TNF ligand receptor. *Science* 1994;264:667.

Feldman M et al: Anti TNFα therapy of rheumatoid arthritis. *Adv Immunol* 1997;64:283.

Gramaglia I et al: Ox-40 ligand: A potent costimulatory molecule for sustaining primary CD4 T cell responses. *J Immunol* 1998;161:6510.

Green EA, Flavell RA: TRANCE-RANK, a new signal pathway involved in lymphocyte development and T cell activation. *J Exp Med* 1999;189:1017.

Grewal IS, Flavel RA: CD40 and CD154 in cell-mediated immunity. *Annu Rev Immunol* 1998;16:111.

Nagata S, Golstein P: The FAS death factor. *Science* 1995;27: 1449.

Nagumo H et al: CD27/CD70 interaction augments IgE secretion by promoting the differentiation of memory B cells into plasma cells. *J Immunol* 1998;161:6496.

Wajant H et al: TNF receptor associated factors in cytokine signaling. *Cytokine Growth Factor Rev* 1999;10:15.

Walczak H et al: Tumoricidal activity of tumor necrosis factor-related apoptosis-inducing ligand in vivo. *Nat Med* 1999;5:157.

Ware CF et al: Tumor necrosis factor-related ligands and receptors. *Cytokine Handbook,* 3rd ed. Thomson AW (Ed), Academic Press 1998.

INTERLEUKIN-2

Brennan P et al: Phosphatidylinositol 3-kinase couples the interleukin-2 receptor to the cell cycle regulator E2F. *Immunity* 1997;7:679.

Kuroda K et al: Implantation of IL-2-containing osmotic pump prolongs the survival of superantigen-reactive T cells expanded in mice injected with bacterial superantigen. *J Immunol* 1996;157:1422.

Leonard W et al: The molecular basis of X-linked severe combined immunodeficiency: the role of the interleukin-

2 receptor γ chain as a common γ chain, γc. *Immunol Rev* 1994;138:61.

Lin J-X et al: Signaling from the IL-2 receptor to the nucleus. *Cytokines Growth Factor Rev* 1997;8:313.

IL-6 FAMILY

Cherel N et al: Molecular cloning of two isoforms of a receptor for the human hematopoietic cytokine interleukin-11. *Blood* 1995;86:2534.

Du X et al.: Interleukin-11: Review of molecular, cell biology, and clinical use. *Blood* 1997;89:3897.

Gadient RA et al: Leukemia inhibitory factor, interleukin 6, and other cytokines using the GP130 transducing receptor: roles in inflammation and injury. *Stem Cells* 1999; 17:127.

Heinrich PC et al: Interleukin-6-type cytokine signaling through the gp130/Jak/STAT pathway. *Biochem J* 1998; 334:297.

Hirano T: Interleukin 6 and its receptor: Ten years later. *Int Rev Immunol* 1998;16:249.

Mosley B et al: Dual oncostatin M (OSM) receptors: Cloning and characterization of an alternative signaling subunit conferring OSM-specific receptor activation. *J Biol Chem* 1996;271:32635.

Pennica D et al: Cardiotrophin-1: Biologic activities and binding to the LIF receptor/gp130 signaling complex. *J Biol Chem* 1995;270:10:915.

Taga T, Kishimoto T: Gp130 and the interleukin-6 family of cytokines. *Annu Rev Immunol* 1997;15:797.

Wallace P et al: In vivo properties of oncostatin M. *Ann N Y Acad Sci* 1995;762:42.

OTHER INTERLEUKINS

Chomarat P et al: Interleukin-4 and interleukin-13: Their similarities and discrepancies. *Int Rev Immunol* 1998; 17:1.

Komastu T et al: IL-12 and viral infections. *Cytokine Growth Factor Rev* 1998;9:277.

Lalani T et al: Biology of IL-5 in health and disease. *Ann Allergy Asthma Immunol* 1999;82:317.

McKenzie GJ et al: Simultaneous disruption of interleukin (IL)-4 and IL-13 defines individual roles in T helper cell type 2-mediated responses. *J Exp Med* 1999;189:1565.

Moore KW et al: IL 10. *Annu Rev Immunol* 1993;11:165.

Mosmann TR, Moore KW: The role of IL 10 in cross-regulation of T_H1 and T_H2 responses. *Immunol Today* 1991; 12:A49.

Muller G et al: Gene targeting in immunology. In: *Immunological Review,* Goran Moller (editor), No 148. Munksgaard Copenhagen, Stockholm, 1995.

Nelms K et al: The IL-4 receptor: signaling mechanisms and biologic functions. *Annu Rev Immuno.* 1999;17:701.

Waldmann TA et al: The multifaceted regulation of interleukin-15 expression and the role of this cytokine in NK cell differentiation and host response to intracellular pathogens. *Annu Rev Immunol* 1999;17:19.

INTERFERONS

Cousens LP et al: Two roads diverged: Interferon α/β- and interleukin 12-mediated pathways in promoting T-cell interferon γ responses during viral infection. *J Exp Med* 1999;189:1315.

Diaz MO et al: Nomenclature of the human interferon genes. *J Interferon Res* 1994;14:221.

Farrar MA, Schreiber RD: The molecular cell biology of interferon-γ and its receptor. *Annu Rev Immunol* 1993; 11:571.

Marrack P et al: Type I interferons keep activated T cells alive. *J Exp Med* 1999;189:521.

Strober W et al: Reciprocal IFN-γ and TGF-β responses regulate the occurrence of mucosal inflammation. *Immunol Today* 1997;17:61.

van den Broek MF et al: Immune defense in mice lacking Type I and/or Type II interferon receptors. *Immunol Rev* 1995;148:5.

Weiner HL: Oral tolerance: immune mechanisms and treatment of autoimmune diseases. *Immunol Today* 1997;18: 335.

Young HA, Hardy KJ: Role of interferon gamma in immune cell regulation. *J Leuk Biol* 1995;58:37.

TRANSFORMING GROWTH FACTOR B

Kingsley D: The TGF-β superfamily: New members, new receptors and new genetic tests of function in different organisms. *Genes Dev* 1994;8:133.

Massague J et al: The TGF-β family and its composite receptors. *Trends Cell Biol* 1994;4:172.

Shull NM et al: Targeted disruption of mouse TGFβ1 gene results in multifocal inflammatory disease. *Nature* 1992; 359:693.

Wahl SM: Transforming growth factor beta: The good, the bad, and the ugly. *J Exp Med* 1994;180:1587.

HEMATOPOIETIC CYTOKINES

Armitage JO: Emerging applications of recombinant human granulocyte-macrophage colony-stimulating factor. *Blood* 1998;92:4491.

DeGroot RP et al: Regulation of proliferation, differentiation and survival by the IL-3/IL-5/GM-CSF receptor family. *Cell Signal* 1998;10:619.

Eder M et al: IL-3 in the clinic. *Stem Cells* 1997;15:327.

Fixe P et al: M-CSF: Haematopoietic growth factor or inflammatory cytokine? *Cytokine* 1998;10:32.

Garland J et al (editors): *Colony Stimulating Factors,* 2nd ed. Marcel Dekker, Inc., 1998.

Kaushansky K: Thrombopoietin. *New Engl J Med* 1998;339: 746.

Lyman SD et al: c-kit ligand and flt3 ligand: Stem/progenitor cell factors with overlapping yet distinct activities. *Blood* 1998;91:1101.

Orlic D et al: *Hematopoietic Stem Cells Biology and Transplantation,* vol 872. New York Academy of Sciences, 1999.

Solar GP et al: Role of c-mpl in early hematopoiesis. *Blood* 1998;92:4.

Weiss M et al: Granulocyte colony-stimulating factor to prevent the progression of systemic nonresponsiveness in systemic inflammatory response syndrome and sepsis. *Blood* 1999;93:425.

Yagi M et al: Sustained ex vivo expansion of hematopoietic stem cells mediated by thrombopoietin. *Proc Natl Acad Sci USA* 1999;96:8126.

CYTOKINE RECEPTORS

Davies DR, Wlodawer A: Cytokines and their receptor complexes. *FASEB J* 1995;9:50.

Massague J: TGF-β signal transduction. *Annu Rev Biochem* 1998;67:753.

Miyajima A et al: Common subunits of cytokine receptors and the functional redundancy of cytokines. *Trends Biol Sci* 1992;17:378.

Sprang SR, Bazan JF: Cytokine structural taxonomy and mechanisms of receptor engagement. *Curr Opin Struc Biol* 1993;3:815.

VIROKINES & VIRORECEPTOR

Lanlani AS, McFadden G: Secreted poxvirus cytokine binding proteins. *J Leuk Biol* 1997;62:570.

McFadden G: DNA viruses that affect cytokine networks. In: *Human Cytokines: Their Role in Disease and Therapy,* Aggarwal B, Puri K (editors). Blackwell Science, 1995.

Smith GL: Virus strategies of evasion of the host response to infection. *Trends Microbiol* 1994;2:81.

Spriggs MK: Virus-encoded modulators of cytokines and growth factors. *Cytokines Growth Factor Rev* 1999;10:1.

Chemokines

11

Joost J. Oppenheim, MD, & Richard Horuk, PhD

In the late 1960s, activated T lymphocytes were found to secrete lymphokines that had potent chemoattractant activity for monocytes and neutrophils. Since that time, over 35 such chemoattractant cytokines, or **chemokines,** have been characterized, and additional members are being discovered at an accelerating rate, making this one of the largest functional groups of cytokines known. Most are small peptides, with molecular weights ranging from 8,000 to 16,000, that share 20–72% amino acid sequence similarity with one another. We now know that virtually all cell types have the capacity to produce one or more chemokines, each of which acts on specific types of target cells bearing the appropriate receptors.

Like other cytokines, chemokines are multifunctional: individual chemokines regulate not only chemotaxis but also adhesion, degranulation, angiogenesis, development of hematopoietic and immune cells, and the genesis of lymphoid organs. Most, however, have little or no effect on cell proliferation. Along with their roles in normal physiology and host defense, chemokines are also implicated in a number of autoimmune or inflammatory disorders, including multiple sclerosis, rheumatoid arthritis, asthma, and organ transplant rejection. In addition, several important human pathogens mimic or inhibit chemokine functions to their own advantage or use chemokine receptors as a means to bind and invade their target cells. These observations have inspired an intensive search for new drugs that could target specific chemokines or their receptors and eventually provide new approaches to treating these disorders.

CLASSIFICATION OF CHEMOKINES

Chemokine nomenclature has not yet been standardized. The first chemokine to be discovered was named interleukin-8 **(IL-8),** but most others are known by abbreviations of one or more historical names, which are often idiosyncratic or unenlightening (Table 11–1). The most meaningful and widely accepted classification scheme recognizes four sub-families of chemokines based on features of their amino acid sequences (Figure 11–1). In particular, most chemokines contain two or three pairs of cysteine (C) residues that form intramolecular disulfide bonds, which help maintain the folded structure of the molecule; one of these disulfides generally forms between C1 and C3, the other between C2 and C4. In one subfamily of chemokines, C1 and C2 are separated by a single amino acid; these are termed the **CXC,** or α, chemokines. Others have no intervening amino acid between C1 and C2, and are called **CC,** or β, chemokines. One unusual human chemokine, called **lymphotactin,** has only a single cysteine pair, and so is the only known member of the **XC,** or γ, subfamily. The largest chemokine, called **fractalkine,** has three residues interposed between C1 and C2, making it the sole **CX3C,** or δ, chemokine. As we shall see, the members of each subfamily often have overlapping functional properties, as they bind to particular subsets of receptors.

CHEMOKINE RECEPTORS & SIGNAL TRANSDUCTION

Sixteen functional **chemokine receptors** have so far been identified (see Figure 11–1). All of them belong to the much larger superfamily of receptors that have **seven transmembrane domains**—a family that also includes the opioid and olfactory receptors, as well as receptors for other chemoattractant substances, such as formylmethionyl peptides and complement protein C5a (see Chapters 2 and 12).

The 16 functional receptors identified so far include five CXCRs, nine CCRs, one CX3CR, and one XCR. Each of these receptors binds only the corresponding subfamily of chemokines, but some are able to bind as many as eight different members of that subfamily with high affinity. By the same token, a given chemokine may bind and signal through several different chemokine receptors of a single type; for example, the CC chemokine MIP-1α binds with high affinity to CCR1, CCR3, or CCR5. Although most or all chemokines can be secreted from the cells that

Table 11–1. Proinflammatory chemokines.

Chemokine	Major Cell Sources	CXCR 1	CXCR 2	CXCR 3	CCR 1	CCR 2	CCR 3	CCR 5	CCR 8	CX3C 1
CXC Subfamily										
ELR+ CXC										
IL-8	M,N,DC,T,NK,F,EC,K,Ep	▓	▓							
GROα, -β, -γ	M,N,DC,T,F,EC,K		▓							
ENA-78	M,F,EC,K		▓							
GCP-2	M,F		▓							
NAP-2	Plt		▓							
ELR− CXC										
IP-10	M,N,DC,T,F,EC,K,Ep			▓						
MIG	M,F,EC,K,Str			▓						
I-TAC	M,T			▓						
CC Subfamily										
MCP-1	M,N,DC,Eo,Mt,F,EC,K					▓				
-2	M,N,T,F					▓				
-3	M,F,EC,K,Ep,Plt				▓	▓	▓			
-4	M,F,EC,Ep					▓	▓			
Eotaxin-1	M,T,F,EC,Ep						▓			
-2	M,T						▓			
RANTES	M,DC,T,Eo,Mt,F,EC,K,Plt				▓		▓	▓		
MIP-1α	M,N,CD,T,Mc,F				▓			▓		
-1β	M,N,DC,T,Mt,F							▓		
I-309	M,T								▓	
MPIF-1	M,DC				▓					
HCC-2	M				▓		▓			
-4	M				▓					
CX3C Subfamily										
Fractalkine	M,DC,T,NK,EC									▓

Abbreviations: ELR = glutamate/leucine/arginine; IL = interleukin; GRO = growth-related peptide; ENA = epithelial-derived neutrophil attractant; GCP = granulocyte chemotactic protein; NAP = neutrophil-activating peptide; IP = interferon γ-inducible protein; MIG = monokine induced by interferon γ; I-TAC = interferon-inducible T-cell alpha chemoattractant; MCP = monocyte chemoattractant protein; RANTES = regulated on activation, normal T expressed and secreted; MIP = macrophage inflammatory protein; M = monocyte/macrophage; N = neutrophil; DC = dendritic cell; T = T cell; B = B cell; Eo = eosinophil; Mt = mast cell; NK = natural killer cell; F = fibroblast; EC = endothelial cell; K = keratinocyte; Sm = smooth muscle cell; Ep = epithelial cell; Plt = platelet; Str = stromal cell.

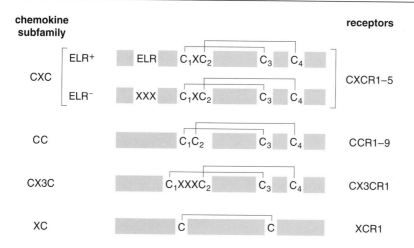

Figure 11–1. Chemokine subfamilies. Schematic structures depict amino acid sequences that define each subfamily. *Abbreviations:* E = glutamate; L = leucine; R = arginine; C = cysteine; X = any amino acid. Brackets linking C residues denote intrachain disulfide bonds.

produce them, they tend to adhere nonspecifically to nearby cell surfaces and components of the extracellular matrix, eventually forming a relatively fixed concentration gradient of immobilized chemokine molecules within the host tissue. As a result, target cells generally recognize these immobilized proteins, rather than free, soluble chemokines, and follow the fixed gradient to its source.

Like other receptors that have seven transmembrane domains, the chemokine receptors are **G-protein-coupled receptors,** meaning that their signaling function depends on interaction with a guanosine triphosphate (GTP)-binding protein, or G-protein, in the cytoplasm. Chemokine receptors interact with a particular class of G-protein (called heterotrimeric G_i-proteins) that are each composed of α_i, β, and γ polypeptides. In the absence of chemokine, a G-protein and its bound GTP associate stably with the cytoplasmic domain of the chemokine receptor. Chemokine binding causes a conformational change in the receptor that leads to hydrolysis of the GTP into guanosine diphosphate (GDP) and dissociation of the G-protein into α_i and β/γ subunits. The latter subunits then activate various cytoplasmic effector enzymes, including phospholipases, which lead to inositol phosphate production, increased intracellular Ca^{2+} concentration, and activation of protein kinases. This signaling cascade, in turn, leads to the biologic effects of the chemokine, which may include actin-dependent locomotion, induction of adhesion proteins, degranulation, leukocyte activation, and other phenomena. Like other signals involving G_i-proteins, chemokine signaling can be blocked by pertussis toxin, an agent widely used in laboratory studies of this signaling pathway.

BIOLOGIC ACTIVITIES OF CHEMOKINES

The biologic properties of chemokines are largely dictated by the conditions under which they are secreted, the receptor they bind, and the cells on which those receptors are expressed (Figure 11–2). Most can be assigned to one of two broad functional categories. **Proinflammatory chemokines** are produced in the course of immune or inflammatory reactions and serve to mobilize host defenses. The **developmental,** or **homeostatic, chemokines,** on the other hand, are produced more or less continually and help guide development, maintain homeostasis, or direct the traffic of circulating cells through normal tissues. The following summary will consider 33 human chemokines as representatives of these two cate-

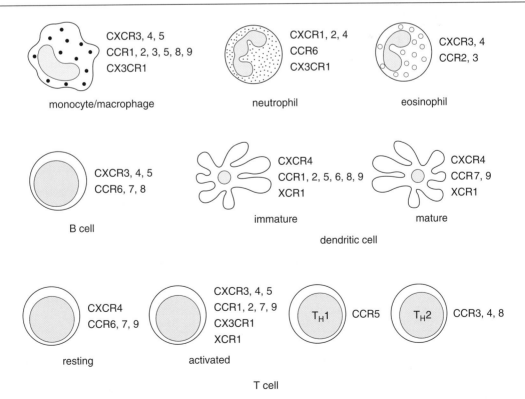

Figure 11–2. Chemokine receptor expression by hematopoietic cells. Only selected receptors are shown.

gories, emphasizing their effects on immune functions; other effects will be briefly noted and are described more fully in the accompanying tables and references.

Proinflammatory Chemokines

Many chemokines from the CC, CXC, and CX3C subfamilies have proinflammatory activity, in that they attract particular leukocytes into sites of injury or infection (see Table 11–1). Nearly all members of this category can be secreted by activated macrophages, but individual members are also produced, after appropriate stimulation, by many other hematopoietic and nonhematopoietic cells. Stimuli that induce their release variously include bacterial lipopolysaccharide (LPS), IL-1, tumor necrosis factor α (TNFα), interferon γ (IFNγ), and other broadly specific signals of tissue injury and distress. Two (NAP-2 and PF-4) are released only by activated platelets. All proinflammatory chemokines of the CC subfamily are encoded on chromosome 17, whereas those of the CXC subfamily are on chromosome 4.

Most known CXC chemokines are proinflammatory, but the type of inflammation they promote varies according to the receptors they bind (Table 11–2). This, in turn, is determined by the presence or absence of the amino acid sequence glutamate-leucine-arginine (abbreviated in single-letter code as ELR) at positions 4, 5, and 6 near their amino termini. Those that have this sequence (called the **ELR$^+$ CXC chemokines**) are able to bind two specific receptors (CXCR2 and, in some cases, CXCR1 as well) that are highly expressed on **neutrophils.** As a result, the ELR$^+$ CXC chemokines (eg, IL-8 and GROα) preferentially attract neutrophils, and so have a prominent role in **acute inflammation.** When they encounter chemokines of this type, circulating neutrophils rapidly adhere to endothelial cells and migrate into the underlying tissue, following the chemokine gradient. At high concentrations, the ELR$^+$ CXC chemokines can also induce neutrophil activation and degranulation, making them key regulators of **innate** cell-mediated immunity. As would be expected, mice that are unable to express receptors for these chemokines have reduced acute inflammatory responses and increased susceptibility to some microbial pathogens.

Most CXC chemokines that lack the ELR sequence (ie, most **ELR$^-$ CXC chemokines**) are also proinflammatory, but do not bind CXCR1 or CXCR2. Instead, they bind to CXCR3, which is expressed predominantly on activated T cells (particularly T_H1 cells), B cells, monocytes, and natural killer (NK)

Table 11–2. Proinflammatory chemokine receptors.

Receptor	Major Receptor-Expressing Cells	Chemokine Ligands	Major Effects
CXCR1	N, rstT, EC	IL-8, GCP-2	Neutrophil attraction
CXCR2	N, rstT, EC	IL-8, GRO, ENA-78, GCP-2, NAP-2	Acute inflammation Mobilize marrow neutrophils Fibroplasia Angiogenesis
CXCR3	actT, M, B, NK, Eo, EC	IP-10, MIG I-TAC	T-cell and macrophage attraction Chronic inflammation Angiostasis
CCR1	actT, M, NK, immDC	MIP-1α, RANTES, HCC-2, MCP-2, -3, -4, MPIF-1	T-cell and macrophage attraction Chronic inflammation Growth, mobilization, and adhesion of monocytes Immature dendritic cell attraction
CCR2	actT, M, immDC, Mt, Eo, Baso	MCP-1 to -4	T-cell and macrophage attraction Chronic inflammation Immature dendritic cell attraction Histamine release
CCR3	actT$_H$2, M, NK, Eo, Baso	Eotaxin-1, -2, RANTES, MIP-1α, MCP-2, -3, -4, HCC-2	Eosinophil attraction Allergic inflammation Histamine release
CCR5	actT$_H$1, M, NK, immDC	MIP-1α, -1β, RANTES, MCP-2	Favors T_H1 responses
CCR8	actT$_H$2, M, B, immDC	I-309, TARC, MIP-1β, HCC-4	Favors T_H2 responses
CX3CR1	N, actT, NK, M	Fractalkine	Leukocyte-endothelial adhesion

All of the indicated processes are enhanced unless otherwise noted. Chemokine acronyms are defined in Table 11–1.
Abbreviations: N = neutrophil; rstT = resting T cell; EC = endothelial cell; actT = activated T cell; M = monocyte–macrophage; B = B cell; NK = natural killer cell; Eo = eosinophil; immDC = immature dendritic cell; Mt = mast cell; E = eosinophil; Baso = basophil; actT$_H$2 = activated T$_H$2 cell; actT$_H$1 = activated T$_H$1 cell.

cells. By chemoattracting these cell types, ELR$^-$ CXC chemokines (eg, IP-10 or I-TAC) promote **chronic inflammation,** particularly the development of T_H1-mediated **acquired** immune responses. The only exceptions are BLC and SDF-1, which are ELR$^-$ CXC chemokines that bind distinct receptors and produce developmental and homeostatic, rather than proinflammatory, effects (see later discussion).

A majority of **CC chemokines** are proinflammatory, and these produce their effects through various combinations of five different receptors (CCR1, -2, -3, -5, and -8) found on activated T cells, immature dendritic cells, and other mononuclear cell types. The proinflammatory CC chemokines (which include RANTES, MIP-1α, and others) generally promote **chronic inflammation** and acquired immune responses. RANTES, for example, preferentially attracts activated memory T cells because these cells express its three receptors (CCR1, -3, and -5), and experimental inhibitors of either RANTES or CCR1 greatly retard progression of autoimmune arthritis in animal models by inhibiting T-cell and macrophage infiltration of the joints. MIP-1α, which uses the same three receptors, has been implicated in chronic pulmonary immune responses, such as those against influenza virus or schistosomal infection. Some CC chemokines tend to favor either T_H1 or T_H2 responses, reflecting differences in receptor expression; I-309, for example, uses CCR8, which is expressed preferentially on T_H2 cells. The MCP chemokines, a subgroup of CC chemokines that act through CCR2, may be important regulators of monocyte function because mice lacking either MCP or CCR2 genes show defective monocyte chemotaxis and increased susceptibility to infections. MCPs and the closely related eotaxin proteins also selectively attract and activate eosinophils, basophils, and mast cells, which are key effector cells in **allergic reactions** (see Chapter 13). Eotaxin-1, which utilizes only CCR3, has especially prominent eosinophil and basophil chemoattractant activity.

Fractalkine is by far the largest chemokine, with a molecular weight of 95,000. It is also the only known **CX3C chemokine** and the sole known ligand for CX3CR1. Its size derives from the fact that its chemokine sequence is only the carboxy-terminal part of a much larger cell surface protein, which also includes a long, heavily glycosylated protein stalk tethered to transmembrane and cytoplasmic domains. Thus, fractalkine is both a chemokine and a mucin. It is expressed on the activated endothelial cells of injured or infected tissues in response to LPS, IL-1, TNFα, or other inflammatory mediators. Because the chemokine sequence projects out from the endothelial surface, it is readily detected by passing neutrophils, activated T cells, monocytes, and NK cells that express CX3CR1. Contact with fractalkine causes these cells to adhere to the endothelial surface, its mucin stalk offering numerous sites for selectin-mediated cell adhesion.

Proinflammatory chemokines exhibit other activities as well. For example, most or all ELR$^+$ CXC chemokines promote **angiogenesis** (the growth of small blood vessels) and chemoattract endothelial cells, whereas many ELR$^-$ CXC chemokines that act on CXCR3 (including IP-10, MIG, and I-TAC) have the opposite effects. The dichotomy is not universal, however, as SDF-1, which lacks the ELR sequence, is both angiogenic and an endothelial-cell chemoattractant. Some solid-tissue cancers express angiogenic chemokines constitutively, which may help support vascularization of these tumors, but mice that lack CXCR1 and CXCR2 develop normally, suggesting that the angiogenic effects they mediate are not essential for life. CXCR2 is also expressed on some neurons and glial cells and has been proposed to have a role in directing neural migration during development.

Developmental Or Homeostatic Chemokines

Individual members of the CC, CXC, and XC chemokine subfamilies exert their primary effects on the development or maintenance of normal tissues, rather than during defensive reactions per se. Most are produced continually, but the cells that produce them vary widely. Common sources include macrophages, T cells, and dendritic cells, but some of these chemokines, such as SDF-1, are derived mainly from stromal cells of nonhematopoietic origin. Properties of these chemokines and their receptors are summarized in Tables 11–3 and 11–4; a few notable examples will be considered in detail.

The CXC chemokine **SDF-1** was initially identified as a growth factor for pre-B cells, but is now known to be critical for lymphocyte homing and angiogenesis. Unlike all other CXC chemokines, whose genes lie on chromosome 4, SDF-1 is encoded on chromosome 10. It is considered a relatively primitive chemokine because its overall sequence resembles the CXC and CC families equally, but it has been highly conserved in evolution, so that the human and mouse proteins differ at only a single amino acid. Small amounts are constitutively present in normal plasma. SDF-1 is expressed by stromal cells of many tissues and chemoattracts a broad spectrum of target cells because its unique receptor (CXCR4) is widely distributed. Deliberate inactivation of the SDF-1 or CXCR4 genes in mice indicates that this chemokine is essential in fetal development: mice lacking these genes die at or before birth with severe defects in the immune, circulatory, and central nervous systems. CXCR4 is also important as one of the two main coreceptors used by the type-1 human immunodeficiency virus (HIV-1) to infect T lymphocytes and neuronal cells (see later section and Chapter 46).

BLC, another CXC chemokine, is the only known ligand for CXCR5 and is primarily involved in lymphocyte homing and in the development of secondary

Table 11–3. Developmental and homeostatic chemokines.

Chemokine	Major Cell Sources	CXCR 4	CXCR 5	CCR 4	CCR 6	CCR 7	CCR 9	CX3CR 1
CXC Subfamily								
SDF-1	Str, EC	■						
BLC	Str, FDC		■					
CC Subfamily								
MDC	M, DC, NK			■				
TARC	M, DC, T			■				
LARC	M, DC, T, Eo, EC				■			
ELC	M, DC, T					■		
SLC	M, DC, T					■		
TECK	DC, T						■	
XC Subfamily								
Lymphotactin	T, NK							■

Abbreviations: SDF = stromal-derived factor; BLC = B-lymphocyte chemoattractant; MDC = macrophage-derived chemokine; TARC = thymus and activation-regulated cytokine; LARC = liver and activation-regulated cytokine; ELC = Epstein-Barr virus-induced molecule 1 ligand chemokine; SLC = secondary lymphoid tissue chemokine; TECK = thymus-expressed chemokine; Str = stromal cell; EC = endothelial cell; FDC = follicular dendritic cell; M = monocyte/macrophage; DC = dendritic cell; NK = natural killer cell; T = T cell; Eo = eosinophil.

lymphoid tissues. BLC is expressed constitutively at a high level by follicular dendritic cells in lymphoid follicles, chemoattracts B cells and a small subset of memory T cells into these follicles, and is required for the formation of **germinal centers.** In mice that lack CXCR5, primary follicles in all types of lymphoid tissues are maldeveloped and activated B cells fail to migrate into them, remaining instead in the surrounding T-cell zones. As a result, germinal centers fail to form, and the mice are unable to mount normal antibody responses to a variety of antigens.

Among the CC chemokines that serve developmental or homeostatic roles, TECK, SLC, ELC, and LARC have been most extensively characterized.

TECK, encoded on chromosome 8, is the only known ligand for CCR9 and is highly expressed by dendritic cells in the fetal spleen, small intestine, and thymic medulla. It appears to be produced by dendritic cells of lymphoid, but not myeloid, origin. TECK chemoattracts monocytes, dendritic cells, and thymocytes and may be particularly important in directing thymocytes from the thymic cortex into the medulla as they mature.

SLC and **ELC** are both encoded on chromosome 9, act through CCR7, and are constitutively expressed in T-cell-rich zones of lymphoid tissues throughout the body. Their target cells include thymocytes, resting or activated T cells, activated B

Table 11–4. Developmental and homeostatic chemokine receptors.

Receptor	Major Receptor-Expressing Cells	Ligands	Major Effects
CXCR4	Virtually all	SDF-1	Lymphocyte homing Angiogenesis Neural and cardiac development
CXCR5	actT, B, M	BLC	B-cell homing to follicles Germinal center formation
CCR4	actT$_H$2, NK	TARC, MDC	Favors T$_H$2 responses
CCR6	rstT, immDC, B, N	LARC, β defensins	Attract immature dendritic cells Activate resting memory T cells
CCR7	T, matDC, B	SLC, ELC	Attract T and mature DC cells to T-cell-rich zones
CCR9	thymocytes, T, DC, M	TECK	Attract T cells and precursors to thymus
XCR1	actT, NK, DC, thymocytes	Lymphotactin	Lymphocyte attraction

All of the indicated effects are enhanced unless otherwise noted. Chemokine acronyms are defined in Table 11–3.
Abbreviations: actT = activated T cell; B = B cell; M = monocyte–macrophage; actT$_H$2 = activated T$_H$2 cell; NK = natural killer cell; rstT = resting T cell; immDC = immature dendritic cell; N = neutrophil; T = T cell; matDC = mature dendritic cell; SDF = stromal-derived factor; BLC = B-lymphocyte chemoattractant; TARC = thymus and activation-regulated cytokine; MDC = macrophage-derived chemokine; LARC = liver and activation-regulated cytokine; SLC = secondary lymphoid tissue chemokine; ELC = Epstein–Barr virus-induced molecule 1 ligand chemokine; TECK = thymus-expressed chemokine.

cells, and mature, antigen-bearing dendritic cells. By attracting these target cells, SLC and ELC maintain the normal populations of, and traffic through, the T-cell zones. Just as importantly, they promote the specific encounters among T cells, B cells, and antigen-presenting cells (APCs) that can initiate acquired immune responses. In addition, SLC is displayed on the surfaces of high endothelial venules and provides a key signal that directs circulating naive T cells and mature dendritic cells to adhere to these vessels and migrate into the lymphoid tissue.

LARC, encoded on chromosome 2, acts through CCR6, and is produced constitutively by the skin and other tissues. One of its main functions is to attract circulating immature **dendritic cells,** which express CCR6, into these tissues, where they take up residence and function as immunologic sentinels. LARC expression also increases in some infected or distressed tissues, attracting additional immature dendritic cells, which can then capture antigens and help launch an immune response. Interestingly, shortly after they capture antigen and becoming mature (Chapter 6), dendritic cells stop expressing CCR6 and instead express CCR7, which makes them responsive to SLC and ELC. This shift in chemokine responsiveness is one of the factors that triggers migration of mature dendritic cells from the site of antigen capture to the T-cell-rich zones of lymphoid tissues.

Defensins as Ligands for Chemokine Receptors

In addition to their direct antimicrobial activities, human α and β defensins function as chemoattractants for resting T lymphocytes and for immature (but not mature) dendritic cells. This provides an important link between innate and acquired immunity, in that α defensins released by neutrophils in the course of an innate, cell-mediated immune response would also serve to attract the cell types needed for an acquired immune response. Although the chemoattractant pathways used by α defensins are not yet clear, the β defensins have been shown to function through CCR6, the receptor for LARC.

MICROBIAL INTERACTIONS WITH THE CHEMOKINE PATHWAYS

Certain microbial pathogens have subverted chemokines or chemokine receptors to their own advantage. The most notorious example is the **human immunodeficiency virus type 1** (HIV-1), which uses chemokine receptors as an essential coreceptor to infect human cells. HIV-1 initially recognizes and binds to its main target cells—macrophages and helper T lymphocytes—by virtue of the CD4 protein on their surfaces, but it is unable to enter or infect these cells unless it simultaneously contacts a surface chemokine receptor. Although a number of chemokine receptors can support

HIV-1 entry in vitro, only two have been proven to play a major role in human disease: CXCR4 is the main coreceptor used by strains that preferentially infect T lymphocytes, whereas those that infect macrophages use CCR5 (see Chapter 46 for details). As a result, the natural ligands of these receptors (RANTES, MIP-1α, MIP-1β, and MCP-2 for CCR5; SDF-1 for CXCR4) can competitively block infection by the corresponding viral strains in vitro, suggesting a possible avenue for development of new antiretroviral drugs.

A number of pox and herpes viruses, on the other hand, encode proteins that target chemokines or chemokine receptors. **Poxviruses** of the myxoma subfamily, for example, encode several proteins that bind and inhibit particular classes of cytokines. **Human herpesvirus 8 (HHV-8),** the causative agent of Kaposi's sarcoma, codes for at least two chemokine-like proteins that bind CC and CXC receptors, and it also encodes a constitutively active (ie, ligand-independent) chemokine receptor that may function as an oncogene in infected cells. Moreover, some viruses benefit indirectly from normal chemokine activities: for example, interferons suppress the production of IL-8, which in turn suppresses the antiviral activity of IFNα and so promotes replication of **cytomegalovirus** and other pathogens.

The Duffy Antigen

In addition to their functional receptors, many CC and CXC chemokines also bind to a membrane molecule called **DARC** (or **Duffy antigen**) found on the surfaces of erythrocytes and certain other cell types. DARC is unable to transmit signals, and its normal function is unknown although it is used by the malarial parasite *Plasmodium vivax* as a receptor to bind and invade human red blood cells. Because of its abundance and wide distribution, DARC is proposed to serve as a nonfunctional "sink" that binds and sequesters chemokines and so limits their effects. Interestingly, however, people with inherited mutations that eliminate DARC expression on erythrocytes (but not on other cells) appear normal, apart from their resistance to *P vivax* malaria. Hence, the significance of DARC for chemokine function, if any, remains obscure.

THERAPEUTIC APPLICATIONS OF CHEMOKINES & THEIR INHIBITORS

An intensive search is underway to identify clinically useful drugs that could target the chemokine pathways. Laboratory studies using modified chemokine proteins, antichemokine antibodies, or specific gene deletions in mice reveal that, despite the redundancy and overlap of these pathways, interfering with chemokine action can produce dramatic antiinflammatory effects. In animal models, for example, inhibiting IL-8 can ameliorate the adult respiratory distress syndrome and minimize reperfusion injury following vascular occlusion, whereas inhibiting MIP-1α can reduce relapses in chronic autoimmune encephalitis. Endogenous cytokines and hormones, such as IL-10, glucocorticoids, and transforming growth factor β (TGFβ) all suppress the production and effects of proinflammatory chemokines. Recently, highly potent and selective nonpeptide antagonists targeting CCR1, CCR2, CCR5, CXCR2, or CXCR4

have been described, and their therapeutic potentials are being explored. An alternative approach might exploit the phenomenon of **desensitization,** in which administration of the ligand for one member of the 7-transmembrane receptor superfamily leads to phosphorylation and inactivation of multiple other members of this superfamily. If the many beneficial effects of the chemokines can be preserved, such efforts hold great promise for uncovering new therapies for inflammatory and immunologic disease.

REFERENCES

Baba M et al: A small-molecule, nonpeptide CCR5 antagonist with highly potent and selective anti-HIV-1 activity. *Proc Natl Acad Sci U S A* 1999;96:5698.

Baggiolini M: Chemokines and leukocyte traffic. *Nature* 1998;392:565.

Bais C et al: G-protein-coupled receptor of Kaposi's sarcoma-associated herpesvirus is a viral oncogene and angiogenesis activator. *Nature* 1998;391:86.

Barnes DA et al: Polyclonal antibody directed against human RANTES ameliorates disease in the Lewis rat adjuvant-induced arthritis model. *J Clin Invest* 1998; 101: 2910.

Cyster JG: Chemokines and cell migration in secondary lymphoid organs. *Science* 1999;286:2098.

Dairaghi DJ et al: HHV8-encoded vMIP-I selectively engages chemokine receptor CCR8. Agonist and antagonist profiles of viral chemokines. *J Biol Chem* 1999;274: 21569.

Dieu MC et al: Selective recruitment of immature and mature dendritic cells by distinct chemokines expressed in different anatomic sites. *J Exp Med* 1998;188:373.

D'Souza MP, Harden VA: Chemokines and HIV-1 second receptors—Confluence of two fields generates optimism in AIDS research. *Nat Med* 1996;2:1293.

Gao JL et al: Impaired host defense, hematopoiesis, granulomatous inflammation and type 1-type 2 cytokine balance in mice lacking CC chemokine receptor 1. *J Exp Med* 1997;185:1959.

Horn F et al: GPCRDB: An information system for G protein-coupled receptors. *Nucleic Acids Res* 1998;26:275.

Horuk R et al: The CC chemokine I-309 inhibits CCR8-dependent infection by diverse HIV-1 strains. *J Biol Chem* 1998;273:386.

Horuk R et al: Expression of chemokine receptors by subsets of neurons in the normal central nervous system. *J Immunol* 1997;158:2882.

Luster AD: Chemokines—Chemotactic cytokines that mediate inflammation. *N Engl J Med* 1998;338:436.

Murphy PM: AIDS—Pirated genes in Kaposi's sarcoma. *Nature* 1997;385:296.

Rothenberg ME et al: Targeted disruption of the chemokine eotaxin partially reduces antigen-induced tissue eosinophilia. *J Exp Med* 1997;185:785.

Sica A et al: Bacterial lipopolysaccharide rapidly inhibits expression of C-C chemokine receptors in human monocytes. *J Exp Med* 1997;185:969.

Sallusto F et al: Flexible programs of chemokine receptor expression on human polarized T helper 1 and 2 lymphocytes. *J Exp Med* 1998;187:875.

Tachibana K et al: The chemokine receptor CXCR4 is essential for the vascularization of the gastrointestinal tract. *Nature* 1998;393:591.

Zingoni A et al: The chemokine receptor CCR8 is preferentially expressed in Th2 but not Th1 cells. *J Immunol* 1998;161:547.

Complement & Kinin

12

Kenji M. Cunnion, MD, MPH, Eric Wagner, PhD, & Michael M. Frank, MD

Complement activation, kinin generation, blood co-agulation, and fibrinolysis are physiologic processes that occur through sequential cascade-like activation of enzymes normally present in their inactive forms in plasma. Although these four distinct systems perform different functions, they interact with one another and with various cell membrane proteins. The first two—complement and kinins—are critical elements of the innate immune system, promoting inflammation and, in the case of complement, providing a first line of defense against infection.

the vessel, in directed migration of phagocytic cells into areas of inflammation, and, ultimately, in clearing infectious agents from the body.

The fourth function of complement is to help regulate the biologic activity of cells. Complement binding to cells may cause their activation and even cause them to divide. Complement binding to antigens may facilitate their binding to receptors on antigen-presenting cells and thereby render them far more "antigenic."

THE COMPLEMENT SYSTEM

Complement is a collective term used to designate a group of plasma and cell membrane proteins that play a key role in the host defense process. Table 12–1 lists the major proteins, their molecular weights, and their serum concentrations.

FUNCTIONS OF COMPLEMENT

This complex system, which now numbers more than 25 proteins, acts in at least four major ways. The first and best known function of the system is to cause **lysis** of cells, bacteria, and enveloped viruses. The second is to mediate the process of **opsonization,** in which foreign cells, bacteria, viruses, fungi, and so forth, are prepared for phagocytosis. This process involves the coating of the foreign particle with specific complement protein fragments that can be recognized by receptors for these fragments on phagocytic cells (see Chapter 2).

The third function of the complement proteins is the generation of peptide fragments that regulate features of the inflammatory and immune responses. These proteins play a role in vasodilatation at the site of inflammation, in adherence of phagocytes to blood vessel endothelium, in egress of the phagocytes from

Table 12–1. Molecular weights and serum concentrations of complement components.

Classical Pathway Component	Molecular Weight	Serum Concentration (μg/mL)
C1q	410,000	70
C1r	85,000	34
C1s	85,000	31
C2	102,000	25
C3	190,000	1,200
C4	206,000	600
C5	190,000	85
C6	128,000	60
C7	120,000	55
C8	150,000	55
C9	71,000	60
Alternative pathway component		
Properdin	53,000	25
Factor B	90,000	225
Factor D	25,000	1
MBL pathway component		
MBL	200–400	0.002–10
MASP-1	93	1.5–13
MASP-2	76	Unknown

Abbreviations: MBL = mannan-binding lectin; MASP = MBL-associated serum protein.

PATHWAYS OF COMPLEMENT ACTIVATION

Most of the early-acting proteins of the complement cascade are present in the circulation in an inactive form. The proteins undergo sequential **activation** to ultimately cause their biologic effects.

Three major pathways of complement activation operate in plasma. A general scheme of the system is shown in Figure 12–1. The first complement activation pathway to be discovered is termed the **classical complement pathway.** Under normal physiologic conditions, activation of this pathway is initiated by antigen–antibody complexes. The second pathway, known as the **alternative complement pathway,** was discovered more recently, although phylogenetically it probably is the older activation pathway. It does not absolutely require antibody for activation. The third and most recently described pathway is known as the **mannan-binding lectin (MBL) pathway.** It is triggered by mannan-binding lectin, a member of the collectin group of proteins that recognize repeating sugar patterns, as might occur on the carbohydrate capsule of bacteria. All three pathways function through the interaction of proteins termed **components,** or **factors.** They proceed by means of sequential activation and assembly of a series of components, leading to the formation of complex enzymes capable of binding and cleaving a key component, C3, which is common to all three pathways. Thereafter, the pathways proceed identically through binding of the terminal components to form a membrane attack complex, which ultimately causes cell lysis.

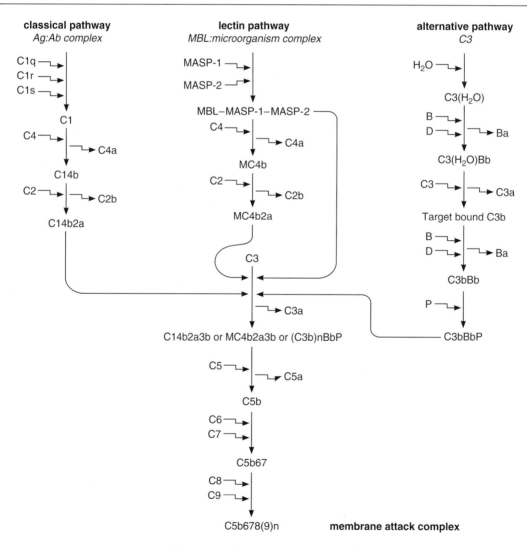

Figure 12–1. The complement cascade.

NOMENCLATURE

The proteins of the classical pathway and the terminal components are designated by numbers following the letter *C*. Proteins of the alternative pathway are generally given letter designations as are other proteins that have major regulatory effects on the system.

The proteins of each pathway interact in a precise sequence. When a protein is missing, as occurs in some of the genetic deficiencies, the sequence is interrupted at that point. The early steps in the activation process are associated with the assembly of complement cleavage fragments to form enzymes that bind the next proteins in the sequence to continue the reaction cascade. These enzymes are designated with a bar placed over the symbol of the component to indicate active enzymatic activity.

THE CLASSICAL COMPLEMENT PATHWAY

Initiation

The sequence of events that take place in the classical complement cascade is depicted in Figure 12–2. In most cases, the classical pathway is initiated by binding of antibody to an antigen. A single molecule of immunoglobulin M (IgM) on an antigenic surface, or two molecules of IgG of appropriate subclass bound side by side (a doublet), can bind and activate the first component of the pathway, **C1.** C1 is a macromolecular complex composed of three different proteins (C1q, C1r, and C1s) held together by calcium ions. Each C1 complex is composed of one C1q, two C1r, and two C1s chains. The enzymatic potential of the complex resides in the C1r and C1s chains, each of which is a proenzymatic form of a serine protease. Antibody binding is mediated by the much larger C1q portion of the complex, which binds the Fc portion of immunoglobulins. C1q can bind to IgM, IgG1, IgG2, or IgG3. It does not bind IgG4, IgE, IgA, or IgD, so these antibody classes cannot activate the classical pathway.

C1q is itself composed of six identical subunits, each containing one copy each of three different polypeptide chains. Portions of these three chains closely resemble collagen and coil around one another to form a triple-helical collagen-like arm that is highly flexible. In the C1q complex, the six subunits are arranged to create a globular central core from which the six arms radiate outward (see Figure 12–2). At the end of each arm is a pod-like structure that is formed by the carboxy termini of all three chains and that mediates binding to the C_{H2} domains in immunoglobulins of appropriate subclasses. The binding specificity of C1q has been exploited in creating clinical assays (called **C1q binding assays**) to detect immune complexes in serum.

If the antibody-binding sites (epitopes) on a target antigen are too low in density for proper arrangement of antibody molecules, C1 binding does not occur. This is seen with erythrocytes coated with anti-Rh0 (D) antibody as a result of maternal–fetal **Rh incompatibility.** Although complement-activating subclasses of IgG are formed against such erythrocytes, complement is not usually activated and has no role in their destruction because the necessary IgG doublets do not form.

Binding of C1 to antibody results in activation of the proteolytic enzyme activities of C1r and, subsequently, C1s. Each of these polypeptides becomes activated on cleavage into two fragments, the shorter of which has protease activity. It is believed that the function of the activated C1r enzyme, $\overline{\text{C1r}}$, is to cleave C1s, which then develops enzymatic activity. $\overline{\text{C1s}}$ then cleaves the next component of the pathway, C4 (see Figs 12–1 and 12—2A).

C4 & C2

C4 is a three-chain molecule. The largest of the three chains, the α chain, is cleaved at a single site by $\overline{\text{C1s}}$, with the release of a small peptide, C4a. The larger peptide, C4b, consisting of most of the α chain together with the β and γ chains of C4, binds to the target cell to continue the complement cascade. Binding involves the formation of a covalent amide or ester bond between the target cell and the α chain of C4 (see the discussion of chemistry under the section on C3). In the presence of magnesium ion, C4b on a target cell is capable of interacting with and binding the next component in the series, a single-chain molecule termed C2. C2 binds to C4b and, in the presence of $\overline{\text{C1s}}$, is cleaved. The larger cleavage fragment of C2 (C2a), which contains the enzymatic site, remains in complex with C4b to continue the complement cascade (see Figure 12–2B). The complex of C4b and C2a develops a new activity: the ability to bind and cleave the next component in the series, C3. For this reason it is termed the **classical pathway C3 convertase.** The peptide complex C4b2a is unstable and may release the C2a peptide as an enzymatically inactive fragment; however, target-bound C4b can accept another C2 and, in the presence of active C1, regenerate a convertase capable of continuing the complement cascade. These early steps in the classical pathway are under tight regulation, as discussed later.

C3

The C3 convertase of the classical pathway binds and activates C3, a glycoprotein present at a concentration of about 1.2 g/L of plasma. C3 consists of two disulfide-linked chains, termed α and β. Two amino acids at positions 988 and 991 in the C3 α chain are linked by a thioester bond that lies buried in a hydrophobic pocket of the protein and twists the α chain into a strained configuration (Figure 12–3).

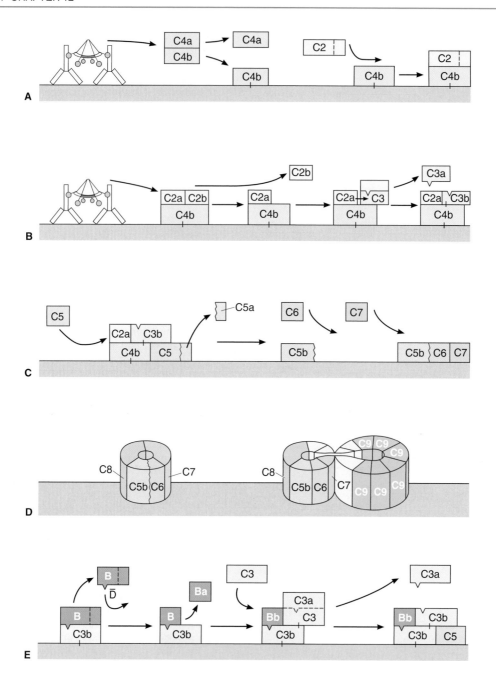

Figure 12–2. Diagram of the complement cascade. **A:** The classical complement pathway. A doublet of IgG antibody molecules on a surface can bind and activate C1, a three-part molecule composed of C1q, C1r, and C1s. C1q has a core and six radiating arms, each of which ends in a pod. The pod recognizes and binds to the Fc fragment of the IgG. On activation the C1 binds and cleaves C4. The small fragment, C4a, is released. The large fragment, C4b, binds to the target to continue the cascade. In the presence of magnesium ion, C2 recognizes and binds to C4b. **B:** Once C2 is bound to C4b, it can be cleaved by C1. A small fragment, C2b, is released, and the large fragment, C2a, remains bound to the C4b. This newly formed complex of two protein fragments can now bind and cleave C3. This molecule is, in turn, cleaved into two fragments: C3a and C3b. The small fragment, C3a, is released, and the large fragment, C3b, can bind covalently to a suitable acceptor. C3b molecules that bind directly to the C4b continue the cascade. **C:** The complex formed of C2a, C4b, and C3b can bind and cleave C5. A small fragment of C5, C5a, is released. The large fragment, C5b, does not bind covalently. It is stabilized by binding to C6. Here for clarity the C4b2a3b complex is no longer shown, although it is still present on the surface. When C7 binds, the complex of C5b, C6, and C7 becomes hy-

When C3 is activated by the convertase, a peptide C3a (MW 9000) is cleaved from the α chain. As a result, the internal thioester on the remaining C3b fragment becomes exposed to the surrounding medium. This highly reactive thioester has a half-life of roughly 30–60 ms and, during this time, reacts to form a covalent bond with any suitable acceptor in its vicinity.

If C3b bonds covalently to the adjacent C4b fragment on the target surface, the two (along with C2a) form a complex that can continue the complement cascade (see Figure 12–2B). In addition, the presence of bound C3b strongly **opsonizes** the target particle, increasing its phagocytosis by cells that carry **C3b receptors** (CR1; see section on C3 Receptors). C3b also has a strong tendency to interact with nearby IgG molecules, and the dimer formed by C3b and IgG is a more potent opsonin than is C3b alone. If, on the other hand, the thioester does not encounter a suitable acceptor, it reacts with water to form the conformationally altered inactive species $C3b(H_2O)$; this rapid inactivation helps to ensure that the reactive form of C3b is destroyed and does not produce unwanted activation.

The regulation and degradation of bound C3b depend on interaction with the circulating factors H and I. In the presence of these factors, C3b is cleaved to iC3b, which continues to act as an opsonin through complement receptor 3 (CR3). However, iC3b can no longer activate the terminal components of the complement cascade. The product iC3b undergoes further cleavage in the presence of CR1 and factor I to C3dg. C3dg and C3d, the final degradation product, interact with complement receptor 2 (see Figure 12–3).

THE CLASSICAL PATHWAY C5 CONVERTASE

The complex on a target surface consisting of C4b, C2a, and C3b (C4b2a3b) has a newly expressed enzymatic activity: It can coordinate with and cleave C5 and so is called the **classical pathway C5 convertase.** Again, two fragments, C5a and C5b, are formed, with C5a being the smaller. The larger fragment (C5b) remains noncovalently associated with the $\overline{C4b2a3b}$ complex and is available to interact with later components. It is C5b that initiates the segment of the complement cascade that leads to membrane attack.

In summary, the early steps of the complement cascade lead to the generation of a series of enzymatically active peptides and peptide complexes. As each complex is formed, it has a different specificity from the preceding complex and interacts with the next protein in the complement cascade. Each enzyme interacts with multiple molecules of the next substrate protein in the cascade of reactions either until it decays, as occurs with the C3 and C5 convertases, or until it is inhibited by regulatory proteins present on cells or in plasma. Thus, there is a potential for considerable biologic amplification: A limited number of antigen–antibody complexes lead to the activation of large numbers of complement molecules.

Nonimmunologic Classical Pathway Activators

A number of nonimmunologic activators of the classical pathway exist. Certain bacteria (eg, certain *Escherichia coli* and *Salmonella* strains of low virulence), viruses (eg, parainfluenza virus, human immunodeficiency virus), and even apoptotic cells interact with C1q directly, causing C1 activation and, in turn, classical pathway activation in the absence of antibody. Such an interaction in most cases aids the natural defense process of the host. Other structures, such as the surface of urate crystals, myelin basic protein, denatured DNA, bacterial endotoxin, and polyanions (such as heparin) also may activate the classical pathway directly. Such activation by urate crystals is thought to contribute to the inflammation and pain associated with gout.

THE ALTERNATIVE COMPLEMENT PATHWAY

C3 not only serves as a pivotal component of the classical pathway but also is the key component of the **alternative complement pathway.** This pathway, which is critically important in the innate immune system, provides yet another means of activating the complement cascade, in this case in the absence of antibody. Circulating plasma C3 undergoes spontaneous hydrolysis of its thioester bond to form a conformationally altered species called $C3(H_2O)$ as wa-

---

drophobic. It is partially lipid-soluble and can insert into the lipid of the cell membrane bilayer. **D:** When the C5b67 binds C8, a small channel is formed in the cell membrane. Multiple molecules of C9 can bind and markedly enlarge the channel. The channel has a hydrophobic outer surface and a hydrophilic central channel that allows passage of water and ions. **E:** The alternative complement pathway. In the presence of magnesium ion, C3b on a surface can bind factor B, just as C4b can bind C2. Factor D, a fluid-phase factor, can cleave bound factor B into two fragments: Ba and Bb. Ba is released. The C3bBb complex can now bind an additional molecule of C3 and cleave it, just as C4b2a can bind and cleave C3. C3a is released, and the new complex of C3bBbC3b, usually written (C3b)2Bb, can bind C5 to continue the cascade.

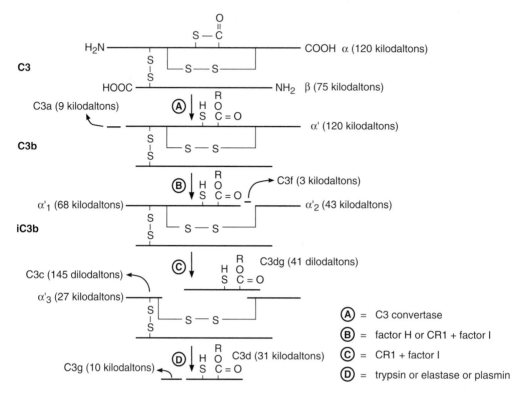

Figure 12–3. The C3 degradation pathway. The α and β chains of C3 are shown. Activation of C3 with the formation of C3a and C3b by the C3 convertases is shown (step A). C3b is degraded to iC3b by the action of factor H or CR1 plus factor I (step B). Two forms of iC3b have been described, differing in loss of a 3-kd fragment. In the presence of CR1 and factor I, C3c is released and C3dg remains target-bound (step C). C3dg can be further degraded to C3d by proteolytic enzymes (step D). Specific cellular receptors exist for each of these fragments.

ter slowly penetrates to the thioester group. Once the thioester group has opened, $C3(H_2O)$ acts like C3b (described earlier). In the presence of magnesium ions it can bind the C2-like protein, factor B, and interact with the C1-like protein, factor D, to form the alternative pathway convertase that cleaves C3, just as the classical convertase cleaves C3. Thus under normal physiologic conditions C3 in plasma undergoes slow hydrolysis, interacts with the alternative pathway proteins and cleaves C3 to form C3a and C3b (see Figure 12–1). Stringent control mechanisms (see later discussion) operate to limit the extent of the reaction and so prevent massive complement activation and damage to host cells. If these reactions happen to occur near a foreign particle, however, some C3b fragments may become covalently bound to its surface (see Figure 12–2E).

Factor B can then be acted on by factor D, forming a complex (C3bBb), the **alternative pathway C3 convertase.** The C3 convertase, in turn, can bind and cleave an additional molecule of C3 to form a larger complex (denoted C3bBbC3b) that has **C5 conver-**tase activity. The latter complex then efficiently triggers subsequent steps in the complement cascade and so promotes an attack on the particle to which it is bound.

The alternative pathway C3 convertase (C3bBb) is extremely unstable and would ordinarily dissociate rapidly. In the blood, however, a protein called **properdin** binds to this convertase and stabilizes it, thus slowing its decay and allowing it to continue the complement cascade.

For many years, investigators have used a protein derived from cobra venom (**cobra venom factor**) to activate complement in the laboratory. Recent studies have shown that this protein is related to cobra C3 and is a physiologic analog of C3b in this reptile. Cobra venom factor, when added to human plasma, functions just like human C3b to activate the alternative pathway. As described later on, endogenous C3b is under tight regulatory control by other plasma proteins. By contrast, cobra venom factor is not inhibited by these regulators and therefore can induce massive complement activation.

THE MANNAN-BINDING LECTIN PATHWAY

The initiating serum protein for the MBL pathway is mannan-binding lectin. MBL is present in mammals and birds and belongs to a family of molecules termed collectins. Like C1q, MBL is composed of chains ending in pod-like structures in this case arranged in dimers to hexamers. MBL recognizes certain carbohydrates expressed on the surface of microorganisms (see Chapter 2). Once bound to a surface, MBL can then activate two MBL-associated serine proteases: MASP-1 and MASP-2. These proteases share structural homology with C1r and C1s. Activated MASP-2 cleaves C4 to generate the C3 convertase, C4b2a. MASP-1 is believed to cleave C3 and may activate the alternative pathway directly. The terminal components of the complement cascade then proceed as in the classical pathway.

There appear to be additional methods of activating the MBL pathway by antigen-antibody complexes and IgG molecules lacking terminal galactose residues, as are found in some patients with rheumatoid arthritis. Preliminary evidence suggests MBL may have a receptor on phagocytes aiding the phagocytic process. The MBL pathway is regulated by C1 inhibitor and α_2-macroglobulin.

THE LATE COMPONENTS C5-9 & THE MEMBRANE ATTACK COMPLEX

The late phase of the complement cascade (see Figure 12–2C) begins when C5 is bound and then cleaved by a convertase of the alternative, classical or MBL pathway, into C5a and C5b. C5a is released and produces biologic effects, which are described in a later section. C5b continues the lytic sequence; however, it does not form a covalent bond with the surface of its target. C5b is rapidly inactivated unless it is stabilized by binding to the next component in the cascade, C6. The C5b6 complex can bind C7, the third protein involved in membrane attack. The C5b67 complex is strongly hydrophobic and interacts with nearby membrane lipids. It is capable of inserting into the lipid bilayer of cell membranes. In that location, one C5b67 complex can accept one molecule of C8 and multiple molecules of C9, ultimately forming a cylindrical transmembrane channel, C5b678(9)n, which has been termed the **membrane attack complex (MAC)** (Figure 12–4). This structure has a hydrophobic outer surface, which associates with the membrane lipid of the bilayer, and a hydrophilic core through which small ions and water can pass. The extracellular fluid then communicates with the fluid inside the cell, so that once this complex is inserted into the membrane, the cell cannot maintain its osmotic and chemical equilibrium. Water enters the cell because of the high internal osmotic pressure, and the cell swells and bursts. The assembly of C5b-C8 appears to form a small membrane channel that is increasingly enlarged and stabilized by the binding of multiple molecules of C9. One such channel penetrating the erythrocyte membrane is sufficient to destroy the cell. Cells with more complex metabolic machinery can, to some extent, internalize and destroy complement complexes that form on the cell surface or shed them as vesicles from the cell surface, thereby providing some protection against complement attack.

FLUID-PHASE REGULATORS

The complement system has evolved to aid in the host defense process by directly damaging invading organisms and by producing tissue inflammation. Strict regulatory control of this system is of critical importance to prevent complement-mediated destruction of the host's own tissues. When complement is involved in causing disease, it usually is functioning normally but is misdirected, that is, damaging to the host tissues. Many fluid-phase and cell-bound control proteins have evolved to defend against such attack (Table 12–2).

The C1 Inhibitor

The first of these, **C1 inhibitor (C1INH),** is a serine protease inhibitor (serpin) that recognizes activated $\overline{C1r}$ and $\overline{C1s}$ and destroys their activity. This glycoprotein also acts as an inhibitor of activated Hageman factor (see section on Proteins of the Kinin Cascade), of activated kallikrein, of clotting protein XIa, and of plasmin. Thus, C1INH regulates enzymes formed during activation of the kinin-generating system, the clotting system, the fibrinolytic system, and the complement cascade. In each of these systems, C1INH binds to the active site of the enzyme to destroy its activity and in the process is consumed. During C1 inactivation the C1 is dissociated, freeing C1q of its subunits. Because C1INH is consumed when acting as an inhibitor, the synthetic product of two active genes is necessary to provide the relatively high plasma concentration of the protein gene product required for effective inhibitor activity. A relative deficiency occurs in patients with **hereditary angioedema,** who have a defect in one of the two genes responsible for formation of C1INH. These patients have one half to one third the normal level of C1INH and have frequent attacks of angioedema—painless swelling of deep cutaneous tissues—whose cause is still uncertain. It may arise from activation of the kinin-generating system or from activation of the complement system, with generation of peptides that cause vascular leakage.

C4-binding Protein, Factor I & Factor H

C4-binding protein **(C4bp)** and a second protein, factor I, are responsible for regulation of C4b. C4bp

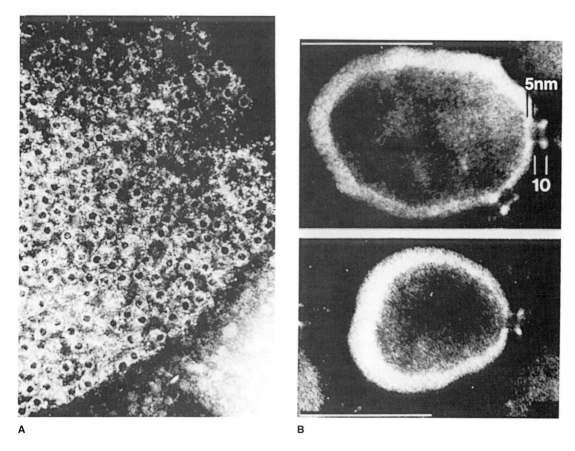

A   B

Figure 12–4. Lysis of cells by C5b-9, the membrane attack complex (MAC). **A:** Surface of cells lysed by antibody and complement. Note the surface lesions. (Micrograph courtesy of R. Dourmashkin.) **B:** Two views of the purified lesions allowed to attach to lipid micelles. The hollow cylinder formed by the C5b-9 has allowed the electron-dense dye to enter the lipid droplet. (Photograph courtesy of S. Bhakdi.)

Table 12–2. Complement regulatory proteins.

Protein	Molecular Weight	Target	Mechanism of Action
Fluid phase			
C1 inhibitor	105	C1	Dissociates C1 complex, inactivates C1r and C1s enzymes
Factor H	150	C3b	Cofactor of C3b cleavage
Factor I	88	C3b, C4b	Cofactor for C3b and C4b cleavage
C4-binding protein	550	C4b	Cofactor for C4b cleavage
S-protein	84	C5b-7	Inhibits MAC insertion
Clusterin	70	C5b-7	Inhibits MAC insertion
Factor J	20	C1, C3, B	Inhibits C1 complex formation, inhibits C3 cleavage by alternative pathway C3 convertase
Cell-associated			
CR1(CD35)	190[a]	C3b, C4b	Cofactor for C3b and C4b cleavage
		C3bBb, C4b2a	Dissociates C3/C5 convertases
DAF(CD55)	70	C3bBb, C4b2a	Dissociates C3/C5 convertases
MCP(CD46)	45–70	C3b (C4b)	Cofactor for C3b cleavage
CD59(protectin)	18–20	C8, C9	Inhibits MAC formation
HRF	65	C8, C9	Inhibits formation of MAC

[a] Most common isoform of CR1.
Abbreviations: CR1 = complement receptor type 1; DAF = decay-accelerating factor; MCP = membrane cofactor protein; HRF = homologous restriction factor; MAC = membrane attack complex, C5b-9.

binds to C4b and facilitates its cleavage by the prote-olytic enzyme **factor I.** On target surfaces, C4bp is not required for C4b cleavage by factor I, but its presence may accelerate the cleavage process.

Factor I also acts proteolytically to inactivate C3b and $C3(H_2O)$ (see Figure 12–3). This activity re-quires a cofactor termed **factor H.** Factor H acts as an obligate cofactor in the fluid phase and as an ac-celerator of C3 cleavage on cell surfaces. In the pres-ence of factors H and I, the C3b or $C3(H_2O)$ α chain is cleaved at two sites to form a partially degraded molecule, **iC3b.** This molecule, although inactive in continuing the complement cascade, is active as an opsonin. Under the appropriate conditions, as dis-cussed later, factor I can cleave iC3b further to form molecules termed C3dg and C3d, which also interact with specific receptors that recognize these C3 degra-dation peptides.

S Protein, Clusterin, & Factor J

Another control protein, **S protein** (also called **vi-tronectin**), interacts with the C5b67 complex as it forms in the fluid phase and binds to its membrane-binding site to prevent the binding of C5b67 to bio-logic membranes. Following binding of S protein to fluid-phase C5b67, binding of C8 and C9 to the fluid-phase complex can proceed, but the complex does not insert into lipid membranes and does not lyse cells.

Clusterin and factor J are two recently described fluid-phase regulators of complement. Clusterin acts by preventing insertion of the C5b67 complex into the cell membrane and protects cells against im-munologic damage. Low levels of clusterin are asso-ciated with some of the manifestations of systemic lupus erythematosus. Clusterin has also been found in the plaques of Alzheimer's disease patients. Factor J is a protein that inhibits C1 complex formation and inhibits C3 cleavage by the alternative pathway C3 convertase.

Protected Site Concept

In the control of complement attack against host tissue, it would be beneficial if complement proteins such as C3b were rapidly degraded when bound to host cells but not degraded when bound to the sur-face of a microorganism. A process for accomplish-ing this goal has evolved. When deposited on a mi-croorganism, C3b is often in a "protected site," which is protected from the action of the control proteins factors H and I. The C3b persists to activate the alternative pathway and destroy the organism. In contrast, on host cells C3b interacts with factors H and I and is degraded. The biochemical basis for this protection of C3b on an organism surface is not yet completely understood but appears to relate to the presence of charged carbohydrates such as sialic acid on mammalian cells, which may facilitate the binding of factor H.

GENETIC CONSIDERATIONS

Most of the genes encoding proteins of the classi-cal and alternative pathways have been cloned, and their amino acid sequences have been determined. Moreover, the activation peptides have been studied in some detail. Allotypic variants of many of the pro-teins have been found that show genetic polymor-phisms, as demonstrated by differences in surface charge. Almost all of the variants of complement pro-teins show autosomal-codominant inheritance at a single locus. The genes for C4, C2, and factor B are located within the major histocompatibility locus on the short arm of chromosome 6 in humans and are termed class III histocompatibility genes. C2 is highly homologous to factor B and may have arisen as a gene duplication of factor B. The significance of the intimate colocalization of histocompatibility genes and complement genes is unknown at present.

Interestingly, there are two C4 loci on chromo-some 6; thus, there are four C4 genes: two on each chromosome 6. The two loci code for proteins termed C4A and C4B, which differ in functional ac-tivity. Individuals with at least one null allele at one of the C4 loci are thought to be prone to the develop-ment of autoimmune disease. Genes for many of the regulatory proteins that interact with C4 and C3 are grouped as a supergene family on chromosome 1. This family is now known to encode factor H, C4-binding protein, decay-accelerating factor, CR1, and CR2. The gene products of this family each have one or more 60-amino-acid domains or short consensus repeats (SCRs) that may repeat multiple times in the molecule. They presumably originated from a com-mon gene precursor. See Chapter 25 for a discussion of inherited complement component deficiencies with associated syndromes.

BIOLOGIC CONSEQUENCES OF COMPLEMENT ACTIVATION IN INFLAMMATION

In general, the larger fragments formed during complement component cleavage tend to continue the complement cascade, whereas the smaller frag-ments mediate aspects of inflammation. For example, the cleavage of C3 and C5 generates C3a and C5a fragments, which consist of the first 77 and 74 amino acids of the C3 and C5 α chains, respectively. Cleav-age of C4 generates C4a from the α chain of C4. All of these small activation peptides have **anaphyla-toxic** activity: They cause smooth muscle contraction and degranulation of mast cells and basophils, with consequent release of histamine and other vasoactive substances that induce capillary leakage. **C5a** is the most potent of these anaphylatoxins.

C5a and C3a also have important immunoregula-tory effects on T-cell function, either stimulating

(C5a) or inhibiting (C3a) aspects of cell-mediated immunity.

C5a has profound effects on phagocytic cells. By interacting with specific cell membrane C5a receptors, (C5aR) it is strongly chemotactic for neutrophils and mononuclear phagocytes, inducing their migration along a concentration gradient toward the site of generation. It increases neutrophil adhesiveness and causes neutrophil aggregation. In addition, it dramatically stimulates neutrophil oxidative metabolism and the production of reactive oxygen species, and it triggers lysosomal enzyme release from a variety of phagocytic cells. Cellophane membranes used in **renal dialysis** machines, and membrane oxygenators may activate the alternative pathway with C5a generation. This, in turn, may lead to neutrophil aggregation, embolization of the aggregates to the lungs, and pulmonary distress. It is suspected that C5a generation plays an important deleterious role in the development of **adult respiratory distress syndrome.**

The life span of these biologically potent peptides, C3a and C5a, is limited by a serum carboxypeptidase that cleaves off the terminal arginine from the peptides, in most cases markedly reducing their activity.

COMPLEMENT RECEPTORS & REGULATORY MEMBRANE PROTEINS

C1q Receptors

The precise function and importance of the following group of C1q receptors has not yet been defined. Cell-associated C1q binding molecules include C1qRp, $C1qR_{02-}$, CR1, gC1qR, and cC1qR. C1qRp is found on myeloid cells, endothelial cells, platelets, and microglial cells. C1qRp binds with C1q as well as MBL and lung surfactant protein A (SP-A). Activation of this receptor enhances CR1 and Fc receptor-mediated phagocytosis. $C1qR_{02-}$ activation triggers the generation of toxic oxygen radicals by neutrophils, eosinophils, and vascular smooth muscle cells. gC1qR is found on phagocytes, platelets, and endothelial cells, and for neutrophils it induces chemotaxis. cC1qR binds C1q and MBL and helps mediate phagocytosis, cytotoxicity, antibody production, and cytokine secretion (Table 12–3).

C3 Receptors

The best studied receptors are those that recognize C3 fragments (see Table 12–3). Importantly, these receptors do not recognize native circulating C3 and are not blocked by the normal plasma protein. C3 receptors can therefore be more effective in mediating the binding of C3-coated particles to phagocytic cells. A series of receptors exist for C3b, iC3b, C3d, and C3dg.

Complement receptor 1, or CR1 (CD35), is expressed on erythrocytes, mononuclear phagocytes, eosinophils, B lymphocytes, some T lymphocytes, glomerular podocytes, follicular dendritic cells, and astrocytes. CR1 is a receptor for C3b and C4b. The most common allelic form of CR1 is composed of 30 repeating units of 60–70 amino acids termed short consensus repeats (SCRs). These are then arranged into four tandem repeats of seven SCRs each, called long homologous repeats (LHRs).

CR1 is a cofactor for factor I-mediated cleavage of C3b into iC3b and promotes further cleavage by factor I of iC3b to C3dg. CR1 also acts to disrupt C3 and C5 convertases by binding C4b and displacing C2a or binding C3b and displacing Bb.

Table 12–3. Complement receptors.

Receptor	Molecular Weight	Ligand	Mechanism of Action
CR1(CD35)	190	C3b,C4b,iC3Bb	Phagocytosis, immune complex clearance, cofactor for C3b and C4b cleavage
CR2(CD21)	140	C3d,C3dg,iC3b	B-cell activation
CR3(CD11b/18)	165(α chain) 95(β chain)	iC3b	Phagocytosis, cellular adhesion
CR4(CD11c/18)	150(α chain) 95(β chain)	iC3b	Cellular adhesion
C3aR	48	C3a	Chemotaxis, mast cell degranulation, increase vascular permeability
C5aR	43	C5a, C5a desArg	Chemotaxis, mast cell degranulation, increase vascular permeability, cellular adhesion
C1qRp	126	C1q,MBL,SP-A	Phagocytosis
$C1qR_{02-}$	Not published	C1q	Oxygen radical generation by neutrophils, eosinophils, and vascular smooth muscle
gC1qR	33	C1q	Chemotaxis
cC1qR	56	C1q,MBL,SP-A	Phagocytosis, cytotoxicity, antibody production, cytokine secretion

Abbreviations: MBL = mannan-binding lectin; SP-A = surfactant protein A.

CR1 plays a role in the opsonization and phagocytosis of particles coated with C3b. CR1 enhances the phagocytosis of IgG and C3b-coated particles by monocytes and neutrophils. Here phagocytosis requires simultaneous triggering of two receptors on the phagocyte surface. Activated monocytes (C3b and Fcγ) can phagocytose C3b-coated targets in the absence of IgG. CR1 expressed on erythrocytes aids in the transport of immune complexes to the liver for degradation by Kupffer cells.

Complement receptor 2, or CR2 (CD21), is a receptor for C3d and C3dg and is found on B lymphocytes, follicular dendritic cells, some T lymphocytes, thymocytes, and astrocytes. The main function of CR2 is thought to be the regulation of B-cell immune responses to antigen. CR2 can also function as a cofactor for factor I-mediated iC3b cleavage.

Complement receptor 3, or CR3 (CD11b/CD18, Mac-1), is member of the leukocyte β_2-integrin family of adhesion molecules. CR3 is primarily a receptor of iC3b and is found on mononuclear phagocytes, granulocytes, natural killer cells, and microglial cells. Like CR1, CR3 enhances the phagocytosis of particles coated with IgG and iC3b. CR3 is also important in the adhesion of monocytes and neutrophils to endothelial cells via its counterligand, ICAM-1. This is an important step in margination prior to inflammatory cells passing from the vasculature to sites of inflammation.

Complement receptor 4, or CR4 (CD11c/CD18), is also a β_2-integrin and an iC3b receptor. It is found on myeloid cells, dendritic cells, natural killer cells, activated B cells, some activated T cells, platelets, and microglial cells. Like CR3, CR4 is believed to assist neutrophil adhesion to endothelium during the inflammatory process. Recently, a number of children with deficiency of all of the CR3-related proteins have been identified. They present with a history of delayed separation of the umbilical cord at birth and frequent soft-tissue and cutaneous infections by a variety of organisms, especially staphylococci and *Pseudomonas aeruginosa*. Neutrophils lacking these receptors do not marginate normally, and affected children have a marked leukocytosis.

Regulatory Molecules

Several other cellular membrane proteins act not as receptors but rather to control untoward complement activation. **Decay-accelerating factor (DAF)** is a single-chain membrane protein that is a potent accelerator of C3 convertase and C5 convertase decay, but, unlike CR1 and CR3, it has no factor I cofactor activity (see Table 12–2). DAF (CD55) mediates C3 and C5 convertase decay through displacement of C2a and Bb. Functionally, the protein acts to limit membrane damage if complement is activated on a host cell surface. Membrane cofactor protein (MCP, CD46) facilitates degradation of C3b and C4b by acting as a cofactor for factor I. MCP is expressed on nearly every cell type except for erythrocytes and is believed to play a significant role in preventing complement-mediated damage to host cells. MCP is of particular interest because it has proven to be the receptor for measles virus, allowing the infection of cells.

C8-binding protein, also known as **homologous restriction factor (HRF),** acts to prevent successful completion and membrane insertion of the MAC. This membrane protein therefore acts to prevent cell lysis at yet another step in the complement cascade.

CD59 is yet another regulatory protein that prevents assembly of the complete C5b-9 complex on target cells and so prevents complement-mediated lysis. Interestingly, DAF, HRF, and CD59 are each bound to the cell surface by a **phosphoinositide glycosidic linkage** rather than by a transmembrane domain within the amino acid backbone of the protein. This phosphoinositide linkage is reported to give the protein far greater lateral mobility within the cell membrane, increasing its ability to intercept damage-causing complement complexes. In patients with **paroxysmal nocturnal hemoglobinuria,** phosphoinositide-linked proteins are incorrectly assembled or inserted into cellular membranes of hematologic cells due to a specific enzyme defect, rendering these cells exquisitely sensitive to complement-mediated lysis.

COMPLEMENT IN THE ACQUIRED IMMUNE RESPONSE

Many cells essential in the acquired immune response have complement receptors. These include macrophages and dendritic cells, all mature B cells, and a subset of T cells. It is believed that complement binding to antigens like those on the surfaces of microorganisms facilitates binding of the antigen to antigen-presenting cells, markedly increasing its antigenicity. It is reported that mice lacking either C4 or CR1/CR2 have a marked increase in autoimmune diseases, and it has been suggested that complement is important in negative selection of self-reactive T cells.

Mimicry of Complement Proteins

Given the stability of the complement proteins and receptors in evolution and their importance in host defense, it is not surprising that microbes have evolved mechanisms for inhibiting activity of the proteins or using them for their own ends. In general, pathogenic organisms have mechanisms for decreasing the effectiveness of complement peptides. These range from the presence of capsules surrounding the outer membrane that prevent the interaction of complement peptides with phagocyte complement receptors, to the synthesis of proteins that aid degradation of complement peptides. Organisms have also subverted the complement peptides to their own ends.

For example, Epstein–Barr virus (EBV) produces a surface protein that mimics the C3 fragment C3d, thereby gaining entry to B cells by binding to CR2 (CD21), the B-cell C3d receptor. Measles virus enters cells by binding to CD46, the membrane cofactor protein (MCP).

THE KININ CASCADE

The kinin-generating system is a second important mediator-forming system in blood. Here, the major final product, **bradykinin,** is a 9-amino-acid peptide with potent ability to cause increased vascular permeability, vasodilatation, hypotension, pain, contraction of many types of smooth muscle, and activation of phospholipase A$_2$ with attendant activation of cellular arachidonic acid metabolism. Bradykinin effects are in most cases mediated by interaction with one of two types of bradykinin receptors (B-1 and B-2) present on many cell types, including vessel endothelial cells, smooth muscle, nerve cells, and synovial lining cells. Specific bradykinin receptor antagonists are now available, and a wide range of physiologic effects of bradykinin are being established. Often interaction with bradykinin causes the release of a variety of cytokines, altering cellular function. Recent studies have suggested an important role for bradykinin in blood pressure homeostasis and aspects of renal function, including glomerular filtration rate and renal plasma flow.

PROTEINS OF THE KININ CASCADE

Four plasma proteins make up the bradykinin-generating system: **Hageman factor, clotting factor XI, prekallikrein,** and **high-molecular-weight kininogen** (Figure 12–5). Factor XI circulates as a complex with high-molecular-weight kininogen in a molar ratio of 2:1. Prekallikrein also circulates in a complex with high-molecular-weight kininogen in a molar ratio of 1:1. In contrast, Hageman factor circulates as an uncomplexed single-chain plasma protein.

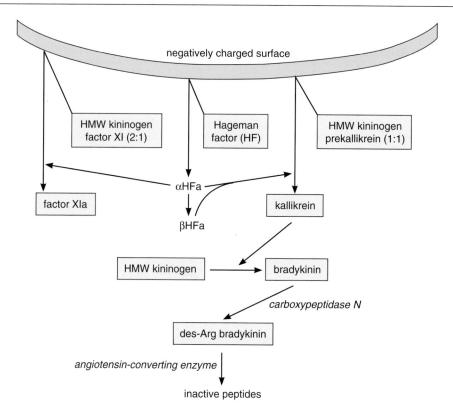

Figure 12–5. The kinin-generating pathway. We emphasize the fact that complexes of high-molecular-weight (HMW) kininogen with both factor XI and prekallikrein associate on a surface with Hageman factor. The Hageman factor is activated and in turn is responsible for the activation of factor XI and prekallikrein. Active kallikrein cleaves HMW kininogen to release bradykinin.

STEPS IN KININ ACTIVATION

On interaction with a negatively charged surface such as is supplied experimentally by glass or naturally by many biologically active materials like the lipid A of bacterial lipopolysaccharide, Hageman factor is cleaved and activated. The cleaved Hageman factor (αHFa) has proteolytic activity and can cleave additional molecules of Hageman factor to generate more αHFa. Cleavage of the single chain of Hageman factor yields heavy and light chains that remain linked by disulfide bonds. The active enzymatic site of Hageman factor resides in its light chain. Cleavage is also catalyzed by other proteolytic enzymes, particularly kallikrein. αHFa can interact with the complex of factor XI and high-molecular-weight kininogen to activate factor XI to factor XIa. This, in turn, can activate the intrinsic coagulation cascade. αHFa can also interact with the high-molecular-weight kininogen/prekallikrein complex to cleave the single-chain prekallikrein into a two-chain molecule (kallikrein), with the chains associated via a disulfide linkage. The cleaved molecule has proteolytic enzymatic activity associated with the lower molecular weight chain. To facilitate these cleavages of both factor XI and prekallikrein, high-molecular-weight kininogen complexes are bound to the surface, presumably near the Hageman factor.

AMPLIFICATION & REGULATION OF KININ GENERATION

Active kallikrein is capable of further cleaving αHFa, with loss of the heavy chain but not the light chain. The resulting molecule, βHFa, remains capable of activating the high-molecular-weight kininogen/prekallikrein complex, but it does not remain surface-bound and does not interact efficiently with the high-molecular-weight kininogen/factor XI complex. Prekallikrein is also a single-chain glycoprotein that is converted to an active form by cleavage within a disulfide bridge, resulting in a two-chain molecule with the chains linked by disulfide bonds. The enzymatic site resides in the light chain, and the surface-binding site in the heavy chain. Active kallikrein can cleave high-molecular-weight kininogen at several sites to release bradykinin from the kininogen. Bradykinin has a short half-life because it is rapidly attacked by carboxypeptidase N, which removes the C-terminal arginine to form the molecule termed des-Arg bradykinin. des-Arg bradykinin no longer has the smooth muscle-contracting activity of bradykinin and cannot induce capillary plasma leakage when injected into skin, but it retains some vascular effects. des-Arg bradykinin is, in turn, cleaved by angiotensin-converting enzyme (ACE) to form low-molecular-weight peptides that lack biologic activity.

PLASMA INHIBITORS OF KININ GENERATION

The inhibitors of this mediator-generating system include C1 inhibitor, α_2-macroglobulin, and α_1-proteinase inhibitor. C1 inhibitor and α_2-macroglobulin are the principal inhibitors of active kallikrein, with C1 inhibitor contributing most to inhibitory activity. C1 inhibitor and α_1-proteinase inhibitor are the major inhibitors of factor XIa, and C1 inhibitor is the principal inhibitor of active Hageman factor.

LOW-MOLECULAR-WEIGHT KININOGEN & TISSUE KALLIKREINS

A low-molecular-weight kininogen also exists in plasma. This protein has an identical heavy chain to that of high-molecular-weight kininogen. Low-molecular-weight kininogen can act as a source of bradykinin, but it is not easily cleaved by kallikrein. Tissue kallikreins (low-molecular-weight kallikreins found in multiple tissues) can cleave low-molecular-weight kininogen to lysyl-bradykinin (bradykinin with an additional linked lysine). Presumably, lysyl-bradykinin undergoes the same degradation pathway as does bradykinin.

FUNCTIONS OF KININS IN DISEASE

The physiologic role of the kinin-generating system is uncertain, and in only a few cases do we understand its role in disease. Free bradykinin and lysyl-bradykinin have been found in nasal secretions during **rhinitis** and viral nasal inflammation, and it is reasonable to believe that both blood and tissue kallikreins contribute to its presence. It is believed that kinins, due to their ability to cause smooth muscle contraction and capillary leakage, contribute to **asthma,** but this is by no means proven. Kinin generation has been found following antigen challenge of human lung fragments passively sensitized with specific IgE antibody, but the exact pathways involved in its generation are still uncertain. It has also been suggested that release of tissue kallikreins and activation of the kinin system is responsible for the severe pain of **pancreatitis** and plays a role in the synovitis of rheumatoid arthritis. The kinin-generating system is believed to be involved in edema formation in **hereditary angioedema,** because kinins are present in fluid from suction-induced blisters over angioedema areas and because levels of circulating prekallikrein fall during attacks of this disease. In addition, ACE is critical in the normal degradation of bradykinin, and ACE inhibitors markedly increase the severity of hereditary angioedema. Nevertheless, the kinin-forming system has not yet been conclusively proved to be responsible for the attacks of edema in hereditary angioedema.

REFERENCES

GENERAL

Frank MM: The complement system. In: *Samter's Immunologic Diseases,* 5th ed. Frank MM et al (editors). Little Brown, 1995.

Morgan BP: Physiology and pathophysiology of complement: progress and trends. *Crit Rev Clin Lab Sci* 1995; 32:265.

Volanakis JE, Frank MM (editors): *The Human Complement System in Health and Disease.* Marcel Decker, 1998.

CLASSICAL PATHWAY

Cooper NR: The classical complement pathway: Activation and regulation of the first complement component. *Adv Immunol* 1985;37:151.

ALTERNATIVE PATHWAY

Pangburn MK, Muller-Eberhard HJ: The alternative pathway of complement. *Springer Semin Immunopathol* 1984;7:163.

MEMBRANE ATTACK COMPLEX

Mayer MM et al: Membrane damage by complement. *Crit Rev Immunol* 1981;2:133.

Nicholson-Weller A, Halperin JA: Membrane signaling by complement S56-9: The membrane attack complex. *Immunol Res* 1993;12:244.

CONTROL MECHANISMS

Liszewski MK et al: Control of the complement system. *Adv Immunol* 1996;61:201.

Ochs HD et al: Regulation of antibody responses: The role of complement and adhesion molecules. *Clin Immunol Immunopathol* 1993;67:533.

Zahedi K et al: Structure and regulation of the C1 inhibitor gene. *Behring Inst Mitt* 1993;93:115.

GENETIC CONSIDERATIONS

Campbell RD et al: Complement system genes and the structures they encode. *Prog Immunol* 1992;5:25.

Perlmutter DH, Colton HR: Complement molecular genetics. In: *Inflammation: Basic Principles and Clinical Correlates,* 2nd ed. Gallin JE et al (editors). Raven Press, 1992.

MANNOSE-BINDING PROTEIN

Epstein J, et al: The collectins in innate immunity. *Curr Opin Immunol* 1996;8:29.

Thompson C: Research news: Protein proves to be a key link in innate immunity. *Science* 1995;269:301.

BIOLOGIC EFFECTS

Gerard C, Gerard NP: C5a anaphylatoxin and its seven transmembrane segment receptor. *Ann Rev Immunol* 1994; 12:775.

Goldstein IM: Complement: Biologically active products. In: *Inflammation: Basic Principles and Clinical Correlates,* 2nd ed. Gallin JE et al (editors). Raven Press, 1992.

Hugli TE: Biochemistry and biology of anaphylatoxins. *Complement* 1986;3:111.

CELL MEMBRANE RECEPTORS & REGULATORY MOLECULES

Brown EJ: Complement receptors, adhesion, and phagocytosis. *Infect Agents Dis* 1992;1:63.

Fearon DT, Carter RH: The CD19/CR2/TAPA-1 complex of B lymphocytes: Linking natural to acquired immunity. *Ann Rev Immunol* 1995;13:127.

Morgan BP, Meri S: Membrane proteins that protect against complement lysis. *Springer Semin Immunopathol* 1994;15: 369.

ADAPTIVE IMMUNE RESPONSE

Carroll MC: The role of complement and complement receptors in induction and regulation of immunity. *Annu Rev Immunol* 1998;16:545.

MOLECULAR MIMICRY

Fishelson Z: Complement related proteins in pathogenic organisms. *Springer Semin Immunopathol* 1994;15:345.

KININS

Kozin F, Cochrane CH: The contact activation system of plasma: Biochemistry and pathophysiology. In: *Inflammation: Basic Principles and Clinical Correlates,* 2nd ed. Gallin JI et al (editors). Raven Press, 1992.

Margolius HS: Kallikreins and kinins: Molecular characteristics and cellular tissue responses. *Diabetes* 1996;45: S14.

Wetsel RA: Structure, function, and cellular expressions of complement anaphylatoxin receptors. *Curr Opin Immunol* 1995;7:48.

Inflammation

13

Abba I. Terr, MD

Immune responses, whether innate or acquired, are often accompanied by other types of physiologic, cellular, or biochemical reactions in the host. Many of these are evolutionarily primitive defensives that can be mobilized either with or without immune activation. For example, acute injury commonly triggers responses in the local vasculature that give rise to redness, warmth, and swelling in the affected tissues (see Chapter 2). Various types of nucleated host cells may migrate into an injured site, becoming visible under the microscope as a cellular infiltrate. Reactions sometimes include local or disseminated blood clotting and coagulation; activation of the complement or kinin cascades; or systemic manifestations such as fever, malaise, or musculoskeletal aching. When a pathogen or irritant contacts a mucosal surface, glandular epithelial cells may dramatically increase their production of mucus or other secretions. If an injury is severe and protracted, fibroblasts and endothelial cells at the site often proliferate and form a permanent scar.

The entire, multifaceted host reaction to injury is termed **inflammation,** or the inflammatory response. There are several distinct inflammatory pathways, each of which proceeds via a sequence of biologic events. Many of the individual events are controlled by cytokines or other small regulatory molecules, which in this context are called **inflammatory mediators.** A given mediator may produce effects directly and also stimulate production of other mediators, giving rise to an integrated response. The particular pathways and events that occur in an inflammatory response depend on many factors, including the nature of the inciting stimulus, its portal of entry, and characteristics of the host. The outcome may be beneficial, detrimental, or both. Although most inflammatory reactions have evolved to inactivate or eliminate injurious substances, or to limit their spread through the body, these same reactions can be deleterious when they injure host tissues or interfere with normal functions. The terms **allergy, atopy, hypersensitivity,** and **anaphylaxis** are used to describe various harmful effects of immunologically mediated inflammatory reactions that are directed against otherwise-innocuous foreign substances, such as dust, pollen, foods, or drugs. The pathogenic consequences of **autoimmune diseases** occur in part because of immunologically mediated inflammation directed against tissues.

In this chapter, we will focus on inflammation that accompanies specific immune responses. Immunologic inflammation occurs in several distinct patterns, each of which arises through a specific mechanism and produces a particular constellation of symptoms and signs. From a clinical standpoint, it is extremely important to recognize these patterns because they offer insight into the pathologic processes at work in a given patient and provide clues that can guide the choice of appropriate therapy.

INFLAMMATORY CELLS

Any cell that participates in inflammatory reactions can be called an **inflammatory cell.** The term is thus applicable to many different cell types (Table 13–1). Some are long-term residents of normal tissues; others are circulating cells that enter tissues only in the course of an inflammatory response. Three types of inflammatory cells—neutrophils, macrophages, and lymphocytes—are the principal effector cells of most acute inflammatory or immune reactions and have been considered at length in earlier chapters. This section focuses on the properties of the other inflammatory cell types. Most of these cells express surface receptors for complement components, for the Fc portions of antibody molecules

Table 13–1. Inflammatory cells.

Circulating	Tissue-Resident
Lymphocytes	Mast cells
Neutrophils	Macrophages
Eosinophils	
Basophils	
Platelets	

(Table 13–2), and for various cytokines. As a result, their activities tend to be controlled directly or indirectly by ongoing immune responses or by activation of the complement cascade.

Eosinophils

Eosinophils are bone marrow-derived granulocytes that share a common progenitor with basophils. Their clinical significance derives from their strong association with **allergic reactions** and with **helminthic parasite infections.** An eosinophil in blood or tissue can be recognized by its bilobed nucleus and by the characteristic eosinophilic granules in its cytoplasm. Human eosinophils are slightly larger than neutrophils, being 13–17 μm in diameter, but they contain substantially fewer specific granules (approximately 200/cell). Eosinophil granules are spherical or oblong and 0.5 μm in diameter; they can be seen under the electron microscope to contain an electron-dense crystalloid core surrounded by a less dense amorphous matrix (Figure 13–1). The major contents of these granules include an **eosinophil peroxidase** (which is biochemically distinct from the myeloperoxidase of neutrophils but mediates the same reaction; see Chapter 2) and other enzymes that can generate toxic oxygen metabolites, a cytotoxic lysophosphatase called **Charcot–Leyden crystal protein,** and at least three other abundant basic proteins. One of the latter, called the **major basic protein,** has a strong affinity for acidic dyes such as eosin and is responsible for the intense red staining of the granules.

Circulating eosinophils normally make up about 1–3% of peripheral white blood cells. These circulating cells, however, represent only a very small proportion of the total eosinophil population: It is estimated that, for every circulating eosinophil, there are approximately 200 mature eosinophils in the bone marrow and 500 in connective tissues throughout the body. Eosinophil production in the bone marrow de-

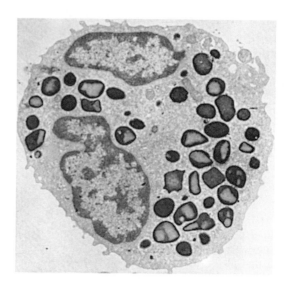

Figure 13–1. Electron micrograph of a mature human eosinophil. The numerous cytoplasmic granules stain darkly owing to the presence of peroxidase and contain characteristic central electron-dense crystalline cores with a surrounding amorphous matrix. The nucleus typically has two lobes. The cell is 15 μm in diameter. (Courtesy of Dorothy F Bainton.)

pends not only on granulocyte–monocyte colony-stimulating factor (GM-CSF) and interleukin-3 (IL-3), which promote differentiation of all types of granulocytes, but also on **IL-5,** which functions as a specific eosinophil growth factor (see Chapter 10). The life span of an eosinophil is relatively short: it has a marrow maturation time of 2–6 days, a circulating half-life of 6–12 hours, and a connective tissue residence time of only a few days. Increased concentrations of eosinophils **(eosinophilia)** in the blood can occur in several clinical settings but are most

Table 13–2. Inflammatory cell immunoglobulin Fc receptors.[a]

Receptor[b]	Present on:					
	Neutrophils	Monocytes	Mast Cells	Basophils	Eosinophils	Platelets
IgM	–	–	–	–	–	–
IgG						
IgG1	+	+	–	?	+	+
IgG2	+	+	–	–	?	+
IgG3	+	+	–	–	?	+
IgG4	+	+	–	–	?	+
IgA	+	+	–	–	?	–
IgD	–	–	–	–	+	–
IgE						
(FcεRI)	–	+	+	+	+	+
(FcεRII)	–	+	+	?	–	–
			?	?	+	+

[a] Symbols: +, receptor present; –, receptor absent; ?, presence unknown.
[b] Immunoglobulin isotype for which the cell has a receptor.

commonly encountered in allergic or parasitic diseases; the increase is thought to be mediated by IL-5. Eosinophilia of solid tissues also can occur in these disorders as a result of chemokines and other mediators released locally by mast cells, macrophages, lymphocytes, and other cells. Intracellular and protozoan parasites do not evoke eosinophilic responses (see Chapter 48).

Eosinophils bear surface immunoglobulin E (IgE) receptors, but these are the low-affinity **FcεRII** (CD23) type and so are largely unoccupied when the serum IgE concentration is within the normal range. Approximately 10–30% of eosinophils from normal individuals also have low-affinity (**FcγRIII**) or intermediate-affinity (**FcγRII**) IgG receptors (see Table 13–2). In addition, 40–50% display receptors for complement components. These various receptor types enable an eosinophil to recognize and bind to particulate antigens that are coated with IgE, IgG, or complement derivatives, much as a neutrophil or macrophage recognizes an opsonized particle. Binding, in turn, leads to eosinophil activation, which is characterized by (1) an increase in the number of surface Fc and complement receptors and certain other surface markers, (2) enhanced oxidative metabolism, (3) de novo synthesis and release of the arachidonate derivative leukotriene C_4 (LTC$_4$; see later discussion) and certain other proinflammatory mediators, (4) production and release of autocrine (IL-3, IL-5, and GM-CSF) and acute inflammatory (IL-1α, IL-6, IL-8, tumor necrosis factor α [TNFα]) cytokines, and (5) increased cytotoxic activity. Activation can also be induced or enhanced by contact with activated endothelial cells, by T-cell-derived lymphokines (GM-CSF, IL-3, and IL-5), or by monokines such as IL-1 and TNFα.

Activation of eosinophils produces changes in their morphology and function. They are called **hypodense** because of their increased size and buoyancy. Activated eosinophils can phagocytose many types of particles in vitro (including bacteria, fungi, mycoplasmas, inert particles, and antigen–antibody complexes), but the evidence that they play a significant role as phagocytes in vivo remains inconclusive. Instead, they appear to act primarily by attaching themselves tightly onto an antibody-coated or complement-coated particle and discharging their granule contents onto its surface through **extracellular degranulation.** This occurs, for example, when eosinophils aggregate around a large tissue parasite, such as *Trichinella, Schistosoma,* or *Fasciola.* The cationic granular proteins may attach themselves to the negatively charged surfaces of these parasites to exert their cytotoxic effects. For example, eosinophil peroxidase tends to attach itself in this manner and so concentrates production of toxic oxygen metabolites onto the target surface. Eosinophils also bind and attack large deposits of antigen–antibody complexes in the tissues (see later discussion). Granular contents released during particu-

larly intense responses can damage host tissues. For example, major basic protein is toxic to respiratory epithelium and is found in elevated concentrations in the sputum and airway secretions of people with asthma. Hexagonal, bipyramidal crystals of granule proteins, called **Charcot–Leyden crystals,** are also found in the sputum of asthmatics; they provide a useful clinical marker for eosinophil-mediated airway reactions.

Mast Cells

Mast cells are marrow-derived, tissue-resident cells that are essential for **IgE-mediated** inflammatory reactions (Table 13–3). Human mast cells are relatively large (10–15 μm in diameter) and heterogeneous in shape but generally are round, oval, or spindle-shaped, and they bear numerous surface projections (Figure 13–2). They possess a single round or oval eccentrically located nucleus. Their most distinctive feature under the light microscope is the presence in each cell of 50–200 densely packed granules that appear to fill the cytoplasm and that exhibit a distinctive purplish (**metachromatic**) coloration in hematoxylin-stained tissue preparations. Each granule is membrane-bounded and 0.1–0.4 μm in diame-

Table 13–3. Properties of human mast cells and basophils.

	Mast Cells	Basophils
Cell diameter	10–15 μm	5–7 μm
Nucleus	Bilobed or multi-lobed	Round or oval; eccentric
Cell surface contour	Smooth with occasional short, broad projections	Numerous narrow projections
Predominant localization	Connective tissues	Blood
Life span	Weeks or months	Days
Terminally differentiated	No	Yes
Major granule contents	Histamine, chondroitin sulfate, neutral proteinases, heparin, TNFα	Histamine, chondroitin sulfate, neutral proteinases, major basic protein, Charcot-Leyden protein
Cytokines produced	Il-4, -5, -6, and -13, and TNFα	IL-4, IL-13, TNFα
Enzymes	Tryptase, chymase	Tryptase (small amount)
Mediators synthesized and released after degranulation	TNFα, LTB$_4$, TLC$_4$, LTD$_4$, PGC$_2$	LTC$_4$, PAF

Abbreviations: IL = interleukin; LT = leukotriene; PAF = platelet-activating factor; PG = prostaglandin.

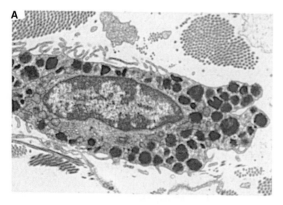

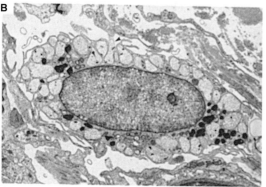

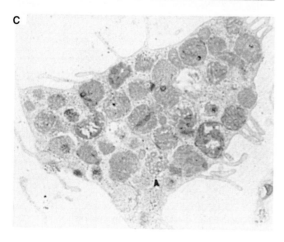

Figure 13–2. Electron micrographs of skin mast cells. **A:** An unstimulated mast cell. (Courtesy of Marc M Friedman.) **B:** A mast cell activated 5 minutes earlier with ragweed antigen. Note the swollen, lucent appearance of the secretory granules. (Courtesy of Marc M Friedman.) **C:** Cytoplasm of an unstimulated mast cell, showing the diverse appearances of the granules, which may contain crystalline, whorled, or granular material. (Courtesy of Karen Oetkon.) Each cell is 10–15 μm in diameter.

ter; the granules contain relatively large amounts of **histamine, heparin, TNFα,** and other preformed inflammatory mediators that are described later in this

chapter. They also contain superoxide dismutase, peroxidase, and numerous acid hydrolases (eg, β-hexosaminidase, β-glucuronidase, and arylsulfatase) that may act to degrade the extracellular matrix. Under the electron microscope, the granules may be seen to contain amorphous electron-dense granular zones as well as highly ordered crystalline arrays (see Figure 13–2).

Mast cells express on their surfaces large numbers of high-affinity Fc receptors for IgE (**FcεRI**). As a result, the surface of each cell is coated with lymphocyte-derived IgE molecules that have been adsorbed from the circulation and serve as receptors for specific antigens. Mast cells are scattered in connective tissues throughout the body but are found in especially large numbers beneath surface tissues such as the skin (which contains 10^4 mast cells/mm^3), lung alveoli (10^6 mast cells/g of tissue), gastrointestinal mucosa, and nasal mucous membranes. They are thus strategically positioned to detect inhaled or ingested antigens. When its surface IgE molecules bind antigens, a mast cell promptly undergoes activation, characterized by granule enlargement, solubilization of the crystalline structures within the granules, and then **degranulation** with release of granule contents into the surrounding tissues. Some of the substances within the granules increase local vascular permeability, smooth muscle contraction, and epithelial mucus secretion, whereas others act as chemotactic factors to attract other inflammatory cells. These regulatory factors are sometimes referred to as **mast cell mediators.** Some of the granular proteinases and other enzymes may have nonspecific effects on an antigen, but otherwise mast cells do not appear to carry out any significant direct effector activities such as phagocytosis.

Histochemical and biochemical analyses indicate that mast cells at various body sites differ in the relative amounts of two neutral proteinases in their cytoplasmic granules. The two proteinases, called tryptase and chymase, together make up 25–70% of granule protein by weight; their physiologic substrates are undetermined. Most mast cells in the lungs and gastrointestinal mucosa contain only tryptase and are called MC$_T$ cells, whereas the majority in the skin and gastrointestinal submucosa contain both tryptase and chymase (MC$_{TC}$ cells). This difference appears to be reversible and depends on factors in the local microenvironment; its functional significance is unknown.

Basophils

Basophils are circulating marrow-derived cells that have many of the same properties as tissue mast cells, although they are a distinct cell lineage. At 5–7 μm in diameter, they are the smallest cells of the granulocyte series and account for no more than 1% of nucleated cells in the marrow or peripheral blood. Like mast cells, basophils bear high-affinity Fc receptors for IgE (approximately 270,000 FcεRI receptors are present on each cell) and contain histamine-rich cytoplasmic granules. These two attributes distinguish mast cells and basophils from all other human cell types and explain their unique role in allergic inflammation. Basophils, however, differ from mast cells morphologically and biochemically in several respects (Figure 13–3; see Table 13–3).

Small to moderate numbers of basophils accumulate in tissues in a variety of inflammatory conditions involving the skin (eg, late-phase cutaneous allergic responses, cutaneous basophil hypersensitivity reactions, and lesions of bullous pemphigoid), the small intestine (Crohn's disease), the kidneys (allergic interstitial nephritis, renal allograft rejection), nasal mucosa (allergic rhinitis), and eyes (allergic conjunctivitis). In view of these associations and the many similarities between basophils and mast cells, it is generally presumed that basophils participate in IgE-mediated reactions in a manner analogous to that of mast cells. Nevertheless, the importance of basophils in immunity and hypersensitivity has yet to be proven.

Although the relative roles of mast cells and basophils have yet to be defined precisely, it is clear that basophils are uniquely involved in the late phase of IgE-associated allergic reactions in tissues (see later section) and in potentiating IgE synthesis by releasing IL-4 and IL-13. In addition to IgE-mediated activation, basophils can also be activated by lectins such as concanavalin A, complement components C3a or C5a, calcium ionophores, or certain enzymes including phospholipase A. The role of these non-IgE activators in clinical disease is uncertain, but may be the basis for nonimmunologic allergic-like reactions to certain agents, as discussed in Chapter 26.

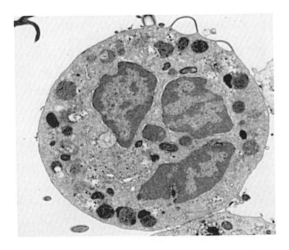

Figure 13–3. Electron micrograph of a peripheral blood basophil. The nucleus is multilobed, and the cytoplasmic surface is smooth with occasional short blunt folds or uropods. The cell is 5–7 μm in diameter. (Courtesy of Marc M Friedman.)

Platelets

Platelets are anucleate cytoplasmic fragments derived from bone marrow megakaryocytes and are the smallest circulating blood cells (2 μm in diameter). They have a 10-day life span in the circulation. Their primary function is in blood clotting, but they also store and can release mediator substances that have important proinflammatory effects. During clot formation, platelets undergo an **activation** response that causes them to aggregate and also to discharge the contents of the three types of storage granules in their cytoplasm (called dense bodies, α granules, and lysosomal granules, respectively) to the exterior. The released products may include various arachidonate metabolites (prostaglandin G_2 [PGG_2], PGH_2, and thromboxane A_2 [TXA_2]; see later discussion), growth factors, and bioactive amines, as well as neutral and acid hydrolases. Occlusion of a blood vessel by platelet aggregates has the useful effects of entrapping leukocytes and preventing the spread of antigen through the circulation. Platelets express surface Fc receptors for IgG and also low-affinity (**FcεRII**) receptors for IgE. The latter receptor allows platelets to bind and secrete cytotoxic products (probably hydrogen peroxide or other oxygen metabolites) onto IgE-coated tissue parasites but without inducing platelet aggregation or degranulation. Antigen binding through the platelet FcεRII also induces production of **platelet-activating factor (PAF)**, a potent inflammatory mediator (see later discussion).

Endothelial Cells

Although not usually classified as inflammatory cells themselves, endothelial cells can participate actively in immune responses by promoting immigration and modulating the responses of circulating inflammatory cells. When endothelial cells are exposed to cytokines (eg, IL-1, TNFα or interferon gamma [IFNγ]) or other products released at the site of an ongoing immune response, they may become activated and acquire increased adhesiveness for monocytes, neutrophils, and other circulating cells. Such increased adhesiveness is important in attracting leukocytes into the involved tissue (see Chapter 2). Activated endothelial cells sometimes express class II major histocompatibility complex (MHC) proteins (and so may function as antigen-presenting cells) and can also secrete the cytokines IL-1 and GM-CSF, which modulate immune responses.

MEDIATORS OF INFLAMMATION

Inflammatory mediators are host-derived compounds that are secreted by activated cells and serve to trigger or enhance specific aspects of inflammation. Such compounds are said to be **proinflammatory,** meaning that they promote inflammation. Many of the **cytokines** act as inflammatory mediators, as detailed in Chapter 10. This section describes some of the other major mediators (Table 13–4), classifying them somewhat arbitrarily into four groups: (1) those with vasoactive and smooth muscle-constricting properties, (2) those that attract other cells and are termed chemotactic factors, (3) enzymes, and (4) proteoglycans. These categories are not mutually exclusive, and several mediators can be assigned to more than one group.

1. VASOACTIVE & SMOOTH MUSCLE-CONSTRICTING MEDIATORS

Histamine

Histamine (Figure 13–4) is an inflammatory mediator found preformed in the granules of mast cells and basophils. It is synthesized within these granules by the action of histidine decarboxylase on the amino acid histidine and may make up as much as 10% of granule contents by weight. Histamine is bound through ionic linkages to proteoglycans and proteins within the granules and is bound particularly tightly to mast cell heparin; however, it dissociates from these ligands when released to the extracellular space by degranulation. Histamine exerts its physiologic effects by interacting with any of three different target cell receptors, designated H_1, H_2, and H_3. The receptors are expressed in a tissue-specific manner and each produces characteristic effects (Table 13–5). Major effects mediated by the **H_1 receptor** include contraction of bronchial, intestinal, and uterine smooth muscles and augmentation of vascular permeability in postcapillary venules. **Antihistamine** drugs used to treat allergies act by selectively blocking H_1 receptor binding. In contrast, binding of **H_2 receptors** augments gastric acid and airway mucus secretion and can be inhibited by such compounds as

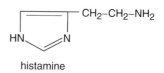

histamine

Figure 13–4. Chemical structure of histamine.

cimetidine and ranitidine, which are useful for treating peptic ulcer disease. **H_3 receptor** binding principally affects histamine synthesis and release.

Arachidonic Acid Metabolites

The prostaglandins and leukotrienes are metabolites produced by enzymatic cyclooxygenation and lipoxygenation, respectively, of arachidonic acid (Figure 13–5). They constitute two major families of inflammatory mediators, whose members exhibit diverse vasoactive, smooth muscle-constricting, and chemotactic properties. Thromboxanes and lipoxins are other arachidonic acid derivatives with additional effects. All of these compounds are known chemically as **eicosanoids.** Their actions are local because they are metabolized close to the site of production. Many **nonsteroidal antiinflammatory drugs,** such as **aspirin,** act primarily by blocking the synthesis of prostaglandins. Selective **leukotriene pathway inhibitors** have some efficacy in the treatment of asthma and may have use in other allergic disorders.

Arachidonic acid is a 20-carbon fatty acid containing four double bonds (Figure 13–6). It can be liberated from membrane phospholipids either through the sequential action of phospholipase C and diacylglycerol lipase or by the direct action of phospholipase A_2 on membrane phospholipids. Once liberated, arachidonic acid can be metabolized by either the cyclooxygenase or lipoxygenase pathway. Each

Table 13–4. Some major inflammatory mediators.[a]

Vasoactive and smooth muscle-constricting mediators
Histamine
Arachidonate metabolites (PGD_2, LTC_4, LTD_4, TXE_4)
PAF
Adenosine
Chemotactic factors
Chemokines
PAF
Complement components, especially C5a
Arachidonate metabolites (LTB_4)
Enzymatic mediators
Tryptase, others
Proteoglycan mediators
Heparin

Abbreviations: PGD_2 = prostaglandin D_2; LT = leukotriene; TXE_4 = thromboxane E_4; PAF = platelet-activating factor.
[a] The limited selection represented here omits many proinflammatory cytokines (see Chapter 10) and other mediators.

Table 13–5. Histamine receptors.

Receptor	Histamine Actions
H1	Increased postcapillary venular permeability
	Smooth muscle contraction
	Pulmonary vasoconstriction
	Increased cGMP levels in cells
	Enhanced mucus secretion
	Leukocyte chemokinesis
	Prostaglandin production in lungs
H2	Enhanced gastric acid secretion
	Enhanced mucus secretion
	Increased cAMP levels in cells
	Leukocyte chemokinesis
	Activation of suppressor T cells
H3	Histamine release inhibition
	Histamine synthesis inhibition

Abbreviations: cGMP = cyclic guanosine monophosphate; cAMP = cyclic adenosine monophosphate.

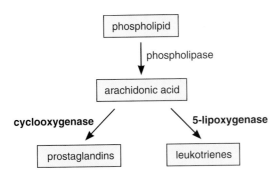

Figure 13–5. Major pathways of arachidonic acid formation and metabolism.

of these pathways can give rise to many alternative products (see Figure 13–6), each with its own spectrum of effects, and any of these metabolites may be produced by many different cell types in response to various stimuli. A complete discussion of the arachidonate metabolites is beyond the scope of this text, which instead considers only a few representative mediators of this class that are involved in inflammation.

A. Cyclooxygenase Products: The main product of the cyclooxygenase pathway in connective tissue mast cells is prostaglandin D_2 (PGD_2). This mediator promotes local vascular dilatation and vascular permeability (although to a lesser extent than does histamine) and also is a chemoattractant for neutrophils. PGD_2 is thought to have a role, along with histamine, in mediating wheal-and-flare reactions in IgE-mediated allergic responses and may be responsible for the systemic flushing and hypotensive episodes that occur in patients with systemic mastocytosis. It enhances release of histamine from basophils, which themselves do not generate cyclooxygenase products.

B. Lipoxygenase Products: The four principal products of the lipoxygenase pathway are the leukotrienes: LTB_4, LTC_4, LTD_4, and LTE_4 (see Figure 13–6). These are the principal arachidonate metabolites released by mucosal mast cells. LTB_4 is a potent chemoattractant (see later discussion). LTC_4, LTD_4, and LTE_4 collectively make up what was once termed "slow-reacting substance of anaphylaxis": they induce smooth muscle contraction, bronchoconstriction, and mucus secretion in the airways and the wheal-and-flare reaction in the skin. When injected intravenously, the last two compounds can cause hypotension and cardiac dysrhythmias. The leukotrienes are several hundred-fold more potent on a molar basis than is histamine and are therefore believed to have an important role in the genesis of allergic disorders.

Platelet-Activating Factor

PAF is a lipophilic organic mediator (Figure 13–7) that has been extensively studied in animal models. It is synthesized and released, along with histamine and leukotrienes, by rabbit, guinea pig, and rat mast cells and platelets. Its actions mimic features of IgE-mediated inflammation, including eosinophil and neutrophil chemoattraction and activation, smooth muscle contraction, and vascular dilatation. Initial enthusiasm for PAF as an important mediator of human allergy and anaphylaxis has been tempered, however, by a number of recent studies. Human mast cells and other cells can synthesize PAF but seem resistant to releasing it, so its role as an extracellular mediator is questionable. Attempts to induce bronchoconstriction using PAF in nonasthmatic human volunteers produced equivocal results, and specific PAF antagonists failed to inhibit bronchoconstriction in response to inhaled allergens in asthmatics or to improve ongoing symptomatic asthma.

Adenosine

The nucleoside adenosine (Figure 13–8) is liberated from degranulating mast cells and can then bind to surface adenosine receptors on many cell types. Its effects include bronchoconstriction and the induction of fluid secretion from intestinal epithelial cells. Blood adenosine concentrations may rise during acute asthmatic episodes.

2. CHEMOTACTIC MEDIATORS

Among the most important chemotactic mediators are the peptides that make up the **chemokine** family of cytokines, which are considered in detail in Chapter 11. Certain complement components, notably **C5a,** are also potent chemoattractants (see Chapter 12). In addition, several nonpeptide inflammatory mediators have been found to have significant chemoattractant activity. These include PAF and LTB_4 (see previous discussion), which, together with C5a, are potent neutrophil chemoattractants that are active at concentrations as low as 10^{-10} M. PAF also has strong chemoattractant effects on eosinophils.

3. ENZYMATIC MEDIATORS

A panoply of enzymes can be found in the storage granules of inflammatory cells and can be released to the exterior on degranulation (Table 13–6). In addition to their effects on antigens and host tissues, a few of these can act to initiate the complement, clotting, or kinin cascade. For example, mast cell tryptase can cleave complement factor C3 to generate C3a, and it also acts on many clotting proteins. Other mast cell proteinases can proteolytically activate kallikrein or kininogen (see Chapter 12).

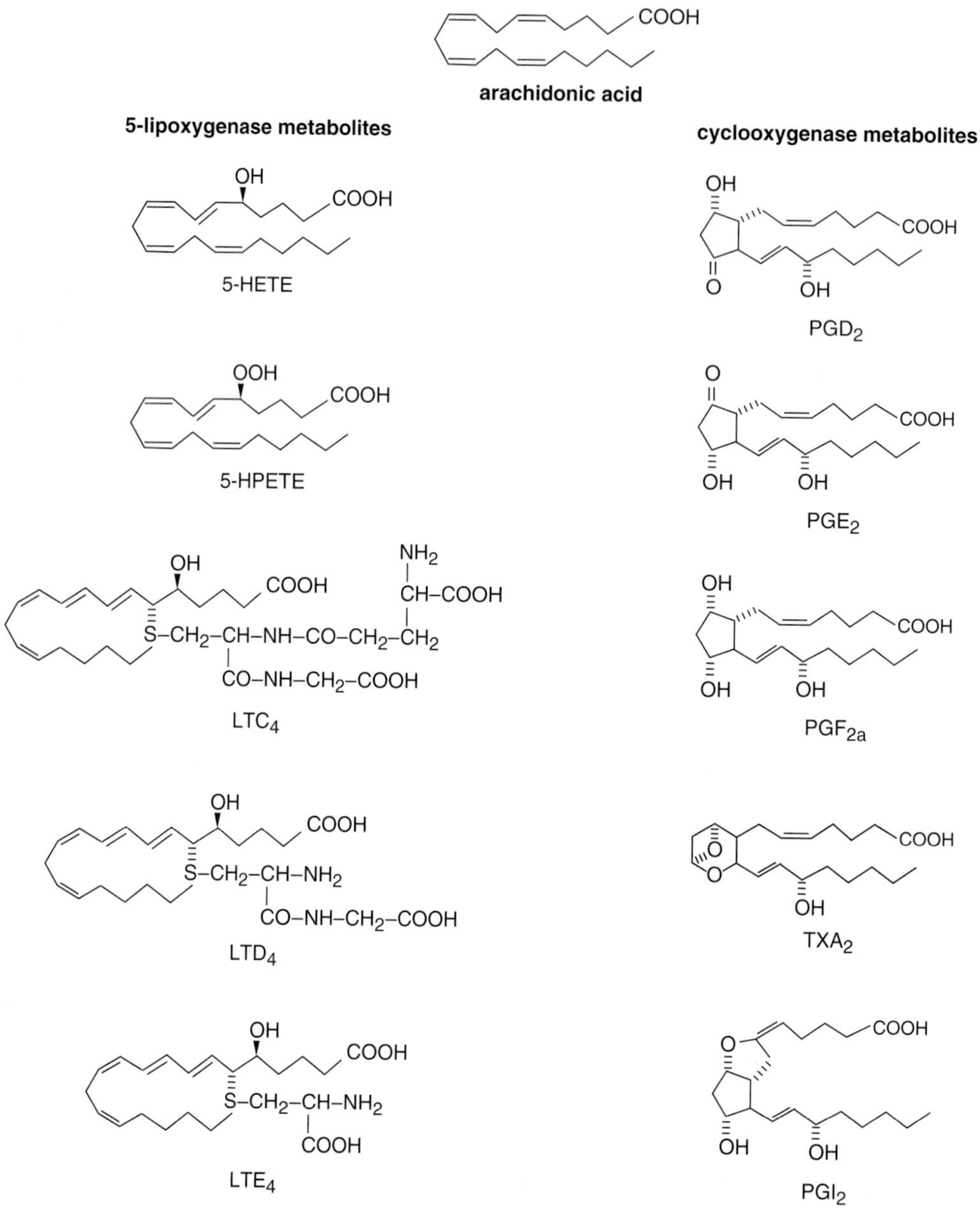

Figure 13–6. Chemical structures of arachidonic acid and of some principal 5-lipoxygenase and cyclooxygenase metabolites. Each of the compounds depicted is a physiologically active inflammatory mediator. *Abbreviations:* 5-HETE = 5-hydroxyeicotetraraenoic acid; 5-HPETE = 5-hydroperoxyeicotetraraenoic acid; LT = leukotriene; PG = prostaglandin; TX = thromboxane.

4. PROTEOGLYCANS

Mast cell and basophil granules are rich in protein–polysaccharide complexes called proteoglycans, which form much of the structural matrix of these granules and also serve as binding sites for heparin and other mediators. These may be the primary functions of the chondroitin sulfate that is present in such granules. Other proteoglycans, however, also have intrinsic regulatory activity. For example, the major granular proteoglycan in human mast cells is heparin (MW 60,000), which has anticoagulant activity and also is capable of modulating tryptase activity (see previous discussion). Each human mast cell contains about 5 pg of heparin.

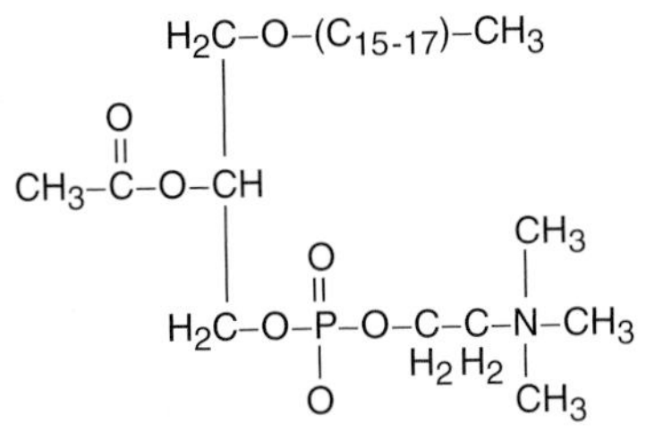

$$H_2C-O-(C_{15-17})-CH_3$$

$$CH_3-\overset{\overset{\displaystyle O}{\|}}{C}-O-CH$$

$$H_2C-O-\overset{\overset{\displaystyle O}{\|}}{P}-O-\underset{H_2}{C}-\underset{H_2}{C}-\underset{CH_3}{\overset{CH_3}{N}}-CH_3$$

$$\underset{O}{|}$$

PAF

Figure 13–7. Chemical structure of the secreted, bioactive form of platelet-activating factor (PAF).

Table 13–6. Major enzymes involved in inflammation.

Enzymes	Representative Effects in Inflammation
Neutral proteases: tryptase, chymase, carboxypeptidase	Fibrosis
Acid hydrolases: β-Hexosaminidase β-glucuronidase	Degradation of ground substance
Oxidative enzymes[a] NADPH oxidase, superoxide dismutase, myeloperoxidase, peroxidase	Oxidative killing of micro-organisms

[a] See Chapter 2 for details.
Abbreviation: NADPH = reduced form of nicotinamide adenine dinucleotide phosphate.

TYPES OF IMMUNOLOGICALLY MEDIATED INFLAMMATORY RESPONSES

Much of what is now known about inflammatory reactions in humans was derived from use of the **skin test**—a procedure in which a small amount of a purified antigen is injected beneath the skin and the response to the injection is then observed. Skin testing is widely used in clinical practice to assess whether patients are hypersensitive to particular antigens. It is also very useful experimentally for studying the mechanisms of immune reactions: for example, biopsies of test sites can be performed to examine the cellular infiltrates induced by an antigen, and fluids extracted from the sites can be assayed for inflammatory mediators.

More than a century of experience with skin testing in humans has revealed at least four distinct patterns of immunologically mediated inflammatory reactions (Table 13–7). Under the somewhat artificial conditions of the skin test, a single pure antigen may induce exclusively one type of reaction in a given patient. By contrast, responses against the more complex, multicomponent antigens encountered in nature often include two or more of these patterns simulta-

neously. Thus, these reaction patterns are not mutually exclusive but, rather, serve to highlight the major integrated pathways by which humans respond to foreign substances.

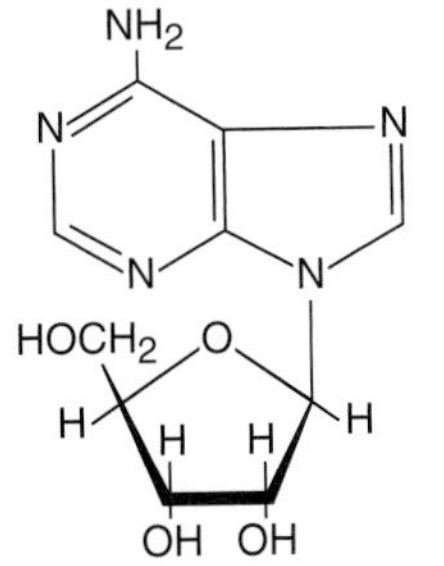

Cell-Mediated Immunity

Cell-mediated immunity (**CMI**) is the term applied to defensive reactions that are mediated primarily by activated T lymphocytes and macrophages. Reactions of this type are very common. They occur through the sequence of events outlined in Chapter 4, in which contact with antigen leads to activation, proliferation, and differentiation of T cells that have the appropriate specificities. Owing to the time required for these events to take place and for significant numbers of cells to be recruited into the response, CMI reactions develop rather slowly. Even in a highly immunized host, CMI responses exhibit a relatively long lag phase and do not achieve their maximal intensity until approximately 36 hours after exposure to the antigen. Consequently, CMI responses are also called **delayed-type hypersensitivity (DTH)** reactions.

The two main effector functions of CMI are cytotoxicity and inflammation. Whereas cytotoxicity is mediated by MHC class I-restricted cytotoxic CD8 T cells, the term DTH refers mainly to the inflammatory effects, which are mediated by class II-restricted CD4 T cells through their release of lymphokines such as IL-2, IFNγ, and TNFα. The evolution of a DTH reaction is schematized in Figure 13–9. The reaction is initiated by activation of an antigen-specific T_H cell, which then releases immunoregulatory and proinflammatory lymphokines and other substances into the surrounding tissues. These compounds, together with bioactive substances released by the antigen-presenting cell, promote clonal expansion of the responsive T_H cell and serve to attract additional inflammatory cells from the circulation. The chemoattracted cells may include antigen-specific and nonspe-

NH_2

HOCH_2

OH OH

adenosine

Figure 13–8. Chemical structure of adenosine.

Table 13–7. Classes of immunologically mediated inflammation.

Type of Inflammation	Skin Test Terminology	Time to Maximal Reaction (hours)	Predominant Cellular Infiltrate	Principal Mediators	Principal Mechanism Inducing the Inflammatory Response
Cell-mediated (CMI)	Delayed (DTH)	36	Lymphocytes, macrophages	Lymphokines	Lymphokines released from activated T_H1 cells induce primarily macrophage and T-cell responses
Immune complex-mediated	Late	8	Neutrophils	Complement factor C5a	Immune complexes fix complement, inducing neutrophil reaction
IgE-mediated Immediate phase	Immediate	0.25	Eosinophils	Histamine, leukotrienes	Antigen binding to surface IgE leads to mast cell degranulation, with release of stored mediators
Late phase	Late	6	Eosinophils, neutrophils	PAF, TNFα, PGD_2, IL-4, leukotrienes	Mediators synthesized and released by mast cells after degranulation
Cutaneous basophil hypersensitivity	Delayed	36	Basophils	Unknown	Unknown

Abbreviations: CMI = cell-mediated immunity; DTH = delayed-type hypersensitivity; PAF = platelet-activating factor; TNF = tumor necrosis factor; PGD_2 = prostaglandin D_2; IL-4 = interleukin-4; IgE = immunoglobulin E.

cific T or B lymphocytes, as well as monocytes, neutrophils, eosinophils, and basophils. Some of the cytokines promote differentiation and activation of macrophages and so enhance the phagocytic, bactericidal, and antigen-presenting functions of these cells. These activated macrophages, in turn, secrete other cytokines including IL-12, which promotes differentiation of the T_H cells toward a T_H1 phenotype, so that eventually the effects of T_H1-derived cytokines come to predominate (see Chapter 9). Local blood vessels are induced to dilate, which further enhances immigration of cells from the bloodstream. The coagulation–kinin systems also become activated, so that fibrin is formed and deposited at the site. Fibrin deposition is

probably important in confining the inflammatory reaction to a discrete location and imparts a firm consistency (**induration**) that is characteristic of tissues undergoing DTH reactions.

Viewed under the light microscope, the site of an ongoing DTH reaction can be seen to contain a tissue infiltrate composed mainly of lymphocytes and macrophages, along with variable numbers of plasma cells and other inflammatory cells. This is sometimes referred to as a **chronic inflammatory infiltrate** to indicate the relatively long time (several days or more) needed for its development and to distinguish it from acute inflammatory infiltrates, which are composed primarily of neutrophils (see Chapter 2).

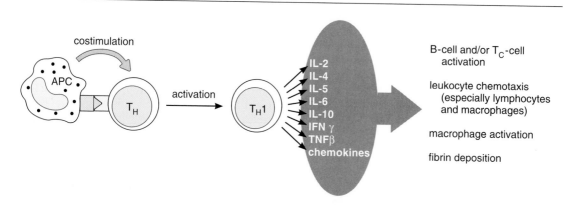

Figure 13–9. Schematic depiction of the immunologic events that give rise to a cell-mediated inflammatory response.

Certain types of antigens induce CMI with an especially pronounced macrophage response, leading to the formation of granulomas (see Chapter 2). Such **granulomatous inflammation** is therefore a subtype of CMI. It develops most commonly in response to particulate antigens that are large, insoluble, and resistant to elimination. These include foreign bodies (eg, suture material, silica, talc, or mineral oil); fungi; metazoan parasites; or mycobacteria, such as *Mycobacterium tuberculosis* or *M leprae.*

CMI reactions are encountered in many clinical settings, including numerous infectious diseases and certain types of vaccination sites, or following contact of many different types of chemicals with the skin or mucous membranes. CMI is also a major mechanism of allograft rejection and graft-versus-host disease and plays a role in some autoimmune disorders and in tumor immunity. Cytotoxic T-cell reactions against virus-infected host cells are another example of this type of response. Indeed, immunity to infection by any type of intracellular pathogen is mediated by CMI; the types of organisms that provoke this type of immunity include viruses; fungi; protozoa; helminthic parasites; and some bacteria, such as *Chlamydia.*

Hypersensitivity diseases mediated by DTH are discussed in Chapter 29. The most common disease in this category is **allergic contact dermatitis.** In this disease, the sensitizing agents are usually haptens that form antigenic complexes when they bind to host proteins in the skin and are then processed and presented by Langerhans' cells. Examples of common substances that act in this manner are pentadecyl catechol (the active immunogen in the oil of **poison ivy**) and **nickel** found in jewelry.

Despite their potential protective effects, prolonged or intense CMI reactions can lead to permanent injury to host tissues. Perhaps for this reason, active feedback inhibition mechanisms exist that limit the intensity of CMI reactions. The mechanisms involved in this inhibition are unknown but appear to be antigenically nonspecific. Thus, persons with severe or widespread diseases that induce CMI are sometimes found to have reduced or absent cellular immunity to various unrelated antigens. This state of generalized, nonspecific depression of cellular immunity is called **anergy.** It is usually defined clinically as the absence of DTH skin test reactivity to commonly encountered antigens or loss of a previously positive DTH skin test. Anergy may occur in individuals with extensive granulomatous disorders, such as miliary tuberculosis, severe coccidioidomycosis, lepromatous leprosy, or sarcoidosis. It also occurs in Hodgkin's disease. A temporary loss of CMI can occur during the acute phase of certain viral infections such as measles. Not surprisingly, CMI is also impaired in the various congenital forms of cellular immunodeficiency and in the acquired immune deficiency syndrome (AIDS).

Immune Complex-Mediated Inflammation

Immune complex-mediated inflammation refers to the inflammatory responses that occur when an antibody binds to antigen and activates the complement cascade. Reactions of this type do not require the active participation of the lymphocytes that originally generated the antibody. Thus, they can occur relatively rapidly in an immunized host who has preformed circulating antibodies of the appropriate specificity (see Table 13–7). The two classic types of immune complex-mediated reactions—the localized **Arthus reaction,** and systemic **serum sickness**—have similar underlying mechanisms. Each occurs through the sequence of immune complex formation and deposition, complement activation, and cellular infiltration.

A. Immune-Complex Formation: The classic complement pathway is activated when antibody molecules of an appropriate class bind to an antigen in a spatial conformation that allows subsequent binding of complement component C1 (see Chapter 12). For this to occur, the chemical nature of the antigen is generally less important than the number and types of antibody molecules it binds. IgM antibodies, or IgG antibodies of any subclass except IgG4, can activate the classical pathway, whereas IgA, IgE, and IgD cannot. As few as one IgM or two IgG molecules can suffice to activate (or "fix") complement when bound to the surface of a particulate antigen, such as a bacterium or a virus-infected host cell.

By contrast, soluble molecular antigens generally fix complement only after they have been incorporated into larger, multimeric **antigen-antibody complexes.** Such complexes (also called **immune complexes**) form because each immunoglobulin four-chain unit contains two independent and identical antigen-binding sites and can therefore bind to two antigen molecules simultaneously. Thus, when soluble antigen and antibody molecules are present in an appropriate molar ratio, they can cross-link one another to form a multimolecular lattice, as depicted in Figure 13–10. Because they contain numerous antibody molecules, immune complexes are often highly efficient at activating complement.

B. Complex Deposition: The physical properties of immune complexes are strongly influenced by the molar ratios of the molecules they contain (see Chapter 15). Complexes formed with a substantial excess of either antigen or antibody are small and relatively soluble, whereas those formed at near-stoichiometric equivalence are larger and have a tendency to precipitate out of solution (the so-called precipitin reaction). Large, insoluble complexes of the latter type can form in the circulation when a large amount of antigen is introduced into the bloodstream of an immunized person. The complexes then tend to be deposited in tissues throughout the body, particularly in the internal elastic lamina of arteries and in perivascular regions. They also tend to be-

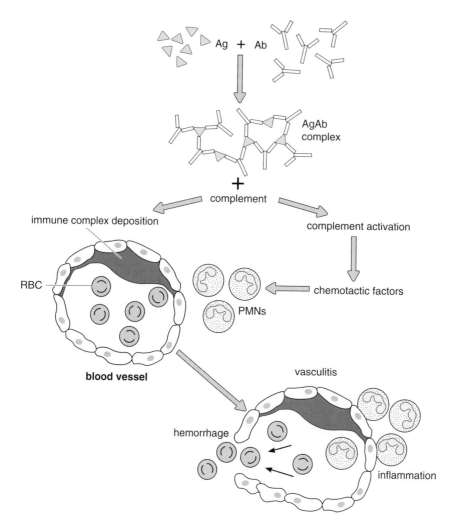

Figure 13–10. Schematic depiction of the immunologic events in immune complex-mediated inflammation. *Abbreviations:* Ag = antigen; Ab = antibody; RBC = red blood cell; PMN = polymorphonuclear leukocyte.

come trapped as the serum is filtered through renal glomeruli, and so they accumulate within the basement membranes of glomerular capillaries. Thus, massive systemic antigen exposure can lead to the widespread deposition of complement-fixing immune complexes. This is the pathogenic mechanism of serum sickness.

Alternatively, high concentrations of antigen–antibody complexes can form at a discrete site where antigen is present in a solid tissue. This can occur, for example, when an antigen is injected into the dermis of an immunized person. The resulting complexes precipitate as focal deposits in the blood vessels and fix complement, producing a localized inflammatory response that is called the **Arthus reaction.**

C. Complement Activation and Cellular Infiltration: The principal inflammatory factor derived from the complement cascade appears to be C5a,

which is a powerful chemoattractant for neutrophils. When immune complexes in and around a blood vessel wall fix complement, C5a is released and stimulates neutrophilic infiltration (ie, acute inflammation) of the vessel. The resulting vasculitis has several components (see Figure 13–10). Neutrophils release lysosomal enzymes and toxic oxygen metabolites while phagocytosing the immune complexes, and these cause destruction of the vessel wall with associated microhemorrhages into the tissues. Endothelial cells swell and proliferate, platelets aggregate in the lumen, and fibrin is deposited in and around the vessel owing to activation of the coagulation cascade. Later in the progression of the injury, macrophages and lymphocytes also infiltrate the area, although the precise factors that attract them have not been determined. One possibility, suggested by recent research, is that antigen–antibody complexes deposited in a tissue can be recognized directly by local mast cells or other resident cells that express low-affinity Fc receptors and so might provoke the secretion of chemokines or other mediators that attract inflammatory cells.

Clinical Manifestations

As is true of all other types of inflammation, immune complex-mediated reactions can be beneficial, detrimental, or both. This type of inflammation often occurs in concert with other antibody-mediated phenomena (eg, opsonization) during normal immune responses. In addition, it is the primary mechanism underlying several types of hypersensitivity. The Arthus reaction, for example, can frequently be observed at inoculation sites in persons who receive subcutaneous antigen injections as a treatment for allergy, and it also occurs occasionally as a response to insect bites or injected medications. These reactions are generally limited to mild edema and cellular infiltration, with little or no vascular destruction. More severe Arthus reactions also occur in two autoimmune disorders—autoimmune thyroiditis and Goodpasture's syndrome—in which the action of antithyroglobulin antibodies and antiglomerular basement membrane antibodies, respectively, can lead to destruction of the involved tissues.

Serum sickness is a systemic vasculitis of variable severity that is characterized clinically by fever, lymphadenopathy, arthralgias, and dermatitis. It once occurred commonly in persons receiving intravenous injections of large quantities of foreign immune serum—a widely used treatment for various infectious or toxic diseases prior to the antibiotic era. Today, it occurs occasionally among transplant patients who receive heterologous serum as a source of antilymphocyte or antithymocyte antibodies to suppress transplant rejection. Serum sickness also can occur as an allergic reaction to penicillin or other drugs or during the prodromal phase of some viral infections, most notably viral hepatitis.

A chronic form of serum sickness can be induced in animals by repeated intravenous infusions of antigen. Depending on the specific animal, antigen, and dosage regimen used, this can result in widespread vasculitis, glomerulonephritis, pulmonary alveolitis, or other lesions. This has been proposed as an experimental model for the immunopathogenesis of the human disorders systemic lupus erythematosus, rheumatoid arthritis, polyarteritis nodosa, and other diseases of unknown etiology that are characterized by the presence of circulating immune complexes and by vasculitis. The serum sickness model, however, does not fully mimic the pathologic and clinical manifestations of these disorders, and the antigens responsible for vasculitis in the human diseases remain unknown.

The presence of circulating immune complexes does not always indicate disease. In fact, small quantities of immune complexes can be found in the serum of normal persons. The antigens responsible for these complexes are not all known, although at least some are antigens from ingested foods. The remainder may be other environmental antigens or autoantigens. Most such complexes are promptly eliminated through phagocytosis by splenic macrophages and other cells, whose surface Fc and complement receptors enable them to bind the IgG and C3 proteins present in these complexes. Immune complex disease thus appears to require (1) large amounts of antigen; (2) generation of immune complexes large enough to activate complement; and (3) in some cases, impaired function of the phagocyte system, possibly because of abnormalities in the Fc or complement receptors.

IgE-Mediated Inflammation

IgE-mediated inflammation occurs when antigen binds to the IgE antibodies that occupy the FcεRI receptor on mast cells. Within minutes, this binding causes the mast cell to degranulate, releasing certain preformed mediators. Subsequently, the degranulated cell begins to synthesize and release additional mediators de novo. The result is a two-phase response: an initial immediate effect on blood vessels, smooth muscle, and glandular secretion, followed a few hours later by cellular infiltration of the involved site. This type of inflammatory reaction is commonly referred to as **immediate hypersensitivity.**

As just mentioned, IgE antibodies bind to mast cells via the numerous high-affinity Fcε receptors on the surface of each cell. The binding is noncovalent and reversible, so that the bound antibodies are in constant equilibrium with the pool of circulating IgE. As a result, each mast cell can bind many different antigens. The events that occur on binding are depicted in Figure 13–11. The response is initiated when a multivalent antigen binds and cross-links two or more IgE antibodies occupying FcεRI receptors. This cross-linking transmits a signal that activates the mast cell, resulting in activation of protein tyrosine kinases and increases in intracellular free calcium levels. These signaling events are complete within 2–3 minutes after antigen binding. Soon thereafter, cytoplasmic granules fuse with one another and with the surface membrane, discharging their contents to the exterior. Basophils are the only other cell type that express FcεRI receptors, but it is not known whether they contribute significantly to immediate hypersensitivity reactions.

The **immediate phase** of the inflammatory response is due mainly to preformed mediators (especially **histamine**) stored in the mast cell granules and also to certain rapidly synthesized arachidonate derivatives. It reaches maximal intensity within about 15 minutes after antigen contact. This phase is characterized grossly by erythema, localized edema in the form of a wheal, and **pruritus** (itching), all of which

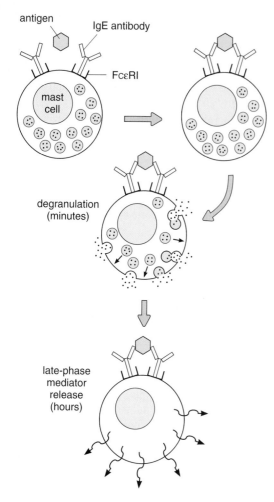

antigen

IgE antibody

FcεRI

mast cell

degranulation (minutes)

late-phase mediator release (hours)

Figure 13–11. Schematic depiction of the immunologic events in an IgE-mediated inflammatory response.

can be attributed to histamine. Microscopic examination at this stage reveals only vasodilation and edema. The granule contents, however, also induce local expression of the vascular addressin VCAM-1 (see Chapter 2), as well as secretion of RANTES and other chemokines (see Chapter 11), which promote subsequent recruitment of inflammatory cells to the site. Manifestations of the **late phase** are due in part to presynthesized TNFα and in part to other mediators (principally PAF, IL-4, and various arachidonate metabolites) whose synthesis begins after the mast cell degranulates. The effects of these mediators become apparent about 6 hours after antigen contact and are marked by an infiltrate of eosinophils and neutrophils. Clinical features of the late phase include erythema, induration, warmth, pruritus, and a burning sensation at the affected site. Fibrin deposition probably occurs transiently, but there is no evidence of significant immunoglobulin or complement deposition. Mast cell-derived IL-4 promotes the production of T_H2 cells (see Chapter 9). TNFα not only functions in the short term as a leukocyte chemoattractant but also can stimulate local angiogenesis, fibroblast proliferation, and scar formation during prolonged hypersensitivity reactions.

IgE-mediated inflammation is the mechanism underlying **atopic allergy** (eg, hay fever, asthma, and atopic dermatitis), systemic **anaphylactic reactions,** and allergic **urticaria** (hives). It is also at least partially responsible for immunity to helminthic parasites. It may normally play a facilitative role as a first line of immunologic defense because it causes rapid vasodilation and thus facilitates the entry of circulating soluble factors and cells to the site of antigen contact. Many serious sequelae of allergic disease can be ascribed to the actions of the chemoattracted leukocytes rather than to the mast cells themselves.

Cutaneous Basophil Hypersensitivity

The physiologic significance of cutaneous basophil hypersensitivity (CBH, previously called Jones-Mote hypersensitivity) is presently unknown. It is elicited by protein antigens that, when injected into the skin, produce a localized area of swelling that develops over the same time course as a DTH reaction but which is softer than a typical DTH lesion and is pruritic. Viewed under the microscope, the lesions reveal a prominent infiltrate of basophils but no granulomas or other features of DTH. Lesions of this type appear to be antibody-mediated, but their mechanism of formation is uncertain. Basophilic infiltrates are sometimes seen in allograft rejection, some viral infections, and allergic contact dermatitis, suggesting that CBH may be a component of DTH in some clinical settings.

REFERENCES

Adarem A, Underhill DM: Mechanisms of phagocytosis in macrophages. *Annu Rev Immunol* 1999;17:593.

Bayon Y et al: Mechanisms of cell signaling in immune-mediated inflammation. *Cytokines Cell Mol Ther* 1998; 4:275.

Church MK, Levi-Schaffer F: The human mast cell. *J Allergy Clin Immunol* 1997;99:155.

Däeron M: Fc receptor biology. *Annu Rev Immunol* 1997; 15:203.

Desreumaux P, Capron M: Eosinophils in allergic reactions. *Curr Opin Immunol* 1996;8:790.

DeVries ME et al: On the edge: The physiological and pathophysiological role of chemokines during inflammatory and immunological responses. *Semin Immunol* 1999; 11:95.

Gallin JI, Snyderman R (editors): *Inflammation: Basic Principles and Clinical Correlates,* 3rd ed. Lippincott Williams & Wilkins, 1999.

Locati M, Murphy PM: Chemokines and chemokine receptors: Biology and clinical relevance in inflammation and AIDS. *Annu Rev Med* 1999;50:425.

Lukacs NW, Ward PA: Inflammatory mediators, cytokines, and adhesion molecules in pulmonary inflammation and injury. *Adv Immunol* 1996;62:257.

Opdenakker G et al: The molecular basis of leukocytosis. *Immunol Today* 1998;19:182.

Sozzani S et al: The role of chemokines in the regulation of dendritic cell trafficking. *J Leukocyte Biol* 1999;66:1.

Suffredini AF et al: New insights into the biology of the acute phase response. *J Clin Immunol* 1999:19:203.

Walport MJ, Davies KA: Complement and immune complexes. *Res Immunol* 1996;147:103.

14

The Mucosal Immune System

Warren Strober, MD, & Ivan J. Fuss, MD

The mucosal immune system is composed of the lymphoid tissues that are associated with the mucosal surfaces of the gastrointestinal, respiratory, and urogenital tracts. It has evolved within an antigenic environment quite distinct from that in the interior of the body and so has a number of features that differentiate it from the systemic lymphoid system. These include production of a mucosa-related immunoglobulin, IgA; a population of T cells with mucosa-specific regulatory properties or effector capabilities; and a mucosa-oriented cell-homing system that allows lymphocytes initially activated in the mucosal follicles to migrate selectively to the diffuse mucosal lymphoid tissues underlying the epithelium. This last feature leads to the partial segregation of mucosal cells from systemic cells and thus qualifies the mucosal immune system as a somewhat separate immunologic entity.

The primary function of the mucosal immune system is to provide for host defense at mucosal surfaces. In this role, it operates in concert with several nonimmunologic protective factors, including (1) resident bacterial flora that inhibit the growth of potential pathogens; (2) mucosal motor activity (peristalsis and ciliary function) that maintains the flow of lumenal constituents and thus reduces the interaction of potential pathogens with epithelial cells; (3) substances such as gastric acid and intestinal bile salts that create a mucosal microenvironment unfavorable to the growth of pathogens; (4) mucous secretions that create a barrier (glycocalyx) between potential pathogens and the epithelial surfaces; and, finally, (5) innate humoral factors, such as lactoferrin, lactoperoxidase, and lysozyme, that have inhibitory effects on one or another specific microorganism. Optimal host defense at the mucosal surface depends on both intact mucosal immune responses and nonimmunologic protective functions. Thus, even with an intact immune system, antibiotic therapy that eliminates normal flora may result in infection by an organism that ordinarily cannot gain a foothold at the mucosal surface. Conversely, mucosal infections are common in patients with congenital or acquired immunodeficiency even in the presence of normal nonimmunologic protective factors.

A second but equally important function of the mucosal immune system is to prevent the entry of mucosal antigens into the circulation and thus to protect the systemic immune system from inappropriate antigenic exposure. This occurs both at the mucosal surface, by preventing the entry of potentially antigenic materials, and in the circulation, by providing for the clearance of mucosal antigens via a specific transport system. In addition, the mucosal immune system contains regulatory T cells that act to inhibit systemic immune responses to antigens that breach the mucosal barrier. This latter aspect of mucosal immune function may be important in the development of autoimmune processes and could conceivably be manipulated to treat a variety of autoimmune diseases.

ANATOMY

The mucosal system can be divided morphologically and functionally into two major parts: (1) the organized lymphoid tissues consisting of mucosal follicles (also called gut-associated lymphoid tissue [GALT] or bronchus-associated lymphoid tissues [BALT]) and (2) a diffuse lymphoid tissue compartment consisting of widely distributed cells located in the mucosal lamina propria (Figure 14–1 and see Chapter 3). The organized tissues are sites of antigen entry and induction of immune response, whereas the diffuse tissues are sites where antigens interact with differentiated cells and cause the secretion of antibodies by B cells or induce helper or cytotoxic activities of T cells. The two parts of the mucosal immune system are linked by a mucosal homing mechanism, so that activated cells from the lymphoid follicles travel to the diffuse lymphoid areas where they can best interact with their cognate antigens. Both the organized and diffuse immune cell populations are exquisitely antigen-dependent in that their numbers are remarkably reduced in germ-free states and are expanded under conditions of antigen overload. The normal state is more or less midway between these

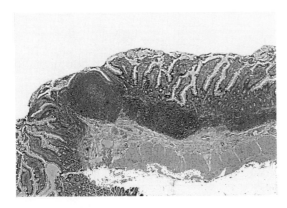

Figure 14–1. Histologic section of primate ileum showing a large lymphoid aggregate (Peyer's patch) and diffuse lymphoid tissue in the lamina propria. B- and T-lymphoid cells contact antigen and are induced to differentiate in the Peyer's patches; they then migrate to the lamina propria, where they perform their effector functions. Antigens enter the Peyer's patches through specialized cells (M cells) in the overlying epithelium.

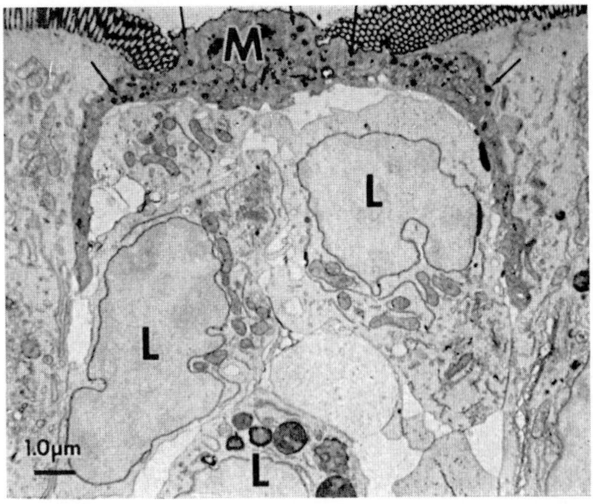

Figure 14–2. Transmission electron micrograph of a mouse M cell (M). Antigens pinocytosed from the mucosal lumen are transported without digestion to the underlying tissue, which includes lymphocytes (L) and dendritic cells. Arrows indicate pinocytotic vesicles in the M-cell cytoplasm.

extremes and is characterized by sufficient antigen stimulation to expand the mucosal population to a size that far exceeds that of the spleen and lymph nodes combined; on this basis, the mucosal immune system is the largest component of the overall lymphoid system.

MUCOSAL LYMPHOID AGGREGATES

The mucosal lymphoid aggregates are morphologically different from those of the systemic lymphoid system in that they receive antigen via the epithelium rather than through the lymphatic or blood circulation. This necessitates a distinct morphology that contains a number of unique elements.

M Cells. M cells are flattened epithelial cells with poorly developed brush borders and a thin overlying glycocalyx; they are distinguished from absorptive epithelial cells by their ability to pinocytose materials in the overlying mucosal lumen and to transport it in an undegraded form to the follicle proper (Figure 14–2). A wide range of substances are taken up by M cells, including soluble proteins, inert particulates, and various microorganisms. Although for the most part this uptake appears to be nonspecific, some degree of selectivity must exist because otherwise transport function would be overwhelmed by bacteria from the normal intestinal flora. One possibility is that secreted IgA antibodies coat bacteria in the normal flora and retard their uptake.

Following transport via M cells, particulates and other substances accumulate in the follicular dome areas or interfollicular areas, where they are taken up by dendritic cells or phagocytic cells. In addition, some materials migrate to other lymphoid organs. M cells have been shown to bear major histocompatibility complex (MHC) class II proteins; nevertheless, it is doubtful that they act as antigen-presenting cells (APC).

Dome Area Cells. The area just below the epithelium in the lymphoid follicle (the so-called dome area) contains a dense band of dendritic cells that are well positioned to take up antigens emerging from the M cells. These MHC class II–expressing cells take up ingested protein antigen and then present it to T cells to elicit T-cell proliferation and cytokine production. Recently, it has been shown that several subpopulations of dendritic cells are present as defined by their cytokine secretions (see later discussion).

Follicular T Cells. T cells are scattered through the dome area and other areas of the follicle, including the germinal centers; however, they are densest in the interfollicular areas, where they frequently bear activation markers such as the IL-2Rα chain. Whereas CD4 T cells are widely distributed throughout the mucosal follicle, CD8 T cells are found exclusively in the interfollicular area.

T cells in mucosal follicles produce a variety of both T_H1- and T_H2-type cytokines, depending on the conditions of immunization. In recent studies it was shown that T_H1-type responses predominate when protein antigen is administered orally in the absence of adjuvants, whereas T_H2-type responses occur when such antigen is given along with certain adjuvants such as cholera toxin. As noted later on, these different T-cell differentiation patterns shape the outcome of the mucosal response.

Follicular B Cells. Below the dome area is the follicular area, which contains the germinal centers. The latter are generally similar to those in other lymphoid tissue except for the fact that the B cells they contain differentiate primarily into surface IgA-expressing (sIgA+) B cells. Thus, whereas the outer zones contain sIgM+/sIgD+ B cells intermixed with numerous T cells, the inner zones contain sIgA+ B cells and relatively few sIgG+ B cells. Interestingly, very few if any IgA plasma cells are present in the follicular tissues because these cells develop only after additional differentiation in the draining mesenteric lymph nodes and in the lamina propria.

DIFFUSE MUCOSAL LYMPHOID TISSUE

The diffuse lymphoid tissues of the mucosal immune system consist of cell populations present in two separate compartments: the **intraepithelial lymphocyte (IEL) compartment** and the **lamina propria lymphocyte (LPL) compartment** (Figure 14–3).

Intraepithelial Lymphocytes

The IEL population, as the name implies, comprises cells lying above the lamina propria and basement membrane, among the epithelial cells. About one of every four to six epithelial cells is an IEL, so that this population is surprisingly large. The IELs form a phenotypically and morphologically distinct population that differs from cell populations in the lamina propria or in other lymphoid organs. For instance, most IELs are CD8 T cells (90% in mice; 50–80% in humans), many of which are granulated and some of which express FcεRI, a receptor typically found on mast cells. Perhaps more strikingly, a significant subpopulation bears the γδ T-cell receptor (TCR) rather than the αβ TCR (20–80% in mice; 5–10% in humans).

The origin of IELs also sets them apart from other cell populations. Studies of thymectomized mice indicate that many of these cells (including both αβ- and γδ-bearing IELs) are not of thymic origin and are instead composed of bone marrow cells that undergo development and selection in association with the intestinal epithelium. The significance of this extrathymic development is unclear, but one possibility is that it ensures that TCR specificities in the IEL are biased toward antigens encountered in the epithelial environment.

The function of IELs is not fully understood. What is clear is that they are mature, differentiated T cells that, on stimulation via the TCR, proliferate poorly yet produce ample amounts of various cytokines. In addition, they display the capacity to mediate cytotoxic function and this, along with the fact that they are CD8 T cells, suggests that they act in vivo as cytolytic effector cells. This applies to both the αβ and

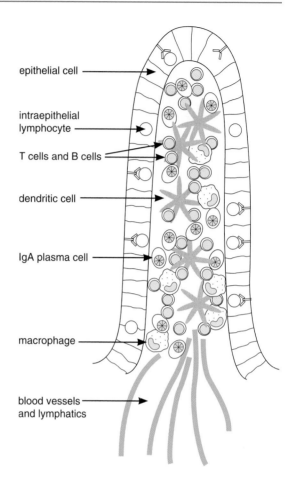

Figure 14–3. Diagrammatic representation of cells in an intestinal villus. Intraepithelial lymphocytes (IELs) are present above the basement membrane and between epithelial cells. The lamina propria lies beneath the basement membrane, and contains a mixture of B cells, T cells, macrophages, dendritic cells, and other cell types.

epithelial cell

intraepithelial lymphocyte

T cells and B cells

dendritic cell

IgA plasma cell

macrophage

blood vessels and lymphatics

γδ TCR-bearing T-cell subpopulations, and it is likely that these subpopulations differ more in their range of antigen specificities than in their overall function. One hypothesis is that IELs respond to a restricted set of "stress" proteins expressed on or released by epithelial cells in response to bound microorganisms; this leads, in turn, to elimination of the epithelial cells along with the bound organisms. Thus, IELs may undercut the ability of pathogens to colonize the mucosa by reacting against the cellular substrate necessary for such colonization, rather than against the organisms themselves.

Lamina Propria Cells

The lamina propria cells contain a complex array of cells, including T cells, B cells, macrophages, dendritic cells, and mast cells. The lamina propria T-cell population is composed mainly of CD4 cells

men. This final step is accompanied by proteolytic cleavage of the SC receptor molecule, so that a portion of this receptor is also incorporated into secreted IgA. Interestingly, the cellular synthesis and translocation of SC are independent of the presence of IgA, and the amount of SC synthesized usually exceeds the amount necessary for transport; this leads to the secretion of free (unbound) SC.

IgA transport mediated by SC occurs in the epithelium of the digestive tract, the salivary glands, the bronchial mucosal, and lactating mammary glands. It also occurs in the uterine epithelium, where SC synthesis is regulated by estrogen. In the human liver, SC is present on biliary epithelial cells but not on hepatocytes, so that SC-mediated transport is a relatively minor process. However, an alternative pathway, mediated by the asialoglycoprotein receptor on hepatocytes, leads to the selective uptake and degradation of monomeric IgA from the blood. This has the important effect of clearing the circulation of IgA-coated antigens that may have penetrated the mucosal barrier and that have the potential of evoking untoward immune responses. This process, together with the ability of IgA to retain bound antigens in the mucus of the lumen, helps prevent mucosal antigens from entering the systemic circulation—a phenomenon called **immune exclusion.** Its importance is shown by the fact that individuals with selective IgA deficiency (ie, those who have low IgA levels and normal IgM and IgG levels) show increased absorption of macromolecules and high levels of circulating immune complexes following ingestion of antigens. Moreover, immune exclusion has the effect of restricting immune responses against mucosal antigens to the mucosal lymphoid system and thus to the unique mucosal regulation of such responses, as discussed later on.

SECRETORY VERSUS CIRCULATING IGA

In humans, most circulating IgA is produced in the bone marrow and is in the form of IgA1 monomers, whereas secretory IgA is produced mainly at mucosal sites (as either IgA1 or IgA2 dimers or polymers). Polymeric IgA (whether IgA1 or IgA2) is more rapidly catabolized than monomeric IgA because polymeric IgA is subject to additional catabolic mechanisms such as SC-mediated transport and a sialoglycoprotein receptor-mediated uptake.

The separate origins of mucosal and circulating IgA in humans have led some investigators to suggest that the IgA system is bipartite, that is, it is composed of two relatively independent synthetic centers that are separately regulated. An alternative view is that the IgA1 B cells that produce IgA in the marrow originate in the mucosa and secondarily colonize the marrow. In any case, the monomeric IgA1 arising from the bone marrow in humans appears better suited than other forms of IgA to mediate the clearance of mucosal antigens from the circulation (as discussed earlier).

PRODUCTION OF OTHER IMMUNOGLOBULINS IN THE MUCOSA

Immunoglobulins other than IgA also play a role in the mucosal immune system. Mucosal synthesis of IgM, which can also be transported across the epithelial cell via an SC-mediated mechanism, occurs normally, and usually serves as an adequate replacement for IgA in individuals with selective IgA deficiency. Synthesis of IgG, on the other hand, is quite low in most mucosal areas, and IgG cannot be transported across the epithelium. Nevertheless, it does have a mucosal role: It is synthesized in substantial amounts in the distal pulmonary tract and is thus an important antibody class in pulmonary secretions. IgE is also synthesized in mucosal tissues, particularly during parasitic infection or in certain allergic states; however, IgE B cells do not localize preferentially to the mucosa, and the proportion of mucosal B cells synthesizing IgE is small, as it is in other tissues.

REGULATION OF IGA SYNTHESIS AT MUCOSAL SITES

The basis of preferential IgA B-cell development in Peyer's patches is not yet fully understood. One factor that has been identified is that IgA class switching requires the presence of transforming growth factor beta (TGFβ) and that T cells capable of producing TGFβ develop in Peyer's patches but not in other B-cell generative sites (Figure 14–5). Thus, at least one reason IgA B cells develop in Peyer's patches is that B cells at this site are under the influence of Peyer's patch-specific T cells that produce TGFβ.

Although TGFβ is necessary for IgA B-cell differentiation, it is not sufficient. Instead, stimulation of the B cells by LPS, CD40L, or antigen also is required, perhaps to prevent apoptotic death of B cells exposed to relatively high concentrations of TGFβ. The effects of cytokines, such as IL-4 and IL-5, may also be critical.

IgA class switching is followed by B-cell development into IgA memory cells or IgA plasma cells. This further development again depends on T cells, which act on B cells via cell-cell interactions, such as those involving OX40 on T cells and OX40-ligand on B cells, as well as by secreting lymphokines such as

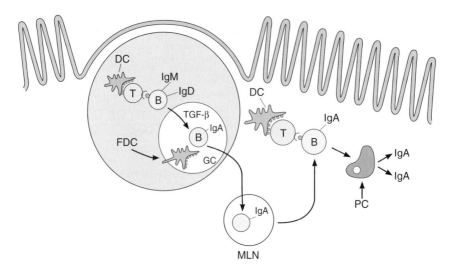

Figure 14–5. Regulation of IgA synthesis at mucosal sites. Dendritic cell (DC)-activated T cells interact with IgM/IgD B cells and induce class-switching to IgA B cells under the influence of transforming growth factor beta (TGFβ). IgA B cells in the germinal centers (GC) are inhibited from further differentiation by contact with antigen on the surface of follicular dendritic cells (FDC) until they migrate via the mesenteric lymph node (MLN) to the lamina propria. There, further contact with T cells expressing CD40L and cytokines (IL-5 and IL-6) leads to IgA plasma cell (PC) formation.

IL-5 and IL-6. Interestingly, cross-linking of surface IgA on B cells inhibits proliferation, whereas cross-linking surface IgM induces proliferation. This may explain the lack of IgA plasma cell development in Peyer's patches, where IgA B cells encounter antigens bound to follicular dendritic cells. It should be noted, however, that antigen-mediated inhibition of IgA B cells can be reversed by a strong T-cell signal delivered via CD40L and perhaps other T-cell surface molecules. Thus, one might hypothesize that IgA B cells developing in Peyer's patches are initially suppressed by exposure to antigen in the germinal centers and are then activated following migration to the lamina propria, where they encounter CD40L-expressing activated T cells. This ensures that IgA B cells do not secrete IgA until they arrive at effector sites where such secretion is needed.

MUCOSAL HOMING

Lymphoid cells that become activated in mucosal follicles preferentially migrate to effector sites in the lamina propria underlying the mucosal surfaces (Figure 14–6). This selective homing ensures that immune responses induced in mucosal tissues are expressed in mucosal sites. In addition it accounts for the fact that antigen contact at one mucosal surface (eg, the intestine) can lead to the production of specific IgA at other mucosal surfaces (eg, the lung).

Although B-cell homing is directed to all mucosal sites, some regional preferences have been noted; thus, bronchial node-derived B cells have a greater tendency to home to the lungs than to the intestines, and Peyer's patch B cells have a greater propensity to home to the intestines than to the lungs. Mucosal T cells developing in mucosal follicles also tend to migrate back to mucosal sites, but in this case the migration is more promiscuous, and one can detect migration to systemic sites as well. This is exemplified by recent studies showing that intrarectal introduction of a virus leads to the appearance of CTLs in both the lamina propria and the spleen.

Mucosal homing is mediated in large part by tissue-specific interactions between integrins and other molecules on the surface of migrating leukocytes and ligands (addressins) on endothelial cells in particular vascular beds (see Chapter 3). With respect to mucosal homing, the most important interaction is that between $\alpha_4\beta_7$ on mucosal cells and its ligand MAdCAM-1 on mucosal endothelial cells. Recently, evidence has accrued indicating that $\alpha_E\beta_7$ may be a second integrin that plays a role in mucosal homing; however, in this case the homing may be restricted to a particular subset of cells.

A second mechanism of mucosal homing is tissue-specific retention of cells at mucosal sites. This mechanism may be particularly important with respect to IELs because the latter express $\alpha_E\beta_7$ integrin, which interacts with E-cadherin on epithelial cells. Because $\alpha_E\beta_7$ is also present on a substantial portion of LPLs it may also mediate retention of these cells in the mucosa via interaction with an as-yet-unidentified ligand.

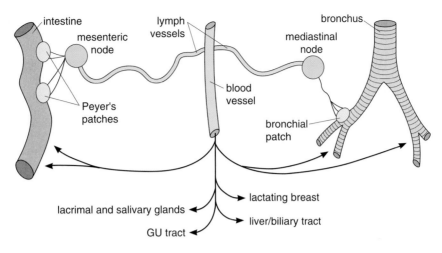

Figure 14–6. Cell traffic in the mucosal immune system. Cells originating in the mucosal follicles localize in subepithelial regions of many mucosal tissues. The ability to do so is governed by specific interactions between homing receptors on lymphoid cells and vascular addressins on endothelial cells. *Abbreviation:* GU tract = genitourinary tract.

ORAL TOLERANCE

Mucosal immune cells are constantly exposed to antigenic substances, including those present in food or associated with the intestinal flora, which have the potential to evoke unnecessary and potentially harmful immune responses. Such responses are normally inhibited, however, by a specialized mechanism, known as oral tolerance, which renders the mucosal immune system unresponsive to oral antigens (Figure 14–7). As a rule, oral tolerance develops in relation to protein antigens and is a T-cell-mediated phenom-

enon. In contrast, polysaccharide antigens do not induce oral tolerance, consistent with the observation that such antigens are T-cell-independent and typically evoke IgM antibody responses that have low pathogenic potential. Other factors that influence the development of oral tolerance include antigen dose, the genetic makeup of the host, prior immunization, and the level of overall immunologic activation. In contrast, certain bacterial toxins, such as cholera toxin, are strong mucosal adjuvants and induce oral immunogenic responses rather than tolerogenic responses.

Of the several mechanisms that have been shown to operate in the development of oral tolerance, per-

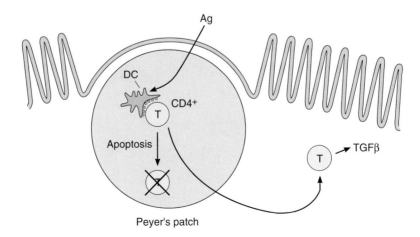

Figure 14–7. Induction of oral tolerance. Protein antigens entering the Peyer's patches are captured by dendritic cells (DC), which then induce antigen-specific T cells to either undergo apoptosis (deletional mechanism) or differentiate into transforming growth factor beta (TGFβ)-producing suppressive T cells (suppressive mechanism).

haps the best established is the induction of suppressor T cells. Thus, mice subjected to oral immunization with relatively small doses of antigen develop T cells in their Peyer's patches and spleen that, when transferred to a second animal, can suppress responses to the same antigen given parenterally in a form that ordinarily is immunogenic. Both CD4 T and CD8 T cells have this capability, though CD4 T cells are more effective. The suppressor T cells (now referred to as Tr-1 cells or T_H3 cells) operate in an antigen-nonspecific fashion by producing TGFβ, IL-10, or possibly other suppressor factors. Because of this antigen-nonspecificity, oral tolerance induced by feeding one antigen (antigen 1) can lead to suppression of responses against a second antigen (antigen 2) if antigen 1 is readministered along with antigen 2 to activate the suppressor cells. Such "bystander" suppression could theoretically enable one to suppress a pathologic immune reaction by inducing oral tolerance with an irrelevant antigen, provided, of course, that the suppressor cells induced by the irrelevant antigen can be delivered to the appropriate site. Attempts to treat various autoimmune diseases via oral antigen-induced bystander suppression are currently underway.

A second mechanism of oral tolerance involves induction of T-cell anergy, T-cell deletion, or both. Thus, mice fed relatively large amounts of an antigen subsequently can be shown to lack cells capable of responding to that antigen, yet they may manifest little or no suppressor activity with respect to that antigen. Such deletional nonresponsiveness occurs over a wide range of oral antigen doses, and is not the exclusive province of high-dose oral antigen administration as initially thought. Only at high doses of oral antigen, however, is the deletional mechanism profound enough to preclude the generation of both T-cell effectors and T-cell suppressors.

Studies in mice also show that feeding of antigen elicits an initial T_H1 response that is then superseded by a tolerogenic response marked by the induction of T_H3 suppressor cells. This appears to reflect the presence of two distinct types of dendritic cells in the dome areas of Peyer's patches (1) a unique dendritic cell that expresses IL-10 rather than IL-12 and may thus favor the development of TGFβ or IL-10-producing suppressor T cells or both; and (2) a dendritic cell similar to those in spleen and other lymphoid tissues that expresses IL-12 and therefore induces a T_H1 effector response. One can hypothesize that oral administration of protein antigens in the absence of a mucosal adjuvant triggers a T-cell induction pathway resulting in the development of tolerogenic T_H3 cells that at the same time suppress the development of immunogenic T_H1 cells. Alternatively, oral administration of protein antigens in the presence of mucosal adjuvants favors the T_H1 immunogenic pathway, which reciprocally suppresses the T_H3 suppressor pathway. This hypothesis finds strong support from the study of mouse models of inflammation, wherein the induction of strong T_H1 responses leads to mucosal inflammation on the one hand and suppression of counterregulatory T_H3 responses on the other, whereas T_H1 responses tempered by T_H3 responses prevent such inflammation. This suggests a possible cause for human inflammatory bowel disease, which may represent a breakdown in oral tolerance or an imbalance in the immunogenic and tolerogenic responses of the mucosa.

ORAL IMMUNIZATION VERSUS ORAL TOLERANCE INDUCTION

If protein antigens are likely to induce oral tolerance, how does the mucosal immune system overcome such tolerance to mount protective IgA antibody and CTL responses? One answer is that mucosal immune responses occur when soluble protein antigens are accompanied by adjuvants or are themselves capable of overcoming mucosal tolerogenic mechanisms. In other words, immune responses result when the initial T_H1 response is vigorous enough to preclude switching to a tolerogenic T_H3 response.

This view of mucosal adjuvant activity describes, at least in part, the mechanism of action of cholera toxin, one of the most potent of the mucosal adjuvants. Cholera toxin is a potent inhibitor of IL-12 production and thus inhibits rather than enhances T_H1 responses in most circumstances. While inhibiting T_H1 responses, however, it favors the increased development of T_H2 and T_H3 responses, leading to the production of IL-4 and IL-5 on the one hand, and TGFβ and IL-10 on the other, all of which are cytokines that support IgA B-cell responses. As a result, cholera toxin is an adjuvant for IgA humoral responses, but not necessarily for cell-mediated responses. Other adjuvants may well have different effects on mucosal immune responses. Indeed, some virulent bacteria express proteins that enhance costimulation of T cells and promote T_H1 responses and so would presumably suppress IgA responses. The overall picture that emerges is that immunogenic mucosal responses and adjuvant activity are closely linked and must be defined in relation to the type of mucosal response that is being elicited.

BREAST MILK IMMUNOLOGY

An important aspect of mucosal immunity is the capacity of IgA B cells to enter the lactating breast and to secrete IgA, which is then transported into breast secretions (ie, the colostrum and milk). This is, in fact, a key means of intergenerational transfer of immunity and is thus a tangible example of the importance of mucosal immune processes in mammalian survival.

IgA B cells home to lactating breast tissue following the secretion of certain gestational hormones that presumably act by inducing the expression of specific addressins on breast tissue endothelial cells. Within breast tissue, IgA B cells differentiate and the IgA subsequently secreted is transported into milk via the SC transport mechanism. The concentration of IgA in initial breast secretions (colostrum) is extremely high (average 50 mg/mL, versus 2.5 mg/mL in adult serum) during the first 4 postpartum days and then rapidly falls to serum levels. Such IgA secretion is accompanied by the secretion of other, less specific host defense factors, such as lysozyme; lactoferrin; cytokines; and various antibacterial glycoproteins, glycolipids, oligosaccharides, and lipids. Together, these various soluble agents act as potent host defense components in the newborn gut.

The breast secretions are also rich in various cellular elements that contribute breast milk immunity. These include activated neutrophils and macrophages, which produce active oxygen radicals and various proinflammatory cytokines, such as TNFα, IL-1β, and IL-6. In contrast, the lymphocyte content of breast secretions is relatively low, and whether such cells survive the environment of the infant intestine is open to question.

The various soluble and particulate immune elements present in breast milk secretion provide critical protection to the newborn against infectious diseases, particularly in the unhygienic environments of less developed countries. Extensive data support the contention that breast feeding offers protection against the development of infant diarrhea, septicemia, lower respiratory tract infection, and necrotizing enterocolitis.

A final possible salutary effect of breast feeding relates to the ability of IgA to prevent absorption of certain environmental proteins early in life, at a time when the infant is susceptible to developing lifelong IgE-mediated allergic reactions. This possibility has, in fact, been used as an explanation for why early dietary exposure to certain antigens leads to allergy, or why transient IgA deficiency has been associated with atopy. It should be noted, however, that the data on this point are conflicting, and the precise role, if any, of breast feeding in allergy development remains to be defined.

REFERENCES

GENERAL
Kelsall BL, Strober W: Host defenses at mucosal surfaces. In: *Clinical Immunology Principles and Practice,* Rich R (editor). Mosby, 1996.

McGhee JR et al: Mucosal Immune Responses: An Overview. In: Mucosal Immunology, Ogra PL (Editor). Academic Press, 1999.

ANTIGEN-PRESENTING CELLS
Blumberg RS et al: Expression of a nonpolymorphic MHC-class I like molecule CD1d, by human intestinal epithelial cells. *J Immunol* 1991;147:2518.

Kelsall BL, Strober W: Distinct populations of dendritic cells are present in the subepithelial dome and T cells regions of the murine Peyer's patch. *J Exp Med* 1996;183:237.

Mayer L, Blumberg RS: Antigen presenting cells: Epithelial cells. In: *Mucosal Immunology,* Ogra PL (editor). Academic Press, 1999.

M CELLS
Tomohiro K, Owen RL: Structure and function of intestinal mucosal epithelium. In: *Mucosal Immunology,* Ogra PL (editor). Academic Press, 1999

INTRAEPITHELIAL LYMPHOCYTE
Lefrancois L, Puddington L: Basic aspects of intraepithelial lymphocyte immunobiology. In: *Mucosal Immunology,* Ogra PL (editor). Academic Press, 1999.

MUCOSAL MAST CELLS
Befus AD et al: Mast cells from the human intestinal lamina propria. *J Immunol* 1987;138:2604.

LAMINA PROPRIA LYMPHOCYTES
Boirivant M et al: Hypoproliferative human lamina propria T cells retain the capacity to secrete lymphokines when stimulated via CD2/28 pathways. *Proc Assoc Am Physicians* 1996;108:56.

James SP, Kiyono H: Gastrointestinal lamina propria T cells. In: *Mucosal Immunology,* Ogra PL (editor). Academic Press, 1999.

London SD, Robin D: Functional role of mucosal cytotoxic lymphocytes. In: *Mucosal Immunology,* Ogra PL (editor). Academic Press, 1999.

IGA STRUCTURE & TRANSPORT
Mestecky J, McGhee JR: Immunoglobulin A (IgA): molecular and cellular interactions involved in IgA biosynthesis and immune responses. *Adv Immunol* 1987;40:153.

Mestecky J et al: Selective transport of IgA: cellular and molecular aspects. *Gastroenterol Clin North Am* 1991; 20:441.

Sanderson IR, Walker WA: Mucosal barrier. In: *Mucosal Immunology,* Ogra PL (editor). Academic Press, 1999.

Underdown BJ et al: Mucosal immunoglobulins. In: *Mucosal Immunology,* Ogra PL (editor). Academic Press, 1999.

REGULATION OF IGA SYNTHESIS

Coffman RL et al: Transforming growth factor-β specifically enhances IgA production by lipopolysaccharide-stimulated murine B cell lymphocytes. *J Exp Med* 1989; 170:1039.

Kawanish H et al: Mechanisms regulating IgA production in murine gut-associated lymphoid tissues. *J Exp Med* 1983;157:433.

McIntyre TM et al: Novel in vitro model for high-rate IgA class switching. *J Immunol* 1995;154:3156.

McIntyre TM, Strober W. Gut-associated lymphoid tissue: Regulation of IgA B-cell development. In: *Mucosal Immunology,* Ogra PL (editor). Academic Press, 1999.

Weinstein PD, Cebra JJ: The preference of switching to IgA expression by Peyer's patch germinal center B cells is likely due to the intrinsic influence of their micro environment. *J Immunol* 1991;147:4126.

ORAL TOLERANCE

Braun MC et al: Cholera toxin suppresses interleukin-12 production and IL-12 receptor beta 1 and beta 2 chain expression. *J Exp Med* 1999;189:541.

Iwasaki A, Kelsall BL: Freshly isolated Peyer's patch but not spleen, dendritic cells produce interleukin 10 and induce the differentiation of T helper type 2 cells. *J Exp Med* 1999;190:229.

Strober W et al: Oral tolerance. *J Clin Immunol* 1998;18:1.

MUCOSAL CELL HOMING

Belyakov IM et al: The importance of local mucosal HIV-specific CD8(+) cytotoxic T lymphocytes for resistance to mucosal viral transmission in mice and enhancement of resistance by local administration of IL-12. *J Clin Invest* 1998;102:2072.

Butcher EC: Lymphocyte homing and intestinal immunity. In: *Mucosal Immunology,* Ogra PL (editor). Academic Press, 1999.

Ludviksson BR et al: Administration of mAb against alpha E beta 7 prevents and ameliorates immunization-induced colitis in IL-2-/- mice. *J Immunol* 1999;162:49.

Springer TA: Traffic signals for lymphocyte recirculation and leukocyte emigration: the multi step paradigm. *Cell* 1994;76:301.

Schon MP et al: Mucosal T lymphocyte numbers are selectively reduced in integrin alpha E (CD103)-deficient mice. *J Immunol* 1999;162:6641.

BREAST MILK

Butler JE: Immunoglobulins and immunocytes in animal milks. In: *Mucosal Immunology,* Ogra PL (editor). Academic Press, 1999.

Hanson LA, Telemo E: Immunobiology and epidemiology of breastfeeding in relation to prevention of infections from a global perspective. In: *Mucosal Immunology,* Ogra PL (editor). Academic Press, 1999.

Koldovsky O, Goldman A: Growth factors and cytokines in milk. In: *Mucosal Immunology,* Ogra PL (editor). Academic Press, 1999.

Section II.
Immunologic Laboratory Tests

Clinical Laboratory Methods for Detection of Antigens & Antibodies

15

Clifford Lowell, MD, PhD

This chapter discusses the tests used for the detection of **antibodies** and **antigens.** The presence of an antibody to a defined protein or compound depends on the immune response of the patient; hence antibody detection is used to quantitatively and qualitatively evaluate normal and abnormal immune responses. The increasing use of molecularly cloned antigens has dramatically improved the precision of antibody detection. In contrast, antigen detection is usually used to determine the presence of foreign proteins or compounds (eg, infectious agents or drugs). Antigen detection as the characterization of the cell surface phenotype (identification of molecules expressed on the cell surface) is a fundamental method for the analysis of cells, particularly hematopoietic cells. The widespread use of **monoclonal antibodies (mAbs)** as specific reagents for defined antigens (either cellular proteins or components of pathogenic organisms) has dramatically improved methods of antigen detection.

Although the technologies for detecting antigens and antibodies have become increasingly automated, the scientific principles that underlie these methodologies remain the same. Fundamentally, detection of antibodies and antigens depends on the formation of antibody–antigen complexes. One of the binding partners (the antibody or the antigen) is defined, often labeled, and is used as a probe to search for the other partner. Hence, we begin this chapter by reviewing the principles of antibody–antigen binding and then provide an overview of the specific methods that depend on these principles.

ANTIGEN-ANTIBODY BINDING

The process of antibody binding to antigen (the formation of immune complexes) underlies much of immunologic testing. In its simplest form, a specific mAb is used to look for a single antigenic epitope, and formation of the complex is monitored by precipitation of the complex or by the presence of a tag (fluorescent, radioactive, or enzymatic) on the antibody. Reciprocally, use of molecularly cloned proteins as model antigens can be used to look for specific antibodies that recognize this protein; furthermore, one can determine the isotype of the reacting antibodies (IgG, IgM, or IgE). More complex mixtures of antibodies-antigens can also be used. For example, the antibodies for a specific test may be the polyclonal sera from an animal immunized with the antigen (or sera from a patient with a known disease or condition), and the antigens may be a complex mixture of proteins, carbohydrates, and nucleic acids from an infectious agent. Often the antibody or antigen is fixed to a solid support that allows the immune complex to be separated from other components of the binding mixture (Figure 15–1). This process, often referred to as immunoprecipitation, is usually used when the antibody or antigen on the solid support is present in vast excess in the mixture. Immunoprecipitation requires some process or method for separation of the immune complexes, such as centrifugation or filtration. The amount of the complex is then determined by a second binding reaction with a labeled reagent.

When the antibodies and antigens are present in equimolar ratios, they form insoluble complexes that precipitate naturally. Light scattering (or formation of turbidity) can be used to monitor accumulation of precipitate in the solution. In this circumstance, the relative concentrations of the antigen and antibody are the most important determinants for formation of the complexes (Figure 15–2). Maximum precipitation occurs when the antibody–antigen concentrations are equivalent (**zone of equivalence)** and decreasing amounts of precipitate (or very small complexes) are formed in zones of antigen or antibody excess. Thus

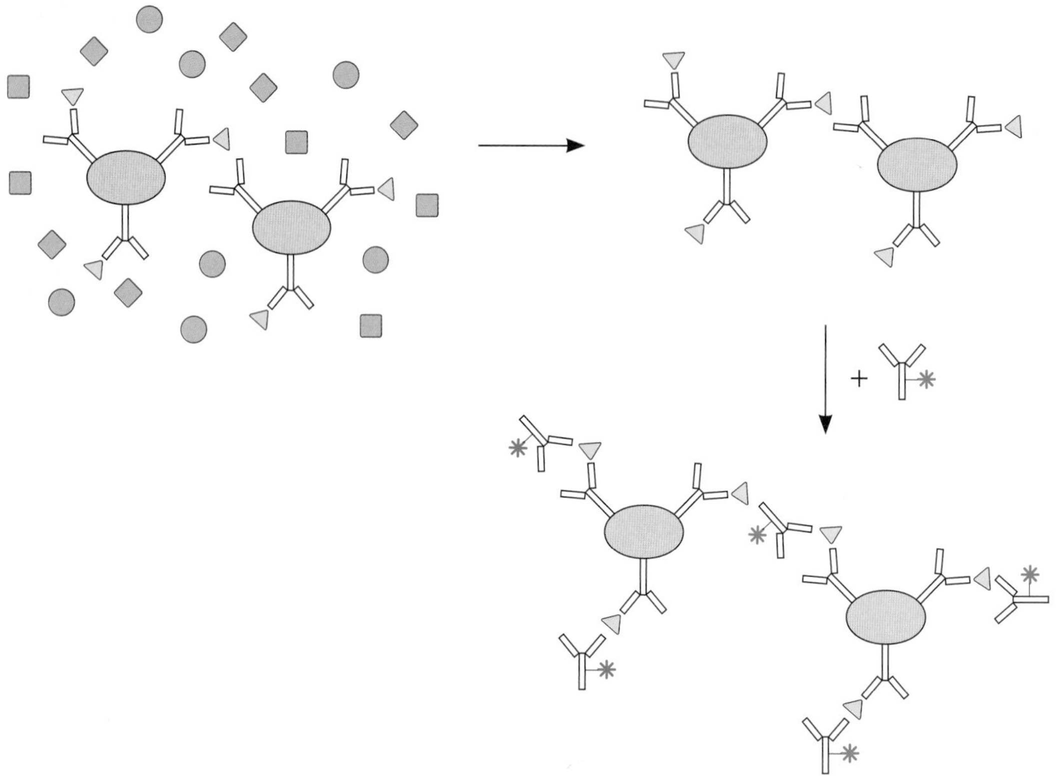

Figure 15–1. Principle of antigen detection using a surface-bound antibody for isolation of antigen–antibody complexes. The antibody, which specifically recognizes one antigen, is bound to the surface of insoluble beads. The beads are mixed with the specimens and antigen–antibody binding occurs. Subsequently, the beads are separated from the antigen solution (often by centrifugation or filtration), and the presence of the bound antigen on the beads is detected with another antibody that is labeled (radioactive, fluorescent, or enzymatic).

formation of insoluble immune complexes can be used to quantify the amount of antigens if a known concentration of antibody is used (or vice versa). The **prozone** phenomenon occurs when antibody or antigen is in vast excess and suboptimal immune complexes form. This phenomenon can lead to misinterpretation of tests when large amounts of antibody are present (eg, in multiple myeloma or polyclonal gammopathies) or when antigens are improperly diluted (eg, in agglutination reactions—see later section).

Testing Methods That Depend on Formation of Immune Complexes

Immunodiffusion. Immunodiffusion is the simple technique by which antigens and antibodies are placed in separate wells within a semisolid support (eg, agar) then allowed to mix through the support by diffusion. When a zone of equivalence is reached, a line of precipitation occurs, which is visible when light is passed through the gel (Figure 15–3). This simple technique launched the field of serology in the first part of the 20th century and remains in use today. Double diffusion in agar, often referred to as

Ouchterlony analysis, characterizes the relationship between different antigens. In this methodology, antigens are placed in wells of agar (poured in small dishes or on glass slides), and antibody is placed in a center well. The reactants are allowed to diffuse together, and the nature of the precipitation lines between the wells is characterized (Figure 15–4). Although simple, immunodiffusion methods are limited by insensitivity and by the requirement for relatively large amounts of precipitating antigens or antibodies. Also the rate of diffusion can make the test time-consuming. This latter problem is often solved by placing the agar matrix in an electric field, which drives the antigens and antibodies together—a technique called **countercurrent immunoelectrophoresis (CIE)**. CIE also increases the efficiency of antigen–antibody complex formation and often increases the sensitivity of the assay. Table 15–1 lists examples of antibodies and antigens that are still assayed by immunodiffusion methods.

Nephelometry. In nephelometry, the formation of immune complexes in solution is monitored by spectrometry. Scattering of an incident light is used to de-

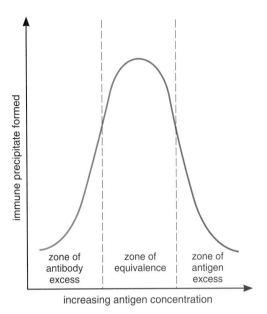

immune precipitate formed

zone of antibody excess | zone of equivalence | zone of antigen excess

increasing antigen concentration

Figure 15–2. Antigen–antibody precipitin curve. Typical precipitin curve resulting from titration of increasing antigen concentration plotted against amount of immune precipitate formed. The amount of antibody is kept constant throughout.

tect complexes in dilute solutions of antigens and antibodies. In more concentrated mixtures of reactants, the immune complexes turn the solution cloudy, which can be measured by light absorption or turbidimetry. Nephelometric determination of antigens is performed by addition of constant amounts of highly purified and optically clear specific antisera to

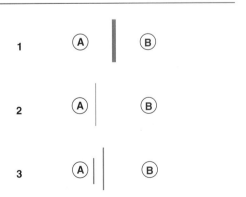

1 (A) | (B)

2 (A) | (B)

3 (A)| | (B)

Figure 15–3. Reactions in simple double diffusion. In (1) antigen A and antibody B react equidistantly and intensely at equivalence. In (2) antigen A is present in reduced concentration or has not diffused as rapidly owing to size or charge, forming a precipitin line closer to the antigen well. In (3) a contaminant or impurity present in antigen A is reacting with antibody B.

varying amounts of antigen. Mixing is performed in a cuvette within a light beam, and the progressive formation of immune complexes is measured in a photoelectric cell as the optical density (Figure 15–5). Accurate measurement of antigens can be made only in the ascending limb of the precipitation curve (see Figure 15–2) where there is a direct linear relationship between antigen concentration and optical density. Thus, samples with high concentrations of antigens may require dilution for accurate measurements. The amount of optical density can be measured at a single instant following addition of antibody to the antigen—the so-called endpoint determination. This method is hampered, however, by the fact that many components in serum samples, such as lipids or preformed immune complexes, can contribute substantially to background light scattering. To avoid this problem, modern nephelometers subtract background light scatter prior to addition of antisera and then measure formation of immune complexes continuously. The determination of the kinetics of immune complex formation, a process called **rate nephelometry,** provides a more accurate quantitation of antigen levels. In this method, the amount of antigen is proportional to the peak rate of immune complex formation as long as the reaction occurs on the ascending limb of the precipitation curve (or at slight antibody excess). Automated nephelometers confirm that the reaction is in antibody excess by adding known amounts of each antigen being analyzed (so-called calibrators) to the reaction and confirming increased immune complex formation. Nephelometry is used to measure the levels of a variety of serum antigens and proteins (Table 15–2).

Complement Fixation. The formation of immune complexes in solution can also be monitored by the ability of these complexes to fix and consume complement proteins. Because of their relative ease and low cost, complement fixation (CF) assays are widely used to detect immune responses to infectious agents (eg, coccidioidomycosis, histoplasmosis, and others [Table 15–3]). Many CF assays have been replaced by more sensitive, enzyme-based methods (see following section) and are now usually used as confirmatory assays. The CF assay is a two-stage reaction: In the first stage the antigen is mixed with patient sera with a known amount of complement. Formation of immune complexes leads to fixation of complement. In the second stage of the reaction, the amount of residual hemolytic complement activity is determined (Figure 15–6). Results are expressed as the dilution of patient sera in which complement consumption is lost. CF assays usually reflect IgG titers against the antigen and are best used to diagnose disseminated disease. Since CF assays work by measuring functional activity (RBC lysis) of complement, they can be complicated by the presence of any anticomplement activity in the patient serum, such as preformed immune complexes, heparin, or chelating agents.

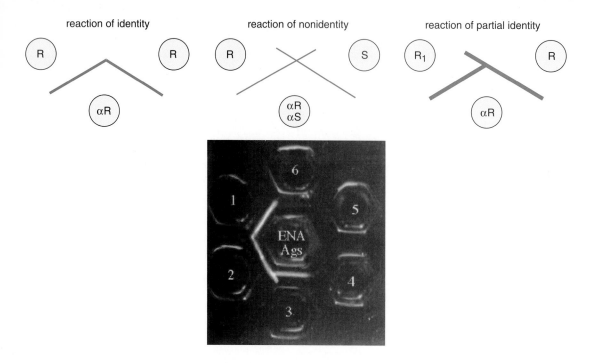

Figure 15–4. Top: Reaction patterns in angular double immunodiffusion (Ouchterlony). Antigens are shown as R, R$_1$, and S, and the reactive antibodies are αR, and αS. As the antibodies and antigens diffuse outward from their spots in the gel, precipitation reactions occur. If the antigens are the same (the reaction of identity), the precipitin lines fail to cross because all the reactive antibody will precipitate. However, if the antigens are unrelated (the reaction of nonidentity) and the antibody mixture contains immunoglobulins that react with both antigens, the precipitin lines cross because the reactions occur independently of one another. If antigenic determinants are partially shared between antigens, in the reaction of partial identity, the precipitin lines cross in only one direction. In the case shown, antigen R$_1$ shares some antigenic determinants with antigen R, but not all. **Bottom:** An example of a screening immunodiffusion assay used to detect the presence of antibodies against extractable nuclear antigens (ENA) in various patients. Patients 1 and 2 have lines of identity with the ENA; patient #3 has only a partial reaction to some of the ENA. Other patients are nonreactive.

Cryoglobulins. Cryoglobulins are serum immunoglobulins (Igs) that precipitate at temperatures less than 37°C. The presence of cryoglobulins in the blood is determined by incubating serum samples at 4°C for several hours, then looking for the formation of a precipitate. The precipitated proteins are then isolated by centrifugation, solubilized in 37°C buffer, and assayed for the presence of immunoglobulins by nephelometry or immunofixation electrophoresis. The three types of cryoglobulins are

Table 15–1. Antibodies routinely assayed by immunodiffusion or electroimmunodiffusion.

Antibodies to extractable nuclear antigens (ENA)–anti-sn RNP, anti-Sm, anti-SSA (Ro), anti-SSB (La), anti-Scl-70 (topoisomerase I)
Antifungal antibodies (Coccdiomycosis, Aspergillus, Histoplasmosis)
Anti-*Entamoeba histiolytica*

Type I: Cryoprecipitatable monoclonal Ig or light chains.

Type II: Monoclonal Igs, most often of the IgM isotype, that bind to normal polyclonal IgG. Antibodies that recognize normal IgG are called **rheumatoid factors (RFs);** hence type II cryoglobulins are cold-precipitable monoclonal RFs bound to their antigen (polyclonal IgG).

Type III: Polyclonal RFs (usually IgM or IgA isotypes) bound to polyclonal IgG.

Type I cryoglobulins usually are associated with malignancy and often are found in high concentrations in the serum (greater than 5 mg/mL). These can cryoprecipitate at physiologically relevant temperatures and, therefore, can present with cold-induced symptoms, such as cold-induced digital ischemia. Type II cryoglobulins are associated with chronic infections, most notably hepatitis C. They generally do not precipitate at physiologic temperatures and usually present as immune complex disease (eg, cutaneous vasculitis, glomerulonephritis). Type III cryo-

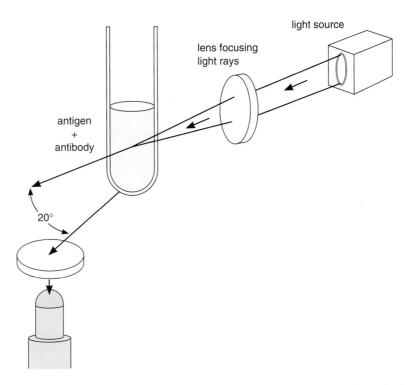

Figure 15–5. The principle of nephelometry for measurement of antigen–antibody reactions. Example shown is for the Beckman Array 360 System. This instrument uses a tungsten halogen lamp with a spectral range of 420–600 nm as a high-intensity light source. The formation of antigen–antibody complexes leads to light scattering, which is measured by silicon photodetectors as a forward angle of 20°. In other tungsten-based systems, the incident light may be filtered to a specific wavelength (610 nm) and scattered light collected at different angles. The rate of formation of the antigen–antibody complexes is represented by increased light scatter.

globulins occur in autoimmune disorders, such as systemic lupus, and a variety of chronic viral, bacterial, and parasitic infections. Type III cryoglobulins typically are found in low concentrations in the serum (less than 1 mg/mL) and basically are circulating immune complexes.

Testing Methods in Which the Antigen or Antibody Is Fixed to a Solid Surface

Agglutination Assays. Agglutination (or aggregation) of antigen-coated particles by reactive antibodies is among the most time-honored of immuno-

assays. Much of this testing technology has now been replaced by more sensitive methods for antibody detection; however, agglutination-based assays are still routinely used in blood bank testing to classify red blood cell (RBC) types and to look for autoimmune anti-RBC antibodies (reviewed in Chapter 17). Although very simple to perform, all agglutination assays suffer from the fact that they are semiquantitative.

Agglutination assays that test for the presence of an antibody depend on the availability of a particle that is coated with the appropriate antigen. The particle can be an RBC displaying its natural blood group antigens or a synthetic particle (eg, a latex bead) which is artificially coated with antigen. In the pres-

Table 15–2. Antigens and antibodies routinely assayed by nephelometry.

Complement proteins (C3 and C4)
Immunoglobulins (IgM, IgG, IgA)
Rheumatoid factor
α_1-Antitrypsin
Ceruloplasmin
Microalbumin
Prealbumin

Table 15–3. Examples of antibodies routinely assayed by complement fixation (most often as a confirmatory test).

Antifungal antibodies (Cocciodiomycosis, Histoplasmosis)
Antiviral antibodies (adenovirus, herpes virus, influenza)
Anti*Mycoplasma pneumoniae*
Antirickettsial antibodies

First Stage:

Second Stage:

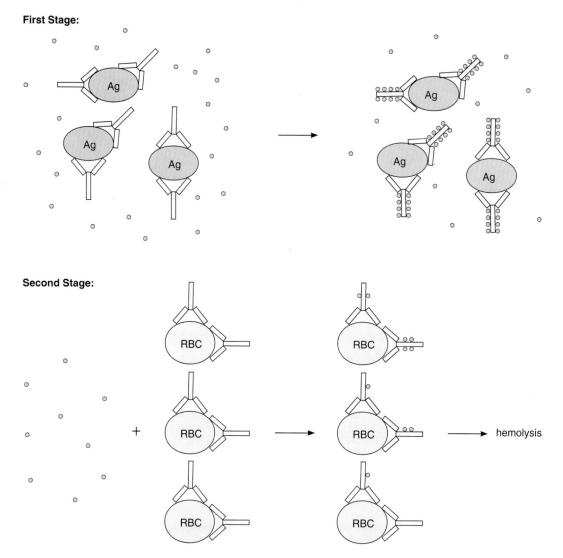

Figure 15–6. The principle of complement fixation assays. In the first stage, antigen and antibody react in the presence of complement (shown as dots). The antigen–antibody complexes fix complement proteins, resulting in the consumption of some but not all of the available complement components. In the second stage, the activity of the residual complement is determined by adding an excess of sensitized sheep red blood cells (RBCs); these fix the residual complement and undergo hemolysis. Thus, a reciprocal relationship exists between the amount of antigen in the first stage and the residual complement left over for the second stage.

ence of specific antibody, the particles aggregate. The formation of aggregates can be seen visually in a tube, in a microtiter well, or even on a simple glass slide (Figure 15–7). This process can be reversed and used to detect antigens. In this case, the particle is coated with specific antibody to look for antigens that are capable of binding and agglutinating the particles. A special category of agglutination involves spontaneous agglutination of RBCs by certain viruses, such as influenza virus. These viruses contain surface proteins that bind to RBC proteins and aggregate the RBCs. One can block this reaction with

antiviral antisera that adsorbs to the viral surface and prevents interaction with the RBCs. This inhibition of viral hemagglutination can be used to titer the antiviral antibody activity of patient sera.

A frequently used hemagglutination assay is the **heterophile antibody** test for acute infectious mononucleosis (often referred to as the **monospot** test). Heterophile antibodies are IgM antibodies that, probably, result from the cross reaction between antigens on the agent of infectious mononucleosis (the Epstein–Barr virus) and equine RBC antigens. Incubation of horse RBCs with sera from patients with infectious mononu-

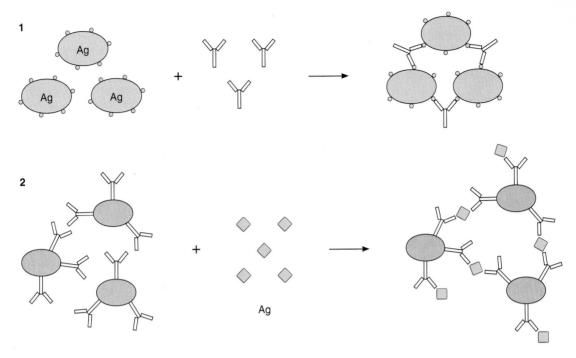

Figure 15–7. Examples of agglutination reactions. In (1) the particles are coated with antigens; for example, latex beads that are artificially coated with antigen or RBCs that are displaying their own natural surface antigens. Following addition of antibodies, the particles are aggregated by bridging antibody reactions. In (2) particles are coated with the test antibody and exposed to the antigen mixtures. If the antigens have multiple epitopes, antibodies on different particles will react with the same antigen molecule and become aggregated.

cleosis leads to agglutination—the presence of anti-EBV antibodies in the patient can then be confirmed by more specific bead-based or immunofluorescent methods.

In **latex agglutination** assays latex beads are coated with either antigen (to look for specific antibody) or a defined antibody (to assay for antigen). Although widely used in the past, most have been replaced by more sensitive, automated methods. Examples include particles coated with human immunodeficiency virus, hepatitis B virus, or various fungal antigens to assay patient sera for evidence of prior infection (as reflected by the presence of specific antibodies). The classic pregnancy test is a latex agglutination assay in which beads coated with antibodies to human chorionic gonadotropin are mixed with patient urine to detect the presence of the hormone.

In response to some infectious agents (most commonly *Mycoplasma pneumoniae*) or during autoimmune reactions, patients produce antibodies that have the particular ability to agglutinate RBCs at 4°C. These antibodies, referred to as **cold agglutinins,** are assayed by incubation of serial dilutions of patient sera with a 1% RBC solution at 4°C overnight and then examined for agglutination. True cold agglutinins go back into solution at 37°C, and therefore reincubation of the sample at 37°C should result in

deagglutination of the RBCs. This simple assay is widely used as a surrogate marker for immune response to *M pneumoniae* infection; indeed, 50–80% of acutely infected patients produce cold agglutinins, which are typically IgM antibodies.

Screening assays to look for antibodies against rare bacterial pathogens continue to be performed using agglutination reactions. Examples include assays for brucellosis or *Francisella* infections. In these cases, the particle is the organism itself—incubation of whole, fixed bacteria with patient sera leads to agglutination of the organisms if the patient is mounting an immune response against the agent. These assays suffer from low sensitivity and cross-reactivity (eg, patients infected with *Tularensis* can have a false-positive test for *Brucella* antibody). They are extremely easy to perform, however, and are very inexpensive; hence they remain in common use today. Positive tests are confirmed by other methods (see later section).

Enzyme-Linked Immunoabsorbent Assays (ELISA). In ELISA, the antibody (or antigen) is fixed to a surface, such as a well of a microtiter plate or a plastic bead. The test sample is applied and bound material is detected by a secondary, enzymatically labeled antibody. These assays are rapid, simple, and easily adaptable to automated analyzers. They require highly purified reagents; use of mAbs and re-combinant antigens have greatly facilitated the wide-spread use of ELISA.

The most common version of the ELISA is the **sandwich assay** (Figure 15–8). A mAb to a specific antigen is fixed to microtiter plates (small plastic plates, treated to maximize protein binding, that contain 96 wells with a volume of 200 μL each). The wells are incubated with serial dilutions of the patient sample to allow binding of the antigen to the surface-bound antibody, then washed. Bound antigen is detected with a secondary antibody that is enzymatically labeled. After another washing, the wells are incubated with a substrate for the enzyme and the enzymatic reaction (appearance of product) is determined. This basic ELISA method can be modified in a variety of ways: Wells can be coated with antigens to detect specific antibodies in patient sera (the isotype of the antibody can be determined by using either anti-IgM or anti-IgG as the second-step reagent). An alternative approach to measuring antibodies to specific antigens is the **antibody capture** assay. Wells are coated with anti-IgM and anti-IgG, resulting in capture of all patient IgM or IgG. The wells are then incubated with a known antigen, followed by a mAb specific for that antigen (Figure 15–9).

Common enzymes used in the detection step are horseradish peroxidase and alkaline phosphatase; these enzymes can be covalently coupled to mAbs without affecting either the antigen-binding capacity of the antibody or inhibiting the activity of the enzyme. A variety of substrates can be incubated with these enzymes to produce colored products that can be quantitated using microtiter plate spectrophotometers. Because the last step of the assay is enzymatic, these assays have the advantage of being extremely sensitive. Many modern autoanalyzers use horseradish peroxidase substrates that produce **chemiluminescent** products, further enhancing sensitivity. Measuring the rate of the reaction, rather than simply the extent of the reaction at a single fixed instant, allows ELISA to be accurate quantitatively. The amount of antigen is determined by comparison to a standard curve generated with known amounts of antigen.

In many situations, the sensitivity of these assays can be further enhanced by use of additional steps in the reaction. Most commonly, this is done by use of secondary antibodies labeled with the vitamin biotin; wells are then incubated with enzymatically labeled avidin (a protein component of egg white), which binds biotin with extremely high affinity (K_D of 10^{-15} M) and specificity (Figure 15–10). **Biotin/avidin-enhanced** immunoassays allow for antigen detection using extremely small samples. Biotin/avidin-enhanced assays are also used in immunofluorescent assays (see later discussion).

The popularity of the **enzyme-linked immunoassays** (EIA) in clinical practice reflects their easy adaptation to automated analyzers that allow substantially increased throughput in the laboratory. Automated machines can handle microtiter plates, using robotic arms to automatically fill and wash the wells and to move the plate to a coupled spectrophotometer.

Microparticle Enzyme Immunoassays. A variation of the ELISA uses small beads (1 mm in size) coated with the appropriate antigen or antibody. The microparticle enzyme immunoassay (MEIA) is an extension of the bead assay. In this case, submicron-sized particles are coated with antibody or antigen. The advantage of these tiny particles is that their relatively large surface area leads to higher concentra-

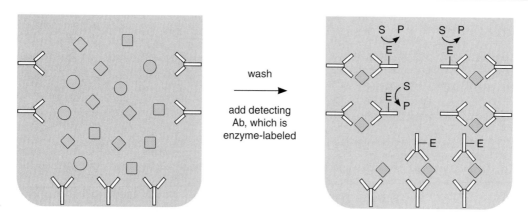

Figure 15–8. Example of a sandwich ELISA assay for antigen detection. Microtiter wells are coated with mAbs and then the wells are incubated with the specimen to allow antigen to bind to the fixed antibodies. Following washing, an enzyme-labeled (shown as E) detecting antibody is used to reveal antigen bound to the surface. Plates are washed free of unbound detecting antibody and substrate (S) is added to the wells. The formation of colored (or fluorescent) product (P) is monitored in a microtiter plate spectrophotometer.

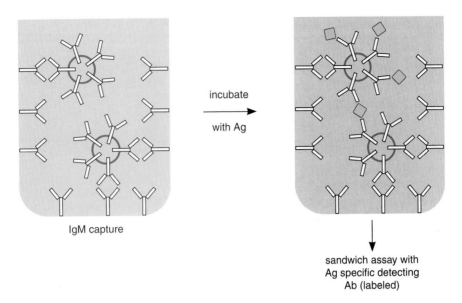

Figure 15–9. Example of antibody capture method. In this method, microtiter plate surfaces are coated with antibodies that bind specifically to patient IgM (shown as pentameric structures) or IgG (not shown). Thus, the entire pool of patient IgM or IgG is immobilized in the well. The wells are washed and mixed with antigens, following which a standard sandwich ELISA is performed. The amount of antigen bound is proportional to the amount of reactive IgM or IgG in the patient sera.

tions of antibody or antigen. As a result, binding reactions can be completed in a very short (15–30 minutes) time. The assay proceeds as a standard sandwich assay, but performed in suspension. The particles then are separated from the unbound reagents by filtration through glass fiber filters, which irreversibly bind the microparticles. The filters are exposed to the appropriate substrate (depending on the enzyme label used), and the extent of the enzymatic reaction is measured using automated analyzers. Table 15–4 provides a partial list of antibodies and antigens measured by MEIA. A number of tests traditionally based on immunodiffusion, CF, or agglutination reactions are now determined by MEIA technology on automated analyzers. In addition to the advantage of automation, these new methods can

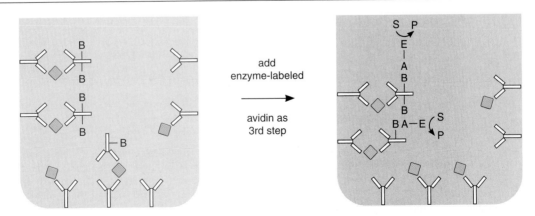

Figure 15–10. Example of biotin/avidin-enhanced ELISA sandwich assay. After the second step of the assay, in which the detecting antibody is labeled with biotin (B), a third step is added in which enzyme-labeled avidin (A) is added. Subsequently, the binding of avidin is monitored by conversion of substrate (S) to product (P). This enhances the signal because of the extremely high affinity and specificity of biotin–avidin interaction. Also, the detecting antibodies can be labeled with many biotin molecules, so that many avidin–enzyme conjugates can bind.

Table 15–4. Examples of antigens and antibodies routinely assayed for by MEIA-based assays (partial list).

Antiviral antibodies (CMV, HBV, HAV, rubella)

Ferritin, B_{12}, folate

IgE

Antitoxoplasma

Tumor markers (PSA, CA-125, CEA, AFP)

Thyroid hormones (TSH, T_3, T_4)

Therapeutic drug monitoring (digoxin, quinidine)

Detection of drugs of abuse (cocaine, barbiturates, THC)

Abbreviations: CMV = cytomeglovirus; HBV = hepatitis B virus; HAV = hepatitis A virus; PSA = prostate-specific antigen; CEA = carcinoembryonic antigen; AFP = α-fetoprotein; TSH = thyroid-stimulating hormone; T_3 = triiodothyronine; T_4 = tetraiodothyronine; THC = tetrahydrocannabinol.

offer a tenfold to 1000-fold increase in sensitivity of detection compared with the older manual methods.

Electrophoresis Methods

The separation of serum proteins in electric fields has been used for generations to characterize human immune responses and disease states. There are two basic procedures: **zone electrophoresis,** which separates proteins based on surface electric charge, and **denaturing electrophoresis,** which separates proteins based on molecular weight. In both methods, serum samples are placed in support media and subjected to an electric field to induce protein migration. Commonly used support media include agarose gels strips, cellulose acetate, or polyacrylamide gel. In clinical applications for routine separation of serum proteins, cellulose acetate strips are most commonly used because they are optically clear, allowing microquantities of proteins to be used and detected by chemical (or immunochemical) staining methods.

Serum Protein Electrophoresis (SPEP). In this assay, a small amount of patient serum (or other biologic fluid) is placed in the center of a shallow well within a strip of cellulose acetate. The film is subjected to an electric field, the proteins migrate based on their charge, and then the film is stained to localize the protein bands (Figure 15–11). The stained film can be scanned by a densitometer to provide an analytical representation of the electrophoretic pattern. Normal human sera is separated into five major bands: albumin, α_1-globulin, α_2-globulin, β-globulin and γ-globulin, which represent mainly IgG. SPEP is useful in the diagnosis of human paraprotein disorders such as multiple myeloma and Waldenström's macroglobulinemia (Figure 15–12). In these disorders, an electrophoretically restricted protein spike usually occurs in the γ-globulin region. The spike represents accumulation of a single type of Ig that has a defined surface charge, versus the normal pattern of multiple different types of Igs that have vary-

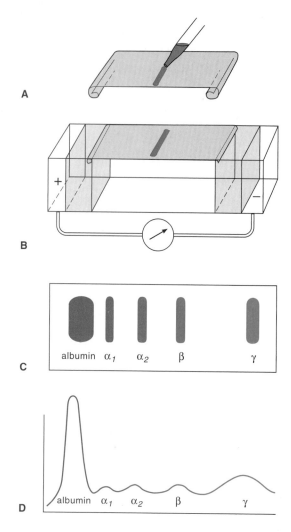

Figure 15–11. Technique of cellulose acetate zone electrophoresis. **A:** Small amount of serum or other fluid is applied to cellulose acetate strip. **B:** Electrophoresis of sample is performed in electrolyte buffer. **C:** Separated protein bands are visualized in characteristic position after being stained. **D:** Densitometer scanning from cellulose acetate strip converts bands to characteristic peaks of albumin, α_1-globulin, α_2-globulin, β-globulin, and γ-globulin.

ing charges (and hence produce a smear in the γ-globulin region of the gel). A marked decrease in serum γ-globulin concentration can sometimes also be detected by this technique. Electrophoresis of urine samples **(UPEP)** analyzes proteins excreted by the kidney. Free immunoglobulin light chains are readily detectable in urine when present in increased amounts, as in the Bence Jones proteinuria of myeloma (Figure 15–13). Zone electrophoresis in agarose gels has also been useful in the diagnosis of

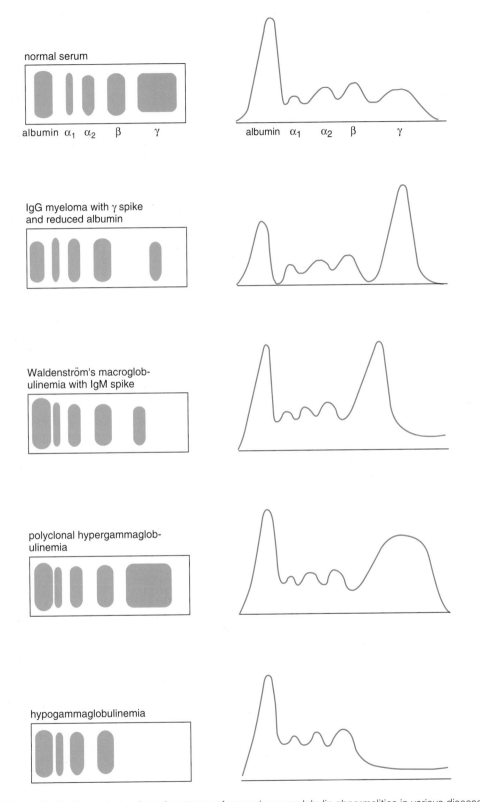

Figure 15–12. Zone electrophoresis patterns of serum immunoglobulin abnormalities in various diseases.

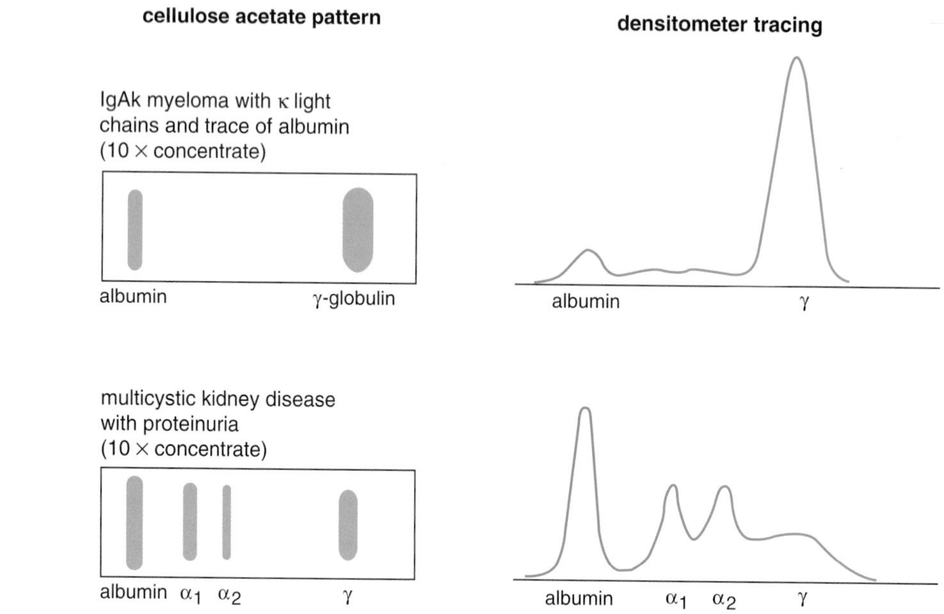

cellulose acetate pattern

densitometer tracing

IgAk myeloma with κ light
chains and trace of albumin
(10 × concentrate)

albumin   γ-globulin

albumin   γ

multicystic kidney disease
with proteinuria
(10 × concentrate)

albumin α₁ α₂   γ

albumin   α₁ α₂   γ

Figure 15–13. Zone electrophoresis patterns of urine abnormalities in various diseases.

certain central nervous system diseases, such as multiple sclerosis, with alterations in cerebrospinal fluid (CSF) proteins (Figure 15–14). Abnormalities in levels of serum proteins other than Igs may also be detected by SPEP. Although very easy to perform, SPEP is considered a screening assay for determination of protein abnormalities; more quantitative or specific assays are performed on samples with an abnormal pattern.

Immunoelectrophoresis. This assay combines electrophoretic separation of serum proteins followed by immunologic detection of particular proteins using specific antisera. This assay is widely used to characterize and quantitate monoclonal paraproteins.

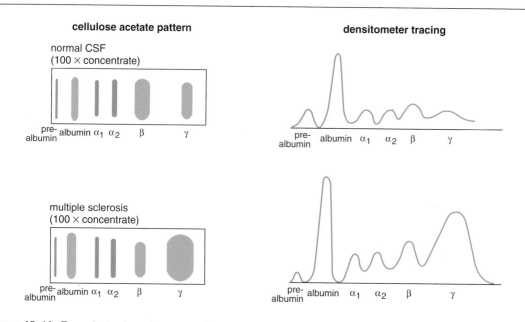

cellulose acetate pattern

densitometer tracing

normal CSF
(100 × concentrate)

pre-   albumin α₁ α₂   β   γ
albumin

pre-   albumin α₁   α₂   β   γ
albumin

multiple sclerosis
(100 × concentrate)

pre-albumin α₁ α₂   β   γ
albumin

pre- albumin   α₁   α₂   β   γ
albumin

Figure 15–14. Zone electrophoresis patterns of cerebrospinal fluid from normal subject and multiple sclerosis patient.

Past methods have used agarose gels as supports for electrophoresis of serum, urine, or CSF proteins, followed by immunodiffusion within the agarose to look for precipitin arcs. This technology has been replaced by **immunofixation electrophoresis** in which the sample proteins are separated in a buffered agarose gel. After electrophoresis, antiserum against antibody heavy or light chains is overlaid directly onto the gel surface along the axis of the electrophoretic migration, and immunoprecipitation in situ is allowed to occur. The resulting antigen–antibody complexes become trapped in the gels pore structure. The gel is then processed to removed excess soluble proteins, dried, and stained with a protein-specific stain to reveal the precipitin bands. Interpretation is made by visually comparing the specific protein bands with the reference protein electrophoretic pattern (Figure 15–15); normal Igs appear as a smear, and monoclonal proteins appear as a specific band. This method is especially helpful in the detection of paraproteins of the IgM and IgA isotypes, which may be undetectable in the excess of normal IgG.

Denaturing Gel Electrophoresis and Western Blotting. In this technique, proteins are denatured by incubation with an ionic detergent (sodium dodecyl sulfate, or SDS) at 100°C, followed by electrophoresis in polyacrylamide gels (SDS-PAGE). Because the detergent uniformly coats all the proteins, rendering the surface charge of the protein negative, the proteins migrate within the electric field based on the amount of SDS molecules bound to them, which in turn is influenced by the size of the protein. This method therefore separates proteins by molecular weight. SDS-PAGE is often combined with immunoblotting to specifically identify particular proteins in a given sample. Following electrophoresis by SDS-PAGE, the proteins are electrophoretically transferred to a piece of filter paper (often nylon or nitrocellulose) to which they adhere by nonpolar interactions. The filter paper can then be incubated with specific antisera to reveal the reactive proteins. This entire process is referred to as Western blotting or immunoblotting. This procedure is used extensively in research laboratories to define specific proteins in biologic samples. A widespread clinical use of immunoblotting is to define the pattern of antibody reactivity of individual patients to certain pathogens, such as human immunodeficiency virus (HIV). In the **HIV Western blot,** viral proteins (isolated by in vitro culture of virus) are separated on SDS-PAGE and transferred to a filter. The filter serves as a solid antigen support for a typical sandwich type ELISA assay. The filter is incubated with patient sera, washed, and then incubated with anti-IgG (which is enzymatically labeled) in order to reveal the presence of patient antibodies to specific HIV proteins. Because the filter can be stored indefinitely, commercial vendors are able to produce and sell these strips with electrophoretically separated HIV viral antigens. This assay is widely used as a confirmatory assay for the presence of HIV infection. Patients are confirmed to have been infected by HIV if they make antibodies that recognize at least two specific viral proteins (Figure 15–16).

SERUM VISCOSITY

The measurement of serum viscosity is a simple and valuable tool for evaluating the likelihood of complications with paraproteinemia. Normally, the formed elements of the blood contribute more significantly to whole-blood viscosity than do plasma proteins. In diseases with elevated concentrations of serum proteins, however, particularly the Igs, the serum viscosity may reach very high levels and result in a characteristic symptom complex, the **hyperviscosity syndrome.** This syndrome is characterized by

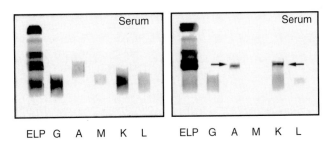

Figure 15–15. Immunofixation electrophoresis. **Left:** Normal serum pattern. In lane 1 (ELP), total serum proteins have been electrophoresed and precipitated onto the cellulose acetate (or plastic in the assay system shown). In lanes 2-6 (G–L) specific antisera reactive with IgG, IgA, IgM, κ-light chains or λ-light chains (designated G A M K L) are reacted with the serum proteins, and then immunoprecipitates are detected on the plastic strip. In the normal pattern, the polyclonal immunoglobulins are represented by a smear of proteins since many different forms of differing electric charge are present. **Right:** Sample from a patient with multiple myeloma and an IgA-κ paraprotein. Note the very heavy and distinct bands present in the IgA and κ-light chain regions (*arrows*) as well as the residual polyclonal immunoglobulins.

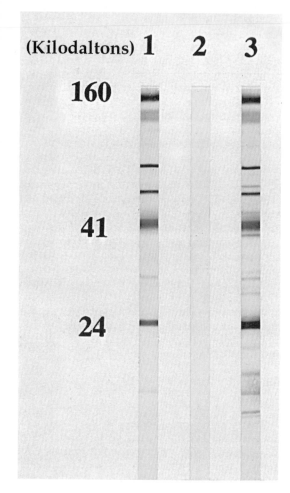

Figure 15–16. HIV Western blot analysis of serum from a patient who tested repeatedly positive on HIV ELISA screening assays. Lane 1 shows the reaction of a known positive control serum sample that contains antibodies that recognize a host of viral proteins—the most clinically significant are p24, p41, and p160 (which are named based on their molecular weights and are viral core, or in the case of p160, envelope proteins). Lane 2 shows the lack of reaction with negative control sera. Lane 3 shows the test patient sera; the patient has a spectrum of antibodies that recognize the same viral structural proteins as the control sample. Hence, this patient is confirmed to be infected with HIV (ie, HIV-positive).

an Ostwald viscosimeter. A few milliliters of serum are warmed to 37°C and allowed to descend through a narrow-bore capillary; the rate of the descent of the serum through the capillary is compared with the rate at which distilled water moves. The ratio of these two numbers provides a measure of the relative serum viscosity. Normal values range from 1.4 to 1.9.

Serum viscosity measurements are primarily of use in evaluating patients with Waldenström's macroglobulinemia, multiple myeloma, and cryoglobulinemia. In myeloma, aggregation or polymerization of the paraprotein in vivo often results in hyperviscosity. The correlation between levels of relative serum viscosity and clinical symptoms is, however, not direct, and thus it can be difficult to predict at what point clinical symptomatology will result. Increased serum viscosity may interfere with various laboratory tests that employ flow-through devices, such as hematology counters and analyzers in clinical chemistry.

IMMUNOHISTIOCHEMICAL METHODS

Immunofluorescence Assays (IFA). In this method, specific antibodies (usually mAbs) conjugated with fluorescent labels are used as probes for the detection of antigens in samples of patient tissues or on patient cells. In each case, the binding of the antibodies to the tissues or cells is visualized directly using a fluorescence microscope. The latter contains a high-intensity light source, excitation filters to produce a wavelength capable of causing fluorescence activation, and a barrier filter to remove interfering wavelengths of light (Figure 15–17). When observed in the fluorescence microscope against a dark background, fluorescent antibodies bound specifically to antigens can be visualized by their bright color. The advantage of this assay is that is allows visualization of the antigen within specific cell types in a tissue or even within specific subcellular compartments of cells. For example, using this method, cytoplasmic antigens can be easily distinguished from nuclear antigens. Use of a fluorescent antibody to detect cellular or tissue antigens is referred to as **direct IFA** (Figure 15–18)

Alternatively, this basic process can be used to detect antibodies within patient sera that are reactive to a specific pathogen or that are cross-reactive to specific tissue antigens. Dilutions of patient sera are incubated with cells or tissues known to be infected with the pathogen. Unbound antibodies are removed by washing, and the specifically bound antibodies are visualized with fluorescently labeled anti-Ig antisera. This method remains in use for detection of antibodies against herpes simplex virus or Epstein–Barr virus (although it is being replaced by MEIA-based detection methods). The detection of reactive antibodies in patient sera using a secondary labeled anti-

very slow flow of blood through the microvasculature, resulting in tissue ischemia. This can be directly visualized in the retina as aggregates of RBCs in the small vessels where blood flow has nearly stopped (referred to as "boxcar" lesions). Serum viscosity is determined by a variety of factors, including protein concentration; the size, shape, and deformability of serum molecules; and the molecular charge or temperature sensitivity of the proteins.

In clinical practice, serum viscosity is measured in

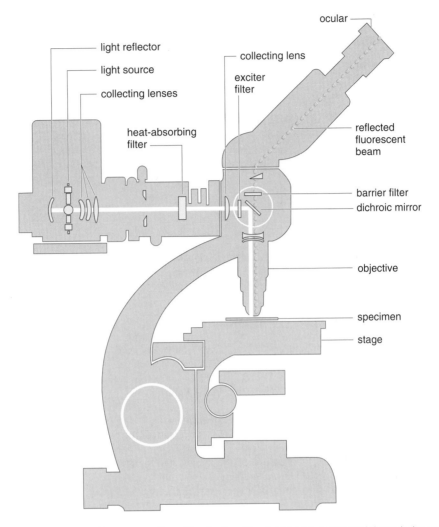

Figure 15–17. Fluorescence microscope with epiillumination. The light beam is directed through the exciter filter and down onto the specimen. A dichroic mirror allows passage of selected wavelengths in one direction but not another. After reaching the specimen, the light is reflected through the dichroic mirror and emitted fluorescent light is visualized at the ocular.

Ig is referred to as an **indirect IFA** (see Figure 15–18). Indirect IFA assays are commonly used to assay for the presence of autoantibodies that react inappropriately to specific cell types or subcellular structures. The classic **antinuclear antibody (ANA)** test is an example (Figure 15–19). In this test, dilutions of patient sera are incubated with tissue culture cells (a human cell line called HepG2 is used), and specifically bound antibodies (of either IgM or IgG isotypes) are detected with labeled secondary antibodies. The pattern of binding of patient antibodies to the nuclear antigens in this cell line (homogenous, speckled, rim pattern, nucleolar) correlate with fine specificity of the ANA and with the presence of specific autoimmune disorders, such as systemic lupus erythematosus (SLE) (see Chapter 31). IFA assays can also take advantage of the biotin–avidin amplification method used in ELISA assays. In this case, the primary antibody is labeled with biotin (for indirect assays the detecting antibody is biotinoylated), and fluorescently labeled avidin is used for detection. Because of the high affinity and specificity of the biotin–avidin interaction, this method significantly improves the sensitivity of IFA assays.

Fluorescence is the emission of light of one color (wavelength) while a substance is irradiated with light of a different color. Several different fluorochromes are used in the clinical laboratory for IFA assays. These same reagents are also heavily used in flow cytometry (fluorescence-activated cell sorter,

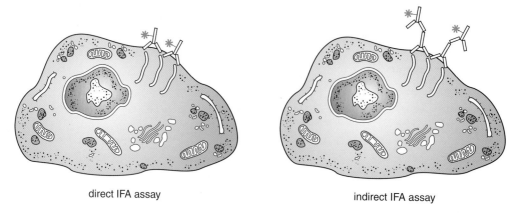

direct IFA assay   indirect IFA assay

Figure 15–18. Direct and indirect immunofluorescence assays (IFA). In the direct assay, a monoclonal antibody (mAb), which is labeled with a fluorescent marker such as fluorescein or rhodamine, of known specificity is reacted directly with a tissue or cell specimen to establish the presence of the antigen. The indirect assay is most often used clinically to determine if a patient's serum has antibodies that cross-react with specific cellular antigens; in this case the binding of the patient's antibodies is revealed by a secondary anti-Ig antibody that is labeled.

FACS) assays (see Chapter 16). The classic fluorochromes are fluorescein and rhodamine. These compounds are linked to isothiocyanate to form reactive agents (called fluorescein isothiocyanate [FITC] or tetramethyl-rhodamine isothiocyanate, respectively) that readily form covalent bonds with the ε-amino residues of lysine and terminal amino groups. Incubation of these agents with proper concentrations of antibodies results in the covalent labeling of the antibody without affecting the ability of the antibody to bind to antigen. When stimulated with light at approximately 480–490 nm, FITC-conjugated antibodies emit at roughly 530 nm (green), whereas rhodamine-labeled mAbs emit at approximately 580 nm (red). Using a microscope with

filters that distinguish these wavelengths, one can use differently labeled antibodies simultaneously to detect different antigens in the same sample or to examine the relationship of different subcellular proteins. The simultaneous use of differently labeled sets of mAbs for antigen detection is routinely used in flow cytometry.

Immunohistochemical Assays. In this method, the primary antibodies used are labeled with enzymes, and their binding is detected by the presence of enzymatic activity. These antibodies can be the same reagents used in ELISA assays. In these cases, the samples are incubated with enzymatic substrates that produce a product that precipitates directly on the tissue section (usually producing a brown- or red-

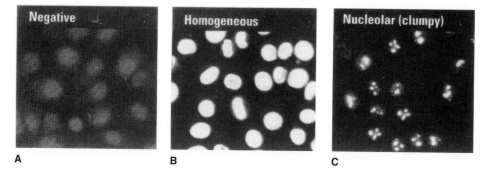

A   B   C

Figure 15–19. Examples of antinuclear antibody (ANA) staining patterns. In these indirect immunofluorescence assays, patient sera are incubated with HepG2 cells, and the binding of patient antibodies is revealed using a fluorescein secondary antibody. Examples of negative control, homogeneous staining, and nucleolar staining patterns are shown. The particular staining pattern for ANA is correlated with the particular nuclear antigen to which the patient makes autoantibodies. In many cases, different ANA patterns reflect different disease states in the patient—homogenous staining is seen in 60–80% of patients with systemic lupus erythematosus, whereas nucleolar staining is more commonly seen in patient with scleroderma.

stained product). This method is useful because binding of the antibody to samples can be visualized directly with a normal light microscope. To enhance signal production, indirect assays often use a horseradish peroxidase-labeled secondary antibody or a biotin/avidin-based antibody to reveal an unlabeled primary antibody. Immunohistochemical staining is used widely to detect tumor antigens or to classify lymphocyte cell types in surgical pathology sections.

COMPLEMENT ASSAYS

Complement is one of the effector mechanisms of immune complex-induced tissue damage. Clinical disorders of complement function have been recognized for many decades. The nine major complement components of the classic pathway (C1–C9), several from the alternative pathway, and various inhibitors can be measured in human serum. Clinically useful assays of complement include those that test pathway function (the total hemolytic assays; CH_{50} and AH_{50}) and tests of the quantities and functions of individual components.

It is worth emphasizing that the collection and storage of serum samples for functional or immunochemical complement assays present special problems as a result of the remarkable lability of some of the complement components. Rapid removal of serum from clotted specimens and storage at temperatures of –70°C or lower is required for preservation of maximal activity. An important source of error in complement determination is poor sample handling.

Hemolytic Assays. The hemolysis of RBCs by antibodies in vitro depends on complement. This requirement forms the basis for widely used assays of complement activity. The hemolytic assay for the classical complement pathway employs sheep RBCs, rabbit antibodies against sheep RBCs, and patient sera as a source of complement. The sheep RBCs are opsonized with the rabbit antibody (at a subagglutinating dose of antibody) and then mixed with dilutions of patient sera; hemolysis is measured spectrophotometrically. The amount of lysis in a standardized system describes an S-shaped curve (Figure 15–20) when plotted against increasing amount of complement (or patient sera). In the midregion of the curve, near 50% hemolysis, a linear relationship exists between the degree of hemolysis and the amount of complement activity present. For clinical purposes, measurement of total hemolytic activity of serum is taken at the 50% hemolysis level; this is called the **CH_{50} unit.** CH_{50} units are standardized by using a defined amount of sheep RBCs, antisheep RBC antibody and guinea pig serum as a source of complement. Standard curves are set up with the known reagents and used to compare with patient samples. Variables that can influence the degree of hemolysis include RBC concentration,

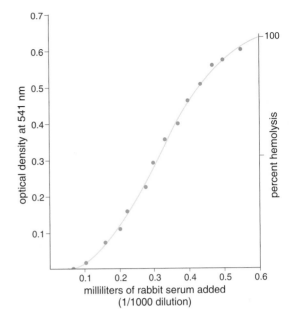

Figure 15–20. Relationship of complement concentration to hemolysis of antibody-sensitized red blood cells (RBCs). In this model experiment, increasing amounts of rabbit serum, as a source of complement, is added to a fixed amount of sensitized RBCs, and the hemolysis of the cells is measured at 541 nm (the absorption maximum of hemoglobin). The curve forms an S shape.

fragility of the RBCs, amount of antibody used for sensitization, the nature of the antibody (IgM versus IgG), and the presence of preformed immune complexes or anticomplement factors in patient sera.

The value CH_{50} units in human serum may be determined by converting the S-shaped curve to a linear curve using the von Krogh equation:

$$X = K(Y/1 - Y)^{1/n}$$

where X = number of milliliters of diluted serum used; Y = percentage of RBC lysis; K = constant; and $n = 0.2 \pm 10\%$ under standard conditions.

Converting this equation to log form allows one to graph the results on a log–log plot, where the values of $Y/(1 - Y)$ are plotted against the serum dilutions X. The reciprocal of the dilution of serum that intersects the curve at the value $Y/(1 - Y) = 1$ is the CH_{50} unit (Figure 15–21). The values for CH_{50} units can vary significantly between different laboratories unless standardized reagents are used.

The alternative pathway of complement activation shares the terminal components (C3 and C5–C9) with the classical pathway but has several unique components (D, B, and P). To measure the function of this pathway, the **AH_{50} assay** is used. This assay depends on the ability of complement to lyse unsensitized sheep RBCs by activation of the initial com-

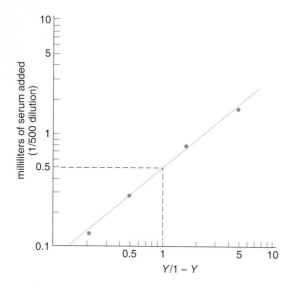

Figure 15–21. Determination of CH_{50} units from serum. Standard curve relating milliliters of serum (1:500 dilution) to $Y/(1 - Y)$ from the von Krogh equation. When $Y/(1 - Y) = 1.0$, the percentage of lysis equals 50%. In the example shown, 0.5 mL of 1:500 serum dilution has produced $Y/(1 - Y) = 1.0$, or 50% lysis. The CH_{50} value for this serum equals 1000 because 1 mL of undiluted serum has 1000 lytic units.

Table 15–5. Diseases associated with reduced hemolytic complement activity.

Systemic lupus erythematosus with glomerulonephritis

Acute glomerulonephritis

Immune complex diseases

Infective endocarditis with immune complexes and glomerulonephritis

Disseminated intravascular coagulation

Hereditary complement deficiencies

Mixed cryoglobulinemia

Advanced cirrhosis of the liver

ponents of the alternative pathway (to ensure that the classical pathway is not activated, these assays are done with ethylene glycol tetraacetic acid (EGTA) to chelate Ca^{2+} ions—the classical pathway is calcium-dependent). Because the alternative pathway and the classical pathway share common terminal components, deficiencies in these proteins result in loss of both CH_{50} and AH_{50} activity. Normal CH_{50} activity with reduced AH_{50} values results from defects in alternative complement components.

The CH_{50}/AH_{50} assays are relatively insensitive assays for total complement activity but are excellent screens to rule out genetic deficiency of complement components. Homozygous deficiency of an individual component totally abrogates hemolytic activity for the pathway tested. For example, patients with homozygous deficiency of C2 have undetectable CH_{50}. Reduced serum complement activity occurs in a variety of acquired disease states (Table 15–5). Reduction in serum complement activity can be due to any one or a combination of (1) complement consumption by in vivo formation of antigen–antibody complexes, (2) decreased synthesis of complement, (3) increased catabolism of complement, or (4) formation of inhibitors (usually autoantibodies). In all cases, however, a significant (80–90%) reduction in one component must occur in order to affect total hemolytic activity. In principle, the activity of each individual component of the complement cascade can be determined using variations of the standard CH_{50}/AH_{50} assay. These assays are done by providing an excess of all the components except for the one tested and then adding serial dilutions of the patient serum until 50% hemolysis is observed. The easiest way to do this is to use serum that is genetically deficient in a specific component (eg, C4-deficient guinea pig serum or C6-deficient rabbit serum) or that is depleted of a given component by chemical means. Sensitized RBCs are mixed with the deficient sera and serial dilutions of the patient sera to determine the point at which 50% hemolysis is observed.

Immunochemical Assays for Complement Components. Because functional assays reflect only major changes in the levels or activity of complement proteins, many laboratories test for the level of individual complement proteins using a number of the standard methods for antigen detection described earlier. The method most commonly used to measure C3, C4, C1-inhibitor, and factor B is rate nephelometry; the other components can be measured by immunodiffusion or ELISA. Although these tests can pick up more subtle changes in complement protein levels than functional assays, improper handling of specimens can also result in erroneous values in these assays. For example, in storage, C3 spontaneously converts to C3c, which has a smaller molecular size than native C3.

REFERENCES

GENERAL

Crocker J, Burnett D: *The Science of Laboratory Diagnosis,* ISIS Medical Media, 1998.

Rose NR, Mackay IR: *The Autoimmune Diseases,* 3rd ed, Academic Press, 1998.

Rose NR et al: *Manual of Clinical Immunology,* 5th ed, American Society for Microbiology, 1997.

Sheehan C: *Clinical Immunology: Principles and Laboratory Diagnosis,* 2nd ed, Lippincott, 1997.

IMMUNODIFFUSION, NEPHELOMETRY, AND CRYOGLOBULINS

Agnello V, Romain P: Mixed cryoglobulinemia secondary to hepatitis C infection. *Rheum Dis Clin North Am* 1996; 22:1.

Beckman Instructions for the Beckman Array 360 System, Beckman Instruments, 1993.

Deverill I, Reeves WG: Light scattering and absorption development in immunology. *J Immunol Methods* 1980; 38:191.

Gorevic PD: Cryopathies: Cryoglobulins and cryofibrinogenemia. In: *Samter's Immunologic Diseases,* Vol 2, 5th ed. Frank MM et al (editors). Little Brown and Co., 1995.

Kaufman L et al: Comparative evaluation of commercial EIA and microimmunodiffusion and complement fixation tests for *Coccidioides immitis. J Clin Microbiol* 1995;33:618.

Ouchterlony O, Nilsson LA: Immunodiffusion and immunoelectrophoresis. In: *Handbook of Experimental Immunology.* Vol 1, Weir BM (editor). Blackwell, 1986.

Shahangian S et al: Concentration dependencies of immunoturbidimetric dose-response curves: Immunoturbidimetric titer, reactivity, and relevance to design of turbidimetric immunoassays. *Clin Chem* 1992;38:831.

AGGLUTINATION, ELISA, & MEIA TECHNIQUES

Charles PJ, Maini RN: Enzyme-linked immunosorbent assay in the rheumatological laboratory. In: *Manual of Biological Markers of Disease.* Kluwer Academic Publishers, 1993.

Jaspers JP et al: Nine rheumatoid factor assays compared. *J Clin Chem Clin Biochem* 1988;26:863.

Kasahara Y: Principles and application of particle immunoassay. In: *Immunological Assays and Biosensors for the 1990s,* Nakamura RM et al (editors). American Society for Microbiology, 1992.

Kemeny DM: *A Practical Guide to ELISA,* Pergamon Press, 1991.

Kricka LJ: Selected strategies for improving sensitivity and reliability of immunoassays. *Clin Chem* 1994;40:347.

Maclin E, Young DS: Automation in the clinical laboratory. In: *Tietz Textbook of Clinical Chemistry,* 2nd ed. W.B. Saunders Co., 1994.

Tijssen P, Adam A: Enzyme-linked immunosorbent assays and developments in techniques using latex beads. *Curr Opin Immunol* 1991;3:233.

ELECTROPHORESIS

Bio-Rad Laboratories. *Protein Blotting. A Guide to Transfer and Detection.* Bio-Rad Laboratories, 1996.

Garfin DE: Electrophoretic methods. In: *Biophysical Methods for Protein and Nucleic Acid Research.* Glasel JA, Deutscher MP (editors). Academic Press, 1995.

Keren DF: *High Resolution Electrophoresis and Immunofixation: Techniques and Interpretations,* 2nd ed. Butterworth-Heinemann, 1994.

Roberts RT: Usefulness of immunofixation electrophoresis in the clinical laboratory. *Clin Lab Med* 1986;6:601.

Timmons TM, Dunbar DS: Protein blotting and immunodetection. *Methods Enzymol* 1990;182:679.

SERUM VISCOSITY

Kwaan HC, Bongu A: The hyperviscosity syndromes. *Semin Thrombosis Hemostasis* 1999;25:199.

Pruzanski W, Watt JF: Serum viscosity and hyperviscosity syndrome in IgG multiple myeloma. Report on 10 patients and review of the literature. *Ann Intern Med* 1972; 77:853.

IMMUNOHISTOCHEMICAL TECHNIQUES

Arndt-Jovin D et al: Fluorescence digital imaging microscopy in cell biology. *Science* 1985;230:247.

Cuello AC: *Immunohistochemistry II.* Wiley and Sons, 1993.

Elias JM: *Immunohistopathology: A Practical Approach to Diagnosis.* ASCP Press, 1990.

Taylor CR: An exaltation of experts: Concentrated efforts in the standardization of immunohistochemistry. *Hum Pathol* 1994;25:1.

Taylor CR, Cote RJ: *Immunomicroscopy: A Diagnostic Tool for the Surgical Pathologist.* W.B. Saunders Co., 1994.

COMPLEMENT ASSAYS

Ahmed AEE, Peter JB: Clinical utility of complement assessment. *Clin Diag Lab Immunol* 1995;2:509.

Dodd G, Sims T: *Complement. A Practical Approach.* Oxford University Press, 1998.

Porcel JM et al: Methods for assessing complement activation in the clinical immunology laboratory. *J Immunol Methods* 1993;157:1.

Rosen FS: Genetic deficiencies of the complement system: An overview. In: *Complement in Health and Disease,* 2nd ed. Whaley K et al (editors). Kluwer Academic Publishers, 1993.

16 Clinical Laboratory Methods for Detection of Cellular Immunity

Clifford Lowell, MD, PhD

The immune system in humans has been divided into two major parts: **humoral immunity** (antibody and complement) and **cellular immunity.** In practical terms, such a division allows one to separate B-lymphocyte function (antibody production) from the activities of T cells and innate immune cells (monocytes and granulocytes). In many ways this separation is artificial; production of antibodies by B cells, for example, is critically dependent on helper T-cell function. Nevertheless, this division of the immune system provides a practical framework for the laboratory evaluation of immunity in clinical practice.

In this chapter we focus on methods to evaluate aspects of immune effector cells not directly related to antibody production. A variety of assays assess the function of these cells, but, in contrast to the evaluation of antibodies, these assays are beset by difficulties in test standardization, biologic variability, imprecision, complexity, and cost. Hence, only a limited number of them are used in routine clinical practice. The most consistent and reproducible of the methods for evaluating cellular immunity employ immunochemical means for detecting cellular antigens or markers. The advent of **monoclonal antibodies (mAbs)** for detecting various leukocyte subsets has provided us with panels of reagents to enumerate and characterize cells of the immune system. As our understanding of the cellular immune system improves, many of the methods used in the research laboratory will make their way into routine clinical use.

The present chapter reviews the tests that have medical application in the detection of immune cell types and their corresponding functions. The intention is to familiarize the reader with the principles, applications, and interpretations of assays in routine clinical use. The topics discussed include (1) assays for leukocyte phenotyping, (2) delayed-type hypersensitivity skin testing, (3) lymphocyte activation assays, (4) assessment of monocyte–macrophage function, and (5) determination of granulocyte function.

LEUKOCYTE PHENOTYPING

Determination of the number and types of cell surface molecules (often referred to as markers) is a widely used method for assessing the cells of the immune system. This method allows us quantify B cells, T cells, monocytes, and granulocytes within different sites in the body (bone marrow, spleen, blood, lymph nodes). In addition, we can enumerate subsets of these cell types. For example, **T-lymphocyte subsets** that differ in their functional properties can be distinguished phenotypically. Moreover, as immune cells develop from precursor cells or respond to external stimuli, they express characteristic patterns of surface molecules. The surface phenotype can also therefore provide clues as to the differentiation state of the cell.

Panels of mAbs have been developed that recognize defined antigenic determinants on the leukocyte surface. The mAbs are conjugated with either fluorescent dyes or enzymes and then are used to stain leukocytes in tissue sections or in fresh cell suspensions. The cell types that are recognized by the mAbs can be counted by immunohistochemical techniques, fluorescence microscopy (Chapter 15) or by flow cytometry (see next section). Precise quantitation of T and B cells in human peripheral blood has made important contributions to our understanding of immunodeficiency disorders, autoimmune diseases, tumor immunity, and immunity to infections. It should be emphasized, however, that the numbers of T or B cells do not necessarily correlate with the functional capacity of these cells. These assays provide a nosologic classification of immunocompetent cells; further evaluation of lymphocyte function may be required to assess immunologic competence in clinical practice.

In 1983, the First International Workshop on Human Leukocyte Differentiation Antigens met and established a new nomenclature for immunologically defined cellular types and subtypes. They defined a series of **clusters of differentiation (CD)** antigens that are expressed on specific cell types of the hematopoietic system. The number of recognized CD antigens has increased steadily over the years and now numbers well over 150 (see Appendix). Of note, CD antigens are not necessarily leukocyte-specific; many are expressed on nonhematopoietic cell types as well. Moreover, the definition of leukocyte surface phenotypes is a work in progress; the list of CD antigens is incomplete.

Flow Cytometry for the Detection of Leukocyte Antigens

Flow Cytometers. The most widely used method for detecting the binding of mAbs to leukocyte surfaces is flow cytometry. The engineering of flow cytometers is extremely complex, and hence only the basic concepts will be reviewed here. In general, a flow cytometer is an instrument capable of analyzing single cells as they pass through an orifice at high velocity. The flow cytometer measures the properties of light scattering by the cells and the emission of light from fluorescently labeled mAb bound to the surface

of the cell (Figure 16–1). The light-scattering properties of cells are related to their size and intracellular content or complexity. In general, larger cells produce more forward light scatter (conceptually similar to a shadow), and cells with more intracellular complexity (ie, granules, vesicles, mitochondria, etc) produce more side light scatter (Figure 16–2). Light-scattering properties can be used to calculate cell volume and have been used by a variety of analyzers to count and characterize different blood cells (neutrophils, basophils, lymphocytes, etc). The flow cytometer also detects fluorescently emitted light of different wavelengths from each cell. Using mAb that are conjugated with different fluorochromes (eg, fluorescein isothiocyanate [FITC] for green light emission, rhodamine for red/orange light emission—see Chapter 15), one can detect the emission of light from single cells that bind these mAbs. More complex flow cytometers have multiple filters and detection systems that allow for analysis of as many as seven different photochrome-conjugated mAbs that

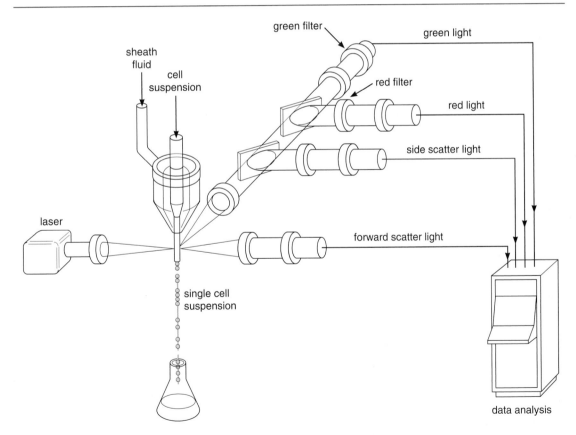

Figure 16–1. Conceptualized components of a simple "four-parameter" flow cytometer. Laser light is scattered by single cells in suspension and collected at approximately 180° and 90° to the incident beam. The reflected light is passed through filters and detected by photomultiplier tubes (PMTs), which convert the light signal to an electronic signal. A computer analyzes the data. Increasingly complex flow cytometers use more than one laser and multiple light filters and PMTs to enable the collection of fluorescent light emitted at a variety of different wavelengths.

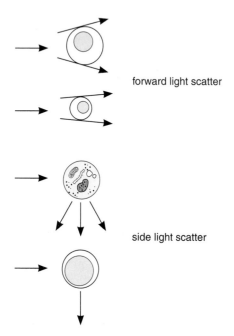

forward light scatter

side light scatter

Figure 16–2. Light scattering of cells in the flow cytometer. Forward scatter is proportional to size; larger cells have greater scatter. Side scatter is proportional to intracellular complexity; cells with more granules (neutrophils) have more scatter than cells with a simple cytoplasm (lymphocytes).

emit light at different wavelengths. Hence, multiple markers on the same cell can be analyzed simultaneously. Modern flow cytometers analyze as many as 2000–4000 cells per second; hence one is able to rapidly collect a large amount of data on different cell populations within a single sample.

Sample Preparation. Cells must be in a single cell suspension for analysis by flow cytometry. Aggregates or clumps of cells, which are often found during isolation of solid tissue, are not amenable to flow cytometry. In contrast, single-cell suspensions produced from bone marrow samples, lymph node biopsies, tissue samples from lymphoid malignancies (made by teasing the tissue apart in a buffered saline solution), or simply from peripheral blood are optimal for flow cytometric analysis. The mononuclear cells from a particular tissue sample can be purified further by density gradient centrifugation on Ficoll-Hypaque. This method results in a yield of 70–90% mononuclear cells with a high degree of purity but may also result in the loss of some lymphocyte subtypes or even of tumor cells. As an alternative, many labs simply stain samples of peripheral blood with labeled mAbs, lyse the red blood cells with commercial lysing reagents, and then analyze the sample on the flow cytometer. By using the ability of the cytometer to electronically gate individual populations of cells, one can determine the cell surface staining of different cell types within a mixed population of cells (see following section). This "whole blood lysis" method is widely used to analyze leukocyte types.

Data Collection and Analysis. The simple type of flow cytometer illustrated in Figure 16–1 collects four pieces of data for every cell that passes through the laser: (1) forward light scatter, (2) side light scatter, (3) green fluorescence, (4) red/orange fluorescence. More complex machines are able to separate red and orange fluorescence. These data are fed into a computer, and the operator can display them in a variety of fashions. Most commonly used are X/Y plots in which light scattering or emitting properties are shown on the different axes. One can then estimate the number of leukocytes that stain for one, both, or neither of the markers.

Figure 16–3 shows a typical example of lymphocyte staining of a normal peripheral blood sample. Based on their forward/side scatter light properties, one can define the lymphocytes (low forward/low side scatter, R1 area in Figure 16–3), the monocytes (medium forward/medium side scatter, R2 area), and the granulocytes (medium forward scatter/high side scatter, R3 area). Using standard flow cytometry analysis, one can "draw" an electronic region (or gate) around each group of these cells (as shown by the regions in Figure 16–3) and then display the fluorescent properties of these based on the mAbs with which the cells were stained. In the sample shown in Figure 16–3, 50% of total white blood cells are lymphocytes (in R1), 10% are monocytes (in R2) and 40% are granulocytes (R3). The T-cell/B-cell marker analysis of the lymphocytes reveals that 70% of the cells are T cells as defined by the CD3 marker, the other 30% of the lymphocytes are B cells as defined by the CD19 marker. Of the T cells, 71% are CD4+ and 29% are CD8+,whereas the B cells are evenly divided into 50% with the κ-light chain immunoglobulin and 50% with λ-light chain. In R2 all the cells are monocytes as defined by the CD14 marker, and in R3 all the cells are granulocytes as defined by the staining with a cocktail of the CD13/33 mAbs. Both the monocytes and granulocytes (and the lymphocytes as well, but not shown) stain with CD45 mAb. By comparison with many other individuals, we would find that the numbers and proportions of T-cell subsets, B-cell subsets, monocytes, and granulocytes in this patient would fall into the normal range. Hence, this patient has no quantitative defects in immune cell development that would result in immunodeficiency (of course, he may have defects in cellular function).

In contrast, the peripheral blood sample shown in Figure 16–4 is from a patient with a severe aberration in his immune system. As can be seen in the forward/side scatter plot, this patient has cells only within the lymphocyte region (R1) and has virtually no monocytes or granulocytes (in R2 or R3, respec-

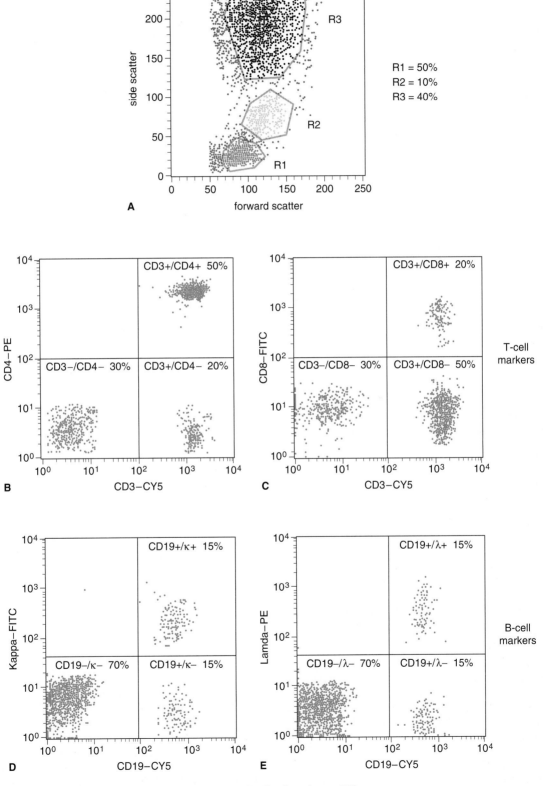

Figure 16–3. *Continued on p. 238*

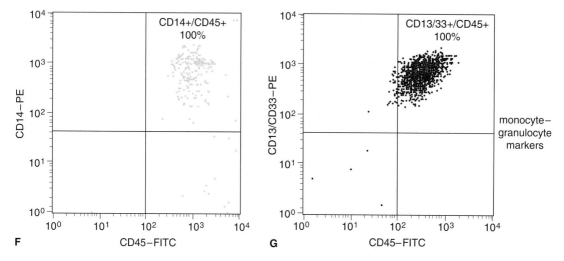

Figure 16–3. (Continued) Monoclonal antibody staining and flow cytometric analysis of normal peripheral blood. The top panel shows an *xy* plot of the forward versus side light scatter of the blood elements, which reflect their size and complexity, respectively. Under the top graph are six panels representing analysis of the cells in the various gated region (T lymphocytes in the first two panels, B lymphocytes in the middle two panels, and monocytes–granulocytes in the lower two panels). The percentage number of each cell type within each quadrant (ie, positive for neither, one or two of the mAbs shown) are shown as a function of the number of cells within the region (R1, R2, or R3) not the total number of leukocytes. To calculate the total number of cells in a given subset one would need to multiply the number of cells in that subset times the total number of cells in that region. For example, CD4 T cells make up a total of 25% of this patient's peripheral leukocytes (50% of the lymphocytes are CD4+ and the lymphocytes in R1 are 50% of all the cells). Shown next to each marker is the type of fluorochrome used to label that mAb: fluorescein isothiocyanate (FITC) for green fluorescence, phycoerythrin (PE) for orange color, and CY5 for red color.

tively). When his cells are stained with a mixture of CD5 and CD19 mAbs, we find that 85% of all his lymphocytes coexpress CD5 and CD19, which is extremely abnormal as CD5 is only found on a small subset of B cells. Costaining with mAbs that recognize the λ and κ Ig-light chains reveals that 85% of all the lymphocytes (or 100% of all the B cells) express only the κ-light chain. Hence, this patient has a monoclonal proliferation of B cells. Analyses with other mAbs reveals that the κ-restricted cells stain for a variety of B-cell markers in a pattern consistent with the disease chronic lymphocytic leukemia. The remaining 15% of non-B cells are normal T cells. Hence, the patient has a hematopoietic malignancy with a severe defect in the cellular arm of his immune system.

As can be seen from these simple cases, flow cytometry has the overwhelming advantage of being a rapid and objective method for the enumeration of the different subsets of various hematopoietic cells. With the continued development of mAbs that recognize an increasing array of cell surface markers, our ability to subclassify blood cells will continue to improve.

Fluorescence-Activated Cell Sorters. Flow sorter machines are more complex versions of standard flow cytometers that can not only detect the flu-

orescence from surface-bound mAbs but can also separate the differentially stained cells (Figure 16–5). The machines direct the flow of single cells into different collection tubes using electric fields that are triggered by the fluorescence of the cells. This results in rapid, accurate, and highly reproducible separation of cells based on their differential staining with mAbs. Viability and sterility can be maintained, so that separated cell populations can be cultured in vitro and used for functional assays. Cell sorters are used extensively in the research setting, but less so in the clinical laboratory.

Clinical Uses of Flow Cytometry

Some of the many clinical applications of flow cytometry are listed in Table 16–1. The most widespread use of the technique is for enumeration of lymphocyte subsets in patients with immune defects (most commonly AIDS—see Chapter 46) and in the classification of hematopoietic malignancies (leukemia/lymphomas—further described in Chapter 43). The most commonly used assays are described as follows.

T-Cell Antigens. HIV infection causes the progressive loss of CD4 T cells, which heralds the onset of frank immunodeficiency. Flow cytometry is used frequently to enumerate the total number of CD4 cells in these patients. This is often done by multiply-

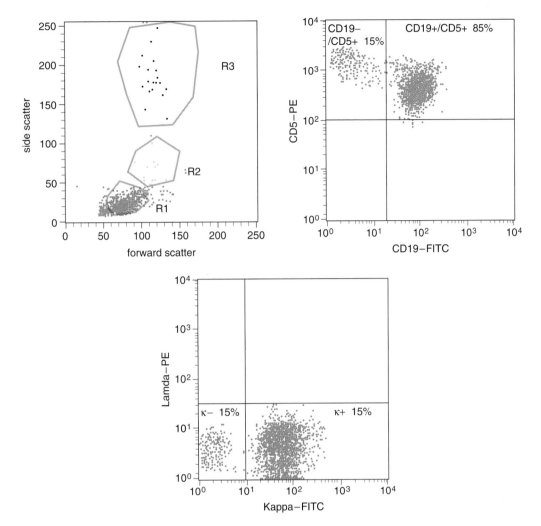

Figure 16–4. Flow cytometric analysis of peripheral blood from a patient with chronic lymphocytic leukemia. This patient has virtually no monocytes or granulocytes in the peripheral blood whereas 85% of his total cells are a monospecific type of B lymphocyte that marks aberrantly with the CD5 antigen. The lack of monocytes and granulocytes indicate that this patient is at great risk for infection.

ing the percentage of CD4 lymphocytes times the total lymphocyte count provided by the hematology laboratory. Commercially available methods of determination of absolute CD4 cell counts by flow cytometry have been recently developed using a known number of fluorescent beads added to the sample to provide a standard against which to compare the cell percentage.

Routine monitoring of T lymphocytes is also performed in the setting of induced immunosuppression in transplantation patients, such as during the treatment of transplant rejection by the administration of T-cell-depleting mAbs. Likewise, recovery of T cells during bone marrow transplantation is routinely followed by flow cytometry. Classification of primary forms of immunodeficiency that result from defects

in T-lymphopoiesis depends on leukocyte phenotyping. Primary T-cell immunodeficiencies include **Wiskott–Aldrich syndrome, DiGeorge syndrome,** and a variety of **severe combined immunodeficiency states (SCID),** all of which result in loss of T-cell subsets. Alterations in the ratio of CD4 to CD8 T cells can also occur in many other diseases, including autoimmune disorders and infectious disease. The diagnosis of T-cell malignancies depends critically on flow cytometry.

B-Cell Antigens. Characterization of B-cell phenotypes has its primary use in diagnosis of hematopoietic malignancy. Different antigenic markers appear at different stages of B-cell differentiation. These different markers can determine the stage of B-cell development at which the malignant transfor-

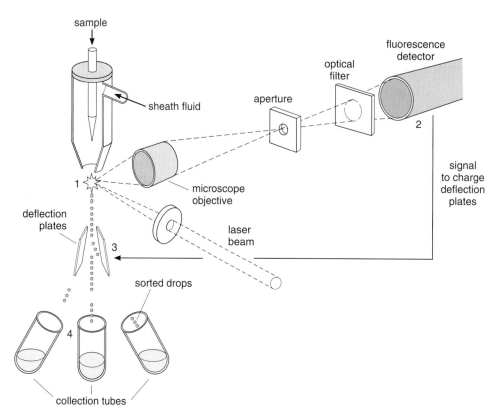

Figure 16–5. Cell purification by flow sorting. **1:** Cells in suspension are stained with fluorescent mAbs then forced out of a small nozzle into the light detection chamber. **2:** A laser beam directed at the cells excites the fluorescence, which is then collected in the detector. **3:** The cell droplets then pass through a high-voltage electric field that is generated by a pair of deflection plates. Signals are relayed to the deflection plates that rapidly alter the field through which the cells pass. **4:** Based on the changes in the electric field, the charged droplets are then electrically deflected into different collection tubes.

Table 16–1. Clinical applications of flow cytometry.

Leukocyte phenotyping
Diagnosis of congenital immunodeficiency diseases
Assessment of prognosis of HIV-positive patients
Monitoring of immunotherapy or chemotherapy in immuno-deficiency diseases
Monitoring of immune reconstitution in bone marrow transplant recipients
Tumor cell phenotyping
Diagnosis and classification of leukemias and lymphomas
Determination of clonality of immunoglobulin-bearing cells from lymphomas and leukemias
Differentiation of hematopoietic from nonhematopoietic tumors or cells
Assessment of prognosis of cancers
DNA analysis
Determination of aneuploidy
Determination of cell cycle kinetics
Neutrophil function analysis
Other applications
Reticulocyte counting
Platelet-associated immunoglobulin detection
Leukocyte crossmatching in transplant recipients
Cytogenetics

mation occurred and can be used to classify the different subtypes of B-cell leukemias and lymphomas. Knowledge of the surface antigen phenotype of these malignancies is important for prognostic and therapeutic decision making.

Enumeration of B cells is also important in evaluating primary immunodeficiency. The most common form of immunodeficiency, **common variable immunodeficiency** can present with reduced immunoglobulin levels and low numbers of B cells. Likewise, the X-linked **Bruton agammaglobulinemia** disorder results from a defect in B-cell development revealed by a profound defect in their numbers. In the **hyper-IgM syndrome** class switching does not occur, and patients fail to express IgG or other isotypes on their cell surface.

Myeloid Antigens. Phenotypic analysis of myeloid antigens is used extensively to characterize **myelodysplastic syndromes** and **myeloid leukemias.**

Hematopoietic stem–progenitor cells express CD34. Detection of these cells by anti-CD34 staining has become a critical component of bone marrow transplantation procedures. This assay allows one to count the number of progenitor cells in a bone marrow sample and thus determine the effective dosage of stem cells being delivered to the recipient during transplantation. In many centers, stem cell transplantation is now performed by treating donors with cytokine cocktails (eg, granulocyte colony-stimulating factor [G-CSF]) that result in the production and release of large numbers of stem–progenitor cells directly into the peripheral blood. These cells can be easily harvested from the blood, concentrated, and enumerated by anti-CD34 staining. Specific doses of CD34 cells can then be delivered to the recipients (whose own hematopoietic systems are usually destroyed following intensive chemotherapy for malignancy) to ensure rapid and complete engraftment by donor cells. Extra donor cells are often stored in liquid nitrogen and can be delivered to the patient at a later date as "salvage" therapy if needed.

A technical problem with staining myeloid cells (and to a lesser extent, B cells) is the nonspecific binding of labeled mAbs to **Fc receptors** on the cell surface. Myeloid cells express abundant levels of the receptors that recognize the Fc region of certain immunoglobulin isotypes (eg, Fcγ receptors bind the Fc portion of IgG). Monocytes–macrophages and granulocytes use these receptor systems to facilitate the uptake and killing of Ig-bound microorganisms (and other foreign particles). However, these receptors can also bind fluorescently labeled mAbs that are used as staining reagents and are readily detected by flow cytometry, giving the false impression that specific binding has occurred. To control for this phenomenon, the staining of the specific mAb is compared with the staining of an **isotype-matched mAb** that is raised against an unrelated antigen, such as a hapten or nonmammalian protein. Alternatively, many laboratories routinely block FcγRs on cell samples by preincubation with large amounts unlabeled rabbit polyclonal antisera. This preincubation step blocks all the Fc receptors and reduces nonspecific staining.

Intracellular Antigens. Flow cytometry can also be used to detect a variety of intracellular antigens. In these circumstances cells must be first treated with agents that make the cells permeable (ie, result in holes in the membrane) without completely breaking them apart. At the same time, the cells are treated with mild fixatives that will lightly cross-link cytoplasmic proteins in place and prevent them from leaking outside the cell. The newly permeable cells are then incubated with mAbs that recognize the intracellular antigens, the mAbs enter the cells and bind directly, after which the cells are analyzed by flow cytometry. This procedure tends to have more technical problems that traditional cell surface staining and is influenced both by the antigen to be studied and the particular mAb used (not all mAbs work). Nevertheless, detection of **intracellular terminal de-**

oxynucleotide transferase (TdT) and **myeloperoxidase** are routinely performed in clinical laboratories to help define early B-cell malignancies and myeloid leukemias, respectively. Tdt, an enzyme expressed during immunoglobulin gene rearrangement, is responsible for addition of random oligonucleotides at the junctions of Ig segments. Hence, its expression in a malignant B-cell population is indicative of a very immature B-cell phenotype. Likewise, myeloperoxidase is a major constituent of primary granules in neutrophils; expression of this protein develops midway through granulocyte maturation and hence is used to classify various subtypes of myeloid leukemias.

Other Uses of Flow Cytometry: DNA-Ploidy, Functional Assays, and Apoptosis. The DNA content of cells is a direct reflection of their position in the cell cycle (Chapter 1). In populations of rapidly dividing cells, a large number are in S, G2, and M phases of the cell cycle and hence have more than 2n chromosomes. Similarly in tumors with a large number of genetic rearrangements, chromosomal duplications, and amplifications **(aneuploidy),** a large percentage of cells have an aberrant amount of DNA. Flow cytometry is routinely used to assay the amount of genetic material in a cell to determine the **S-phase fraction** or amount of aneuploidy in a population of cells. This technique is often applied to solid tumors (breast, colon, prostate cancers) because in many circumstances the number of highly replicative cells and the degree of genetic rearrangement correlate with prognosis. DNA analysis is performed by incubation of permeabilized cells with fluorescent dyes (eg, propidium iodide) that will intercalate into the DNA and fluoresce when bound; the amount of fluorescence is directly proportional to DNA content.

A number of leukocyte functional assays use flow cytometric detection methods. The production of O_2^- (superoxide) as an assay for chronic granulomatous disease is routinely performed in clinical laboratories (see under Neutrophil Function Assays). Other assays tend to be restricted to the research laboratory, but include methods for measuring phagocytic uptake of fluorescent particles, degranulation assays, determination of intracellular Ca^{2+} mobilization (during leukocyte activation), and changes in cytoskeletal structure.

Cell viability is routinely determined in the clinical laboratory by flow cytometry. In the simplest method, cells are incubated directly with propidium iodide, and the proportion of fluorescent (dead) cells is directly counted. Because the dye will only enter cells that already have broken membranes and a disrupted nuclear structure, only dead cells fluoresce. Because the fluorescence of propidium iodide is in the far red portion of the spectrum, this method is often combined with regular mAbs staining in mixed cell populations. The dead cells can be identified in the population, and their staining properties can be ignored during data analysis. A number of other fluorescent markers have been developed to detect cells undergoing **apoptosis** (the process of active cell death), including binding proteins (eg, annexin V) that recognize abnormal lipids on apoptotic cell membranes. The binding of these proteins is usually detected by flow cytometry.

The number of different methodologies that use flow cytometry continues to grow. The preceding is only a partial list—other assays include bacterial determination, viral assays, and nucleic acid sequence detection. Basically, any assay that has a fluorescent readout and that can be performed on single-cell suspension is amenable to detection by flow cytometry. Flow cytometry is one of the most heavily used and rapidly growing methodologies (perhaps second only to molecular nucleic acid based assays) in the clinical laboratory.

DELAYED-TYPE HYPERSENSITIVITY SKIN TESTING

Delayed-type hypersensitivity (DTH) skin testing is used clinically for two primary reasons: (1) to assess immune competence and (2) to determine whether a patient has memory T cells that recognize a particular pathogen (ie, evidence of prior infection). Testing is performed by intradermal (not subcutaneous) injections of sterilely prepared antigens into the forearm or other easily accessible skin site. The degree of induration (swelling due to inflammation) is measured 48 hours after injection. The DTH skin response requires antigen-specific memory T cells and produces inflammation that peaks approximately 48 hours after the injection. Inflammation results from the production of local cytokines and chemokines at the injection site, which results in the recruitment of large numbers of neutrophils and mononuclear cells. The DTH response is a true measure of the cellular-dependent arm of the immune response.

The timing and induration help to distinguish DTH reactions from two other inflammatory responses to the intradermal injection of antigen. IgE-mediated (mast cell-dependent) hypersensitivity responses produce immediate weal and flare at the site of injection and, occasionally, late-phase responses after several hours. Inflammatory reactions that result from the formation of immune complexes at the skin site—the so-called Arthus reaction—develop 12–24 hours after injection. This response is indicative of high levels of preexisting IgG to the test antigen.

Skin testing with a battery of antigens against common fungal agents (some pathogenic, others not) can be used to validate the general competence of the cellular immune system. Common test antigens (also known as recall antigens) are listed in Table 16–2. In some cases, competence testing can be done using

Table 16–2. Examples of common antigen preparations used for DTH testing.

Antigen	Comments
Candida albicans	Common, nonpathogenic organism against which normal patients should respond
Trichophyton (dermatophyton)	As with *C albicans*, used as control
Coccidioidin	Antigen of coccidiodomycosis
Histoplasmin	Antigen of histoplasmosis
Tuberculin purified protein derivative (PPD)	Antigen of *Mycobacterium tuberculosis*
Mumps	Used to validate prior vaccination
Tetanus toxoid	As with mumps testing

antigens to which most patients in the United States have been immunized as children and hence should mount vigorous responses. Patients who fail to respond to common antigens are referred to **anergic** and have some defect in cell-mediated immune responses. Clinical situations that may result in anergy are outlined in Table 16–3.

In the United States, the DTH test most commonly used to determine prior infection with a particular pathogen is the response to **purified protein deriva-**

Table 16–3. Clinical conditions associated with anergy.

I Pharmocologic Treatments
  Corticosteroids
  Immunosuppressive drugs (cyclosporine, anti-T-cell Ab treatment)
  Chemotherapeutics for malignancy
  Some nonsteroidial therapies (in some patients)

II Immunologic Deficiencies
  Congenital immunodeficiency (SCID, Wiskott–Aldrich, DiGeorge)
  Ataxia–telangiectasia
  AIDS

III Coexistent Diseases
  Carcinoma
  Chronic lymphocytic leukemia
  Lymphomas (Hodgkins and non-Hodgkins)
  Sarcoidosis
  Uremia
  Liver disease (cirrhosis)
  Autoimmune disorders—rheumatoid arthritis

IV Coexistent infectious diseases
  Influenza, measles, mumps
  Miliary or active tuberculosis
  Disseminated mycotic infections
  Lepromatous leprosy

V Technical errors in skin testing
  Improper Ag concentrations (too dilute)
  Injection too deep into skin
  Improper interpretation of test results

tive (PPD), which assesses past infection with tuberculosis. The PPD test permits the identification and treatment of latently infected individuals prior to the onset of clinical disease. Obviously, anergic patients who fail to respond to recall test antigens may have false-negative results with PPD (or any other DTH test).

Repeated PPD testing may produce a so-called booster effect. This phenomenon is seen in individuals, particularly the elderly, who have had prior infection with tuberculosis but whose cell-mediated immune response to tuberculosis has waned over the years such that it does not produce induration when first challenged with PPD. The initial test, however, "boosts" the patient's immune response to PPD antigens, and, as a result, a positive skin test occurs on subsequent challenge with PPD. Unless one is aware of the booster effect, the combination of an initial negative PPD test and a subsequent positive test can lead to the incorrect conclusion that the patient has been infected with tuberculosis in the interim. To avoid being misled by the booster effect, many nursing homes employ a two-stage test in which PPD is administered twice, one month apart.

DTH skin testing is of relatively little value in assessing cellular immunity during the first year of life. Infants may have limited exposure to the various recall antigens used, so control results are difficult to interpret. Consequently, leukocyte phenotyping and in vitro assays for T-cell function are much more useful in the diagnosis of congenital immunodeficiency.

A variant form of DTH testing is used in the diagnosis and evaluation of dermatitis—so-called **contact hypersensitivity** testing. Contact hypersensitivity develops as a result of cutaneous exposure to a sensitizing antigen. Upon reexposure to the antigen, inflammation develops at the skin contact site 48–72 hours later. A classic form of contact hypersensitivity is the skin inflammatory responses to the antigens of plants such as poison oak or poison ivy. **Patch testing** is commonly employed by allergists and dermatologists to detect cutaneous hypersensitivity to various substances thought to be responsible for contact dermatitis. The test substance is applied in a low concentration and the area covered with an occlusive dressing. After 48–96 hours, the dressing is removed and the site is examined for the presence of inflammatory reactions. Patch testing is commonly done with panels of known and common antigens, which can often reveal the presence of unsuspected clinical sensitivity to various agents. False-positive reactions can result from too high a concentration of the test substance, irritation rather than allergy, and allergy to the adhesive used in the dressing. False-negative tests usually result from too low a concentration of the test substance and inadequate skin penetration. The results of patch testing must be weighed with clinical history—the combination of a positive test in the setting of a strong history of exposure is best for reliable diagnosis.

Occasionally, patients who are highly sensitive to various antigens have marked local reactions to skin testing. These severe reactions include marked induration and even skin necrosis at the challenge site. This can occur in patients with robust immune response to PPD antigens. Injection of corticosteroids into the site of severe induration will significantly abort the immune response. If unusual sensitivity is suspected (ie, if there is a high probability that the patient may have been exposed to the test antigen or may have had a strong positive result in the past), preliminary testing with dilute solutions of antigen are indicated. Similarly, painful blistering and inflammation can sometimes occur following surface application of contact sensitizers during patch testing; this is also adequately treated by topical steroid application.

LYMPHOCYTE ACTIVATION ASSAYS

The two primary general types of assay of lymphocyte activation are (1) determination of changes in cell surface phenotype (ie, acquisition of "activation" markers on the cell surface) and (2) the ability of lymphocytes to proliferate following stimulation. In most cases, lymphocyte activation assays evaluate mainly T-cell responses, but under certain circumstances evaluation of B-cell activation may also be important. Related to these methods are assays that measure the products of activated lymphocytes (T-cell cytokines or B-cell-produced immunoglobulins) or the acquisition of effector function by cytolytic T cells. Most of these assays are performed by in vitro culture of lymphocytes isolated from various body sites. Determination of the ability of lymphocytes to become activated is used principally to characterize immunodeficiency states. Lymphocyte activation measures the *functional* capability of lymphocytes to respond to antigenic or mitogenic stimulation and is therefore a more direct test of immunocompetence than simple enumeration of lymphocyte numbers. Most of these assays are not directly amenable to standardization between different laboratories, and, although they appear to be quantitative, they should be viewed more as qualitative assessments of immune response. Furthermore, activation type assays demonstrate the greatest biologic variation between individuals.

Activation Markers. Activated T cells undergo a series of morphologic and phenotypic changes. This includes an expansion in size, the manifestation of open chromatin by histologic staining, and the expression of surface proteins not found on small resting cells. The expression of activation markers by T cells can be determined in fresh cells directly isolated from inflammatory sites or in cultured cells that have been stimulated in vitro. In both circumstances, determination is made by flow cytometry. The activation of T cells in vitro can be accomplished either with specific antigens (plus antigen presenting cells) or through use of general lymphocyte mitogens. The low frequency of T cells specific for a particular antigen can render these cells difficult to detect in many samples. The number of activated T cells isolated from an inflamed site, however, may be much greater than the number of such cells circulating in the peripheral blood. For example, activated T cells can be isolated by bronchoalveolar lavage from sarcoidosis patients or from the cerebrospinal fluid of patients with active multiple sclerosis.

Lymphocyte Proliferation. Lymphocyte proliferation is usually determined using polyclonal activators of lymphocytes or lymphocyte mitogens. The most commonly used T-cell stimuli are lectins, such as phytohemagglutinin (PHA) and concanavalin A (Con A); bacterial toxins that act as superantigens; chemical compounds, such as phorbol myristate acetate (PMA) and calcium ionophores; cytokines; and mAbs to surface receptors (especially CD3). B-cell proliferation is often induced with pokeweed mitogen (PWM—although this will also activate T cells), superantigens, lipopolysaccharide (LPS), or mAbs that cross-link the surface immunoglobulin (B-cell receptor). The mixed lymphocyte reaction, which assesses responses to histocompatibility antigens, is reviewed in Chapter 19.

Proliferation responses are measured using purified lymphocytes cultured in vitro in small 96-well microtiter plates. Cells are stimulated for defined periods (usually 48 hours), after which DNA synthesis is measured by pulse labeling the cultures with tritiated thymidine (^{3}H-Tdr). The incorporation of ^{3}H-Tdr into chromosomal DNA reflects the rate of cell proliferation. One can also use nonradioactive assays to determine cell proliferation, such as using fluorescent dyes that incorporate into DNA or dyes that measure oxidative respiration such as MTT (a tetrazolium substrate that is converted to an insoluble product and is measured in the spectrophotometer). Bromodeoxyuridine (BrdU) is also often used to assay proliferation—like ^{3}H-Tdr it will be incorporated into DNA in highly replicative cells—and it can be detected in DNA using mAb staining (similar to the methods used for other intracellular antigens) followed by flow cytometry. The advantage of BrdU staining is that it can be delivered to patients in vivo, hence one can directly follow the proliferative fraction of a lymphocyte subset during a natural immune response. BrdU staining has also found a clinical use in grading the proliferative fraction of tumors in vivo. Patients are given an injection of BrdU after which tumor tissue is removed and the proliferative fraction is determined by flow cytometry.

Both the culture time and the dose response can affect the interpretation of lymphocyte proliferation assays. Since clinically important defects in cellular responses are rarely absolute, quantitative relationships

between normal control samples and patient samples need to be established as much as possible. Using both microtiter culture systems and semiautomated cell harvesters, one can attempt to determine both the dose and time response kinetics of either mitogen-activated or antigen-stimulated T cells. Altered lymphocyte function can result in shifts in either time or dose response curves. Such comparison may allow one to tease out subtle or partial defects in lymphocyte responsiveness that may occur in different disease states. Considerable controversy exists in the literature concerning the form in which data are presented. Many laboratories report simply the counts per minute of incorporated ^{3}H-Tdr. It is also common, however, to use a "stimulation index"—the ratio of the incorporated ^{3}H-Tdr in stimulated versus resting cultures. Neither method is entirely satisfactory. Because the stimulation index is a ratio, marked differences between patient and control samples can result simply from changes in the low levels of ^{3}H-Tdr incorporated by resting cells.

Antigen-dependent proliferative responses can be assessed using antigens to which the patient mounts a vigorous DTH response. In general, normal subjects show agreement between the results of skin tests and antigen-induced lymphocyte activation. In certain conditions, however, the in vitro technique may be a more sensitive index of cell-mediated immunity to a specific antigen. As in the case of mitogen-induced activation, time and dose response kinetics are crucial in generating reliable data. Compared with mitogen-induced lymphocyte activation, antigen stimulation results in lower total DNA synthesis because only a fraction of the T cells respond, and the time to maximal response is usually delayed.

Cytolytic T-Cell Responses. Assays for cytolytic T lymphocytes (CTL) in patients can be performed as a variant of a mixed lymphocyte culture using allogeneic cells (see Chapter 19) or can be done using autologous target cells that express the antigen of interest and are loaded with ^{51}Cr. Cytotoxicity is measured as the percentage of ^{51}Cr released from specific target cells compared with the percentage released from control (nonspecific) targets. Because CTL responses are restricted by MHC class I molecules, CTL assays require the generation of custom target cells for each patient and thus are almost exclusively limited to research applications.

Cytokine Production. Activated T cells produce a large repertoire of cytokine products. One can assay cytokine production to assess the type of immune response occurring within a given site in the body, for example, to distinguish T_H1 versus T_H2 type responses. In the simplest system, T cells isolated from inflammatory sites are cultured in vitro, and the spectrum of cytokines they release into the media is determined by enzyme-linked immunosorbent (ELISA)-type assays (see Chapter 15). Alternatively, resting T cells can be activated in culture and cytokine production determined. These methods measure the total amount of any given cytokine produced by a T-cell population, but do not allow one to judge the percentage of T cells within the population that are producing a given cytokine. To determine this, the enzyme-linked immunospot (ELISPOT) assay can be used. Activated lymphocytes are incubated in a semisolid agar that limits diffusion of the cytokine products to the immediate area of the cell. The agar is then dried and probed with labeled anticytokine mAbs, producing spots that represent T cells producing the cytokine of interest. Finally, one can determine cytokine production cell by cell by mAb staining for intracellular cytokines followed by flow cytometric analysis. Currently, assays of cytokine responses remain primarily a research tool.

MONOCYTE-MACROPHAGE ASSAYS

Monocytes and macrophages, which are considered part of the innate immune system, coordinate adaptive immune responses through cytokine production, act as effectors to remove specific types of pathogens, and play a central role in clearing apoptotic cells during tissue remodeling and development. One can readily identify these cell types in tissue samples or cell suspensions using mAb staining. As shown in Figure 16–3, identification of monocytes in the peripheral blood by flow cytometry is most reliably performed using CD14 mAb staining combined with appropriate forward and side scatter gating. Mononuclear cells also express a host of other markers (CD11b, CD11c, CD16, CD32, CD64, and scavenger receptors of various types) that facilitate their identification. Histochemical staining for nonspecific esterase (α-naphthol esterase) is commonly performed on leukemic samples to define monocyte-derived disease. Remember that the great heterogeneity in the types of tissue macrophages (Langerhans' cells, Kupffer cells, osteoclasts, alveolar macrophages, bone marrow macrophages, lymph node dendritic cells) is also reflected in the variety of surface markers expressed by these cells.

NEUTROPHIL FUNCTION ASSAYS

Polymorphonuclear neutrophils (PMNs) are the primary effector cells of the innate immune system. These cells have a finite life span (a relatively short 24 hours) and are constantly being produced in the bone marrow. PMNs are the first cells to enter an inflammatory site, where, following activation by a variety of stimuli, they undergo respiratory burst to release superoxide, degranulate to release antimicrobial peptides and proteins, and produce limited numbers of proinflammatory cytokines. PMN deficiency results in susceptibility to bacterial (or other pathogen)

infection. Such deficiencies are due either to reduced numbers of PMNs (as occurs with bone marrow suppression following chemotherapy) or to defects intrinsic to the PMN. This discussion will focus on the latter and review methods to evaluate intrinsic defects that are clinically significant. These include assays to evaluate adhesion, chemotaxis, phagocytosis, production of superoxide, and bacterial killing. Many of the methods to evaluate PMN function use nonstandardized procedures; hence, different methods are often used by different laboratories.

Neutrophil Adhesion. The ability of PMNs to adhere to endothelial surfaces and migrate into inflammatory sites is critical for their ability to control bacterial infections. PMNs use a host of cell surface receptors, including **selectins** and **integrins,** to carry out this function. The major leukocyte-associated selectin, L-selectin, acts in concert with endothelial selectins to allow PMNs to roll along the endothelial surface. In the presence of inflammatory mediators (chemokines, TNFα, or bacterial products such as LPS), the PMNs become activated and firmly attach to the endothelial surface using their integrin receptors. Deficiency of either selectins or integrins results in a specific deficiency of leukocyte adhesion (socalled **leukocyte adhesion deficiency** or LAD). In such patients, PMNs fail to enter into inflammatory sites, and bacterial infections rapidly spread. Clinically these patients are recognized by their inability to make pus at the site of an infection. Lack of these surface molecules can be readily determined by mAb staining and flow cytometry: LAD I patients lack the β_2-subunit (CD18) of the major leukocyte integrins, and LAD II patients lack a fucosyl transferase enzyme involved in the expression of selectin ligands on the leukocyte surface. The inability of these PMNs to adhere to appropriate surfaces can be evaluated using in vitro adhesion assays. PMNs are activated with various agents and allowed to bind to ligand-coated surfaces, and the strength of binding is determined by resistance to removal with washing. Neutrophils also use a variety of cell surface receptors to bind opsonized pathogens. These include FcγRs and various sugar-binding proteins (scavenger receptors). One can determine the expression of these receptors by mAb staining or by determining the binding of fluorescently labeled particles, coated with the appropriate ligands, to the surface of the PMNs. Clinically recognized immunodeficiency resulting from the lack of these receptor systems has yet to be defined. The ability of PMNs to respond to inflammatory stimuli, however, is manifested by up-regulation of these receptors on the cell surface. Hence, increased expression of many of these adhesion receptors can be used as activation markers for PMNs.

Chemotaxis. Directional motility of PMNs to inflammatory sites is mediated by a host of chemotactic molecules (bacterial products such as formylated peptides or host-derived chemokines). The inability of PMNs to respond to these stimuli results in defective migratory responses. This can be quantitated in the laboratory by use of the modified Boyden chamber assay. Cells to be tested are placed in the upper chamber and are separated from the lower chamber containing a chemotactic substance by a filter membrane with small pore size. Cells enter the filter and are either trapped in it or migrate all the way through. The extent of migration is determined by counting cells in filter and lower chamber (by flow cytometry or using labeled cells). A more rigorous method of determining PMN chemotaxis involves the use of semisolid agarose media formed in a small Petri dish, into which a holes are cut that contain the cells, the chemotactic stimulus, or control nonchemotactic proteins. The dish is incubated for several hours, and the migration of the PMNs under the agarose toward the well containing chemotactic factors is determined microscopically. Migration toward the nonchemokine-containing wells represents random motion of PMNs (so called **chemokinesis**). Defects in chemotactic responses are used to evaluate idiopathic immunodeficiencies.

Phagocytosis. Ingestion of microorganisms by neutrophils is an active process that requires energy production by the phagocytic cell. Internalization of antibody-coated and complement-coated microorganisms occurs rapidly following their surface contact with PMNs and macrophages. Because subsequent intracellular events, such as superoxide production and degranulation into the phagocytic vesicle, depend on successful ingestion, assays that evaluate phagocytosis allow one to determine the step at which potential functional defects may occur. The term *phagocytosis* is usually limited to evaluation of this initial step of bacterial killing. Assays of phagocytosis are very simple—as easy as incubating cells directly with opsonized (IgG or complement-bound) particles and microscopically observing the cells for uptake of the particles. One must have a method to distinguish between surface-bound but not internalized particles. This can be accomplished using chemical means to remove surface-bound particles (acid treatment) or by staining with dyes that obscure the surface-bound but not the intracellular particle. More quantitative assays have been developed that use fluorescently labeled or radioactive particles that permit direct counting of phagocytosis in larger cultures of PMNs or macrophages. One can test the effect of various cellular activators (or the ability of different opsonins) to stimulate phagocytosis. A variety of particles can be used, including yeast, bacteria, and various types of red blood cells.

Determination of Respiratory Burst and Degranulation. Perhaps the most frequently applied test of PMN function is the determination of the ability of these cells to produce superoxide (O_2^-). This test is used as a functional assay to screen for **chronic granulomatous disease (CGD),** a well-recognized disorder of phagocytes caused by inherited deficiency of one of several subunits of the oxidase that acts on the reduced form of nicotinamide adenine dinucleotide phosphate (NADPH), most commonly the p91^{phox} and p47^{phox} proteins (Figure 16–6). Two assays are used to determine the ability of activated PMNs to produce superoxide: (1) the slide **nitroblue tetrazolium (NBT) test** and (2) the flow cytometric 2′,7′-**dichlorofluorescein (DCF) test.** NBT is a clear, yellow, water-soluble compound that forms formazan, a deep blue dye, on reduction. Incubation of activated PMNs (achieved by treatment with PMA, exposure to LPS, or incubation with opsonized particles to stimulate phagocytosis) with NBT results in production of O_2^- and reduction of the dye. The activated PMNs then appear blue when visualized under simple light microscopy. This simple screening test can be performed on as little as a single drop of blood. This qualitative assay can be quantitated by extraction of the blue precipitate from the PMNs and measurement by spectroscopy. Children with complete deficiency of NADPH oxidase activity have striking defects in the slide NBT test, but mutations that result in only partial loss of function are better detected using the quantitative assay. The flow cytometric DCF assay provides a simpler and more reproducible method for CGD screening. This assay actually measures the formation of H_2O_2, which is

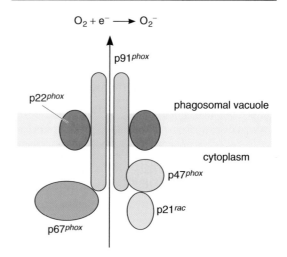

$$O_2 + e^- \longrightarrow O_2^-$$

Figure 16–6. Subunits of the active NADPH oxidase complex of phagocytes. The protein subunits p22^{phox} and p91^{phox} are membrane-bound, but the p47^{phox}, p67^{phox}, and p21^{rac} subunits are cytosolic. Activation of the NADPH oxidase depends on the assembly of these components during PMN activation; signaling events provided by the p21^{rac} subunit drive cytoskeletal changes that are required for complex assembly. Although chronic granulomatous disease (CGD) can result from loss of any one of these subunits, more than 90% of all cases can be accounted for by mutations in p47^{phox} (autosomal-recessive) or p91^{phox} (X-linked).

derived from O_2^- by the enzyme superoxide dismutase. H_2O_2 can be measured by the oxidation of the nonfluorescent compound 2',7'-dichlorodihydrofluorescein (DCFH) to the fluorescent compound DCF, which is easily detected by flow cytometry. PMNs are incubated with DCFH, which readily enters the cells, and are then activated by incubation with PMA (or other agents). Soon thereafter, the cells are analyzed by flow cytometry, and the increase in mean fluorescence of the PMN population is determined. Because the DCF assay is based on flow cytometry, it has the tremendous advantage of enabling the visualization of individual cellular differences, thereby allowing for detection of partial defects in NADPH oxidase function or for screening for heterozygous carriers of the X-linked forms of the disease. Because about two thirds of all cases of CGD are due to mutations in the X-linked p91^{phox,} women who are heterozygous for the disease will have a population of PMNs that have randomly inactivated the normal X chromosome (by the process of Lyonization) during their differentiation from stem cells. These cells will fail to undergo respiratory burst, while other cells within the carrier will behave normally because they have inactivated the mutant allele. Hence, carriers will demonstrate two populations of reactive PMNs using the DCF or similar assays (Figure 16–7).

Degranulation assays are usually used for the diagnosis of immunodeficiency due to lack of granule constituent proteins. Degranulation is the process of fusion of lysosomes and phagosomes, with the subsequent discharge of intralysosomal contents into the phagolysosome. Degranulation is an active process and requires energy expenditure by the cell. Thus, impairment of normal metabolic pathways of the neutrophil—especially oxygen consumption and the metabolism of glucose through the hexose monophosphate shunt—interferes with degranulation and subsequent intracellular bacterial killing. Degranulation of PMNs can be induced in suspended cells by treatment with various activating agents and compounds that affect the actin cytoskeleton of the cell (eg, cytochalasin B). The cells will release mainly contents of secondary and tertiary granules, and these components can be measured directly by ELISA assay. The most common marker protein of secondary granules is lactoferrin, and albumin is used as a marker for tertiary granule release. Assays for release of primary granules are best done by looking for release of these granules into enclosed spaces. The "frustrated-phagocytosis system" (Figure 16–8) provides such as assay. Heat-aggregated IgG or immune complexes are fixed to a tissue culture dish, and PMNs are then incubated on the dish. The cells bind the IgG complexes through FcγR and attempt to phagocytose the particles. At the same time, primary granules fuse with the phagosomes, which remain at the cell surface, resulting in the release of primary granule constituents into media. The rate of release of primary granule proteins, such as myeloperoxidase (MPO) and β-glucuronidase, is used to estimate degranulation. These assays are used to search for functional defects in granule release. Deficiency in either secondary or primary granule proteins can also be diagnosed by intracellular mAb staining and flow cytometry. Surprisingly, although absence of secondary granules produces severe immunocompromise, lack of MPO (a common disorder found in 1 in 2000 people) has relatively mild effects on immune function.

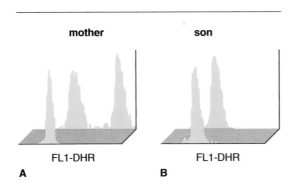

mother **son**

FL1-DHR FL1-DHR

A **B**

Figure 16–7. Three-dimensional flow-cytometric display of dihydrorhodamine (DHR) fluorescence in a patient with chronic granulomatous disease and his mother, a carrier. DHR reduction occurs by the same mechanism as DCF, although most laboratories prefer to use DCF. **A:** Fluorescent intensity of DHR (horizontal axis) of neutrophils from the mother. The peak in the foreground shows the histogram of unstimulated cells. After stimulation with phorbol myristate acetate (PMA), two peaks are shown (background of panel **A**). The population to the left are neutrophils that did not reduce the DHR and thus show no increase in fluorescence. The peak to the right demonstrates an increase in fluorescence of PMNs that have reduced the DHR. In panel **B** the patient's PMNs do not reduce the DHR and thus there is no difference in fluorescence intensity of unstimulated (peak in foreground) versus PMA-stimulated cells (peak in background).

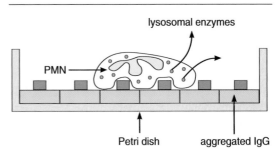

lysosomal enzymes

PMN

Petri dish aggregated IgG

Figure 16–8. Assay of granulocyte degranulation by the "frustrated phagocytosis" method. The neutrophil is attached to aggregated IgG fixed to the bottom of a Petri dish. Lysosomal enzymes are discharged into the supernatant as the cell attempts to phagocytose the IgG but is "frustrated." (Courtesy of S Barrett.)

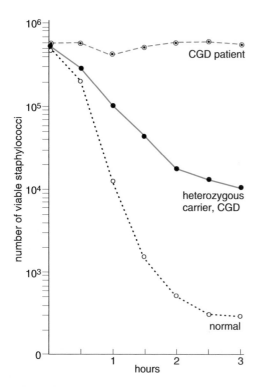

Figure 16–9. Bactericidal assay of granulocytes. Curves represent the number of viable intracellular organisms that survive after being ingested by granulocytes. Note the marked decline in bacterial survival in normal cells compared with reduced to absent killing by cells from patients and relatives with chronic granulomatous disease (CGD).

Table 16–4. Disorders of neutrophil function.

Leukocyte adherence deficiency
Chronic granulomatous disease (X-linked or autosomal-recessive)
Job's syndrome
Chédiak–Higashi syndrome
Myeloperoxidase deficiency
Glucose-6-phosphate dehydrogenase deficiency
Acute leukemia
Down syndrome
Premature infants

Transient neutrophil dysfunction
    Acute infections
    Ataxia–telangiectasia

Bacterial Killing. The microbicidal assay has long been considered the best functional assay for the evaluation of potential PMN disorders. Because efficient killing of bacteria requires all the steps described earlier, a defect in microbicidal activity can result from a defect in any of these systems. It would therefore be logical to assume that this assay is performed first in the evaluation of patients with defects in innate immune responses. This is not the case, however, because microbicidal assays are difficult to perform and labor-intensive. Microbicidal assays are usually used only when other simpler assays of PMN function (eg, respiratory burst and immunophenotyping) have failed to reveal a diagnosis.

Many strains of bacteria and fungi are effectively engulfed and killed by human neutrophils in vitro. The bactericidal capacity of PMNs for the test strain 502A of *Staphylococcus aureus* is commonly performed. Bacteria growing in log phase are incubated with human serum (to provide a source of complement proteins and IgG as opsonins) and freshly isolated PMNs at a ratio of roughly five to ten bacteria per PMN. After a short time (30 minutes), the extracellular bacteria are killed by addition of gentamicin. Because the antibiotic does not enter the cells, intracellular organisms survive. Aliquots of PMNs are sampled following addition of antibiotic and at 30-minute intervals thereafter. Intracellular bacteria are liberated by lysis of neutrophils with sterile water, and the number of viable organisms is determined by plating serial dilutions of the lysates on blood agar bacterial plates. Results are plotted as in Figure 16–9. Normal PMNs show a two-log reduction in viable intracellular *S aureus* after 1 hour incubation, but killing is virtually absent in PMNs derived from CGD patients. Carriers can show an intermediate phenotype. By varying the test organism or the source of opsonin, this assay can be used to measure a wide range of microbial killing activities. Because failure to ingest bacteria results in complete loss of all viable organisms following addition of the antibiotics, the laboratory must be aware of how to interpret what may appear as extremely rapid killing.

Examples of the commonly recognized neutrophil functional disorders are shown in Table 16–4.

REFERENCES

GENERAL

Coligan JE et al: *Current Protocols in Immunology,* John Wiley and Sons, 1999.

Lefkovits I: *Immunology Methods Manual,* Academic Press, 1997.

Rich R: *Clinical Immunology—Principles and Practice,* Mosby Press, 1995.

Rose NR et al: *Manual of Clinical Immunology,* 5th ed. American Society for Microbiology, 1997.

LEUKOCYTE PHENOTYPING & FLOW CYTOMETRY

Barclay I et al: *The Leukocyte Antigen Facts Book,* Academic Press, 1997.

Given AL: *Flow Cytometry: First Principles,* Wiley-Liss, Inc., 1992.

Jaroszesk MJ et al: *Flow Cytometry Protocols,* Humana Press, 1998.

Jennings CD, Foon KA: Recent advances in flow cytometry: Application to the diagnosis of hematologic malignancy. *Blood* 1997;90:2863.

Ormerod MG: *Flow cytometry: A practical approach,* 2nd ed. IRL Press, 1994.

DELAYED-TYPE HYPERSENSITIVITY SKIN TESTING

Blatt SF et al: Delayed-type hypersensitivity skin testing predicts progression to AIDS in HIV-infected patients. *Ann Intern Med* 1993,119:177.

Dannenberg AM: Delayed-type hypersensitivity and cell-mediated immunity in the pathogenesis of tuberculosis. *Immunol Today* 1991;12:228.

De Bruin-Weller MS et al: Atopy patch testing—A diagnostic tool? *Allergy* 1999;54:784.

Lein AD, Von Reyn CF In vitro cellular and cytokine responses to mycobacterial antigens: Application to diagnosis of tuberculosis infection and assessment of response to mycobacterial vaccines. *Am J Med Sci* 1997; 313:364.

LYMPHOCYTE ACTIVATION ASSAYS

Ahmed SA et al: A new rapid and simple nonradioactive assay to monitor and determine the proliferation of lymphocytes: An alternative to [³H]thymidine incorporation assay. *J Immunol Methods* 1994,170:211.

Bach FH, Van Rood JJ: The major histocompatibility complex: Genetics and biology. *N Engl J Med* 1976,295:806.

Gupta, S et al: *Mechanisms of lymphocyte activation and immune regulation VII : Molecular determinants of microbial immunity,* Plenum Press, 1998.

Sfikakis PP, Tsokos GC: Lymphocyte adhesion molecules in autoimmune rheumatic diseases: Basic issues and clinical expectations. *Clin Exper Rheum* 1995,13:763.

Viedma-Contreras JA: Leukocyte activation markers in clinical practice. *Clin Chem Lab Med* 1999,37:607.

MONOCYTES & MACROPHAGES

Kuhns DB et al: Endotoxin and IL-1 hyporesponsiveness in a patient with recurrent bacterial infections. *J Immunol* 1997,158:3959.

Springer TA: Traffic signals for lymphocyte recirculation and leukocyte emigration: The multistep paradigm. *Cell* 1994,76:301.

Wright SD: Toll, a new piece in the puzzle of innate immunity. *J Exp Med* 1999,189:605.

NEUTROPHIL FUNCTIONAL ASSAYS

Bogomolski-Yahalom V, Matzner Y: Disorders of neutrophil function. *Blood Reviews* 1995,9:183.

Borregaard N, Cowland JB: Granules of the human neutrophilic polymorphonuclear leukocyte. *Blood* 1997,89: 3503.

Casimir CM, Teahan CG: The respiratory burst of neutrophils and its deficiency. In *Immunopharmacology of Neutrophils,* Hellewell and Williams (eds). Academic Press, London, 1994.

Malech HL, Nauseef WM: Primary inherited defects in neutrophil function: Etiology and treatment. *Semin Hematol* 1997,34:279.

Malech HL: Progress in gene therapy for chronic granulomatous disease. *J Infect Dis* 1999,179:S318.

17

Blood Banking & Immunohematology

Maurene Viele, MD, & Elizabeth Donegan, MD

The ability to successfully transfuse whole blood, or more specific blood components, has saved countless lives and supported the advance of modern surgery and cancer chemotherapy. The first lifesaving transfusion was performed almost 200 years ago by James Blundell in 1818. Today, more than 20 million blood components, prepared from approximately 12.6 million blood donations, are transfused in the United States annually. The safety of blood transfusion has steadily improved since the first US blood bank was founded in the 1940s. Tests were developed and implemented to detect the infectious diseases recognized as transmitted in blood products. New molecular diagnostic techniques are now being investigated to improve the sensitivity of the tests used for donor blood analysis.

Nevertheless, transfusion continues to require the removal of blood from one human being for infusion into another. This "living transplant" carries with it the complexities of its human source and thereby brings with it the potential of undesirable side effects in the recipient. Some risks of transfusion are now known, and others have yet to be described. Consequently, the need for transfusion must be judged carefully in light of these risks.

BLOOD GROUPS

The first blood group system was described at the turn of the 20th century by Karl Landsteiner. He observed that erythrocytes from some individuals clumped when mixed with the serum of others but not with their own. Using this agglutination technique, he classified an individual's erythrocytes into four types: A, B, AB, and O. It is now recognized that A and B represent carbohydrate antigens on the erythrocyte. Group O individuals have neither of these antigens on their erythrocytes, whereas erythrocytes from AB individuals have both A and B antigens. The ABO system is the most important blood group system for transfusion purposes.

Knowledge about blood groups has expanded to include a diverse and numerous array of antigenic determinants on erythrocytes. Approximately 600 erythrocyte antigens are known, of which 207 belong to 23 recognized blood group systems. Each blood group system has members, each of which may be composed of one or more different antigens. Each antigen is controlled by one gene. The antigenic determinants of a blood group are produced either directly (for proteins) or indirectly (for carbohydrates) by alleles at a single gene locus or at other gene loci so closely linked that crossing over is extremely rare. For any antigen of a blood group, a single allele is present at that locus and other alleles are therefore excluded. A specific antigen on the erythrocyte surface is usually detected in the blood bank laboratory by reacting erythrocytes with sera known to contain antibodies reactive with that antigen. This test defines a phenotype.

ERYTHROCYTE ANTIGENS

H & ABO

Antigenic determinants of the H and ABO systems are carbohydrate moieties whose specificity resides in the terminal sugars of an oligosaccharide. On erythrocyte and endothelial surfaces, most of the antigens are bound to glycosphingolipids. Genetic control is via the production of transferase enzymes that conjugate terminal sugars to a stem carbohydrate. The H and ABO systems have separate gene loci and are independent of each another (Figure 17–1).

The H gene codes for a fucosyl transferase enzyme that adds fucose to precursor chains and completes the stem chain. The H gene is rarely absent; this phenotype (*hh*) is called O$_h$, or Bombay, type. In the absence of a complete stem chain, additional sugars cannot be added despite the presence of A or B transferase, and high-titer anti-H is produced.

The ABO blood groups are determined by allelic genes A, B, and O (Table 17–1). The A-group transferase adds *N*-acetylglucosamine to the completed stem chain. The B-group transferase adds a terminal D-galactose. The *O* gene produces no transferase to modify the blood group substance (see Figure 17–1).

Both groups A and B can be divided into subgroups. Many subgroups of A have been described,

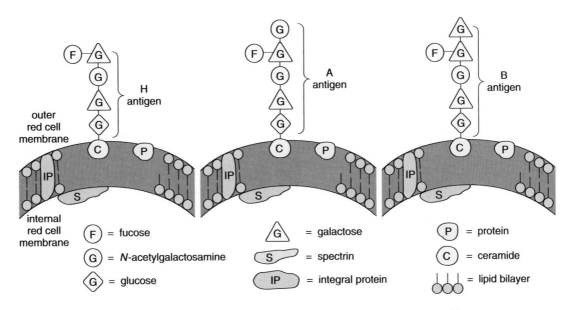

Figure 17–1. Chemical structure of A, B, and H blood groups.

but most are rare. The most important are A_1 and A_2. Differences between subtypes of group A appear to be quantitative, that is, in the number of antigenic sites per erythrocyte surface. AB blood can also be divided into A_1B and A_2B types. Although less frequently detected, subgroups of group B can also be distinguished. Subgroups of group B, like those of group A, demonstrate a continuum in the number of antigenic sites per erythrocyte.

The naturally occurring antibodies to groups A and B are thought to be stimulated by very common substances. Intestinal bacteria are known to have substances chemically similar to and therefore antigenically cross-reactive with A and B. Antibodies to A or B antigens (or both) are first detected in children at 3–6 months of age, peaking at 5–10 years of age and falling with age and in some immunodeficiency states.

Two other systems directly interact with the ABO and H systems: Lewis and secretor. Secretion of ABH substances in body fluids (saliva, sweat, milk, etc) is controlled by the allelic genes *Se* and *se*. These genes are independent of ABO and are inherited in a mendelian dominant manner. Eighty percent of people are *Se;* they secrete Lewis antigens in addition to ABH substances. Typing of body fluids for these antigens has been useful in forensic investigations.

Rh (Rhesus)

The Rhesus blood group system is second in importance only to the ABO system. Anti-Rh antibodies are the leading cause of hemolytic disease of the newborn (HDN) and may also cause delayed hemolytic transfusion reactions.

Recent investigations have elucidated the genetic basis of the primary Rh antigens: D, C, c, E, e. The Rh locus on chromosome 1 consists of two adjacent structural genes designated *RHD* and *RHCE*. The *RHD* gene encodes the D polypeptide present on the erythrocyte in Rh-positive individuals. The *RHD* gene is completely absent in the genome of Rh-negative individuals, which explains why no D antigen counterpart (d) has ever been found in Rh-negative people. The *RHCE* gene encodes for both C/c and E/e proteins via alternative splicing events.

Previous theories explaining the genetic basis of the Rh system gave rise to different nomenclatures.

Table 17–1. Routine ABO groupings.

			Frequency (%) in US Population			
Blood Group	Erythrocyte Antigens	Serum Antibody	White	Black	Native American	Asian
O	H	Anti-A, Anti-B	45	49	79	40
A	A	Anti-B	40	27	16	28
B	B	Anti-A	11	20	4	27
AB	A and B	—	4	4	<1	5

In the Wiener nomenclature, multiple Rh alleles were designated as either R or r with one of many superscripts. R alleles produced the antigen $Rh_o(D)$ in a particular phenotype in addition to two other antigens; r alleles denote the absence of Rh_o. In the Fisher and Race system (Table 17–2), three allelic gene pairs were thought to commonly produce five antigens (the remaining antigens are rare variants). Each antigen (D, C, c, E, and e) has a corresponding designation in the Wiener system (ie, D = Rh_o, C = rh′, etc). C and c, as well as E and e, function as alleles. No d antigen was known, so d describes the absence of D. The Rh antigens were believed to be inherited as two sets of three, one from each parent.

Clinically, Rh-positive (Rh+) means the presence of D (Rh_o) and Rh-negative (Rh–) indicates the absence of D (Rh_o). D is the most immunogenic of the Rh antigens. Slightly less than half of Rh+ people are homozygous for D. Because there are no antisera to detect the absence of D, determination of zygosity depends on family studies or gene amplification techniques. Roughly 15% of whites are Rh–. Rh-negativity is less common in other races. Erythrocytes with less than the normal number of D antigen sites are described and designated weak D (previously termed D^u). A weak D can appear as D negative (Rh–) in testing if blood is typed only with routine anti-D antisera but is detected if the indirect antiglobulin test is used. Blood-banking standards require all donor blood to be tested using methods that detect weak D antigen. If weak D is detected, the blood unit is labeled Rh-positive.

Other Erythrocyte Antigens

Many of the remaining 20 blood group systems are rarely implicated in transfusion reactions. Antibodies to the Kidd, Duffy, Kell, and MNS systems, however, are known for their ability to cause hemolysis if antigen-positive blood is transfused into a sensitized recipient. In general, hemolytic antibodies are IgG and react at 37°C (body temperature). IgM antibodies rarely cause hemolysis.

Antibodies to Kidd antigens are a frequent cause of delayed hemolytic transfusion reaction and can cause HDN. These antibodies are often difficult to

identify in test systems because of poor reactivity. Four antigenic phenotypes have been described: Jk(a+ b–), Jk(a– b+), Jk(a+ b+), and Jk(a– b–).

The antigens of the Duffy system (Fy^a and Fy^b) are controlled by codominant alleles. Antibodies to Fy^a are more commonly associated with delayed hemolytic transfusion reactions than are those to Fy^b. Many blacks have a third allele, which produces the Fy(a– b–) phenotype. Duffy antigens on erythrocytes serve as receptors for the entry of *Plasmodium vivax* into the erythrocytes. Fy(a– b–) individuals who lack Duffy antigens are resistant to *P vivax* infection.

The Kell system, as first described, included the allelic pair K and k, k antigen being the more frequent. The system now includes two additional allelic pairs and several variants. The K antigen is highly immunogenic, with one of 20 individuals transfused with K+ cells developing antibody. Antibodies to Kell antigen cause HDN, hemolytic transfusion reactions, and, occasionally, autoimmune hemolytic anemia. Individuals of the McLeod phenotype lack Kx antigen, which is a precursor in the synthesis of Kell antigens. These individuals have erythrocyte and neuromuscular system abnormalities. The McLeod phenotype is also associated with some cases of chronic granulomatous disease (see Chapter 24).

METHODS FOR DETECTION OF ANTIGEN & ANTIBODIES TO ERYTHROCYTES

Antiglobulin Tests

Antibody or complement adsorbed onto erythrocytes is detected by using antibodies to human serum globulins (AHG). AHG reagents are produced either in animals or in tissue culture by using monoclonal antibody techniques (see Chapter 15). These reagents may be polyspecific (a mixture of antibodies to IgG, complement, and heavy and light chains) or monospecific (antibodies to specific immunoglobulin or components of complement). The direct antiglobulin test (DAT) detects antibody or complement coating the surface of erythrocytes, whereas the indirect antiglobulin test (IAT) identifies antibody in serum or plasma.

To perform the DAT (Figure 17–2) erythrocytes are washed with saline to remove unbound antibody or complement and then AHG is added. If antibody is present on the erythrocytes, the Fab portion of AHG attaches to the Fc portion of the erythrocyte-bound antibody. Bridging of AHG Fab molecules between erythrocytes results in visually detectable agglutination. The DAT is used in the investigation of autoimmune or drug-induced hemolytic anemia, HDN, and suspected hemolytic transfusion reactions.

The IAT detects **serum** or **plasma antibodies,** which can attach in vitro to erythrocytes (see Figure

Table 17–2. Rh blood group terminology.

Fisher–Race	Wiener	Common Genotypes
Rh-Positive		White
DCe	R_1	R_1
DcE	R_2	R_2
Dce	R_0	r
DCE	R_z	Black
Rh-Negative		R_0
dce	r	R_1
dCe	r'	r
dcE	r''	Asian
dCE	r^y	R_1
		R_2

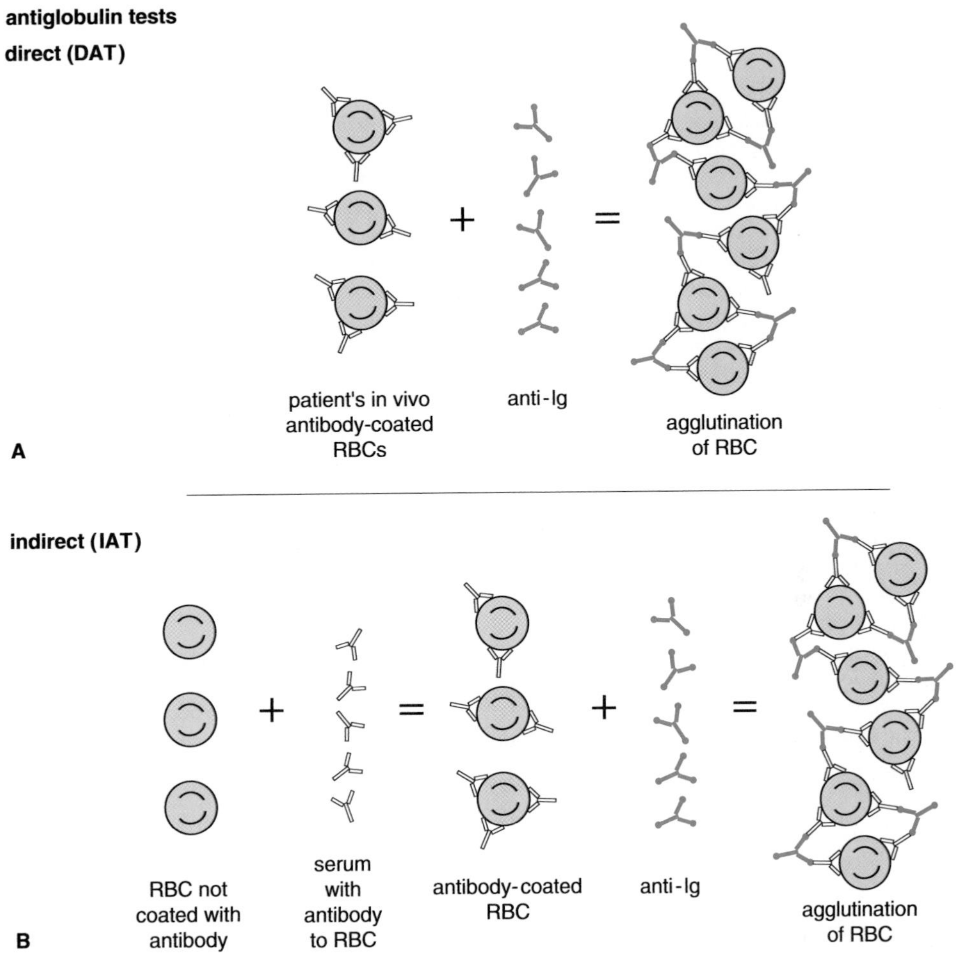

antiglobulin tests

direct (DAT)

A

indirect (IAT)

B

Figure 17–2. A: Schematic illustration of the technique for the direct antiglobulin test (DAT). **B:** Schematic illustration of the technique for the direct antiglobulin test (IAT).

17–2). This test differs from the DAT in that before an IAT is performed, the serum or plasma to be tested is incubated with erythrocytes so that antibody, if present, binds to erythrocyte antigen. The erythrocytes are then washed to remove any unbound globulin, and AHG is added. If agglutination is observed, antibodies to erythrocyte antigens are present. The IAT is used by blood banks in three ways. First, to identify the presence and specificity of recipient plasma antibody, plasma is tested using panels of reagent erythrocytes with known antigens on their surface. Second, to select donor blood that is free of specific erythrocyte antigens, commercial reagents, containing known erythrocyte antibodies, are used to test donor blood for the absence of the antigen. Third, to confirm the absence of an antigen–antibody reaction, recipient plasma is tested against donor blood cells (crossmatch).

Pretransfusion Testing

Blood is tested prior to transfusion to prevent clinically significant destruction of the transfused erythrocytes. Clinically significant antibodies are those known to have caused unacceptably shortened erythrocyte survival in vivo or frank hemolysis. Generally, these antibodies react at 37°C (body temperature) and in the indirect antiglobulin test. Prior to transfusion, the recipient's erythrocytes and plasma are tested for ABO and Rh_o (D) types and for antibodies to erythrocyte antigens, often called the "type and screen." Additionally, the recipient's plasma is tested for compatibility with the erythrocytes from the intended donor (crossmatch).

Type & Screen

ABO and Rh_o (D) **types** are determined by mixing the recipient's erythrocytes with anti-A, anti-B, and anti-D antisera. The ABO group is then confirmed by testing the recipient's plasma against commercial reagent A and B cells to detect isoagglutinins.

The recipient's plasma is **screened** for alloantibodies that may not be demonstrated in the crossmatch. In antibody screens, suspensions of reagent O erythrocytes that contain known erythrocyte antigens on their surface are incubated at 37°C with the recipient's plasma. If antigen–antibody complexes are formed, hemolysis or agglutination of erythrocytes is observed. The screen is completed by the IAT and again observed for agglutination.

In the **crossmatch,** compatibility between donor and recipient is determined. Donor cells are combined with recipient plasma, centrifuged, and observed for hemolysis or agglutination (called the "immediate spin" crossmatch). If the recipient either has a history of previous erythrocyte antibody or has had antibody detected during the antibody-screening procedure, the IAT using recipient plasma and donor red cells must be performed before a crossmatch may be considered compatible.

A variety of methods to increase the sensitivity of the IAT has been developed. These methods add albumin, low-ionic-strength solution (LISS), polybrene, or polyethylene glycol (PEG) to the test system. Reagent erythrocytes can also be treated with proteolytic enzymes to enhance the reactivity of some erythrocyte antigens (Rh and Kidd) and to abolish the reactivity of others (M, N, Fy^a, and Fy^b).

TRANSFUSION REACTIONS

Blood transfusion has become increasingly safe, but a variety of adverse reactions, only some of which are preventable, continues to occur (Table 17–3). Patients who are transfused must be monitored during infusion for immediate reactions and over time to detect delayed reactions.

Hemolytic Reactions

The transfusion of incompatible blood may cause immediate hemolysis. Immediate hemolytic transfusion reactions, which are fatal in approximately 10–40% of cases, generally occur when ABO-incompatible blood is transfused. The cause is most often managerial or clerical error, such as transfusing patients with units intended for other recipients. Two thirds of these errors occur in areas other than the hospital blood bank. Incompatible transfusions involving other blood groups are usually less severe, but deaths have been reported. The most common presentation of a hemolytic transfusion reaction is fever or fever with chills. Other signs or symptoms are chest pain, hypotension, nausea, flushing, dyspnea, and hemoglobinuria. The hemolytic transfusion reaction may progress to shock, disseminated intravascular coagulation (DIC), and renal failure.

Delayed hemolytic transfusion reactions occur 3–10 days after transfusion and may be clinically undetected. This reaction occurs from an anamnestic immune response to transfused erythrocytes in a previously sensitized person with undetectable antibody in pretransfusion testing. Presenting symptoms are fever, anemia, and jaundice. The patient's transfused erythrocytes are coated with antibody demonstrated by a positive DAT. The antibody specificity is identified by removing it from the surface of the coated transfused erythrocytes by a procedure called elution. The eluted antibody is then tested against a panel of reagent erythrocytes by the IAT. The frequency of delayed hemolytic transfusion reactions is 1 per 4000

Table 17–3. Transfusion reactions.

Cause	Incidence	Manifestations	Treatment
Erythrocyte antibodies			
Hemolytic (acute)	<0.02%	Fever, chills, hypotension. Pain in back or infusion site. Hemoglobin in blood and urine.	Stop transfusion; blood/urine to blood bank. Hydrate. Monitor hematocrit, liver, and renal function.
Hemolytic (delayed)		Lowered hematocrit, increased bilirubin; elevated LDH days to weeks posttransfusion.	Monitor hematocrit, also liver and renal function if severe.
Cytokines, WBC	<2%	Temperature raised ≥1°C, chills.	Stop transfusion: rule out hemolytic reaction blood/urine to blood bank; premedicate with antipyretics; give leukocyte-reduced products if available.
Donor WBC antibodies	<0.2%	Noncardiac pulmonary edema, bronchospasm.	Stop transfusion, treat symptoms.
Plasma proteins	2–3%	Itching, urticaria, rarely asthma, bronchospasm, anaphylaxis.	Stop transfusion; give antihistamines for urticaria; treat symptoms.

Abbreviations: LDH = lactate dehydrogenase; WBC = white blood cells.

units of blood transfused. Mortality from delayed hemolytic transfusion reactions is uncommon.

Febrile Reactions

In the past, febrile nonhemolytic transfusion reactions (FNHTR) were thought to be caused by cytotoxic or agglutinating antibodies in the recipient, directed against donor leukocyte antigens. Leukocyte reduction filters used at the time of red cell or platelet transfusion decreased the amount of leukocytes transfused and should have eradicated FNHTRs. When this anticipated effect was not observed, researchers looked for other causes to explain the fever, chills, and rare rigors that describe a FNHTR. It was observed that during storage, cytokines (IL-1β, IL-6, TNFα) are released from leukocytes present in red cell and platelet components. These cytokines are known to have pyrogenic activity and thus may be the cause of this adverse reaction. FNHTR must be distinguished from fever associated with hemolytic transfusion reactions and from the high fever (>40°C) and rigors associated with bacterial contamination of blood components. Only one in eight patients with a febrile reaction has another reaction on subsequent transfusion. Recurrent febrile reactions are often controlled with antipyretics, leukocyte-reduced components, or recently collected components.

Transfusion-Related Acute Lung Injury

High-titer leukocyte antibodies in donor plasma can cause pulmonary edema (see Chapter 40). Donor antibodies bound to recipient granulocytes (or infrequently, recipient antibodies bound to donor granulocytes) activate complement. Complement activation leads to the sequestration of antibody–granulocyte complexes in the lung microvasculature. The presence of activated complement fragments and leukocyte enzymes or free radicals are thought to cause lung injury with resultant pulmonary edema. The sequelae are fever, dyspnea, and marked hypoxemia. The acute respiratory distress occurs within 1–6 hours of a transfusion and often requires aggressive respiratory support. Although some deaths have been reported, most patients with transfusion-related acute lung injury (TRALI) improve within 48–96 hours if promptly treated. The risk of TRALI is approximately 1 per 5000 units transfused.

Allergic Reactions

Allergic reactions to transfusion are characterized by itching, hives, and local erythema. Rarely are they accompanied by cardiopulmonary instability. They are thought to be caused by infused plasma proteins and occur in 1–2% of transfusions. Patients with a history of allergy more frequently have allergic reactions to blood. Mild reactions can be treated with antihistamines and the transfusion continued. Pretreatment with antihistamines often prevents recurrent allergic reactions. If the allergic reaction is severe,

washed erythrocytes may be indicated. After transfusion of as little as 10–15 mL of a blood component, some IgA-deficient recipients with anti-IgA experience anaphylactic reactions. Fortunately, these reactions are rare. The reaction is due to the IgA present in transfused plasma and is prevented by transfusing plasma-free or IgA-deficient components.

Other transfusion reactions include those caused by bacterial contamination of blood components, congestive heart failure due to intravascular volume overload, and donor erythrocyte destruction prior to infusion. Erythrocytes may be destroyed by inadvertent overheating, improper freezing technique, or mixing with nonisotonic solutions.

Transfusion-Transmitted Infection

Transfusion may be complicated by a variety of infectious microorganisms, only some of which can be detected by current donor-screening methods (Table 17–4). The most frequently reported posttransfusion infections in developed countries are various bacterial contaminants, hepatitis, cytomegalovirus (CMV), human immunodeficiency virus-1 (HIV-1), and human T-cell lymphotrophic virus I/II (HTLV-I/II). Elimination of potentially infected blood depends on successful donor screening by medical history, aseptic blood collection, and adequate laboratory testing of the donated blood. The presence of hepatitis B surface antigen (HBsAg), antibody to hepatitis B core antigen (anti-HBc), antibody to hepatitis C virus (anti-HCV), anti-HIV 1/2, HIV-1 antigen (p24), anti-HTLV I/II, and syphilis (STS) is currently tested in all US blood donors.

The prevalence of posttransfusion hepatitis (PTH) is estimated to be <1%. PTH is caused by hepatitis B virus in 5% of cases and by hepatitis C virus in 95% of cases. Of transfusion recipients who develop posttransfusion hepatitis, 50% develop chronic hepatitis; 10% of these develop cirrhosis. All blood components can potentially transmit hepatitis, except those that can be pasteurized, such as albumin and other plasma proteins.

CMV is transmitted to CMV-seronegative transfusion recipients by leukocytes contaminating erythrocyte and platelet components. Roughly 50% of blood donors are infected with CMV, which limits avail-

Table 17–4. Transfusion-transmitted infection.[a]

Infection	Risk/Unit Transfused
Hepatitis C	1:103,000
Hepatitis B	1:63,000
HTLV-I/II	1:640,000
HIV-1 infection	1:675,000

Abbreviations: HTLV-I/II = human T-cell lymphotrophic virus-I/II; HIV-1 = human immunodeficiency virus-1.

[a] Rare infections include syphilis, malaria, Epstein–Barr virus infection, delta hepatitis, brucellosis, Chagas' disease, babesiosis, and leishmaniasis.

ability of CMV-negative blood. CMV disease causes significant morbidity and mortality in severely immunocompromised patients. When possible, CMV-seronegative blood should be given to low-birth-weight infants (<1250 g), CMV-seronegative pregnant women, and CMV-seronegative recipients of CMV-seronegative bone marrow or organ transplants.

HIV-1 infection due to transfusion is rare since implementation of donor HIV-1 antibody testing (March 1985). HIV-1 can be transmitted by erythrocytes, platelets, cryoprecipitate, fresh-frozen plasma, and possibly other blood components. The risk of infection by transfusion is now estimated to be about 1 in 675,000 per unit transfused. The virus can be transmitted by blood collected from donors who have been recently infected but don't yet have detectable levels of HIV antigen or antibodies (called the "window period"). Even though HIV-2 infection is rare in the United States, isolated cases are reported in parts of Europe and West Africa. Consequently, all US blood donations are screened for antibodies to both HIV-1 and HIV-2 as well as to HIV p24 antigen. To date 3 US blood donors were found to have been infected with HIV-2 since HIV-2 testing was implemented in 1992.

Human T-lymphotrophic viruses type I and type II (HTLV-I and HTLV-II) are also retroviruses known to be transmitted by transfused blood products. Donor screening histories and serologic testing for evidence of HTLV-I/II infection has reduced the risk of transfusion-transmitted HTLV-I/II infection to 1:641,000. Both viruses are associated with a slowly progressive spinal cord disorder known as tropical spastic paraparesis/HTLV-associated myelopathy (TSP-HAM). Blood donors found to be infected with HTLV-I or HTLV-II by serologic testing have been shown to have an increased incidence of infections (bladder–kidney infections with HTLV-I and bladder–kidney infections, bronchitis, and oral herpes with HTLV-II) when compared with seronegative donor controls. In addition, HTLV-I can cause adult T-cell leukemia (See Chapter 43).

Other Diseases Transmitted by Transfusion

Bacterial contamination of blood products is an important cause of morbidity and mortality. The source of blood product contamination is either silent bacteremia in the donor or skin contaminants at the venipuncture site. Storage of products at standard refrigerator temperatures (4°C) retards the growth of most bacteria so the risk of transfusion-transmitted bacteria in red blood cells is about 1:500,000 units transfused. In stark contrast, platelet products carry a much higher bacterial contamination risk of 1:12,000 units transfused due to their storage at room temperature. Gram-negative organisms are more often found in refrigerated products, whereas in platelets stored at ambient temperature the organisms are gram-posi-

tive. The mortality rate from transfused bacterially contaminated blood products has been estimated to be as high as 25%.

Epstein–Barr virus (EBV) may be transmitted by transfusion. In most cases it results in asymptomatic seroconversion, but it can cause a mononucleosis syndrome.

Posttransfusion syphilis is now rare. There is a low prevalence of syphilitic infection in blood donors, and all donors are screened for antibody. Since the organism does not survive cold storage for more than 96 hours, it can be transmitted only by fresh blood or platelets.

Malaria remains a disease of major worldwide importance. The parasite can be present in erythrocytes of carriers for years after infection. No available laboratory tests are simple and sensitive enough to screen the blood donor population; therefore, blood banks in the United States rely on histories taken at the time of donation. Donors who have traveled to areas where malaria is endemic are deferred for 12 months.

Other parasites are transmitted by transfusion. In the United States, *Babesia microti,* the causative agent of babesiosis, is the second most common parasitical infection transmitted by blood products. *Trypanosoma cruzi,* which causes Chagas' disease, is a very rare cause of transfusion-transmitted parasitic infection in the United States; however, in the endemic countries of Central and South America, blood transfusion is a common source for this infection. Microfilariasis is a transfusion risk in the tropical areas of the world where *Wuchereria bancrofti, Loa loa,* and other filarial parasites are found. Transfusion-transmitted leishmaniasis is also reported.

Immunologic Mechanisms of Transfusion Reactions

Hemolytic transfusion reactions are caused by antigen–antibody complexes on the erythrocyte membrane. These complexes activate Hageman factor (factor XIIa) and complement and induce the production of several cytokines. Hageman factor activates the kinin system (see Chapter 12). Bradykinins thus generated increase capillary permeability and dilate arterioles, causing hypotension. Complement is activated and leads to intravascular hemolysis as well as to histamine release from mast cells. Hageman factor and free incompatible erythrocyte stroma activate the intrinsic clotting cascade, with consequent DIC. Systemic hypotension with renal vasoconstriction and the formation of intravascular thrombi lead to renal failure. When complement activation is incomplete, the reaction is less severe. Erythrocytes coated with C3b are cleared from the circulation by phagocytes, resulting in extravascular hemolysis.

The mechanism of graft-versus-host disease (GVHD) depends on the engraftment and clonal expansion of donor lymphocytes in the recipient. Donor lymphocytes recognize recipient tissue antigens as "foreign" and cause a clinical syndrome characterized by fever, skin rash, hepatitis, and diarrhea. In transfusion-associated GVHD (TA-GVHD), bone marrow is also a target of donor lymphocytes, and a significant aplasia results. Most cases of TA-GVHD are poorly responsive to treatment and result in death. Gamma irradiation of lymphocyte-containing blood components to preclude lymphocyte activation and expansion prevents TA-GVHD. Patients at risk for TA-GVHD are fetuses receiving intrauterine transfusions, patients transfused with HLA-matched platelets, newborns undergoing exchange transfusion, patients with T-cell immunodeficiencies, and patients severely immunosuppressed by intensive irradiation and chemotherapy (see Chapter 53). There are rare reports of graft-versus-host disease following transfusion of blood from a haploidentical donor into an immunocompetent recipient. Consequently, designated blood donations collected from blood relatives are now irradiated before transfusion.

RH ISOIMMUNIZATION

The D antigen is a common, strongly immunogenic antigen, 50 times more immunogenic than the other Rh antigens. The prevalence of antibody formation to Rh+ blood depends on the dose of Rh+ cells: 1 mL of cells sensitizes 15% of individuals exposed; 250 mL sensitizes 60–70%. After the initial exposure to Rh+ cells, weak IgM antibody can be detected as early as 4 weeks. This is followed by a rapid conversion to IgG antibody. A second exposure to as little as 0.03 mL of Rh+ erythrocytes may result in the rapid formation of IgG antibodies.

The majority of potential transfusion reactions to Rh can be prevented by transfusing Rh– individuals with Rh– blood. Immunization and antibody formation to D antigen still occur owing to occasional Rh sensitization during pregnancy or to transfusion errors, particularly during emergencies. Immunization to other Rh antigens may occur because donor blood is typed routinely for D but not for other Rh antigens.

Hemolytic disease of the newborn occurs with the passage of Rh+cells from the fetus to the circulation of the Rh– mother. Once anti-D antibody is formed in the mother, IgG but not IgM anti-D antibodies cross the placenta, causing hemolysis of fetal erythrocytes. Rh– mothers become sensitized during pregnancy or at the time of delivery as a result of transplacental fetal hemorrhage. Following delivery, 75% of women will have had transplacental fetal hemorrhage. Some obstetric complications increase the risk of transplacental fetal hemorrhage: antepartum hemorrhage, toxemia of pregnancy, cesarean section, external version, and manual removal of the placenta. Transplacental fetal hemorrhage can also occur following spontaneous or therapeutic abortion, amniocentesis, chorionic villus sampling (CVS), or percutaneous umbilical cord sampling (PUBS). Overall Rh immunization occurs in 8–9% of Rh– women following the delivery of the first Rh+ ABO-compatible baby and in 1.5–2.0% of Rh– women who deliver Rh+ ABO-incompatible babies.

Rh Prophylaxis

Rh immunization can now be suppressed almost entirely in antepartum or postpartum Rh– women if high-titer anti-Rh immunoglobulin (RhIg) is administered within 72 hours after the potentially sensitizing dose of Rh+ cells.

The protective mechanism of RhIG administration is not clear. RhIG does not effectively block Rh antigen from immunosuppressive cells by competitive inhibition, since effective doses of RhIG do not cover all D antigen sites. Intravascular hemolysis and rapid clearance of RhIg-coated erythrocytes is also unlikely. Although this mechanism appears to explain the 90% protective effect of ABO incompatibility between mother and fetus, RhIG-induced erythrocyte hemolysis is extravascular. Rh+ fetal cells are removed primarily by highly phagocytic cells in the spleen and liver. The most likely mechanism is a negative modulation of the primary immune response, which thereby depresses antibody formation. Antigen–antibody complexes are bound to cells bearing Fc receptors in the lymph nodes and spleen. These cells presumably stimulate suppressor T-cell responses, which prevent antigen-induced B-cell proliferation and antibody formation.

A prophylactic dose of 300 µg of RhIG intramuscularly prevents Rh immunization following exposure to up to 15 mL of Rh+ erythrocytes, which corresponds to 30 mL of fetal whole blood. Initial recommendations were that 300 µg of RhIG be given to nonimmunized Rh– mothers within 72 hours after delivery of an Rh+ infant. The postpartum dose of RhIG decreased the incidence of anti-D development to 1% in Rh– women giving birth to Rh+ infants. To further decrease the chances of developing anti-D in this population of women, antepartum RhIG is also now administered at 28 weeks' gestation. A dose of RhIG is also indicated for an Rh– woman after any terminated pregnancy, amniocentesis, CVS, PUBS, and fetal surgery or manipulation. Additional doses may have to be given in cases of massive transplacental fetal hemorrhage.

Large doses of RhIG can effectively suppress immunization following inadvertent transfusion of Rh+ blood into Rh– patients if given within 72 hours of transfusion. Once Rh immunization is demonstrated by the IAT, administration of RhIG is ineffective.

BLOOD COMPONENT THERAPY

Improvements in the medical care of previously fatal illnesses has placed increasing demands on the blood supply. As the need for blood products has expanded, the pool of eligible blood donors has decreased due to more intensive screening and testing. The separation of a whole-blood donation into its component parts (fresh-frozen plasma, platelets, and erythrocytes) has helped stretch a limited blood supply.

Erythrocytes

During acute blood loss, 1 hour or more is required for equilibration of intravascular and extravascular fluids and an accurate assessment of the fall in the hemoglobin level. Generally, a loss of 20% of blood volume can be corrected with crystalloid (electrolyte) solution alone, which can then be supplemented with colloid (protein) solution. Whole blood is indicated if blood loss exceeds one third of blood volume. Operative blood loss of 1000–1200 mL rarely requires transfusion in an otherwise healthy adult. If increased oxygen-carrying capacity is required, erythrocyte transfusion is indicated (Table 17–5).

A decreased hemoglobin level is tolerated better in a patient with chronic anemia than in a patient with acute blood loss. Patients with a slow decline in their hemoglobin level compensate for the decreased oxygen-carrying capacity by increasing their cardiac output. 2,3,-Diphosphoglycerate is also increased in patients with chronic anemia, shifting the oxyhemo-globin dissociation curve to the right. This rightward shift enhances oxygen release to the tissues.

All erythrocyte components should be administered through blood filters. Medications, especially solutions containing calcium or glucose, should not be infused with blood components.

Platelets

Platelets function to control bleeding by acting as hemostatic plugs on vascular endothelium. Platelet abnormalities that require platelet transfusion may be either quantitative or qualitative. The vast majority of platelet transfusions are given to supplement decreased numbers of circulating platelets due to suppressed production, pooling, or dilution.

Platelets are available as either platelet concentrates (recovered from a whole-blood donation) or as plateletpheresis (collected by using a cytopheresis instrument). The transfusion of one platelet concentrate is expected to increase the platelet count of a 70-kg adult by 5000–10,000/μL. A plateletpheresis is equivalent to four to eight platelet concentrates because both have the same number of platelets. The survival of transfused platelets decreases in patients who are actively bleeding; who have splenomegaly, fever, infection, or DIC; or who are sensitized to platelet antigens. The transfusion of ABO-incompatible platelets may be associated with slightly decreased platelet survival.

Much discussion ensues whenever the subject of indications for the appropriate use of platelet transfusions arises. Little good clinical evidence addresses the indications for platelet therapy. General guidelines suggest that stable, afebrile thrombocytopenic

Table 17–5. Guidelines for component therapy.

Component	Indications for Use
Red blood cells	Use to increase O_2-carrying capacity; 1 unit increases hemoglobin 1 g/dL in a 70-kg patient. Consider the degree of anemia, intravascular volume, and presence of coexisting cardiac, pulmonary, or vascular conditions. 1. If hemoglobin >10 g/dL, transfusion is rarely indicated. 2. If hemoglobin <7 g/dL, transfusion is usually indicated. 3. If hemoglobin is 7–10 g/dL, assess clinical status, mixed venous pO_2, and O_2 extraction ratio.
Platelets	Use to control or prevent bleeding due to low platelet count or abnormal platelet function; one concentrate increases platelet count by approximately 5000 platelets/μL. 1. Generally, patients with platelet counts <50,000–10,000 should receive platelets to prevent bleeding. 2. Actively bleeding patients with platelet counts <50,000 may benefit from platelets.
FFP	Used to increase clotting factors in patients with documented deficiencies (PT >1.5 × normal, 1 unit increases the level of any factor 2–3%. 1. FFP should not be used as a volume expander or nutritional source. 2. FFP is useful for treatment of factor II, V, VII, X, XI, or XIII deficiencies when specific concentrates are not available. 3. FFP is useful for patients with warfarin overdose who have life-threatening bleeding or who require emergency surgery. 4. FFP may be useful in massive blood transfusion (>1 blood volume within a few hours). 5. FFP is useful as a source of C1-esterase inhibitor in deficient patients with life-threatening angioedema and in patients with thrombotic thrombocytopenic purpura.

Source: Data used with permission, from the following sources: Fresh frozen plasma—indication and risks, *JAMA* 1985;**253**:551; Platelet transfusion therapy, *JAMA* 1987;**257**:1777; and Perioperative red blood cell transfusion, *JAMA* 1988;**260**:2700.
Abbreviations: PT = prothrombin time; FFP = fresh-frozen plasma.

adults and older children are not at high risk of serious bleeding unless their platelet counts fall below 5,000–10,000 μL. Indications for transfusion of unstable patients are more problematic. Bleeding patients should be more aggressively transfused, and many experts suggest transfusion when platelet counts fall below 30,000–50,000 μL. Thrombocytopenic patients undergoing invasive procedures do not generally experience increased complications unless their platelet counts are <50,000 μL; however, the patient's clinical situation and the site of the procedure or surgery should influence the decision to transfuse. Patients undergoing surgery on the eye, brain, spinal cord, or airway are at higher risk of serious sequelae due to bleeding and may require higher platelet counts for safety.

Plasma Products

Fresh-frozen plasma (FFP), stored plasma, and cryoprecipitate are valuable sources of coagulation factors. Stored plasma and FFP may often be used interchangeably. Levels of factors V and VIII in stored plasma are half those in FFP, but levels of other factors are equivalent. Cryoprecipitate was initially produced to provide therapeutic doses of factor VIII and von Willebrand's factor. This use has been greatly supplanted by the development of recombinant or treated factor VIII, which have lower infectious risks to recipients. Cryoprecipitate is now most often used to treat bleeding in patients with fibrinogen less than 100 mg/dL.

FFP is used for treating isolated congenital factor deficiencies, for which a safer factor concentrate product is not available. It is also used to correct warfarin overdoses in patients with significant bleeding. FFP is also used to treat thrombotic thrombocytopenic purpura and C1 esterase inhibitor deficiency. Massively transfused patients with a prothrombin time or partial thromboplastin time greater than 1.5 times normal and platelet counts above 50,000/μL may benefit from FFP treatment. FFP or plasma should never be used for volume expansion because colloid solutions without infectious risk are available (ie, albumin).

REFERENCES

American College of Physicians Clinical Guideline: Practice strategies for elective red blood cell transfusion. *Ann Intern Med* 1992;116:403.

Anderson KC, Weinstein HJ: Transfusion-associated graft-versus-host disease. *N Engl J Med* 1990;323:315.

Capon SM, Goldfinger D: Acute hemolytic transfusion reaction, a paradigm of the systemic inflammatory response: New insights into pathophysiology and treatment. *Transfusion* 1995;35:513.

Colin Y et al: Genetic basis of the RhD-positive and RhD-negative blood group polymorphism as determined by Southern analysis. *Blood* 1991;78:2747.

Goodnough LT et al: Transfusion medicine blood transfusion. *N Engl J Med* 1999;340:438.

Hartwell, EA: Use of Rh immune globulin ASCP practice parameter. *Am J Clin Pathol* 1998;110:281.

Heddle NM et al: The role of the plasma from platelet concentrates in transfusion reactions. *N Engl J Med* 1994; 331:625.

Issitt PD, Anstee DJ: *Applied Blood Group Serology,* 4th ed. Montgomery Scientific, 1998.

Mollison PL: *Blood Transfusion in Clinical Medicine,* 10th ed. Blackwell, 1997.

Mourant AE et al: *The Distribution of Human Blood Groups and Other Polymorphisms,* 2nd ed. Oxford University Press, 1976.

Murphy EL et al: Increased incidence of infectious diseases during prospective follow-up of human T-lymphotropic virus type II- and I-infected blood donors. *Arch Intern Med* 1999;159:1485.

NIH Consensus Conference: Platelet transfusion therapy. *JAMA* 1987;257:1777.

NIH Consensus Conference: Perioperative red blood cell transfusion. *JAMA* 1988;260:2700.

NIH Consensus Conference: Fresh-frozen plasma. *JAMA* 1985;253:551.

Petz LD et al (editors): *Clinical Practice of Transfusion Medicine,* 3rd ed. Churchill Livingstone, 1996.

Pineda AA et al: Hemolytic transfusion reaction: Recent experience in a large blood bank. *Mayo Clin Proc* 1978; 53:378.

Popovsky MA et al: Transfusion-related acute lung injury: A neglected, serious complication of hemotherapy. *Transfusion* 1992;32:589.

Rudmann SV: *Textbook of Blood Banking and Transfusion Medicine.* W. B. Saunders Company, 1995.

Sazama K: Reports of 355 transfusion-associated deaths: 1976 through 1985. *Transfusion* 1990;30:583.

Schreiber GB et al: The risk of transfusion-transmitted viral infections. *N Engl J Med* 1996;334:1685.

Snyder EL (editor): *Transfusion Medicine Topic Update. Platelet Transfusion: A Consensus Development Conference.* Yale University, 1994.

Vengelen-Tyler V (editor): *Technical Manual for the American Association of Blood Banks,* 13th ed. American Association of Blood Banks, 1999.

Welch HG et al: Prudent strategies for elective red blood cell transfusion. *Ann Intern Med* 1992;116:393.

18

Molecular Genetic Techniques for Clinical Analysis of the Immune System

Tristram G. Parslow, MD, PhD

Genetic information in humans and most other organisms is encoded in the linear sequence of four nucleotide bases (abbreviated A, T, G, and C) along the strands of a DNA molecule. The sequence of the human genome is more than 3 billion DNA bases long, is divided among 23 chromosomes, and is present twice in each diploid nucleus. The human genome contains an estimated 100,000 genes, each comprising, on average, no more than a few thousand bases of coding sequence that specify a particular protein or structural RNA. The coding information of a typical human gene is rarely contained in a single, uninterrupted stretch of DNA but, instead, is divided into shorter coding segments called **exons,** which are separated by noncoding regions called **introns.** Individual genes are also widely separated from one another along the DNA, with noncoding sequences in between. Altogether, coding sequences are thought to make up only 5–10% of the human genome, and the function of the remaining sequences is, for the most part, unknown. The complete sequences of many human genes have been determined (by using techniques that lie outside the scope of this chapter), and the sequence of the entire human genome is likely to become known within a few years.

During the past two decades, advances in nucleic acid chemistry and recombinant DNA technology have made it practical to analyze individual genes rapidly and precisely. The techniques involved are now commonplace in research and are gradually being adapted for use in clinical laboratories as well. DNA offers numerous advantages as a substrate for clinical analysis: It is a remarkably sturdy biomolecule that is fairly easy to handle; it can be obtained from either fresh or fixed tissue or blood specimens; and it can be manipulated and dissected in ways that are not possible with proteins. Most importantly, access to the information contained in DNA enables us to diagnose and investigate many disease processes at the most fundamental level. This chapter summarizes the basic concepts and practical techniques for analyzing DNA from clinical specimens, along with some specialized applications to the immune system. At the end of the chapter, related techniques for studying cellular RNA are briefly discussed.

NUCLEIC ACID PROBES

Underlying the complexity of DNA is a simple but profound symmetry. Each DNA molecule is composed of two linear strands of bases, which are bound to each other side by side and coiled to form a double helix (Figure 18–1). The two strands are held together by hydrogen bonding between adjacent bases: A on one strand always binds to T on the other, and similar binding occurs between G and C. In normal DNA, the two strands are said to be **complementary** in that every base is appropriately paired to the corresponding position on the opposite strand. Bases within a strand are held together by strong covalent bonds, but the base-pairing bonds between strands are relatively weak, so that the two strands can easily be separated (**"denatured"** or **"melted apart"**) by heat or alkaline pH. When slowly returned to physiologic conditions, the strands reanneal spontaneously and in perfect alignment to re-form the original double-stranded helix.

This spontaneous pairing between complementary strands provides the basis for many of the techniques that are used to detect and characterize genes. These techniques employ short strands of known sequence as **probes** to detect strands with the complementary sequence. Probes of any desired sequence can readily be obtained in abundant quantities and at very high purity: Single DNA strands up to about 100 bases long are easily prepared by using automated chemical synthesizers, whereas larger DNA sequences are generally introduced ("cloned") into bacteria to be replicated biologically. It is also possible to use probes made of RNA—a molecule that, for the purposes of this chapter, can be considered equivalent to single-stranded DNA—since these also anneal specifically to a complementary DNA strand. RNA probes are most often prepared enzymatically by cloning the corresponding DNA sequence and using this as a template for in vitro transcription, that is, producing a complementary RNA strand from the template DNA.

Cellular DNA can be isolated by chemical extraction from a blood or tissue specimen followed by enzymatic treatment to remove traces of contaminating

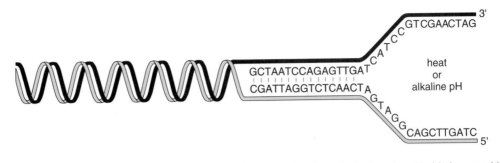

Figure 18–1. Structure of DNA. The molecule consists of two strands of covalently linked nucleotide bases, which are coiled around each other to form a double helix. The two strands are held together by relatively weak hydrogen bonds between bases. The strands dissociate from each other when exposed to heat or alkaline pH but spontaneously reassociate when returned to physiologic conditions.

RNA or protein. Unless special precautions are taken, the extremely long strands of chromosomal DNA are usually sheared by mechanical forces into random fragments of roughly 50,000–100,000 bp during the purification process. To use a nucleic acid probe, this target DNA is first heated or exposed to alkali in order to separate the strands and then mixed with the labeled probe and returned to normal temperature and pH. As the molecules reassociate, some of the target strands anneal (**"hybridize"**) to the probe rather than to the unlabeled complementary strand, forming labeled duplexes. To maximize the likelihood that a target strand will anneal to the probe rather than to its original partner, the hybridization reaction is usually carried out with a great molar excess of probe. The stability of the complex formed by a probe and its target is influenced by many factors, the most important of which are temperature, salt concentration, the length and base composition of the probe, and the presence of any mismatched bases. Under the conditions used in most assays, two strands must share at least 16–20 consecutive bases of perfect complementarity to form a stable hybrid. The probability of such a match occurring by chance is less than one in a billion (10^{-9}). Thus, nucleic acid probes possess an extraordinary degree of specificity: A typical probe is capable of recognizing and binding selectively to a single copy of its complementary sequence among the 3 billion bp in the human genome. DNA or RNA probes can easily by tagged with radioisotopes, fluorochromes, or enzymatic markers prior to use (Figure 18–2) and can then act as "molecular stains" that recognize and bind only to the exact complementary sequence.

HYBRIDIZATION ASSAYS

Several different methods can be used to test whether a DNA specimen contains sequences com-

plementary to a particular probe. One common approach takes advantage of the fact that, under certain conditions (eg, when exposed to ultraviolet light or when heated in a high concentration of salt), DNA strands can be made to bind tightly onto nylon or nitrocellulose membranes. In a procedure called **dot blot hybridization** (Figure 18–3A), a solution of target DNA is denatured, spotted onto the surface of such a membrane, and then treated so that the separated DNA strands adhere irreversibly to the membrane. When immobilized in this manner, the target strands remain accessible on the membrane surface but are prevented from reannealing with one another. The membrane is then incubated with labeled probes under conditions in which the probe does not adhere to the membrane but may hybridize with the target strands. Afterward, the filter is washed extensively to remove unhybridized probe. Any probe that has hybridized to the bound DNA can then be detected by autoradiography or enzymatic assay, depending on the particular label that it carries.

In an alternative approach, called a **nuclease protection** assay, target and probe DNAs are denatured, allowed to anneal together in solution, and then treated with an enzyme that specifically cleaves single-stranded but not double-stranded DNA. A probe survives this enzymatic digestion only if it has become stably hybridized to the target DNA (Figure 18–3B).

The interaction between probe and target occurs with one-to-one stoichiometry, and this tends to limit the sensitivity of hybridization assays. One way of maximizing the signal obtained is to incorporate multiple labels into a single probe, such as by radioactively labeling many bases in the probe (Figure 18–4). It may also be appropriate to use multiple probes that each recognize adjacent regions of a longer target sequence or to attach secondary probes onto a long, unhybridized "tail" on the primary probe (see Figure 18–4). A recent innovation is to attach

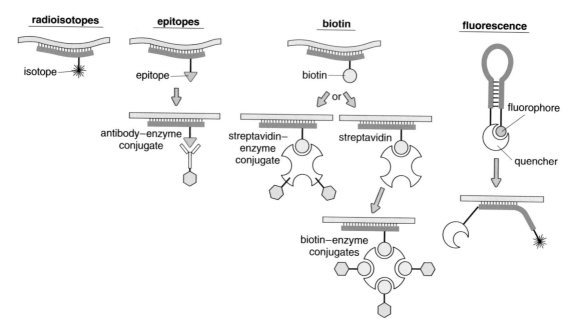

Figure 18–2. Some methods for labeling and detecting DNA or RNA probes. Radioisotopes, small epitopes, or biotin can be incorporated covalently into one or more positions in a probe at the time of synthesis. The most commonly used radioisotopes for this purpose are ^{32}P and ^{35}S, which can be detected by autoradiography or scintillation counting. Probes labeled with epitopes or biotin can be detected by secondary labeling with an enzyme conjugated to a specific antibody or to the polyvalent biotin-binding protein, streptavidin. One variation on the latter technique uses unconjugated streptavidin alone, which is then detected by binding of a biotin-enzyme conjugate. The enzyme used most commonly in these procedures is alkaline phosphatase, which can readily be assayed by its ability to generate chromogenic or chemiluminescent products. The fluorescent probe shown is a molecular beacon—a single-stranded probe whose sequence is designed to be self-complementary and that has a fluorophore attached to one end and a fluorescence quencher on the other. The unhybridized molecular beacon folds into a hairpin conformation, bringing the fluorophore and quencher together so that fluorescence is suppressed; hybridization separates the two ends, allowing the probe to fluoresce.

short DNA sidechains onto the primary probe by means of synthetic chemistry, creating an artificial **branched DNA** molecule that can interact with many copies of a secondary probe. Still another approach is to use probes that form polyvalent complexes with an enzyme or fluorochrome marker, similar to those used in immunohistochemistry (see Chapter 15). For example, hybrids containing a probe that has been labeled with biotin can first be incubated with the polyvalent biotin-binding protein streptavidin and then secondarily tagged with many copies of a biotinylated marker enzyme (see Figure 18–2). The use of enzymatic detection systems that produce colored or chemiluminescent products can greatly amplify the signal obtained, as can the use of molecular beacons—probes that become fluorescent only after they hybridize (see Figure 18–2). Even when such measures are taken, however, about 10^4–10^5 copies of a target sequence must usually be present in a sample to be detectable by routine hybridization.

SOUTHERN BLOT

The simplest hybridization assays, such as the dot blot assay, indicate whether a particular sequence is present in the target DNA and may also give an estimate of its abundance. These assays are rarely used clinically, because easier and more sensitive tests can provide the same information (see the section, Target Amplification Techniques). Nucleic acid probes, however, offer special advantages when they are used in conjunction with **restriction enzymes,** a class of bacterial enzymes that cut both strands of a linear DNA molecule at specific short recognition seuences, usually 4–6 bp long. For example, the enzyme *Eco*RI cuts only within the sequence GAATTC, whereas the enzyme *Bam*HI cleaves only GGATCC. Each restriction enzyme therefore cleaves long target DNA molecules into specific smaller segments called **restriction fragments,** whose number and length are determined by the sequence of the substrate DNA.

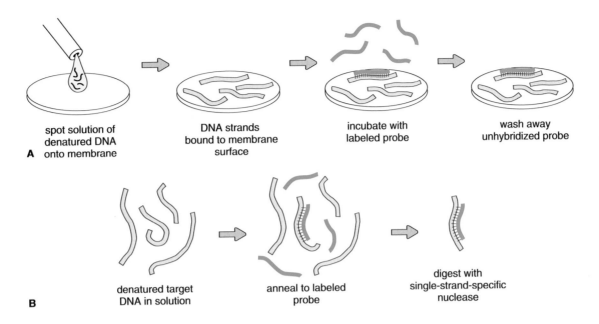

Figure 18–3. Two simple hybridization assays using nucleic acid probes. **A:** In the dot blot assay, denatured target DNA is attached to the surface of a nylon or nitrocellulose membrane and then incubated with a solution of labeled probe. **B:** In the nuclease protection assay, the reaction between probe and denatured target DNA takes place in solution; probes that have annealed to a target strand are detected by their ability to resist digestion by an enzyme (eg, nuclease S1) that specifically digests single-stranded but not double-stranded nucleic acids.

Because of the enormous size and complexity of the human genome, cleaving human DNA with a restriction enzyme yields millions of unique restriction fragments ranging up to tens of thousands of bases long. Nevertheless, the fragment that carries any particular gene can readily be identified, provided that a DNA probe complementary to the gene is available. The technique used for this purpose (Figure 18–5A) is called the **Southern blot,** after its inventor, E. M. Southern. DNA extracted from a tissue or blood specimen is first cleaved with one or more restriction enzymes, and the resulting DNA fragments are then subjected to electrophoresis through an agarose gel, which separates them according to length. Afterward, the gel is immersed in alkali solution to melt apart the complementary strands of each fragment. A sheet of nylon or nitrocellulose is then pressed firmly against the gel; the denatured DNA fragments bind tightly to this sheet and are drawn out of the gel. When the sheet is peeled away, it retains on its surface the immobilized DNA fragments, still arranged according to length as they had been in the gel but now exposed and accessible to further analysis. The sheet is then incubated with the labeled probe, which binds only to the fragment bearing its complementary sequence. Unbound probe is washed away, and the location of the remaining hybridized probe is determined by virtue of the label it carries. The size of the

bound target fragment can then be deduced from its location on the membrane because this corresponds to the distance it migrated in the agarose gel.

The Southern blot reveals not only the presence of a particular sequence but also the size of the restriction fragment on which it lies. This size, in turn, is determined by the distribution of nearby restriction sites and so reflects the local DNA sequence.

GENE REARRANGEMENT ASSAY FOR LYMPHOCYTE CLONALITY

If all the cells in a population contain identical DNA, the restriction fragment carrying any given gene will have the same length in every cell, and all of these fragments will appear together as a single band on a Southern blot. This is the case for most cellular genes, including the immunoglobulin (Ig) and T-cell receptor (TCR) genes of nonlymphoid cells. In lymphocytes, however, the Ig and TCR genes undergo specific rearrangements (see Chapter 7), which markedly alter the DNA sequences in and around these loci. Such rearrangements can be detected on the Southern blot by a shift in the size of the restriction fragment that carries an Ig or TCR gene. Moreover, because the size of the shifted fragment depends on the exact rearrangement that has

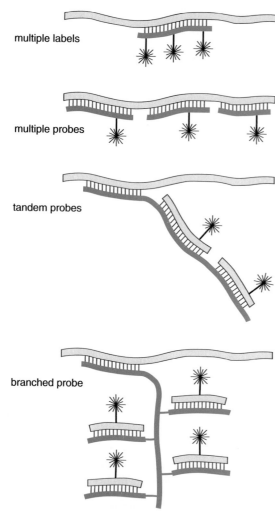

multiple labels

multiple probes

tandem probes

branched probe

Figure 18–4. Some approaches for increasing the sensitivity of nucleic acid hybridization assays. These can be used singly or in combination.

occurred, it represents a unique and characteristic property of each lymphocyte clone—a molecular fingerprint that can be used to distinguish one lymphoid clone from another.

This provides a powerful means of estimating the clonal composition of lymphocyte populations (Figure 18–5B). In normal polyclonal lymphocyte populations, each of the innumerable clones contributes its own distinctively sized Ig or TCR fragment, but none of these is abundant enough to be detectable. Only when large numbers of clonally related cells are present do the rearranged genes appear in sufficient quantity to produce a detectable band. The presence of abnormally sized Ig or TCR bands on the Southern blot thus suggests the presence of a predominant clone of lymphoid cells, and this, in an appropriate

setting, can be taken as evidence of lymphoid malignancy.

By using the Southern blot assay, clonal rearrangements of the Ig heavy-chain genes can be found in the neoplastic B cells in essentially all cases of B-cell lymphoma regardless of histologic type. The clinical utility of this approach is somewhat limited, however, because B-cell clonality can often be assessed more easily and cheaply by comparing the ratio of kappa (κ) and lambda (λ) light-chain proteins, using immunohistochemical stains (see Chapter 15). Nevertheless, the rearrangement assay is invaluable for demonstrating clonality in cases when malignant B cells either fail to express Ig protein or are heavily contaminated with polyclonal lymphocytes. Ig heavy-chain gene rearrangements are usually demonstrable in the lymphoid blast crisis of chronic myelogenous leukemia, in hairy cell leukemia, in "non-T, non-B" acute lymphoblastic leukemia, and in most null large-cell lymphomas (see Chapter 43).

The analysis of TCR rearrangements has even greater potential usefulness because no other practical method is available for assessing T-cell clonality. For technical reasons, most clinical assays focus on the TCR β-chain genes, which have been found to be clonally rearranged in nearly all cases of T-cell leukemia and lymphoma, including plaque- or tumor-stage mycosis fungoides, Sézary syndrome, and adult T-cell leukemia-lymphoma. The assay is especially useful for distinguishing reactive lymphadenopathy from T-cell lymphoma (see Chapter 43).

Although Ig and TCR gene rearrangements are generally confined to the B- and T-cell lineages, respectively, the correlation is not absolute. Roughly 15% of poorly differentiated lymphoid malignancies harbor rearrangements of both TCR β- and Ig heavy-chain genes—an example of lineage infidelity. Ig light-chain rearrangements, which occur later in normal ontogeny than heavy-chain rearrangements (see Chapter 7), are more specific for the B lineage but less sensitive for detecting clonality. Absence of any rearrangements argues strongly that a tumor is not of lymphoid origin. Specimens from separate lymphomatous lesions in a single patient usually show identical rearrangements. Because the rearrangements in recurrent cancers are identical to those seen prior to treatment, the Southern blot technique offers special advantages in monitoring remission and recurrence, since it may reveal persistence of a malignant clone that is not yet detectable morphologically.

The Southern assay for lymphocyte clonality has several limitations. Although it is potentially more sensitive than histologic examination (a clonal subpopulation can be detected even when diluted 100-fold with polyclonal cells), this degree of sensitivity requires prior knowledge of the position of an abnormal band on the gel. Faint bands seen in a case being analyzed de novo must be interpreted with great care because they may represent technical artifacts. To

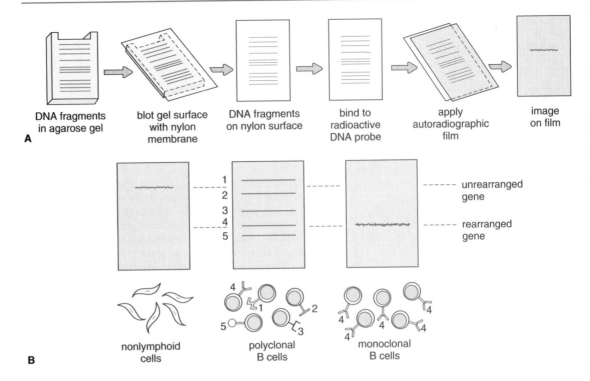

Figure 18–5. The Southern blot technique and an application of this technique for determining clonality of lymphoid cell populations. **A:** The blotting technique is described in the text; it can be used to determine the size of DNA restriction fragments that encompass a specific gene. **B:** DNA rearrangement in lymphocytes alters the sizes of fragments bearing the immunoglobulin or T-cell receptor genes: The sizes of the rearranged fragments are characteristic of each B-cell or T-cell clone. This provides a means of detecting B or T cells and of assessing the clonal composition of lymphoid populations. The approach is illustrated for B cells by using an immunoglobulin gene. DNA isolated from nonlymphoid cells contains only unrearranged immunoglobulin genes, whereas DNA from normal lymphocyte populations reveals many different rearranged genes—one from each of the many independent B-cell clones. Detection of only a single rearranged gene suggests that a lymphocyte population is monoclonal and therefore possibly malignant.

minimize degradation of the DNA, fresh or frozen tissue must be used, and processing must begin promptly. The method has been applied successfully to specimens obtained during fine-needle biopsies of lymph nodes, but obtaining sufficient DNA for a complete analysis generally requires a blood or tissue specimen that contains at least 25 million leukocytes.

It is also important to recognize that the TCR β locus includes far fewer V-gene segments than are found in the Ig loci. This greatly increases the probability that unrelated T-cell clones will coincidentally have the same rearrangement. Moreover, benign inflammatory responses to some antigens have been shown to use a particular TCR β V region preferentially and so might appear monoclonal by this assay. These facts may ultimately limit the validity of TCR rearrangements for diagnosing T-cell neoplasia. More fundamentally, it is unclear that monoclonality signifies malignancy in every case. Therefore, as with any other single test, results from gene rearrangement analyses must always be interpreted in the context of all other available clinical and laboratory data.

IN SITU HYBRIDIZATION

Another specialized hybridization technique, called **in situ hybridization,** is based on the ability of labeled probes to bind target DNA in thin tissue sections or cytologic smears (Figure 18–6). This technique reveals not only the presence of a specific sequence but also its spatial distribution within tissues or individual cells. In brief, cells or tissues attached to the surface of a glass microscope slide are fixed, incubated with a labeled probe, and then washed to remove unbound probe. The specimen is then coated with a thin layer of photographic emulsion or chromogenic substrate that reveals the location of any bound radiolabeled or enzymatically labeled probe. The assay is technically arduous and not very sensitive. It is very useful for detecting abundant RNA species or viral DNA, which may be present in large amounts in a single infected cell It can also be used cytogenetically to map the chromosomal locations of individual genes or to identify large-scale chromosomal anomalies.

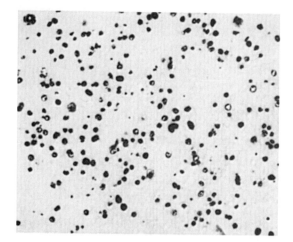

Figure 18–6. Detection of viral DNA in human cells by in situ hybridization. A lymph node biopsy specimen from a patient with Hodgkin's disease was fixed onto the surface of a glass slide and then hybridized with a biotinylated nucleic acid probe specific for sequences from Epstein–Barr virus. Hybridized probe was detected with streptavidin-conjugated alkaline phosphatase. The nuclei of cells that harbor the viral DNA stain darkly. (Courtesy of Lawrence M Weiss.)

TARGET AMPLIFICATION TECHNIQUES: POLYMERASE CHAIN REACTION

In the past, a major drawback of hybridization assays was their need for relatively large amounts of sample DNA to compensate for their low sensitivity. This problem has been surmounted in recent years by the development of powerful enzymatic techniques that can exponentially replicate specific DNA sequences in the test tube. With these techniques, it is now possible to analyze vanishingly small samples that initially contain fewer than ten copies of the sequence of interest. The new methods take advantage of the chemical properties of nucleic acids and of highly specialized enzymes that can repair and replicate DNA in vitro.

Every single-stranded DNA molecule has two ends, called the 5′ and 3′ ends, whose chemical and biologic properties differ. In double-stranded DNA, the two strands are always antiparallel (ie, their 3′ and 5′ ends are in opposite orientation to each other). Cellular enzymes known as **DNA polymerases,** which elongate these strands during DNA replication, can do so only by adding new nucleotide bases sequentially onto the 3′ end of a preexisting strand, which serves as a **primer.** Moreover, most DNA polymerases function only when the primer is annealed to a longer second strand, which serves as a **template** for DNA synthesis; the enzyme adds nu-

cleotides in a sequence complementary to that of the template, producing a base-paired double helix.

These properties of DNA polymerases are exploited in a technique called the **polymerase chain reaction (PCR)**, which can be used to replicate a particular region of target DNA selectively in vitro (Figure 18–7). Beginning with sample DNA from a very small number of cells, PCR can be used to synthesize multiple copies of a particular gene or gene segment that is present in those cells. PCR works best for copying regions less than about 2000 bp, and the DNA sequences flanking the region of interest must be known in advance. To use PCR, two short DNA primers (usually at least 16–20 bases long) are synthesized whose sequences are complementary to those of the flanking regions but on opposite strands; the two primers must be chosen so that their 3′ ends are directed toward each other (see Figure 18–7). A vast molar excess of these primers is added to the sample DNA, which is then denatured by heating and

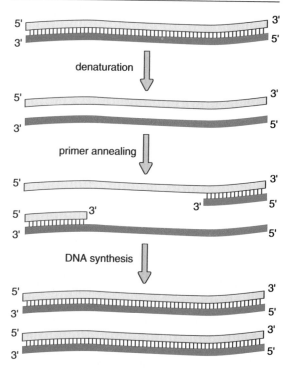

Figure 18–7. One cycle of DNA amplification by PCR. Each cycle consists of sequential heat denaturation, primer annealing, and DNA synthesis steps. Two different primers are used and must be oriented as shown with respect to each other. DNA synthesis is performed with a thermostable DNA polymerase and proceeds unidirectionally from each primer. After one cycle, the region between the primers has been duplicated. If the process is repeated, the number of copies of this region increases exponentially, doubling with each cycle until the supply of primers is exhausted.

allowed to anneal with the primers. A bacterial DNA polymerase is then added, which initiates synthesis at the 3′ end of each annealed primer and produces a new strand complementary to a portion of the adjacent template strand. Synthesis is continued for long enough that the newly synthesized strands extend through the entire region of interest. When the mixture is then denatured and reannealed again, each newly synthesized strand provides a new template for synthesis from the opposite primer. By repeated cycles of denaturation annealing, and synthesis, the region between the two primers is amplified exponentially, with the number of double-stranded copies of this region doubling at each cycle. The thermal cycling is performed in automated, programmable instruments that can accommodate many samples, and using thermostable DNA polymerases, isolated from thermophilic bacteria because these can better withstand exposure to high temperatures. Under ideal conditions, 220,000 copies should theoretically be produced from a single original DNA molecule after only 20 cycles of PCR. This is enough copies to allow detection by routine hybridization techniques.

Perhaps the most common problem encountered when using PCR is cross-contamination: Because the method is so sensitive, extreme care must be taken to avoid transferring even a trace of target DNA from one specimen to another. Another limitation of this technique arises from the fact that the bacterial polymerases frequently make errors when synthesizing new strands and so can introduce mutations that are not present in the original sample.

The basic technique of PCR amplification has been adapted in a great many ways to serve particular purposes. For example, it is widely used to facilitate detection of minute amounts of viral or bacterial DNA in clinical specimens because it can often identify these microorganisms much more rapidly than conventional culture techniques. A similar approach can be used to monitor lymphoid cancers; if primers are chosen that selectively amplify only a uniquely rearranged Ig or TCR V/(D)/J gene segment in the malignant clone, this can be used as an extremely sensitive assay for detecting persistence or regrowth of that clone in blood or tissues after cancer therapy. The PCR reaction can be monitored quantitatively by using primers designed as molecular beacons (see earlier section); each beacon that is used to prime DNA synthesis unfolds and becomes fluorescent, so that the rate at which fluorescence increases over successive PCR cycles reflects the original concentration of template DNA in the sample. Methods have also been developed that allow **in situ PCR** on tissue sections so that cells harboring a distinctive DNA sequence, such as a viral genome, can be identified morphologically. The amplifying power of PCR is so great that it allows analysis of genes from individual cells, which can be excised from frozen tissue sections using laser-capture microdissection. This has

made it possible, for example, to detect clonal Ig gene rearrangements in the rare Reed–Sternberg cells of Hodgkin's disease, confirming their B-cell origin.

It is also possible to search for single-point mutations within a target sequence by testing PCR-amplified DNA for **single-strand conformational polymorphisms (SSCP).** For this purpose, the amplified product is treated with alkali to separate the DNA strands and is then quickly applied to an electrophoretic gel under nondenaturing conditions (Figure 18–8). Because the individual strands are not given the opportunity to reanneal with other strands, they tend instead to fold up on themselves by forming base pairs at short regions of intrastrand complementarity. Even subtle mutations can greatly affect the folding pattern and, hence, the three-dimensional shape of the folded strand, causing it to migrate anomalously on the gel relative to the normal sequence. One advantage of this technique is that it can detect many alternative mutations within an amplified region, even if their identities are not known in advance.

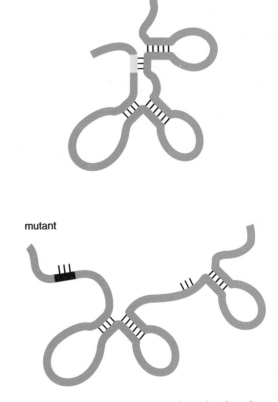

Figure 18–8. Single-strand conformational polymorphism. Under suitable conditions, a single strand of DNA often anneals with itself to form a complex folded structure as a result of regions of internal complementarity. Mutations may alter the folding pattern, and so change the electrophoretic mobility of the strand on a gel.

METHODS OF ANALYZING RNA

DNA and RNA probes can also be used to analyze the RNAs from a clinical specimen, and this can be highly advantageous for some purposes. Whereas DNA analysis can reveal the presence and structure of a particular gene sequence, RNA analysis indicates whether, and how strongly, it is being expressed. Another important advantage is sensitivity: A cell that expresses a particular gene often contains hundreds of copies of the RNA derived from it, and this RNA may be readily detectable even though the gene itself is not. Techniques such as in situ or dot blot hybridization can easily be adapted to search for specific sequences in cellular RNA. In a modified form of the Southern blot, called the **Northern blot,** a mixture of cellular RNAs can be separated according to length by agarose gel electrophoresis, transferred to the surface of a nylon or nitrocellulose membrane, and then hybridized to a labeled nucleic acid probe to determine the size and abundance of any particular RNA species.

RNA analysis has some inherent limitations, however. Because expression of a given RNA varies widely depending on the lineage and physiologic state of a cell, it is critical to sample the right tissues at the right time. RNA is less durable than DNA (eg, it degrades rapidly and irreversibly at alkaline pH) and must be handled with correspondingly greater care. In addition, the number and types of enzymes that are available to manipulate RNA sequences are very limited. For some applications, it is necessary to begin by making a DNA copy of the target RNA, which then serves as the substrate for further analysis. For example, PCR amplification of RNA is carried out by a two-stage procedure known as **reverse transcriptase PCR (RT-PCR).** The first stage employs an enzyme called reverse transcriptase, which synthesizes a DNA strand complementary to the RNA of interest by using one of the PCR primers as its primer. This complementary DNA **(cDNA)** is then used, in the second stage, as the starting material for PCR amplification by a conventional thermostable DNA polymerase.

GENOMIC ARRAYS

As an increasing proportion of all human genes are discovered and sequenced, techniques are being developed that allow vast numbers of these genes to be examined simultaneously in a single tissue specimen. These techniques are variations on the dot-blot hybridization assay described earlier, but involve the use of a **genomic array**—a large collection of different DNA probes individually displayed in a pattern of tiny spots on a glass microscope slide or other two-dimensional surface. One common type of probe (called an **expressed sequence tag,** or **EST**) is a short sequence complementary to part of the coding region from a particular gene whose function may or may not be known. Genomic arrays can be prepared either by painting a minute amount of each probe onto a slide robotically or by synthesizing each probe directly on the surface using microlithographic technology similar to that used in manufacturing computer chips. Either approach yields a high-density array of as many as hundreds of thousands of short, defined DNA probes immobilized on a small surface. The array is then incubated with fluorescently labeled DNA prepared from a tissue specimen, under conditions that allow each tissue DNA fragment to hybridize only to a perfectly complementary probe. Afterward, the amount of tissue DNA bound to each spot in the array is measured fluorometrically. Depending on the probes used, a single array can scan for a multitude of human or pathogen genes, or can screen individual genes to detect specific sequence variations or mutations in the chromosomes. Alternatively, RNA extracted from a tissue sample can be used to prepare labeled cDNA, which can then be screened against an array of EST probes to determine which genes are active in the tissue and at what levels they are expressed.

Genomic arrays have already proven their ability to provide enormous amounts of information, but the challenge of interpreting and applying that information remains. Nevertheless, one can envision a future in which, for example, routine evaluation of biopsies using such chips could detect, classify, and reveal the etiology of a lymphoid cancer and simultaneously provide information on metabolic phenotype and drug sensitivities to guide individualized therapy.

OVERVIEW & PROSPECTS

Tests based on nucleic acid technology are a relatively new addition to the armamentarium of the clinical immunology laboratory, and it is not yet clear to what extent they will supplement or replace conventional assays. They are particularly well suited to the detection of viruses and other microorganisms in tissue specimens because such organisms can often be recognized and positively identified by their unique RNA or DNA sequences much more quickly and inexpensively than by culture. Hence, PCR-based tests have already assumed an important role in microbiologic diagnosis, and it seems likely that this role will increase in the future. Immunologically important organisms that are currently assayed in this manner include Epstein–Barr virus, human immunodeficiency viruses, and human T-cell leukemia viruses (see Chapters 43 and 46).

DNA-based assays are also very useful for detecting large-scale chromosomal deletions or rearrangements that occur at fairly constant locations in the genome and that characterize several types of hematologic malignancies. Examples include the Philadelphia chromosome of chronic myelogenous leukemia, the t(14,18) of follicular lymphoma, and the t(8,14) and related anomalies of Burkitt's lymphoma (see Chapters 7 and 43). Detection of these rearrangements can be a useful adjunct in diagnosis and also provides a simple means to monitor disease progression or to search for minimal residual disease after therapy. The Southern blot assay for lymphocyte clonality has similar potential utility and may be especially useful for evaluating poorly differentiated malignancies; however, it is currently too labor-inten-

sive and technically demanding to be adopted by many clinical laboratories. PCR, LCR, and related techniques can detect extremely subtle DNA anomalies, including single-base point mutations, and are likely to be used increasingly for the diagnosis of congenital immunodeficiencies and of hereditary predispositions to cancer or other disorders. The emerging technologies for genomic analysis will certainly help identify genes that have diagnostic and prognostic value for individual patients and may also yield new and unexpected insights into disease biology.

REFERENCES

THEORY & PROTOCOLS

Duggan DJ et al: Expression profiling using cDNA microarrays. *Nat Genet* 1999;21:10.

Graves DJ: Powerful tools for genetic analysis come of age. *Trends Biotechnol* 1999;17:127.

Lipshutz RJ et al: High density synthetic oligonucleotide arrays. *Nat Genet* 1999;21:20.

McNicol AM, Farquharson MA: In situ hybridization and its diagnostic applications in pathology. *J Pathol* 1997; 182:250.

Simone NL et al: Laser-capture microdissection: Opening the microscopic frontier to molecular analysis. *Trends Genet* 1998;14:272.

Wagener C: Molecular diagnostics. *J Molec Med* 1997;75: 728.

SPECIFIC APPLICATIONS

Cleary ML et al: Monoclonality of lymphoproliferative lesions in cardiac-transplant recipients. *N Engl J Med* 1984; 310:477.

Cossman J et al: Gene rearrangements in the diagnosis of lymphoma/leukemia: Guidelines for use based on a multiinstitutional study. *Am J Clin Pathol* 1991;95:

347.

Davey MP, Waldmann TA: Clonality and lymphoproliferative lesions. *N Engl J Med* 1986;315:509.

Haase AT et al: Quantitative image analysis of HIV-1 infection in lymphoid tissue. *Science* 1996;274:985.

Kuppers R, Rajewsky K: The origin of Hodgkin and Reed/Sternberg cells in Hodgkin's disease. *Annu Rev Immunol* 1998;16:471.

Shibata D et al: Detection of specific t(14;18) chromosomal translocations in fixed tissues. *Hum Pathol* 1990;21:199.

Tang YW et al: Molecular diagnostics of infectious diseases. *Clin Chem* 1997;43:2021.

Tawa A et al: Rearrangement of the T-cell receptor beta chain gene in non-T-cell non-B-cell acute lymphoblastic leukemia of childhood. *N Engl J Med* 1985;313:1033.

Weiss LM et al: Clonal rearrangements of T-cell receptor genes in mycosis fungoides and dermatopathic lymphadenopathy. *N Engl J Med* 1985;313:539.

Weiss LM et al: Frequent immunoglobulin and T-cell receptor gene rearrangements in "histiocytic" neoplasms. *Am J Pathol* 1985;121:369.

Histocompatibility Testing

19

Lee Ann Baxter-Lowe, PhD, & Beth W. Colombe, PhD

Today most histocompatibility laboratories provide human leukocyte antigen (HLA) typing and perform a variety of tests to support allogeneic transplantation, including assays to detect humoral and cellular responses to alloantigens. HLA typing plays an important role in contemporary medicine because HLA molecules are (1) the primary targets of immune responses to allogeneic transplants, (2) critical for responses to antigenic stimuli, and (3) implicated in genetic susceptibility to autoimmune disease. During the last decade histocompatibility laboratories have developed many new techniques that have supplemented, and sometimes supplanted, conventional methods for HLA typing and other tests for compatibility.

HLA molecules were first recognized as the "major transplantation antigens" that determine compatibility of allogeneic grafts. Although these molecules were first recognized for their antigenic qualities, it is now known that HLA molecules play a pivotal role in intercellular communication with T and natural killer (NK) cells (see Chapters 4, 6, and 9).

One of the hallmarks of HLA molecules is their diversity in the human population. HLA typing detects and classifies this diversity. HLA typing emanated from observations made by scientists using an agglutination technique to study leukocyte antigens in patients who had received multiple blood transfusions. The first HLA specificities (types) were defined when statistical methods were applied to complex patterns of agglutination reactions with sera containing alloantibodies. Over the ensuing years many technical advances occurred in HLA typing, including complement-dependent lymphocytotoxicity, microlymphocytotoxicity, and molecular typing. Application of these methods has resulted in continuous discovery of novel HLA molecules, which, by 1999, surpassed 1000 officially recognized HLA alleles.

Many patients who are candidates for allogeneic transplantation have developed alloantibodies in response to foreign HLA molecules encountered from pregnancy, transfusion, or prior allografts. These antibodies can cause rejection of allogeneic organ and tissue grafts. Crossmatching was developed to detect donor-specific alloantibodies in the serum of patients who are candidates for allogeneic transplants. Use of sensitive crossmatch techniques to assess compatibility of patients and kidney donors has virtually eliminated hyperacute rejection of renal grafts and made a major contribution to improved graft and patient survival.

Current practices in histocompatibility testing for allogeneic transplantation are influenced by the organ or tissue to be transplanted as well as the transplant protocol. Although the routine tests performed by histocompatibility laboratories are fundamentally similar, the tests are often customized for each transplant program (eg, variation in the sensitivity of lymphocytotoxicity tests, the use of flow cytometric methods for detection of antibodies, and the differences in the level of resolution for HLA typing).

During the last decade, high-resolution HLA typing methods have become available that can define HLA polymorphism at an allele level. High-resolution HLA typing methods are now routinely used for selection of unrelated donors for hematopoietic stem cell transplantation and sometimes for disease association. These methods are rarely used for solid organ transplantation, in which donor limitations preclude the ability to search for well-matched unrelated donors.

This chapter describes the histocompatibility tests most frequently used today and new methods that offer potential for improved histocompatibility testing in the future. Internet sites that provide useful information about HLA polymorphism, histocompatibility, and transplantation are listed in Table 19–1.

HISTOCOMPATIBILITY TESTING FOR TRANSPLANTATION

The primary goal of pretransplant histocompatibility testing is to optimize compatibility between organ or tissue donors and recipients in order to prevent rejection of the graft and to prevent graft-versus-host disease (GvHD) for grafts that potentially transfer sufficient numbers of lymphoid cells (eg, bone marrow, liver) to cause GvHD. HLA matching between donor and recipient is desirable for allogeneic trans-

Table 19–1. Useful Websites for histocompatibility testing and transplantation.

Anthony Nolan HLA Informatics	http://www.ashi-hla.org	IMGT/HLA database; HLA sequence data; official HLA nomenclature
American Society for Histocompatibility and Immunogenetics	http://www.ashi-hla.org	Histocompatibility information for general readers and another for patients; news updates; useful links; laboratory standards
British Society for Histocompatibility and Immunogenetics	http://www.umds.ac.uk/tissue/bshil.html	Introduction to tissue typing and blood groups; laboratory standards
National Marrow Donor Program Home Page	http://www.marrow.org	Sections for patients, donors; news; information for HLA typing labs and transplant coordinators
United Network for Organ Sharing Home Page	http://www.unos.org	Information for transplant patients; transplant statistics
Immunogenetics (IMGT) database	http://www.ebi.ac.uk/imgt/hla/	HLA sequence database information, documentation, nomenclature, query tools, and submission forms for novel alleles
Sanger Centre Home Page	http://www.sanger.ac.uk/	Human genome project and related databases; chromosome 6 maps
MHCPEP	http://wehih.wehi.edu.au/mhcpep/	Database of peptides that bind to HLA molecules

Abbreviations: HLA = human leukocyte antigen; IMGT = immunogenetics.

plantation. In practice, however, the extensive polymorphism of HLA makes it difficult to locate HLA-matched donors for transplants unless an HLA-matched sibling donor exists. Based on Mendelian inheritance, 25% of offspring will inherit the same HLA type. Thus, family size influences the likelihood of having an HLA-identical sibling. In the United States approximately 30% of patients have an HLA-identical sibling donor. In contrast, in Japan approximately 12% of patients have an HLA-identical sibling donor. The majority of patients therefore require transplants from donors who are not HLA-identical (partially HLA-matched related donors or unrelated donors). Routine tests used to assess histo-

compatibility for allogeneic transplants are summarized in Table 19–2.

The method and resolution of HLA typing or tissue typing that is optimal for donor selection depends on several factors, including the extent of HLA matching required for transplant (eg, organ, transplant protocol), relationship to the recipient (ie, relative or unrelated), time constraints, and specimen characteristics (eg, cell source, quality, quantity). For example, for solid organ transplants from cadaver donors in which HLA disparity usually occurs between donor and recipient, low-resolution typing is adequate and turnaround time must be minimal. HLA matching is most important for transplantation of

Table 19–2. Selection of histocompatibility tests.

Typing Method / Transplant	Low-resolution AB	Low-resolution DR/DQ	High-resolution AB	High-resolution DR/DQ	C	DP	ABO	XM
Blood or bone marrow, sibling or related donor	U	U	R	R	R	V	V	V
Blood or bone marrow, unrelated donor	U	U	I	U	V	V	V	V
Kidney	U	U	R	R	V	R	U	U
Pancreas	U	U	R	R	V	R	U	U
Heart/lung	U	U	R	R	V	R	U	U
Liver	V	V	R	R	V	R	V	V
Cornea	V	R	R	R	V	R	R	R

Abbreviations: U = usually; V = variable, depends on transplant center practice; R = rarely; I = increasing use.

lymphohematopoietic cells. Large registries of volunteer donors are now available to locate well HLA-matched unrelated donors for patients who lack a suitably matched family donor. High-resolution molecular HLA typing is often used for evaluation of these donors. Typical HLA typing requirements are listed in Table 19–2.

Some patients have existing antibodies directed toward HLA mismatches of potential donors. These antibodies are formed after contact with foreign HLA molecules (eg, pregnancy, transfusion, transplantation). The formation of specific antibodies to alloantigens is referred to as **sensitization.** Preformed antibodies directed against mismatched antigens of the donor can cause hyperacute rejection of certain solid organ grafts and have been associated with increased rates of rejection following blood and marrow transplants. A **crossmatch** is used to test for the presence of donor-specific preformed antibodies in the patient's serum. Crossmatches can be performed using lymphocytotoxicity sometimes supplemented with more sensitive flow cytometry assays. A positive crossmatch attributable to specific antibodies toward donor HLA mismatches is considered to be a contraindication for most transplants.

Antibody screening is used to detect alloantibodies and attempt to define the specificity of alloantibodies in patients who are transplant candidates who are at risk for preformed alloantibodies. Lymphocytotoxicity is the traditional method for antibody screening, and a number of alternative methods for detecting alloantibodies have been used during recent years (eg, flow cytometry, enzyme-linked immunosorbent assay [ELISA]).

Functional assays that detect T-cell responses to alloantigens are sometimes used to supplement HLA typing. These include the mixed lymphocyte culture (MLC) and the cell-mediated lympholysis test (CML). Assays that measure the precursor frequency of helper and cytolytic T cells are available but are primarily used in research settings.

HLA POLYMORPHISM & TYPING

HLA Genetics

The genetics of the HLA system is described in detail Chapter 6. Briefly, the gene products detected by HLA typing are encoded by a cluster of related genes located in the major histocompatibility complex (MHC) on the short arm of chromosome 6 (Figure 19–1). Historically the MHC has been considered to encompass about 4 megabases that are subdivided into three regions: The class I region of approximately 2000 kilobases includes the polymorphic HLA-A, B, and C loci, the class II region of approximately 1000 kilobases includes the HLA-DR, -DQ, and -DP loci, and the class III region of approximately 1000 kilobases encodes genes with diverse functions. Recent discovery of genes that are homologous to HLA genes (eg, HFE) or that play a role in HLA function (eg, tapasin) has defined an extended MHC that spans 8 megabases. These genes are not currently included in HLA typing, but it is conceivable that certain HLA-like genes may be included in the future.

In addition to the expressed HLA genes, numerous class I and class II pseudogenes are located in the MHC. These pseudogenes provided challenges in the development of molecular typing methods because it is necessary to type the expressed genes without detecting the closely related pseudogenes. Rarely, the

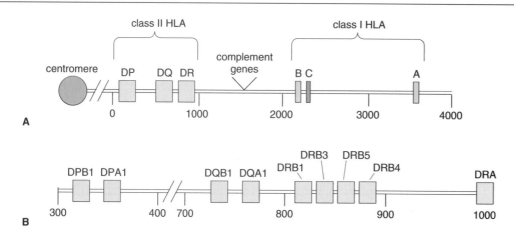

Figure 19–1. MHC genes on chromosome 6. **A:** Schematic representation of genes of the class I and II HLA regions. The region containing complement genes and genes for other factors, such as tumor necrosis factor (TNF), is indicated. **B:** Expanded view of class II HLA region showing genes for α and β chains of class II molecules. Pseudogenes have been omitted. The presence of genes for DRB3, DRB4, and DRB5 depends on the haplotype.

presence of a pseudogene can confound molecular HLA typing.

HLA Polymorphism & Nomenclature

The extensive polymorphism of HLA was initially shown by the large number of serologic specificities (types) defined by alloantibodies (Table 19–3). Functional assays suggested that a cells with the same HLA specificity could have differences that are recognized by T cells. The molecular basis for these observations was revealed by sequencing the genes encoding these antigens. This investigation demonstrated that cells with the same serologic specificity may have different amino acid sequences. By 1999, the number of known HLA alleles exceeded 1000, and the number continues to increase. The number of known alleles corresponding to particular specificity ranges from 1 to more than 50. This is demonstrated Figure 19–2, which shows the number of alleles for each HLA-A specificity that were known in October 1999.

Establishing the nomenclature for HLA alleles has been challenging because HLA is extremely polymorphic. The first sequenced alleles were assigned names with two digits that corresponded to their serologic specificity followed by two digits that indicated the chronologic order of naming by the World Health Organization (WHO) Nomenclature Committee for Factors of the HLA System. For example, the first allele sequenced from an HLA-A2 gene was named HLA-A*0201, and the second was named HLA-A*0202. Discovery of polymorphism that does not alter the protein sequence was addressed by adding from one to three numbers and a letter to names to identify synonymous (silent) mutations and polymorphism located in noncoding regions of the genes (Figure 19–3). By October 31, 1999, 40 alleles had been named in the HLA-A2 group, including 5 distinguished by silent mutations in the coding regions and 2 null alleles (no protein expressed).

Today, HLA typing may be performed by serologic typing methods that report specificities listed in Table 19–3 or molecular types that are derived from the allele names (Figure 19–3). The genetic diversity of HLA, HLA nomenclature, and use of a variety of HLA typing methods has reached such complexity that the subject is rarely understood by individuals outside the histocompatibility field.

The relationship between serologic specificities and molecular types is not always straightforward. For example, many recently discovered alleles have not been typed by serologic methods and, therefore, have no defined serologic specificity. These alleles were assigned names using homology for certain key sequences located in previously named alleles. Thus, the first two digits of a name currently considered to belong to an "allele group" rather than a particular serologic specificity. The relationship between alleles and serologic specificities is sometimes complicated

Table 19–3. HLA antigen specificities.[a]

A	B	C	DR	DQ	DP
A1	B5	Cw1	DR1	DQ1	DPw1
A2	B7	Cw2	DR103	DQ2	DPw2
A203	B703	Cw3	DR2	DQ3	DPw3
A210	B8	Cw4	DR3	DQ4	DPw4
A3	B12	Cw5	DR4	DQ5(1)	DPw5
A9	B13	Cw6	DR5	DQ6(1)	DPw6
A10	B14	Cw7	DR6	DQ7(3)	
A11	B15	Cw8	DR7	DQ8(3)	
A19	B16	Cw9(w3)	DR8	DQ9(3)	
A23(9)	B17	Cw10(w3)	DR9		
A24(9)	B18		DR10		
A2403	B21		DR11(5)		
A25(10)	B22		DR12(5)		
A26(10)	B27		DR13(6)		
A28	B35		DR14(6)		
A29(19)	B37		DR1403		
A30(19)	B38(16)		DR1404		
A31(19)	B39(16)		DR15(2)		
A32(19)	B3901		DR16(2)		
A33(19)	B3902		DR17(3)		
A34(10)	B40		DR18(3)		
A36	B4005				
A43	B41		DR51		
A66(10)	B42				
A68(28)	B44(12)		DR52		
A69(28)	B45(12)				
A74(19)	B46		DR53		
A80	B47				
	B48				
	B49(21)				
	B50(21)				
	B51(5)				
	B5102				
	B5103				
	B52(5)				
	B53				
	B54(22)				
	B55(22)				
	B56(22)				
	B57(17)				
	B58(17)				
	B59				
	B60(40)				
	B61(40)				
	B62(15)				
	B63(15)				
	B64(14)				
	B65(14)				
	B67				
	B70				
	B71(70)				
	B72(70)				
	B73				
	B75(15)				
	B76(15)				
	B77(15)				
	B7801				
	B8101				
	B8201				
	Bw4				
	Bw6				

[a] Antigens as recognized by the World Health Organization. Antigens listed in parentheses are the broad antigens; antigens followed by broad antigens in parentheses are the antigen splits. Antigens of the Dw series are omitted.

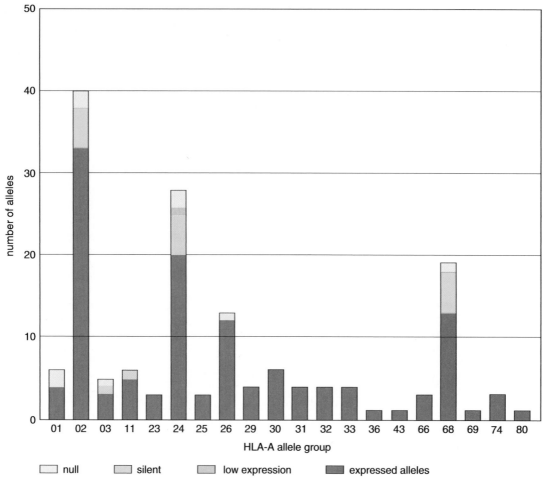

Figure 19–2. Number of HLA alleles known in 1999.

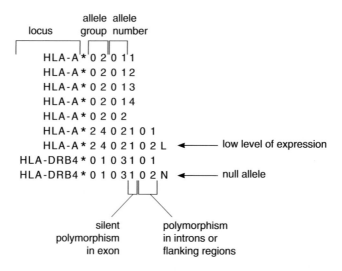

Figure 19–3. Naming of HLA alleles.

by the presence of epitopes associated with two or more serologic specificities in a single allele. Some alleles lack epitopes corresponding to the known specificities and cannot be assigned a specificity using conventional typing sera. These are called blanks. These circumstances and others confound the relationship between certain serologic specificities and molecular types. For example HLA-B*1522 is consistently typed as HLA-B35 by serologic methods. A major effort is underway to establish a correlation between known alleles and defined serologic specificities; updates of these correlations are routinely published. In practice, these relationships can be important because it is often necessary to compare molecular types for one individual with serologic specificities determined for another (eg, typing data from both methods in unrelated donor registries).

In contrast to serologic typing methods that depend on detection of epitopes that are recognized by alloantibodies, molecular HLA typing methods can detect any polymorphic nucleotide sequence. This provides the opportunity to perform typing at different levels of resolution ranging from groups of alleles to individual alleles. Typing that defines groups of alleles, usually approximating serologic specificities, is referred to as **low-resolution,** or **generic,** typing (eg, HLA-DRB1-04). Typing methods that resolve all known alleles are often referred to as **high-resolution** HLA typing (eg, HLA-DRB1*0401). Typing that resolves HLA types beyond serologic specificities but that does not achieve allele level is described as intermediate-resolution tying (eg, HLA-DRB1-0401/09/13/16/21/26/33). The National Marrow Donor Program has created codes to facilitate management of these complex intermediate resolution data. In this system, the name for HLA-DRB1-0401/09/13/16/21/26/33 is DRB1-04EJV.

Further complexity is caused by differences in molecular HLA typing methods and the continual need to update interpretation of molecular typing data as the number of known HLA alleles increases. Several molecular methods detect key polymorphic sequences and use these data to predict the allele. The interpretation of these data is influenced by the library of HLA sequences used for interpreting these data. For example, in 1987 five sequences were known for the HLA-DRB1-04 group. At that time, a probe for a polymorphic sequence at codon 71 was used to assign DRB1-0401 because this polymorphism was believed to be unique to this allele. By 1999, six additional HLA-DRB1*04 alleles had been discovered that shared this polymorphic sequence. Thus data that would have been typed as DRB1*0401 in 1987 may be interpreted as DRB1*0401, 0409, 0413, 0416, 0421, 0426, or 0433 in 1999.

There are more complicated examples in which the assignment of HLA types based on detection of key polymorphic sequences is affected by knowledge of HLA polymorphism. For example, certain reagents used to detect HLA-A-03 in 1998 would also detect HLA-A*3204, which was discovered in 1999. Thus a sample containing HLA-A*3204 might be typed as HLA-A*03 before 1998 and with appropriate adjustments in reagents, typed as HLA-A*32 after the discovery in HLA-A*3204 in 1999. Situations such as this have stimulated interest in use of automated nucleotide sequencing for molecular HLA typing because this approach minimizes the likelihood that the presence of an unknown allele will produce an HLA typing assignment.

The continual discovery of additional HLA alleles also complicates use of National Marrow Donor Program (NMDP) codes. The same molecular typing data may have different code depending on when the sample was typed because the sequence libraries used for data interpretation differed. In practice this discrepancy can be important because a potential donor that is not matched to the patient may actually be matched if a patient's allele is not included in the type because the allele was unknown at the time of the typing. One potential solution currently under investigation is to store typing data in registries as the polymorphic sequences rather than the HLA types.

Inheritance

One of the consequences of the clustering of HLA genes on chromosome 6 is that most individuals inherit a set of nonrecombined HLA alleles from each parent. These genes are codominantly expressed. Thus, if the HLA types of family members are determined, segregation of HLA types within the family can be used to construct the HLA types from each chromosome. The set of HLA alleles found on one chromosome is called a **haplotype.** Determination of haplotypes is important for identification of HLA-identical siblings because sharing of antigens from different haplotypes is common. Determining the inheritance of haplotypes within the family permits identification of HLA-identical siblings with a high degree of confidence. If haplotypes are unknown, some antigens may appear to be matched using low-resolution HLA typing but differ at high-resolution typing. This circumstance is particularly important for certain types of transplants that are strongly influenced by the extent of HLA matching (eg, bone marrow transplant).

SEROLOGIC METHODS IN HISTOCOMPATIBILITY TESTING

Serologic techniques provide one of the simplest and fastest methods for histocompatibility testing. These methods use serum that contains antibodies to HLA antigens. Anti-HLA antibodies are highly specific for the individual structural determinants that characterize the different antigens of the HLA system. Thus, when sera containing HLA antibodies are mixed with lymphocytes, the antibodies bind only to their specific target antigens (Figure 19–4).

When the antigen–antibody complex is formed on the cell surface in the presence of complement, complement activation leads to cell lysis. Thus, cell death is an indicator of the shared specificity of antigen and antibody and is a "positive" test result. Detection of this specificity between antibody and antigen provides the answer to several fundamental questions in histocompatibility testing: (1) What are the HLA antigens of a particular cell? When the antibody specificity is known, as for the HLA typing reagents, and the cell is of unknown phenotype, the positive test results with specific antisera identify the antigens of the cell. (2) Are there anti-HLA antibodies in a particular serum? When the serum is being tested for the presence of HLA antibodies, a positive test indicates antilymphocyte activity in the serum. From the pattern of positive and negative reactions with a panel of HLA-typed cells, the specificity of the antibodies may be inferred. If the patient's serum reacts with the donor cell, the two individuals are incompatible.

Thus, through an iterative process of testing serum and typing cells, HLA antigens are defined, panels of typed lymphocytes are generated, and collections of HLA typing sera of known specificity are created.

TISSUE TYPING BY THE LYMPHOCYTOTOXICITY TEST

Serologic HLA typing is accomplished by exposing the unknown cell to a battery of antisera of known HLA specificity (see Figure 19–4). The typing sera are selected to give unequivocally strong positive scores to ensure reproducibility. If the cells are killed in the presence of antiserum and complement, the cell is presumed to have the same HLA antigen as the specificity of the antibody.

Cell Isolation

Lymphocytes are the preferred cell type for serologic HLA typing, antibody screening, and crossmatching. Traditionally lymphocytes were isolated from whole peripheral blood by buoyant density gra-

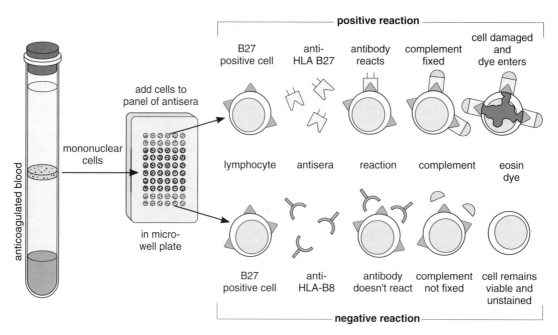

Figure 19–4. Microcytotoxicity testing for HLA antigens. Peripheral blood lymphocytes (PBLs) are isolated by Ficoll-Hypaque centrifugation and adjusted to 2×10^6 cells/mL. Then 1 μL of cells is added to each well of a tissue-typing plate that has been predispensed with a panel of HLA typing sera, each containing alloantibodies to specific HLA antigens. Illustrated are the reactions of HLA B27 cells with antisera specific for B27 (*upper*) and B8 (*lower*). B27 antibodies bind to B27 antigens on the cell surface, the antigen–antibody complex activates and fixes serum complement, the cell membrane is damaged, and the cell dies. Eosin dye penetrates the dead cells, staining them dark red under phase-contrast microscopy, giving a positive test result. In contrast, the anti-B8 antibodies do not complex with the B27 antigen, the complement components are not activated, the cells remain undamaged, and eosin dye is excluded, resulting in a negative test. The cell is thus typed as B27-positive and B8-negative. Each test well is scored as percent dead cells (see Table 19–4), and the overall reaction pattern of the typing sera is interpreted to give the HLA antigen phenotype of the individual (see Table 19–5).

dient separation, from buffy coat, or, in cadaveric testing, from lymph nodes and spleen. Care must be taken to prepare a cell suspension of excellent viability as well as one that is free of erythrocyte and platelet contamination. Although other cell types that bear HLA molecules, such as platelets, amniocytes, and fibroblasts, can be used for HLA typing in special circumstances, lymphocytes are the most responsive and reproducible target for the standard cytotoxicity assay. HLA typing for class II HLA antigens, HLA-DR and -DQ, is performed on lymphocyte preparations enriched for B lymphocytes. Special isolation procedures are required because approximately 80% of normal peripheral blood lymphocytes (PBL) are resting T cells that lack class II HLA antigens on their surface.

Isolation of T and B lymphocytes by magnetic beads is now the most common method for HLA typing and crossmatching. The antibody-coated beads offer versatility, speed of cell recovery, and relative purity of the final cell preparation. Beads with anti-CD2 or anti-CD8 are used to isolate T cells and anti-CD19 for B cells. The beads can be used to obtain adequate numbers of cells from whole blood, buffy coats, or PBL preparations. Cells with bound beads also become more sensitive as targets, possibly due to disturbance of their cell membranes, and thus tests require less incubation time than the standard cytotoxicity assays.

The Complement-Dependent Lymphocytotoxicity Test: NIH Standard Method

Individual HLA antisera are predispensed in 1-μL quantities into the microtest wells of specifically designed plastic trays composed of 60 or 72 wells of 15-μL capacity. An array of anti-HLA sera is chosen with specificities covering the full range of HLA types. Usually each type is represented by at least two antisera. Today most laboratories obtain frozen typing trays from commercial sources. Some laboratories continue to prepare batches of typing trays that are stored for use over several months or years.

For HLA typing, the sera in a test tray are thawed, approximately 2000 lymphocytes are dispensed per well, and the tray is incubated for 30 minutes at room temperature to allow anti-HLA antibodies to bind to their specific target HLA antigens. Complement (5 μL) is added, usually as rabbit serum, and the tray is incubated for another 60 minutes. The complement-dependent cytotoxicity assay for HLA-DR and -DQ typing is performed with appropriate class II typing sera but is modified as follows for B cells isolated over nylon wool: Initial incubation of cells and serum is performed at 37°C or 22°C for 60 minutes; after addition of complement, the mixture is incubated for 120 minutes at room temperature. The extended incubation times are used to promote binding of antibodies and complement. The temperature increase is used to avoid the false-positive reactions that can result from the binding of cold-reactive nonspecific antibodies. When immunoabsorbent beads are used for class II typing, the incubation times are generally decreased by approximately half, possibly because of the weakening of the cell membrane by attachment to the beads.

To visualize the dead and live cells under phase-contrast microscopy, a vital dye, eosin Y, is added, followed by formalin to fix the reaction. Live cells exclude the dye and appear bright and refractile, but dead cells take up the dye and are swollen and dark (see Figure 19–4). In an alternative method known as fluorochromasia, the cells are prelabeled with a fluorochrome such as fluorescein diacetate (green) prior to plating. When the cells are killed in the positive test, the fluorescein leaks out, and the cells "disappear." Positive results are compared with a negative well where all the cells are visible. A second fluorochrome of contrasting color such as ethidium bromide (red) may be added to visualize the dead cells.

Each test well is scored individually by inspection, with the percentage of dead cells per well being noted. The test is unequivocally positive when at least half of the cells are killed (Table 19–4).

An HLA type is assigned by interpreting the patterns of reactivity of the individual sera and their specificities. The typing sera that reacted positively with the test cells should have antibody specificities in common. For an HLA type to be assigned, the majority of sera of that specificity must be unequivocally positive. In phenotyping an individual for class I HLA, one expects to find patterns with two antigens each from the A, B, and C loci. When only a single antigen is identified at a locus, the individual may be homozygous for that type, or the laboratory has failed to identify the second antigen, because the sera may not contain antibodies for the epitopes present on the target cells or there is low expression of the HLA molecules. Table 19–5 shows a representation of a subset of HLA-typing test results.

Serologic Typing Reagents

An ideal HLA-typing serum should be monospecific, that is, would have specificity for a single HLA antigen; however, in reality, the observed alloanti-

Table 19–4. Scoring the lymphocytotoxicity test for HLA typing.

% Dead Lymphocytes in Test Well	Score	Interpretation
0–10	1	Negative
11–20	2	Doubtful positive
21–50	4	Weak positive
51–80	6	Positive
81–100	8	Strong positive

Table 19–5. An example of HLA typing test results.[a]

Serum Name	Specificities	Score
A-001	A1	1
A-002	A1, A36	1
A-003	A1, A11	1
A-004	A2	1
A-005	A2, A28	6
A-006	A2, A28, B7	8
A-007	A3	8
A-008	A3	6
A-009	A3, A10, A11, A19	8
A-010	A11	1
A-011	A10, A11	1
A-012	A11, A1, A3 (weak)	4
B-001	B51, B52, B35	1
B-002	B51, B52	1
B-003	B51, B52, B53	1
B-004	B7, B42	8
B-005	B7, B27	8
B-006	B7, B55	8
B-007	B8	1
B-008	B8, B59	2
B-009	B44, B45, B21	6
B-010	B44, B45	8
B-011	B44	8
B-012	B45	1

[a] Interpretation: HLA phenotype is: A28, A3, B7, B44.

bodies in a single serum are usually polyspecific. An alloantiserum can contain antibodies to multiple determinants on the immunizing antigen(s). Some determinants are the classic HLA **private** specificities that characterize each HLA type (see Table 19–3). Others are **public,** that is, are shared by several antigens that collectively constitute a cross-reacting antigen group (CREG group). Some complex sera can be rendered monospecific by dilution, whereas others lose all activity for all specificities simultaneously.

To determine the specificities of HLA antibodies, sera are tested against panels of cells of known HLA phenotype, a process termed "screening." The cell panel, usually from 40 to 60 cells, is preselected to provide a minimum of two to three representations of the most frequent HLA antigens. The antigens must be distributed among the cells so that the reaction pattern for one antigen is not entirely included within the pattern for a second antigen; for example, all of the HLA-A1 cells must not also be the only HLA-B8 cells. If they were, the reaction patterns for both antibodies would be identical and the determination of A1 or B8, or both, could not be made with certainty. When the sera react with a subset of the panel, the specificity of the antibody is deduced by inspecting the HLA phenotypes of the positive cells.

The majority of HLA antisera are complex sera obtained from multiparous women. Maternal exposure to the mismatched paternal HLA antigens in the fetus gives rise to a polyclonal antibody response that frequently results in sera with multiple specificities. Consequently, several different antisera are used to

type for a specific antigen. It is not unusual for a laboratory to use typing trays composed of more than 200 different sera to type a single individual for HLA-A, -B, -C, and -DR, -DQ antigens.

Placental fluid, a mixture of serum and tissue fluids, has proved to be a valuable second source of alloantisera for tissue typing. Antibodies of high titer can be recovered from the fluid shed from fresh placentae that have been refrigerated for 24 hours after delivery.

HLA antibodies are also found in the sera of patients exposed to HLA antigens through transfusions of blood and organ grafts. Generally, patients are not used as sources of HLA-typing sera, since the quantities obtainable would be limited by their medical conditions.

Attempts to immunize other animals, such as rabbits, for production of HLA antisera have largely failed. The xenoantisera reacted primarily with common human antigens such as the HLA-DR constant region. Efforts in numerous laboratories have produced monoclonal antibodies to certain HLA specificities. It was hoped that hybridoma cell lines (see Chapter 15) would produce inexhaustible quantities of monospecific antibodies to HLA antigens. In reality, many murine monoclonal antibodies have been directed against human monomorphic framework determinants or to common epitopes rather than to the private polymorphic determinants of the individual HLA antigens. Unfortunately, most murine monoclonal antibodies do not fix complement. Noncomplement-fixing antibodies can be used in assays that require only antigen binding, such as ELISA (Chapter 15) and flow cytometry (Chapter 16). Many monoclonal antibodies are reactive with more than one HLA specificity, consistent with the existence of common antigenic determinants on HLA molecules.

As use of molecular HLA typing has increased, serum screening efforts have diminished. A small number of laboratories currently maintain serum screening programs. New methods for producing monoclonal antibodies may be used for preparation of serologic typing reagents if serologic typing is not supplanted by molecular typing methods. The majority of histocompatibility laboratories currently use molecular methods for HLA-DR and -DQ typing, and the use of molecular methods for class I typing is increasing each year. The ease, speed, and technical similarity to crossmatch tests are factors that favor continuation of serologic HLA typing. Another strength of serologic typing methods is that expression of the HLA molecules is determined.

Variability in Serologic Typing Results

HLA-typing sera are not uniform because the complexity of HLA polymorphism and scarcity of the defining antisera make it impossible to create a standard reagent for each specificity. Each tissue-typing laboratory has the responsibility of obtaining the appropriate antisera and monitoring their performance (including commercial products). Results with the laboratory's routine typing trays may be compared with those of other collections of sera for confirmation of an HLA phenotype. All tissue-typing laboratories are required by the standards set by the American Society for Histocompatibility and Immunogenetics (ASHI) to control the quality of serologic and cellular reagents used for clinical testing (see Table 19–1). International and national quality control programs are available for typing, crossmatching, and serum analysis, and satisfactory performance is mandatory for ASHI accreditation of the laboratory.

A second variable in tissue typing is the serum complement, a reagent commercially available as the pooled serum from several hundred rabbits. Rabbit serum contains heterophile antibodies with antihuman lymphocyte activity that enhances its effectiveness in the cytotoxicity assay. Overabundance of these antihuman antibodies render the complement innately cytotoxic and therefore produces false-positive results. As with typing sera, each laboratory must screen its source of complement to find one that promotes strong cytotoxic reactions without causing nonspecific toxicity. Because there is no standard complement source, the same serum tested in different laboratories has the potential to yield disparate results.

Other variables are the method used to visualize the live and dead cells, incubation times, and the definition of the end of the test period. Table 19–6 illustrates the type of reaction patterns obtained on reagent or patient serum screens.

ANTIBODY SCREENING

Antibody screening is used to detect the presence of HLA antibodies in patients who are candidates for transplant. Screening has traditionally been performed using complement-dependent lymphocytotoxicity methods. Most laboratories perform monthly screens for patients on waiting lists for solid organ donors. Sera from each patient are tested for the presence of antibodies against a panel of cells that contain the most frequent HLA types in the donor population present in several different HLA-A and -B combinations (or DR and DQ for class II) to allow determination of the specificities of alloantibodies. The format may be designed as a batch test for all patients or a test for a single patient.

The percent panel reactive antibody (PRA) is calculated as the ratio of the number of positive cells to the number of total panel cells multiplied by 100. PRA is indicative of the extent of sensitization of the patient to HLA. Note that the antibody specificities of sera with high PRA cannot be determined. Special procedures must be used, such as dilution or treatment of the sera, or both, to determine antibody specificities.

HLA Antibody Screening by the ELISA Method

A rapid and highly sensitive solid-phase method for the detection of antibodies to HLA has been commercially developed using the ELISA technique. Purified preparations of HLA antigens affixed to plastic plates are used to capture anti-HLA antibodies in patient sera, thereby avoiding the use of whole cells with their complex array of surface markers. False-positive reactions due to antibody binding to non-HLA antigens is avoided with the use of this technology. Affinity-purified HLA antigens are isolated from platelets or from lymphoblastoid cell lines, pooled, and fixed to the bottom of test wells in a plastic test plate. Antigens derived from platelets are HLA class I only, whereas antigens from cell lines may be class I, class II, or a combination of both types of antigens. Advantages of the ELISA assay over conventional lymphocyte panel testing by cytotoxicity include the ease of rapid batch processing via automated plate readers and the elimination of the need for viable lymphocytes and complement for the assay.

An aliquot of the patient's serum is incubated in the test well where any HLA-reactive antibody of appropriate avidity binds to the fixed antigen. After removal of unbound antibody, an enzyme-linked antibody that is directed against human IgG is added. Addition of enzyme substrate develops positive tests. The readout of the basic ELISA antibody test is either positive (antibody present) or negative (antibody absent). No PRA can be calculated, nor can specificity be assigned to the antibody. Further testing with standard lymphocyte panels (or with newly developed flow cytometry methods, see section on HLA Antibody Detection by Flow Cytometry) is necessary to obtain these parameters. The ELISA test is formulated to detect only IgG, the HLA antibody iso-

Table 19–6. An example of results of serum screening for class I HLA antibodies.[a]

Panel Cell HLA Antigens	Cytotoxicity Test Score for Patient Serum Number				
	1	2	3	4	5
A, A, B, B (locus)					
1, 2, 7, 60	1	1	8	1	8
2, 3, 8, 51	1	8	8	8	8
3, 29, 35, 44	1	8	1	6	8
30, 33, 55, 60	1	1	1	1	8
1, 30, 13, 51	1	1	1	8	8
24, 28, 35, 55	1	1	4	6	4
3, 28, 7, 44	1	8	4	1	6
2, 28, 35, 38	1	1	8	8	8

[a] PRA (panel-reactive antibody) was 0, 38, 50, 63, and 100%, for patient sera 1 through 5, respectively. PRA is calculated as (number of positive tests/number of cells tested) × 100. Analyzed antibodies were as follows (patient sera 1 through 5, respectively): None; A3; A2, weak A28; B51; B35; and Unknown (autoantibody?).

type that is considered to be the most deleterious to solid organ transplant outcome. Consequently, standard ELISA cannot detect cytotoxic IgM and non-HLA antibodies and detects noncomplement-fixing IgG antibodies that cytotoxicity assays miss. ELISA may fail to detect an antibody with specificity for a rare HLA antigen that may be absent or at low levels in the antigen pool. Recently, ELISA products have been developed to provide antibody identification and PRA capability, and an IgM-specific second antibody is available.

Antibody Detection (PRA) by Flow Cytometry

Antibodies binding to non-HLA cell surface antigens can generate false-positive results in both the standard complement-dependent lymphocytotoxicity assay and the flow cytometry crossmatch test, both of which are routinely used to detect antibodies to HLA antigens. A recent product for general HLA antibody detection (measurement of PRA) takes advantage of the additional sensitivity afforded by the flow cytometer. Microbeads are coated with HLA antigens extracted from a cell panel of HLA-typed cell lines. The beads are available with either purified HLA class I or class II HLA antigens or as a mixture of both. The class II particles are distinguishable from the class I particles by fluorescence, making it possible to detect both types of antibody in a single flow cytometer run. The microparticles are incubated with the patient's serum and then stained with an anti-human IgG-fluorescent conjugate that binds to those IgG- anti-HLA antibodies that formed a complex with the beads. The percentage of the beads that stain above background provides a measure of the patient's PRA. This assay can measure noncomplement-fixing HLA antibody but is limited to antibodies of the IgG isotype. Other isotype-specific anti-human Ig conjugates can be used if detection of, for example, IgM HLA antibodies is desired. An additional product of coated microbeads offers several separate bead panels of HLA class I and class II antigens that allow characterization of the specificity of the antibody detected. In addition to the measurement of PRA, the microspheres can be used as a diagnostic test to confirm that the antibody detected by the cell-based assays is indeed anti-HLA. This information can be critical to the decision to transplant in the event of an equivocal positive crossmatch.

CROSSMATCHING

The purpose of the crossmatch test is to detect the presence of antibodies in the patient's serum that are directed against the HLA antigens of the potential donor. If present, the antibodies signal that the immune system of the recipient has been sensitized to donor antigen(s) and is primed to vigorously reject any graft bearing the antigen(s). In the transplanted kidney, the main target of these antibodies is probably the HLA antigens on vascular endothelium of capillaries and arterioles. HLA antigen-antibody complexes on endothelium activate complement and lead to cell damage. Platelets then aggregate, eventually producing fibrin clots, which clog the vessels and cause ischemic necrosis. Even weak, low-titer antibodies, particularly those directed against class I antigens, can contribute to graft rejection. The ultimate goal of the crossmatch is a test of both great sensitivity and specificity for HLA antigens.

PBL Lymphocytotoxicity Crossmatching

A simple crossmatch by the standard cytotoxicity method (see earlier discussion) may be performed with donor PBL as targets. PBL crossmatches are usually included in the preliminary evaluation of potential living related donors for renal graft recipients. PBL are normally about 80% T cells, which carry class I HLA antigens only, and 20% B cells and monocytes, which bear both class I and class II antigens. A strongly positive crossmatch by cytotoxicity (50% or more cell death per well) clearly indicates the presence of antibodies to class I antigens. However, 10–20% cell killing could result from an antibody specific for class II or could be due to a weak anticlass I antibody. To resolve the specificity of the antibody, crossmatching is then performed on cell preparations enriched for either T or B lymphocytes.

T-Cell Lymphocytotoxicity Crossmatching

T-cell crossmatches depicted in Figure 19–5 are performed at room temperature and also at 37°C in some laboratories to avoid the binding of cold-reactive antibodies, presumed to be autoreactive. A positive T-cell crossmatch by any method contraindicates transplantation, no matter how weak the reaction level; that is, a reaction of 4+ (20–50% dead cells per well above background) is considered just as positive a result as 6+ or 8+ (51% dead cells or greater). Some laboratories even consider a reaction of 2 (10–20% dead over background) as a positive crossmatch result.

Several methods to improve the sensitivity of T-cell crossmatches by complement-dependent cytotoxicity have been developed. These include

1. Extended incubation—The simplest modification in the cytotoxicity assay to increase sensitivity is to extend the incubation time of cells, serum, and complement.

2. The Amos wash step—This method interjects a wash step after the incubation of cells and serum and prior to the addition of complement to remove anticomplementary factors in the serum.

3. Antihuman globulin—The cytotoxicity of some antibodies may be enhanced by the addition of a second-step antibody, usually a polyclonal antihuman immunoglobulin (AHG) reagent.

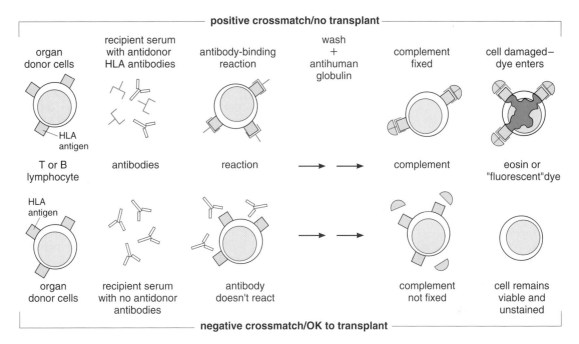

positive crossmatch/no transplant

negative crossmatch/OK to transplant

Figure 19–5. Lymphocytotoxicity T-cell crossmatch test for compatibility between recipient and donor. 1 µL of recipient serum is plated into multiple wells of a microtest plate. For sensitized patients, multiple sera of known panel reactive antibody (PRA) are plated. Donor T cells (2–3 × 10^6) are added, and the test is incubated for 30–60 minutes. To increase sensitivity of the test, the sera are washed from the wells before complement is added, leaving the cells behind. The addition of a second, developing antibody such as goat antihuman IgG (AHG) increases the sensitivity further. After several minutes of incubation with AHG, complement is added and the test incubated for another 60 minutes. A long complement incubation of up to 3 hours is sometimes performed instead of AHG addition. If the recipient serum contains antibodies that react with donor cells, the cells are killed and penetrated by dyes such as eosin or ethidium bromide, indicating a positive crossmatch. A positive serologic T-cell crossmatch is a contraindication to transplantation.

B-Cell Lymphocytotoxicity Crossmatching

Crossmatching for antibodies to class II HLA antigens requires the use of B lymphocytes as targets and the same extended incubation times as HLA-DR and -DQ serologic typing for nylon-wool isolated B cells. A positive B-cell crossmatch may result from antibodies binding to class I or class II HLA antigens. Moreover, B cells are a more sensitive indicator for weak class I antibodies because they carry class I molecules in greater density than T cells. Crossmatching by flow cytometry can readily distinguish between "true B" antibodies and weak class I antibodies of a positive B-cell cytotoxicity crossmatch. The significance for transplant outcome of preformed antibodies to class II antigens is not yet clear. Successful transplantation into patients with low-titer anticlass II antibodies (titer of 1:1 or 1:2) has been reported, as has the acute rejection of grafts transplanted in the face of high-titer (1:8) antibodies. It is possible that the loss of grafts transplanted in the face of T-negative, B-positive crossmatches is due to the anticlass I component of these alloreactive sera.

Flow-Cytometry Crossmatching

Cross-matching by flow cytometry (FCC) (see Chapter 16) has been shown to be 30–250 times more sensitive than visual serologic methods for the detection of IgG HLA antibodies on lymphocytes (Figure 19–6). In this crossmatching application, T cells can be separated from B cells electronically through the use of a fluoresceinated antibody to a T-cell surface antigen such as the CD3 T-cell receptor complex. An electronic "gate" can be created so that only the fluorescently labeled T cells are selected. Donor lymphocytes are incubated with patient's serum to allow binding of any antidonor antibodies. Antibody bound to the selected T-cell population is detected by addition of an antihuman IgG anti-Fc-specific F(ab′)$_2$ antibody labeled with a fluorochrome of a different color from the T-cell marking antibody (eg, green, if the anti-CD3 was red). The flow cytometer counts the number of labeled T cells and creates a histogram displaying the number of cells versus fluorescence intensity (see Figure 19–6). Unlabeled cells lie near the origin, and labeled cells lie

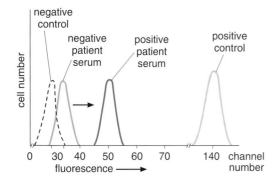

serum	mean channel number	channel shift
negative control	27	—
negative patient	33	6
positive patient	50	23
positive control	140	113

Figure 19–6. Flow cytometry crossmatch (FCC) with patient serum and donor T cells. A schematic composite tracing of an FCC fluorescence histogram illustrating representative peak positions for a negative and positive T-cell FCC in relation to negative and positive control peaks. Peaks represent the number of cells (*y*-axis) at a given fluorescence level (*x*-axis) expressed as channel numbers. Donor lymphocytes are incubated with patient serum, and then a fluorescein isothiocyanate-labeled antihuman immunoglobulin is added, which fluorescently labels donor T cells that have bound patient antibody. When compared with the peak of T cells having no antibody bound, the fluorescent T-cell peak is brighter and shifted to the right on the *x*-axis. When the mean channel fluorescence of the T-cell peak shifts to the right by more than 10 channels on a 256-channel scale, the crossmatch is considered to be positive.

to the right of the origin on the *x*-axis. A shift to the right of the T-cell peak in the experimental test compared with the negative control indicates that anticlass I HLA antibody from the patient serum has bound to the donor T cells. FCCs can also be performed on gated B cells labeled with a B-cell-specific antibody.

FCC is generally performed with the most recent serum and a selection of historically reactive sera for all patients who are on the waiting list for cadaver donors and who have increased risk of rejection (eg, rejected prior transplants, high PRA, living related donors with a negative T-cell and positive B-cell serologic crossmatch).

Occasionally, positive FCC crossmatches occur when both the serologic T- and B-cell crossmatches are negative. The indications for transplant remain controversial. Two possible explanations for these observations are the presence of HLA antibodies that are not cytotoxic or the presence of blocking antibodies that interfere with testing. One alternative for fur-

ther testing is use of HLA-bound beads (described earlier) to clarify the presence of HLA-specific antibodies. Clinical decisions concerning transplantation of the patient can then be made including this finding.

Crossmatching for Autoantibodies

In crossmatching patient serum for donor compatibility, it is most important to distinguish nonspecific antilymphocyte antibodies, referred to as autoantibodies, from the specific antidonor antibodies. The presence of autoantibodies is detected by the autocrossmatch, in which the patient's own serum and cells are combined in the standard cytotoxicity test. Autoantibodies can give a false-positive result in a donor crossmatch, leading to the erroneous disqualification of that donor. Alternatively, preexisting autoantibodies can mask the presence of specific antidonor antibodies. Autoantibody crossmatches are routinely performed in conjunction with all living-donor crossmatches for each serum that is tested. Auto FCC crossmatches are also recommended, particularly in the case of a negative serologic crossmatch coupled with an unexpectedly positive FCC. False-positive FCCs can occur when the patient has autoantibodies of undetermined specificity. Such autoantibody-positive FCCs are not considered to be a contraindication to transplantation.

HISTOCOMPATIBILITY TESTING BY MOLECULAR-BIOLOGIC METHODS

Introduction

The serologic specificities have been identified through the binding patterns of antibodies in serologic tests and from the activation of lymphocytes by disparate MHC antigens in the mixed lymphocyte culture (MLC) test. With the advent of gene cloning and DNA sequencing, HLA antigen specificities are now known to derive from sequence differences localized to several hypervariable regions in the MHC molecules. Most of the differences have arisen from intragene and intergene conversion events that have resulted in the complex polymorphism that characterizes the HLA system. In the HLA class II genes, the variable regions are found mainly in exon 2 and in class I genes; the polymorphisms are concentrated in exons 2 and 3. These variations in sequence are localized in the antigen-binding cleft and to the alpha-helical regions facing the T-cell receptor, locations strategic to the ability of the immune system to recognize and respond to pathogenic (and possibly autoimmunogenic) endogenous and exogenous antigens.

HLA alleles share many of the same sequence motifs but in different combinations. Consequently, HLA class I and class II antigens can be thought of as a patchwork of combinations of these various sequence polymorphisms occurring on a background of shared (consensus) nucleotide base sequences. The long-observed phenomenon of crossreactivity of anti-sera and, more recently, the cross-hybridization of oligonucleotide probes, can be explained by the fact that several antigens can share the same sequence motifs. For example, the concept of the "public" (ie, held in common) HLA antigen specificity, such as antigens Bw4 and Bw6 that are associated with all HLA B locus specificities, is confirmed by finding a polymorphic amino acid sequence located at residues 77–83 in all B locus antigen sequences. An even greater degree of sharing of specific polymorphic sequences takes place among the class I alleles, even occurring across the class I loci, making typing for class I alleles more technically demanding than for class II alleles. An important consequence of these shared sequence motifs is that certain heterozygous combinations of alleles cannot always be distinguished from a second, different combination. All DNA typing methods must take this into consideration when proposing schema for allele identification. Clearly, the most definitive HLA typing method would be to carry out a complete sequence analysis of the DNA of the HLA genes of each individual. Automated nucleotide sequencing is currently regarded as the gold standard for HLA typing, but this technology is currently limited to laboratories that support hematopoietic stem cell transplant programs that frequently use unrelated donors.

Table 19–7 compares major features of molecular and serologic typing methods. Molecular typing methods offer several advantages over serologic methods, including improved accuracy, higher resolution, and specimen flexibility. Molecular typing methods can be particularly advantageous for typing samples containing HLA molecules that are in the same cross-reactive group. Several publications document the clinical benefits of molecular typing that have been attributed to improved accuracy or higher resolution typing. The sequence data provided by molecular methods along with knowledge of the structure and function of HLA are currently being used to better understand the molecular basis for allorecognition and HLA-associated diseases.

Molecular Typing Methods

The first molecular typing method detected restriction fragment length polymorphism (RFLP) in genomic DNA and was primarily used for class II HLA typing. A few reports also described the use of sequence-specific oligonucleotide probe (SSOP) hybridization to RNA templates. After the discovery of the polymerase chain reaction (PCR), several easier and more powerful molecular typing methods were rapidly developed. The first used SSOP hybridization to amplify templates. This was followed by typing by sequence-specific priming (SSP), which relies on the specificity of the amplification to determine HLA types. The most recent development has been sequence-based typing (SBT), which takes advantage of automated nucleotide sequencing. These methods are summarized in Table 19–8.

Table 19–7. Comparison of HLA typing methods: DNA-based and serologic.

Method	Serologic	DNA:SSP/SSOP	DNA:SBT
Number of identifiable types			
HLA-A	21	21–151	151
HLA-B	43	43–301	301
HLA-C	10	10–83	83
HLA-DR	18	18–282	282
HLA-DQ	9	9–43	43
HLA-DP	—	6–87	87
Sample material	2–3 million live lymphocytes	Minute amount of DNA	Minute amount of DNA
Reagents	Alloantisera (supply exhaustible) some monoclonals	Synthetic oligonucleotide primers/probes (supply unlimited)	Synthetic digonudeo tide primers (supply unlimited)
Power to identify new alleles	Very limited: depends on availability and specificity of sera	Limited: based on knowledge of sequences and on novel reaction patterns	Unlimited: new alleles identified by their sequences
Level of resolving power for known alleles	Generic level	Generic to allele level	Allele level
Important factors	Expression of HLA on cell surface Viability of test cells	Quality and quantity of genomic DNA and amplification factors Stringency of test conditions	Quality and quantity of genomic DNA and amplification factors

Abbreviations: SSP/SSOP = sequence-specific priming/sequence-specific oligonucleotide probing; SBT = sequence-based typing; HLA = human leukocyte antigen; PCR = polymerase chain reaction.

Table 19–8. Molecular histocompatibility testing techniques.

Name	Characteristic Reagents	Characteristic Processes	Polymorphisms Detected
RFLP	Bacterial restriction endonucleases	Southern blotting	Restriction fragment length
SSP	Sequence-specific PCR primers	PCR/gel electrophoresis	Generic to allele-level
SSOP	Sequence-specific oligonucleotide probes	PCR/hybridization of probes to PCR product	Generic to allele-level
SBT	Labeled primers/labeled sequence terminators	PCR/nucleotide sequencing of PCR product	Allele-level
Heteroduplex analysis RSCA	Denatured, single-strand DNA/Artificial universal hetero-duplex generator (UHG)	Reannealing of strands of DNA/electrophoresis of recombined DNA	DNA complexes characteristic of alleles

Abbreviations: RFLP = restriction fragment-length polymorphism; SSP = sequence-specific priming; SSOP = sequence-specific oligonucleotide probing; SBT = sequence-based typing; PCR = polymerase chain reaction; HLA = human leukocyte antigen; RSCA = Reference Strand Conformational Analysis.

Gene Amplification

The majority of molecular HLA typing methods use PCR to selectively amplify the segments of HLA genes that are required for typing. The specificity of the amplification can be **locus-specific** (eg, HLA-A, HLA-B, HLA-DRB1), **group-specific** (eg, DRB1-01, DRB1-02), or **allele-specific** (eg, DRB1-0401, DRB1*0402). For PCR, the specificity is determined by the sequence of the primers and amplification conditions (eg, thermal cycling, [Mg^{2+}]). Most typing schemes require conditions that avoid coamplification of pseudogenes.

SSP Typing

One of the most frequently used molecular typing methods takes advantage of sequence-specific priming (SSP), which is depicted in Figure 19–7. Primer pairs are designed to specifically amplify each polymorphic sequence that must be detected to provide the desired level of typing resolution. A primer pair that amplifies a different segment of DNA is usually included in the same tube as a positive control. Target DNA is added to a tube containing the primers and the other reaction components (eg, DNA polymerase, buffer, Mg^{2+}), and thermal cycling is performed. PCR products are usually detected by separating the amplified DNA on an agarose gel. After electrophoresis, the DNA is stained (eg, ethidium bromide), and the reaction is scored for the presence of the product of the internal control primers and the presence or absence of the HLA-specific product.

The combination of positive and negative HLA reactions is used to assign the HLA type. If no HLA-specific products and no internal control products are present, the reaction is scored as a failure and must be repeated. The number of primers included in the test varies according to the locus and level of resolution required. For a low-resolution HLA-DRB typing, typically about 20–30 reactions are needed; for an ABC typing usually about 100–200 reactions are required. Sets of typing primers are currently provided by several commercial vendors. As the number of known HLA alleles increases, the minimum number of reactions required for SSP typing also increases. Variations on this method include use of multiplex PCR and different techniques for detecting positive reactions (eg, hybridization with labeled probes).

The major advantages of this method are that equipment requirements are minimal, the time required for testing is short, and it is fairly easy to learn. Major disadvantages are requirements for a large number of reactions and for high-purity DNA to ensure that reaction specificity is not compromised. One weakness in the formats that are currently in use is that the HLA typing primers are not internally controlled. Thus, a false-negative result can be obtained if the internal control (a different primer pair) is positive, but the HLA-specific primers are dysfunctional. Although it is theoretically possible to construct more appropriate internal controls, to date, this has not been accomplished.

SSOP Typing

Sequence-specific oligonucleotide probe hybridization was the first PCR-based HLA typing method. This method involves the selective amplification of the HLA target followed by hybridization to a panel of oligonucleotide probes. The two most frequently used formats are depicted in Figure 19–8: (1) dot or slot blots with amplified DNA bound to a solid support (eg, membrane) and hybridized to probes in solution and (2) reverse dot or slot blots with probes bound to a solid support hybridized to amplified DNA in solution. The dot blot format is favorable for typing large numbers of samples. Some high-volume laboratories use this approach for typing batches of 96 or 384 samples. The reverse dot blot is favorable for testing small numbers of samples. In general, if the number of probes exceeds the number of sam-

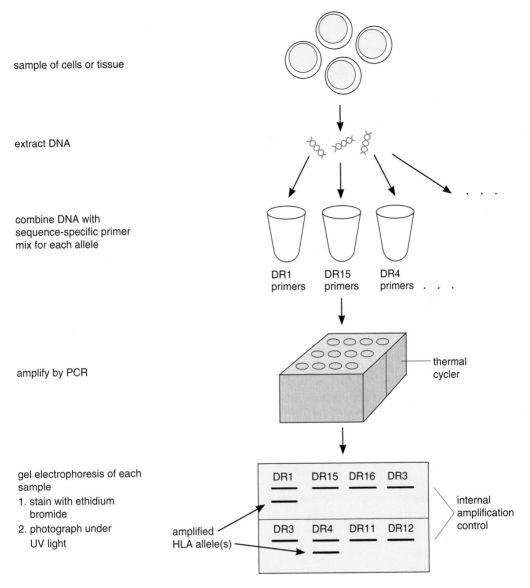

sample of cells or tissue

extract DNA

combine DNA with
sequence-specific primer
mix for each allele

DR1 primers   DR15 primers   DR4 primers . . .

amplify by PCR

thermal cycler

gel electrophoresis of each sample
1. stain with ethidium bromide
2. photograph under UV light

amplified HLA allele(s)

DR1   DR15   DR16   DR3

DR3   DR4   DR11   DR12

internal amplification control

Figure 19–7. Typing for HLA class II by sequence-specific priming (SSP). DNA is extracted from the specimen (cells, tissue) and mixed with primers having specificity for the sequences characteristic of each type. Aliquots of the sample are placed in separate tubes, each containing a specific primer set, and amplified in the thermal cycler. The amplified products are electrophoresed and the gels stained with ethidium bromide and photographed under UV light. The presence of the band indicates that the sample DNA had the sequence corresponding to the particular HLA type. No amplification implies the absence of that particular allelic sequence in the sample DNA. All tubes contain an additional primer to serve as a control on PCR amplification. This sample types as DR1, DR4 by SSP.

ples, the reverse dot blot is most efficient, and if the number of samples exceeds the number of probes, the reverse dot blot is most efficient.

Reagents for dot/slot blots are commercially available or made by individual laboratories. Typically 1–5 μL of amplified DNA from each sample is applied to nylon membranes using a manifold with dots or slots. Certain high-volume procedures transfer less than 2 μL of amplified DNA directly to the membrane without use of a manifold. Probes can be synthesized by standard methods or purchased in HLA typing kits that are available from several vendors. In 1999, the approximate minimum number of probes required for low-resolution typing was 30 for HLA-A, 60 for HLA-B, and 30 for DRB1. After hybridization with probes, the membranes are washed to re-

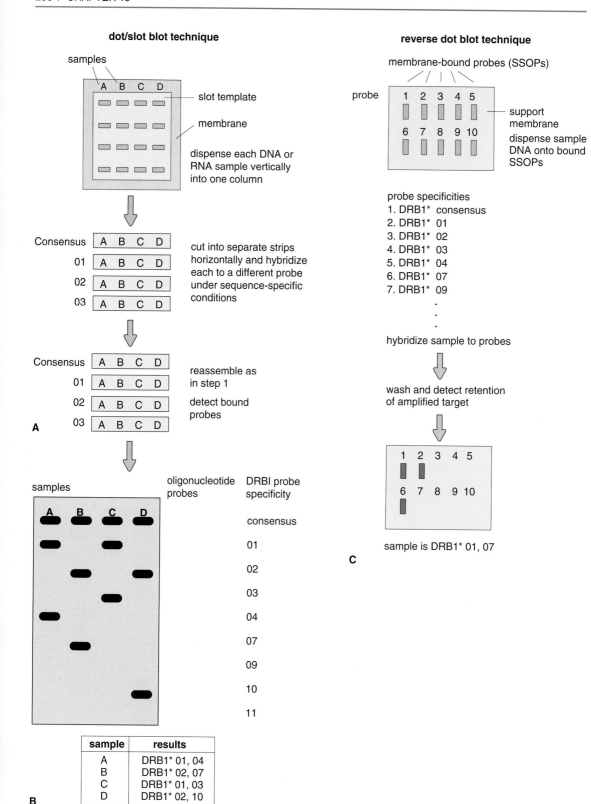

dot/slot blot technique

samples

A B C D

— slot template

— membrane

dispense each DNA or RNA sample vertically into one column

Consensus A B C D
01 A B C D
02 A B C D
03 A B C D

cut into separate strips horizontally and hybridize each to a different probe under sequence-specific conditions

Consensus A B C D
01 A B C D
02 A B C D
03 A B C D

reassemble as in step 1

detect bound probes

A

samples

A B C D

oligonucleotide probes

DRBI probe specificity

consensus

01

02

03

04

07

09

10

11

sample	results
A	DRB1* 01, 04
B	DRB1* 02, 07
C	DRB1* 01, 03
D	DRB1* 02, 10

B

reverse dot blot technique

membrane-bound probes (SSOPs)

probe

1 2 3 4 5

6 7 8 9 10

— support membrane

dispense sample DNA onto bound SSOPs

probe specificities
1. DRB1* consensus
2. DRB1* 01
3. DRB1* 02
4. DRB1* 03
5. DRB1* 04
6. DRB1* 07
7. DRB1* 09
.
.
.

hybridize sample to probes

wash and detect retention of amplified target

1 2 3 4 5

6 7 8 9 10

sample is DRB1* 01, 07

C

Figure 19–8. HLA typing by sequence-specific oligonucleotide probes. **A:** Samples of DNA (or RNA) (A, B, C, or D) are dotted directly onto a support membrane by using a slotted template (the slot blot). Replicates of a single sample are placed into a single column of slots. After all samples have been dispensed, the membrane is cut horizontally into

move nonspecifically bound probes. Labels attached to the probe are detected (eg, chemiluminescence, enzymatic methods with colorimetric detection, radioactivity), and the patterns of positive and negative hybridization are used to assign HLA types. One major advantage of this format is that positive and negative controls can be included for each probe.

Reverse dot blots require a substantial investment to develop conditions that maintain sequence specificity for a large number of probes under the same hybridization and wash conditions. This format is therefore generally limited to use of commercial products. Initially the probes were applied as dots, and more recently some companies apply the probes in lines. In this format, reading the type is analogous to reading a bar code.

Several variations of the SSOP format have been reported. One method uses probes bound to the bottom of 96-well trays, and hybridization of amplified DNA to the probes is detected using ELISA methods. This variation of the reverse dot blot provides an opportunity to include positive and negative controls for each probe and takes advantage of automated systems for ELISA methods.

SBT

Sequence-based HLA typing involves determining the nucleotide sequence of an amplified segment of an HLA gene. This is usually accomplished using an automated nucleotide sequencer. Briefly, the HLA gene segment is amplified, the excess nucleotides and primers are removed, the amplified DNA is used as a template for a sequencing reaction, and the products of the sequencing reactions are purified and applied to a sequencing gel.

Sequencing reactions contain a mixture of normal and modified nucleotides (dideoxynucleotides) that terminate polymerization when they are incorporated into the replicating strand of DNA. A primer is used to initiate DNA synthesis using DNA polymerase. When a dideoxynucleotide is incorporated into the new DNA molecule, the polymerization is terminated. Thus, primer extension products are generated that are terminated at every position of the DNA molecule. Fluorescent labels are used to distinguish chains terminated by each base (A, C, G, or T). The labels are incorporated using a dye-labeled primer (dye primer chemistry) or dye-labeled dideoxynucleotide terminators (dye terminator chemistry).

Custom dye primers can be purchased in kits or obtained by custom synthesis (expensive). Another alternative is to use PCR primers that contain a tail that can be hybridized to a labeled primer. Drawbacks of dye primer chemistry include detection of premature termination products, which can cause substantial problems during interpretation of the sequencing data, and cumbersome set up (four reactions per sequence). These problems are eliminated by using dye-labeled dideoxyterminators that are insensitive to premature termination products because these are unlabeled and therefore not detected by the sequencer. Dye-terminator reactions are performed in a single tube (Figure 19–9). One disadvantage of the dye–terminator method is that the signal from the dye-labeled products can be significantly decreased by the presence of primers and nucleotide remaining from the PCR reactions (present in unpurified template). Early dye-labeled primer chemistries suffered from variable peak heights caused by enzymatic differences in nucleotide incorporation. This is now minimized with new enzymes that reduce discrimination against dideoxynucleotides (eg, AmpliTaq, FS which has a point mutation in the active site).

The primer extension products are separated on a gel that resolves single base differences in DNA (or sequencing gels). The gel is run in an automated sequencer that usually contains a laser that excites the dye molecules and a detector that records the emissions from each dye. Software converts the primary data into a chromatogram format and automates nucleotide assignments for each position. The data are manually edited, and the sequence is compared with a library containing all known sequences to assign the allele(s) in the sample. One advantage of this method is that the sequence of each of the DNA strands can be determined to confirm the types. This is recommended because technical artifacts can cause the occasional loss of a particular nucleotide, which can cause incorrect interpretation of the data from heterozygotes.

Limitations of Molecular Typing Methods

Methods that detect a few key polymorphic sequences to deduce an HLA type can sometimes assign an incorrect type if an unknown allele is present. These methods cannot detect novel alleles that are distinguished by sequences that are not present at the polymorphic sites tested. Furthermore problems arise with different interpretations of the data depending on the list of HLA sequences used for assignment of HLA types (detailed earlier). This circumstance makes it difficult to compare typings

---

strips. Individual probes that are specific and diagnostic for individual HLA alleles, such as DR1 and DR2, are prepared. Each strip is hybridized with a different lableled sequence-specific oligonucleotide probe (SSOP). The probes hybridize only to an exactly complementary nucleotide sequence in the sample. **B:** The membrane is reassembled and probes are detected. A band indicates the presence in the sample of the sequence of the corresponding HLA type. **C:** In the reverse dot blot, the sequence-specific probes are bound to the membrane support, and the sample DNA is hybridized with amplified DNA. The membrane is washed, and the hybridized DNA is detected by colorimetric methods.

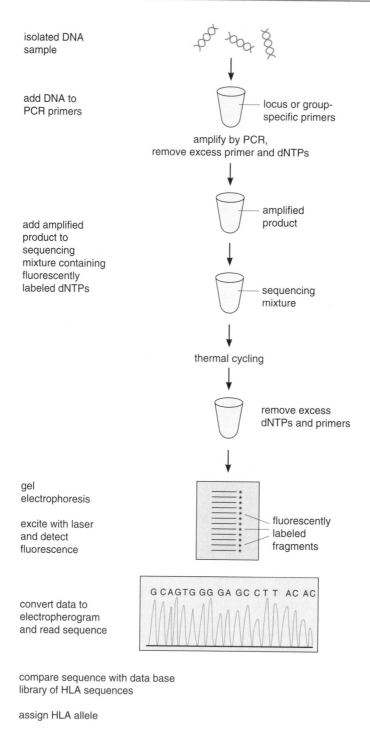

isolated DNA
sample

add DNA to
PCR primers

locus or group-
specific primers

amplify by PCR,
remove excess primer and dNTPs

amplified
product

add amplified
product to
sequencing
mixture containing
fluorescently
labeled dNTPs

sequencing
mixture

thermal cycling

remove excess
dNTPs and primers

gel
electrophoresis

excite with laser
and detect
fluorescence

fluorescently
labeled
fragments

convert data to
electropherogram
and read sequence

G CAGTG GG GA GC CT T AC AC

compare sequence with data base
library of HLA sequences

assign HLA allele

Figure 19–9. Automated DNA sequence-based HLA typing using dye–terminator chemistry. DNA is isolated from a cell or tissue sample and amplified by PCR, using locus-, group-, or allele-specific primers. The amplified product is distributed into four tubes, each one a polymerase, dNTPs, and sequencing mixtures. Each of the four sequencing mixtures is labeled with a fluorescently tagged sequence terminator: tube 1 with labeled cytosine (C*), tube 2 with labeled guanine (G*), tube 3 with labeled thymine (T*), and tube 4 with labeled adenine (A*). The product is amplified by PCR to incorporate the labeled terminators. The four sample tubes are pooled and electrophoresed to separate prime extension products according to size. The sequencer detects the fluorescence in each band and software converts the data into nucleotide sequences. Software compares the sequence to the library of HLA sequences and assigns the HLA type.

performed at different dates. In addition, the extrapolation from limited sequence data to a type can sometimes cause assignment of different types depending on the method and reagents used for the typing.

A major limitation that affects typing of heterozygous amplicons is that multiple interpretations of the data are possible for certain combinations of alleles. This situation can be resolved by performing the typing on selectively amplified alleles. Sometimes ambiguities can be resolved by using a combination of data from two methods (eg, SSOP and SSP or SBT and SSP).

Sometimes novel alleles that are distinguished by different patterns of SSOP or SSP data can be missed if the data are consistent with the presence of known alleles. A major limitation is that interpretation of the data is influenced by the library of sequences used to interpret the data.

SBT, which typically determines the sequence of a segment representing substantial portions of the HLA gene, is less susceptible to these problems. If the sequence is determined for a selectively amplified allele, the sequence is precise. Because most laboratories do not determine the sequence for the entire HLA gene, polymorphism outside the sequenced region is not detected. Many laboratories perform SBT using heterozygous templates (eg, two HLA-A alleles that are coamplified). These data are typically interpreted by comparing the determined sequence with the sequences of all possible combinations of known alleles. Sometimes these results are ambiguous (ie, multiple interpretations of the sequence data of the heterozygous data). If the library of HLA sequences is increased in number, the number of ambiguities or alternative interpretations of the data increases.

Other Molecular Testing Methods

Molecular HLA typing per se may not be required when only a preliminary assessment of HLA identity is desired, (eg, multiple donors are available for unrelated bone marrow transplantation).

Heteroduplex Methods. Heteroduplex formation is a rapid method that uses the property that denatured DNA strands reanneal into heteroduplexes (ie, to form a double helix in alternative combinations that are less than perfectly matched at all base pairs). If the individuals are genetically disparate for HLA alleles, mismatching at the polymorphic bases modifies the bending or increases the superhelical diameter of the DNA and causes a retardation in its electrophoretic mobility (see Chapter 15). When denatured DNA from two genetically disparate individuals is mixed, novel heteroduplexes form, generating new band patterns in electrophoresis. Thus, the genetic identity between two individuals can be quickly assessed by mixing PCR DNA from their

HLA genes. Alternatively, a reference DNA for a single allele or a synthetic universal heteroduplex generator (UHG) molecule can be added to a PCR sample. This forms heteroduplex complexes that are unique for each allele, thus generating unique diagnostic bands and, that can be used to assign an HLA type.

Chimerism Testing—Posttransplant monitoring of hematopoietic stem cell transplants includes testing to monitor the engraftment process. Increasing use of nonmyeloablative conditioning regimens has stimulated use of chimerism testing to evaluate the relative proportions of donor cells after transplant. Historically, engraftment was detected using serologic methods to detect donor-specific HLA molecules. Today, chimerism testing is usually accomplished using molecular methods. If HLA disparities exist between donor and recipient, a test can be designed to quantify the relative amounts of HLA genes that are unique to donor and recipient (ie, the HLA mismatches). If the donor and recipient have different gender, Y chromosome-specific sequences can be detected using in situ hybridization (Chapter 18) or amplification-based methods. Because these approaches are applicable to only a subset of patients, most centers use tests that detect other polymorphic loci that can be used for all donor-recipient pairs (including HLA and gender-identical pairs). These tests discriminate between donor and recipient cells using highly polymorphic loci that have polymorphism in the number of tandemly repeated sequences. One type of target, termed variable number tandem repeats (VNTR), typically detects repeats of 30–100 bp. Another type, termed short tandem repeats (STR), detects repeats of 2–6 bp.

Usually a large number of STR or VNTR loci are examined for each donor–recipient pair, and the most informative (donor and recipient-specific alleles that are easily resolved) loci are selected for testing. The relative amount of donor-and-patient-specific alleles are determined to monitor engraftment. The methods used for this analysis vary substantially in sensitivity, which typically is between 1 and 10%, but can be as low as 50% for certain methods. Some methods are quantitative and others are qualitative.

CELLULAR ASSAYS FOR HISTOCOMPATIBILITY

In vivo, recognition of nonself antigens and destruction of cells bearing such markers is accomplished by cells of the immune system. Some of the clinically relevant HLA molecules that can trigger the immune response are not readily detected by the serologic methods discussed previously. Instead, lymphocytes are used as discriminatory reagents to detect histoincompatibility between donor and recipient.

Cellular tests include the MLC (described in Chapter 16), the CML (described in Chapter 16), primed lymphocyte typing (PLT), and measurement of cytotoxic T cell precursors (CTLp) and helper T cell precursors (HTLp). In general, these tests are cumbersome and expensive, most laboratories have replaced cellular tests with high-resolution molecular typing.

For many years the MLC was considered to be an in vitro model for detecting histoincompatibility that is not revealed by serologic typing methods. Several studies involving bone marrow transplantation have failed to show a significant association between MLC reactivity and rejection or GvHD. For blood or marrow transplants, most centers have replaced MLC tests with high-resolution molecular HLA typing. The MLC continues to be used by some centers to monitor induction of tolerance following hematopoietic stem cell and solid organ transplants. The PLT test involves use of homozygous typing cells in an MLC to determine the type of the responder cell. This test is rarely used today because it has been supplanted by molecular class II HLA typing.

Limiting dilution analysis is used to measure CTLp (measurement of cytotoxicity or interferon secretion) and HTLp (measurement of IL-2 secretion). The clinical value of CTLp and HTLp tests, which have been investigated in the bone marrow transplant setting, remains controversial. It has been suggested that this test may be most useful to T-cell-depleted transplants.

A summary of the serologic and cellular methods for histocompatibility testing is presented in Table 19–9. These methods are in current use and are accepted as appropriate (in some instances mandatory) procedures for clinical histocompatibility testing.

HLA Typing for Allogenic Transplantation

The routine selection of tests for histocompatibility testing is summarized in Table 19–2. HLA typing currently plays an important role in selection of compatible donors for hematopoietic stem cell transplants. In general, HLA matching is associated with decreased rates of rejection and GvHD and increased survival. Large studies reported in 1998 and 1999 suggest that there are advantages for matching HLA-A, -B, -C, -DR, -DQ, and -DP at a high-resolution level. Nevertheless, issues related to the relative importance of mismatching for each locus as well as permissible HLA disparities are unresolved. Other histocompatibility tests (eg, cellular assays and crossmatching) are sometimes used.

In general, the association between HLA matching and solid organ transplants is influenced by the organ(s) transplanted and the transplant protocol. In re-

Table 19–9. Serologic and cellular methods used in histocompatibility testing.

Test	Test Type and Components	Time	Application
Tissue typing			
Complement-dependent lymphocytotoxicity	Serologic (HLA, antisera; complement; test cells)	3 h	Identification of class I and II HLA antigens.
Crossmatching			
PBL crossmatch	Serologic (recipient serum; donor cells; complement; AHG optional)	3 h	Detection of preformed antidonor antibodies in patient serum.
TB-cell crossmatch	Serologic (purified donor T or B cells; recipient serum; AHG optional with T cells)	3–6 h	T cells: detection of antidonor class I HLA antibodies; B cells: detection of antibodies to class I and II HLA.
MLC test	Cellular (donor and recipient cells combined in tissue culture)	6 d	Class II HLA antigen compatibility.
CML test	Cellular (patient cells from primary MLC; fresh donor stimulators as targets)	4 h	Detection of anti-donor CTL.
FCC	Serologic (patient serum; donor cells; fluorescent antihuman immunoglobulin)	3–4 h	Detection of very weak and non-cytotoxic antidonor antibodies.
Autocrossmatch	Serologic (patient PBL, T and B cells, and serum) and FCC.	3–4 h	Detection of nonspecific antilymphocyte antibodies (autoantibodies).
Screening			
Screening for class I HLA antibodies	Serologic (patient serum; panel of HLA-typed T cells or PBL)	3 h × 60 cells	Detection of class I HLA antibodies; identification of antibody specificity.
Screening for class II HLA antibodies	Serologic (patient serum absorbed; B-cell panel typed for HLA-DR, DQ)	4 h × no. of cells plus absorption time	Detection of class II HLA antibodies; identification of antibody specificity.

Abbreviations: PBL = peripheral blood lymphocyte; MLC = mixed leukocyte culture; CML = cell-mediated lympholysis test; FCC = flow cytometry crossmatch; HLA = human leukocyte antigen; AHG = antigen to human serum globulins; CTL = cytotoxic T lymphocyte.

nal transplantation numerous reports show that HLA matching (low resolution) is associated with increased graft and patient survival. Evidence for an anti-class I antibody determined using positive T-cell lymphocytotoxicity crossmatch is a contraindication for transplant. Other more sensitive crossmatch tests (flow cytometry) or B-cell crossmatches are subject to practices at individual transplant centers. At the other extreme, there is little support for histocompatibility in liver transplantation, and testing is usually minimal.

A positive effect of HLA matching on kidney graft outcome has been clearly documented in reports from the two largest studies of renal transplant data: the UCLA Transplant Registry, Los Angeles, California, which has collected data on 106,000 transplants, and the Collaborative Transplant Study (CTS), Heidelberg, Germany, with data on 107,500 renal transplants. Both of these studies agree that the main factor that improves long-term (up to 10-year) renal allograft survival is donor–recipient matching for HLA antigens (Table 19–10). Table 19–10 indicates the decreasing graft survival rates obtained in primary renal transplants when the donor is HLA-identical (sibling), half identical (parent), and completely mismatched and unrelated (cadaver).

Beneficial effects of HLA matching on short-term graft survival (1 year) are no longer apparent in the results from many individual transplant centers. Immunosuppression with cyclosporine has improved first-transplant graft survival of cadaver and living related transplants to near that of HLA-identical transplants: approximately 80–85% after 1 year.

Matching for the splits (subtypes) of HLA broad antigens may be even more significant for graft outcome than simple matching of the "generic" HLA antigens (eg, matching for B51 or B52 rather than for the broad B5 antigen). As shown in Table 19–11, from a CTS review of 33,000 transplants, matching for A and B locus antigen splits in conjunction with HLA-DR shows a striking correlation with graft survival. Table 19–11 shows percent graft survival for patients with 0, 3, and 6 mismatches for HLA-A, -B, and -DR antigens and the estimated half-life survival time for those grafts. Well-matched grafts (zero mismatches) survive approximately 60% longer than do completely mismatched (six mismatches) grafts

Table 19–11. Effect of HLA-A, -B, and -DR mismatches on primary renal graft survival.[a]

Number of Mismatches	Estimated 10-year Graft Survival(%)		Half-Life of Graft (years)	
	Study 1	Study 2	Study 1	Study 2
0	53	65	12.3	20.3
1–2	—	47	—	10.4
3–4	42	38	9.4	8.4
5–6	32	32	7.5	7.7

Sources: Study 1 data from G. Opelz: *Collaborative Transplant Study,* Newletter personal communication, May 1992; Study 2 data from Zhou & Cecka: in *Clinical Transplants,* 1993 (see References).
[a] Matching for split HLA-A and -B locus antigens.

(half-life of 12.3 and 7.5 years, respectively). Corroborative data is provided by the UCLA Transplant Registry showing graft half-lives of 20.3, 8.4, and 7.7 years for zero, three to four, and five to six antigen mismatches, respectively.

Despite the dramatic improvement in 1-year survival, however, the ensuing rate of graft loss due to chronic rejection remains essentially unchanged; that is, half of cadaver grafts are still lost by 9 years, compared with 7.3 years in 1978. Thus, the use of cyclosporine has not established an operational state of long-term organ tolerance. It is estimated that if all kidneys were shared nationally, 25% of all waiting patients could be transplanted with kidneys with no HLA-A, -B, or -DR mismatches. These statistics argue in favor of sharing organs on a regional and national scale to promote the most beneficial usage of scarce organ resources. To achieve this end, the National Organ Transplant Act of 1987 established the United Network for Organ Sharing (UNOS). UNOS links local and regional transplant procurement centers with a national registry of waiting recipients and establishes mandatory criteria for selection of recipients based on a point system for the following attributes: quality of HLA matching, degree of sensitization (panel-reactive antibody [PRA]), time on the waiting list, medical emergency status, and geographic factors.

In heart transplantation, distribution of hearts based on HLA matching is impractical because of the lack of availability of the organ. Retrospective analysis indicates that HLA matching offers a benefit to graft survival, although there are few well-matched grafts to evaluate. For those prospective heart recipients who are sensitized to HLA antigens, a pretransplant crossmatch is routinely performed using preorgan-harvest donor blood where possible to minimize ischemia time of the heart.

For liver transplantation, better HLA-matched livers are associated with fewer rejection episodes, but, paradoxically, liver graft survival results show no advantage from HLA matching and, possibly, a detri-

Table 19–10. Effect of HLA matching on long-term renal allograft survival.

Organ Donor	Number of Haplotypes Matched[b]	% Graft Survival (10 year)	Transplant Half-Life (years)
HLA-identical sibling	2	74	24
Parent	1	54	12
Cadaver[a]	0	40	9

Source: Data from Terasaki PI (editor): *Clinical Transplants 1992.* UCLA Tissue Typing Laboratory, 1993, p. 501.
[a] Recipient treated with cyclosporine.
[b] N = 40,765 transplants.

mental effect. Those patients who suffer recurrence of an autoimmune-type disease in the new, well-matched liver grafts presumably express the autoantigen better with shared rather than with disparate HLA antigens, thereby encouraging renewed disease. Some liver patients are transplanted despite positive crossmatches, whereas others receive no pretransplant testing. No consensus has been reached regarding the utility of crossmatching liver patients prior to transplant.

Data on over 2100 pancreas plus kidney transplants from the UNOS transplant registry indicates the beneficial effect of matching for HLA antigens. Patients with technically successful transplants who were mismatched for zero or one HLA antigens had significantly better ($p < 0.05$) 5-year graft survival than did those mismatched for from two to six HLA antigens. Preliminary data for cornea transplantation show that patients with previously rejected transplants benefit from a well-matched transplant.

REFERENCES

GENERAL
Arnett KL, Parham P: HLA class I nucleotide sequences, 1995. *Tissue Antigens* 1995;46:217.
Bodmer JG et al: Nomenclature for factors of the HLA system, 1998. *Tissue Antigens* 1999;53:407.
Dyer P, Middleton D: *Histocompatibility Testing: A Practical Approach.* Oxford University Press, New York, 1993.
Marsh SGE, Bodmer JG: HLA class II region nucleotide sequences, 1995. *Tissue Antigens* 1995;46:258.
Marsh SGE et al. *The HLA Facts Book.* Academic Press, 2000.
McCluskey J (editor). Immunobiology of the major histocompatibility complex. *Rev Immunogenet* 1999;1:1. (entire issue).
Phelan DL et al (editors): *ASHI Laboratory Manual,* 3rd ed. American Society for Histocompatibility and Immunogenetics, 1994.

SPECIAL METHODS
Böyum A: Separation of leukocytes from blood and bone marrow. *Scand J Clin Lab Invest* 1968;21(suppl):97.
Cook DJ et al: Flow cytometry crossmatching (FCXN4) in the UNOS kidney transplant registry. In: *Clinical Transplants 1998.* Cecka JM, Terasaki PI (editors). UCLA Tissue Typing Laboratory, 1999.
Fuller TC et al: HLA alloantibodies and the mechanism of the antiglobulin-augmented lymphocytotoxicity procedure. *Hum Immunol* 1997;56:94.
Hirschberg H et al: Cell mediated lymphocytes: CML. A microplate technique requiring few target cells and employing a new method of supernatant collection. *J Immunol Methods* 1977;16:131.
Lee P, Garovoy MR: Flow cytometry crossmatching. The first 10 years. In: *Transplantation Reviews 1994* Tilney N, Morris P (editors), Vol 8:1.
Rudy T, Opelz G: Dithiothreitol treatment of crossmatch sera in highly immunized transplant recipients. *Transplant Proc* 1987;19:800.
Terasaki PI et al: Microdroplet testing for HLA-A, -B, -C and -D antigens. *Am J Clin Pathol* 1978;69:103.

HLA & TRANSPLANTATION
Hata Y et al: Effects of changes in the criteria for nationally shared kidney transplants for HLA-matched patients. *Transplantation* 1998;65:208.
Mahoney RJ et al: The flow cytometry crossmatch and early renal transplant loss. *Transplantation* 1990;49:527.
Sutherland DER et al: Pancreas transplant results in United Network for Organ Sharing. In: *Clinical Transplants 1993.* Terasaki PI, Cecka JM (editors). UCLA Tissue Typing Laboratory, 1994.
Terasaki PI et al: A ten-year prediction for kidney transplantation survival. In: *Clinical Transplants 1992.* Terasaki PI, Cecka JM (editors). UCLA Tissue Typing Laboratory, 1993.
Thorsby E (editor). Immunogenetics of allorecognition. *Rev Immunogenet* 1999;1:279.
Zhou YC, Cecka JM: Effect of HLA matching on renal transplant survival. In: *Clinical Transplants 1993.* Terasaki PI and Cecka JM (editors). UCLA Tissue Typing Laboratory, 1994.

MOLECULAR TYPING
Baxter-Lowe LA: HLA testing using molecular genetic tools. In *Molecular Genetics in Diagnosis and Research.* Allen R, AuBuchon J (editors). American Association of Blood Banks, Bethesda, MD, 1995.
Bidwell JL et al: A DNA RFLP typing system that positively identifies serologically well-defined and ill-defined HLA-DR and -DQ alleles, including DRw10. *Transplantation* 1988;45:640.
Bugawan TL et al: A method for typing polymorphism at the HLA-A locus using PCR amplification and immobilized oligonucleotide probes. *Tissue Antigens* 1994;44:137.
Dyer P, Middleton D (editors): Histocompatibility Testing: A Practical Approach. IRL Press, 1993.
Jeffreys AJ et al: Hypervariable "minisatellite" regions in human DNA *Nature* 1985;314:67.
Hansen J (editor): The detection and application of DNA polymorphisms. *Rev Immunogenet* 1999;1:125.
Mytilineos J et al: Comparison of serological and DNA PCR-SSP typing results for HLA-A and HLA-B in 421 black individuals: A collaborative transplant study report. *Hum Immunol* 1998;59:512.
Olerup O, Zetterquist H: HLA-DR typing by PCR amplification with sequence-specific primers (PCR-SSP) in 2 hours: An alternative to serological DR typing in clinical practice including donor–recipient matching in cadaveric transplantation. *Tissue Antigens* 1992;39:225.
Opelz G et al: Analysis of HLA-DR matching in cadaver kidney transplants. *Transplantation* 1993;55:782.

Petersdorf EW et al: Optimizing outcome after unrelated marrow transplantation by comprehensive matching of HLA class I and II alleles in the donor and recipient. *Blood* 1998;92:3515.

Prasad VK et al: DNA typing for HLA-A and HLA-B identifies disparities between patients and unrelated donors matched by HLA-A and HLA-B serology and HLA-DRB1. *Blood* 1999;93:399.

Sasazuki T et al: Effect of matching of class I HLA alleles on clinical outcome after transplantation of hematopoietic stem cells from an unrelated donor. Japan Marrow Donor Program. *N Engl J Med* 1998;339:1177.

Sintasath DM et al:Analysis of HLA-A and -B serologic typing of bone marrow registry donors using polymerase chain reaction with sequence-specific oligonucleotide probes and DNA sequencing. *Tissue Antigens* 1997;50: 366.

Tonks S et al: Molecular typing for HLA class I using ARMS-PCR: further developments following the 12th International Histocompatibility Workshop. *Tissue Antigens* 1999;53:175.

Yu N et al: Accurate typing of HLA-A antigens and analysis of serological deficiencies. *Tissue Antigens* 1997;50: 380.

Laboratory Evaluation of Immune Competence

20

Clifford Lowell, MD, PhD

The integrity of the human immune system depends on a complex interplay of cells (lymphocytes, monocytes, neutrophils), secreted factors (immunoglobulins, cytokines, chemokines), and serum proteins (complement, acute phase reactants). Defects in the production or function of any of these components can result in impairments that range from catastrophic immunodeficiency to subtle increases in the frequency of infections with specific classes of organisms.

The indications for testing immune competence are listed in Table 20–1. Of these the most important is suspected immunodeficiency. Clinical clues to the presence of an immunodeficiency syndrome include (1) increased frequency of infections, (2) failure to clear infections rapidly despite adequate therapy, (3) dissemination of local infections to distant sites, (4) occurrence of opportunistic infections, and (5) development of certain types of cancer (eg, Kaposi's sarcoma in AIDS patients).

The clinical presentation or initial test results may strongly suggest a certain syndrome or defect, allowing the physician to focus on a particular aspect of the immune system. In other cases, the evaluation proceeds by examining the four major components of the immune system (1) B cells (humoral immunity) (2) T cells (cellular immunity) (3) phagocyte function, and (4) complement components.

VARIABLES & LIMITATIONS IN IMMUNOLOGIC TESTING

The results of immunologic tests should always be interpreted within the context of the clinical history and presentation. A number of limitations warrant emphasis. Results of tests of cellular immunity can vary between different laboratories for technical reasons. There also can be biologic causes for variability. Genetic polymorphisms, gender, age, and environmental influences affect normal immune function, sometimes rendering it difficult to assess the clinical significance of differences in test results between individuals. Intercurrent infections, exacerbation of autoimmunity, and medications can affect the evaluation of immune competence. For example, nitroblue tetrazolium (NBT) slide or 2′,7′-dichlorofluorescein (DCF) flow cytometric testing for **chronic granulomatous disease (GCD)** (see Chapter 16) should not be performed in patients who have severe ongoing infections because many of the polymorphonuclear neutrophils (PMNs) in these patients are already fully active or have degranulated. These PMNs will fail to respond to further stimulation in the tests, giving the misleading impression that the patient has a primary defect in PMN function. Nearly all the simple assays of immune function use cells or serum isolated from the peripheral blood, even though the blood in not the most common site of immunologic activity. Immune responses ongoing in lymph nodes, the spleen, or even the bone marrow may not be reflected by changes in the blood. Finally, bear in mind that the presence of normal numbers of cells or normal levels of immunoglobulins does not exclude the possibility of immune dysfunction. A normal serum IgG level does not necessarily mean that the patient's antibody repertoire is adequate to recognize all pathogens. The same is true for T-cell responses. Functional assays can help to address this problem, but our inability to

Table 20–1. Indications for laboratory testing for immune competence.

Clinical diagnosis, therapeutic monitoring, or prognosis of[a]:

Congenital and acquired immunodeficiency diseases (see Chapters 20–25, 46)

Immune reconstitution following bone marrow or other lymphoid tissue grafts (see Chapter 52)

Immunosuppression induced by drugs, radiation, or other means (see Chapter 53) for transplant rejection, cancer treatment, or autoimmune diseases

Autoimmune disorders as a possible adjunct to diagnosis (rarely useful) or to monitor therapy

Immunization to monitor efficacy or immune status

Clinical or basic research

[a] Tests must be interpreted in the clinical context, particularly in conjunction with a thorough history and physical examination.

fully evaluate the immunologic repertoire of individual patients is perhaps our greatest limitation in the assessment of the immune system.

ASSESSMENT OF IMMUNOLOGIC COMPETENCE

A brief summary of one approach to evaluating the basic elements of the immune system is described in the following steps. Most of this discussion focuses on the evaluation and diagnosis of an immunodeficiency, but some of the individual tests described play a role in diagnostic work-ups in other diseases. More complete descriptions of testing procedures and methods are provided in Chapters 15 and 16.

Initial Evaluation. The patient's age, general clinical history, history of infections, and findings on physical examination help guide the evaluation of immune competence. Identification of the specific types of pathogens to which a patient is susceptible can provide significant insight into the type of immunodeficiency involved. For example, patients with deficiencies in the late-acting components of the complement cascade are uniquely susceptible to *Neisseria* infections. Likewise, defects in T-cell function often manifest as susceptibility to viruses and intracellular pathogens.

The initial evaluation of childhood immunodeficiency should include chest radiographs to rule out thymic agenesis (especially if lymphopenia is present). Simple analyses, such as a complete blood count and morphologic examination, often are adequate to recognize major deficiencies in hematopoietic lineages or leukemia. Normal values for lymphocyte, monocyte, and neutrophil levels are very different in children versus adults; results must therefore be viewed in the context of age. True lymphopenia is seen in **severe combined immunodeficiency** (SCID), in **common variable immunodeficiency** (CVID), in major histocompatibility (MHC) class II deficiency (**bare lymphocyte syndrome),** and in **X-linked agammaglobulinemia** (XLA). In contrast, lymphocytosis may suggest **X-linked lymphoproliferative syndrome (Duncan's syndrome)** or malignancy. Leukocytosis (both lymphocytes and granulocytes) is a feature of the **leukocyte adhesion deficiency** (LAD) syndromes as well as hyperresponsive immune states. Abnormal appearing neutrophils are often seen in patients with **chronic granulomatous disease** (CGD) and are a hallmark of **Chèdiak–Higashi syndrome.** Abnormal platelet morphology is seen in **Wiskott–Aldrich syndrome.**

Evaluation of Humoral Immunity. Evaluation of virtually any abnormality in the immune system requires determination of immunoglobulin levels and subtypes. Indeed, the most common form of primary immunodeficiency, **selective IgA deficiency,** is readily recognized by low levels of this immunoglobulin, especially in mucosal secretions. XLA patients usually have IgG levels of less than 100 mg/dL unless studies are performed in the first few months of life when maternal IgG persists. Patients with **hyper-IgM syndrome** (congenital deficiency of CD40L) are recognized by the combination of extremely high levels of IgM and virtually absence of other immunoglobulin types. High IgE levels are seen in many allergic and hypersensitivity syndromes. **Paraproteins** (monoclonal immunoglobulins) can be indicative of malignancy, such as lymphoma or multiple myeloma. Consideration of the patient's age is critical in interpreting immunoglobulin levels because normal levels differ with age.

Specific testing for IgG subclasses (IgG1, IgG2, IgG3, or IgG4) may also be useful in some patients. Deficiency of certain subtypes, such as IgG2, may be associated with recurrent infections and an inability to respond to polysaccharide antigens. Clinical features of selective deficiency of specific IgG subclasses is reviewed in Chapter 21.

Immunophenotyping by flow cytometry is a key part of the evaluation of immune function. Surface staining for all leukocyte subsets is performed simultaneously. Alterations or defects in B-cells are revealed by staining for a host of B-cell-surface markers (Chapter 16).

Determining the levels of antibodies specific for particular antigens can provide an estimate of the ability of the individual to make a humoral immune response. One approach is to examine serum for the presence of antibodies directed against antigens to which the individual should have been exposed. For example, antibodies against tetanus and diphtheria toxoids should be present in individuals who have received the appropriate vaccinations. Alternatively, development of a specific humoral immune response can be examined directly by deliberate immunization with agents such as pneumococcal polysaccharide, capsular antigens of *Haemophilus influenzae,* and keyhole limpet hemocyanin (KLH). Serum is collected at 2- to 3-week intervals and specific antibody titers measured by ELISA assay.

Antibody function can also be assessed by measurement of naturally occurring isohemagglutinins. These IgM antibodies are directed against microbial polysaccharides but cross-react with the human A and B antigens present on red blood cells. Although isohemagglutinin titers usually rise with age, testing is still useful in infants, because newborns can make IgM, and maternally derived IgG does not interfere with measurement of isohemagglutinins.

Additional assessments of humoral immunity include in vitro proliferation and immunoglobulin production by B cells in response to mitogenic stimulation. A variety of agents can be used, most of which nonspecifically activate B cells (eg, **bacterial lipo-**

polysaccharide [LPS] or infection with Epstein–Barr virus). Often, patients with CVID manifest defects in Ig production in these in vitro assays.

Evaluation of Cellular Immune Function. The simplest evaluation of cellular (T-cell) immunity is enumeration of T-cell numbers and subtypes by mAb staining and flow cytometry. A large number of mAbs that recognize and distinguish immature, mature, resting, and activated T cells have been developed. Using this methodology, T-cell deficiency is easily recognized in diseases such as SCID and AIDS. Indeed, the quantitation of CD4 T cells is widely used to monitor disease progression in AIDS and the response to therapy.

The major in vivo functional assay for evaluation of T-cell responses is **delayed-type hypersensitivity (DTH) testing.** The ability to mount DTH responses to intradermally injected antigens depends on the ability of antigen-specific, memory T cells to secrete the appropriate cytokines and chemokines to initiate mononuclear infiltration (see Chapter 16). Responses are assessed to test antigens to which the patient either has been immunized or should have been exposed (see Table 16–2). Lack of response to a wide range of antigens suggests a T-cell defect. The reliability of the test is influenced by several factors (Chapter 16), including the antigen used, injection technique, medication, and the age of the patient. DTH reactions are often minimal in young infants because of lack of exposure to the test antigen.

The simplest in vitro analysis of T-cell function is the measurement of proliferation induced with nonspecific **mitogenic lectins,** such as phytohemagglutinin (PHA) or concanavalin A (Con A). Proliferative responses are measured by incorporation of radiolabeled nucleotides into DNA or by other means (Chapter 16). Patients with defects in signaling molecules (eg, forms of SCID lacking the tyrosine kinase ZAP-70) have reduced numbers of T cells that fail to proliferate in these assays. Additional evaluation of lymphocyte responses in vitro may be indicated, such as tests for antigen-specific responses, cytolytic function, or cytokine responses.

Evaluation of Phagocyte Function. Assessment of phagocyte function is indicated in patients with chronic bacterial infections, repeated pneumonias, or abnormal blood counts. Like all assays of immune function, the first step is enumeration and marker analysis by staining for known surface antigens and flow cytometry. Certain markers are immediately informative for phagocytic defects, such as the absence of CD11b/CD18 (αm/β_2-integrin) in **leukocyte adhesion deficiency 1 (LAD1).** In contrast to lymphocyte disorders, careful morphologic examination of myeloid cells is important—various **myelodysplastic syndromes, granule deficiencies** or disorders such as **Chèdiak-Higashi syndrome** can be recognized by alterations in neutrophil morphology. Similarly, bone marrow biopsy and examination of myeloid precursors (as well as other hematopoietic elements) play a more central role in evaluation of phagocyte disorders than lymphocyte defects. In particular, defects in myeloid cell production, presenting as neutropenia, are recognized in this fashion. Defects in cytokine production or receptors (**granulocyte colony-stimulating factor [G-CSF]** receptor) are known causes of congenital neutropenia (**Kostmann's syndrome).** These patients have varying levels of peripheral blood neutropenia and an accumulation of immature myeloid forms in the marrow that are recognized morphologically and by flow cytometry. Histochemical staining is helpful in the recognition of granule disorders, such as **myeloperoxidase deficiency.** Of course, neutropenia due to malignancy (from either infiltration of the marrow by nonhematopoietic cells or as a result of leukemia) is also diagnosed by bone marrow biopsy and analysis.

A number of functional tests of myeloid cells are helpful in characterizing phagocyte defects (see Chapter 16). Of these, tests for superoxide production (to rule out CGD) and microbicidal function are central. CGD is caused by congenital deficiency of one of the subunits of reduced nicotinamide adenine dinucleotide phosphate (NAPDH) oxidase. As a result, myeloid cells (both neutrophils and macrophages) fail to undergo respiratory burst to produce O_2^- following activation. This respiratory burst is assayed by reduction of NBT (a simple screening test) or, more quantitatively, by the flow DCF assay. Bactericidal function is tested by quantitative assessment of killing of *Staphylococcus aureus* that has been opsonized with serum proteins (complement). Specific defects in fungicidal responses can also be evaluated. These functional methods result in abnormal tests if any one of the steps of bacterial phagocytosis and killing are defective. Usually these assays are performed on neutrophils, but in research protocols, monocyte-macrophage function can be separately determined.

Evaluation of Complement Deficiencies. Assays for complement function often are performed prior to extensive evaluation of lymphocyte and phagocyte function. Hereditary deficiencies leading to the complete absence of individual components of the classical pathway can be associated with a breakdown in host resistance to certain bacteria and with autoimmune disease (systemic lupus erythematosus and glomerulonephritis; Chapter 25). The CH50 (Chapter 15) is an excellent screening test for the hereditary deficiencies of the classical pathway, because detectable CH50 activity requires the presence of at least some of each component of the pathway. If there is detectable CH50 activity, then a homozygous deficiency in the classical pathway is excluded. When the clinical picture suggests a homozygous complement deficiency, a CH50 of zero should prompt evaluation of individual complement components. Note that a reduction in the CH50 to zero is not specific for homozygous deficiencies and can result from disease activity in lupus and other immune complex-mediated disorders.

Subsequent Evaluation. Results of initial testing guide the laboratory immunologist in deciding about subsequent testing. Research protocols tailored to the individual patient may be needed to define the defect leading to immunodeficiency. Alternatively, initial results may lead to testing for known mutations that result in immunodeficiency, such as mutation in the *BTK* gene (leading to XLA), the *WASP* gene (leading to **Wiskott-Aldrich syndrome**), or various kinase genes associated with SCID syndromes (*ZAP-70* or *JAK-3*). Indeed, as the molecular understanding of immunodeficiency improves, genetic test-ing may become a routine part of screening.

REFERENCES

GENERAL

Noroski LM, Shearer WT: Screening for primary immunodeficiencies in the clinical laboratory. *Clin Immunol Immunopathol* 1998,86:237.

Rosen FS et al: The primary immunodeficiencies. *N Engl J Med* 1995,333:431.

Rosen FS, Geha RS: *Cases Studies in Immunology: A Clinical Companion.* Current Biology Ltd/Garland Publishing, 1996.

LYMPHOCYTES

Lawton AR, Hummell, DS: Primary antibody deficiencies. In *Clinical Immunology, Principles and Practice.* Mosby, 1995.

Powderly WG et al: Recovery of the immune system with antiretroviral therapy: The end of opportunism? *JAMA* 1998,280:72.

Virella G: Diagnostic evaluation of humoral immunity. *Immunol Ser* 1993,58:275.

PHAGOCYTES

Etzioni AM et al: Recurrent severe infections caused by a novel leukocyte adhesion deficiency. *N Engl J Med* 1992, 327:1789.

Holland SM, Gallin JI: Neutrophil disorders. In *Santer's Immunological Diseases,* 5th ed. Little, Brown & Co., 1995.

COMPLEMENT

Ahmed, AE, Peter JB: Clinical utility of complement assessment. *Clin Diag Lab Immunol* 1995,2:509.

Colten HF, Rosen FS: Complement deficiencies. *Annu Rev Immunol* 1992,10:809.

OTHER

Brooks EG et al: T-cell receptor analysis in Omenn's syndrome: Evidence for defects in gene rearrangement and assembly. *Blood* 1999;93:242.

He XS et al: Quantitative analysis of hepatitis C virus-specific CD8(+) T cells in peripheral blood and liver using peptide-MHC tetramers. *Proc Natl Acad Sci U S A* 1999;96:5692.

Lee PP et al: Characterization of circulating T cells specific for tumor-associated antigens in melanoma patients. *Nature Med* 1999;5:677.

Smith CI et al: X-linked agammaglobulinemia: Lack of mature B lineage cells caused by mutations in the Btk kinase. *Springer Semin Immunopathol* 1998;19:369.

Sullivan JL: The abnormal gene in X-linked lymphoproliferative syndrome. *Curr Opin Immunol* 1999;11:431.

Uribe L, Weinberg KI: X-linked SCID and other defects of cytokine pathways. *Semin Hematol* 1998;35:299.

Section III.
Clinical Immunology

Antibody (B-Cell) Immunodeficiency Disorders

21

Robert L. Roberts, MD, PhD, & E. Richard Stiehm, MD

MECHANISMS OF IMMUNODEFICIENCY

Four major components of the immune system protect the individual against a constant assault by viral, bacterial, fungal, and protozoal pathogens. These components include antibody-mediated (B-cell), cell-mediated (T-cell), phagocytic, and complement systems. Each system may act independently or in concert with one or more of the others.

Deficiency of one or more of these systems may be congenital, acquired, secondary to an embryologic abnormality or enzymatic defect, or of unknown cause (Table 21–1).

The clinical findings of immunodeficiency are related to the degree of deficiency and the particular system that is deficient in function (Table 21–2). The types of infections provide an important clue to the type of immunodeficiency disease. Recurrent bacterial otitis media and pneumonia are common in hypogammaglobulinemia. Patients with defective cell-mediated immunity are susceptible to fungal, protozoal, and viral infections that may present as pneumonia or chronic infection of the skin and mucous membranes or other organs. Systemic infection with uncommon bacterial organisms, normally of low virulence, is characteristic of chronic granulomatous disease. Other phagocytic disorders are associated with superficial skin infections or systemic pyogenic infections.

Numerous advances continue to be made in the identification and diagnosis of specific immunodeficiency disorders (Table 21–3). Screening tests are available for each component of the immune system (Table 21–4). These tests enable the physician to diagnose more than 75% of immunodeficiency disorders. The remainder can be diagnosed with more advanced studies (see Chapters 15 and 16) not available in all hospital laboratories. There remain a number of

Table 21–1. Causes of immunodeficiency.

Genetic patterns
Autosomal-recessive
Autosomal-dominant
X-linked
Gene deletions and rearrangements

Biochemical and metabolic deficiency
Adenosine deaminase deficiency
Purine nucleoside phosphorylase deficiency
Biotin-dependent multiple carboxylase deficiency
Deficient membrane glycoproteins

Vitamin or mineral deficiency
Biotin
B_{12}
Iron
Vitamin A
Zinc (acrodermatitis enteropathica)

Arrest in embryogenesis
DiGeorge syndrome
Asplenia

Autoimmune diseases
Passive antibody (neonatal neutropenia due to maternal antibody)
Active antibody (antibody to neutrophils or T cells)
Active T cell (thymoma)

Acquired immunodeficiency
Postviral infection
Posttransfusion
Multiple transfusions
Metabolic disorders
Hemoglobinopathies
Chronic infection
Nutritional deficiency
Drug abuse
Medications
Protein-losing states (enteropathy, severe burns)
Maternal alcoholism
Radiation therapy
Immunosuppressive therapy
Cancer
Chronic renal disease
Splenectomy
Trauma

Table 21–2. Clinical features associated
with immunodeficiency.

Features frequently present and highly suspicious
Chronic infection
Recurrent infection (more than expected)
Unusual microbial agents or opportunist infections
Incomplete clearing between episodes of infection or
incomplete response to treatment

Features frequently present and moderately suspicious
Skin lesions (eczema, cutaneous candidiasis, rash,
seborrhea, alopecia, severe warts, etc)
Diarrhea (chronic)
Growth failure
Hepatosplenomegaly
Hematologic abnormalities (leukopenia, abnormal
morhphology)
Recurrent abscesses
Recurrent osteomyelitis
Evidence of autoimmunity
Failure to thrive

**Features associated with specific immunodeficiency
disorders**
Ataxia
Telangiectasia
Short-limbed dwarfism
Cartilage-hair hypoplasia
Idiopathic endocrinopathy
Partial albinism
Thrombocytopenia
Eczema
Tetany
Periodontitis
Failure of umbilical cord to separate

Table 21–3. Classification of primary immunodeficiency
disorders.

Antibody (B-cell) immunodeficiencies[a]
X-linked agammaglobulinemia
Transient hypogammaglobulinemia of infancy
Common variable immunodeficiency
Hyper-IgM immunodeficiency (T-cell defect)
IgA deficiency
IgM deficiency
IgG subclass deficiencies
Polysaccharide unresponsiveness
Transcobalamin deficiency
Immunodeficiency with thymoma
Netherton syndrome

Cellular (T-cell) immunodeficiencies[b]
DiGeorge anomaly
Chronic mucocutaneous candidiasis
Biotin-dependent multiple cocarboxylase deficiency
Natural killer cell deficiency
Idiopathic CD4 lymphopenia

**Combined B-cell (antibody) and T (cellular)-cell
deficiencies**[c]
Severe combined immunodeficiency (including X-linked
SCID, Nezelof syndrome, etc)
Combined immunodeficiency with T-cell membrane or sig-
naling defects
Wiskott–Aldrich syndrome
Ataxia–telangiectasia
Nijmegen breakage syndrome
Immunodeficiency with short-limbed dwarfism/cartilage
hair hypoplasia
Immunodeficiency with enzyme deficiency; adenosine
deaminase or nucleoside phosphorylase deficiency
Graft-versus-host disease
Bare lymphocyte syndrome
Omenn syndrome
Reticular dysgenesis
X-linked lymphoproliferative syndrome

Phagocytic dysfunction diseases[d]
Neutropenic syndromes
Chronic granulomatous disease
Leukocyte glucose-6-phosphate dehydrogenase deficiency
Chédiak–Higashi syndrome
Myeloperoxidase deficiency
Specific granule deficiency
Glycogen storage disease type 1b
Hyper-IgE/Job's syndrome
Leukocyte adhesion defect (types I and II)
Schwachman syndrome
Tuftsin deficiency
Periodontitis syndromes

[a] Described in Chapter 21.
[b] Described in Chapter 22.
[c] Described in Chapter 23.
[d] Described in Chapter 24.

individuals with an immunodeficiency disorder of unknown etiology or mechanism. The discovery of genes associated with specific immunodeficiencies has allowed for detection of the carrier state and intrauterine diagnosis of many disorders.

In addition to antimicrobial treatment of specific infections, new forms of immunotherapy are available to assist in the control of immunodeficiency or perhaps even to cure the underlying disease (Table 21–5). Some treatments, such as bone marrow transplantation, are limited by the availability of suitable donors although haploidentical, matched unrelated and umbilical cord blood stem cell transplants have enlarged the donor pool. The enzyme deficiencies (eg, adenosine deaminase deficiency) associated with immunodeficiency offer a potential new avenue of therapy, that is, enzyme replacement. The most recent successful approach to treatment is that of gene therapy. Several patients with adenosine deaminase deficiency have been treated with their own cells transfected with the gene coding for adenosine deaminase. A number of recombinant cytokines are also used in clinical trials for treatment of immune disorders, such as interferon gamma for treating chronic granulomatous disease and granulocyte colony-stimulating factor for treating the neutropenia associated with some forms of immunodeficiency.

This chapter discusses antibody (B-cell) deficiency.

The next three chapters cover cellular (T-cell) deficiency; combined T-cell, B-cell deficiency; and phagocytic dysfunction. Complement factor deficiencies are discussed in Chapter 25. Chapter 46 is devoted to AIDS. The terminology used for specific deficiencies is based on the classification proposed by a committee of the World Health Organization (see Table 21–3).

Table 21–4. Initial immunologic screening evaluation.

Antibody-mediated immunity
Quantitative immunoglobulin levels: IgG, IgM, IgA
Isohemagglutinin titer (anti-A and anti-B): measures IgM antibody function primarily
Specific antibody levels following immunization

Cell-mediated immunity
Leukocyte count differential: measures total lymphocytes
Total T cells, helper T cells, and suppressor T cells
Delayed hypersensitivity skin tests: measure specific T cell and inflammatory response to antigens
Natural killer cell number and function

Phagocytic activity
Leukocyte count with differential: measures total neutrophils and assesses morphology
Nitroblue tetrazolium (NBT), chemiluminescence, superoxide production: measures neutrophil oxidative function

Complement
Total hemolytic complement

Table 21–5. Treatment of immunodeficiency.

Disorder	Treatment	Comments
B-cell (antibody deficiency)	Gamma globulin replacement (intramuscular or intravenous)	Not effective for selective IgA deficiency. Risk of anaphylaxis
	Hyperimmune gamma globulin (varicella, CMV, RSV)	For specific exposure in immunodeficient patients and prophylactically in transplant recipients (anti-CMV) and infants with BPD (RSV)
T-cell (cellular deficiency)	Erythrocyte infusion (irradiated blood)	May benefit certain enzyme deficiencies (ADA)
	ADA–PEG	Specifically for ADA deficiency; replaces erythrocyte infusion
	Cultured thymus transplantation	For DiGeorge syndrome (very restricted use)
	Thymic factors: thymosin, thymopentin	May improve T-cell function but lack of documented effectiveness
Combined B and T deficiency	Interleukin-2 (May be conjugated to polyethylene glycol)	For selected patients with SCID and defect in IL-2 synthesis. Increases CD4 cell numbers in AIDS
	IFNγ	Patients with partial defect in IFNγ receptor expression and in IL-12 deficiency
	Bone marrow transplantation	Only viable treatment for many conditions. High risk for GVH disease and infections
	Cord blood cell transplantation	Probably best alternative when no HLA-identical related donor available
	Gene therapy	Has been used for ADA deficiency, but effectiveness not proven
Phagocytic cell deficiency	Granulocyte transfusions	Used successfully in very severe infections in CGD
	IFNγ	Prophylactically for CGD and in high dose to treat infections
	Granulocyte colony-stimulating factor	For increasing numbers and neutrophil function in CGD and other neutrophil disorders
	Stem cell transplantation (bone marrow or cord blood)	For CGD, LAD, and Chédiak–Higashi
	Gene therapy	Trials in progress for CGD and considered for other disorders

Abbreviations: CMV = cytomegalovirus; RSV = respiratory syncytial virus; BPD = bronchopulmonary dysplasia; ADA = adenosine deaminase; PEG = polyethylene glycol; IL = interleukin; SCID = severe combined immunodeficiency; AIDS = acquired immunodeficiency disorder; IFN = interferon; GVH = graft-vs-host; HLA = human leukocyte antigen; CGD = chronic granulomatous disease; LAD = leukocyte adhesion deficiency.

ANTIBODY (B-CELL) IMMUNODEFICIENCY

The primary antibody immunodeficiency disorders range from complete absence of all classes to selective deficiency of a single class or subclass. Selective antibody deficiency with normal immunoglobulin levels also occurs, and morbidity depends chiefly on the degree of antibody deficiency. Screening tests for the specific diagnosis of antibody deficiency disorders are readily available in most hospital laboratories (see Table 21–4 and Chapter 15). Other more sophisticated procedures, such as quantitation of B cells in peripheral blood, determination of in vitro immunoglobulin production, and suppressor cell assays, may yield more precise diagnosis and insight into the cause or mechanism of the observed deficiency (Table 21–6).

X-LINKED AGAMMAGLOBULINEMIA

Major Immunologic Features
- Symptoms of recurrent pyogenic infections usually by 5–6 months of age.
- IgG less than 200 mg/dL, with absence of IgM, IgA, IgD, and IgE.

Table 21–6. Evaluation of antibody-mediated immunity.

Test	Comment
Protein electrophoresis	For presumptive diagnosis of hypogammaglobulinemia or to evaluate for paraproteins
Quantitation of immunoglobulins	Best procedure for quantitation of IgG, IgM, IgA, and IgD
Enzyme-linked immunosorbent assay (ELISA)	IgE quantitation
Isohemagglutinins	For evaluation of IgM function. Expected titer of >1:4 after 1 year of age
Specific antibody response	For evaluation of immunoglobulin function. Immunize with tetanus or diphtheria toxoid or pneumococcal polysaccharide. Do not immunize with live virus if immunodeficiency is suspected
B-cell quantitation with monoclonal antibody	Normally 10–20% (total IgG-, IgM-, IgD-, and IgA-bearing cells) of total circulating lymphocytes
IgG subclass levels	Use for patients with IgA deficiency and symptomatic patients with normal IgG levels

- B cells absent in peripheral blood.
- Good response to treatment with immunoglobulin replacement.

General Considerations
In 1952, Ogden Bruton described the first case of X-linked agammaglobulinemia (XLA), a boy with recurrent pneumococcal infections who had no γ-globulin peak on serum electrophoresis and responded well to gamma-globulin injections.

The disorder is easily diagnosed by the marked deficiency or complete absence of all five serum immunoglobulin classes. Infants with this disorder usually become symptomatic following the natural loss of transplacentally acquired maternal immunoglobulin at about 5–6 months of age. They suffer from severe chronic bacterial infections, which can be controlled readily with gamma globulin and antibiotic treatment. The prevalence of this disorder is one case per 100,000 population. Two female siblings with congenital hypogammaglobulinemia have been reported.

Immunologic Pathogenesis
Extirpation of the bursa of Fabricius in birds results in complete agammaglobulinemia. The human equivalent of the bursa, the source of B-cell precursors, is thought to be either the gastrointestinal tract–associated lymphoid tissue (tonsils, adenoids, Peyer's patches, and appendix), the stem cells in fetal liver, and bone marrow. In XLA, an absent stem cell population presumably causes the complete absence of B lymphocytes and plasma cells. There is evidence of pre-B cells in the marrow and peripheral blood of patients, however, suggesting that the defect may be at a later stage of B-cell differentiation. These pre-B cells do not secrete immunoglobulin. The genetic defect has recently been defined as a deficiency of the enzyme B-cell progenitor kinase (BPK), a cytoplasmic tyrosine kinase. The gene encoding this enzyme is on the long arm of the chromosome at Xq22. This results in a more precise diagnosis, the ability to detect the carrier state, and eventual gene therapy.

The individual immunoglobulin isotypes are a result of immunoglobulin heavy (H)-chain diversity. Individual H chains form by the somatic rearrangement of variable (V), diversity (D), and joining (J) segment genes, as described in Chapters 7 and 8. In some cases of XLA, a truncated μ chain is produced as a consequence of premature transcription prior to D-J segment rearrangement. In others, failure of V_H gene rearrangement results in the production of truncated μ and α H chains.

Clinical Features
A. Symptoms and Signs: Patients with XLA remain asymptomatic until 5–6 months of age, when the passively transferred maternal IgG reaches its lowest level. The loss of protection from maternal an-

tibodies usually coincides with the age at which these children are increasingly exposed to pathogens. Initial symptoms consist of recurrent bacterial otitis media, bronchitis, pneumonia, meningitis, dermatitis, and, occasionally, arthritis or malabsorption. Many infections respond promptly to antibiotic therapy, and this response occasionally delays the diagnosis of hypogammaglobulinemia. The most common organisms responsible for infection are *Streptococcus pneumoniae* and *Haemophilus influenzae;* other streptococci and certain gram-negative bacteria are occasionally responsible. Although patients normally have intact T-cell immunity and respond normally to viral infections such as varicella and measles, there have been reports of paralytic poliomyelitis and progressive enterovirus encephalitis following immunization with live vaccines or exposure to wild virus. The encephalitis in a few patients has responded to treatment with intravenous immunoglobulin. Fatal echovirus infection has been reported. A relationship of echovirus infection, dermatomyositis, and agammaglobulinemia has been proposed. These observations suggest that some patients with agammaglobulinemia may also be unusually susceptible to some viral illnesses.

An important clue to the diagnosis is the failure of infections to respond completely or promptly to appropriate antibiotic therapy. In addition, many patients with agammaglobulinemia have a history of continuous illness with no periods of well-being between bouts of illness.

Occasionally, patients may not become symptomatic until early childhood. Some may present with other complaints, such as chronic conjunctivitis, abnormal dental decay, or malabsorption. The malabsorption may be severe and may retard growth in both height and weight. Frequently, the malabsorption is associated with *Giardia lamblia* infestation. A disease resembling rheumatoid arthritis has been reported in patients with agammaglobulinemia, principally in untreated infants. It may indicate the need for more intensive immunoglobulin therapy.

Physical findings usually relate to recurrent pyogenic infections. Chronic otitis media and externa, serous otitis, conjunctivitis, an abnormal degree of dental decay (Figure 21–1), and eczematoid skin infections are frequently present. Despite the repeated infections, the tonsils and lymph nodes are absent and the spleen is of normal size.

B. Laboratory Findings: The diagnosis of XLA is based on the absence or marked deficiency of all five immunoglobulin classes. Although the diagnosis is suspected from serum protein electrophoresis and established by immunoelectrophoresis (see Chapter 15), specific quantitation of immunoglobulins is necessary, especially during early infancy. Total immunoglobulin levels are usually below 250 mg/dL. The IgG level is usually below 200 mg/dL, and IgM, IgA, IgD, and IgE levels are extremely low or unde-

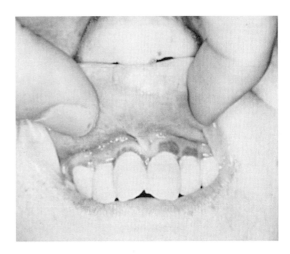

Figure 21–1. Early periodontal disease in a child with agammaglobulinemia. Recurrent ear infections and dental disease were the first manifestations of susceptibility to infection.

tectable. Rarely, patients have complete absence of IgG, IgA, IgM, and IgD but normal amounts of IgE. It is unusual for patients with agammaglobulinemia to have depressed levels of IgG and normal levels of IgM or IgA. Before a diagnosis of immunodeficiency is established in such patients, failure to make antibody following antigenic stimulation should be demonstrated. The diagnosis is difficult in infants under 6 months of age because of maternal IgG in the serum, but an absence of IgM, IgA, and B cells suggests the diagnosis.

Isohemagglutinins from natural immunization are normally present in infants of the appropriate blood group by 1 year of age. Titers of anti-A and anti-B should be greater than 1:4 in normal individuals. Antibody to a specific antigen may be measured following immunization, but a patient suspected of having an immunodeficiency disorder should never be immunized with live attenuated viral vaccine. Rarely, an intestinal biopsy to determine the presence or absence of plasma cells may be necessary to assist in the diagnosis in difficult cases. In XLA, there are no plasma cells in the lamina propria of the gut, no circulating B cells, but normal to increased numbers of T cells. T-cell immunity is intact. Delayed hypersensitivity skin tests are usually positive; isolated peripheral blood lymphocytes respond normally to phytohemagglutinin (PHA) and to allogeneic cells in mixed leukocyte culture (MLC).

C. Other Tests: Radiography of the lateral nasopharynx to show the lack of lymphoid tissue rarely adds significant information to the findings on physical examination. X-ray films of the sinuses and chest should be obtained at regular intervals to monitor the patient's course and to determine the adequacy of treatment. Pulmonary function studies should also be performed regularly, when the patient is old enough to cooperate. Gastrointestinal tract symptoms should be investigated for the presence of *G lamblia* and other causes of malabsorption.

Immunologic Diagnosis

Total immunoglobulin levels are below 250 mg/dL; the IgG level is below 200 mg/dL, and IgM, IgA, IgD, and IgE levels are markedly reduced or absent. B cells are absent in peripheral blood and lymph nodes, and there are no plasma cells containing immunoglobulins in tissue and lymph nodes. No antibodies are formed following specific immunization. T-cell numbers and functions are intact. Natural killer (NK) cell activity is normal.

Molecular Diagnosis

XLA results from a mutation of a gene at Xq22 termed *Btk,* which encodes a tyrosine kinase that is a component of the signal transduction pathway permitting pre B-cells to differentiate to B cells. Multiple unique mutations are observed in different patients. Mutation analysis can be used to make a definitive diagnosis or identify the carrier state.

Differential Diagnosis

A diagnosis of XLA may be difficult to establish in the age range of 5–9 months. The majority of normal infants during this time have IgG levels below 350 mg/dL but usually show some evidence of IgM and IgA production (usually >20 mg/dL) as well as specific antibody production. If the diagnosis appears uncertain, several approaches may be taken. Immunoglobulin levels may be determined again 3 months after the initial values. If IgG, IgM, or IgA levels increase, XLA is highly unlikely. Alternatively, the patient may be immunized with killed vaccines, and specific antibody levels determined. Patients suspected of having XLA should never be immunized with live vaccines. Finally, B-cell number can be assayed; their absence is strong evidence for XLA.

Other illnesses that can mimic XLA include transient hypogammaglobulinemia of infancy (see next section), early onset of common variable immunodeficiency, or severe congenital HIV infection. In all of these disorders, B cells are present.

A significant number of familial syndromes of agammaglobulinemia and neutropenia have been described, but whether this is an association or a consequence of recurrent infection is uncertain. Some patients with XLA and growth hormone deficiency have also been described.

Patients with severe malabsorption—particularly protein-losing enteropathy—may have severely depressed levels of immunoglobulins because of enteric loss. In most instances, a diagnosis of protein-losing enteropathy can be established by the demonstration of a concomitant deficiency of serum albumin. Occasionally, however, patients with severe malabsorption and primary agammaglobulinemia also lose albumin through the intestinal tract. Under these circumstances, a diagnosis can best be made by intestinal biopsy. Patients with protein-losing enteropathy have normal numbers of plasma cells containing intracellular immunoglobulins in the gut and in other lymphoid tissues, and they also have normal numbers of circulating B cells.

Polyarthritis may be a presenting feature in patients with agammaglobulinemia; they usually respond promptly to immunoglobulin therapy. Most patients with juvenile rheumatoid arthritis have elevated levels of immunoglobulins. Patients with chronic lung disease should be investigated for cystic fibrosis, asthma, α_1-antitrypsin deficiency, or immotile cilia syndrome.

Treatment

Immunoglobulin therapy consists primarily of the use of intravenous immunoglobulin (IVIG). Although manufacturing techniques may vary for the different preparations, all contain almost exclusively IgG, with only trace amounts of IgM and IgA.

IVIG preparation is similar to that of intramuscular immunoglobulin, but with added steps to remove aggregates that stimulate the complement pathway in vivo. Intramuscular immunoglobulin (IG) should not be given intravenously. IVIG is preferable to IG because larger amounts can be safely given. Slow subcutaneous infusions of IVIG or IG can also be given in case of poor intravenous access or reactions to IVIG and are very well tolerated. The usual dose by this route is 100 mg/kg at weekly intervals.

The usual dose of intravenous immunoglobulin is 400 mg/kg given intravenously once each month. If symptoms are not controlled, the total dose or the frequency should be increased, even as often as every week. During an acute illness, such as meningitis or pneumonia, immunoglobulin may be given as frequently as every day if the patient fails to respond appropriately to antibiotics and standard doses of immunoglobulin. If a patient with an acute illness has not received immunoglobulin for 2 weeks, it is advisable to provide a repeat maintenance dose.

The half-life of intravenous immunoglobulin is between 15 and 25 days. Serum levels of IgG approaching normal can be achieved for the first 2–4 days following intravenous administration, but they return to abnormal values after 2–3 weeks.

Reactions to intravenous immunoglobulin are rare. Patients occasionally experience dyspnea, sweating, increased heart rate, or abdominal pain. In most instances these symptoms subside when the infusion rate is temporarily reduced. More serious reactions include anaphylactoid reactions, aseptic meningitis, and renal insufficiency.

Anaphylactoid reactions to immunoglobulin administration are usually not mediated through the IgE allergic pathway because most patients with hypogammaglobulinemia do not form IgE antibodies. The chief causes of these reactions are aggregate formation in the immunoglobulin preparation and inadvertent intravenous administration of intramuscular preparations. Patients who have repeated reactions to immunoglobulin should first be treated with an alternative preparation obtained from a different commercial source. If reactions continue, it may be necessary to remove aggregates by centrifugation prior to administration.

Therapeutic immunoglobulin is prepared from pools of serum obtained from donors screened for hepatitis or acquired immunodeficiency syndrome (AIDS). A few cases of hepatitis C but no HIV have been reported as a result of IVIG. Hepatitis C transmission is now eliminated by solvent detergent treatment or pasteurization of IVIG.

Additional therapy may be necessary in patients who fail to respond to maximum doses of immunoglobulin. Continuous use of antibiotics may be necessary. Physical therapy with postural drainage should be used for patients with chronic lung disease or bronchiectasis.

Occasionally, a patient with agammaglobulinemia has minimal or no symptoms. Treatment should be immunoglobulin therapy, even without a history of repeated infection, to avoid future infections that may cause permanent complications.

Malabsorption in patients with agammaglobulinemia usually responds to immunoglobulin treatment. If *G lamblia* is found, the treatment is metronidazole in doses of 35–50 mg/kg/day in three divided doses for 10 days (for children) or 750 mg orally three times a day for 10 days (for adults).

Complications & Prognosis

Although patients with XLA have survived to the second and third decades, the prognosis must be guarded. Despite apparently adequate immunoglobulin replacement therapy, many patients develop chronic lung disease. Severe infection early in infancy may result in irreversible lung damage. Patients with severe pulmonary infection frequently develop bronchiectasis and chronic lung disease. Patients who recover from meningitis may have severe neurologic handicaps. Regular examinations and prompt institution of therapy are necessary to control infections and to prevent complications. Fatal echovirus infections of the central nervous system have been reported even in patients receiving immunoglobulin therapy. Some of these infections have been associated with dermatomyositis or arthritis. Some patients may develop leukemia or lymphoma. Vaccine-related poliomyelitis may occur. Their household contacts should also not receive live oral poliovirus vaccine.

TRANSIENT HYPOGAMMAGLOBULINEMIA OF INFANCY

All infants develop physiologic hypogammaglobulinemia at approximately 5–6 months of age. At this time, the serum IgG level reaches its lowest point (approximately 350 mg/dL), and many normal infants begin to experience recurrent respiratory tract infections. Occasionally, an infant may fail to initiate IgG synthesis at this time, resulting in a prolonged period of hypogammaglobulinemia termed **transient hypogammaglobulinemia of infancy (THI).** This is more pronounced and prolonged in premature infants because of decreased transplacental maternal IgG at birth. The normal serum levels of IgM and IgA and the presence of B cells exclude XLA.

Patients with clinically significant THI have recurrent infections and poor or absent antibody responses to vaccine antigens. Some of these infants may benefit from IVIG infusions or continuous antibiotic treatment. Most will recover by age 18–24 months. IVIG inhibits antibody formation and is contraindicated if the infant is making antibodies. The cause of THI is unknown. A single study suggested that patients with THI have a transient defect in the number and function of helper T cells.

COMMON VARIABLE IMMUNODEFICIENCY (Acquired Hypogammaglobulinemia)

Major Immunologic Features

- Recurrent pyogenic infections, with onset at any age.
- Increased incidence of autoimmune disease.
- Total immunoglobulin level less than 300 mg/dL, with the IgG level below 250 mg/dL.
- B-cell numbers usually normal.

General Considerations

Patients with common variable immunodeficiency (CVID) present clinically like patients with XLA, except that they usually do not become symptomatic until 15–35 years of age. In addition to increased susceptibility to pyogenic infections, they have a high prevalence of autoimmune disease. These patients may also have subtle abnormalities in T-cell immunity, which in most instances progressively deteriorates with time. The disease affects both males and females and may occur at any age, even in infancy.

Immunologic Pathogenesis

The cause of CVID is unknown and probably multifactorial. Most patients have an intrinsic defect in B cells. Peripheral blood lymphocytes from some patients with CVID have an inhibiting effect on the immunoglobulin synthesis in cells from normal patients, suggesting that the course of this disorder may reside at the level of suppressor T cells. Other patients have diminished numbers of helper T cells. Some studies have shown a heterogeneity of arrested B-cell development, ranging from normal proliferative B-cell responses and IgM-secreting cells to absent proliferative responses. Two enzymatic abnormalities have been described. In some patients there is a failure of glycosylation of the heavy-chain IgG. In others, a deficiency of 5'-nucleotidase has been found. The latter abnormality is most probably secondary to alterations in T-cell:B-cell ratios rather than being a primary defect.

Genetic studies of CVID have demonstrated an autosomal-recessive mode of inheritance in certain families. IgA deficiency and autoimmunity may occur in family members. CVID patients are more susceptible to the development of lymphatic and gastrointestinal malignancies.

Clinical Features

A. Symptoms and Signs: Recurrent sinopulmonary infections are the initial presentation of CVID in most cases. These may be chronic rather than acute and overwhelming, as in XLA. Infections may be caused by pneumococci, *H influenzae,* or other pyogenic organisms. Chronic bacterial conjunctivitis may be an additional presenting complaint. Some patients develop severe malabsorption prior to the diagnosis of agammaglobulinemia. The malabsorption may be severe enough to cause protein loss sufficient to produce edema. Giardiasis, cholelithiasis, and achlorhydria are additional findings.

Autoimmune disease has been a presenting complaint in some patients with CVID. A rheumatoid arthritis-like disorder, systemic lupus erythematosus (SLE), thrombocytopenic purpura, dermatomyositis, hemolytic anemia, hypothyroidism, Graves' disease, inflammatory bowel disease, and pernicious anemia have been reported in association with CVID.

In contrast to patients with X-linked infantile agammaglobulinemia, those with CVID may have marked lymphadenopathy and splenomegaly. Intestinal lymphoid nodular hyperplasia has been described in association with malabsorption. Other abnormal physical findings relate to chronic lung disease or intestinal malabsorption.

B. Laboratory Findings: Immunoglobulin measurements may show slightly higher IgG levels than are reported in XLA. Total immunoglobulin levels are usually below 300 mg/dL, and the IgG level is usually below 250 mg/dL. IgM and IgA may be absent or present in significant amounts. Blood group isohemagglutinins are absent or present in low titers (<1:10). The failure to produce antibody following specific immunization establishes the diagnosis in patients who have borderline immunoglobulin values. Live attenuated vaccines should not be used for immunization. Peripheral blood B lymphocytes are usually present in normal numbers in patients with CVID.

Although most patients have intact cell-mediated immunity, a significant number demonstrate subtle abnormalities as evidenced by absent delayed hypersensitivity skin test responses, depressed responses of isolated peripheral blood lymphocytes to PHA and allogeneic cells, and decreased numbers of T cells. Many patients have reduced in vitro production of cytokines and interleukins (IL), including IL-2, IL-4, and IL-5, and interferon gamma. On the other hand, some patients have elevated levels of IL-4 and IL-6. Others have reduced CD4/CD8 ratios. NK cell activity is normal. A few patients have abnormal macrophage/T-cell interaction. Repetition of these tests is important, because the immunodeficiency appears to progressively involve cell-mediated immunity, resulting in additional immunologic deficiencies.

Biopsy of lymphoid tissue reveals a lack of plasma cells. Although some lymph node biopsies may reveal lymphoid hyperplasia, the absence of cells in the B-cell-dependent areas is strikingly similar to that seen in congenital agammaglobulinemia.

C. Other Tests: Other test abnormalities may relate to associated disorders. The chest roentgenogram usually shows evidence of chronic lung disease, and sinus films show chronic sinusitis. Pulmonary function studies are abnormal. Patients with malabsorption may have abnormal gastrointestinal tract biopsies, with blunting of the villi similar to that seen in celiac disease. Studies for malabsorption may indicate a lack of normal intestinal enzymes and an abnormal D-xylose absorption test. Occasionally, autoantibodies are found in patients who have an associated autoimmune hemolytic anemia or SLE. Autoantibodies are not found in those with an associated pernicious anemia, but biopsies of the stomach demonstrate marked lymphoid cell infiltration.

Immunologic Diagnosis

The total immunoglobulin level is below 300 mg/dL, with the IgG level below 250 mg/dL. IgM and IgA may be absent or present in reduced or normal amounts. The antibody response following specific immunization is absent.

Natural antibodies such as blood group isohemagglutinins are absent or present in low titers. The failure to produce antibody following vaccine administration establishes the diagnosis in patients who have borderline immunoglobulin values. Live attenuated vaccines should not be given. Peripheral blood B lymphocytes are usually present in normal numbers.

Cell-mediated immunity may sometimes be depressed, with negative hypersensitivity skin tests, depressed responses of peripheral blood lymphocytes to PHA and allogeneic cells, and decreased numbers of circulating peripheral blood T cells. The CD4/CD8 ratio may be reduced. The number of B cells in the peripheral blood may be normal or diminished. Occasionally, the number of null cells (lymphocytes lacking surface markers for either T or B cells) increases.

Differential Diagnosis

XLA can be differentiated from CVID by the deficiency of B cells in the former. Severe malabsorption in protein-losing enteropathy may cause hypogammaglobulinemia, but these patients always have a concomitant deficiency of serum albumin and often a selective loss of CD4 lymphocytes. When the presenting feature of CVID is an autoimmune disease, there may be a delay in recognizing and treating the immune deficiency. In most instances, however, patients with autoimmune disease have normal or elevated immunoglobulin levels. Patients with chronic lung disease should also be investigated for possible CVID. If HIV infection is suspected in a patient with hypogammaglobulinemia, HIV should be sought by means of viral culture or polymerase chain reaction (PCR) techniques rather than antibody testing.

Treatment

The treatment of CVID is identical to that of XLA (see Table 21–5). Immunoglobulin and frequent use of antibiotics are usually required. IVIG (400 mg/kg) is given once each month. Additional immunoglobulin should be given during an acute illness. Patients should be monitored at regular intervals with chest radiographs and pulmonary function tests. Pulmonary physical therapy is an essential part of treatment in patients with chronic lung disease.

Complications & Prognosis

Patients with CVID may survive to the seventh or eighth decade. Women with this disorder have had normal pregnancies and delivered normal infants (albeit agammaglobulinemic until 6 months of age). The major complication is chronic lung disease, which may develop despite adequate immunoglobulin replacement therapy. An increased prevalence of malignant disease, including leukemia, lymphoma, and gastric carcinoma, has been observed.

IMMUNODEFICIENCY WITH HYPER-IGM

Major Immunologic Features

- Levels of IgG and IgA low; elevated or normal IgM.
- Antibody function poor; cellular immunity impaired.
- Variable neutropenia in X-linked form.
- Sclerosing cholangitis, hepatitis, and hepatoma in adults.

Immunodeficiency with hyper-IgM (HIM) is characterized by high levels of IgM (ranging from 150 to 1000 mg/dL) associated with a deficiency of IgG and IgA and poor antibody function. In most instances it is inherited in an X-linked manner, but several cases have been reported of an acquired form that affects both sexes. Normal sequential development of immunoglobulins is initiated by IgM synthesis followed by IgG and IgA synthesis. HIM is usually caused by a mutation of the gene for CD40 ligand (CD154) on T cells, which regulates switching from IgM to IgG and IgA in B cells. The normal sequence of IgM to IgG antibody production depends on the binding of the B-cell CD40 to the CD40 ligand on T cells.

The disease presents with recurrent pyogenic infections, including otitis media, pneumonia, and septicemia. *Pneumocystis carinii* pneumonia is a frequent initial infection. Some patients have recurrent neutropenia, hemolytic anemia, or aplastic anemia. Those who survive past 20 years often develop sclerosing cholangitis, chronic liver disease, or hepatoma.

Laboratory evaluation may reveal a marked increase in the serum IgM level, with absence of IgG, IgA, and IgE. Isohemagglutinin titers may be elevated, and the patient may form antibodies following specific immunization. Detailed studies of cell-mediated immunity may show subtle abnormalities. Patients with this disorder may develop an infiltrating neoplasm of IgM-producing plasma cells.

A tentative diagnosis can be made by the absence of CD40 ligand on activated T cells as assessed by flow cytometry. A precise diagnosis can be made by mutation analysis of the CD40 ligand gene. Nearly every patient has a unique mutation. The carriers can also be identified.

Treatment with IVIG is similar to that for XLA (see Table 21–5). Granulocyte colony-stimulating factor (G-CSF) can be used for neutropenia, and liver transplantation has also been used in liver failure. Stem cell transplantation has been performed successfully.

SELECTIVE IGA DEFICIENCY

Major Immunologic Features

- IgA level below 15 mg/dL, with other immunoglobulin levels normal or increased.
- Cell-mediated immunity usually normal.
- Increased association with allergies, recurrent sinopulmonary infection, gastrointestinal tract disease, and autoimmune disease.
- IgA absent in secretions.

General Considerations

Selective IgA deficiency is the most common immunodeficiency disorder. The prevalence in the normal population has been estimated to be between

1:800 to 1:400. Although many patients are asymptomatic, IgA deficiency predisposes to a variety of diseases. The diagnosis of selective IgA deficiency is established by finding a serum IgA level of less than 15 mg/dL.

Immunologic Pathogenesis

The cause of selective IgA deficiency is usually unknown. An arrest in the development of B cells has been suggested on the basis of the observation that these patients have increased numbers of B cells with both surface IgA and IgM or surface IgA and IgD. An associated IgG2 subclass deficiency has been found in some patients, and this may accentuate their predisposition to infections. Usually, the number of IgA B cells is decreased; however, the presence of normal numbers of circulating IgA-bearing B cells in many patients suggests that this disorder is associated with decreased synthesis or release of IgA or impaired differentiation to IgA plasma cells rather than with the absence of IgA B lymphocytes. Using the concept of sequential immunoglobulin production (IgM to IgG to IgA), selective IgA deficiency could result from an arrest in the development of immunoglobulin-producing cells following the normal sequential development of IgM to IgG. The increased prevalence of infections, autoantibodies, autoimmune diseases, and cancer may arise from the defective mucosal immunity to environmental microbial and other pathogens. An increased prevalence of HLA-A1, -B8, and -Dw3 has been found in patients with IgA deficiency and autoimmune disease.

Cultured IgA lymphocytes from IgA-deficient patients synthesize but fail to secrete IgA. Suppressor T cells from some patients selectively inhibit IgA production by normal lymphocytes.

Acquired IgA deficiency occurs frequently in patients treated with penicillamine, phenytoin, and other drugs. In at least some instances, spontaneous recovery of IgA levels occurs when the drug is discontinued.

Clinical Features

A. Symptoms and Signs:

1. Recurrent sinopulmonary infection—Recurrent sinopulmonary bacterial or viral infections are the usual presenting features, occasionally showing as recurrent or chronic right middle lobe pneumonia. Pulmonary hemosiderosis occurs with increased frequency and may be erroneously diagnosed as chronic lung infection.

2. Allergy—In surveys of selected atopic populations the prevalence of selective IgA deficiency is 1:400 to 1:200, compared with a prevalence of 1:800 to 1:400 in the normal population, possibly because patients who lack IgA in their secretions may more readily absorb allergenic proteins, thereby enhancing the formation of IgE antibodies. Allergic diseases in patients with selective IgA deficiency are often diffi-

cult to control. Allergic symptoms in these patients may be "triggered" by infection as well as by other environmental agents.

An increase in circulating antibody to bovine proteins, sometimes with circulating immune complexes, has been found in patients with selective IgA deficiency. This has been interpreted as additional evidence for abnormal gastrointestinal tract absorption. Removal of cow's milk from the diet, however, is usually not effective in ameliorating symptoms.

A unique form of allergy exists in certain patients with selective IgA deficiency who develop high titers of antibody directed against IgA. Anaphylactic reactions from infusion of blood products containing IgA occur in some of them. The prevalence of antibodies directed against IgA in patients, however, is much higher (30–40%) than the prevalence of such anaphylactic transfusion reactions. Most patients who have anti-IgA antibodies have not had a history of immunoglobulin or blood administration, suggesting that these antibodies are autoantibodies or that they arise from sensitization to breast milk, passive transfer of maternal IgA, or cross reaction with bovine immunoglobulin from ingestion of cow's milk.

3. Gastrointestinal tract disease—An increased prevalence of celiac disease occurs in patients with selective IgA deficiency. It may present at any time and is similar to celiac disease unassociated with IgA deficiency. Intestinal biopsies show an increase in the number of IgM-producing cells. The incidence of an antibasement membrane antibody increases. Ulcerative colitis and regional enteritis have also been reported in association with selective IgA deficiency. A significant number of patients have pernicious anemia and antibodies to both intrinsic factor and gastric parietal cells.

4. Autoimmune disease—A number of autoimmune disorders are associated with selective IgA deficiency. They include SLE, rheumatoid arthritis, dermatomyositis, pernicious anemia, thyroiditis, Coombs-positive hemolytic anemia, Sjôgren's syndrome, and chronic active hepatitis. Although the association may be fortuitous, the increased prevalence of IgA deficiency in patients with SLE and rheumatoid arthritis (1:200 to 1:100) is statistically significant.

The clinical presentation in patients with autoimmune disease associated with selective IgA deficiency does not differ significantly from that of individuals with the identical disorder and normal or elevated levels of IgA. Because patients with selective IgA deficiency are capable of making normal amounts of antibody in the other immunoglobulin classes, they usually have the autoantibodies that characterize the specific autoimmune disease (antinuclear antibody, anti-DNA antibody, antiparietal cell antibody, etc).

5. Selective IgA deficiency in apparently healthy adults—Patients with selective IgA deficiency are capable of making normal amounts of antibody of the IgG and IgM classes. Many are entirely asymptomatic, although some may develop significant disease with time. The reasons for this are unclear, but the IgA deficiency may affect exposures to pathogens and other agents in the environment.

6. Selective IgA deficiency and genetic factors—Both an autosomal-recessive and an autosomal-dominant mode of inheritance of IgA deficiency have been postulated. IgA deficiency appears with greater than normal frequency in families with other immunodeficiency disorders such as hypogammaglobulinemia. Partial deletion of the long or short arm of chromosome 18 (18q syndrome) or ring chromosome 18 has been described. Many patients with abnormalities of chromosome 18, however, have normal levels of IgA in their serum. Selective IgA deficiency has been reported in one identical twin but not the other. In a study of familial IgA deficiency, an association with HLA-A2, -B8, and -Dw3 was described. Other studies have shown an increase in association with HLA-A1 and -B8.

7. Selective IgA deficiency and cancer—Selective IgA deficiency has been reported in association with thymoma, reticulum cell sarcoma, and squamous cell carcinoma of the esophagus and lungs. Several patients with IgA deficiency and cancer also had concomitant autoimmune disease and recurrent infection.

8. Selective IgA deficiency and drugs—Phenytoin and many other anticonvulsants have been implicated as a possible cause of selective IgA deficiency or hypogammaglobulinemia in some patients, who are frequently symptomatic with recurrent sinopulmonary infections. Withdrawal of the drug does not always result in a return to normal IgA levels. In vitro production of IgA by peripheral blood lymphocytes in these patients may be normal or deficient. Deficient T-cell/B-cell interaction is found in some patients.

B. Laboratory Findings: Selective IgA deficiency is defined as a serum level of IgA below 15 mg/dL, with normal or increased levels of IgG, IgM, IgD, and IgE. Some patients with IgA deficiency may also have IgG2 subclass deficiency. B cells from these patients are capable of forming normal amounts of antibody following immunization. In most instances, absence of IgA in the serum is accompanied by absent IgA in the secretions but with normal secretory component. Increased amounts of 7S IgM may be found in the serum and secretions. As discussed earlier, some patients have autoantibodies, including antibodies directed against IgG, IgM, and IgA. The number of circulating peripheral blood B cells (including IgA-bearing B cells) is normal. Increased numbers of suppressor T cells have been found in some patients.

Cell-mediated immunity is usually normal as assessed by delayed hypersensitivity skin tests, the response of isolated peripheral blood lymphocytes to PHA and allogeneic cells, and the number of circulating T cells. A few patients have low levels of T cells, diminished production of T-cell interferon, and decreased lymphocyte mitogenic responses.

Other laboratory abnormalities relate to the associated diseases. Individuals who have chronic sinopulmonary infection may have abnormal roentgenograms and pulmonary function. Those with celiac disease show appropriate pathology in gastrointestinal tract biopsies, impaired D-xylose absorption, and antibasement membrane antibody in some cases. Patients with autoimmune disease have characteristic autoantibodies, such as anti-DNA, antinuclear, antiparietal cell, and a positive Coombs test. An increase in circulating immune complexes has been described.

Differential Diagnosis

Selective IgA deficiency must be distinguished from other more severe immunodeficiency disorders with a concomitant deficiency of IgA. Forty percent of patients with ataxia-telangiectasia have IgA deficiency. If IgA deficiency is found during the first years of life, a definitive diagnosis may not be possible because the complete ataxia-telangiectasia syndrome may not be present until the patient is 4–5 years old. Selective IgA deficiency occurs in chronic mucocutaneous candidiasis and cellular immunodeficiency with abnormal immunoglobulin synthesis (Nezelof's syndrome) and selective deficiency of IgG2. A careful history should be obtained to rule out IgA deficiency secondary to drugs, especially anticonvulsants or penicillamine.

Treatment

Patients with selective IgA deficiency should not be treated with gamma globulin. Therapeutic gamma globulin contains only a small quantity of IgA, and this is not likely to reach mucosal secretions through parenteral administration. Furthermore, IgA-deficient patients are capable of forming IgG or IgE anti-IgA antibodies and subsequently experiencing anaphylactic transfusion reactions. Patients with combined IgA and IgG subclass deficiency with documented impaired antibody formation have been treated with gamma globulin without risk of anaphylaxis. Patients with recurrent sinopulmonary infection should be treated aggressively with broad-spectrum antibiotics to avoid permanent pulmonary complications. Those with SLE, rheumatoid arthritis, celiac disease, and so on are treated in the same fashion as patients with the same diseases without IgA deficiency.

Transfusion reactions in patients with selective IgA deficiency may be minimized by several means. Packed washed (three times) erythrocytes should be used to treat anemia. This decreases but does not eliminate the risk. Alternatively, patients may be given blood from an IgA-deficient donor whose blood type matches the recipient's. Patients should carry medical identification indicating they are IgA-deficient.

Complications & Prognosis

IgA-deficient patients have survived to the sixth or seventh decade without severe disease, but most become symptomatic during the first decade of life. Prompt treatment of complications and associated diseases increases longevity and reduces morbidity. This requires regular follow-up examinations. A very few patients have developed normal IgA levels after years of IgA deficiency.

SELECTIVE IGM DEFICIENCY

Selective IgM deficiency is a rare disorder associated with the absence of IgM and normal levels of other immunoglobulin classes. IgM-bearing B cells are present in normal numbers. Some patients are capable of normal antibody responses in the other immunoglobulin classes following specific immunization, whereas others respond poorly. Cell-mediated immunity appears to be intact, based on limited study.

The cause of selective IgM deficiency is unknown. As a developmental disorder, absent IgM with normal IgG and IgA contradicts the theory of sequential immunoglobulin development. It is found in both males and females.

Patients with selective IgM deficiency are susceptible to autoimmune disease and to overwhelming infection with polysaccharide-containing organisms (eg, pneumococci, *H influenzae*). They may also have chronic dermatitis, diarrhea, and recurrent respiratory infections. It would appear logical to treat these patients in a manner similar to the way an infant is treated following splenectomy, that is, either immediate antibiotic (penicillin or ampicillin) treatment of all infections or continuous antibiotic treatment. If patients are unable to form antibody to specific antigens, gamma-globulin therapy should be given.

SELECTIVE DEFICIENCY OF IGG SUBCLASSES

Major Immunologic Features

- Total serum IgG normal, but one or more IgG subclasses deficient.
- T-cell immunity normal.
- Recurrent bacterial and respiratory infections.
- Sometimes associated with other immunodeficiencies, such as selective IgA deficiency or ataxia–telangiectasia.

General Considerations

IgG antibodies exist in four isotypic variants identified by antigenic differences of the Fc portion of the immunoglobulin molecule. These are termed IgG1, IgG2, IgG3, and IgG4 and make up approximately 65, 20, 10, and 5% of the total serum immunoglobulin levels, respectively (Figure 21–2). IgG subclasses develop independently, with IgG1 and IgG3 maturing more rapidly than IgG2 or IgG4. Deletion of constant heavy-chain genes or abnormalities of isotype switching may result in deficiencies of one or more of the IgG subclasses with normal or near normal levels of total IgG.

Clinically, patients have recurrent respiratory tract infections and repeated pyogenic sinopulmonary infections with *S pneumoniae, H influenzae,* and *Staphylococcus aureus.* Some patients develop or present with evidence of autoimmune diseases, such as SLE or pulmonary hemosiderosis.

IgG1 deficiency is usually associated with other subclass deficiencies and low total IgG, and therefore these patients have common variable immunodeficiency.

IgG2 deficiency is associated with recurrent sinopulmonary infections and an inability to respond to polysaccharide antigens (such as pneumococcal or *H influenzae* polysaccharide). The patient does respond normally, however, to protein antigens such as tetanus or diphtheria toxoid.

IgG2/IgG4 deficiency is usually found in individuals with recurrent infections or autoimmune disease who are either normoglobulinemic or hypergamma-

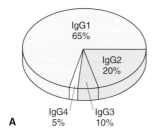
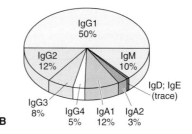

Figure 21–2. Normal distribution of serum immunoglobulins. **A:** Percentages of IgG subclasses relative to total IgG. **B:** Percentages of immunoglobulin classes and subclasses relative to total immunoglobulin.

globulinemic. A few healthy individuals with this deficiency have been described. It is also found in some patients with ataxia-telangiectasia.

IgG3 deficiency is found in a small percentage of those individuals with recurrent infections who are screened by specific IgG subclass determinations for antibody deficiency. Familial occurrence of IgG3 deficiency has been reported.

IgG3 deficiency is also associated with recurrent respiratory infections or manifestations of autoimmune disease. IgG4 is low or absent in a significant number of asymptomatic (normal) individuals.

A diagnosis of one or more IgG subclass deficiencies is made by the finding of significantly low levels (>2 standard deviations below age-adjusted geometric means) of one or more IgG subclasses. For children older than 2 years, IgG1 levels should be <250 mg/dL, IgG2 <50 mg/dL, and IgG3 <25 mg/dL. The total IgG concentration may be normal, low, or elevated. The response to immunization may be variable, ranging from normal to a selective inability to respond to polysaccharide antigens. T-cell immunity is usually intact.

Patients with selective IgG subclass deficiency respond to treatment with immunoglobulin administered in a manner similar to that used in the treatment of CVID or XLA. The decision to commit a patient to lifelong treatment is a difficult one, however, and should not be based on immunoglobulin levels alone. The antibody response following immunization and the clinical course should be assessed before IVIG is given.

Impaired Polysaccharide Responsiveness

These patients, similar to those with IgG subclass and IgA deficiency, have recurrent respiratory infections, sinusitis, or asthma. Most are children younger than age 5. They respond normally to protein antigens but have impaired responses to polysaccharide antigens such as pneumococcal vaccine. This may be maturational, and the child may grow out of the problem by age 5–10, but in others it persists for a lifetime. Management includes frequent and sometimes continuous antibiotics and, very rarely, IVIG.

IMMUNODEFICIENCY WITH THYMOMA (Good's Syndrome)

Major Immunologic Features
- Recurrent infections.
- Acquired hypogammaglobulinemia may precede or follow thymoma.

General Considerations

Recurrent infection may be the presenting sign if the thymoma is associated with immunodeficiency. This takes the form of sinopulmonary infection, chronic diarrhea, dermatitis, septicemia, stomatitis, and urinary tract infection. Thymoma has also been associated with muscle weakness (when found in conjunction with myasthenia gravis), aplastic anemia, thrombocytopenia, diabetes, amyloidosis, chronic hepatitis, and the development of nonthymic cancer.

Patients with acquired hypogammaglobulinemia should be observed at regular intervals for the development of thymoma, which is usually detected on routine chest roentgenograms. Occasionally, the thymoma is detected prior to the development of immunodeficiency. Marked hypogammaglobulinemia is usually present. The antibody response following immunization may be abnormal. Some patients have deficient T-cell immunity as assayed by delayed hypersensitivity skin tests and peripheral blood lymphocyte response to PHA. Increased activity of suppressor cells has been found in some patients. In patients who have aregenerative anemia, pure erythrocyte aplasia is seen on marrow aspiration. Thrombocytopenia, granulocytopenia, and autoantibody formation are occasionally observed. In 75% of cases, the thymoma is of the spindle cell type. Some tumors may be malignant.

In no instance has the removal of the thymoma resulted in improvement of immunodeficiency. This is in contrast to pure erythrocyte aplasia and myasthenia gravis, which may improve following removal of the thymoma. IVIG is beneficial in controlling recurrent infections and chronic diarrhea.

The overall prognosis is poor, and death secondary to infection is common. Death may also be related to associated abnormalities such as thrombocytopenia and aplastic anemia.

5′-NUCLEOTIDASE DEFICIENCY

There have been several reports of decreased activity of 5′-nucleotidase and immunodeficiency. This enzyme deficiency has been described in association with acquired hypogammaglobulinemia, X-linked hypogammaglobulinemia, Wiskott–Aldrich syndrome, AIDS, and selective IgA deficiency. 5′-Nucleotidase, however, may be a differentiation marker of lymphocytes—in particular B lymphocytes—in the peripheral circulation of these patients and the deficiency may therefore reflect a diminished number of B cells or an abnormality of their maturation.

TRANSCOBALAMIN II DEFICIENCY

Several patients have been described with a deficiency of transcobalamin II, a vitamin B_{12}-binding protein necessary for the transport of vitamin B_{12} into cells. These patients have hypogammaglobulinemia, macrocytic anemia, lymphopenia, granulocytopenia, thrombocytopenia, and severe intestinal malabsorption. Vitamin B_{12} treatment resulted in the reversal of all of the manifestations of the disorder. Specific antibody synthesis occurred following administration of vitamin B_{12}.

REFERENCES

MECHANISMS OF IMMUNODEFICIENCY

Noroski LM, Shearer WT: Screening for primary immunodeficiencies in the clinical immunology laboratory. *Clin Immunol Immunopathol* 1998;86:239.

Ochs HD, Smith CIE, Puck JM (editors): *Primary Immunodeficiency Diseases.* Oxford University Press, 1999.

Rosen FS, Cooper MD, Wedgewood RJP: The primary immunodeficiencies. *N Engl J Med* 1995;333:431.

Stiehm ER: *Immunologic Disorders in Infants and Children,* 4th ed. WB Saunders, 1996.

Stiehm ER: New and old immunodeficiencies. *Pediatr Res* 1993;33(suppl):S2.

WHO Scientific Group: Primary Immunodeficiency Diseases. Clin Exp Immunology. 1995; Supplement

X-LINKED AGAMMAGLOBULINEMIA

Marx J: Tyrosine kinase defect also causes immunodeficiency. *Science* 1993;259:897.

Monafo V et al: X-linked agammaglobulinemia and isolated growth hormone deficiency. *Acta Paediatr Scan* 1991; 80:563.

Tsukada et al: Deficient expression of a B cell cytoplasmic tyrosine kinase in human X-linked agammaglobulinemia. *Cell* 1993;72:279.

Van Maldergem L et al: Echovirus meningoencephalitis in X-linked hypogammaglobulinemia. *Acta Paediatr Scand* 1989;78:325.

TRANSIENT HYPOGAMMAGLOBULINEMIA OF INFANCY

Tiller Jr, TL, Buckley RH: Transient hypogammaglobulinemia of infancy: Review of the literature, clinical and immunologic features of 11 new cases, and long term followup. *J Pediatr* 1978;92:347.

COMMON VARIABLE IMMUNODEFICIENCY

Cunningham-Rundles C: Clinical and immunologic analyses of 103 patients with common variable immunodeficiency. *J Clin Immunol* 1989;9:22.

Eisenstein EM et al: Evidence for a generalized signaling abnormality in B cells from patients with common variable immunodeficiency. *Adv Exper Med Biol* 1995;371B: 699.

Hermans PE et al: Idiopathic late-onset immunoglobulin deficiency: Clinical observations in 50 patients. *Am J Med* 1976;61:221.

X-LINKED IMMUNODEFICIENCY WITH HYPER-IGM

Arrufo A et al: The CD40 ligand, gp39, is defective in activated T cells from patients with X-linked hyper IgM syndrome. *Cell* 1993;72:291.

Levy J et al: Clinical spectrum of X-linked hyper-IgM syndrome. *J Pediatr* 1997;131:47.

Stiehm ER, Fudenberg HH: Clinical and immunologic features of dysgammaglobulinemia type 1. *Am J Med* 1966; 40:895.

SELECTIVE IGA DEFICIENCY

Ammann AJ, Hong R: Selective IgA deficiency: Presentation of 30 cases and a review of the literature. *Medicine* 1971;50:223.

Ferreira A et al: Anti-IgA antibodies in selective IgA deficiency and in primary immunodeficient patients treated with gamma-globulin. *Clin Immunol Immunopathol* 1988; 47:199.

Oxelius VA et al: Linkage of IgA deficiency to Gm allotypes: The influence of Gm allotypes on IgA-IgG deficiency. *Clin Exper Immunol* 1995;99:211.

SELECTIVE IGM DEFICIENCY

Guill MF et al: IgM deficiency: Clinical spectrum and immunologic assessment. *Ann Allergy* 1989;62:547.

IGG SUBCLASS DEFICIENCY

Heiner DC: Recognition and management of IgG subclass deficiencies. *Pediatr Infect Dis J* 1987;6:235.

Inone R et al: IgG2 deficiency associated with defects in production of interferon gamma. *Scan J Immunol* 1995; 41:130.

Ochs HD, Wedgwood RJ: IgG subclass deficiencies. *Ann Rev Med* 1987;38:325.

Schur PH et al: Selective gamma-G globulin deficiencies in patients with recurrent pyogenic infections. *N Engl J Med* 1970;283:631.

IMPAIRED POLYSACCHARIDE RESPONSIVENESS

Ambrisino DM et al: An immunodeficiency characterized by impaired antibody responses to polysaccharides. *N Engl J Med* 1987;316:790.

IMMUNODEFICIENCY WITH THYMOMA

Hermaszewsk RA, Webster AD: Primary hypogammaglobulinemia: A survey of clinical manifestations and complications. *Quart J Med* 1993;86:31.

Soppi E et al: Thymoma with immunodeficiency (Good's syndrome) associated with myasthenia gravis and benign IgG gammopathy. *Arch Intern Med* 1985;145:1704.

Waldmann TA et al: Thymoma, hypogammaglobulinemia and absence of eosinophils. *J Clin Invest* 1967;46:1127.

T-Cell Immunodeficiency Disorders

22

Robert L. Roberts, MD, PhD, & E. Richard Stiehm, MD

Immunodeficiency disorders with isolated defective T-cell immunity are rare because of the collaboration between T and B cells in the process of antibody formation. Some patients with T-cell deficiency have normal levels of immunoglobulin but fail to produce specific antibody following immunization.

Patients with cellular immunodeficiency disorders are susceptible to a variety of acute and chronic viral, fungal, and protozoal infections. They may also have unusual susceptibility to malignancy.

Screening tests to evaluate T-cell immunity are listed in Table 22–1. Additional tests permit precise diagnosis in many instances.

Table 22–1. Evaluation of cell-mediated immunity.

Test	Comment
Total lymphocyte count	Normal at any age: >1200/µL
Delayed cutaneous hyper-sensitivity skin test	Used to evaluate specific immunity to antigens. Suggested antigens are *Candida,* mumps, tetanus toxoid, purified protein derivative
Lymphocyte response to mitogens (PHA), antigens, and allogeneic cells (mixed leukocyte culture)	Used to evaluate T-cell function. Results are expressed as stimulated counts divided by resting counts (stimulated index)
Total T cells using monoclonal antibodies to CD3	Used to quantitate the number of circulating T cells. Normal: >60% of total lymphocytes
Monoclonal antibody T-cell subsets (CD4 and CD8)	Determines T-cell subsets, eg, helper/suppressor
Cytokine production (IL-1, IL-2, lymphotoxin, tumor necrosis factor, etc)	Used to detect specific cytokine production from subsets of mononuclear cells as an index of function
Cytotoxic function	Determines general and specific T-cell effector function

Abbreviations: PHA = phytohemagglutinin; IL = interleukin.

DIGEORGE ANOMALY
(Congenital Thymic Aplasia, Immunodeficiency With Hypoparathyroidism, Third & Fourth Pouch/Arch Syndrome)

Major Immunologic Features
- Congenital aplasia or hypoplasia of the thymus and parathyroid glands.
- Hypocalcemia.
- Variable degree of T-cell deficiency.
- Immunoglobulin levels and antibody function usually normal.
- Characteristic facial abnormalities.
- Congenital heart disease common.

General Considerations
DiGeorge anomaly is one of the few immunodeficiency disorders with symptoms immediately following birth. The complete syndrome consists of the following features: (1) abnormal faces consisting of low-set ears, "fish-shaped" mouth, hypertelorism, notched ear pinnae, micrognathia, and an antimongoloid slant of eyes (Figure 22–1); (2) hypoparathyroidism with hypocalcemia; (3) congenital heart disease; and (4) cellular immunodeficiency. Initial symptoms are related to associated abnormalities of the parathyroids and heart and may result in hypocalcemia and congestive heart failure, respectively. If the diagnosis of DiGeorge anomaly is suspected because of these early clinical findings, confirmation may be obtained by demonstrating decreased numbers of T cells and a 22 q11 chromosomal deletion.

Immunologic Pathogenesis
During weeks 6–8 of intrauterine life, the thymus and parathyroid glands develop from epithelial evaginations of the third and fourth pharyngeal pouches (Figure 22–2). The thymus begins to migrate caudally during week 12 of gestation. At the same time, the philtrum of the lip and the ear tubercle become differentiated along with other aortic arch structures. It is likely that DiGeorge anomaly is the result of interference with normal embryologic development at approximately 12 weeks of gestation. In some pa-

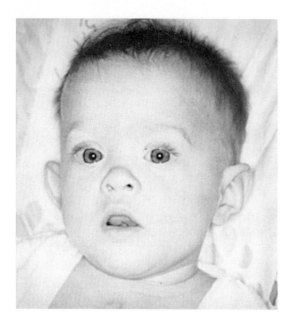

Figure 22–1. Infant with DiGeorge anomaly. Prominent are low-set and malformed ears, hypertelorism, and fish-shaped mouth. Also note the surgical scar from cardiac surgery.

tients, the thymus is not absent but is in an abnormal location or is extremely small, though the histologic appearance is normal. It is possible that such patients have "partial" DiGeorge anomaly, in which hypertrophy of the thymus may take place with subsequent development of normal immunity.

Genetic Pathogenesis

Up to 90% of patients with DiGeorge anomaly have a hemizygous deletion of 22q11, a region termed the DGCR (DiGeorge critical region) that can be readily detected by fluorescent in situ hybridization (FISH) using probes for this region and an undeleted chromosome 22 region near this locus. Patients have similar cardiac defects and the Spritzen (velocardiofacial) syndrome have a similar deletion. This deleted region includes a DiGeorge candidate gene termed *Ufd1* (ubiquitin fusion degradation) that encodes for a transcription factor regulating cell death in the neural crest, branchial arches, the heart, and the thymus. One or the other parent of a few patients with the DiGeorge anomaly may also carry the deletion, and then the disorder is inherited in an autosomal-dominant fashion. Maternal alcoholism may be a risk factor in some patients with the DiGeorge anomaly.

Clinical Features

A. Symptoms and Signs: The most frequent presenting sign in patients with DiGeorge anomaly occurs in the first 24 hours of life with hypocalcemia

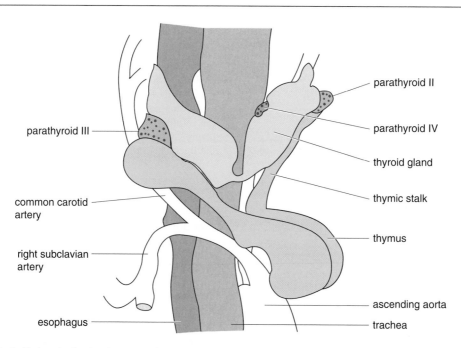

Figure 22–2. Embryologic development of the thymus and parathyroid glands from the third and fourth pharyngeal pouches.

that is resistant to standard therapy. Various types of congenital heart disease have been described, including interrupted aortic arch, septal defects, patent ductus arteriosus, and truncus arteriosus. Renal abnormalities may also be present. Most patients have the characteristic facial appearance described earlier. Patients who survive the immediate neonatal period may then develop recurrent or chronic infection with various viral, bacterial, fungal, or protozoal organisms. Pneumonia, chronic infection of the mucous membranes with *Candida,* diarrhea, and failure to thrive may be present.

Spontaneous improvement of T-cell immunity often occurs, particularly when initial T cell counts are low but not absent. These patients are considered to have "partial" DiGeorge anomaly, but the reason for the spontaneous improvement in T-cell immunity is unknown. Patients should also be suspected of having DiGeorge anomaly on the basis of hypocalcemia and congenital heart disease with or without the abnormal facies or T-cell defects. Some of these patients develop severe T-cell deficiency.

B. Laboratory Findings: T-cell immunity can be evaluated immediately after birth in a patient suspected of having DiGeorge anomaly. The lymphocyte count is usually low (<1500/μL) but may be normal or elevated. A chest x-ray film of the anterior mediastinum may reveal absence of the thymic shadow, indicating failure of normal development. Delayed hypersensitivity skin tests to recall antigens are of little value during early infancy, because sufficient time has not elapsed for sensitization to occur. T cells are markedly diminished in number, and the peripheral blood lymphocytes fail to respond to phytohemagglutinin (PHA) or allogeneic cells.

Immunoglobulin evaluation is not useful because of passive maternal immunoglobulin. Most DiGeorge patients can produce adequate specific antibody responses. Sequential studies of both T-cell and B-cell immunity are necessary because either improvement or deterioration of immunity can occur spontaneously.

Hypoparathyroidism is diagnosed by low serum calcium, elevated serum phosphorus, and an absence of parathyroid hormone. Congenital heart disease may be diagnosed immediately following birth and may be mild or severe. Other congenital abnormalities include esophageal atresia, bifid uvula, and urinary tract abnormalities.

Immunologic Diagnosis

T-cell immunity may be markedly depressed, as indicated by lymphocytopenia, depressed numbers of circulating T cells, and diminished proliferative responses to PHA and allogeneic cells. Normal T-cell immunity may develop with time, particularly if the initial CD4 cell count exceeds 400 cells/μL and there is some proliferative response to mitogens.

Many patients with DiGeorge anomaly have normal B-cell immunity as indicated by normal levels of immunoglobulins and a normal antibody response following immunization. Others, however, have low immunoglobulin levels and fail to make specific antibody following immunization. Live attenuated viral vaccines should not be used for immunization in these patients. Natural killer (NK) cell activity is normal.

Differential Diagnosis

Infants with severe congenital heart disease and subsequent congestive heart failure who develop transient hypocalcemia should be suspected of having DiGeorge anomaly. When the characteristic facial features are found, suspicion should be even stronger. Studies of T-cell immunity usually establish a diagnosis, except in infants with DiGeorge anomaly who have effective T-cell immunity. It is essential that all infants with congenital heart disease and hypocalcemia be monitored until they are at least 1 year old.

The hypocalcemia associated with DiGeorge anomaly is usually permanent, in contrast to that seen in congenital heart disease with congestive heart failure. Parathyroid hormone levels are low to absent, and the patients are resistant to the standard treatment for hypocalcemia. Low parathyroid hormone levels may also be found in transient hypocalcemia in infancy.

Immunologic studies in DiGeorge anomaly and in severe combined immunodeficiency disease may be identical in the newborn period. Patients with the fetal alcohol syndrome may have facial and cardiac abnormalities similar to those in patients with DiGeorge anomaly, as well as recurrent infections associated with decreased T-cell immunity.

Treatment

Patients with T-cell deficiency should receive *Pneumocystis carinii* prophylaxis.

General care includes management of hypocalcemia and correction of cardiac abnormalities. The hypocalcemia is controlled by calcium supplementation orally in conjunction with vitamin D or parathyroid hormone. Congenital heart disease frequently results in congestive heart failure and may require immediate surgical correction. If surgery is performed prior to the availability of a fetal thymus or bone marrow transplantation, blood transfusion products should be irradiated with 3000 R to prevent a graft-versus-host (GVH) reaction.

Transplantation of fetal thymus, postnatal thymus, and HLA-matched bone marrow have all been used for permanent reconstitution of T cell immunity. No attempts at immunologic reconstitution are warranted if T-cell immunity is normal. Most patients undergo spontaneous resolution of the T-cell immunodeficiency. Intravenous immunoglobulin therapy should be used if antibody deficiency exists and to control recurrent infection.

Complications & Prognosis

Prolonged survival has been reported following successful thymus transplantation or spontaneous remission of immunodeficiency. Sudden death may occur in untreated patients or in patients initially found to have normal T-cell immunity. Congenital heart disease may be severe, and the infant may not survive surgical correction. Death from GVH disease following blood transfusions has been observed in patients in whom a diagnosis of DiGeorge anomaly was not suspected. Most patients who survive long term have minimal heart disease.

CHRONIC MUCOCUTANEOUS CANDIDIASIS (With & Without Endocrinopathy)

Major Immunologic Features

• Chronic candidal infection of skin, nails, and mucous membranes with or without endocrinopathy.
• Negative delayed hypersensitivity skin tests to *Candida* antigen despite chronic candidal infection.
• Intact T-cell immunity to most antigens.

General Considerations

Chronic mucocutaneous candidiasis affects both males and females. A familial occurrence has been reported in some instances, suggesting an autosomal-recessive or -dominant inheritance. The disorder is a selective defect in T-cell immunity, resulting in susceptibility to chronic candidal infection. B-cell immunity is intact, resulting in a normal antibody response to *Candida* and, in some patients, the development of autoantibodies associated with idiopathic endocrinopathies. The disorder may appear as early as

1 year of age or may be delayed until the second decade.

Various theories have been proposed to explain the association of chronic candidal infection and the development of endocrinopathy. Initially it was believed that hypoparathyroidism predisposed to candidal infection. Subsequently it was found that many patients developed severe candidal infection without evidence of hypoparathyroidism. A basic autoimmune disorder has been postulated, with the suggestion that the thymus also functions as an endocrine organ and that the thymus and other endocrine glands are involved in an autoimmune destructive process.

Clinical Features

A. Symptoms and Signs: The initial presentation of chronic mucocutaneous candidiasis may be either chronic candidal infection or idiopathic endocrinopathy. If candidal infection appears first, several years to decades may elapse before endocrinopathy occurs. Candidal infection may involve the mucous membranes, skin, nails, and, in older patients, the vagina. In severe forms, infection of the skin occurs in a "stocking-glove" distribution and of granulomatous lesions (Figure 22–3). Patients are usually not susceptible to systemic candidiasis. Rarely, they may develop other infections.

Other findings are related to the specific endocrinopathy. The autoimmune polyendocrinopathy-candidiasis ectodermal dystrophy (APECED) syndrome is inherited as an autosomal-recessive disorder. Hypoparathyroidism with hypocalcemia and tetany is the most common endocrinopathy. Addison's disease is the next most common.

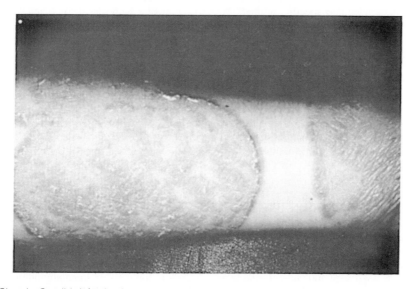

Figure 22–3. Chronic *Candida* infection in a patient with mucocutaneous candidiasis. Note the well-demarcated areas of involvement.

Other patients not fitting this syndrome may also have hypothyroidism, diabetes mellitus, hypogonadism, adrenocorticotropic hormone (ACTH) deficiency, and pernicious anemia. Occasionally, there is a history of acute or chronic hepatitis. Associated disorders include pulmonary fibrosis, keratoconjunctivitis, vitiligo, alopecia, enamel dysplasia, hematologic disorders, and myopathy.

B. Laboratory Findings: Studies of T-cell immunity reveal a specific, although variable, defect. Patients usually have a normal total lymphocyte count. Peripheral blood lymphocytes respond normally to PHA, allogeneic cells, and antigens other than *Candida* antigens. Delayed hypersensitivity skin test response to *Candida* antigen is absent in the presence of documented chronic candidiasis. Some patients may have additional defects, including the inability to form migration inhibitory factor (MIF) or other cytokines in response to *Candida* antigens or the inability of lymphocytes to be activated by *Candida* antigens and decreased suppressor T-cell activity.

B-cell immunity is intact, as evidenced by normal or elevated levels of immunoglobulins, increased amounts of antibody directed against *Candida,* and autoantibody formation. Occasionally, IgA is absent. Plasma inhibitors of T-cell function and increased numbers of suppressor T cells have been reported in some cases. Isolated cases have neutrophil chemotaxis or macrophage abnormalities.

Other laboratory abnormalities are related to the endocrinopathies. Hypoparathyroidism causes decreased serum calcium, elevated serum phosphorus, and low or absent parathyroid hormone. Increased skin pigmentation may herald the onset of Addison's disease prior to disturbances in serum electrolytes, which can be documented by an ACTH stimulation test. Other abnormalities of endocrine function include hypothyroidism, abnormal vitamin B_{12} absorption, and diabetes mellitus. Abnormal liver function studies may indicate chronic hepatitis. Occasionally, iron deficiency is present, which, when treated, results in improved resistance to the candidal infection. Autoantibodies associated with specific endocrinopathy are usually present before and during the development of endocrine dysfunction and may be absent when endocrine deficiency is complete. Endocrine function should be evaluated on a yearly basis because the endocrinopathies are progressive.

Immunologic Diagnosis

Major indices of T-cell immunity—response of peripheral blood lymphocytes to PHA and allogeneic cells, activation of lymphocytes and cytokine production in response to antigens other than *Candida* antigens, and T-cell numbers—are normal. In some patients, only the delayed hypersensitivity skin test response to *Candida* antigens is absent. Others have absent cytokine production or absent lymphocyte activation by *Candida* antigens. Plasma inhibitors of cellular immunity may also occur. B-cell immunity is intact with normal production of antibody to *Candida.*

Differential Diagnosis

Children with chronic candidal infection of the mucous membranes may have a variety of immunodeficiency disorders. Detailed studies of T-cell immunity differentiate between chronic mucocutaneous candidiasis, in which there is a selective deficiency of T-cell immunity to *Candida* antigens, from other disorders in which T-cell immunity may be completely deficient. DiGeorge anomaly (thymic aplasia and hypoparathyroidism) presents early in infancy, whereas chronic mucocutaneous candidiasis with hypoparathyroidism is a disorder of later onset and progressive nature. Patients with late-onset idiopathic endocrinopathies should be considered to have chronic mucocutaneous candidiasis, even though candidal infection is not present at the time of diagnosis. These patients may develop chronic candidal infection as late as 10–15 years after the onset of endocrinopathy. A patient with chronic candidiasis, especially involving the mucous membranes, may have secondary immunodeficiency from immunosuppressive therapy or HIV infection.

Treatment

Topical treatment with a variety of antifungal drugs is only minimally successful for skin infection. Oral antifungals, such as ketoconazole, fluconazole, and itraconazole are the mainstay of therapy and often control candidal infections. Intravenous amphotericin can be used if oral antifungal therapy is ineffective.

Treatment does not prevent the development of endocrinopathies. The physician must be alert to the gradual development of endocrine dysfunction—particularly Addison's disease and hypothyroidism. Bone marrow transplantation was successful in a single case.

Complications & Prognosis

Patients may survive to the second or third decade but usually experience extensive morbidity. Individuals with severe candidal infection of the mucous membranes and skin develop serious psychologic difficulties. Systemic infection with *Candida* usually does not occur. Rarely, patients may develop systemic infection from other fungi. Hypoparathyroidism is difficult to manage, and complications are frequent. Patients may succumb at an early age from endocrinopathy, bronchiectasis, or chronic hepatitis.

NATURAL KILLER CELL DEFICIENCY

NK cells are non-B/non-T-cell (CD3$^-$) lymphocytes but have receptors for the Fc portion of the immunoglobulin molecule (CD16). In addition, they have the NKH-1 (CD56[+], CD16[+]) determinant, which identifies the NK cells as large granular lymphocytes morphologically. NK cells spontaneously lyse a number of target cells, including tumor cells, a broad range of virus-infected cells when activated by interleukin-2 (IL-2) or interferon gamma. It is therefore believed that these cells play a role in host defense against cancer and microbial infection.

Deficiency of NK cells is not confined to a single defined immunodeficiency disorder, although there are isolated case reports of what appear to be selective NK deficiencies. NK-cell deficiency has been documented in the Chèdiak–Higashi syndrome, the X-linked lymphoproliferative syndrome, and leukocyte adhesion defect (CD11/CD18 deficiency). NK-cell deficiency has also been detected in primary immunodeficiency diseases, primarily in severe combined immunodeficiency disease and other T-cell disorders, suggesting an association between NK- and T-cell defects.

Although NK-cell deficiency has been detected most consistently in the X-linked lymphoproliferative syndrome (see Chapter 23), there are reports of patients with recurrent severe infections with herpes viruses, including varicella, cytomegalovirus infection, and herpes simplex in whom immunologic evaluation was normal, except for deficient NK-cell numbers and function. Thus, isolated defects in NK-cell function occur, but no specific treatment exists to correct the NK-cell defect.

IDIOPATHIC CD4 LYMPHOCYTOPENIA

Idiopathic CD4 lymphocytopenia possibly caused by an as yet unidentified virus or viruses varies from minimal abnormalities to fatal opportunistic infection in both males and females between the ages of 17 and 70 years. The defect is reversible in some patients. The syndrome can be differentiated from HIV-associated CD4 lymphocytopenia by the absence of evidence of HIV-1 infection, using HIV-1 polymerase chain reaction (PCR) or antibody testing, and the absence of hypergammaglobulinemia. In many cases CD4 lymphopenia may be a normal variant.

BIOTIN-DEPENDENT CARBOXYLASE DEFICIENCIES

Patients with infantile chronic mucocutaneous candidiasis, ataxia, alopecia, intermittent lactic acidosis, and increased excretion of β-hydroxypropionate, methylcitrate, β-methylcrotonylglycine, and 3-β-hydroxyisovalerate in the urine have been described. They have immunologic abnormalities in both B-cell and T-cell function. A second (neonatal) form has been described with severe acidosis and multiple episodes of sepsis. An intrauterine diagnosis has been made, and intrauterine therapy with biotin has been given. Treatment with biotin, 10 mg/day, reduced the abnormal metabolites in the urine and reversed the alopecia, ataxia, and chronic candidiasis. Multiple biotin-dependent carboxylase deficiencies may be one of several causes of the chronic mucocutaneous candidiasis syndrome with abnormal T-cell function or severe recurrent sepsis. Biotin deficiency and immunodeficiency may also result from nutritional deficiencies; hyperalimentation without biotin supplementation; and diets high in avidin (raw eggs), which binds biotin and prevents its absorption.

REFERENCES

DiGEORGE ANOMALY

DiGeorge AM: Congenital absence of the thymus and its immunologic consequences: Concurrence with congenital hypoparathyroidism. In: *Immunologic Deficiency Diseases in Man.* Bergsma D, McKusick FA (eds). National Foundation-March of Dimes Original Article Series. Williams & Wilkins, 1968.

Iamagishi H et al: A molecular pathway revealing a genetic basis for human cardiac and craniofacial defects. *Science* 1999;183:1158.

Markert ML et al: Complete DiGeorge syndrome: Persistence of profound immunodeficiency. *J Pediatr* 1998; 132:15.

Radford DJ et al: Spectrum of DiGeorge syndrome in patients with truncus arteriosis: Expanded DiGeorge syndrome. *Pediatr Cardiol* 1988;9:95.

CHRONIC MUCOCUTANEOUS CANDIDIASIS

Ahonen P et al: Clinical variation of autoimmune polyendocrinopathy-candidiasis-ectodermal dysplasia (APECED) in a series of 68 patients. *N Engl J Med* 1990; 322:1829

Herrod HG: Chronic mucocutaneous candidiasis in childhood and complications of non-*Candida* infection: A report of the Pediatric Immunodeficiency Collaborative Group. *J Pediatr* 1990;116:377.

Kirkpatrick CH: Chronic mucocutaneous candidiasis. Antibiotic and immunologic therapy. *Ann N Y Acad Sci* 1988; 544:471.

Mobacken H, Moberg S: Ketoconazole treatment of 13 patients with chronic mucocutaneous candidiasis: A prospective three-year trial. *Dermatologica* 1986;173: 229.

NATURAL KILLER CELL DEFICIENCY

Biron CA et al: Severe herpes virus infections in an adolescent without natural killer cells. *N Engl J Med* 1989;320: 1731.

Komiyama A et al: Impaired natural killer cell recycling in childhood chronic neutropenia and morphological abnormalities and defective chemotaxis. *Blood* 1985;66:99.

Ritz J: The role of natural killer cells in immune surveillance. *N Engl J Med* 1989;320:1789.

Stiehm ER: New and old immunodeficiencies. *Pediatr Res* 1993;33(suppl):S2.

IDIOPATHIC CD4 LYMPHOCYTOPENIA

Smith DK et al: Unexplained opportunistic infections and CD4 T lymphocytopenia without HIV infection. An investigation of cases in the United States. *N Engl J Med* 1993;328:373.

Sneller MC et al: A unique syndrome of immunodeficiency and autoimmunity associated with absent T cell CD2 expression. *J Clin Immunol* 1994;14:359.

BIOTIN-DEPENDENT MULTIPLE COCARBOXYLASE DEFICIENCY

Cowan MJ, Ammann AJ: Immunodeficiency associated with inherited metabolic disorders. *Clin Haematol* 1981; 10:139.

23

Combined Antibody (B-Cell) & Cellular (T-Cell) Immunodeficiency Disorders

E. Richard Stiehm, MD, Robert L. Roberts, MD, PhD

Combined immunodeficiency diseases vary in cause and severity. Defective T- and B-cell immunity may be **complete,** as in severe combined immunodeficiency disease (SCID), or **partial,** as in ataxia–telangiectasia. Several of the disorders have distinctive clinical features that permit a clinical diagnosis, as for example, Wiskott–Aldrich syndrome (WAS). **Enzymatic deficiencies** in the purine pathway have been described in association with combined immunodeficiency, and specific **genetic mutations** of single amino acids are responsible in many instances. These discoveries have provided additional evidence for a diverse origin of combined immunodeficiency disease.

Studies of both T- and B-cell immunity are necessary to completely evaluate patients with combined immunodeficiency disorders (see Tables 21–1, 21–4, 21–6). In addition, analysis of erythrocyte and leukocyte enzymes (adenosine deaminase and nucleoside phosphorylase, respectively) can assist appropriate classification.

The onset of symptoms in patients with combined immunodeficiency diseases is usually early in infancy. These patients are susceptible to a very wide spectrum of microorganisms. Prognosis is poor unless stem cell transplantation can be accomplished.

RETICULAR DYSGENESIS

Reticular dysgenesis is a form of SCID in which a profound deficiency of myeloid elements of the hematopoietic system occurs. As a result, marked **leukopenia** is present in addition to B- and T-cell immunodeficiency, and onset of infection is very early. Bone marrow transplantation has been used successfully.

SEVERE COMBINED IMMUNODEFICIENCY (SCID)

Major Immunologic Features
- Onset of viral, bacterial, fungal, or protozoal infections before 3 months of age.

- X-linked, autosomal, and sporadic forms.
- T- and B-cell immunity severely impaired.
- Heterogeneity of immunologic defects.
- Stem cell transplantation treatment of choice.

Severe combined immunodeficiency (SCID) is a phenotypic term for a wide variety of congenital and hereditary immunologic defects characterized by early onset of infections, defects in both B- and T-cell systems, lymphoid aplasia, and thymic dysplasia. Inheritance can be X-linked, autosomal-recessive, or sporadic. The illness occurs in both sexes and all racial groups.

Clinical Manifestation
In most patients illness begins within the first 3 months of life with respiratory infections, pneumonia (often due to *Pneumocystis carinii*), thrush, diarrhea, and failure to thrive. The infections are resistant to treatment, and shedding of a virus (eg, respiratory syncytial virus, cytomegalovirus) from the respiratory or gastrointestinal tract is persistent. Erythematous or maculopapular skin rashes may be present. Vomiting, fever, and persistent diaper rash are common.

Physical examination reveals evidence of the aforementioned infections (rales, thrush, rash, etc) as well as a complete absence of tonsils and lymph nodes. Occasionally the liver and spleen are enlarged.

Diagnosis
Screening laboratory tests reveal marked lymphopenia (total lymphocyte count <1500 cells/µL). Neutropenia and thrombocytopenia may be present. Immunoglobulin levels are usually low, but maternal IgG may mask a lack of IgG synthesis in an infant younger than 6 months old. IgM and IgA levels are usually absent or low.

A thymic shadow is absent on chest x-ray films, but a stressed immunologically normal infant may also have the same finding.

The most useful test is a blood T-cell analysis (CD3, CD4, CD8). Most SCID patients have marked CD4 lymphopenia (CD4 cells <200 cells/µL). Assessment of B cells (CD19) and natural killer (NK) cells (CD16/56) is useful in subdividing the illness into genetic subtypes. Proliferative assays with phytohemagglutinin (PHA) and antigens, enzyme assays for adenosine deaminase and nucleoside phosphorylase, signal transduction assays, and mutation analysis are often needed to identify the precise genetic or immunologic defect.

Pathogenesis

As noted, most patients with SCID have profound deficiency of lymphocytes, but most have B cells, albeit nonfunctioning, and NK cells may or may not be absent. The presence or absence of these markers is used to classify SCID. The most common form of SCID (50% of cases) is **X-linked SCID** (T$^-$B$^+$NK$^-$), caused by mutations in the gene encoding the γ_c **chain of the IL-2 receptor.** The γ_c chain, also a component of the receptors for IL-4, IL-7, IL-9, and IL-15, transmits an intracellular activation signal into the nucleus through phosphorylation of Janus kinase-3 (JAK-3), leading to T-cell activation.

Another form of SCID (10% of cases) results from mutation of **JAK-3 kinase** and is inherited in an autosomal-recessive pattern. It closely resembles X-linked SCID, that is, it is T$^-$B$^+$NK$^-$. JAK-3 kinase is immediately downstream from the γ-chain of the IL-2 receptor in the signal transduction pathway for T-cell activation. A less common form of T$^-$B$^+$ SCID is caused by mutations of the α-**chain of the IL-7 receptor,** a cytokine necessary for T-cell development. NK cells are present.

About a third of SCID patients have defects in genes encoding **recombinase activity proteins** (RAG1 and RAG2) that affect V-D-J recombination in B and T cells. These autosomal defects are usually NK$^+$ (ie, T$^-$B$^-$NK$^+$). Another T$^-$B$^-$NK$^+$ form of autosomal-recessive SCID is termed Athabascan SCID and occurs among Navajo, Apache, and Northwest Territory native Americans; the gene defect is unknown.

Other forms of SCID include **surface receptor/transduction** defects, **ZAP-70** deficiency with isolated absence of CD8, defective **cytokine synthesis** (IL-1, IL-2), defects of the **T-cell receptor ε and γ chains,** and an **IL-2 α-chain** deficiency production.

Variants of SCID with incomplete defects of B- and T-cell synthesis include the **bare lymphocyte syndrome, Omenn syndrome,** and **short-limbed dwarfism.** Another variant is **Nezelof's syndrome** (combined immunodeficiency with immunoglobulins), which may present after age 5. These patients have poor antibody function despite the presence of immunoglobulin. **Griscelli's syndrome** is a combined immunodeficiency in patients with fine silvery hair, hepatosplenomegaly, and lymphoid hyperplasia. They resemble patients with Chédiak–Higashi syndrome but without the giant granulocyte azurophilic granules. **OKT4 epitope deficiency** is quite common, identified by the absence of reactivity with the OKT4 monoclonal antibody to CD4 lymphocytes. CD4 cells are present when assessed by another monoclonal antibody (eg, Leu-3b). These patients have only mild susceptibility to infection.

Treatment

Aggressive diagnostic measures are necessary to establish the cause of chronic infection before treatment can be instituted. Open lung biopsy or bronchoscopy should be performed if *Pneumocystis carinii* infection is suspected. Therapy includes pentamidine, trimethoprim–sulfamethoxazole, or both. Specific antibiotic treatment is necessary for suspected bacterial infection. Superficial candidal infection is treated with topical antifungal drugs, but systemic infection requires intravenous amphotericin B or other antifungal drugs.

Complications must be avoided. Live attenuated virus should not be used for immunization. Blood products containing potentially viable lymphocytes should be irradiated with 2500 R prior to administration (see the discussion of graft-versus-host [GVH] disease in the following paragraphs). Prophylactic trimethoprim–sulfamethoxazole should be used to prevent *P carinii* infection.

Intravenous immunoglobulin (IVIG) should be administered in doses of 400 mg/kg every 1–4 weeks, but this regimen does not correct the T-cell deficiency. Definitive treatment consists of **stem cell transplantation.** The ideal donor is a human leukocyte antigen (HLA)-identical sibling. The donor and recipient must be matched by HLA typing and histocompatibility confirmed by a nonreactive mixed leukocyte reaction (MLR). Despite careful matching, a GVH reaction may develop. Transplantation of unmatched cells results in a fatal GVH reaction.

The use of haploidentical (half-matched) bone marrow from a parent, prepared by removing mature T cells by lectins or by monoclonal antibody-complement combination can be done at various centers. Many of these patients need to be immunosuppressed to ensure engraftment of the depleted marrow. This procedure is nearly as successful as HLA-identical transplantation. Another type of transplant is a matched unrelated donor, selected through the national registry of HLA-typed donors. Matched or partially matched banked cord blood can also be used. Immunosuppression of the recipient is usually necessary.

Other considerations in stem cell transplantation are the cytomegalovirus (CMV) and Epstein–Barr virus (EBV) status of the donor; antiviral drugs are sometimes used to prevent CMV infection or EBV immunoproliferative disease. Prophylaxis with cyclosporine is usually necessary to prevent or minimize GVH.

COMBINED IMMUNODEFICIENCY WITH T-CELL MEMBRANE OR SIGNALING DEFECTS

Major Immunologic Features

- Phenotypic characteristics of other combined immunodeficiency disorders.
- Mild to severe infections.
- Structurally abnormal T-cell receptor or abnormal signal transduction.

T cells are activated following interaction with an antigen-presenting cell (APC), a step that is dependent on cell-to-cell contact. The T-cell receptor (TCR) binds to the major histocompatibility complex (MHC) of the APC, resulting in the expression of cytokine receptors and cytokine secretion. Multiple intracellular events, including the accumulation of phosphorylated substrates (especially tyrosine phosphorylation) and increases in concentrations of Ca^{2+}, also are necessary for cell activation. These events lead to secretion of cytokines, such as IL-2, tumor necrosis factor, interferon gamma, and transforming growth cell proliferation, and differentiation into cytotoxic cells.

Most patients have normal or near-normal T-cell numbers but deficient or absent proliferative responses to mitogens, antigens, or anti-CD3 monoclonal antibody. Most have moderate susceptibility to infection, but in some patients this is mild. A defective TCR (eg, the lack of the CD3 ζ chain) or an abnormality of signal transduction (such as a G-protein or a tyrosine kinase abnormality) have been identified in a few of these patients. Only a few research laboratories have the methods to evaluate these patients' biochemical defects.

MAJOR HISTOCOMPATIBILITY COMPLEX (MHC) CLASS II DEFICIENCY (Bare Lymphocyte Syndrome)

Major Immunologic Features

- Leukocyte class I or class II HLA antigens (or both) absent or markedly decreased.
- Immunologic features usually similar to those of combined immunodeficiency disease.
- A few patients asymptomatic or only minimally symptomatic.

General Considerations

Patients with the MHC Class II Deficiency have deficient expression of HLA molecules with resultant combined immunodeficiency. A description of the HLA genes of the MHC on the short arm of chromosome 6, the families of cell surface proteins encoded by these genes, their expression on cells of the immune system, and their role in the immune response is found in Chapter 6.

This autosomal-recessive disease occurs primarily in families from the Mediterranean area and is often associated with consanguinity. The first case was discovered by an inability to HLA type the patient's cells. From detailed investigation of subsequent patients, it is clear that the bare lymphocyte syndrome represents a collection of at least four genotypic abnormalities with differing phenotypic expressions. In all patients expression of class I or class II HLA antigens, or both, is abnormally low or absent. In patients with deficient cell surface class II antigens, both the presence and absence of the class II gene has been found. In some instances, when the gene is present, class II antigens can be induced following stimulation of cells in vitro with antigens or interferon gamma. In others, there is an abnormality of the transactivating class II regulatory gene (CIITA) that lies outside the major histocompatibility locus. In still others, there is a deficiency in a DNA-binding protein referred to as the X-box-binding protein (RF-X), implicated in regulation of class II gene transcription.

Clinical Features

Most patients have clinical features similar to those present in severe combined immunodeficiency. These include early onset of opportunistic infections, chronic diarrhea, recurrent viral infections, oral candidiasis, central nervous system viral infection, aplastic anemia, and growth failure.

Laboratory Findings: T cells are near normal, but CD8 cells are increased and CD4 cells decreased. Lymphocytes proliferate normally to PHA but poorly to antigen. Immunoglobulins are usually decreased, and antibody responses are poor.

Routine typing for histocompatibility antigens reveals the absence or decreased expression of HLA class I or class II antigens, or both. An intrauterine diagnosis can be established in the presence of a family history by analyzing fetal blood cells or chorionic villus biopsy material. To assist in bone marrow transplantation and matching, HLA genotyping is done with restriction enzyme fragments and specific HLA probes. The bare lymphocyte syndrome should not be confused with other combined immunodeficiency diseases because no other syndrome lacks HLA antigens. In rare instances, severe leukopenia associated with other forms of immunodeficiency may make HLA typing difficult.

Pathogenesis

At least three genetic defects, localized on different chromosomes, cause MHC class II deficiency, all of which affect transcription of MHC class II genes. These genes are termed CIITA (transactivating protein deficiency), RFX-J (promoter X-box regulatory factor 5 deficiency), and RFXAP (regulatory factor X associated protein deficiency) and are localized on chromosomes 16p13, 1q21, and 13q, respectively. Atypical patients have been described.

Treatment

Severe forms of this syndrome require bone marrow transplantation. Determining an appropriate donor for transplantation may be difficult and may require special techniques such as DNA hybridization. Supportive therapy, with the use of IVIG and prophylactic trimethoprim-sulfamethoxazole, is similar to that for SCID.

MHC CLASS I DEFICIENCY

Bare lymphocyte syndrome-class I is less common and less severe than MHC class II deficiency and is manifested by recurrent respiratory infections, particularly sinusitis. A few patients are asymptomatic. Inheritance is autosomal-recessive. The diagnosis is made by the inability to type lymphocytes at the class I loci (eg, HLA-A, B, and C) but the presence of class II HLA antigens (DR, DP, DQ). The defect is associated with mutations of a gene on chromosome 6 that encodes a peptide transporter (TAP, transporter associated with antigen processing) needed for class I expression.

A few patients have both class I and class II MHC deficiencies. These patients clinically resemble the patients with MHC class II deficiency.

OMENN SYNDROME

This is an autosomal-recessive variant of combined immunodeficiency characterized by the early onset of a seborrheic pruritic skin eruption, hepatosplenomegaly, and lymphadenopathy. Eosinophilia is present, serum IgE level is usually elevated, and other immunoglobulin levels are low. CD8 cytotoxic cells attacking the skin has been suggested as a possible immunologic abnormality. Engrafted maternal cells may be implicated in some patients, causing an Omenn-like syndrome.

The cause of the illness is a defect of V-D-J recombination of antigen receptor gene loci secondary to mutations of RAG 1 and RAG 2 genes (recombination activity genes 1 and 2) on 11p13. Bone marrow transplantation is curative.

WISKOTT–ALDRICH SYNDROME
(Immunodeficiency With Thrombocytopenia & Eczema)

Major Immunologic Features
- X-linked syndrome of eczema, recurrent pyogenic infection, and thrombocytopenia with decreased platelet volume.
- Decreased antibody responses to polysaccharide antigens with decreased IgM and elevated IgA and IgE levels.
- Decreased T-cell function with increased susceptibility to autoimmunity and malignancy.

General Considerations

Male infants with Wiskott-Aldrich syndrome (WAS) may become symptomatic early in life, with bleeding secondary to thrombocytopenia. Subsequently they develop recurrent bacterial infection in the form of otitis media, pneumonia, and meningitis. Eczema usually appears by 1 year of age. The disease is progressive, with increasing susceptibility to infection and cancer. At autopsy, the thymus and lymph nodes have an abnormal architecture, with depletion of lymphoid cells, poor follicle formation, and poor corticomedullary differentiation.

Immunologic Pathogenesis

Two of the earliest abnormalities are thrombocytopenia and hypercatabolism of immunoglobulin. Several hypotheses link thrombocytopenia, eczema, and recurrent infection. It has been suggested that abnormal α granules of platelets and macrophages occur in patients and carriers. Another suggestion is that the inability of patients to respond to polysaccharide antigens results in immunologic attrition. This, however, does not explain the thrombocytopenia or eczema. A 115-kilodalton surface glycoprotein termed sialophorin (CD43) involved in lymphocyte activation and differentiation is decreased or absent on WAS lymphocytes; however, this is not the primary defect because CD43 is encoded on chromosome 16. Decreased expression of B-cell CD23 has been described. CD23 is involved in the differentiation of immune cells, inhibition of monocyte migration, B-cell proliferation, and IgE production. Thus, an abnormality of CD23 might result in many of the hematologic and immunologic defects.

The cause of WAS is a mutation of the WASP gene on Xp11.22 that encodes the Wiskott-Aldrich syndrome protein (WASP). WASP is present in all hematopoietic-derived cells and plays a role in signal transduction regulating cytoskeletal reorganization. Multiple mutations exist and the phenotype may include X-linked thrombocytopenia without immunologic or cutaneous abnormalities.

Clinical Features
A. Symptoms and Signs: Recurrent infection usually does not start until after 6 months of age. Patients are susceptible to infection with capsular polysaccharide-type organisms (eg, *Pneumococcus, Meningococcus,* and *Haemophilus influenzae*), which cause meningitis, otitis media, pneumonia, and sepsis. As the patients become older, they become susceptible to infection with other types of organisms and may have recurrent viral infection. Eczema is usually present by 1 year of age and is typical in distribution

(Figure 23–1) and often associated with other allergic manifestations. Thrombocytopenia is present at birth and may result in severe bleeding, particularly during episodes of infection. The bleeding tendency becomes less severe as the child becomes older.

B. Laboratory Findings: Thrombocytopenia at birth is helpful in diagnosis. The platelet count may range from 5000 to 100,000/μL. Platelets are small in WAS, in contrast to most other thrombocytopenic disorders. Megakaryocytes are present in the bone marrow. Anemia is frequently present and may be Coombs'-positive. An increased incidence of chronic renal disease has been reported.

Immunologic Diagnosis

The earliest immunologic abnormality is hypercatabolism of immunoglobulin G. Studies of B-cell immunity show normal IgG, decreased IgM, increased IgA and IgE levels; or absent isohemagglutinin levels, normal numbers of B cells, and an inability to respond to immunization with polysaccharide antigen. Paraproteins are frequent. T-cell immunity is usually intact early in the disease but declines with advancing years.

Differential Diagnosis

When the complete syndrome is present, there is little doubt about the diagnosis. Idiopathic thrombocytopenia in a male child may be difficult to differentiate from WAS. In idiopathic thrombocytopenic purpura (ITP), the immunoglobulins, isohemagglutinins, and response to polysaccharide antigens are normal. Small platelets favor the diagnosis of WAS. Unaffected male patients with eczema and recurrent infection have normal immunologic studies and normal platelet counts, although they may have elevated levels of serum IgA and IgE.

Treatment

Infections should be treated promptly and aggressively with antibiotics effective against the most common organisms. Corticosteroids should not be used to treat the thrombocytopenia because they enhance the susceptibility to infection. Splenectomy has been fatal in this disease, but when combined with continuous antibiotic prophylaxis, it may control both bleeding and infectious complications. Treatment of immunodeficiency is difficult. Intramuscular gamma globulin is contraindicated because of the thrombocytopenia and potential bleeding at injection sites, but IVIG can be given (see Chapter 21). Successful bone marrow transplantation with immunosuppression to achieve both a lymphoid and a hematopoietic cell engraftment is curative.

Complications & Prognosis

With aggressive therapy, the long-term prognosis has improved. Immediate complications are related to bleeding episodes and acute infection. Autoimmune phenomena such as vasculitis and Coombs'-positive hemolytic anemia may require corticosteroid therapy. As patients become older, they become susceptible to a wider spectrum of microorganisms. Chronic keratitis secondary to viral infection is frequent. Lymphoreticular cancers, especially of the central nervous system, occur in older patients. Myelogenous leukemia occurs more frequently in this disorder than in other immunodeficiency disorders.

ATAXIA-TELANGIECTASIA

Major Immunologic Features

- Clinical onset by 2 years of age.
- Ataxia, telangiectasia, and recurrent sinopulmonary infection in the complete syndrome.
- Selective IgA deficiency, cutaneous anergy, and decreased T-cell function in most patients.
- Hypersensitivity to ionizing radiation with chromosome breakage.
- Predisposition to malignancies, including lymphoma, leukemias, and epithelial cell malignancies.
- Autosomal-recessive with abnormal gene ataxia–telangiectasia mutated (ATM) on 22q22-23.

General Considerations

Ataxia-telangiectasia, an autosomal-recessive disorder, is associated with ataxia, telangiectasia, recurrent sinopulmonary infection, and abnormalities in both T- and B-cell immunity. The disorder was first considered to be primarily a neurologic disease; it is now known to involve the neurologic, vascular, endocrine, and immune systems.

Immunologic Pathogenesis

No unifying theory explains the multisystem abnormalities present in ataxia-telangiectasia. A fundamental immunologic defect is unlikely. Rather, the multisystem abnormalities may be a result of a spe-

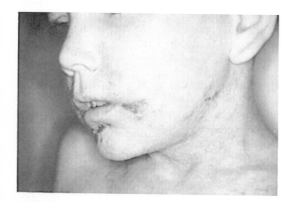

Figure 23–1. Chronic facial eczema in a child with Wiskott–Aldrich syndrome.

cific genetic defect that affects DNA repair and alters the function of many organ systems. The result may be an abnormal collagen (deficient in hydroxylysine); elevated α-fetoprotein level, indicative of a defect in organ maturation; enhanced susceptibility of cells to radiation damage; and defective DNA repair. Clones of lymphocytes with structural rearrangements of band q11 of chromosome 14 and bands q32–35 and p13–15 of chromosome 7 have been consistently found. These chromosome markers may be found in malignant cell lines isolated from ataxia–telangiectasia patients. It is of interest that the structural rearrangements are at the locations that bear the TCR genes. Spontaneously occurring chromosomal translocations involving break points in T-cell receptor genes have been described and suggest a possible defect in recombination. The disorder is progressive, with both the neurologic abnormalities and the immunologic deficiency becoming more severe over time.

Clinical Features

A. Symptoms and Signs: The onset of ataxia may occur at 9 months to 1 year of age or may be delayed to as long as age 4–6 years. Telangiectasia is usually present by 2 years of age but has been delayed until 8–9 years of age. Additional neurologic symptoms—choreoathetoid movements, dysconjugate gaze, and extrapyramidal and posterior column signs—develop with time. Telangiectasia may appear first in the bulbar conjunctiva and subsequently on the bridge of the nose, on the ears, or in the antecubital fossae (Figure 23–2). Recurrent sinopulmonary infections may begin early in life or not until age 10 or older. Susceptibility to both viral and bacterial infections is increased. Secondary sexual characteristics rarely develop at puberty, and most patients develop mental retardation with time.

B. Laboratory Findings: Various degrees of abnormalities in T- and B-cell immunity have been described. Lymphopenia may be present. T-cell numbers may be normal or decreased, and the response of lymphocytes to phytohemagglutinin (PHA) and allogeneic cells may be normal or decreased. There usually is no response to delayed hypersensitivity skin tests. IgG2, IgG4, or IgA2 subclass deficiency is present in some patients. In other patients, IgE may be absent. Antibody responses to specific antigens may be depressed. CD4 cell numbers are usually decreased, and there are decreased α/β and increased γ/δ T cell numbers. The number of circulating B cells is usually normal. Natural killer (NK) cell activity is normal.

Other laboratory abnormalities relate to associated findings. Abnormalities have been shown on pneumoencephalography and imaging of the central nervous system. Decreased 17-ketosteroids, increased follicle-stimulating hormone (FSH) excretion, and insulin-resistant diabetes have been found. There may be cytotoxic antibodies to brain and thymus and elevated titers to EBV antigens. Elevated levels of α-fetoprotein are characteristic and help to differentiate this disorder from the Nijmegen breakage syndrome (see later section).

Immunologic Diagnosis

Selective IgA deficiency (40% of patients); IgA2, IgG2, or IgG4 subclass deficiency; IgE deficiency; and variable deficiencies of other immunoglobulins may be found. The antibody response to specific antigens may be depressed. Variable degrees of T-cell deficiency are observed and usually become more severe with advancing age.

Differential Diagnosis

If the onset of recurrent infection occurs before the development of ataxia or telangiectasia, it may be difficult to differentiate this disorder from cellular immunodeficiency with abnormal immunoglobulin synthesis. If cerebellar ataxia unassociated with telangiectasia and immunologic abnormalities begins gradually, it may take years before the diagnosis can be certain. Usually, by age 4, the characteristic recurrent sinopulmonary infections, immunologic abnormalities, ataxia, and telangiectasia are present simultaneously. Because selective IgA deficiency is the most common immunodeficiency disorder and many such patients have no symptoms, it may take several years before a diagnosis of ataxia-telangiectasia can be excluded. α-fetoprotein levels are normal in IgA deficiency. Chromosomal instability is also present in the Nijmegen breakage syndrome. Exact diagnosis can be established by identifying a mutation of the ataxia telangiectasia mutated (ATM) gene on chromosome 11q22.3.

Treatment

Early treatment of recurrent sinopulmonary infections is essential to avoid permanent complications. Some patients may benefit from continuous broad-

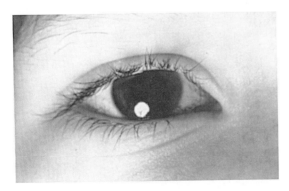

Figure 23–2. Telangiectasis of the conjunctiva and over the bridge of the nose in a child with ataxia–telangiectasia.

spectrum antibiotic therapy. Aggressive physical therapy is beneficial for those with chronic lung disease. Successful bone marrow transplantation has not been performed but probably would not benefit the neurologic problem. Fetal thymus transplantation and thymic hormone therapy have had limited use without clear evidence of efficacy. Intravenous immunoglobulin may decrease the number of infections if the antibody deficiency is severe.

Attenuated viral vaccines should not be given. All blood products should be irradiated prior to administration.

Complications & Prognosis

Long-term survivors develop progressive deterioration of neurologic and immunologic functions. The oldest patients have reached the fifth decade of life. The chief causes of death are overwhelming infection and lymphoreticular or epithelial cell cancer (carcinoma of the stomach, liver, and ovaries). Leukemias, some with associated abnormalities of chromosome 14, have been reported in 24% of patients (Figure 23–3), and non-Hodgkin's lymphomas have been reported in 45%. As these patients reach the second decade, morbidity becomes severe, especially from chronic lung disease, mental retardation, and physical debility. Heterozygote carriers as well as family members have an increased incidence of cancer.

NIJMEGEN BREAKAGE SYNDROME

The Nijmegen breakage syndrome (NBS) is an autosomal-recessive distinct chromosomal instability syndrome characterized by microcephaly, growth retardation, susceptibility to infection, and high risk of malignancy. As with ataxia-telangiectasia, the cells of patients with this syndrome are unusually sensitive to ionizing radiation leading to chromosome breakage; however, these patients do not have ataxia, telangiectasia, or elevated α-fetoprotein levels. The cause is a mutation of the NBS gene at chromosome 8q21; the function of the gene product is unknown.

GRAFT-VERSUS-HOST DISEASE

Graft-versus-host disease (GVHD) occurs when an unopposed attack of histoincompatible cells from the graft takes place in an individual who is unable to reject foreign cells. The requirements for the GVHD reaction are (1) histocompatibility differences between the graft (donor) and host (recipient), (2) immunocompetent graft cells, and (3) immunodeficient host cells. A GVHD reaction may result from the infusion of any blood product containing viable lymphocytes, as may occur in maternal-fetal blood transfusion; intrauterine transfusion; therapeutic whole-blood transfusions or transfusions of packed erythrocytes, frozen cells, platelets, fresh plasma, or leukocyte-poor erythrocytes; or from transplantation of fetal thymus, fetal liver, or bone marrow. The onset of the GVHD reaction occurs 7–30 days following infusion of viable lymphocytes. Once the reaction is established, little can be done to modify its course. In the majority of immunodeficient patients, a GVHD reaction is fatal. The exact mechanism by which a GVHD reaction is produced is unknown. Biopsy of active GVHD lesions usually demonstrates infiltration by mononuclear cells and eosinophils as well as phagocytic and histiocytic cells. The GVHD reaction may appear in three distinct forms: acute, hyperacute, and chronic.

In the **acute** form of GVHD reaction, the initial manifestation is a maculopapular rash, which is frequently mistaken for a viral or allergic rash (Figure 23–4). Initially, it blanches with pressure and then becomes diffuse. If the rash is persistent, it begins to scale. Diarrhea, hepatosplenomegaly, jaundice, cardiac irregularity, central nervous system irritability, and pulmonary infiltrates may occur during the height of the reaction. Enhanced susceptibility to in-

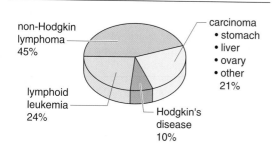

Figure 23–3. Relative percentages of cancers reported in patients with ataxia–telangiectasia.

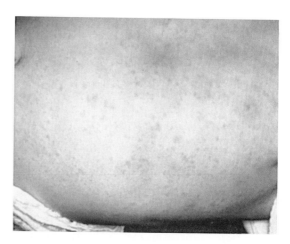

Figure 23–4. Maculopapular rash in early GVHD disease in an infant with severe combined immunodeficiency disease.

fection is also present and may result in death from sepsis.

In the **hyperacute** form of GVHD, the rash may also begin as a maculopapular lesion, but then it rapidly progresses to a form resembling toxic epidermal necrolysis, usually associated with severe diarrhea. This has not been associated with staphylococcal infection. Clinical and laboratory abnormalities similar to those found in the acute form may be observed. Death occurs shortly after the onset of the reaction.

The **chronic** form of GVHD may be a result of maternal-fetal transfusion or attempts at immunotherapy with histocompatible bone marrow transplantation. The clinical and laboratory features may be markedly abnormal or only slightly so. Interference with normal nail growth results in a dysplastic appearance. Chronic desquamation of the skin is usually present. Hepatosplenomegaly may be prominent, along with lymphadenopathy. Chronic diarrhea and failure to thrive are common. Secondary infection is a frequent complication. On biopsy of skin or lymph nodes, histiocytic infiltration may be found, leading to an erroneous diagnosis of Letterer-Siwe disease. Patients with Letterer-Siwe disease have normal immunoglobulin levels and normal T-cell immunity, but patients with chronic GVHD have severe immunodeficiency. Chronic GVHD has also been confused with acrodermatitis enteropathica.

The diagnosis is suggested by the diffuse clinical abnormalities present in a patient who is known to have cellular immunodeficiency and who has received a transfusion of potentially immunocompetent cells in the preceding 5–30 days. The diagnosis is established by the demonstration of sex chromosome or HLA chimerism (Figure 23–5). On occasion, patients with known GVHD fail to have detectable chimerism. Incubation of peripheral blood mononuclear cells with interleukin-2 may result in detectable chimerism.

Management

Prevention of GVHD is essential. Patients with suspected T-cell immunodeficiency should receive only irradiated blood products (at least 2500 R) so as to prevent lymphocyte proliferation and resultant GVHD. Blood products to be irradiated include whole blood, packed erythrocytes, lymphocyte-poor erythrocytes, platelets, and fresh and fresh-frozen plasma.

Following bone marrow transplantation when GVHD is likely, the patients can be given cyclosporin or corticosteroids prophylactically for 3–6 months. Intravenous immunoglobulin therapy can ameliorate some of the symptoms of posttransplant GVHD.

There is no adequate treatment of GVHD once it is established. Corticosteroids serve to enhance the susceptibility to infection. Antilymphocyte globulin or anti-CD3 (OKT3) monoclonal antibody are of lim-

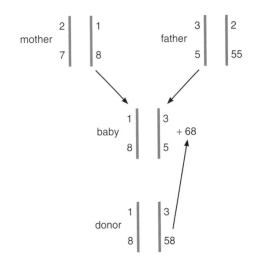

Figure 23–5. Inheritance of HLA antigens from the parents of a child with graft-versus-host disease (GVHD) and detection of additional antigen from the blood donor.

ited value. Cyclosporin and other immunosuppressive agents may be useful. Experimentally, treatment with monoclonal antibody to tumor necrosis factor or interferon gamma reduces the severity of GVHD.

Interestingly, GVHD has not yet been described in patients with AIDS despite their severe T-cell immunodeficiency. This may be a result of HIV-1 infection of the engrafting T cells, preventing the establishment of a graft.

SHORT-LIMBED DWARFISM WITH IMMUNODEFICIENCY AND CARTILAGE–HAIR HYPOPLASIA

Major Immunologic Features

- Skeletal dysplasia with dwarfism and fine hair
- T-cell immunodeficiency with or without B-cell immunodeficiency
- Autosomal-recessive
- Enhanced susceptibility to varicella-zoster infection

Short-limbed dwarfism with immunodeficiency is an autosomal-recessive predominantly T-cell immunodeficiency associated with metaphyseal or spondylo-epiphyseal dysplasia. **Cartilage–hair hypoplasia** is a variant in which fine, sparse hair is persistent.

Dwarfism is recognized at birth. The head size is normal and the hands are short and pudgy (Figure 23–6). Redundant skin folds of the neck occur, and elbow extension is limited. The hair, if abnormal, is light, with a decreased diameter and lacking a central pigmental core. Neutropenia is not uncommon. Radi-

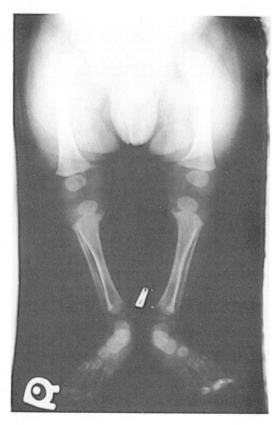

Figure 23–6. X-ray film of extremities in a child with cartilage–hair hypoplasia and immunodeficiency. Note the redundant skin folds.

ologic abnormalities consist of scalloping, irregular sclerosis, and cystic changes of the widened metaphyses (see Figure 23–6). Megacolon and malabsorption may occur.

Immunologic abnormalities can range from severe deficiency of B- and T-cell numbers and function (similar to SCID), a moderate T-cell immunodeficiency, or, occasionally, isolated B-cell deficiency with hypogammaglobulinemia.

Treatment depends on the degree of immunodeficiency. Intravenous immunoglobulin therapy is indicated for antibody deficiency. Successful bone marrow transplantation (HLA-identical and -haploidentical) has been accomplished. *Pneumocystis carinii* prophylaxis is indicated for patients with low CD4 numbers. Varicella-zoster immunoglobulin or acyclovir should be given following exposure to chicken pox. Varicella vaccine or other live virus vaccines are contraindicated.

IMMUNODEFICIENCY WITH ENZYME DEFICIENCY

ADENOSINE DEAMINASE & NUCLEOSIDE PHOSPHORYLASE DEFICIENCY

Major Immunologic Features
- Recurrent and severe viral, bacterial, fungal, and protozoal infections
- Varied degrees of T- and B-cell immunodeficiency
- Purine enzyme activity absent or reduced

General Considerations
Patients with enzyme deficiency and immunodeficiency may have clinical and laboratory abnormalities identical to those of immunodeficient patients with normal enzyme activity. Enzyme deficiency probably accounts for less than 15% of immunodeficiency disorders currently, but additional enzyme deficiencies will likely be discovered.

Adenosine deaminase (ADA) and purine nucleoside phosphorylase (PNP) are necessary for the normal catabolism of purines (Figure 23–7). ADA catalyzes the conversion of adenosine and deoxyadenosine to inosine and deoxyinosine. Nucleoside phosphorylase catalyzes the conversion of inosine, deoxyinosine, guanosine, and deoxyguanosine, to hypoxanthine and guanine. Several mechanisms have been postulated to explain the means whereby these enzyme deficiencies result in immunodeficiency. Experimental evidence indicates that increased amounts of adenosine may result in increased cyclic adenosine monophosphate (cAMP) activity with inhibition of lymphocyte function. Adenosine has also been shown to be toxic to cells in culture as a result of pyrimidine starvation. There is also evidence that exogenous adenosine can lead to the intracellular accumulation of S-adenosylhomocysteine, a potent inhibitor of DNA methylation. The most likely mechanism of inhibition of lymphocyte function, however, is the accumulation of deoxyadenosine and subsequently deoxyadenosine triphosphate (deoxyATP), which then inhibits ribonucleotide reductase and depletes deoxyribonucleoside triphosphates. In PNP deficiency, deoxyguanosine causes the accumulation of deoxyguanosine triphosphate (GTP), which most probably inhibits ribonucleotide reductase. These mechanisms have great importance in devising potential biochemical treatment for these disorders.

The degree of combined immunodeficiency is variable. The spectrum of immunologic aberrations varies from complete absence of T- and B-cell immunity, as in patients with SCID (85–90% of patients), to mild abnormalities of T- and B-cell function. Clinically, the phenotypic expression correlates with the degree of enzyme deficiency. Patients with the most

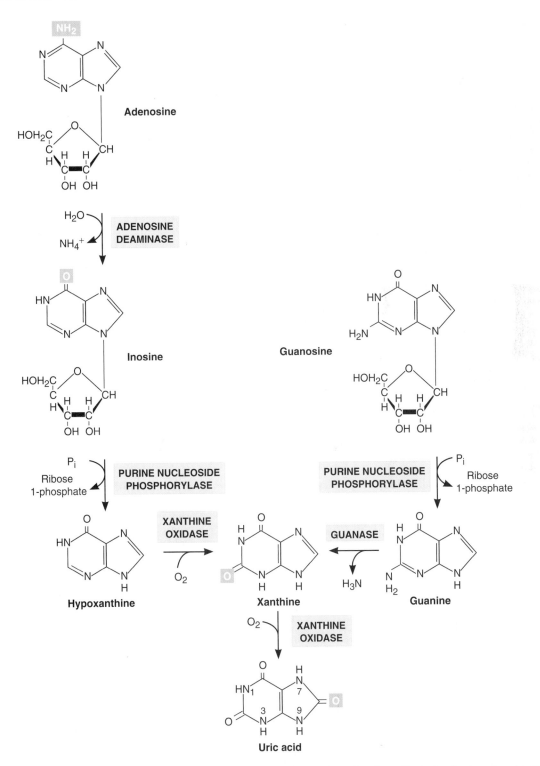

Figure 23–7. Schematic representation of purine metabolic pathway illustrating the critical role of adenosine deaminase and purine nucleoside phosphorylase. (Reproduced, with permission, from Murray RK et al: *Harper's Review of Biochemistry.* 22nd ed. Norwalk, CT, Appleton & Lange, 1990.)

complete form of enzyme deficiency have SCID. About 10–15% of patients have a delayed onset, some until 5–8 years of age. Routine neonatal screening has resulted in the detection of "partial" ADA deficiency in immunologically normal individuals. Patients with enzyme deficiencies should be evaluated completely to determine the extent of the immunologic deficiency. The marked variability in immunodeficiency results in considerable variation in age at onset, severity of symptoms, and eventual outcome. Patients with ADA deficiency and SCID may have radiologic abnormalities that include concavity and flaring of the anterior ribs, abnormal contour and articulation of posterior ribs and transverse processes, platyspondylosis, thick growth arrest lines, and an abnormal bony pelvis. Patients with nucleoside phosphorylase deficiency and T-cell immunodeficiency have normal bone roentgenograms, absent T-cell immunity, normal B-cell immunity, a history of recurrent infection, and autoantibody formation. They are susceptible to fatal varicella and vaccinia infections.

The mode of inheritance of these enzyme defects appears to be autosomal-recessive. The **carrier state** can be demonstrated in both sexes by diminished adenosine deaminase or nucleoside phosphorylase activity. With the identification of the precise genetic defects in these disorders, intrauterine and carrier diagnosis will be more precise. The enzymes are absent in erythrocytes, leukocytes, tissues, and cultured fibroblasts in these patients. An **intrauterine** diagnosis of ADA deficiency can be made. Patients may not be immunodeficient at birth.

The specific genetic defect(s) of both adenosine deaminase and nucleoside phosphorylase have been described. In most instances a mutation in a single nucleotide, which results in a single amino acid change, is responsible.

Treatment

Treatment of this disorder is similar to that for SCID or combined immunodeficiency. Several successful bone marrow transplants have restored immunologic function, although the patients' cells continue to lack enzyme activity.

Some patients with ADA deficiency benefited from monthly infusions of irradiated erythrocytes as a source of ADA enzyme; other patients responded partially or not at all. Biochemical treatment of a single nucleoside phosphorylase-deficient patient with oral uridine was unsuccessful. Deoxycytidine therapy was attempted unsuccessfully in one patient.

Many ADA-deficient patients have been successfully treated with bovine ADA conjugated to polyethylene glycol (PEG-ADA) to prolong the half-life and reduce the immunogenicity of the enzyme. This treatment, given two or three times per week reduces the levels of toxic metabolites, and markedly improves B- and T-cell functions, particularly in patients who have some residual immunity.

Since 1990, several children and three newborns have received gene therapy for ADA deficiency. Their peripheral blood cells or their cord blood cells were transfected with the ADA gene and returned to the patients. Initial evaluation indicates that gene expression has occurred with some clinical benefit; however, these patients continue to receive PEG-ADA.

X-LINKED LYMPHOPROLIFERATIVE SYNDROME (Duncan's Disease)

Major Immunologic Features
- Exquisite susceptibility to Epstein-Barr virus (EBV) infection.
- Fatal infectious mononucleosis following EBV infection in most patients.
- Lymphoma, hypogammaglobulinemia, or aplastic anemia after EBV infection in others.
- Possible cure with bone marrow transplantation.

General Considerations

The X-linked lymphoproliferative (XLP) syndrome is characterized by a hereditary exquisite susceptibility to EBV infection, which can result in (1) severe progressive infectious mononucleosis, with liver failure and death; (2) infectious mononucleosis followed by lymphoproliferation; and (3) immunodeficiency, lymphoma, or aplastic anemia. About 73% of patients develop fatal acute infectious mononucleosis. The mortality rate of XLP is 75% by age 10 and nearly 100% by age 40. The defective gene is on the long arm of the X chromosome (Xq25-26).

Immunologic abnormalities include inverted helper-suppressor T-cell ratios, deficient proliferative responses to mitogenic stimulation, defective interferon gamma production, and decreased NK-cell activity. B-cell abnormalities include hypogammaglobulinemia, failure to switch from IgM- to IgG-specific antibody following immunization with bacteriophage, and weak antibody responses to EBV antigens, especially to EBV nuclear antigen (EBNA). These abnormalities are found primarily in EBV-infected long-term survivors. In contrast, patients who are identified prior to EBV infection usually are immunologically normal, although some may have hypogammaglobulinemia.

The cause of XLP may be a mutation of *DHSP*, a gene which inhibits cellular activation following T-cell activation with antigens such as Epstein–Barr virus; the defective *DHSP* gene may thus permit unregulated T-cell activation.

Management

Intravenous immunoglobulin to prevent EBV infection has been used with limited success. Management once EBV infection has occurred is similar to that of other combined immunodeficiencies, that is, immunoglobulin, antibiotics, *Pneumocystis carinii* infection (PCP) prophylaxis, and so on. Antiviral drugs (eg, acyclovir) are ineffective. Identification of at-risk uninfected carriers using DNA restriction fragment-length polymorphisms (RFLP) of genes at the XLP locus should be done so as to offer bone marrow or cord blood cell transplantation before EBV infection. Bone marrow transplantation, even after EBV infection, has been curative in a few patients, particularly if done before age 12.

REFERENCES

RETICULAR DYSGENESIS

Ownby DR et al: Severe combined immunodeficiency with leukopenia (reticular dysgenesis) in siblings: Immunologic and histopathologic findings. *J Pediatr* 1976;89: 382.

SEVERE COMBINED IMMUNODEFICIENCY DISEASE

Castigli E et al: Severe combined immunodeficiency with selective T-cell cytokine genes. *Pediatr Res* 1993;33:52.

Chu ET et al: Immunodeficiency with defective T-cell response to interleukin 1. *Proc Natl Acad Sci U S A* 1984;81: 4945.

Conley ME: Molecular approaches to analysis of X-linked immunodeficiencies. *Ann Rev Immunol* 1992;322:1063.

Hong R: Disorders of the T cell system. In: *Immunologic Disorders in Infants and Children*, 4th ed. Stiehm ER (editor). WB Saunders, 1996.

Lawlor EJ et al: The syndrome of cellular immunodeficiency with immunoglobulins. *J Pediatr* 1974;84:183.

Pahwa R et al: Recombinant interleukin-2 therapy in severe combined immunodeficiency disease. *Proc Natl Acad Sci U S A* 1989;86:5069.

Puck JM et al: The interleukin-2 receptor gamma chain maps to Xq13.1 and is mutated in X-linked severe combined immunodeficiency. *Hum Mol Genet* 1993;2:1099.

ATAXIA-TELANGIECTASIA

Baxter GD et al: T cell receptor gene rearrangement and expression in ataxia-telangiectasia B lymphoblastoid cells. *Immunol Cell Biol* 1989;67:57.

Boder E, Sedgwick RP: Ataxia-telangiectasia: A familial syndrome and progressive cerebellar ataxia, oculocutaneous telangiectasia and frequent pulmonary infection. *Univ South Cal Med Bull* 1957;9:15.

Savitsky K et al: A single ataxia telangiectasia gene with a product similar to PI-3 kinase. *Science* 1995;268:1749.

Swift M et al: Breast and other cancers in families with ataxia–telangiectasia. *N Engl J Med* 1987;316:1289.

Taylor AMR et al: Fifth International Workshop on Ataxia-Telangiectasia. *Cancer Res* 1993;53:438.

NIJMEGEN BREAKAGE SYNDROME

Weemaes CMR et al: A new chromosomal instability disorder: The Nijmegen breakage syndrome. *Acta Paediatr Scand* 1981;70:557.

WISKOTT-ALDRICH SYNDROME

Cooper MD et al: Wiskott-Aldrich syndrome: Immunologic deficiency disease involving the afferent limb of immunity. *Am J Med* 1968;44:489.

Derry JMJ et al: Isolation of a novel gene mutated in Wiskott-Aldrich syndrome. *Cell* 1994;78:635.

Ochs HD. The Wiskott-Aldrich syndrome. *Semin Hematol* 1998;35:332.

Parkman R et al: Complete correction of the Wiskott–Aldrich syndrome by allogeneic bone marrow transplantation. *N Engl J Med* 1978;298:921.

Shelly CS et al: Molecular characterization of sialophorin (CD43), the lymphocyte surface sialoglycoprotein defective in Wiskott-Aldrich syndrome. *Proc Natl Acad Sci U S A* 1989;86:2819.

Sullivan KE et al: A multi-institutional survey of the Wiskott-Aldrich syndrome. *J Pediatr* 1994;125:876.

IMMUNODEFICIENCY WITH SHORT-LIMBED DWARFISM

Ammann AJ et al: Antibody mediated immunodeficiency in short-limbed dwarfism. *J Pediatr* 1974;84:200.

Lux SE et al: Chronic neutropenia and abnormal cellular immunity in cartilage-hair hypoplasia. *N Engl J Med* 1970; 282:234.

Polmar SH, Pierce GF: Cartilage hair hypoplasia: Immunological aspects and their clinical implications. *Clin Immunol Immunopathol* 1986;40:87.

COMBINED IMMUNODEFICIENCY WITH ENZYME DEFICIENCY

Blaese RM et al: T lymphocyte-directed gene therapy for ADA SCID: Initial trial results after 4 years. *Science* 1995; 270:475.

Giblet ER et al: Nucleoside phosphorylase deficiency in a child with severely defective T cell immunity and normal B cell immunity. *Lancet* 1975;1:1010.

Hershfield MS. Adenosine deaminase deficiency: Clinical expression, molecular basis and therapy. *Semin Hematol* 1998;35:291.

Hershfield MS et al: Enzyme replacement therapy with polyethylene glycol adenosine deaminase in adenosine deaminase deficiency: Overview and case reports of three patients, including two now receiving gene therapy. *Pediatr Res* 1993;33:S42.

Levy Y et al: Adenosine deaminase deficiency with late onset of recurrent infections: Response to treatment with polyethylene glycol-modified adenosine deaminase. *J Pediatr* 1988;113:312.

Meuwissen HJ et al: Combined immunodeficiency disease associated with adenosine deaminase deficiency. *J Pediatr* 1975;86:169.

BARE LYMPHOCYTE SYNDROME
Marcadet A et al: Genotyping with DNA probes in combined immunodeficiency syndrome with defective expression of HLA. *N Engl J Med* 1985;312:1287.

Reigh W et al: Congenital immunodeficiency with a regulatory defect in MHC class II gene expression lacks a specific HLA-DR promoter binding protein, RF-X. *Cell* 1988; 53:897.

COMBINED IMMUNODEFICIENCY WITH T-CELL MEMBRANE OR SIGNALING DEFECTS
Alarcon B et al: Familial defect in the surface expression of the T-cell receptor-CD3 complex. *N Engl J Med* 1988; 319:1203.

Chatila T et al: An immunodeficiency characterized by defective signal transduction in T lymphocytes. *N Engl J Med* 1989;320:696.

Elder ME et al: Human severe combined immunodeficiency due to a defect in ZAP-70, a T cell tyrosine kinase. *Science* 1994;264:1596.

OMENN SYNDROME
Cederbaum SD et al: Combined immunodeficiency presenting as the Letterer-Siwe syndrome. *J Pediatr* 1974;85: 466.

Omenn GS: Familial reticuloendotheliosis with eosinophilia. *N Engl J Med* 1965;273:427.

X-LINKED LYMPHOPROLIFERATIVE SYNDROME
Purtilo DT et al: Epstein–Barr virus infections in the X-linked recessive lymphoproliferative syndrome. *Lancet* 1978;1:798.

Seemayer TA et al: X-linked lymphoproliferative disease: Twenty-five years after the discovery. 1995;38:471.

GRAFT-VERSUS-HOST DISEASE
Glucksberg H et al: Clinical manifestations of graft-versus-host disease in human recipients of marrow from HLA-matched sibling donors. *Transplantation* 1974;18:295.

Kadowaki J et al: XX/XY lymphoid chimerism in congenital immunological deficiency syndrome with thymic alymphoplasia. *Lancet* 1965;2:1152.

Sullivan KM et al: Cyclosporine treatment of chronic graft-versus-host disease following allogeneic bone marrow transplantation. *Transplant Proc* 1990;22:1336.

Phagocytic Dysfunction Diseases

24

Robert L. Roberts, MD, PhD, E. Richard Stiehm, MD

Phagocytic disorders may be divided into extrinsic and intrinsic defects. The **extrinsic** defects include opsonic abnormalities secondary to deficiencies of antibody and complement factors, suppression of the total number of neutrophils or granulocytes, suppression of phagocytic function by drugs, and suppression of the number of circulating neutrophils by autoantibody directed against neutrophil antigens. Other extrinsic disorders may be related to abnormal neutrophil chemotaxis secondary to complement deficiency or abnormal complement components.

Intrinsic disorders of phagocytic function include chronic granulomatous disease, several enzyme defects, glycogen storage disease type 1b, Chédiak-Higashi syndrome, and specific granule deficiency. Intrinsic disorders of directed phagocytic movement (chemotaxis) include the hyper-IgE/Job's syndrome, two leukocyte adhesion defects, Shwachman syndrome, tuftsin deficiency, and several syndromes with periodontitis. Defects of phagocytic movement may also occur secondary to diabetes mellitus, metabolic storage disease, splenic deficiency, malnutrition, immaturity, and burns.

Susceptibility to infection from phagocytic dysfunction ranges from mild recurrent skin infections to severe, overwhelming, fatal systemic infection. Generally, these patients are susceptible to bacterial, but not viral or protozoal infections. Some of the more severe disorders cause overwhelming fungal infections.

Numerous tests can now be performed to evaluate phagocytic dysfunction (see Chapter 16). Screening tests are discussed in Chapter 20, and definitive studies are listed in Table 24–1.

NEUTROPENIA

Neutropenia (circulating neutrophils <500 cells/ μL), when persistent, is associated with a number of primary disorders, including congenital neutropenia (Kostmann's syndrome), cyclic neutropenia, glycogen storage disease type 1b, and myelokathexis (failure of release of neutrophils from the marrow).

Acquired antibody-mediated autoimmune (including Felty's syndrome with rheumatoid arthritis) and isoimmune neutropenias (neonatal) have also been described. Neutropenia is common in several primary immunodeficiencies, including X-linked hyper-IgM, X-linked agammaglobulinemia, and reticular dysgenesis. Treatment with granulocyte colony-stimulating factor (G-CSF) is effective in reversing the neutropenia in some of these disorders.

Table 24–1. Evaluation of phagocytosis.

Test	Comment
Nitroblue tetrazolium tests (NBT)	Used for diagnosis and screening of chronic granulomatous disease (CGD) and for detection of x-linked carrier
Quantitative intracellular killing curve	Used for diagnosis of chronic granulomatous disease and other disorders
Chemotaxis	Abnormal in various disorders associated with frequent bacterial infection. Does not provide a specific diagnosis. Several methods
Chemiluminescence	Abnormal in chronic granulomatous disease and myeloperoxidase deficiency
Superoxide production	Absent in CGD and defective in some other syndromes
Enzyme tests	Glucose-6-phosphate dehydrogenase, myeloperoxidase
Membrane glycoproteins	Deficient in leukocyte adhesion (integrin) disorders and associated with abnormal leukocyte adherence and movement
Genetic analysis	Available for CGD, LAD1, Chédiak–Higashi syndrome

Abbreviations: LAD = leukocyte adhesion deficiency.

CHRONIC GRANULOMATOUS DISEASE

Major Immunologic Features

- Susceptibility to infection with catalase-positive microbes such as *Staphylococcus aureus* and organisms normally of low virulence, such as *Staphylococcus epidermidis, Serratia marcescens, Aspergillus.*
- X-linked (65%) or autosomal-recessive (35%) inheritance
- Onset of symptoms usually in infancy or early childhood: draining lymphadenitis, hepatosplenomegaly, pneumonia, osteomyelitis, and abscesses.
- Diagnosis established by abnormal nitroblue tetrazolium (NBT) test, superoxide generation, chemiluminescence, or flow cytometry.
- Gene identification available.

General Considerations

Chronic granulomatous disease (CGD) is usually inherited as an X-linked disorder, with clinical manifestations appearing during the first 2 years of life. Three autosomal variants of the disease have also been described. All patients are susceptible to infection with some common pathogens as well as a variety of normally nonpathogenic and unusual organisms. The NBT test readily identifies CGD patients and female carriers of the X-linked form of the disease. Carriers of a single CGD gene usually do not have increased susceptibility to infections, but the female carriers of X-linked CGD are highly susceptible to discoid lupus. Early diagnosis and aggressive therapy have improved the prognosis for these patients with CGD, which was originally termed "fatal granulomatous disease of childhood."

Pathogenesis

The four different genetic forms of CGD are based on different biochemical abnormalities and patterns of inheritance. The functional defect, however, which occurs in the respiratory burst, is similarly abnormal in the various forms and results in characteristic clinical abnormalities. The normal respiratory burst in neutrophils and monocytes is triggered by opsonized microorganisms or other appropriate stimuli, resulting in an increase in intracellular oxygen consumption with conversion of oxygen to hydrogen peroxide, oxidized halogens, and superoxide and hydroxyl radicals (Figure 24–1). Patients with CGD are unable to generate a respiratory burst after stimulation of granulocytes and monocytes and are therefore unable to kill microorganisms.

The central enzyme in the respiratory burst is the oxidase of the reduced form of nicotinamide adenine dinucleotide phosphate (NADPH). Without this enzyme, hydrogen peroxide, superoxide, and other microbicidal reactive oxygen species cannot be generated. NADPH is composed of a plasma membrane

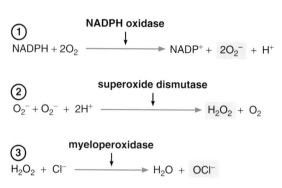

$$\text{①} \quad NADPH + 2O_2 \xrightarrow{\text{NADPH oxidase}} NADP^+ + 2O_2^- + H^+$$

$$\text{②} \quad O_2^- + O_2^- + 2H^+ \xrightarrow{\text{superoxide dismutase}} H_2O_2 + O_2$$

$$\text{③} \quad H_2O_2 + Cl^- \xrightarrow{\text{myeloperoxidase}} H_2O + OCl^-$$

Figure 24–1. Respiratory burst resulting in the generation of superoxide (O_2^-), hydrogen peroxide (H_2O_2), and hypochlorite (OCl^-). *Abbreviations:* NADPH = reduced form of nicotinamide adenine dinucleotide phosphate.

cytochrome b_{588}, consisting of a 91-kilodalton protein (gp91-phox) and a 22-kilodalton (p22-phox), and two cytosolic proteins, a 47-kilodalton (p47-phox), and a 67-kilodalton (p67-phox) component (gp = glycoprotein; p = protein; phox = phagocyte oxidase). Mutations of gp91-phox, termed the X91 variant, is responsible for the X-linked form of the disease, and constitutes 63% of the reported cases. Other variants are autosomal-recessive, including mutations of (1) p47-phox (type A47, on chromosome 7, 33% of cases; (2) p22-phox (type A22, on chromosome 16, 5% of cases); and (3) p67-phox (type A67, on chromosome 1, 5% of cases). These types can be distinguished by Western blot analysis of leukocyte lysates using antibodies to the specific proteins.

Clinical Features

A. Symptoms and Signs: In the majority of patients, the diagnosis can be established before 2 years of age. The most frequent abnormalities are marked lymphadenopathy, infected skin lesions with ulcerations, hepatosplenomegaly, draining lymph nodes, and episodes of pneumonia. Other manifestations include rhinitis, conjunctivitis, dermatitis, ulcerative stomatitis, perianal abscess, osteomyelitis, chronic diarrhea with intermittent abdominal pain, esophageal stenosis, and intestinal and genitourinary tract obstruction. Chronic and acute infection occurs in lymph nodes, skin, lungs, intestinal tract, liver, and bone. A major clue to early diagnosis is the finding of normally nonpathogenic or unusual organisms. Organisms responsible for infection include *Staphylococcus aureus, S epidermidis, Serratia marcescens, Pseudomonas, Escherichia coli, Burkholderia cepacia, Candida,* and *Aspergillus.*

B. Laboratory Findings: The most widely available diagnostic test is the nitroblue tetrazolium (NBT) test, which detects CGD patients as well as female carriers of X-linked CGD. Patient leukocytes cannot reduce NBT dye reduction nor generate appreciable light in chemiluminescence assays. Highly sensitive flow cytometric assays can also detect autosomal carriers of CGD by decreased oxidative burst activity in individual cells. These flow cytometric assays employ fluorescent probes that change emission when exposed to reactive oxygen intermediates. Patients with CGD are unable to kill certain intracellular bacteria at a normal rate. The leukocyte-killing curves for organisms to which these individuals are susceptible (catalase-positive) usually indicate little or no killing over a period of 2 hours (Figure 24–2). Other abnormal findings include decreased oxygen uptake during phagocytosis and abnormal bacterial iodination. Natural killer (NK)-cell activity and T lymphocyte-mediated killing is normal in CGD patients as lymphocyte-mediated killing is not dependent on oxidative burst activity.

Most CGD patients have normal blood leukocyte counts and sedimentation rates when they do not have an active infection. An elevated leukocyte count or sedimentation rate should therefore initiate an investigation for the source of infection. Hypergammaglobulinemia had previously been reported in CGD patients but is not that common today, possibly because earlier diagnosis and aggressive treatment has decreased the infection rates. B- and T-cell function are normal in CGD patients. Complement function is also normal but elevation of complement components might indicate an active infection. Chest films usually identify pneumonias although CT scans are better for identifying lung abscesses, which may be difficult to locate in some patients.

Liver function tests may be abnormal as a result of liver abscesses, characteristic of CGD. Pulmonary function tests are usually abnormal following episodes of pneumonia and may not return to normal for several months. Gastric emptying or barium studies may be used to diagnose GI obstruction due to granulomas. Likewise, intravenous pyelograms and ultrasound may be used to identify sites of urinary tract obstruction. Several X-linked patients have the rare Kell blood type, K_0 (K null), allowing them to be sensitized to Kell antigens following blood transfusion. Histologic examination of the infected area often reveals an accumulation of pigmented histiocytes.

Immunologic Diagnosis

A diagnosis can be established by NBT dye reduction assay or flow cytometric assays and confirmed by identifications of the gene mutation. These genetic assays may also be used to identify the carrier state and to establish an intrauterine diagnosis. Intrauterine diagnosis can be accomplished by NBT testing of fetal blood cells, although genetic analysis of amniotic cells allows the diagnosis to be made much earlier in the pregnancy.

Differential Diagnosis

Few clinical disorders are confused with CGD. Leukocyte glucose-6-phosphate deficiency and myeloperoxidase deficiency have clinical symptoms and laboratory features similar to those of CGD and an abnormal NBT test. Any child presenting with osteomyelitis, pneumonia, liver abscess, or chronic draining lymphadenopathy associated with a normally nonpathogenic or unusual organism should be suspected of having CGD.

Treatment

Long-term survival and reduced morbidity require aggressive, early, intensive therapy. Blood cultures, aspiration of draining lymph nodes, liver biopsy, and open-lung biopsy should be used to obtain a specific bacterial diagnosis. Therapy should be instituted immediately while results of cultures are pending. The choice of antibiotics should be appropriate for the spectrum of bacterial infections likely to be present. Treatment with antibiotics must be prolonged, 5–6 weeks total. Most investigators use prophylactic anti-infective therapy such as trimethoprim-sulfamethoxazole. *Candida* or *Aspergillus* infections require amphotericin B, and itraconzaole may also be added. Many CGD patients now take itraconazole prophylactically to prevent fungal infections.

A controlled trial showed that interferon gamma (IFNγ) reduced the frequency and severity of infections in all types of CGD. The mechanism of action is unclear because oxidase activity is usually not significantly affected; possibly neutrophil and macrophage nonoxidative defense mechanisms are enhanced. The usual dose is 60 µg/m² subcutaneously three times a week.

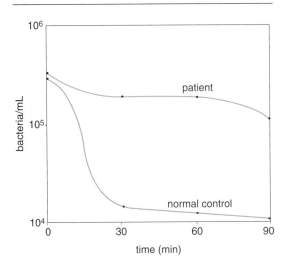

Figure 24–2. Bacterial killing curves in normal control and in patient with chronic granulomatous disease. The patient's phagocyte cells are unable to kill significant numbers of bacteria following an in vitro incubation period of 90 minutes.

Therapy has also included leukocyte infusions for severe infections with an apparent synergistic effect between the normal transfused granulocytes and the CGD granulocytes in the killing of microorganisms. Granulocyte colony stimulating factor (G-CSF) has also been used to treat infected CGD patients by increasing both the number and function of CGD granulocytes. G-CSF has also been used to pretreat the donors for granulocyte transfusions to greatly increase the number of granulocytes available for transfusion. Obstructive lesions respond to corticosteroids. Recently, the number of bone marrow and cord stem cell transplants to treat CGD has increased although these procedures still carry great risks. A number of gene therapy trials are now in progress, but their effectiveness is yet to be proven.

Complications & Prognosis

Chronic organ dysfunction may result from severe or chronic infection. Examples are abnormal pulmonary function, chronic liver disease, chronic osteomyelitis, and malabsorption secondary to gastrointestinal tract involvement. Growth retardation is common. The mortality rate in CGD has been considerably reduced by early diagnosis and aggressive therapy. Survival into the second decade and beyond has been recorded. Female carriers of the X-linked form of CGD have an increased prevalence of systemic and discoid lupus erythematosus.

GLUCOSE-6-PHOSPHATE DEHYDROGENASE DEFICIENCY

Patients with leukocyte glucose-6-phosphate dehydrogenase (G6PD) deficiency have defective generation of hydrogen peroxide and susceptibility to *S aureus* and *E coli,* similar to patients with chronic granulomatous disease. The NBT test is abnormal, but the clinical severity is less than in CGD. The illness is rare and **not** present in patients with **erythrocyte** G6PD deficiency.

Chédiak-Higashi Syndrome

Chédiak-Higashi syndrome (CHS) is a multisystem autosomal-recessive disorder with recurrent bacterial infections from a variety of organisms, hepatosplenomegaly, partial albinism, central nervous system abnormalities, and a high incidence of lymphoreticular cancers.

The characteristic abnormality of giant cytoplasmic granular inclusions in leukocytes and platelets is visible on routine peripheral blood smears under ordinary light microscopy. Additional abnormalities include elevated Epstein-Barr virus (EBV) antibody titers, abnormal neutrophil chemotaxis, decreased NK-cell activity, and abnormal intracellular killing of organisms (including streptococci and pneumococci as well as the organisms found in CGD). The killing defect is manifested in vitro by delayed intracellular killing. Oxygen consumption, hydrogen peroxide formation, and hexose monophosphate shunt activity are normal. Abnormal microtubule function, abnormal lysosomal enzyme levels in granulocytes, and proteinase deficiency in granulocytes have been described and are associated with increased levels of leukocyte cyclic adenosine monophosphate (cAMP). Abnormal leukocyte function has been corrected in vitro by ascorbate, but the results of treatment in vivo are contradictory. Improved granulocyte function in vitro has also been observed after treatment with anticholinergic drugs.

Definitive cure with bone marrow transplantation has been accomplished. Without transplantation, the prognosis is poor because of progressive increased susceptibility to infection and neurologic deterioration. Patients with CHS also risk developing lymphohistiocytic infiltration of the liver, spleen, and lymph nodes associated with pancytopenia and high fever. This condition is referred to as the **accelerated phase** of CHS and is usually fatal. Most patients die during childhood, but survivors to the second and third decades have been reported.

MYELOPEROXIDASE DEFICIENCY

Several patients with complete deficiency of leukocyte myeloperoxidase have been described. Myeloperoxidase is one of the enzymes necessary for normal intracellular killing of certain organisms. It catalyzes the oxidation of microorganisms by intracellular H_2O_2 in the presence of halides (see Figure 24–1). The leukocytes have normal oxygen consumption, hexose monophosphate shunt activity, and superoxide and hydrogen peroxide production. The intracellular killing of organisms is delayed but may reach normal levels with increased in vitro incubation times. Chemiluminescence as enhanced by luminol is decreased because it measures primarily the production of hypochlorous acid. Increased susceptibility to candidal and staphylococcal infections has been reported, but many patients are asymptomatic. The diagnosis can be established by a peroxidase stain of peripheral blood. No specific treatment is available other than appropriate antibiotics.

SPECIFIC GRANULE DEFICIENCY

This is an autosomal-recessive disorder with recurrent mucous membrane and skin infections. The neutrophils are bilobed or kidney-shaped, and secondary granules are lacking under electron microscopy. As a result, certain antimicrobial enzymes, such as lactoferrin and vitamin B_{12}-binding protein, are missing, but the levels of azurophilic granule proteins (eg, myeloperoxidase, lysozyme) are normal. Their neutrophils are very defective in chemotaxis and microbial killing.

GLYCOGEN STORAGE DISEASE (GSD) TYPE 1B

This disorder is a defect in glucose-6-phosphate translocase with resulting hypoglycemia. Patients with GSD type 1b (but not type 1a) have defects in neutrophil chemotaxis, intermittent neutropenia, a defective respiratory burst, and increased susceptibility to bacterial infection. Treatment with G-CSF greatly reverses the neutropenia and improves neutrophil function.

HYPER IGE SYNDROME/JOB'S SYNDROME

Major Features
- Recurrent staphylococcal infections of skin, subcutaneous tissues, lungs, upper airways, and bones.
- Coarse facies.
- Exceptionally high serum IgE levels (>2000 IU/mL).
- Blood and tissue eosinophilia.
- Intermittent chemotactic defects.

These patients have an early onset of cutaneous infections and deep-seated staphylococcal infections, including pneumonia with pneumatocele formation; mastoiditis; and (less commonly) bone, joint, and visceral infection. The skin resembles recurrent severe eczema, but infection is more prominent and pruritus less common. The rash is usually not exacerbated by allergens as would occur in atopic dermatitis. Many patients have coarse facial features (Figure 24–3). Some patients have osteopenia with frequent fractures due to increased osteoclastic activity. The original report of this disorder described two redhaired girls with "cold," nontender, cutaneous abscesses—a condition given the eponym of "Job's" syndrome, probably a mild form of the hyper-IgE syndrome. Both sexes and all major racial groups are affected. A few familial cases have been described, but a clear genetic pattern has not emerged.

All patients have extremely elevated levels of serum IgE (>2000 IU/mL and up to 40,000 IU/mL), blood and tissue eosinophilia, and moderately increased serum IgD levels. Other abnormalities include a variable chemotactic defect (usually during infections), and decreased antibody and T-cell proliferative responses to antigens. IgG, IgM, and IgA levels are normal or elevated, and lymphocyte subsets are within normal limits. The NBT test and complement levels are also normal.

An immunoregulatory T-cell abnormality with excessive IL-4 production has been suggested as the immunologic defect. This does not explain the propensity toward staphylococcal infection, however.

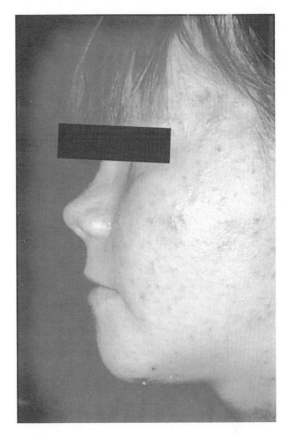

Figure 24–3. Coarse facial features, multiple small abscesses, and "saddle" nose in a female with Job's syndrome.

Treatment consists of optimal antistaphylococcal antibiotics intravenously for infections. Continuous trimethoprim-sulfamethoxazole therapy is of value in controlling cutaneous infection. Topical corticosteroids improve the eczematous rash, and antihistamines may benefit some patients. Topical antibiotics such as mupirocin and topical antifungal drugs may help prevent more deep-seated infections. Levamisole is without benefit. IFNγ and IVIG have also been used.

LEUKOCYTE ADHESION DEFECT-TYPE 1 (LFA-1/Mac-1/p150,95 [CD11/CD18] Deficiency)

Major Immunologic Features
- Leukocytosis and delayed umbilical cord detachment
- Autosomal-recessive mode of inheritance
- Recurrent necrotic soft tissue infections and periodontitis

- Defective leukocyte chemotaxis and cytotoxic function (CTL, NK, and ADCC)
- Deficient expression of leukocyte adhesion proteins CD11a/CD18 (LFA-1), CD11b/CD18 (CR3, Mac-1) and CD11c/CD18 (p150,95)

General Considerations

Patients with leukocyte adhesion defect-type 1 (LAD-1) have recurrent pyogenic infections, often with onset in the first weeks of life, and usually from *Staphylococcus aureus, Pseudomonas aeruginosa, Klebsiella, Proteus,* and enterococci. Delayed separation of the umbilical cord (greater than 3 weeks) is common. As patients become older, they develop recurrent skin infections, sinusitis, vaginitis, perianal abscesses, periodontal disease, tracheobronchitis, pneumonia, recurrent progressive necrotic soft tissue infections, and septicemia. The disease may be fatal in the first years of life, or it may follow a more protracted course, suggesting two clinical phenotypes: moderate and severe. The inheritance pattern of both is autosomal-recessive.

The genetic basis of LAD-1 is mutations of the common beta subunit (CD18) of an integrin gene leading to deficiency of three leukocyte adhesion molecules: LFA-1(CD11a/CD18), CR3 or Mac-1(CD11b/CD18), and p150,95 or CR4(CD11c/CD18) (Figure 24–4). These adhesion molecules are present on lymphocytes, monocytes, granulocytes, and NK cells, mediating cellular interactions, cell movement, and interaction with complement fragments.

Deficiency of these integrins results in several immunologic abnormalities. In vivo and in vitro chemotaxis of granulocytes and in vitro cell spreading are abnormal. Zymosan-induced, but not phorbol myristate acetate-induced, chemiluminescence, is abnormal. Antibody-dependent cellular cytotoxicity, natural killer cytotoxicity, and T-lymphocyte cytotoxicity are abnormal because all require cell interaction.

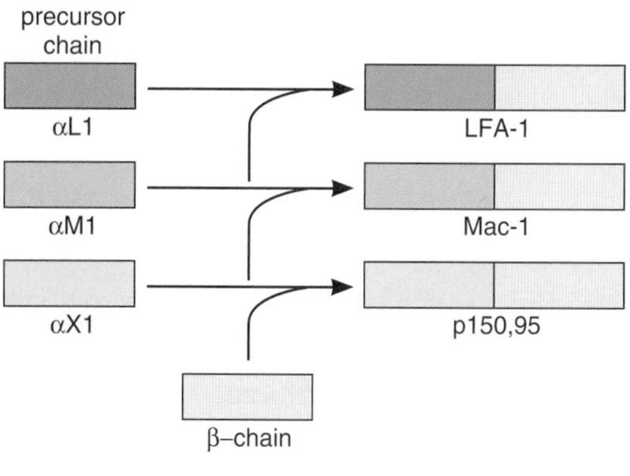

Treatment of LAD-1 is directed toward the specific infectious agents involved. As patients are infected with common pathogenic, but not opportunistic, organisms, they should respond to appropriate antibiotic therapy. Early aggressive treatment should be used, and prophylactic therapy should be given under certain circumstances, such as dental procedures. Bone marrow transplantation has been successful in many LAD-1 patients as they engraft readily. Patients with LAD1 are also candidates for gene therapy.

LEUKOCYTE ADHESION DEFECT (LAD) TYPE 2

LAD type 2 is a rare defect of fucose metabolism, resulting in the absence of the neutrophil receptor [Sialyl-Lewis X (CD15s)] for E-selectin, thereby severely impairing neutrophil adhesion to activated endothelial cells of blood vessels. This deficiency (leukocyte adhesion defect-type 2 [LAD-2]) results in a lack of neutrophil rolling and a chemotactic defect similar to that in LAD-1. These children have periodontitis, recurrent bacterial infections, neutrophilia, and mental and physical retardation. Unlike LAD-1, CD11/CD18 expression on their leukocytes is normal.

SHWACHMAN SYNDROME

Patients with Shwachman syndrome have pancreatic insufficiency, malabsorption, dyschondroplasia, eczema, and recurrent infection. They have neutropenia and decreased neutrophil chemotaxis. The disease is similar to cystic fibrosis because of the pancreatic insufficiency, but the sweat test is normal.

TUFTSIN DEFICIENCY

Tuftsin disease has been reported as a familial deficiency of a phagocytosis-stimulating tetrapeptide that is cleaved from a parent immunoglobulin-like molecule (termed leukokinin) in the spleen. Tuftsin also appears to be absent in patients who have been splenectomized and those receiving total parenteral nutrition. Local and severe systemic infections occur with *Candida, S aureus,* and *Streptococcus pneumoniae.* Tuftsin levels can be measured in only a few specialized laboratories. There is no treatment, and the prognosis is uncertain. Gamma globulin therapy appeared to be beneficial in the two families in which it was tried.

Figure 24–4. Comparative structure of leukocyte adhesion molecules, showing unique α chains and a common (b) chain.

PERIODONTITIS SYNDROMES

Several syndromes of severe periodontitis with chemotactic defects have been described, including localized juvenile periodontitis, rapidly progressive periodontitis, acute necrotizing ulcerative gingivitis, and the Papillon-Lefèvre syndrome (early-onset periodontitis with palmar-plantar hyperkeratosis). Each syndrome has a characteristic oral location, bacterial flora, and hereditary pattern. Oral antibiotics and intensive dental hygiene may aid some patients, but most of them experience loss of all teeth at an early age.

REFERENCES

CHRONIC GRANULOMATOUS DISEASE

Curnutte JT et al: Chronic granulomatous disease due to a defect in the cytosolic factor required for nicotinamide adenine dinucleotide phosphate oxidase activation. *J Clin Invest* 1988;81:606.

Fischer A et al: The management of chronic granulomatous disease. *Eur J. Pediatr* 1993;152:896.

Forrest CB et al: Clinical features and current management of chronic granulomatous disease. *Hematol Oncol Clin North Am* 1988;2:253.

Hobbs JR et al: Chronic granulomatous disease 100% corrected by displacement bone marrow transplantation from a volunteer unrelated donor. *Eur J Pediatr* 1992; 151:806.

International Chronic Granulomatous Disease Cooperative Study Group. A controlled trial of interferon gamma to prevent infection in chronic granulomatous disease. *N Engl J Med* 1991;324:509.

Malech HL et al: Prospects for gene therapy for neutrophil defects. *Semin Hematol* 1997;34:355.

Mills EL et al: X-linked inheritance in females with chronic granulomatous disease. *J Clin Invest* 1980;66:332.

Roos D: The genetic basis of chronic granulomatous disease. *Immunol Rev* 1994;138:121.

GLUCOSE-6-PHOSPHATE DEHYDROGENASE DEFICIENCY

Cooper MR et al: Complete deficiency of leukocyte glucose-6-phosphate dehydrogenase with defective bactericidal activity. *J Clin Invest* 1972;51:769.

MYELOPEROXIDASE DEFICIENCY

Nauseef WM: Myeloperoxidase deficiency. *Hematol Oncol Clin North Am* 1988;2:577.

Parry MF et al: Myeloperoxidase deficiency. *Ann Intern Med* 1981;95:293.

Romano M et al: Biochemical and molecular characterization of hereditary myeloperoxidase deficiency. *Blood* 1997;90:4126.

CHÉDIAK-HIGASHI SYNDROME

Ganz T et al: Microbicidal/cytotoxic proteins of neutrophils are deficient in two disorders: Chédiak-Higashi syndrome and specific granule deficiency. *J Clin Invest* 1988; 82:552.

Haddad E et al: Treatment of Chédiak-Higashi syndrome by allogenic bone marrow transplantation : Report of 10 cases. *Blood* 1995;85:3328.

Haliotis T et al: Chédiak-Higashi gene in humans. 1. Impairment of natural-killer function. *J Exp Med* 1980;151: 1039.

Nagle DL et al: identification and mutation analysis of the complete gene for Chédiak-Higashi syndrome *Nat Genet* 1996;14:307.

TUFTSIN DEFICIENCY

Constantopoulos A: Congenital tuftsin deficiency. *Ann N Y Acad Sci* 1983;419:214.

Phillips JH et al: Tuftsin, a naturally occurring immunopotentiating factor. 1. In vitro enhancement of murine natural cell-mediated cytotoxicity. *J Immunol* 1981; 126: 915.

Zoli G et al: Impaired splenic function and tuftsin deficiency in patients with intestinal failure and long term intravenous nutrition. *Gut* 1998;43:759.

HYPER IgE/JOB'S SYNDROME

Buckley RH et al: Extreme hyperimmunoglobulinemia E and undue susceptibility to infection. *Pediatrics* 1972; 49:59.

Claassen JL et al: Mononuclear cells from patients with the hyper-IgE syndrome produce little IgE when stimulated with recombinant interleukin-4 in vitro. *J Allergy Clin Immunol* 1991;88:713.

Garrand O et al: Regulation of immunoglobulin production in hyper-IgE (Jobs syndrome). *J Allergy Clin Immunol* 1999;103:333.

Hill HR, Quie PG: Raised serum IgE levels and defective neutrophil chemotaxis in three children with eczema and recurrent bacterial infections. *Lancet* 1974;1:183.

Matter L et al: Abnormal immune response to *Staphylococcus aureus* in patients with *Staphylococcus aureus* hyper-IgE syndrome. *Clin Exp Immunol* 1986;66:450.

PERIODONTITIS SYNDROMES

Nisengard RJ, Newman MG (editors): *Oral Microbiology and Immunology,* 2nd ed., W.B. Saunders, 1994.

Quie PG et al: Disorders of polymorphonuclear phagocytic system. In: *Immunologic Disorders in Infants and Children,* 4th ed. Stiehm ER, W.B. Saunders, 1996.

LEUKOCYTE ADHESION DEFECTS

Arnaout MA: Molecular basis for leukocyte adhesion deficiency. In: *Biochemistry of Macrophages and Related Cell Types,* Horton M (editor). Plenum, 1993.

Bauer TR et al: Retroviral-mediated gene transfer of leukocyte integrin CD18 into peripheral blood CD34$^+$ cells derived from a patient with LAD type I. *Blood* 1998;91:1520.

Etzioni A et al: Recurrent severe infections caused by a novel leukocyte adhesion deficiency. *N Engl J Med* 1992;327:1789.

Fischer A et al: Bone marrow transplantation (BMT) in Europe for primary immunodeficiencies other than severe combined immunodeficiency: A report from the European Group for BMT and the European Group for Immunodeficiency. *Blood* 1994;83:1149.

GLYCOGEN STORAGE DISEASE-TYPE 1B

Gitzelmann R, Boshare NU: Defective neutrophil and monocyte functions in glycogen storage disease type Ib: A literature review. *Eur J Pediatr* 1993;152(Suppl I):533.

Kilpatrick L et al: Impaired metabolic function and signaling defects in phagocytic cells in glycogen storage disease type 1b. *J Clin Invest* 1990;86:196.

SHWACHMAN SYNDROME

Aggett PJ et al: An inherited disorder of neutrophil mobility in Shwachman syndrome. *J Pediatr* 1979;94:391.

SPECIFIC GRANULE DEFICIENCY

Ambruso DR et al: Defective bactericidal activity and absence of specific granules in neutrophils from a patient with recurrent bacterial infections. *J Clin Immunol* 1984;4:23.

Lomax KJ, et al: Selective defect in myeloid cell lactoferrin gene expression in neutrophil specific granule deficiency. *J Clin Invest* 1989;83:514.

Complement Deficiencies

25

Eric Wagner, PhD, & Michael M. Frank, MD

INTRODUCTION

As discussed in Chapter 12, complement is activated through three major pathways: the **classical,** the **alternative,** and the newly discovered **mannan-binding lectin (MBL)** pathway. In each, protein fragments derived from several complement component proteins assemble to form an enzymatic complex that has the ability to bind and cleave C3, the central component of the complement system. Once all pathways have converged at the level of **C3,** they proceed in common to interact with the late-acting complement components: C5, C6, C7, C8, and C9. The assembly of these five terminal complement components on a cell surface forms the **membrane attack complex** that is responsible for the lysis of heterologous erythrocytes, some antibody-sensitized autologous erythrocytes, certain bacteria, and viruses, or, in some cases, induction of various cellular responses in nucleated cells. With the exception of MBL deficiency, genetic deficiency in one of the complement components is uncommon. Only limited numbers of patients have a deficiency in a component of the classical pathway, alternative pathway, or the late-acting components. More common are patients with defects in control proteins that regulate a number of steps in the complement activation cascade.

Defects of all but three complement components behave as autosomal-recessive traits (Table 25–1). Usually, **heterozygous** individuals have about **half** the normal levels of the protein for which one of the two alleles of the encoding gene is defective. Because the range of plasma concentrations is broad for many of the complement proteins in normal individuals, however, it is often impossible to distinguish heterozygous individuals from normal individuals on the basis of plasma concentration measurement alone. In most cases, heterozygous individuals are phenotypically normal, except in some instances, which will be discussed later. Affected individuals are those with little or no gene product; their parents are heterozygous. A few complement components are composed of subunits that are encoded by multiple genes. The C1 complex is composed of C1q, C1r, and C1s, each

encoded by a specific gene. C8 is the result of the assembly of the products of two genes encoding for the C8α–γ chain and the C8β chain. Deficiency in one of these complement protein subunits also follows an autosomal-recessive pattern.

When an individual is **homozygous** for deficiency in either a component of the classical pathway or one of the late-acting complement components, the lytic activity of complement is interrupted at the point at which that component functions. In this case, the complement titer, as assessed by the ability of serum to cause the lysis of antibody-sensitized sheep erythrocytes (CH_{50} assay), is **zero.** Similarly, a defect in one of the alternative pathway components or one of the late-acting complement components leads to an alternative pathway titer, as assessed by the ability of serum to cause lysis of unsensitized rabbit erythrocytes (AH_{50} assay), of **zero.**

The major clinical features of each complement deficiency are listed in Table 25–1. Clinical observations in complement-deficient individuals give insights into the role complement plays in various immunologic reactions.

C3 DEFICIENCY

C3 plays a central role in all three complement activation pathways. In addition to being the component at which all three pathways converge, C3 is important in opsonization–phagocytosis of foreign particles, solubilization and elimination of immune complexes, generation of inflammatory peptides, and B-cell activation leading to antibody production. Patients with C3 deficiency suffer from **recurrent infections** caused by encapsulated pyogenic bacteria, such as *Neisseria meningitidis, Streptococcus pneumoniae,* and *Haemophilus influenzae.* Infections are severe in these patients and involve the upper respiratory tract, meninges, and the bloodstream. Some C3-deficient patients also develop immune complex diseases, such as membranoproliferative glomerulonephritis and systemic lupus erythematosus. Some patients have an acquired C3 deficiency caused by an autoantibody termed **C3 nephritic factor** (C3NeF).

Table 25–1. Inherited complement and complement-related protein deficiency states.

Protein	Pattern of Inheritence	Reported Major Clinical Correlates[a]
Common to all pathways:		
C3	Autosomal-recessive	ACUD, PID
Classical pathways:		
C1q	Autosomal-recessive	ACUD, PID
C1r	Autosomal-recessive	ACUD
C1s	Autosomal-recessive	ACUD
C4[b]	Autosomal-recessive	ACUD
C2	Autosomal-recessive	ACUD, PID
Alternative pathway:		
Factor B	Autosomal-recessive	Meningococcemia
Factor D	Autosomal-recessive	Recurrent pyogenic infections
Properdin	X-linked-recessive	Recurrent pyogenic infections, fulminant meningococcemia
MBLectin pathway		
MBL	Autosomal-dominant	Recurrent infections
Membrane attack complex:		
C5	Autosomal-recessive	Recurrent disseminated neisserial infections, SLE
C6	Autosomal-recessive	Recurrent disseminated neisserial infections
C7	Autosomal-recessive	Recurrent disseminated neisserial infections, Raynaud's disease
C8 (β or α–γ chains)	Autosomal-recessive	Recurrent disseminated neisserial infections
C9	Autosomal-recessive	PID
Fluid-phase control proteins:		
C1 inhibitor	Autosomal-dominant or acquired	Hereditary angioedema, autoimmune diseases[c]
C4bp	Autosomal-recessive	Angioedema, Behçet-like syndrome
Factor I	Autosomal-recessive	Recurrent pyogenic infections, ACUD
Factor H	Autosomal-recessive	Recurrent pyogenic infections, ACUD
Cell-bound proteins:		
CR1	Acquired	Association between low erythrocyte expression and SLE
CR3	Autosomal-recessive[d]	Recurrent pyogenic infections, leukocytosis
DAF/CD59/HRF	Acquired	Paroxysmal nocturnal hemoglobinuria

Abbreviations: ACUD = autoimmune collagen vascular disease (SLE, glomerulonephritis); SLE = systemic lupus erythematosus; PID = propensity to infectious diseases; MBL = mannan-binding lectin; C4bp = C4-binding protein; CR1 = complement receptor type 1; CR3 = complement receptor type 3; DAF = decay-accelerating factor; CD59 = protectin; HRF = homologous restriction factor.
[a] A significant number of individuals with complement deficiencies, especially of C2 and the terminal components, are clinically well. Some patients with defects in C5-9 have had autoimmune disease.
[b] Two genes exist in humans that code for C4 (C4A, C4B). Individuals lacking C4A or C4B are designated "Q0" (quantity 0). Thus, individuals can be C4AQ0 or C4BQ0. Such individuals are reported to have an increased incidence of autoimmune disease. Similarly, C2-deficient individuals are reported to have an increased incidence of autoimmune disease.
[c] Includes approximately 85% of cases with silent alleles and 15% with alleles encoding for dysfunctional variant C1 inhibitor protein.
[d] Low but not absent leukocyte CR3 is detectable in both parents of most CR3-deficient children.

C3NeF binds to Bb in the alternative pathway C3 convertase, C3bBb (see Chapter 12), and stabilizes it. This leads to prolongation of the convertase's half-life and continuous activation of C3, resulting in its depletion. C3NeF is associated with membranoproliferative glomerulonephritis and partial lipodystrophy.

CLASSICAL PATHWAY DEFICIENCIES

The classical pathway is mainly activated by antigen-antibody complexes (immune complexes) or antibody-coated targets like bacteria and viruses. Deficiency in one of the classical pathway components leads to a slight increased risk of infections. Because of the presence of the MBL and alternative complement pathways, however, the risk is minor. However, patients with deficiency in some of the early-acting classical pathway components have a marked increase in the incidence of **autoimmune disease.**

Patients deficient in C1q are at an increased risk of developing infections caused by encapsulated bacteria, such as *N meningitidis, S pneumoniae,* and *H influenzae*. These infections are usually less severe than in patients with C3 or alternative pathway component deficiencies. A striking clinical observation in these patients is the development of autoimmune diseases, such as systemic lupus erythematosus and glomerulonephritis. Autoimmune disease in these patients is often severe.

Genes that encode for C1r and C1s are closely linked; therefore, combined C1r and C1s deficiency has been reported in a low number of individuals. As in C1q-deficient patients, patients with C1r/C1s deficiency experience severe lupus erythematosus and glomerulonephritis.

Two genes code for C4: C4A and C4B. The thiolester group of C4A reacts preferentially with amino groups on an activator surface, whereas that of C4B reacts preferentially with hydroxyl groups. Complete C4 deficiency is a rare event in the general population, but a null allele for either the C4A or C4B gene is observed with high frequency. Like patients with C1q deficiency, patients with complete C4 deficiency experience upper respiratory tract infections caused by encapsulated pyogenic bacteria and are at increased risk of *N meningitidis* infection. Generally, these patients develop either discoid or systemic lupus erythematosus. Immune complex disease involving the kidney is also a feature of C4 deficiency. A certain number of patients lack the product of either the C4A or the C4B gene. Deficiency in either gene product is termed C4AQ0 or C4BQ0 (for quantity 0). It has been postulated that there is a strong association between C4A deficiency and systemic lupus erythematosus and between C4B deficiency and an increased risk of infections.

Following mannan-binding lectin deficiency, C2 deficiency is the most common complement deficiency among whites, with an estimated frequency of about 1:20,000. As in C1q-deficient patients, infections observed in C2-deficient patients involve the upper respiratory tract and are caused by encapsulated pyogenic bacteria. No striking increase in infection rates occurs in these individuals, however. About half of the patients experience systemic or discoid lupus erythematosus, lupus-like disease, or immune complex disease that mostly affects the skin and joints. Again, the disease may be mild. Surprisingly, many C2-deficient individuals (more than 25%) appear healthy. The reason for this is uncertain at present but might be explained by the so-called **C2-bypass pathway.** This complement activation pathway is relatively inefficient and has been studied only in vitro in humans. It uses C1, C4, and components of the alternative pathway but allows activation of C3 and late-acting components. It therefore bypasses C2 and may compensate for C2 deficiency.

Interestingly, patients with deficiency in one of the above-mentioned classical pathway complement components have an impaired ability to mount an adequate antibody response to an antigenic challenge. They possess low concentrations of serum IgG2 and IgG4, two IgG isotypes believed to be important in host defense against encapsulated bacteria. This may, in part, explain why patients with classical complement pathway component deficiencies are more susceptible to infections caused by these bacteria. As C3 is known to be important in the regulation of B-cell responses, deficiency in an early classical pathway complement component impairs C3 deposition on an antigenic surface and, therefore, interferes with efficient antibody production.

ALTERNATIVE PATHWAY DEFICIENCIES

The alternative pathway is believed to be important in the primary host defense against microorganisms. This is exemplified by the high prevalence of severe pyogenic infections in C3-deficient patients. Similarly, deficiency in the three other components of the alternative pathway leads to severe infections.

Factor B binds to C3b [or C3(H$_2$O)] and is cleaved by factor D. The enzymatic site on Bb functions in the alternative pathway C3 convertase to cleave C3 and in the alternative pathway C5 convertase to cleave C5. Only one patient with complete factor B deficiency has been described. This patient presented with sepsis caused by *N meningitidis.*

Factor D is the enzyme that cleaves factor B once it has bound to C3b to generate the alternative pathway C3 convertase (C3bBb). Very few patients have factor D deficiency. These patients experience recurrent neisserial infections that involve the lungs, the meninges, and the blood.

Properdin stabilizes the alternative pathway C3 convertase (C3bBb), thereby prolonging its half-life and allowing more efficient alternative pathway activation on an activator surface. **Properdin deficiency** is unique in that it is inherited in an X-linked fashion. Individuals with properdin deficiency have a very high incidence of meningitis caused by *N meningitidis.* Infections that involve the blood and the upper respiratory tract are also observed. Infections are usually not recurrent in these patients; this may be accounted for by the presence of an intact classical pathway that could mediate efficient opsonization and bacterial lysis once specific antibodies to the bacterial strain have developed. Immune complex diseases are not a general feature of alternative pathway complement component deficiencies although discoid lupus erythematosus has been documented in some properdin-deficient patients.

MANNAN-BINDING LECTIN DEFICIENCY

Recently, a third pathway of complement activation was identified. In this pathway, MBL interacts with carbohydrates on the surface of various microorganisms. Mannan-binding lectin is a protein present at very low concentrations in plasma (~1.5 μg/mL). It shares structural homology with C1q and triggers complement activation via components of the classical or the alternative pathways on activation of two serine proteases termed mannan-binding lectin-associated proteases-1 and -2 (MASP-1 and MASP-2). This pathway of complement activation is believed to be important in **early childhood,** especially during the period when maternal antibody protection is lost and an efficient antibody repertoire has yet to be developed (6–18 months of age). It is estimated that as many as 5% of individuals in the general population have a gene defect that leads to substantially reduced levels of MBL in plasma (>10-fold reduction). Mannan-binding lectin deficiency is inherited as an autosomal-dominant trait. Heterozygous individuals have very low levels of the protein in plasma. Patients with MBL deficiency are reported to experience frequent infections, such as recurrent lung infections, recurrent otitis media, diarrhea, and septicemia caused by various bacteria. An increased incidence of *N meningitidis* infections is observed in MBL-deficient patients. In addition to increased susceptibility to infections, it is suggested that MBL deficiency is associated with susceptibility to HIV infection, development of autoimmune disease such as systemic lupus erythematosus, and risk of recurrent miscarriage. It was recently reported that, in patients with cystic fibrosis, MBL deficiency is associated with far more severe disease.

TERMINAL COMPONENT DEFICIENCIES

Late-acting complement components (C5–9) form a complex that inserts in a cell membrane to cause physiologic alterations in nucleated cells or lysis in some bacteria, viruses, and heterologous or abnormal erythrocytes. Patients with terminal complement component deficiencies have intact opsonic function. Nevertheless, with the notable exception of C9 deficiency, many of the patients deficient in C5, C6, C7, or C8 experience recurrent *N meningitidis* meningitis, meningococcemia or disseminated gonococcal disease. Interestingly, these infections occur at an older age than in the complement-sufficient popula-

tion, are caused by untypable and Y-type *N,* and are less lethal than in the normal population. It is possible that such complement-deficient individuals develop specific antibody to the organism that offers partial protection. Individuals with no antibody to the organisms are far more likely to die of overwhelming sepsis than are individuals with circulating antibody. It is of interest that the membrane attack complex is known to induce physiologic changes in nucleated cells that ultimately can lead to tissue damage. Absence of one of the terminal complement components might offer some protection against the tissue-damaging effects of neisserial infections on complement activation. Some cases of systemic lupus erythematosus and other autoimmune diseases have been reported among patients with terminal component deficiencies. An association between C8β chain deficiency and systemic lupus erythematosus has been proposed. The role of late component deficiencies in the development of autoimmunity is still quite unclear. Interestingly, deficiency in the C8α–γ gene occurs mostly in individuals of African, Hispanic, and Japanese origin, whereas deficiency in the C8β gene is mostly observed in those of European heritage and among Sephardic Jews.

The function of C9 in the membrane attack complex is to enlarge the lesion formed in the cell membrane following the binding of C5b, C6, C7, and C8, thereby allowing more rapid osmotic lysis of cells. Lysis of heterologous erythrocytes, however, as well as some bacteria has been shown to occur in the absence of C9, yet at a slower rate. A large number of C9-deficient individuals have been identified in the Japanese population. Although the risk of *N meningitidis* meningitis is clearly increased in these patients, they do not, in general, experience recurrent infections. Furthermore, many C9-deficient individuals are asymptomatic. This suggests that the formation of the C5b-8 complex on the bacterium is sufficient to offer marked protection from recurrent infection. Presumably, C9 improves bacterial killing, explaining why these patients have a higher than normal incidence of meningitis. This higher incidence of meningitis may be contributed to by low levels of complement components in the cerebrospinal fluid, being less effective in killing *N meningitidis* and preventing meningitis in these patients than is the higher level of complement proteins in blood.

CONTROL PROTEIN DEFICIENCIES

Regulatory proteins that control complement activation may also be deficient, and their absence is accompanied by a variety of clinical manifestations. The most common and best studied of these deficiencies is the partial deficiency of C1 inhibitor (also termed C1 esterase inhibitor). C1 inhibitor functions to inactivate the C1 complex by interacting with two of its subcomponents: C1r and C1s. C1 inhibitor also dissociates the C1 complex and inhibits C1 autoactivation in the fluid phase and by weak activators of the classical pathway. In addition, C1 inhibitor is the main regulatory protein of the contact system of the clotting cascade and the kinin-generating system. It inhibits the enzymatic activity of activated factor XII (factor XIIa) and activated factor XI (factor XIa) of the intrinsic coagulation pathway, kallikrein (kinin-generating system), and plasmin (fibrinolytic pathway).

Partial genetic deficiency in C1 inhibitor leads to **hereditary angioedema,** a disease characterized by recurrent episodes of edema of subcutaneous and submucosal tissues. It particularly affects the extremities and the gastrointestinal tract. Typically, attacks last for 1–4 days and are harmless, although they usually induce severe abdominal pain when they involve the bowel wall. Occasionally, attacks affect subcutaneous and submucosal tissue in the region of the upper airway. In this case, they may be associated with respiratory obstruction and asphyxiation. Attacks are sporadic, but may be induced by emotional stress or physical trauma in about half of the patients. Attacks seldom become severe before puberty, although they typically begin in childhood. It is postulated that the clinical manifestations of hereditary angioedema arise from a lack of regulation of the contact system rather than from a lack of regulation of C1, but this issue is still under investigation.

Deficiency of C1 inhibitor is unique because it is inherited as an autosomal-dominant trait. Individuals with hereditary angioedema have defective C1 inhibitor production encoded for by one of the two genes present on chromosome 11. Approximately 85% of patients have one **nonproductive gene** and have one third to one half the normal plasma levels of C1 inhibitor. The product of one normal gene does not appear to be sufficient to control activation of the various mediator pathways. The other 15% of patients have a **gene mutation** in one of the two C1 inhibitor genes that leads to production by that gene of an abnormal C1 inhibitor with no functional activity. Diagnosis of hereditary angioedema is established by the demonstration of low antigenic or functional levels of C1 esterase inhibitor. Such patients usually have normal levels of C1, low levels of C4 and C2, and normal levels of C3. Identification of these patients is of particular importance because the disease may be life-threatening. Most patients are treated effectively with oral substituted methylated androgen preparations, which appear to cause increased synthesis of the natural gene product.

Rarely, patients have an **acquired form** of C1 inhibitor deficiency and present with clinical findings of recurrent angioedema similar to patients with the inherited form of the disease. There are two types of acquired C1 inhibitor deficiency. In the first, which is usually associated with lymphoproliferative disorders and other **malignancies,** excessive C1 activation occurs as a result of complement-activating factors being produced by malignant cells, thereby utilizing C1 inhibitor at a rate higher than that of synthesis. This subtype of acquired C1 inhibitor deficiency may also occur in the course of an **autoimmune disease** such as systemic lupus erythematosus. In the second, a **monoclonal autoantibody** directed against C1 inhibitor is formed. This autoantibody blocks C1 inhibitor function. In contrast to patients with the inherited form of C1 inhibitor deficiency, patients with acquired C1 inhibitor deficiency have profoundly depressed serum C1 titers, reflecting the marked activation and utilization of C1 that, in turn, depletes C1 inhibitor.

Deficiency in C4-binding protein has been observed in a limited number of patients. C4-binding protein serves as a cofactor for factor I-mediated cleavage of C4b, thereby controlling classical pathway activation. C4-binding protein-deficient patients have been reported to experience a Behçet-like syndrome and angioedema.

Factor I is an important enzyme that cleaves and inactivates C3b and C4b in association with cofactors: factor H and C4-binding protein, respectively. A crucial regulatory protein of the alternative pathway blocks C3 autoactivation in the fluid phase. Factor I deficiency leads to secondary C3 deficiency because it allows uncontrolled C3 activation and, thereby, C3 depletion. Patients with factor I deficiency experience recurrent severe infections caused by encapsulated pyogenic bacteria, such as *S pneumoniae* and *N meningitidis*. Infections occur in the upper respiratory tract, the meninges, and the bloodstream. As in C3-deficient patients, factor I-deficient patients have a higher than normal incidence of immune complex diseases such as glomerulonephritis.

Factor H is the cofactor for factor I-mediated cleavage of C3b. Deficiency of factor H leads to secondary C3 deficiency. Factor H-deficient patients, like C3-deficient and factor I-deficient patients, experience recurrent pyogenic infections. *N meningitidis* is the main causative infectious agent associated with infections in these patients. Factor H-deficient patients also develop immune complex diseases, such as membranoproliferative glomerulonephritis. Presumably, these patients, like factor I-deficient patients, lack effective C3b degradation.

Cell membrane-bound proteins also regulate complement activation at the cell surface to prevent complement-mediated cellular damage of host cells. Three of these regulatory molecules are attached to the cell membrane via a glycosyl phosphatidylinositol anchor. They are decay-accelerating factor **(DAF),** protectin **(CD59),** and homologous restriction factor **(HRF).** Mutation in the gene that produces the enzyme necessary for the formation of such an anchor (phosphatidylinositol glycan A gene, *pig*-A gene) leads to acquired deficiency in DAF, CD59, and HRF as well as in all other glycosyl phosphatidylinositol-linked proteins. This occurs as an acquired defect in stem cells of the bone marrow in patients with **paroxysmal nocturnal hemoglobinuria (PNH).** One of the features of PNH is episodic marked intravascular hemolysis. This is thought to result from the lack of complement regulation on the surface of the patient's erythrocytes with subsequent complement-mediated lysis caused by the formation of the membrane attack complex when complement is activated. It is proposed that the sensitivity of erythrocytes to complement-mediated lysis results mainly from lack of cell surface CD59, which regulates complement activation at the level of the membrane attack complex, rather than from lack of DAF.

COMPLEMENT RECEPTOR DEFICIENCIES

Complement receptor type 1 (CR1) is an important complement protein receptor that binds C3b and C4b. It also serves as a cofactor for factor I-mediated cleavage of C4b and C3b, and it inactivates both C3 and C5 convertases of the classical and alternative pathways. On erythrocytes in the circulation, it acts to capture immune complexes that have bound activated complement components and to transport these immune complexes to degradation sites within the liver and the spleen. Some believe that low erythrocyte CR1 numbers result from an inherited partial deficiency, which would predispose individuals to the development of systemic lupus erythematosus. It is more likely that low erythrocyte CR1 number is a consequence rather than a cause of systemic lupus erythematosus. Erythrocyte CR1 may bind circulating immune complexes with attached complement proteins and be removed from the circulating erythrocyte by proteolysis along with these immune complexes when the erythrocytes circulate to sites of immune complex degradation.

Deficiency in complement receptor type 3 (CR3, CD11b/CD18) is also reported. CR3 is a member of the **β$_2$-integrin** family. It is a receptor for iC3b and to a lesser extent for C3d and C3b. CR3 plays an important role in the phagocytosis of particles that are coated with iC3b fragments. CR3 acts in conjunction with IgG Fc receptors on phagocytes to trigger efficient phagocytosis. In addition, it is important for the adhesion of neutrophils to activated endothelial cells in the course of inflammatory reactions. The counterligand for CR3 is intercellular adhesion molecule-1 (ICAM-1). CR3, like the two other members of the β$_2$-integrin family, leukocyte functional antigen-1 (LFA-1, CD11a/CD18) and complement receptor type 4 (CR4, CD11c/CD18), is a heterodimer that contains a unique α chain (CD11b) and a β chain that is common to the other molecules of the family (CD18). Genetic deficiency of CR3 results from a

mutation in the gene that codes for the α chain. The nature of the mutation, in part, affects the severity of the defect. CR3-deficient patients, mostly children, suffer from a severe host defense defect. They experience recurrent severe pyogenic infections that can be life-threatening. Mild cutaneous infections can also be observed in these patients. The infectious agents associated with infections in CR3-deficient patients often include *Staphylococcus aureus* and *Pseudomonas* sp. Wound healing is usually delayed as is the separation of the umbilical cord. Interestingly, β$_2$-integrins are important in normal margination of circulating neutrophils through the endothelium of peripheral blood vessels. Patients with CR3 deficiency (also termed leukocyte adhesion deficiency) therefore have a consistently **elevated leukocyte count.**

COMPLEMENT & AUTOIMMUNE DISEASE

As discussed earlier in this chapter, patients with complement deficiencies, especially of one of the classical pathway components, C3, factor H, or factor I, have an unexpectedly high prevalence of autoimmune disease, particularly systemic lupus erythematosus and glomerulonephritis. Three lines of experimental evidence may explain why this is so. Once antigen–antibody complexes form, complement is activated via the classical pathway, which leads to the deposition of C3 fragments. Complement activation prevents the formation of large immune complex aggregates by interfering with Fc-Fc interactions between immunoglobulins in a process called **solubilization** of immune complexes. Furthermore, immune complexes coated with C3b adhere to circulating erythrocytes that express complement receptor type 1 (CR1). Erythrocytes transport immune complexes from the circulation to immune complex degradation sites, such as the liver and spleen. Deficiency in one of the complement components that function prior to C3, C3, or one of the proteins that regulate C3, prevents C3b from being deposited on immune complexes. Thus, large immune complex aggregates form, are not solubilized, and are not cleared from the circulation, therefore allowing accumulation in sites such as the kidney or joints. Another explanation for the high prevalence of autoimmune disease in complement-deficient animals comes from experiments in mice genetically deficient in C1q. It was recently proposed that autoimmunity in C1-deficient patients may arise from an inability to properly clear apoptotic cells. C1q was shown to bind directly to apoptotic cells and to activate the classical complement pathway. Failure to efficiently clear apoptotic cells from the circulation may expose the immune system to cellular debris against which an autoimmune antibody response could be generated. Another possibility for the high incidence of autoimmune disease in complement-deficient patients is that complement may play a role in the maintenance of self-tolerance in B cells. Based on experimental data from mouse models of complement deficiency, it appears that C4 and the complement receptors CR1 and CR2 may be important in down-regulating autoreactive B cells. Mice deficient in C4 also have a defect in the maintenance of B-cell tolerance to self-antigens.

MANAGEMENT OF COMPLEMENT DEFICIENCIES

Patients with hereditary angioedema usually respond poorly to drugs such as epinephrine, antihistamines, and glucocorticoids that are used to treat episodic angioedema. Two classes of drugs provide effective therapy. Anabolic steroids or impeded androgens are most effective. These agents cause an increase in C1 inhibitor concentration in plasma, presumably owing to increased protein synthesis by hepatocytes. This leads to a rise in C4 and C2 levels toward normal and, in most patients, the drug completely alleviates symptoms. All the useful oral androgens appear to have similar clinical activity, although the effect on levels of C1 inhibitor, C4, and C2 is much less striking with some. Anabolic steroids and androgens markedly diminish the frequency and severity of angioedema attacks. Plasmin inhibitors, like ε-aminocaproic acid (EACA), are fairly effective in improving the clinical manifestations of the disease, although they do not correct the biochemical abnormality (low C4 and C2 levels). Their mode of action is unknown. Although untoward clotting is one concern with this therapeutic strategy, EACA, at the doses used, has not produced this side effect in patients with hereditary angioedema. Muscle toxicity has been noted, however. Infusion of concentrated human C1 inhibitor has proved useful in preventing and treating acute attacks of angioedema.

Patients with PNH can be treated with glucocorticoids to reduce episodes of intravascular hemolysis, although the treatment is often only minimally effective. In some patients with thrombocytopenia, androgens increase platelet counts. Antithymocyte globulin (ATG) is also used to treat patients with PNH who experience thrombocytopenia. Because of its associated hematopoietic stem cell defect, the only cure for PNH is bone marrow transplantation.

Recurrent pyogenic infections is a feature of many complement component deficiencies. Antibiotic therapy is mandatory treatment for these severe infections. Normal human plasma infusions aimed at correcting the complement deficiency have been used and are reported to offer some degree of protection against recurrent infections. The half-life of most complement components is relatively short, however, such that repeated plasma infusions are required. Also, antibody responses to non-self plasma components, in patients with a complete deficiency in one complement plasma protein, may impair the long-term efficacy of this therapy. Because *N meningitidis* infections are so common in complement-deficient individuals, vaccination with the tetravalent meningococcal capsular polysaccharide vaccine is expected to offer a degree of protection against repeated episodes of infection. Vaccination with the pneumococcal and conjugate *H influenzae* vaccines is also recommended, especially in patients with a deficiency in one of the classical pathway complement components or C3. Purified human MBL has been used to restore normal levels in a deficient child, and it is reported to prevent recurrent infections. Such treatment, however, is unlikely to be useful as long-term therapy.

REFERENCES

GENERAL REVIEWS
Colten HR, Rosen FS: Complement deficiencies. *Annu Rev Immunol* 1992;10:809.

Frank MM: Complement in disease: Inherited and acquired complement deficiencies. In: *Samter's Immunologic Diseases,* 5th ed. Frank MM et al (editors). Little Brown, 1995.

Lokki M-L, Colten HR: Genetic deficiencies of complement. *Ann Med* 1995;27:451.

Morgan BP, Walport MJ: Complement deficiency and disease. *Immunol Today* 1991;12:301.

C3 DEFICIENCY
Singer L et al: Complement C3 deficiency: Human, animal, and experimental models. *Pathobiology* 1994;62:14.

ALTERNATIVE PATHWAY DEFICIENCIES
Densen P et al: Functional and antigenic analysis of human factor B deficiency. *Mol Immunol* 1996;33(Suppl 1):68.

MANNAN-BINDING LECTIN DEFICIENCY
Garred P et al: Association of mannose-binding lectin gene heterogeneity with severity of lung disease and survival in cystic fibrosis. *J Clin Invest* 1999;104:431.

Hibberd ML et al: Association of variants of the gene for mannose-binding lectin with susceptibility to meningococcal disease. *Lancet* 1999;353:1049.

Turner MW: Mannose-binding lectin (MBL) in health and disease. *Immunobiol* 1998;199:327.

Valdimarsson H et al: Reconstitution of opsonizing activity by infusion of mannan-binding lectin (MBL) to MBL-deficient humans. *Scand J Immunol* 1998;48:116.

TERMINAL COMPONENTS DEFICIENCIES

Würzner R et al: Inherited deficiencies of the terminal components of human complement. *Immunodef Rev* 1992;3:123.

C9 DEFICIENCY IN POPULATION STUDIES

Fukumori Y, Horiuchi T: Terminal complement component deficiencies in Japan. *Exp Clin Immunogenet* 1998;15:244.

Nagata M et al: Inherited deficiency of the ninth component of complement: An increased risk of meningococcal meningitis. *Pediatr* 1989;14:260.

COMPLEMENT DEFICIENCY AND INFECTION

Densen P et al: Familial properdin deficiency and fatal meningococcemia: Correction of the bactericidal defect by vaccination. *N Engl J Med* 1987;316:922.

Densen P: Complement deficiencies and infection. In: *The Human Complement System in Health and Disease.* Volanakis JE, Frank MM (editors). Marcel Dekker, 1998, p 409.

Figueroa JE, Densen P: Infectious diseases associated with complement deficiencies. *Clin Microbiol Rev* 1991;4:359.

Fijen CAP et al: Protection against meningococcal serogroup ACYW disease in complement-deficient individuals vaccinated with the tetravalent meningococcal capsular polysaccharide vaccine. *Clin Exp Immunol* 1998;114:362.

HEREDITARY ANGIOEDEMA AND ACQUIRED C1 INHIBITOR DEFICIENCY

Cugno M et al: Activation of the coagulation cascade in C1-inhibitor deficiencies. *Blood* 1997;89:3213.

Davis AE III: C1 inhibitor gene and hereditary angioedema. In: *The Human Complement System in Health and Disease.* Volanakis JE, Frank MM (editors). Marcel Dekker, 1998, p 455.

Frank MM et al: Epsilon aminocaproic acid therapy of hereditary angioneurotic edema: A double-blind study. *N Engl J Med* 1972;286:808.

Frank MM et al: Hereditary angioedema: The clinical syndrome and its management. *Ann Intern Med* 1976;84:580.

Frank MM: Acquired C1 inhibitor deficiency. *Behring Inst Mitt* 1989;84:161.

Gelfand JA et al: Treatment of hereditary angioedema with danazol: Reversal of clinical and biochemical abnormalities. *N Engl J Med* 1976;295:1444.

Van Dellen RG: Long-term treatment of C1 inhibitor deficiency with ε-aminocaproic acid in two patients. *Mayo Clin Proc* 1996;71:1178.

Waytes AT et al: Treatment of angioedema with a vapor-heated C1 inhibitor concentrate. *N Engl J Med* 1996;334:1630.

Whaley K et al: Autoimmune C1-inhibitor deficiency. *Clin Exp Immunol* 1996;106:423.

PAROXYSMAL NOCTURNAL HEMOGLOBINURIA

Nakamura H: Mechanism of intravascular hemolysis in paroxysmal nocturnal hemoglobinuria (PNH). *Am J Hematol* 1996;53:22.

Rosse WF: Paroxysmal nocturnal hemoglobinuria and complement. In: *The Human Complement System in Health and Disease.* Volanakis JE, Frank MM (editors). Marcel Dekker, 1998.

COMPLEMENT DEFICIENCY & AUTOIMMUNITY

Botto M et al: Homozygous C1q deficiency causes glomerulonephritis associated with multiple apoptotic bodies. *Nat Genet* 1998;19:56.

Carroll MC: The role of complement and complement receptors in induction and regulation of immunity. *Annu Rev Immunol* 1998;16:545.

Davies KA, Walport MJ: Processing and clearance of immune complexes by complement and the role of complement in immune complex diseases. In: *The Human Complement System in Health and Disease.* Volanakis JE, Frank MM (editors). Marcel Dekker, 1998.

Korb LC, Ahearn JM: C1q binds directly and specifically to surface blebs of apoptotic human keratinocytes. *J Immunol* 1997;158:4525.

Prodeus AP et al: A critical role for complement in maintenance of self-tolerance. *Immunity* 1998;9:721.

Ratnoff WD. Inherited deficiencies of complement in rheumatic diseases. *Clin Immunol Rheumatol* 1996;22:75.

Walport MJ et al: Complement deficiency and autoimmunity. *Ann N Y Acad Sci* 1997;815:267.

The Atopic Diseases

26

Abba I. Terr, MD

GENERAL CONSIDERATIONS

Definitions

Allergy refers to certain diseases in which immune responses to environmental antigens cause tissue inflammation and organ dysfunction. **Hypersensitivity** and **sensitivity** are synonyms for allergy. Table 26–1 compares the distinguishing features of allergic diseases. An **allergen** is any antigen that causes allergy. The term refers to either the antigenic molecule itself or its source, such as pollen grain, animal dander, insect venom, or food product. **Atopy** is the inherited propensity to respond immunologically to such common naturally occurring allergens with the continual production of IgE antibodies. Allergic rhinitis and allergic asthma are the most common manifestations. Atopic dermatitis is less common, and allergic gastroenteropathy is rare. These manifestations may simultaneously coexist in the same patient or at different times. Atopy can also be asymptomatic (Figure 26–1).

Rhinitis, asthma, and eczematous dermatitis occur in a significant number of patients without atopic IgE-mediated allergy. Furthermore, IgE antibodies also cause **nonatopic allergic diseases**—anaphylaxis and urticaria-angioedema (see Chapter 17) IgE antibodies are also important in acquired immunity to parasites.

Thus, atopy is a condition with certain specific immunologic and clinical features. It affects a significant portion of the general population, estimated at 10–30% in developed countries. The etiology of atopy involves complex genetic factors that are not yet well understood. There is epidemiologic evidence that allergy—particularly atopic diseases—are affecting a higher proportion of the population of developed countries over the past several decades. Explanatory hypotheses include an adjuvant effect of air pollutants and deviation of the immune response because of the marked diminution of childhood infectious diseases. Clinical disease requires both genetic predisposition and environmental allergen exposure.

Immunology

A detailed description of the immunopathogenesis of IgE-mediated diseases is given in Chapter 13. Both **mast cells** and **basophils** have high-affinity IgE cell membrane receptors for IgE **(FcεRI).** Mast cells are abundant in the mucosa of the respiratory and gastrointestinal tracts and in the skin, where atopic reactions localize. The physiologic effects of the mediators released from or activated by these cells cause the pathophysiology of the immediate and late phases of atopic diseases. The important mediators of IgE allergy are histamine, chemotactic factors, prostaglandins, leukotrienes, and platelet-activating factor.

Atopic patients typically have multiple allergies; that is, IgE antibodies to, and symptoms from, many environmental allergens. The total serum IgE level is higher on average in the atopic population than in a comparable nonatopic population, although the overlap is sufficient that a normal serum IgE concentration does not rule out the diagnosis of atopy. In general, total IgE in serum is higher in allergic asthma than in allergic rhinitis and higher still in atopic dermatitis. Some nonatopic diseases are associated with a high serum total IgE (Table 26–2). For these reasons, measurement of total serum IgE is not a dependable diagnostic indicator of atopy and does not identify specific IgE antibodies. Mast cell-bound and not circulating IgE antibodies initiate atopic reactions on exposure to allergen.

It has been suggested that antibodies of the IgG4 subclass may also fix to mast cells and basophils. The mast cell affinity for IgG4 appears to be low, and evidence that IgG4 antibodies can trigger mediator release in the presence of allergens is controversial. Their production in fact is enhanced by specific allergen immunotherapy.

Etiology

The etiology of atopy is unknown. There is substantial evidence for a complex of genes with variable degrees of expression encoding protein factors, some of which are pathogenic and others protective.

These genes and gene clusters occupy positions on

Table 26–1. Comparison of allergy with other responses.

Disease	Mechanism	Antigen Source	Result
Allergy	Immunologic	Foreign	Disease
Immunity	Immunologic	Foreign	Prophylaxis
Autoimmunity	Immunologic	Self	Disease
Toxicity	Toxic	Foreign	Disease

Table 26–2. Diseases associated with elevated total serum IgE.

Disease	Possible Explanation of Elevated IgE
Allergic rhinitis	Multiple atopic allergies
Allergic asthma	Multiple atopic allergies
Atopic dermatitis	Multiple allergies and linkage to a non-MHC gene
Allergic bronchopulmonary aspergillosis	Unknown; varies with disease activity
Parasitic diseases	IgE antibodies associated with protective immunity
Hyper-IgE syndrome	Unknown
Ataxia-telangiectasia	T-suppressor cell defect?
Wiskott–Aldrich syndrome	Unknown
Thymic alymphoplasia	Unknown
IgE myeloma	Neoplasm of IgE-producing plasma cells; IgE is mono-clonal
Graft-versus-host reaction	Transient T-suppressor cell defect?

at least 11 different chromosomes in the human genome. These are the ones that influence the propensity for atopy through the regulation of total IgE production and specific IgE antibodies to allergen epitopes, cytokines and their receptors, enzymes and receptors for mast cell mediators, and undoubtedly other factors involved in disease pathogenesis (Table 26–3).

One theory suggests that atopic allergy results from an abnormal regulation by T lymphocytes of the B cells committed to IgE production through the secretion of IgE-binding factors that either enhance or suppress B-cell differentiation.

A second theory proposes a defect in absorption of environmental allergens at respiratory and gastrointestinal surfaces prior to processing of the allergen for the immune response.

A third theory attributes both the enhanced production of allergen-specific IgE antibodies and the hyperreactivity of target tissues to the mediators released from mast cells to an inherited (or perhaps acquired) **autonomic imbalance** with a β-adrenergic blockade or cholinergic overactivity or both. There is some experimental and clinical evidence for each theory; none that is compelling.

Substantial evidence points to the critical role of **cytokines** in the ability of CD4 T lymphocytes to induce IgE antibody production by B cells. Interleukin-4 (IL-4) and IL-13 enhance but interferon gamma

(IFNγ) suppresses IgE responses. The currently popular paradigm recognizes two T_H cell subsets—T_H1 and T_H2—and that a reciprocal balance between the numbers of these cells locally in tissues influences the development of atopy and other diseases through the profile of cytokines that they synthesize and release. Extensive experimental evidence suggests that IgE production and atopic disease require the presence of IL-4, IL-5, IL-13, and granulocyte-macrophage colony-stimulating factor (GM-CSF) production by T_H2 cells. Thus, a fourth theory would involve up- or

Table 26–3. Candidate genes identified to date in atopy.

Chromosome	Candidate Genes
1p	IL-12
2q	CD28
3p24	bcl-6, IL-3, IL-4, IL-5, IL-13, GM-CSF, LTC4 synthase; receptors for macrophage-CSF, β₂-adrenergic agonists, corticosteroids
6p21-23	MHC, TNF, TAP-1, TAP-2, 5-lipoxygenase, FcεR1 β chain
12q14-24	IFNγ, stem cell factor, NFκB, Stat-6, LTA4 hydrolase
14q11-13	TCR α/β chains, NFκB inhibitor
16p11-12	IL-4 receptor

Abbreviations: CSF = colony-stimulating factor; MHC = major histocompatibility complex; TNF = tumor necrosis factor; TAP = transporter of antigenic peptide; IFN = interferon; TCR = T-cell receptor; IL = interleukin.
Source: Modified with permission from Borish L. *Ann Allergy Asthma Immunol. 1999;82,413.*

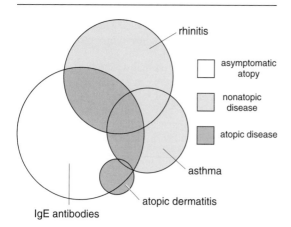

Figure 26–1. Interrelationships of atopy, atopic diseases, and IgE antibodies to environmental allergens.

down-regulation of these and other cytokines by as yet unidentified etiologic factors in atopy.

Environmental factors play a role in etiology. An accumulation of clinical experience suggests that the initial age of exposure to a particular food or pollen may determine the intensity of the subsequent IgE antibody response. A concurrent viral respiratory infection during environmental allergen exposure may have an adjuvant effect on both specific and total IgE production. Tobacco smoking may exert a similar effect.

Finally, the relationship between IgE-mediated atopic allergy and IgE-mediated immunity in **helminthiasis** offers an interesting opportunity to speculate about etiology. Atopic allergy is a prominent clinical problem in developed countries, which are largely free of helminthic infestation. In populations in which these infections are endemic, serum IgE levels are typically high because of ongoing IgE stimulation, and it can be assumed that tissue mast cells are chronically saturated with parasite-specific IgE antibodies. The IgE mast cell-mediated immune mechanism has a selective advantage for the host under these circumstances. In a population free of parasitic infections, however, the IgE immune system may be vestigial for immunity but still available to react adversely to innocuous environmental allergens.

ATOPIC ALLERGENS

The allergens responsible for atopic disease are derived principally from natural airborne organic particles, especially plant pollens, fungal spores, and animal and insect debris, and, to a lesser extent, from ingested foods. The ability of different pollens, molds, or foods to sensitize for IgE allergy varies and is determined both by genetic predilection and by the geographic and cultural factors responsible for exposure to the allergen.

Pollen Allergens

The allergenic pollens are from wind-pollinated (anemophilous) flowering plants. Unlike insect-pollinated (entomophilous) plants, they discharge large numbers of lightweight, buoyant pollen grains that are dispersed over a wide area by wind currents. Within each local geographic area the common allergenic plants pollinate during specific and predictable seasons, producing seasonal respiratory symptoms in allergic patients.

The number of pollen-producing plants is enormous, but those of proven allergenicity are limited. The major taxa and representative examples are listed in Table 26–4. Within each botanic subclass many species cause allergy, including natural, cultivated, and ornamental plants. Those with attractive flowers are generally insect-pollinated, producing small

Table 26–4. Botanic classifications of pollinating plants frequently associated with atopic respiratory allergy.

Botanic Classification[a]	Common Names of Typical Plants
Division Microphyllophyta	Club mosses
Division Pteridophyta	Ferns
Division Pinophyta	
Subdivision Pinicae	Conifers
Division Magnoliophyta	Flowering plants
Class Liliopsida	
Subclass Commelinidae	Grasses, sedges
Subclass Arecidae	Palms, cattails
Class Magnoliopsida	
Subclass Hamamelididae	Nettles, beeches
Subclass Caryophyllidae	Chemopods, sorrels
Subclass Dilleniidae	Willows, poplars
Subclass Rosidae	Maples, ashes
Subclass Asteridae	Ragweeds, sages

Source: Adapted and reproduced, with permission, from Weber RW, Nelson HS: Pollen allergens and their interrelationships. *Clin Rev Allergy* 1985;**3**:291.
[a] Classification system of Takhtajan.

amounts of heavy pollen that does not become airborne, and thus they are usually not the cause of inhalant allergy.

Allergenic pollen grains are mostly spherical, 15–50 μm in diameter, and they can usually be identified morphologically by light microscopy (Figure 26–2). Air sampling for identifying and quantitating pollens is done by volumetric impaction devices, such as the rotorod or rotoslide sampler (Figure 26–3). Several representative examples of pollen seasons are shown in Figure 26–4.

Mold Allergens

Fungi are abundant, ubiquitous multicellular eukaryotic organisms. They are saprophytic, growing on a variety of dead or decaying organic material, where they flourish in direct relation to temperature and humidity. They reproduce sexually or asexually, producing airborne spores, some of which are allergenic. Over 20,000 species have been identified, of which a limited number produce airborne spores containing allergens.

Allergy to fungal spores is an important cause of disease in many atopic patients. Specific diagnosis, however, is hampered by the confusing taxonomic classification and nomenclature because of the enormous biologic complexity of fungi in their morphologic, reproductive, and ecologic behavior. Although it is difficult to obtain pure spores of many species for immunologic testing, some of the clinically important allergens have been isolated, sequenced, and expressed as recombinant proteins G. Seasonal patterns of spores in air samples are poorly defined, making clinical correlation especially problematic. Mold spores range in size from 1 to 100 μm in diameter (see Figure 26–2). Volumetric impaction samplers used for pollen counting are inefficient in trapping spores and do not yield quantitative data for

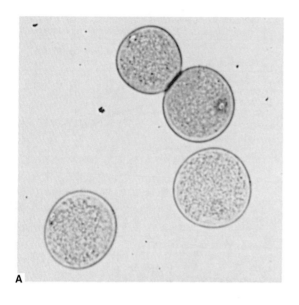
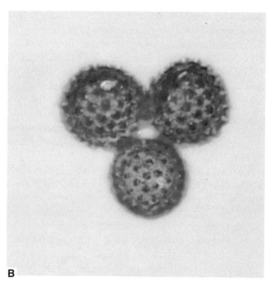
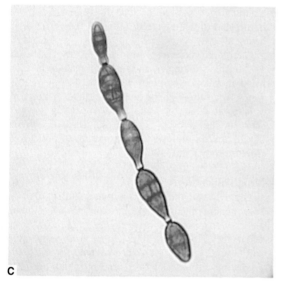
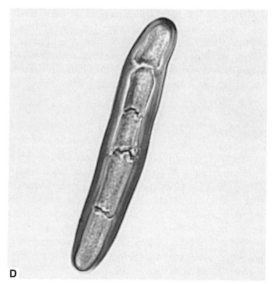

Figure 26–2. Photomicrographs of several common pollens. **A:** grass (30 μm in diameter); **B:** ragweed (20 μm in diameter); **C:** *Alternaria* mold spores (70 μm in length); **D:** *Helminthosporium* mold spores (80 μm in length). (Courtesy of William R Solomon, MD)

spores. Table 26–5 lists some of the fungi most frequently associated with atopic allergy.

Arthropod Allergens

There are more than 50,000 species of mites. The house dust mites, *Dermatophagoides pteronyssinus* and *D farinae,* are the most common of all of the known atopic allergens. These tiny arachnids, barely visible to the naked eye, are found in house dust samples throughout the world but are most prevalent in warm, humid climates. They are especially abundant in bedding, upholstery, and blankets, where their natural substrate, desquamated human skin scales, are likely to be found. The two species cross-react extensively but not completely. House dust contains other uncharacterized allergens of minor importance. IgE antibodies and environmental exposure to these mite allergens correlate especially well with atopic asthma and atopic dermatitis, because exposure is by inhalation and dermal contact, respectively.

Other allergenic mites such as *Euroglyphus maynei, Lepidoglyphus destructor,* and *Acarus siro*—storage mites that infest grains—may cause occupational allergy in grain handlers.

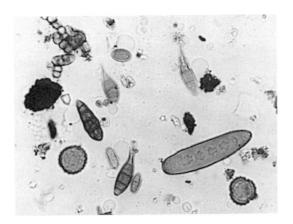

Figure 26–3. Typical "catch" of a volumetric air sampler showing pollen grains, mold spores, insect debris, plant particles, dust, and unidentified particles. (Courtesy of William R Solomon, MD)

Table 26–5. Common fungal aeroallergens.

Basidiomycetes	Botrytis
Ustilago	Helminthosporium
Ganoderma	Stemphylium
Alternaria	Cephalosporium
Cladosporium	**Phycomycetes**
Aspergillus	Mucor
Sporobolomyces	Rhizopus
Penicillium	**Ascomycetes**
Epicoccum	Eurotium
Fusarium	Chaetomium
Phoma	

Various species of cockroaches are insect pests in homes and restaurants, especially in large cities where overcrowding and poor hygiene is common. The rate of sensitivity to cockroach allergen among allergic patients in inner-city populations is high, often as an isolated allergy. Other "endemic" causes of respiratory allergy are the emanations and debris of certain insects that swarm in huge numbers seasonally in specific locales. Examples of such insects include caddis fly and mayfly at the eastern and western ends, respectively,

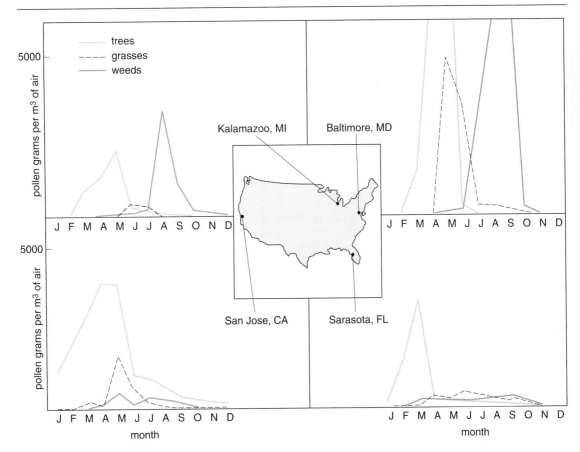

Figure 26–4. Representative examples of quantitative pollen counts at four different locations in the United States during the same year (1984). Data from the American Academy of Allergy and Immunology Pollen and Mold Committee.

of Lake Erie; the green nimitti midge, *Cladotanytarsus lewisi,* in the Sudan; and Lepidoptera in Japan.

Animal Allergens

Atopic allergy to household pets, especially cats and dogs, has always been easily recognized because patients sensitive to these animals experience immediate intense attacks of asthma when in the same house with an animal to which they are allergic. Other animals encountered in domestic, occupational, and recreational settings also cause allergy. The source of the allergen may be in the dander (horse, dog, cat) or urine (rodents).

Food Allergens

Allergenic components of foods can induce IgE antibodies that cause either atopic or nonatopic (anaphylactic) reactions. IgE antibodies to foods frequently exist in atopic patients without causing any reaction when the food is eaten. The factors that operate to convert asymptomatic sensitivity to symptomatic disease are currently unknown. Nonpathogenic IgG antibodies to food antigens occur in many people.

Virtually any food is capable of causing allergy, but certain foods are more likely than others to be allergenic. Seafoods are a prominent cause of allergy in areas where fish is a staple in the diet. Ingested crustaceans and mollusks are an important cause of anaphylaxis and anaphylactoid reactions. Based on definitive challenge studies, about 8% of children younger than 3 years of age are allergic to foods, most often milk, egg, peanuts, fish, and tree nuts. Three percent of adults have food allergy, most commonly to tree nuts, fish, and shellfish. Wheat, corn, chocolate, and citrus fruits, on the other hand, are often believed to cause a variety of symptoms that are not allergic.

The allergenicity of a particular food protein can be changed by heating or cooking. A reaction can occur to the raw food only or to the cooked form only, or to both.

Occupational allergy, especially asthma from the inhalation of airborne food allergens, is a significant problem for many food handlers.

Allergen Extracts

Pollens, molds, foods, and animal and insect emanations are biologically complex materials made up of a mixture of numerous chemicals, many of which have allergenic potential. Aqueous extracts used in testing for IgE antibodies in allergic patients may contain a number of allergens in addition to nonallergenic compounds. The effort to isolate, purify, analyze, characterize, name, and standardize every important atopic allergen is ongoing. To date, almost 100 allergen proteins causing human IgE-mediated disease have been isolated and purified, and the genes for many have been cloned and are being used increasingly for clinical diagnosis, skin testing and immunotherapy. Purified allergens are essential reagents for research studies on structure-function relationships and for genetic studies. For many years, standardization of extracts was based on weight/volume or total protein content, neither of which reflects the allergen content accurately. Currently, allergen content is expressed either by skin test titration or by **radioallergosorbent test (RAST)** inhibition, and the term **allergen unit** (AU) is used to denote bioequivalence. A comparison of these methods is shown in Table 26–6.

DIAGNOSTIC TESTING

Cutaneous & Intradermal Allergy Testing

The cutaneous test (prick test, puncture test, epicutaneous test) is used for routine diagnosis in atopic and anaphylactic diseases. A single drop of concentrated aqueous allergen extract placed on the skin, which is then pricked lightly with a needle point at the center of the drop (Figure 26–5A). After 20 minutes the reaction is graded and recorded as indicated in Table 26–7. Negative (diluent) and positive (histamine) controls should be included. Negative results, especially to nonpollen allergens should be repeated using the intradermal skin test (intracutaneous test), in which a measured quantity of allergen is injected into the skin (see Figure 26–5B) through a 27-gauge needle.

The recommended volume ranges from 0.005 to 0.02 mL, but is usually 0.01 mL. Negative and positive controls are used. In most cases, intradermal testing in suspected IgE-mediated diseases is performed only for allergens giving negative or at most 1+ responses to prior prick-testing because the intradermal test is approximately a thousand times more sensitive. The reaction is read in 20 minutes (see Table 26–7). A 1:500 (wt/vol) dilution of most common inhalant allergens is satisfactory for diagnosis of atopic allergy.

After the immediate wheal-and-erythema response subsides, a late-phase 6-12-hour reaction appears in some cases. The diagnostic significance of the late-phase skin reaction is currently uncertain.

Antihistaminic drugs inhibit IgE-mediated wheal-and-flare skin tests and must be discontinued prior to testing.

Table 26–6. Approximate equivalence of different methods for expressing allergen content in extracts used for testing and immunotherapy.

Method	Units
Weight/volume (W/V)	1:20
Protein nitrogen units/mL (PNU/mL)	10,000
Allergy units/mL (AU/mL)	100,000
Noon units/mL	100
Micrograms of protein/mL	100

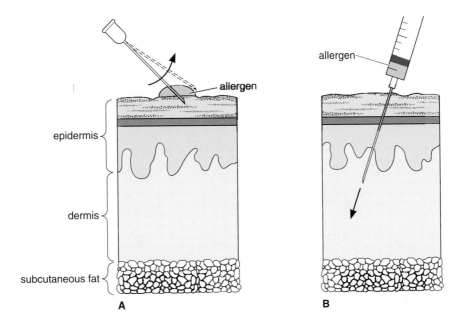

Figure 26–5. The technique of allergy skin testing. **A:** Cutaneous test. **B:** Intradermal test.

In Vitro Tests for IgE Antibodies

Quantitative measurement of allergen-specific IgE antibodies in serum requires special methods to detect the extremely minute quantities (picograms per milliliter) found in allergic patients. The standard technique is the RAST. This is a two-phase (solid-liquid) system using an insolubilized allergen that is incubated first in the test serum to react with allergen-specific antibodies and then in radiolabeled heterologous antihuman IgE to detect the allergen-specific antibodies of the IgE isotype. The method is diagrammed and described in Figure 26–6. The test requires purified preparations of allergens and antihuman IgE. The RAST uses a cellulose disk as the insoluble immunosorbent to which protein allergens are coupled covalently with cyanogen bromide. In a

number of modifications of this method other immunosorbents and other detection labeling systems (various chemicals detected by fluorescence or colorimetry) are used.

Disadvantages of these in vitro methods are both biologic and technical. The quantity of serum IgE antibody is not necessarily a direct reflection of the biologically relevant mast cell-fixed antibody. The test result may be falsely positive in patients with a high total IgE level because of nonspecific binding of allergen to some immunosorbents, and it may be falsely low in desensitized patients with high levels of IgG antibody. Like all other allergy tests, results must be interpreted in the context of the clinical history and examination.

Provocation Testing

Occasionally it is desirable to test the target (respiratory, gastrointestinal, or cutaneous) tissue responsiveness to the allergen under controlled conditions. The patch test for immediate contact urticaria or delayed contact dermatitis is such a procedure. In the nasal provocation test, changes in nasal airway resistance and visible signs of congestion and rhinorrhea are observed after exposure to quantitative allergen challenge. Timed changes in bronchial airway flow rate or resistance are measured by bronchial provocation. Oral challenge with food or drug may be done to observe subjective gastrointestinal symptoms, appearance of skin eruptions, or objective changes in airway resistance.

A positive provocation test does not prove an immunologic basis for the disease, and except for patch

Table 26–7. Wheal-and-erythema skin tests.

Test	Reaction	Appearances
Prick	Neg	No wheal or erythema
	1+	No wheal; erythema <20 mm in diameter
	2+	No wheal; erythema >20 mm in diameter
	3+	Wheal and erythema
	4+	Wheal with pseudopods; erythema
Intracutaneous	Neg	Same as control
	1+	Wheal twice as large as control; erythema <20 mm in diameter
	2+	Wheal twice as large as control; erythema >20 mm in diameter
	3+	Wheal 3 times as large as control; erythema
	4+	Wheal with pseudopods; erythema

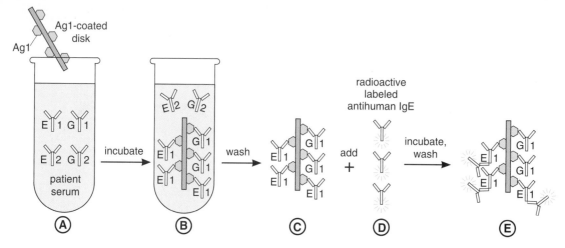

Figure 26–6. Diagram of radioallergosorbent test (RAST). **A:** A disk coated with the test allergen (Ag1) is incubated with serum of a patient with allergy to Ag1, as well as to other allergens (Ag2). **B:** IgE antibodies to Ag1 (E1) and IgG antibodies to the same allergen (G1) react with the Ag1-coated disk, whereas IgE and IgG antibodies (E2, G2) do not, and they remain in the serum. **C,D:** After being washed, the disk is incubated with a radiolabeled heterologous antibody to human IgE. **E:** After the disk is washed to remove unreacted labeled anti-IgE, the amount of radioactivity measured in a gamma counter is proportionate to the quantity of specific IgE antibody (E1) in the patient's serum. IgG antibodies to the same allergen (G1) on the disk do not react with the antihuman IgE antibody.

testing, it is not used for routine diagnosis. Provocation testing is, however, an invaluable research tool for studying pathogenetic mechanisms and drug efficacy in allergic disease.

ALLERGIC RHINITIS

Major Immunologic Features
- Most common clinical expression of atopic hypersensitivity.
- IgE-mediated allergy localized in the nasal mucosa and conjunctiva.
- Pollens, fungal spores, dust, and animal danders usual atmospheric allergens.

General Considerations
Allergic rhinitis (allergic rhinoconjunctivitis or hay fever) is the most common manifestation of an atopic reaction to inhaled allergens. More than 20 million persons in the United States suffer from this disease. It is a chronic disease with onset usually during childhood or adolescence.

Epidemiology
Allergic rhinitis occurs in 10–12% of the US population. It accounts for 80% of rhinitis in children and 30% in adults. The prevalence and morbidity rate are influenced by the geographic distribution of the common allergic plants and dust mite. The disease affects both sexes equally. It persists for many years if untreated and causes considerable morbidity and time lost from school or work.

Clinical Features
A. Symptoms: A typical attack consists of profuse watery rhinorrhea, paroxysmal sneezing, nasal obstruction, and itching of the nose and palate. Postnasal mucus drainage causes sore throat, clearing of the throat, and cough. An accompanying allergic blepharoconjunctivitis usually occurs, with intense itching of the conjunctivae and eyelids, redness, tearing, and photophobia. In some patients, conjunctivitis may occur in the absence of nasal symptoms. The disease occurs seasonally in patients with pollen allergy or year-round if the sensitivity is to a perennial allergen such as house dust. Perennial symptoms may occur with seasonal exacerbations in patients with multiple allergies. Diurnal variation may suggest a household allergen, and symptoms that disappear on weekends suggest an occupational allergy. Severe attacks are often accompanied by systemic malaise, weakness, and fatigue. Fever is absent. Swelling of the nasal mucosa may lead to headache because of obstruction of the ostia of the paranasal sinuses.

B. Signs: Rhinoscopy shows a pale, swollen nasal mucosa with watery secretions. The conjunctivae are hyperemic and edematous. Eyelid swelling from edema may occur. Lower eyelid ecchymoses—probably from eye-rubbing—are called "allergic shiners." Examination is normal when no allergen exposure has taken place and the patient is asymptomatic.

C. Laboratory Findings: Eosinophils are numerous in the nasal secretions, but this is not diagnostic because nasal eosinophilia is found in some patients with nonallergic rhinitis and in those with asthma. Blood eosinophilia is present during symptomatic periods. The presence of any eosinophils in conjunctival scrapings, however, is probably diagnostic. Sinus imaging, tympanometry, and audiometry may be indicated if an associated sinusitis or otitis media is suspected.

Immunologic Diagnosis

The diagnosis of allergic rhinitis is established by the history and physical findings present during the symptomatic phase. Diagnosis of the specific allergic sensitivities in each case is then determined by skin testing for a wheal-and-flare response or by in vitro testing. Selection of allergens for detection of specific IgE antibodies by skin or in vitro test is based on the patient's history and on the known local environmental allergens.

Differential Diagnosis

Chronic nonallergic (vasomotor) rhinitis is a common disorder of unknown cause in which the primary complaint is nasal congestion, usually associated with postnasal drainage. It differs from allergic rhinitis by the absence of sneezing paroxysms or eye symptoms, and rhinorrhea is minimal. Congestion may be unilateral or bilateral, and it often shifts with position. Symptoms occur year-round and are generally worse in cold weather or in dry climates. The nasal mucosa is unusually sensitive to irritants such as tobacco smoke, fumes, and smog. Symptoms usually begin in adulthood. The disease is more common among women, and it may begin during pregnancy. Examination shows swollen, erythematous nasal mucosa and strands of thick, mucoid postnasal discharge in the pharynx. Allergy skin tests are negative or unrelated to the symptoms. The nasal secretions may or may not contain eosinophils. The therapeutic response to nasal glucocorticoids, oral decongestants and humidification is good, but antihistamines are usually not effective.

Rhinitis medicamentosa is the severe congestion from the rebound effect of excessive use of sympathomimetic nasal sprays or nose drops. The mucosa is often bright red and swollen. It reverses with complete avoidance of nose drops or sprays, even if they have been used excessively for many years.

Infectious rhinitis is almost always due to a virus. Most patients with allergic rhinitis can distinguish their allergic symptoms from those of the common cold, which usually produces fever, an erythematous nasal mucosa, and a polymorphonuclear exudate in the nasal secretions. Primary bacterial or fungal infections of the nasal passages are rare.

Some hormones may produce nasal congestion. This is common in pregnancy or with the use of oral contraceptive drugs. Nasal congestion occurs frequently in myxedema. Certain drugs produce nasal congestion (Table 26–8).

Table 26–8. Drugs that may cause nasal congestion.

Drug	Presumed Mechanism
Oral contraceptives	Unknown
Reserpine	Norepinephrine depletion
Guanethidine	Norepinephrine release blockade
Propranolol	Adrenergic blockade
Thioridazine	Beta-adrenergic blockade
Tricyclic antidepressants	Norepinephrine uptake blockade
Aspirin (rarely)	Idiosyncratic generation of vasodilating arachidonate metabolite?

Anatomic nasal obstructions may occur from foreign bodies, tumors, nasal septal deviation or spurs, and polyps. Nasal polyposis is independent of atopy and allergic rhinitis, but it is associated with asthma, aspirin sensitivity, sinusitis, and eosinophilia. Nasal polyps also occur in children with cystic fibrosis. Anatomic lesions are best detected by fiberoptic rhinoscopy after the application of a topical decongestant.

Vernal keratoconjunctivitis is a disease of unknown cause that usually affects children. The symptoms include giant papillary excrescences of the palpebral conjunctivae with intense itching and a stringy exudate containing eosinophils, mast cells, basophils, and plasma cells. A search for an allergic cause is usually unrewarding. Reversible giant papillary conjunctivitis is caused in some patients by the use of soft contact lenses.

Immunologic Pathogenesis

Soluble allergens from inhaled pollens, spores, and other aeroallergenic particles are rapidly eluted on contact with the moist mucous membranes of the nasal mucosa and conjunctivae. Reaction with the corresponding IgE antibody on local mast cells and basophils releases the various mast cell-associated mediators described in Chapter 13. IgE antibodies have a unique configuration on the Fc portion of the molecule for fixation to mast cells and basophils (Figure 26–7). Fixation occurs at a high-affinity cell surface receptor, **FcεRI.** The allergic reaction is initiated when the polyvalent allergen molecule reacts with antibodies occupying these receptors. The result is a bridging of FcεRI molecules, thereby altering the cell surface membrane. This, in turn, signals intracellular events causing release and activation of mediators of inflammation: histamine, leukotrienes, chemotactic factors, and proteinases. Mast cell activation is modulated by intracellular cyclic nucleotides and is accompanied by cell degranulation. The released activated mediators act locally to cause increased vascular permeability, vasodilation, smooth muscle contraction, and mucous gland secretion. These biologic events account for the salient clinical features of the **immediate phase,** occurring in the

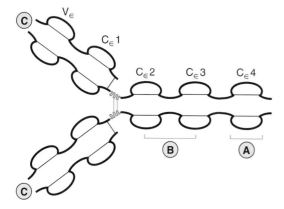

Figure 26–7. Schematic diagram of the IgE antibody molecule. **A:** The structure is similar to that of IgG, but there is an additional H-chain domain, accounting for its higher molecular weight. **B:** The regions of the molecule containing the site for fixation to mast cell FcεRI and **C:** the allergen-binding sites are indicated.

first 15–30 minutes following allergen exposure. Over the succeeding 12 hours progressive tissue infiltration of inflammatory cells occurs, proceeding from neutrophils to eosinophils to mononuclear cells in response to other chemical mediators and biochemical events not yet fully delineated. The period of 6–12 hours after allergen exposure is designated the **late phase** of the IgE response and is characterized by clinical manifestations of cellular inflammation.

Symptoms of sneezing, rhinorrhea, congestion, and pruritus appearing within minutes of exposure are caused by the effects of endogenously liberated histamine, leukotrienes, and prostaglandin D_2 in the early-phase allergic response. Chemotactic factors produce an inflammatory exudate that creates the more persistent congestion and nonspecific tissue hyperirritability of the late-phase response. The hyperirritability lowers the nasal threshold to both allergic and irritant stimuli, such as temperature changes, irritant particles and gases, sunlight, and ingested alcohol, thereby accentuating the effect of other allergens and prolonging symptoms after cessation of the allergen exposure.

A significant number of patients with allergic rhinitis have a coexisting bronchial hyperreactivity in the absence of clinical signs of asthma. It is not known whether this is an intrinsic abnormality related to atopy or an acquired defect from allergen exposure, possibly a component of the late allergic response.

Treatment

Treatment consists of environmental measures to avoid allergen exposure, drugs, and desensitization. Prophylactic avoidance of allergens is usually the most effective means of treatment. Avoidance is not always possible or practical, however, and so medications are needed to control symptoms. In some cases, the immune response itself can be altered by desensitization therapy.

A. Environmental Measures: Avoidance of an allergen is recommended for allergy and not because of a positive skin test alone. Appropriate measures may be the removal of household pets, control of house dust exposure by frequent cleaning, and avoidance of dust-collecting toys or other objects in the bedroom. Air-cleaning devices with high-efficiency particle filters may be helpful. Dehumidification and repair of leaking pipes or roofs may be necessary to prevent mold growth. Avoidance of pollen and outdoor molds is not possible unless the patient is able to stay in an air-conditioned home or office.

In cases of occupational allergy, every effort should be made to modify the patient's work routine and to employ industrial hygiene measures to avoid allergen exposure; however, if these measures fail, a change in the patient's job may be necessary.

B. Drug Treatment: Antihistamines are the most commonly used drugs in allergic rhinitis, although their use is restricted by side effects. The newer nonsedating antihistamines avoid the most troublesome side effects. Orally administered nasal decongestants may be helpful, either alone or in combination with antihistamines. Sympathomimetic and antihistaminic eye drops are useful for allergic conjunctivitis. Cromolyn by nasal sprays or conjunctival drops four times daily is beneficial and virtually free of immediate or long-term toxicity.

Systemic corticosteroids can be extremely effective in relieving symptoms of allergic rhinitis, but because the disease is benign, these drugs should be used with extreme care. Very severe symptoms lasting for only a few days or several weeks each year not relieved by antihistamines can be treated with oral prednisone for 1 or 2 weeks in a dosage just high enough to suppress symptoms. Glucocorticoids by nasal spray may be equally effective without causing significant systemic toxicity. Side effects of nasal burning and epistaxis from nasal corticosteroid sprays are more annoying than dangerous, but the potential for mucosal atrophy and septal perforation with prolonged use requires periodic monitoring. Corticosteroid eye drops to control acute severe allergic conjunctivitis should be used very sparingly for brief periods only, with careful monitoring by an ophthalmologist. Recent studies suggest that chronic high-dose topical glucocorticoids may cause some growth suppression in children.

C. Desensitization: Allergen injection therapy has been shown in many prospective double-blind controlled trials to be effective in treating allergic rhinitis. Because of the length of treatment required and the potential danger of serious systemic reactions, it is reserved for patients whose symptoms are uncontrolled despite appropriate environmental measures and symptomatic medications. The procedure, discussed more fully in Chapter 51, must be individualized and coordinated with environmental and drug treatment to be most effective; therefore, it should be initiated and monitored by a trained allergist.

Complications

Sinusitis may complicate allergic rhinitis. The diagnosis is difficult because of frequent discrepancies between paranasal sinus symptoms and radiographic evidence of pathology. Mild sinus membrane thickening (< 6 mm) is frequent in allergic rhinitis. Significant thickening, opacification, and air-fluid levels usually indicate an infectious sinusitis. Obstruction of the sinus ostia by swollen nasal membranes, whether caused by allergy, a common cold, or nonallergic vasomotor rhinitis, can cause secondary sinus infection, or the sinus mucosa per se may be a target organ in atopy.

Otitis media with or without effusion is common in children, and its causes are multifactorial, usually involving eustachian tube dysfunction and anatomic factors. It is not more prevalent in atopic than in nonatopic children or adults. It is unlikely that inhaled allergen reaches the middle ear or eustachian tube, although tubal obstruction by swollen nasopharyngeal allergic mucosa or dysfunction caused by the allergic mediators could prolong or exacerbate the disease.

Nasal polyps are also of similar frequency in atopic and normal individuals. Although polyposis is not a complication of allergic rhinitis, successful management can be hampered by untreated nasal allergy, and vice versa.

Prognosis

No definitive studies have been done on the course of untreated allergic rhinitis, but it can be expected to recur or persist for many years if not for life. The severity depends on the degree of exposure to the allergen. A patient with a pollen allergy who moves to an area where that pollen-producing plant does not grow will no longer be symptomatic.

ASTHMA

Major Immunologic Features

- IgE-mediated allergy in the bronchial mucosa
- Immunologically released or activated mediators of inflammation: histamine, leukotrienes, and eosinophil chemotactic factor
- Hyperirritability of bronchial mucosa amplified by bronchoconstricting and inflammatory mediators

Definition

Asthma (also known as reversible obstructive airway disease) is characterized by hyperresponsiveness of the tracheobronchial tree to respiratory irritants and bronchoconstrictor chemicals, producing attacks of wheezing, dyspnea, chest tightness, and cough. These are reversible spontaneously or with treatment. The disease is chronic, but it varies in severity from occasional mild transient episodes to severe, chronic, life-threatening bronchial obstruction. An associated eosinophilia occurs in the blood and in respiratory secretions. Episodes of asthma are triggered immunologically by allergen inhalation in patients with atopic allergy.

General Considerations

It is important to understand the role of atopic allergy in asthma. Asthma and atopy may coexist, but not all asthmatics are atopic and only some atopic patients have asthma. All asthmatic patients—regardless of the presence or absence of atopy—have the cardinal features that define asthma: airway hyperreactivity, reversible airway obstruction, and eosinophilia. In those with allergic asthma, attacks are triggered by allergen exposure as well as by other nonallergic factors.

Asthma and atopy are not wholly independent, however, because asthma occurs more frequently among atopic than among nonatopic individuals, especially during childhood. It is not known whether predisposition to the two conditions is genetically linked or if atopy enhances the clinical expression of an undefined asthmatic predisposition. One epidemiologic study showed a positive statistical correlation of asthma and IgE antibodies in all age groups. Nonetheless, by tradition and clinical usefulness, asthma is often classified into extrinsic and intrinsic subgroups.

A. Extrinsic Asthma (allergic, atopic, or immunologic): As a group, these patients generally develop the disease early in life, usually in infancy or childhood. Other manifestations of atopy—eczema or allergic rhinitis—often coexist. A family history of atopic disease is common. Attacks of asthma occur on exposure to allergens, depending on the patient's particular allergic sensitivities. Skin tests show positive wheal-and-flare reactions to the causative allergens. Total serum IgE concentration is frequently elevated but is sometimes normal.

B. Intrinsic Asthma (nonallergic or idiopathic): This characteristically appears first during adult life, usually after an apparent respiratory infection, so that the term **adult-onset asthma** is sometimes applied but is misleading, because some nonallergic asthmatics first develop the disease during childhood and some allergic asthmatics become symptomatic for the first time as adults when first sensitized and exposed to the relevant allergen. Intrinsic asthma pursues a course of chronic or recurrent bronchial obstruction. Skin tests are negative to the usual atopic allergens. The serum IgE concentration is normal. Blood and sputum eosinophilia is present. Personal and family histories are usually negative for other atopic diseases. Other schemes for classifying asthma into subgroups (eg, aspirin-sensitive, exercise-induced, infectious, and psychologic) merely define external triggering factors that affect certain patients more so than others.

Epidemiology

Asthma is a worldwide disease that has been recognized for centuries, but prevalence figures vary, in part because of differences in definition and methods of case finding. It is a common disease, which affects approximately 5% of the population of Western countries. Onset during childhood is predominantly before the age of 5 years, and it affects boys more than girls (by about 3:2). This form is usually of the allergic variety. Adult onset may be at any age, but typically it occurs in the fifth decade. Ordinarily it is of the intrinsic type, and it affects women more than men (by about 3:2).

Many recent studies suggest that the prevalence is increasing. Death caused by asthma—about 2000–3000 cases per year in the United States—is relatively infrequent, but recent reports from the many countries note increasing asthma mortality rates and some evidence of increasing morbidity rates, despite substantial advances in therapy.

Although not a major cause of mortality, asthma remains a leading cause of time lost from work and school.

Clinical Features

A. Symptoms: Asthma is characterized by attacks of wheezing and dyspnea ranging in severity from mild discomfort to life-threatening respiratory failure. Some patients are symptom-free between attacks, whereas others are never entirely free of airway obstruction. The asthmatic attack causes shortness of breath, wheezing, and tightness in the chest, with difficulty in moving air especially during expiration. Coughing is usually present, and with prolonged asthma the cough may produce thick, tenacious sputum that can be either clear or yellow. In children, coughing, especially at night, may be the only symptom to suggest the diagnosis. Fever is absent, but fatigue, malaise, irritability, palpitations, and sweating are occasional systemic complaints.

B. Signs: Physical examination during the attack shows tachypnea, audible wheezing, and use of the accessory muscles of respiration. The pulse is usually rapid, and blood pressure may be elevated. Pulsus paradoxus indicates severe asthma. The lung fields are hyperresonant, and auscultation reveals diminished breath sounds, wheezes, and rhonchi but no rales. The expiratory phase is prolonged. In a severe attack with high-grade obstruction, breath sounds and wheezing may both be absent. These are ominous signs, especially if accompanied by pallor and peripheral cyanosis, excitement or anxiety, and inability to speak. Chronic severe asthma in young children may lead to a structural barrel chest deformity.

C. Laboratory Findings: An increased total eosinophil count in the peripheral blood is almost invariably present unless suppressed by corticosteroids or sympathomimetic drugs. Eosinophilia is present in nasal secretions. Sputum examination reveals eosinophils, Charcot-Leyden crystals, and Curschmann's spirals.

The chest x-ray film may be normal during the attack or show signs of hyperinflation. Transient scattered parenchymal densities indicate focal atelectasis caused by mucus plugs in scattered portions of the airway. Total serum IgE is usually elevated in childhood allergic asthma and normal in adult intrinsic asthma, but this test lacks specificity for diagnosis of asthma or atopy (Figure 26–8).

Pulmonary function tests reveal reversible airway obstructive disease. Flow rates and 1-second forced expiratory volume (FEV_1) are decreased, vital capacity is normal or decreased, and total lung capacity and functional residual capacity are usually normal or slightly increased but may be decreased with extreme bronchospasm. Following administration of an aerosolized sympathomimetic bronchodilator, ventilation improves with significant increase in flow rates and FEV_1. The lack of response in a patient already receiving large doses of sympathomimetic drugs does not rule out reversibility, and the test should be repeated at a later date after improvement from other forms of treatment.

Repeated tests of ventilatory function are helpful in the long-term management of asthma. Serial determinations of FEV_1, maximal expiratory flow rate, or peak flow rate are easily done in the examining room or at home, and they often detect airway obstruction not apparent to the patient or on auscultation of the chest.

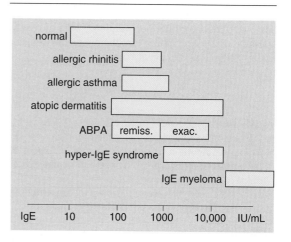

Figure 26–8. Total serum IgE levels in normal individuals and patients with various allergies and IgE disorders. *Abbreviations:* ABPA = allergic bronchopulmonary aspergillosis; remiss. = remission; exac. = exacerbation.

Bronchial provocation testing is not necessary for routine diagnosis but helpful in special circumstances. Nonspecific bronchial hyperirritability is shown by using quantitative challenges with methacholine, histamine, cold air, or exercise. These tests are almost always positive in asthma, but they are not by themselves diagnostic because bronchial hyperirritability occurs in a significant number of patients with allergic rhinitis, in normal subjects following viral respiratory infections, and in a small percentage of normal individuals. Because the procedure provokes an asthma attack, it should not be used in the presence of significant bronchial obstruction or if asthma can be diagnosed by other criteria.

Allergen Bronchoprovocation Testing

Inhalational challenge with aerosolized allergen extracts to provoke a bronchial reaction under controlled conditions in the laboratory is of limited use in clinical practice. Aqueous allergen extracts in several dilutions are prepared in buffered saline. An initial titration skin testing is necessary to determine a safe starting dose for bronchial challenge. A measurement sensitive to acute airway obstruction, usually FEV_1, is used. A fall in FEV_1 begins in 10 minutes or less, peaks at 20–30 minutes, and then returns to baseline. A decrease of 20% or greater is considered significant. A late-phase asthmatic response may occur, beginning at 4–6 hours, peaking at 8–12 hours, and clearing by 24 hours. Allergen challenges may cause isolated early or late responses, or both. Therefore, allergen bronchoprovocation should be performed in a hospital with appropriate facilities for detecting and treating these reactions. A positive late-phase response may increase the patient's nonspecific bronchial hyperirritability for several days, so if a second allergen is to be tested, this should be done no sooner than 1 week later.

The **indications** for provocation testing in clinical practice are limited. For routine diagnosis of atopic asthma, bronchoprovocation with allergen gives results that correlate well with skin tests, but patients with only allergic rhinitis may also have a specific bronchial response to inhaled allergen extract. A positive test to a suspected causative agent of occupational asthma does not necessarily mean that the asthma is immunologic. For example, bronchoprovocation with isocyanates produces specific immediate and late asthmatic responses in workers with clinical isocyanate asthma, even though the illness does not correlate well with an IgE (or other) immune response to this chemical. Allergen bronchoprovocation may be useful to monitor desensitization therapy.

Pathology

Autopsy on individuals with fatal asthma shows hyperinflation of the lungs, hypertrophy and hyperplasia of bronchial smooth muscle, and excessive mucus secretion. Death is usually caused by asphyxiation from mucus plugging the airways. Microscopic examination shows hypertrophy and hyperplasia of submucosal glands and bronchial smooth muscle, mucosal infiltration with an edematous and mixed cellular inflammatory response especially rich in eosinophils, and epithelial desquamation within mucous plugs. Similar but less intense pathology exists during asymptomatic periods. The pathology therefore reflects both the early phase (smooth muscle contraction, edema, hypersecretion) and late phase (cellular inflammation) of the IgE-mediated allergic response. The gross and microscopic pathology of allergic asthma is indistinguishable from that of nonallergic asthma.

Immunologic Pathogenesis

The cause of asthma is unknown. Pathogenesis of the asthmatic attack involves both allergic and nonallergic mechanisms. Some evidence suggests that bronchoconstriction is mediated by an autonomic (vagal) reflex mechanism involving afferent receptors in the bronchial mucosa or submucosa that respond to irritants or chemical mediators and efferent cholinergic impulses, causing bronchial muscle contraction and hypersecretion of mucus. The mast cell-associated mediators (histamine, leukotrienes, prostaglandins, kinins, platelet-activating factor, and chemotactic factors) have properties that can explain the pathologic and functional abnormalities of the asthmatic attack. In the asthmatic patient, the afferent receptors appear to be sensitized to respond to a low threshold of stimulation. Bronchial hyperirritability is enhanced further during the late phase of the asthmatic reaction.

The linkage between allergen/IgE antibody interaction and release, activation, and secretion of mediators from the mast cell is now firmly established. The means by which nonallergic stimuli, such as irritants and viral infections, stimulate mast cells is unknown at present, and it is possible that other cells and mediators are involved in nonallergic asthma.

The variety of nonspecific agents that initiate an asthma attack is extensive. Some of these factors are listed in Table 26–9. Some of these items have been shown to increase the underlying bronchial hyperirritability as well, making the patient more sensitive to the effects of other triggers.

Approximately 10% of asthmatic patients have **aspirin sensitivity.** In these patients, ingestion of aspirin is followed in 20 minutes to 3 hours by an asthmatic attack, which is caused by an idiosyncratic pharmacologic response to the drug (see Chapter 30).

The clinical significance of immediate and late phases of the IgE response is especially clear in asthma. Bronchospastic episodes that occur within minutes after exposure to the allergen and are promptly relieved by bronchodilators correspond to the immediate-phase response. Chronic asthma that is poorly responsive to β-adrenergic agonists and

Table 26–9. Nonspecific triggers of asthma.

Infections
  Viral respiratory infections
Physiologic factors
  Exercise
  Hyperventilation
  Deep breathing
  Psychologic factors
Atmospheric factors
  SO_2
  NH_3
  Cold air
  O_3
  Distilled water vapor
Ingestants
  Propranolol
  Aspirin
  Nonsteroidal antiinflammatory drugs
  Sulfites
Experimental Inhalants
  Hypertonic solutions
  Citric acid
  Histamine
  Methacholine
  Prostaglandin $F_{2\alpha}$
Occupational Inhalant
  Isocyanates

theophylline, associated with enhanced nonspecific airway hyperirritability, and dependent on corticosteroids for reversal, is characteristic of the late-phase allergic response. Bronchial provocation challenge with many of the usual inhaled aeroallergens, such as pollens, fungi, and dust mite, produce dual early and late asthmatic reaction in untreated allergic asthma.

Exercise-induced and hyperventilation-induced bronchoconstriction in asthmatic patients is a consequence of water loss from the airway, which increases the osmolarity of fluid overlying the mucosal epithelial cells. This stimulates mast cells to release mediators, which, in turn, contract bronchial smooth muscle either directly or indirectly through vagal afferent receptor stimulation. Airway cooling, which occurs from inhaling cold air, exaggerates the effect of water loss.

The conceptual model of allergen/IgE antibody-induced allergic disease requires direct contact of the allergen molecule with antibodies fixed to tissue mast cells, which then release mediators locally in the target tissues, where the inflammatory pathology and clinical symptoms and signs localize. In atopy the allergen molecule is often encountered as a component of an airborne particle, such as a pollen grain or mold spore, which is too large when inhaled to penetrate as far as the tracheobronchial tree. Recent immuno-chemical air-sampling methods, however, have shown that pollen and spore fragments and even droplets containing allergen are inhaled as a significant portion of the ambient allergen load inhaled by the allergic patient.

The allergens commonly associated with allergic asthma and allergic rhinitis are generally similar. In-dividual patients, however, may tend to react with rhinitis to pollens and with asthma to molds and animal dander. Very young asthmatic children frequently have food-induced asthma without rhinitis.

Allergic asthma is the usual manifestation of IgE-mediated occupational disease. New occupational inhalant allergens are continually being discovered. A partial list is shown in Table 26–10. Occupational asthma may also arise from nonimmunologic sensitivity or irritation to many other substances that fail to induce IgE antibody or other immune responses. In these cases, the cause and pathogenesis are unknown, but possible mechanisms include toxic chemical injury to the bronchial mucosa, irritant stimulation of mast cells or vagal irritant receptors, and β-adrenergic blockade. Most cases of occupational asthma, however—both IgE-mediated and nonimmunologic—occur in nonatopic workers.

Immunologic Diagnosis

The diagnosis of asthma is made by history, physical examination, and pulmonary function tests to show reversible bronchial obstruction. Blood and sputum examination for eosinophilia is confirmatory. Chest radiography is useful primarily to exclude other cardiopulmonary diseases. The methacholine challenge test is reserved for instances in which the history is equivocal and pulmonary function is normal.

The history is the primary diagnostic tool for evaluating the presence of allergy and identifying the relevant allergens. In general, inhalant allergens that are important in allergic rhinitis are also implicated in allergic asthma. These include pollens, fungi, animal danders, house dust, and other household and occupational airborne allergens. In young children and infants, allergy to foods may also cause asthma. History and physical findings of other atopic diseases—atopic dermatitis or allergic rhinitis—as well as a family history of atopy increase suspicion that the patient's asthma may involve atopic allergy. Skin testing for wheal-and-flare reactions verifies the specific sensitivities. RAST or other in vitro tests may be used instead when skin testing is contraindicated. Bronchoprovocation allergen testing is used primarily in difficult diagnostic cases of suspected occupational lung disease.

Differential Diagnosis

Chronic bronchitis and emphysema (chronic obstructive lung disease) cause airway obstruction that does not respond to sympathomimetic bronchodilators or corticosteroids and in which there is no associated eosinophilia in the blood or sputum. Bronchiolitis, cystic fibrosis, aspiration of a foreign body, and congenital vascular anomalies cause airway obstruction in children. Benign or malignant bronchial tumors or external compression from an enlarged substernal thyroid, thymus enlargement, aneurysm,

Table 26–10. Occupational allergens causing IgE-mediated allergic asthma.

Allergen	Occupational Exposure
Animal products	
Cows, pigs, poultry, mice, hamsters, rabbits, rats, guinea pigs, bats, dogs, cats, horses	Animal/insect breeders, laboratory workers, veterinarians, breeders
Insect dusts	
Mealworms, storage mites, silk filatures, locusts, bees, cockroaches, flies	Grain handlers, sewerage workers, beekeepers
Sea creatures	
Crabs, shrimp, seasquirt body fluid, fish feed, *Echinodorus plamosus* larvae	Processors, breeders
Plant products	
Dusts, flours, cotton dust, grain dusts, grain flours	Cotton mill and textile workers, grain elevator and bakery workers
Fruits, seeds, leaves, pollens	
Castor beans, green coffee beans	Coffee processors, seamen, laboratory workers
Weeping fig, sunflower pollen, tobacco	Producers, agricultural workers
Organic dyes and inks	
Vegetable, dusts, gums, extracts	
Western red and eastern white cedar (plicatic acid), California redwood, exotic woods	Carpenters, sawmill workers
Colophony (abietic acid)	Electronics workers
Microbial agents	
Alginates, fungal allergens, humidifier contaminants, protozoa, fungi, bacteria	Biotechnology industry, laboratory, office workers
Enzymes	
Subtilisin, papain, pineapple bromelain, pepsin, hog trypsin, pancreatic extracts	Detergent manufacturers, pharmaceutical workers, food processors
Therapeutic agents	
Antibiotics and related compounds, penicillins, cephalosporins, tetracycline, phenylglycine acid chloride, sulfonamides, spiramycin	Pharmaceutical workers, poultry chick breeders
Pharmaceuticals and related compounds	
α-Methyldopa, amprolium hydrochloride, cimetidine, furanbased binder, glycyl compound (salbutamol intermediate), psyllium (bulk laxative)	Pharmaceutical workers, nurses
Piperazine	Medical and veterinary workers
Sterilizing agents	
Chloramine, sulfone chloramides, hexachlorophene	Abattoir, kitchen, hospital workers
Inorganic chemicals	
Metal fumes and salts	Metalworkers
Aluminum, chromium, cobalt, fluoride, nickel, platinum, stainless steel, welding fumes, vanadium, zinc	Chemical industry workers, metal refiners, platers, grinders, welders
Ammonium persulfate	Beauticians
Organic chemicals	
Amines (diamines, ethanolamines, tetramines)	Chemical, electronic, plastic, rubber industry workers, photographers, beauticians, fur handlers
Anhydrides (phthalic, tetrachlorophthalic, trimellitic), azobisformamide, azodicarbonamide	Plastics industry workers, food wrappers

Source: Modified and reproduced, with permission, from Butcher BT, Salvaggio JE: Occupational asthma. *J Allergy Clin Immunol* 1986;**78:**547.

or mediastinal tumor may produce wheezing. Acute viral bronchitis with wheezing is often termed **asthmatic bronchitis. Cardiac asthma** refers to intermittent dyspnea (resembling allergic asthma) caused by left ventricular failure. Carcinoid tumors may occasionally cause attacks of wheezing because of release of serotonin or activation of kinins by the neoplasm.

Treatment

The cause of asthma is unknown, so the aim of treatment is symptomatic control. Environmental measures, drugs, and allergen desensitization may be required.

A. Environmental Control: Irritants such as smoke, fumes, dust, and aerosols should be avoided. If the diagnostic evaluation indicates allergy to animal danders, feathers, molds, or house dust, these should be eliminated from the house.

B. Drug Treatment:

1. Sympathomimetics— Beta-adrenergic bronchodilator drugs are effective in the acute attack or for long-term management. Epinephrine has both α- and β-adrenergic effects, but it has a long history of efficacy in acute asthma attacks. It acts rapidly but briefly and is given intramuscularly in a dose of 0.2–0.5 mL of 1:1000 aqueous solution. Albuterol, pirbuterol, metaproterenol, and isoetharine are selective β-adrenergic bronchodilators inhaled in aerosol by a hand-held nebulizer, in an intermittent positive-pressure breathing device, or in metered-dose pressurized inhalers. Overuse can lead to paradoxic bronchial constriction and worsening of asthma. Terbutaline, metaproterenol, and albuterol are available as oral sympathomimetic drugs for sustained bronchodilation in chronic asthma.

Salmeterol, an inhaled β₂-adrenergic bronchodilator, is effective for long-term prophylaxis. It is not useful for relief of an acute attack, because of an extremely long latent period before its action takes place.

2. Xanthines— Although currently out of favor, theophylline and related compounds are bronchodilators especially effective when used with sympathomimetic drugs. Intravenous aminophylline, 250–500 mg, can be administered fairly rapidly in an acute asthmatic attack, and various oral forms of theophylline are available for long-term use. Absorption varies with the drug preparation, age of the patient, and other factors, such as smoking and heart failure. Serum theophylline determination should be used to obtain a therapeutic level of 10–20 µg/mL.

3. Corticosteroids— Glucocorticoids are remarkably effective in the treatment of asthma. Even when all other forms of treatment have failed, the effect is so dependable that failure of response might be considered grounds for questioning the diagnosis of asthma. The therapeutic mechanism in asthma is antiinflammatory. Systemic corticosteroids should be given only when other forms of treatment prove inadequate, beginning at high dosage and continued until the obstruction is alleviated, with return of physical findings and flow rates to normal. The dose necessary to achieve this varies with the individual patient, but 30–60 mg of prednisone daily is usually sufficient. An occasional steroid-resistant patient may require a much higher dose because of an abnormally accelerated rate of drug catabolism. After complete clearing of the attack, the daily dose is reduced by slow tapering over many days or weeks to avoid a recurrence of asthma.

Long-term inhalant glucocorticoid therapy is now accepted as the cornerstone of asthma prophylaxis. Beclomethasone, triamcinolone, flunisolide, fluticasone, and budesonide—highly potent corticosteroid drugs—are available in aerosolized, micronized, or dry powder form for inhalation. Adrenocortical suppression and systemic side effects are usually minimal. Inhaled corticosteroids should not be used for treatment of an acute asthma attack.

4. Cromolyn and Nedocromil— These drugs are believed to inhibit the release of mediators of immediate hypersensitivity in the lung. They are given by inhalation for long-term prophylaxis but are more effective in younger patients with allergic asthma than in adults. They may prevent exercise-induced bronchospasm but do not reverse an acute attack.

5. Other drugs— Antibiotics are required for secondary bacterial bronchitis or pneumonia. Expectorants and hydration are helpful for thick, tenacious sputum. Inhaled ipratropium bromide, an anticholinergic drug with minimal side effects because of poor absorption, may help to eliminate the asthmatic cough.

Leukotriene pathway inhibitors (zafirlukast, montelukast) are prophylactic oral medications especially effective in controlling nocturnal asthma.

C. Desensitization: The advantages of injection treatment in pollen-induced allergic asthma have been shown in several controlled studies (see Chapter 51).

D. Treatment of Status Asthmaticus and Respiratory Failure: A severe attack of asthma unresponsive to repeated use of sympathomimetic drugs, termed "status asthmaticus," is a medical emergency requiring immediate hospitalization and prompt treatment. Factors leading to this condition include respiratory infection, excessive use of respiratory-depressant drugs such as sedatives or opiates, overuse of aerosolized bronchodilators, rapid withdrawal of corticosteroids, and ingestion of aspirin in aspirin-sensitive asthmatic patients.

Arterial blood gas and pH measurements help to assess the effect of treatment. Injections of terbutaline or epinephrine, intravenous aminophylline, and intravenous corticosteroids are indicated if significant CO_2 retention exists. Intravenous hydrocortisone at 4 mg/kg or methylprednisolone at 1 mg/kg, repeated every 2–4 hours, should be given until the patient can be maintained on oral prednisone at 60–80 mg daily in divided doses.

Dehydration usually accompanies status asthmaticus and may give rise to inspissated mucus plugs that further impair ventilation. During the first 24 hours, up to 3–4 L of intravenous fluid may be necessary for rehydration. Oxygen should be supplied by tent, face mask, or nasal catheter to maintain arterial P_{O_2} at about 80–100 mm Hg. Expectorants and chest physical therapy are helpful adjuncts to eliminate mucus plugs. Sedatives should be avoided even in the anxious patient because of the danger of respiratory depression. Antibiotics are used only for concomitant bacterial infection.

Respiratory failure, indicated by an arterial P_{O_2} level above 65 mm Hg and arterial blood pH below 7.25, may require mechanical assistance of ventilation. This should be performed by a team of physicians, nurses, and technicians experienced in this form of respiratory therapy.

Complications & Prognosis

Asthma is a chronic disease, and its severity may change in an unpredictable fashion. Some children apparently "outgrow" asthma in the sense of becoming asymptomatic, but they may continue to show evidence of bronchial lability, and symptoms can reappear later in life. The acute attack can be complicated by pneumothorax, subcutaneous emphysema, rib fractures, atelectasis, or pneumonitis. Although there is no evidence that emphysema, bronchiectasis, pulmonary hypertension, and cor pulmonale result from long-standing uncomplicated asthma, there is substantial evidence that irreversible changes in bronchial mucosa, called "airway remodeling," result from prolonged asthmatic inflammation.

Allergic Bronchopulmonary Aspergillosis

This disease occurs almost exclusively in patients with a history of asthma who harbor *Aspergillus* endobronchially and who develop a heterogeneous form of hypersensitivity with both IgE and IgG antibodies to *Aspergillus* antigens (see Chapter 28).

ATOPIC DERMATITIS

Major Immunologic Features
- Often accompanies atopic respiratory allergy
- Clinical course usually independent of allergen exposure
- Possible very high serum levels of IgE

Definition

Atopic dermatitis (eczema, neurodermatitis, atopic eczema, Besnier's prurigo) is a chronic skin disorder specific to a subset of atopic patients. The essential feature is a pruritic dermal inflammatory response, which induces a characteristic symmetrically distributed skin eruption with predilection for certain skin sites. There is frequent overproduction of IgE by B lymphocytes, possibly caused by abnormal T-lymphocyte regulation. Patients often have multiple IgE antibodies to environmental inhalant and food allergens, but the role of these allergens in the dermatitis is uncertain.

General Considerations

Atopic dermatitis is classified as a cutaneous form of atopy because it is associated with allergic rhinitis and asthma in families (and frequently in the same patient) and the serum IgE concentration is often high. The severity of the dermatitis, however, does not always correlate with exposure to allergens to which the patient reacts positively on skin testing, and allergy desensitization is not effective in this disease. There is evidence for an underlying target organ (ie, skin) abnormality, possibly linked genetically to the high level of serum IgE. Some studies also suggest a partial deficiency in T-cell immunity. Atopic dermatitis may begin at any age.

Clinical Features

A. Symptoms: Onset at 3–6 months of age is typical, but it may first appear during childhood or adolescence and occasionally during adult life. Many cases of infantile eczema clear by 2 years of age. Persistence into later childhood and adult life is marked by frequent cycles of remission and exacerbation. Itching is the cardinal symptom. It often worsens at night and is provoked by temperature changes, sweating, exertion, and emotional stress. Scratching and rubbing cause the eczematous skin eruption to flare. Itching is also exacerbated by irritants such as wool and by drying agents such as soap and defatting solvents. Ingestion of allergenic foods may cause acute exacerbations. The disease may improve spontaneously during the summer.

B. Signs: The skin is dry and scaly. Active skin lesions are characterized by intensely pruritic inflamed papules (prurigo), erythema, and scaling. Scratching produces weeping and excoriations. Chronic lesions are thickened and lichenified. Distribution of the lesions depends on age. In infancy, the forehead, cheeks, and extensor surfaces of the extremities are usually involved. Later, the lesions show a flexural pattern of distribution, with predilection for the antecubital and popliteal areas and the neck. The face, especially around the eyes and ears, is often affected when distribution is more widespread. Staphylococcal pustules are common. Stroking of the skin produces white dermographism, in contrast to the normal erythema and whealing (the triple response of Lewis).

C. Laboratory Findings: Elevated total serum IgE, sometimes extremely high, occurs in 60–80% of cases. A normal level does not rule out the diagnosis.

Epidemiology

Approximately 0.7% of the US population have active disease. Prevalence in children is 4–5%, equally distributed between the sexes. Racial predilection and geographic distribution have not been studied.

Pathology

Grossly, the lesion begins acutely as an erythematous edematous papule or plaque with scaling. Itching leads to weeping and crusting, then chronic lichenification. Microscopically, the acute lesion shows intercellular edema and dermal infiltration with mononuclear cells and CD4 lymphocytes. Neutrophils, eosinophils, plasma cells, and basophils are rare, and vasculitis is absent, but degranulated mast cells can be seen. The chronic lesion features epidermal hyperplasia, hyperkeratosis, and parakeratosis. The dermis is infiltrated with mononuclear cells, Langerhans' cells, and mast cells. Focal areas of fibrosis may occur, including involvement of the perineurium of small nerves.

Immunologic Diagnosis

The history and physical examination are almost always sufficient to make the diagnosis. Marked elevation of serum IgE is confirmatory, but a normal IgE level does not rule out atopic dermatitis. Biopsy is not required.

Skin or in vitro allergy tests usually produce positive results that may reflect concomitant respiratory allergies or asymptomatic sensitivities rather than allergic causes of the skin disease. House dust mite and foods are clinically relevant specific allergens in some children with atopic dermatitis.

Differential Diagnosis

Localized neurodermatitis (lichen simplex chronicus) and allergic or irritant contact dermatitis produce similar eczematous changes of the skin. Seborrhea and dermatophytoses are occasionally confused with atopic dermatitis. Pompholyx (dyshidrosis) with secondary eczema may simulate atopic dermatitis of the hands.

Immunologic Pathogenesis

Atopic dermatitis is an intrinsic skin abnormality, perhaps analogous to the hyperirritable airway in asthma. Some evidence suggests hyperreactivity to cholinergic stimuli, which might relate to the reduced threshold of the itch response. Increased numbers of mast cells and histamine content in the skin have been reported. Blood basophil counts are normal. Intradermal methacholine initially produces a wheal and erythema followed in 2–5 minutes by blanching. This delayed blanch response is typical but not diagnostic of atopic dermatitis.

A. Defective Lymphocyte Regulation: Much indirect information suggests a defect in cell-mediated immunity. Delayed hypersensitivity skin test responses to recall antigens, in vitro lymphocyte responses to mitogen and allergen, and the autologous mixed lymphocyte reaction have all been reported to be deficient. Decreased prevalence of naturally acquired and experimentally induced allergic contact dermatitis and increased susceptibility to herpes simplex virus, vaccinia virus, warts, molluscum contagiosum, and dermatophyte skin infections are consistent with a T-cell effector defect. Many studies document the association of high levels of IgE production with the presence of a predominant population of T helper cells with the T_H2 cytokine profile. Other studies show that excessive production of IgE by peripheral blood B lymphocytes in this disease can be accounted for by deficiency in CD8 T lymphocytes. It has been suggested that a defective CD4 helper T-lymphocyte population could explain the failure of CD8 T lymphocytes to function as suppressors of IgE production and to achieve sufficient cytotoxicity for effective immunity against secondary skin infections.

B. The Role of Allergy: Atopic respiratory diseases with hypersensitivity to environmental allergens, eosinophilia, elevated serum IgE levels, and a family history of allergy are frequently associated with atopic dermatitis. Nevertheless, it is often difficult to attribute the dermatitis to allergy. The skin lesions rarely flare during pollen seasons, although in some patients there is an association with exposure to house dust, animals, or other environmental allergens. More commonly, food allergy is implicated in the dermatitis in children, especially milk, corn, soybeans, fish, nuts, and cereal grains. Controlled food challenges have shown clear-cut exacerbations of the early inflammatory pruritic lesions in selected cases.

C. Association with Systemic Disorders: Eczema indistinguishable from atopic dermatitis is found in children with phenylketonuria and similar skin lesions of Letterer–Siwe disease. Atopic dermatitis without allergy is a feature of several immunologic deficiency disorders, especially Wiskott-Aldrich syndrome, ataxia–telangiectasia, and X-linked hypogammaglobulinemia (see Chapters 21–23).

Treatment

Atopic dermatitis is a chronic disease requiring constant attention to proper skin care, environmental control, drugs, and avoidance of allergens when indicated. Because dry skin enhances the tendency to itch, frequent application of nonirritating topical lubricants is the most important preventive measure. Small areas of active eczema respond well to topical glucocorticoids, but acute involvement of large areas of skin may warrant a brief course of systemic corticosteroids beginning with a high dose and tapering slowly after the acute eruption clears. Oral antihistamines help to control itching. Frequent bathing or washing, irritating fabrics such as wool, and harsh detergents should be avoided. The hands and fingernails must be kept clean to prevent secondary infection, and if infection does occur, an appropriate antibiotic should be prescribed.

Complications & Prognosis

Atopic dermatitis that persists beyond childhood has an unpredictable tendency to remit spontaneously, even after years of involvement. This is not related to the severity, presence or absence of allergy, or treatment. Allergic rhinitis and asthma are not complications but manifestations of the underlying atopic disease.

The most frequent complication is secondary infection, almost always by *Staphylococcus,* as a result of scratching. In the past, the most serious complication was eczema vaccinatum from exposure to vaccinia virus by inadvertent vaccination or contact with a recently vaccinated person in the family or classroom. Eczema herpeticum is a similar condition caused by herpes simplex virus. Topical antibiotics or antihistamines may cause secondary contact dermatitis. Hand dermatitis occurs from excessive contact with water, soap, and solvents in the home and the workplace.

Ophthalmic complications include atopic keratoconjunctivitis, keratoconus, and atopic cataracts.

ALLERGIC GASTROENTEROPATHY

Major Immunologic Features
- Localized IgE reactions in the gut to an ingested food
- Gastrointestinal loss of serum proteins and blood possibly leading to edema and anemia
- Rare in adults; more common but transient in infants

Definition & General Considerations
Allergic gastroenteropathy (also known as eosinophilic gastroenteropathy) is an unusual atopic manifestation in which multiple IgE food sensitivities elicit a local gastrointestinal tract mucosal reaction. Ingested food allergen reacting with local IgE antibodies in the jejunal mucosa liberates mast cell mediators, causing gastrointestinal symptoms shortly after the meal. Continued exposure to the food produces chronic inflammation, resulting in gastrointestinal protein loss and hypoproteinemic edema. Blood loss through the inflamed intestinal mucosa may be significant enough to cause iron deficiency anemia. In some patients, extraenteric manifestations of atopy may be produced by the same food allergen.

Epidemiology
Only a few cases have been reported, but the disease has been described in infants, children, and adults. It is a very rare cause of gastrointestinal symptoms.

Immunologic Pathogenesis
The condition may occur more commonly in infants than in adults because of the much greater permeability of the infantile gastrointestinal mucosa to intact proteins. This may account for the transient nature of allergic gastroenteropathy in infants and young children. The allergic reaction occurs locally in the upper gastrointestinal mucosa. Ingested food allergens react with IgE antibodies fixed to mucosal mast cells, thereby liberating mediators responsible for hyperemia, increased vascular permeability, and smooth muscle contraction.

Clinical Features
A. Symptoms and Signs: Nausea, vomiting, diarrhea, and abdominal pain occur within 2 hours after ingestion of the allergenic food. Symptoms resolve on avoidance of the food. Rhinitis, asthma, or urticaria may accompany the intestinal symptoms. Chronic or repeated exposures to allergenic foods in undiagnosed disease may lead to blood loss anemia, abdominal distension, and voluminous foul stools from steatorrhea, edema from hypoalbuminemia, and systemic symptoms of anorexia, weight loss, and weakness. Children may experience growth retardation. Most patients have other manifestations of and a family history of atopy.

B. Laboratory Findings: Blood counts show hypochromic microcytic iron deficiency anemia and eosinophilia. Stool examination reveals gross or occult blood and Charcot–Leyden crystals. Serum albumin is low, and total serum IgE may be elevated. Gastrointestinal radiography may show mucosal thickening and edema of the small bowel.

Immunologic Diagnosis
A history of chronic or recurrent gastrointestinal symptoms associated with specific foods in an atopic patient should raise a suspicion of this diagnosis, especially if there is accompanying evidence of gastrointestinal blood loss, iron deficiency anemia, intestinal malabsorption, protein-losing enteropathy, other manifestations of atopy, or high serum total IgE.

In reported cases the causative food allergens have been single or multiple. Milk is the usual cause in children. Nursing infants may react to food allergens in breast milk from the maternal diet. IgE antibodies to the suspected food allergens can be identified by skin test or RAST. If necessary, the allergy can be confirmed by elimination and challenge, preferably performed double-blind. Peroral jejunal biopsy may be necessary in difficult cases.

Pathology
An eosinophilic inflammatory infiltrate in the lamina propria of the upper gastrointestinal tract mucosa is present following allergen exposure and resolves with allergen avoidance.

Differential Diagnosis
Gastrointestinal allergy is overdiagnosed. Patients with food-related gastrointestinal symptoms—even atopic patients—are much more likely to have nonallergic food intolerance. Primary gastrointestinal diseases, reactions to food contaminants, and psychologic food aversion must be considered. Inflammatory bowel diseases, intestinal lymphangiectasia, and primary immunoglobulin deficiencies may produce similar symptoms. In children, deficiency of lactase and other carbohydrate-splitting enzymes, phenylketonuria, pancreatic deficiency from cystic fibrosis, and maple syrup urine disease should be ruled out by appropriate tests.

Treatment
Elimination of the allergenic food from the diet is curative. In some cases of milk allergy, boiled milk may be tolerated if the protein allergen is heat-labile. Corticosteroid treatment usually inhibits the reaction, but long-term steroid therapy should be necessary only for patients who do not respond to the elimination diet. There are reports that oral cromolyn in a dose of 200–400 mg given before the allergenic food is eaten inhibits the gastrointestinal allergic reaction, but there are no long-term studies on this form of treatment.

Complications

The major complications are edema and anemia. Unlike intestinal lymphangiectasia, significant gastroenteric loss of plasma immunoglobulins and lymphocytes does not occur, so susceptibility to infection is usually not a problem. Persistent disease activity may lead to secondary reversible lactose intolerance. Malnutrition can result from undiagnosed disease.

Prognosis

The infantile form of allergic gastroenteropathy is usually transient, but the duration of the disease is unpredictable and is not related to severity of the reaction. No long-term follow-up studies on adults are available.

REFERENCES

GENERAL

Hopkin JM: Genetics of atopy. *Clin Exp Allergy* 1989; 19:263.

Ishizaka K: IgE-binding factors and regulation of the IgE antibody response. *Annu Rev Immunol* 1988;6:513.

Marsh DG et al: The epidemiology and genetics of atopic allergy. *N Engl J Med* 1981;305:1551.

ALLERGENS

Anderson JA, Sogn DD (editors): *Adverse Reactions to Foods*. NIH Publication no. 84-2442. US Department of Health and Human Services, 1984.

Anderson MC et al: A comparative study of the allergens of cat urine, serum, saliva, and pelt. *J Allergy Clin Immunol* 1985;76:563.

Korner WE et al: Fungal allergens. *Clin Microbiol Rev* 1995;8:161.

Platts-Mills TAE et al: Problems in allergen standardization. *Clin Rev Allergy* 1985;3:271.

Solomon WR: Aerobiology of pollinosis. *J Allergy Clin Immunol* 1984;74:449.

Weber RW, Nelson HS: Pollen allergens and their interrelationships. *Clin Rev Allergy* 1985;3:291.

ALLERGIC RHINITIS

Allansmith MR, Ross RN: Ocular allergy. *Clin Allergy* 1988; 18:1.

Busse WW: Role of antihistamines in allergic disease. *Ann Allergy* 1994;72:281.

Druce HM, Kaliner MA: Allergic rhinitis. *JAMA* 1988; 259:260.

Fireman P: Newer concepts in otitis media. *Hosp Pract* 1987;22:85.

Friedlaender MH: Ocular allergy. *J Allergy Clin Immunol* 1985;76:645.

Naclerio RM et al: Basophils and eosinophils in allergic rhinitis. *J Allergy Clin Immunol* 1994;94:1303.

Norman PS: Allergic rhinitis. *J Allergy Clin Immunol* 1985; 75:531.

Meltzer EO: An overview of current pharmacotherapy in perennial rhinitis. *J Allergy Clin Immunol* 1995;95:1097.

Philip G, Togias AG: Nonallergic rhinitis. Pathophysiology and models for study. *Eur Arch Otorhinolaryngol Suppl* 1995;1:S27.

Todd NW: Allergy as a cause of otitis media. *Immunol Allergy Clin North Am* 1987;7:371.

ASTHMA

Barnes PJ: New concepts in the pathogenesis of bronchial hyperresponsiveness and asthma. *J Allergy Clin Immunol* 1989;83:1013.

Busse WW: The relationship between viral infections and the onset of allergic diseases and asthma. *Clin Exp Allergy* 1989;19:1.

Chan-Yeung M, Lam S: Occupational asthma. *Am Rev Respir Dis* 1986;133:686.

Chapman ID et al: The relationship between inflammation and hyperreactivity of the airways in asthma. *Clin Exp Allergy* 1993;23:168.

Cherniak RM: Continuity of care in asthma management. *Hosp Pract* 1987;22:119.

Fahy JV, Boushey HA: Controversies involving inhaled beta-agonists and inhaled corticosteroids in the treatment of asthma. *Clin Chest Med* 1995;16:715.

Fireman P: β_2-agonists and their safety in the treatment of asthma. *Allergy Proc* 1995;16:235.

Freedman AN: Models and mechanisms of exercise-induced asthma. *Eur Respir J* 1995;8:1770.

Hargreave FE et al: The origin of airway hyperresponsiveness. *J Allergy Clin Immunol* 1986;78:825.

König P: Inhaled corticosteroids-their present and future role in the management of asthma. *J Allergy Clin Immunol* 1988;82:297.

Lenfant C, Sheffer AL: Guidelines for the diagnosis and management of asthma. *J Allergy Clin Immunol* 1991; 88(suppl):425 [Entire issue].

Mathison DA et al: Precipitating factors in asthma: Aspirin, sulfites, and other drugs and chemicals. *Chest* 1985; 87(suppl):S50.

McFadden ER: Therapy of acute asthma. *J Allergy Clin Immunol* 1989;84:151.

Ohman JL: Allergen immunotherapy in asthma: Evidence for efficacy. *J Allergy Clin Immunol* 1989;84:133.

Pattemore PK et al: Viruses as precipitants of asthma symptoms. I. Epidemiology. *Clin Exp Allergy* 1992;22:325.

Rachelefsky GS, Siegel SC: Asthma in infants and children—treatment of childhood asthma. Part II. *J Allergy Clin Immunol* 1985;76:409.

Siegel SC, Rachelefsky GS: Asthma in infants and children. Part I. *J Allergy Clin Immunol* 1985;76:1.

Spector SL: Leukotriene inhibitors and antagonists in asthma. *Ann Allergy* 1995;75:463.

Summer WR: Status asthmaticus. *Chest* 1985;87(suppl):S87.

Wasserfallen JB, Baraniuk JN: Clinical use of inhaled corticosteroids in asthma. *J Allergy Clin Immunol* 1997; 97:177.

ATOPIC DERMATITIS

Burks AW et al: Atopic dermatitis and food hypersensitivity in children. *Allergy Proc* 1992;13:285.

Businco L, Sampson HA (editors): International symposium on atopic dermatitis: An update. *Allergy* 1989; 44(suppl 9):1.

Charlesworth EN: Practical approaches to the treatment of atopic dermatitis. *Allergy Proc* 1994;15:269.

Friedmann PS et al: Pathogenesis and management of atopic dermatitis. *Clin Exp Allergy* 1995;25:799.

Hanifin JM: Atopic dermatitis. *J Allergy Clin Immunol* 1984; 73:211.

Jones SM, Sampson HA: The role of allergens in atopic dermatitis. *Clin Rev Allergy* 1993;11:471.

Kapp A: Atopic dermatitis-The skin manifestations of atopy. *Clin Exp Allergy* 1995;25:210.

Leung DY: Atopic dermatitis: The skin as a window into the pathogenesis of chronic allergic diseases. *J Allergy Clin Immunol* 1995;96:302.

Morren MS et al: Atopic dermatitis: Triggering factors. *J Am Acad Dermatol* 1994;1:467.

ALLERGIC GASTROENTEROPATHY

Gryboski JD: Gastrointestinal aspects of cow's milk protein intolerance and allergy. *Immunol Allergy Clin North Am* 1991;11:773.

Min K-U, Metcalfe DD: Eosinophilic gastroenteritis. *Immunol Allergy Clin North Am* 1991;11:799.

Scudamore HH et al: Food allergy manifested by eosinophilia, elevated immunoglobulin E level, and protein-losing enteropathy: The syndrome of allergic gastroenteropathy. *J Allergy Clin Immunol* 1982;70:129.

27 Anaphylaxis & Urticaria

Abba I. Terr, MD

The atopic diseases, discussed in the previous chapter, are characterized by a genetic predisposition to the production of IgE antibodies to common environmental antigens. Anaphylaxis and urticaria also are caused by **IgE antibodies,** but they lack the genetically determined propensity and the target organ hyperresponsiveness of atopy, and they have no special predilection for the atopic individual. The immunologic pathogenesis for all IgE-mediated diseases is the same, but separate consideration of atopic and nonatopic diseases is important clinically. Differences exist in the allergens, mode of exposure to the allergen, genetic factors that influence etiology, diagnostic methods, prognosis, and treatment.

Allergic gastroenteropathy, described in Chapter 26, has features of anaphylaxis, but it is included in the chapter on atopic diseases because it occurs almost exclusively in patients with other atopic manifestations.

ANAPHYLAXIS

Major Immunologic Features
- Occurrence of an acute IgE-mediated reaction simultaneously in multiple organs.
- Usual allergen is a drug, insect venom, or food.
- Reaction can be evoked by a minute quantity of allergen; potentially fatal.

General Considerations
A. Definitions: Anaphylaxis is an acute, generalized allergic reaction with simultaneous involvement of several organ systems, usually **cardiovascular, respiratory, cutaneous,** and **gastrointestinal.** The reaction is immunologically mediated, and it occurs on exposure to an allergen to which the subject had previously been sensitized. **Anaphylactic shock** refers to anaphylaxis in which hypotension, with or without loss of consciousness, occurs. **Anaphylactoid reaction** is a condition in which the symptoms and signs of anaphylaxis occur in the absence of an allergen–antibody mechanism. In this case, the endogenous mediators of anaphylaxis are released in vivo through a nonimmunologic mechanism.

B. Epidemiology: Anaphylaxis has no known geographic, racial, or sex predilection. It occurs at the rate of 0.4 cases per million per year in the general population. In the hospitalized population the prevalence is reported to be 0.03–0.06 per 1000 patients, showing that medications and biologic products are a major cause. The disease causes an estimated 500 deaths per year in the United States.

C. Pathology: Grossly, urticaria and angioedema occur. The lungs are diffusely hyperinflated, with mucus plugging of airways and focal atelectasis. The **microscopic** appearance of the lungs is similar to that in acute asthma, with hypersecretion of bronchial mucus, mucosal and submucosal edema, peribronchial vascular congestion, eosinophilia in the bronchial walls, pulmonary edema and hemorrhage, bronchial muscle spasm, hyperinflation, and even rupture of alveoli. Other important features are edema, vascular congestion, and eosinophilia in the lamina propria of the larynx, trachea, epiglottis, and hypopharynx. Myocardial ischemia has been found in a high proportion of cases, probably secondary to shock. Occasionally, myocardial infarction occurs. A direct effect of anaphylaxis on the myocardium or coronary arteries has not been shown. The liver, spleen, and other visceral organs are often grossly congested and microscopically hyperemic and edematous with eosinophilia. Eosinophils are found in the splenic sinusoids, liver, and elsewhere.

Death is usually attributable to asphyxiation from upper airway edema and congestion, irreversible shock, or a combination of these factors. Death may occur after many hours of shock from the effects of the failure of other organs.

D. Immunologic Pathogenesis: Anaphylaxis requires the presence of IgE antibodies and exposure to the allergen, but it is clear that it occurs in only a very small proportion of patients satisfying these requirements. In some cases the mode and quantity of allergen exposure are important, as in the inadvertent injection of allergens to atopic persons.

Anaphylaxis is the systemic manifestation of the allergen–IgE antibody mast cell-mediator release mechanism detailed in Chapter 13. The result is a sudden profound and life-threatening alteration in functioning of the various vital organs. Vascular collapse, acute airway obstruction, cutaneous vasodilation and edema, and gastrointestinal and genitourinary muscle spasm occur almost simultaneously, although not always to the same degree.

E. Anaphylactic Shock: Hypotension and shock in anaphylaxis reflect generalized vasodilatation of arterioles and increased vascular permeability with rapid transudation of plasma through postcapillary venules. This shift of fluid from intravascular to extravascular spaces produces hypovolemic ("distributive") shock with edema (angioedema) in skin and various visceral organs, pooling of venous blood (especially in the splanchnic bed), hemoconcentration, and increased blood viscosity. Low cardiac output diminishes cardiac return and produces inadequate coronary artery perfusion. Low peripheral vascular resistance can lead to myocardial hypoxia, dysrhythmias, and secondary cardiogenic shock. Stimulation of histamine H_1 receptors in coronary arteries may cause coronary artery spasm. Some patients experience anginal chest pains and, occasionally, myocardial infarction during anaphylaxis. After a prolonged period of shock, organ failure elsewhere may ensue, particularly of the kidneys and central nervous system. In some cases shock occurs rapidly before extensive fluid shifts would be expected to take place, suggesting that neurogenic reflex mechanisms might be involved.

F. Urticaria and Angioedema: Histamine and other mediators stimulate receptors in superficial cutaneous blood vessels, causing the swelling, erythema, and itching that characterize urticaria, a hallmark cutaneous feature of systemic anaphylaxis. Increased permeability of subcutaneous blood vessels causes the more diffuse swelling of angioedema, which may account for a substantial volume of fluid loss from the intravascular compartment.

G. Lower Respiratory Obstruction: Bronchial muscle spasm, edema and eosinophilic inflammation of the bronchial mucosa, and hypersecretion of mucus into the airway lumen occur in some patients with anaphylaxis. Histamine and leukotrienes are bronchoconstrictors, the former affecting the larger proximal airways preferentially, and the latter the peripheral airways. Airway obstruction leads to impaired gas exchange and hypoxia. If untreated, acute cor pulmonale and respiratory failure may ensue.

H. Other Effects: Histamine causes gastrointestinal and uterine smooth muscle spasm. Hageman factor-dependent pathways may be activated by basophil and mast cell enzymes during anaphylaxis. One such enzyme has kallikrein activity and has been called basophil kallikrein of anaphylaxis, cleaving bradykinin from high-molecular-weight kininogen. Bradykinin has potent vascular permeability, vasodilating, smooth muscle-contracting, and pain-inducing properties, and it is occasionally found in anaphylactic states. Hageman factor activation of the intrinsic clotting mechanism may explain some of the coagulation abnormalities found in systemic anaphylaxis.

Clinical Features

A. Symptoms and Signs: Exposure to the allergen may be through ingestion, injection, inhalation, or contact with skin or mucous membrane. The reaction begins within seconds or minutes after exposure to the allergen. An initial feeling of fright or sense of impending doom may occur, followed rapidly by symptoms in one or more target organ systems: cardiovascular, respiratory, cutaneous, and gastrointestinal.

The **cardiovascular** response may be peripheral or central. Hypotension and shock occur from generalized arteriolar vasodilatation and increased vascular permeability, thereby lowering blood volume. In some patients without previous heart disease, cardiac arrhythmias may occur. Without prompt intravascular fluid replacement, prolonged shock may lead to the failure of vital organs. Death can result from blood volume depletion and irreversible shock or from a cardiac arrhythmia.

The **respiratory** tract at all levels may be involved. Nasal congestion from swelling and hyperemia of the nasal mucosa and profuse watery rhinorrhea with itching of the nose and palate simulate an acute hay fever reaction. The hypopharynx and larynx are especially susceptible, and obstruction of this critical portion of the airway by edema is responsible for some of the respiratory deaths. Bronchial obstruction from bronchospasm, mucosal edema, and hypersecretion of mucus results in an asthma-like paroxysm of wheezing dyspnea. Obstruction of the smaller airways by mucus may lead to respiratory failure.

The **skin** is a frequent target, with generalized pruritus, erythema, urticaria, and angioedema (especially the eyelids, lips, tongue, pharynx, and larynx). The conjunctival and oropharyngeal mucosae are erythematous and edematous. Urticaria may persist for many weeks.

Gastrointestinal involvement causes crampy abdominal pain and sometimes nausea or diarrhea. Similarly, **uterine** muscle contraction may cause pelvic pain. Spontaneous abortion can result if the patient is pregnant.

Hemostatic changes can occur but are not often detected clinically. The intrinsic coagulation pathway is activated, resulting in the possibility of disseminated intravascular coagulation (DIC) and depletion of clotting factors. Thrombocytopenia may occur, possibly because platelets aggregated by platelet-activating factor (PAF) are sequestered from the circulation. In some cases, circulating heparin or other anticoagulants have been demonstrated.

Convulsions, with or without shock, have been reported rarely. In cases of fatal anaphylaxis, death usually occurs within 1 hour of onset.

B. Laboratory Findings: Laboratory tests are seldom necessary or helpful initially, although certain tests may be used later to assess and monitor treatment and to detect complications. Immediate emergency treatment should never be delayed pending results of laboratory studies. The blood cell counts may be elevated because of hemoconcentration. Eosinophil counts may be elevated but are usually normal or low because of compensatory mechanisms. Chest x-ray films shows hyperinflation, with or without atelectasis caused by airway mucus plugging. The electrocardiogram may show a variety of abnormalities, including conduction abnormalities, atrial or ventricular dysrhythmias, ST-T wave changes of myocardial ischemia or injury, and acute cor pulmonale. Myocardial infarction may be evidenced by electrocardiographic and serum enzyme changes. Plasma histamine and serum tryptase levels may be elevated.

Clinical Diagnosis

The diagnosis in a patient observed during an acute attack should be established or suspected as rapidly as possible by the symptoms and physical findings. Appropriate treatment should be instituted as soon as the condition is suspected. After the reaction is successfully treated, diagnostic efforts are directed at finding the cause.

Immunologic Diagnosis

The history is essential in determining the allergen responsible for an anaphylactic reaction. Skin testing or in vitro tests establish the presence of an IgE immune response to an allergen consistent with the history. Ingestion of a food or drug; parenteral administration of a drug, vaccine, blood product, or other biologic material; or an insect sting occurring shortly (usually 1 hour or less) before the onset of symptoms are likely causes. If the patient has experienced more than one episode, evidence of exposure to a common allergen should be sought.

Identification of the specific allergen may require persistent detective work. A reaction to drinking milk may be caused by penicillin contamination. A reaction to a viral vaccine may be caused by egg white from the egg embryo in which the virus was cultured.

The diagnosis is confirmed by detecting the presence of **IgE antibody** to the suspected allergen. In most cases, the immediate wheal-and-flare skin test is the most reliable procedure, especially if the allergen is a protein (see Chapter 21). Systemic reactions to skin tests have occurred in highly sensitive individuals, so testing should be done initially by the cutaneous prick method. If the test is negative, intradermal testing to diluted sterile extracts of known potency can then be done.

To minimize the risk of anaphylaxis from the skin test itself, serial titration testing with tenfold-increasing concentrations of allergen is recommended when testing with protein allergens. Table 27–1 lists several recommended starting concentrations.

Skin testing in cases of suspected anaphylaxis from venom of Hymenoptera insects has been shown

Table 27–1. Starting intracutaneous skin test concentrations.

Allergen	Starting Concentration
Hymenoptera venoms	0.001 µg/mL
Insulin	0.001 U/mL
Horse serum	1:1000 dilution

to be reliable if freshly reconstituted lyophilized venom extracts are used for testing. Testing with standard food extracts may yield false-negative reactions if the allergen is labile. Prick testing with direct application of the food itself to the skin may yield a positive test, but some foods contain vasoactive chemicals that may produce false-positive reactions.

Skin testing with haptenic drugs is generally not reliable except for penicillin (see Chapter 30). Certain drugs cause nonspecific histamine release, producing a wheal-and-flare reaction in normal individuals (Table 27–2). Immunologic activation of mast cells requires a polyvalent allergen, so a negative skin test to a univalent haptenic drug does not rule out anaphylactic sensitivity to that drug.

In vitro tests to detect the presence of circulating IgE antibody may be helpful if the test is positive, but a negative result does not rule out anaphylactic sensitivity, because the high affinity of IgE antibodies for mast cell receptors may result in a level of circulating IgE antibodies too low for detection by in vitro methods. The radioallergosorbent test (RAST) is the most frequently used in vitro test for IgE antibody, but it can be used only for protein allergens. Technical factors account for a significant number of false-positive and false-negative results (see Chapter 26).

The presence of IgE antibodies detected by skin or in vitro test does not diagnose the cause of anaphylaxis without correlation with the patient's history.

Allergens

The allergens responsible for anaphylaxis are different from those commonly associated with atopy. They are usually encountered in a food, a drug, or an insect sting. Foods and insect venoms are complex mixtures of many potential allergens. In only a few cases have the allergens been identified chemically. The same allergen or allergenic epitope may exist naturally in more than one food, drug, or venom, resulting in cross-reactivity.

A. Foods: Any food can contain an allergen that could cause anaphylaxis. Table 27–3 lists some of the more common ones. The most frequent are peanut,

Table 27–2. Some drugs that cause nonspecific wheal-and-flare skin reactions.

Aspirin	Meperidine
Codeine	Morphine
Curare	Polymyxin B
Histamine	Stilbamidine
Hydralazine	

Table 27–3. Some foods that cause anaphylaxis

Crustaceans	Seeds
Lobster	Sesame
Shrimp	Cottonseed
Crab	Caraway
Mollusks	Mustard
Clams	Flaxseed
Fish	Sunflower
Legumes	**Nuts**
Peanut	Berries
Pea	Egg white
Beans	Buckwheat
Licorice	Milk

tree nuts, and shellfish in adults; and milk, egg, and peanut in children.

B. Drugs: Any drug is capable of causing anaphylaxis, although the risk is minimal for most people. Table 27–4 lists drugs and diagnostic agents reported most frequently. Heterologous proteins and polypeptides are the most likely to induce this type of sensitivity. Most drugs used today are organic chemicals, however, which function immunologically as haptens. The rapid and uncontrolled use of herbal and other "natural" remedies that contain foreign proteins of plant source can be expected to produce more allergic—including anaphylactic—reactions. Anaphylaxis can occur from parenteral, oral, or topical drug administration. In some cases the amount needed to cause a systemic reaction can be extremely small; for example, a reaction in penicillin-allergic patients has been produced by minute amounts of

Table 27–4. Some drugs and diagnostic agents that cause anaphylaxis.

Heterologous proteins and polypeptides	Haptenic drugs
Hormones	Antibiotics
Insulin	Penicillin
Parathormone	Streptomycin
Adrenocorticotropic	Cephalosporin
hormone	Tetracycline
Vasopressin	Amphotericin B
Relaxin	Nitrofurantoin
Enzymes	Diagnostic agents
Trypsin	Sulfobromophthalein
Chymotrypsin	Sodium dehydrocholate
Chymopapain	Vitamins
Penicillinase	Thiamine
Asparaginase	Folic acid
Vaccines	Others
Toxoids	Barbiturates
Allergy extracts	Nonsteroidal antiinflammatory drugs
Polysaccharides	Corticosteroids
Dextran	Diazepam
Iron-dextran	Phenytoin
Acacia	Protamine
	N-Acetylcysteine
	Methotrexate
	Cisplatin
	Cyclosporine
	Azathioprine

penicillin in the milk obtained from penicillin-treated cows.

Anaphylaxis to blood and blood components may be caused by food allergens in donor blood or, rarely, by passive transfer of IgE antibodies to a food or drug when the transfusion recipient ingests that allergen shortly before or after the transfusion.

C. Insect Venoms: Anaphylaxis occurs from stings of Hymenoptera insects (Table 27–5), occasionally from biting insects such as ticks, deer flies, kissing bugs, and bedbugs, and rarely from snake venom. The venom of Hymenoptera insects is a complex biologic fluid containing several enzymes and other active constituents. There are multiple allergens for human anaphylaxis, some specific to a particular species and others cross-reactive among species and genera. Allergens in honeybee venom include phospholipase A, hyaluronidase, phosphatase, and melittin.

The sting of a single insect is sufficient to produce a severe, even fatal, anaphylactic reaction in sensitive patients. Sensitization occurs from prior stings, and if patients are allergic to a common or cross-reacting antigen they may have an anaphylactic reaction after being stung by any species of Hymenoptera insect. There is no evidence that other allergic diseases, including atopy and drug anaphylaxis, predispose to Hymenoptera anaphylaxis. Anaphylaxis immediately following the sting of one or a few Hymenoptera insects is easily distinguished from the toxic effect of envenomation by hundreds of insect stings occurring simultaneously. Toxicity from the large quantities of venom in the latter circumstance causes hemolysis, rhabdomyolysis, and acute renal failure.

D. Other Allergens: Several cases of anaphylaxis have occurred in women during intercourse because of allergy to a glycoprotein allergen in the partner's seminal fluid. There is one report of a woman sensitized to exogenous progesterone administered as a drug. She subsequently had anaphylaxis to endogenous progesterone and was cured by oophorectomy.

Latex allergy is now a recognized cause of anaphylaxis, as well as urticaria, asthma, and allergic contact dermatitis. First reported in 1927, prevalence has rapidly increased since 1989, probably because of the increasing need for universal precautions by medical and dental personnel for protection against HIV infection, as well as the occupational use of latex gloves by food handlers and others. High-risk groups are those who require contact with the allergen: all health care workers, some rubber industry

Table 27–5. Hymenoptera insects.

Honeybee (*Apis mellifera*)
Yellow jacket (*Vespula* spp)
Hornet (*Dolichovespula* spp)
Wasp (*Polistes* spp)
Fire ant (*Solenopsis* spp)

workers, and patients who have had multiple surgical operations, especially children with spina bifida, myelomeningocele, and urogenital defects.

Natural rubber latex allergens are derived from the rubber tree *Hevea brasiliense*. Sensitization is detected by either skin testing or enzyme-linked immunosorbent assay (ELISA), but the diagnosis requires confirmation of the test results by the patient's history. Current estimates are that 1% of the general population and 10–17% of health care workers are sensitized. Powdered latex gloves provide a source for airborne allergen because the allergen adheres to the corn starch powder. Inhaling the airborne allergen-containing powder may cause asthma. Some patients react also to eating certain fruits such as kiwi and avocado because of cross-reacting allergens.

Anaphylactoid Reactions

A reaction clinically and pathologically identical to anaphylaxis can occur without the participation of an IgE antibody and corresponding allergen. This phenomenon is called an anaphylactoid reaction. (The term *anaphylactoid* is sometimes used inappropriately to refer to a mild IgE-mediated anaphylactic reaction.)

A. Exercise-Induced "Anaphylaxis": A number of cases have been described. In some, the reaction occurs only in association with eating, sometimes related to a specific food. During exercise the plasma histamine level rises, suggesting that nonimmunologic mast cell stimulation might be triggered by an endogenous factor, possibly endorphin. The reason for individual susceptibility is unknown, although a familial tendency has been reported, possibly because of a genetic defect. Many cases, however, are transient, suggesting a role for acquired factors.

B. Cholinergic Anaphylactoid Reaction: Exercise, emotions, and overheating provoke reactions in patients with this rare condition. The plasma histamine level rises when the core body temperature increases. Patients may have a positive methacholine urticarial skin test. A proposed mechanism is an abnormal reactivity of mast cells to the compensatory cholinergic response in thermoregulation when the core body temperature is elevated. This disease is an exaggerated form of cholinergic urticaria, described later in this chapter.

C. "Aggregate Anaphylaxis": Administration of immunoglobulins for prophylaxis in patients with common variable immunodeficiency or other immunodeficiency diseases can cause anaphylactoid reactions. High-molecular-weight aggregated gamma globulin is probably responsible because immunoglobulin aggregates can activate complement through the classic pathway. Ultracentrifugation of the preparation to eliminate aggregates prevents such reactions. Aggregated immunoglobulins generate anaphylatoxins C3a, C4a, and C5a from the parent complement components C3, C4, and C5, respec-

tively, in a manner similar to the effect of antigen and corresponding specific IgG or IgM complement-activating antibodies. Anaphylatoxins can activate mast cells for mediator release, thereby producing the reaction.

D. Non-IgE Anaphylaxis: Some patients with selective absence of IgA produce IgG anti-IgA antibodies following transfusion of IgA-containing plasma in whole blood or blood products. In such patients, subsequent administration of transfused IgA may cause anaphylaxis, presumably from complement activation and anaphylatoxin generation by circulating complexes of IgA and anti-IgA. An alternative explanation involves antibodies of the IgG4 subclass. It has been reported that IgG4 antibodies can activate mast cells for mediator release in the presence of antigen. There is no direct proof yet that IgG4 "short-term sensitizing" antibodies are involved in systemic anaphylaxis.

E. Anaphylactoid Reactions from Ionic Compounds: Radiographic iodinated contrast media, especially that used for intravenous pyelography or cholangiography, produce anaphylactoid reactions that are frequently mild, causing only hives or itching. They may be severe, however, causing shock. In one case in 100,000, these reactions are fatal. The reaction can occur on first exposure and does not necessarily recur on subsequent exposure. Attempts to demonstrate specific antibodies to the compounds have been unrewarding. The reaction may be related to the ionic nature of these compounds because newer nonionic contrast media appear less likely to cause such reactions.

The antibiotic polymyxin B is also a highly charged ionic compound that causes anaphylactoid reactions in some patients.

F. Other Causes: Polysaccharides such as dextran, gums, and resins produce anaphylactoid reactions by unknown mechanisms, probably through direct mast cell activation. Certain drugs, especially the opiates, curare, and *d*-tubocurarine, behave similarly (Table 27–6).

G. Idiopathic Anaphylaxis: A few patients experience recurrent attacks of anaphylaxis without evidence of exposure to an antecedent allergen. Exhaus-

Table 27–6. Drugs and additives that cause anaphylactoid reactions.

Nonsteroidal antiinflammatory drugs	Opiate narcotics
Aspirin	Morphine
Aminopyrine	Codeine
Fenoprofen	Meperidine
Flufenamic acid	
Ibuprofen	Mannitol
Indomethacin	Radiographic iodinated contrast media
Mefenamic acid	Curare and *d*-tubocurarine
Naproxen	Dextran
Tolmetin	
Zomepirac	

tive exploration of the history and careful observation of subsequent attacks sometimes reveal an unsuspected allergen, but most of these cases appear to be truly idiopathic. Recurrent idiopathic anaphylaxis, like idiopathic chronic urticaria–angioedema, occurs predominantly in women between 20 and 60 years of age.

Differential Diagnosis

Anaphylactic and anaphylactoid reactions are identical in presentation. The former is produced by an antigen–antibody reaction, whereas the latter is caused by nonimmunologic release of mediators, so that the distinction must be determined by demonstrating whether the causative substance is an allergen.

Other causes of circulatory failure include primary cardiac failure, endotoxin shock, and reflex mechanisms. The most common one misdiagnosed as anaphylactic shock is **vasovagal collapse,** which may occur from the injection of local anaesthetics, particularly during dental procedures. In this case, presentation includes pallor without cyanosis, nausea, bradycardia, and an absence of respiratory obstruction and cutaneous manifestations.

The **Jarisch–Herxheimer reaction** takes place several hours after antimicrobial treatment of syphilis or onchocerciasis. It is characterized by fever, shaking chills, myalgias, headaches, and hypotension. Unlike anaphylaxis, it can be prevented by pretreatment with corticosteroids.

Aspirin and nonsteroidal antiinflammatory drugs affect a certain subset of asthmatic patients, producing an acute asthmatic reaction that may include nasal congestion, erythema, facial swelling, and shock. Sulfite additives in certain foods and drugs may affect some asthmatics with a similar anaphylactic-like reaction. Exercise-induced anaphylaxis must be differentiated from the exertional collapse that occurs in some patients with sickle cell trait.

Treatment

Treatment of anaphylaxis and anaphylactoid reactions is the same. It must be started promptly, so a high index of suspicion is necessary, and the diagnosis must be made rapidly. Once suspected, **aqueous epinephrine,** 1:1000 solution, is injected intramuscularly or subcutaneously in a dose of 0.2–0.5 mL for adults or 0.01 mL/kg of body weight for children. The dose is repeated in 15–30 minutes, if necessary. If the reaction was caused by an insect sting or injected drug, 0.1–0.2 mL of epinephrine, 1:1000 solution, can be infiltrated locally to retard absorption of the residual allergen. In a patient receiving a β-adrenergic-blocking drug, anaphylaxis may be resistant to epinephrine, so that higher doses may be required. A tourniquet should be applied proximally if the injection or sting is on an extremity. The patient should then be examined quickly but thoroughly to assess the involved target organs, so that subsequent treatment is appropriate to the pathophysiologic abnormalities.

A. Shock: The aim is similar to treating any patient in shock: support of the circulation and maintenance of the airway. The patient should be recumbent with the legs elevated in Trendelenberg's position. An intravenous line, preferably by catheter, facilitates drug administration. Intravenous epinephrine can be given in a dose of 1–5 mL, 1:10,000 solution, for adults and 0.01–0.05 mL/kg for children if systolic blood pressure is below 60 mmHg. Other vasopressor drugs, such as dopamine or glucagon, can be administered while blood pressure and pulse rate are being monitored. Patients who are taking β-blockers, even in the form of eyedrops, are refractory to sympathomimetic drugs such as epinephrine, but they will respond to glucagon. The specific treatment for shock, however, is fluid infused rapidly. Normal saline may be satisfactory, although as much as 6 L or more in 12 hours may be necessary. Initially, 1 L should be given every 15–30 minutes while vital signs and urine output are monitored. Plasma or other colloid solutions might be required. It may be necessary to monitor fluid replacement by measuring central venous pressure.

B. Laryngeal Edema: Examination of the airway for the presence of laryngeal obstruction should be done early. Establishing an effective airway is lifesaving. Passage of an endotracheal tube may be difficult because of the swelling. Puncture of the cricothyroid membrane with a 14- or 16-gauge short needle provides an airway, but it is too dangerous to attempt in a child. Cricothyrotomy is the preferred method if treatment must be done outside a hospital. In the hospital, surgical tracheostomy is preferred.

C. Bronchial Obstruction: Epinephrine is a highly effective and rapid bronchodilator, but if bronchospasm persists, nebulized β-adrenergic bronchodilators can be given by intermittent positive-pressure breathing. Hydrocortisone or methylprednisolone injections intramuscularly or intravenously are used if the patient has recently received steroid therapy. Oxygen by nasal catheter at 4–6 L/min is necessary if Pa_{CO_2} is less than 55 mm Hg. In the event of respiratory failure with Pa_{CO_2} above 65 mm Hg, intubation and mechanical assistance of ventilation are necessary.

D. Urticaria, Angioedema, and Gastrointestinal Reactions: These manifestations are not lifethreatening and respond well to antihistamines. If they are mild, an oral antihistamine tablet is adequate. If they are severe, diphenhydramine, 50 mg (1–2 mg/kg for children), can be given intramuscularly or intravenously.

Monitoring treatment is vital in severe cases of anaphylaxis. Measurement of vital signs, examination of upper and lower airway potency, measurement of arterial blood gases and pH, and electrocardiography are best accomplished in the emergency room or intensive care unit. All patients should be observed for 24 hours after satisfactory treatment, except in very mild cases. Histamine H_2 receptor-blocking drugs, such as cimetidine or ranitidine, have been advocated as an adjunct to H_1 receptor antagonists, but their effectiveness has yet to be proved. Corticosteroid drugs have no anti-anaphylactic actions and should not be expected to alleviate the immediate acute life-threatening manifestations, although there may be special indications, as already noted. Complications such as cardiac arrhythmias, hypoxic seizures, and metabolic acidosis are treated in the usual way.

The management of anaphylaxis from a Hymenoptera insect sting is the same as for any anaphylactic reaction. In honeybee stings, the venom sac and stinger usually remain in the skin and should be removed promptly by scraping with a knife or fingernail. Local reactions usually require only cold compresses to ease pain and reduce swelling, but extensive local inflammation may require brief corticosteroid therapy.

Prevention

A. Avoidance: Once the diagnosis of anaphylaxis has been established and the cause has been determined, prevention of future episodes is essential. In the case of food or drug allergy, the allergen and potential cross-reacting allergens must be thoroughly avoided. Hospitals and other health care facilities can institute measures to reduce airborne latex allergens in the workplace. Insect-sensitive patients should avoid outdoor food and garbage, flowers, perfumes, mowing the lawn, and walking barefoot outdoors. Pretreatment with antihistamines and corticosteroids prior to radiography requiring administration of a contrast medium reduces the risk of a reaction in patients who have experienced a prior radiographic anaphylactoid reaction. Patients with IgA deficiency who require blood products should be transfused from donors with absent IgA (see Chapter 21).

Any physician or nurse who administers drugs by injection should be prepared to treat a possible anaphylactic reaction by having appropriate drugs available, and patients should remain under observation for 15–20 minutes after any injection.

B. Anaphylaxis Kit: Patients with anaphylactic sensitivity to Hymenoptera insects or food should carry at all times a preloaded syringe of epinephrine in one of the commercially available preparations. Epinephrine or a β-adrenergic drug in a metered-dose inhaler is not a reliable means of protection for anaphylactic shock.

C. Desensitization: Hymenoptera venom desensitization has been shown to be highly effective, as judged by responses to subsequent natural stings. Treatment is recommended for patients who have experienced systemic anaphylaxis after a sting and who have a significant positive skin test to one or more venoms. The maintenance dose for venom desensitization, 100 µg of each venom, is usually achieved in 12 weeks or less on a weekly, or "rush," schedule. It should be continued at intervals of 4–6 weeks. Most patients maintain long-lasting protection after discontinuing the injections following a 5-year course of desensitization.

Insulin-allergic diabetic patients and the occasional penicillin-sensitive patient may require desensitization.

Complications

Death from laryngeal edema, respiratory failure, shock, or cardiac arrhythmia usually occurs within minutes after onset of the reaction, but in occasional cases irreversible shock persists for hours. Permanent brain damage may result from the hypoxia of respiratory or cardiovascular failure. Urticaria or angioedema may recur for months after penicillin anaphylaxis. Myocardial infarction, abortion, and renal failure are other potential complications.

Prognosis

It is usually assumed that in anaphylaxis each succeeding exposure results in a more severe reaction. Experience with cases of anaphylaxis to penicillin, Hymenoptera venom, and food indicates that this not necessarily the case, however. If sufficient time elapses without allergen exposure, some patients may experience a decrease or loss of sensitivity. There is no method to predict changes in sensitivity, but it can sometimes be documented by periodic testing. Immunotherapy for stinging-insect sensitivity is strikingly effective in favorably altering the prognosis, and desensitization can occasionally abrogate penicillin anaphylaxis for a short time to permit the drug to be used safely. The prognosis must always be guarded by the knowledge that IgE immunologic memory may be lifelong. Anaphylactoid drug reactions follow various courses. Patients who react adversely to radiographic iodinated contrast media usually tolerate subsequent exposure to the same contrast medium without reaction, but statistically a reaction is more likely to occur in a patient who had experienced a prior reaction.

URTICARIA & ANGIOEDEMA

Major Immunologic Features

- Acute form usually from IgE-mediated allergies to foods or drugs.
- Chronic or recurrent disease usually nonimmunologic and of unknown cause.

General Considerations

Urticaria (also known as hives) and angioedema (also known as angioneurotic edema) can be considered a single illness characterized by vasodilatation and increased vascular permeability of the skin (urticaria) or subcutaneous tissues (angioedema). It is a localized cutaneous form of anaphylaxis and is one of the manifestations of systemic anaphylaxis. The same **IgE antibody** mechanism is responsible for the pathogenesis of allergic urticaria–angioedema and for that of systemic anaphylaxis, and the causative allergens are very similar. Idiopathic (nonallergic) urticaria–angioedema is analogous to the anaphylactoid reaction. In contrast to anaphylaxis, urticaria is a benign condition and is much more common.

A. Epidemiology: Urticaria affects about 20% of the population at least once during a lifetime, usually as a single or occasional acute attack.

B. Pathology: A variety of histopathologic lesions have been described, but these correlate poorly with the clinical presentation. They include edema, nonnecrotizing vasculitis, necrotizing vasculitis, perivasculitis, and a variety of different inflammatory reactions in the skin.

C. Pathogenesis: Urticaria and angioedema are the visible manifestations of localized cutaneous or subcutaneous edema from the increased permeability of blood vessels, probably postcapillary venules. Because injection of histamine into the skin produces the spontaneous wheal, erythema, and pruritus similar or identical to a typical urticarial lesion, it is generally accepted that endogenous histamine liberation is the mechanism responsible for the disease. The fact that subcutaneous tissue is looser and contains fewer nerve endings explains the more diffuse swelling and less severe itching in angioedema. Elevated levels of histamine in venous blood draining areas of induced urticaria have been repeatedly demonstrated. Other mediators from mast cells, particularly leukotrienes, are also believed to contribute to the pathophysiology. The role of cytokines and other endogenous chemicals in mediating and modulating the disease has yet to be explored.

D. Immunologic Pathogenesis: Many cases of acute urticaria and angioedema have been shown to have an allergic cause. In these cases, allergen-specific IgE antibody fixed to local mast cells triggers mediator release or activation when allergen is encountered. Other potential immunologic pathways for mast cell mediator liberation, for example, the complement-derived anaphylatoxin pathway, have not been shown to operate in this disease. Idiopathic urticaria–angioedema and the various physical urticarias described later on lack an allergen–antibody etiology. The precise means by which cutaneous mast cells are stimulated under these circumstances is unknown.

Clinical Features

A. Symptoms and Signs: Urticaria appears as multiple areas of well-demarcated edematous plaques that are intensely pruritic. They are either white with surrounding erythema or red with blanching when stretched. Individual lesions vary in diameter from a few millimeters to many centimeters. They are circular or serpiginous. Regardless of the duration of the illness, individual lesions are evanescent, lasting from 1 to 48 hours. They may appear anywhere on the skin surface but often have a predilection for areas of pressure. Angioedema appears as diffuse areas of nondependent, nonpitting swelling without pruritus, with predilection for the face, especially the periorbital and perioral areas. Swelling can occur in the mouth and pharynx as well. Abdominal pain may indicate angioedema of the gut.

Acute urticaria lasts for a few hours or at most a few days and is most likely to be associated with an identifiable cause, including allergy, nonspecific drug effect, infection, or physical factors. Chronic or recurrent urticaria persists with a variable course over a period of many weeks to years. Urticaria and angioedema may appear together in the same patient.

B. Laboratory Findings: There are no abnormal laboratory tests, except for the specific procedures described in a later section.

Clinical Diagnosis

The diagnosis is immediately apparent on inspection of the skin.

Immunologic Diagnosis

A complete medical and environmental history and physical examination are usually necessary to determine the cause. Allergic urticaria may arise from exposure to allergens by ingestion or injection (most commonly), direct skin contact (less frequently), and inhalation (rarely). The discussion on common allergies in anaphylaxis earlier in this chapter applies to acute allergic urticaria.

Food allergy is diagnosed by careful dietary history, use of elimination diets, and appropriate food challenges. Drug allergy requires close scrutiny of the patient's recent drug history, elimination of suspected drugs, and occasionally deliberate challenge, although skin testing is helpful for certain drugs such as penicillin. The diagnosis of cold urticaria is made by applying an ice cube to the forearm for 5 minutes and observing localized urticaria after the skin has been rewarmed. Similar tests with application of heat, ultraviolet light, vibration, pressure, or water to a test area of the skin are appropriate if the history suggests these causes.

Cholinergic urticaria is suggested by the typical appearance of the lesions and exercise provocation. The methacholine skin test is positive in only one third of patients.

Diagnostic tests for parasitic or other infections, lymphomas or other neoplasms, or connective tissue diseases are generally indicated if the history and physical examination would have suggested such diseases in the absence of urticaria. It should be emphasized that in most cases of chronic recurrent urticaria, no cause is found even with the most diligent search.

Causes

A. Allergy: Ingestant allergens are much more frequent causes of urticaria than are inhalants. Any food or drug can cause hives. Occult sources of drugs including proprietary medications, such as laxatives, headache remedies, and vitamin preparations, must be considered. Food and drug additives are occasionally responsible. Insect sting allergy may cause urticaria without any other signs of systemic anaphylaxis.

Skin contact urticaria is an uncommon response in which localized urticaria is provoked on contact with the allergen, such as a food or the house dust mite. The urticaria may then become generalized.

B. Physical Causes: Dermographism, the whealing reaction that is an exaggerated form of the triple response of Lewis, occurs following scratching or stroking of the skin in 5% of the population. Another common phenomenon, unrelated to dermographism, is the appearance of hives after showering.

Cold urticaria may be induced locally by cooling of the skin on contact with cold. The hives often appear only on rewarming. Occasionally generalized hives are provoked by cooling a portion of the body. Patients are in danger of shock when swimming in cold water. The diagnostic ice cube test was described earlier. Occasionally the reaction can be passively transferred by serum to the skin of an unaffected individual.

Familial cold urticaria is a rare autosomal-dominant disorder in which cold produces fever, chills, joint pains, and hives.

Urticaria and angioedema induced by heat, sunlight, water, or vibration are different syndromes and are rare. **Pressure urticaria** is a common feature of all forms of urticaria. Delayed-pressure urticaria resulting from prolonged sustained pressure producing painful swelling is a distinct entity, however.

Cholinergic urticaria is a disease of unknown cause in which small (1–3 mm) wheals with prominent surrounding flare appear after exercise, heat, or emotional stress. Elevated body temperature is necessary for the reaction, which is believed to be initiated by a cholinergic response that triggers mast cell release. Other symptoms, including hypotension and gastrointestinal cramping, may accompany the urticaria and angioedema.

C. Vasculitis: Urticaria is reported as a symptom in some patients with systemic lupus erythematosus (SLE), systemic sclerosis, polymyositis, leukocytoclastic vasculitis, palpable purpura, hypocomplementemia, or cryoglobulinemia, but there is as yet no clear explanation for the association.

Because urticaria is so common, its relationship with the primary disease in these cases is most likely coincidental.

D. Neoplasms: Urticaria or angioedema is occasionally reported in a patient with neoplasm, especially Hodgkin's disease and lymphomas, but a cause-and-effect relationship is difficult to document. Rarely, angioedema from C1 esterase inhibitor deficiency is caused by a lymphoma. This is discussed in Chapter 25.

E. Cyclooxygenase Inhibitors: Aspirin and nonsteroidal antiinflammatory drugs frequently precipitate acute or chronic urticaria. They also potentiate idiopathic urticaria or urticaria from other causes. The mechanism is unknown. The belief that food and drug additives, most notably tartrazine yellow dye and the preservative sodium benzoate, also cause or exacerbate hives is not supported by controlled studies.

F. Emotions: Precipitation of hives by emotional stress or other psychologic factors is a frequent clinical observation. Explanation of this phenomenon requires further study.

G. Idiopathic Urticaria-Angioedema: This category encompasses most cases of chronic urticaria-angioedema, because exhaustive diagnostic studies are unrevealing in the large majority of patients with recurrent urticaria lasting for more than 6 weeks.

Differential Diagnosis

The characteristic appearance of urticaria and angioedema, coupled with a history of rapid disappearance of the individual lesions, leaves little chance of incorrect diagnosis.

Multiple insect bites may evoke wheals, but careful inspection shows the bite punctum at the center of the lesion. Angioedema can be distinguished from ordinary edema or myxedema by its absence from dependent areas of localization and by its evanescent appearance.

Hereditary angioedema is a rare condition that produces periodic swelling and may be accompanied by abdominal pain and laryngeal edema. Urticaria does not occur in this disease. The disease is suspected when there is a similar family history of recurrent episodes unrelated to exposure to allergens. The diagnosis is made by finding decreased serum C4 and is confirmed by the absence of C1 esterase inhibitor activity in the serum. It is described in greater detail in Chapter 25.

Urticaria pigmentosa is an infiltration of the skin with multiple mast cell tumors that appear as tan macules that urticate when rubbed or stroked. It may be accompanied by visceral mast cell tumors (systemic mastocytosis).

Treatment

Urticaria caused by foods or drugs is treated by avoidance of the offending agents, although hyposensitization to a drug might be attempted in the rare instances in which no alternative drug is available. Urticaria associated with infection is self-limited if the infection is adequately treated. In cases of physical allergy, protective measures to avoid heat, sunlight, or cold must be advised.

Drug therapy is a useful adjunct in the treatment of all patients, whether or not the cause has been found, but a good response to symptomatic treatment should not deter the physician from efforts to find an underlying cause. Antihistamine drugs are the principal method of treatment, but they must be given in adequate dosage. H_1 receptor antagonists have a proven but inconsistent effectiveness in treating urticaria. The combined use of H_1 and H_2 receptor blockers is frequently recommended but of unproven value for this disease. Epinephrine injections may relieve hives transiently and should be used in treating angioedema involving the pharynx or larynx. Corticosteroids are usually ineffective and should not be used to treat urticaria of unknown cause.

Complications & Prognosis

Urticaria per se is a benign disease. Because allergic urticaria is a cutaneous form of anaphylaxis, it is possible that an excessive dose of allergen could result in life-threatening systemic anaphylaxis. This is also possible in certain cases of physical urticaria. Angioedema can obstruct the airway if localized in the larynx or adjacent structures.

REFERENCES

ANAPHYLAXIS
Briner WW Jr, Sheffer AL: Exercise-induced anaphylaxis. Med Sci Sports Exerc 1992;24:840.

Ditto AM et al: Idiopathic anaphylaxis: A series of 335 cases. Ann Allergy Asthma Immunol 1996;77:285.

Nicklas RA et al: The diagnosis and management of anaphylaxis. J Allergy Clin Immunol 1998;101:S465.

Slater J: Latex allergy-what do we know? J Allergy Clin Immunol 1992;90:3.

Smith PL et al: Physiologic manifestations of human anaphylaxis. J Clin Invest 1980;66:1072.

Steiner DJ, Schwager RG: Epidemiology, diagnosis, precautions, and policies of intraoperative anaphylaxis to latex. J Am Coll Surg 1995;180:754.

Valentine MD: Insect venom allergy: Diagnosis and treatment. J Allergy Clin Immunol 1984;73:299.

URTICARIA & ANGIOEDEMA
Hirschmann JV et al: Cholinergic urticaria. Arch Dermatol 1987;123:462.

Howes LG et al: Angiotensin receptor antagonists and ACE inhibitors. Aust Fam Physician 1998;27:914.

Kauppinen I et al: Yearbook: Urticaria in children: Retrospective evaluation and follow-up. Allergy 1984;39:469.

Leznoff A: Chronic urticaria. Can Fam Physician 1998;44:2170.

Soter NA, Wasserman SI: Physical urticaria/angioedema: An experimental model of mast cells activation in humans. J Allergy Clin Immunol 1980;66:358.

Wanderer AA et al: Clinical characteristics of cold-induced systemic reactions acquired in cold urticaria syndromes: Recommendations for prevention of this complication and a proposal for a diagnostic classification of cold urticaria. J Allergy Clin Immunol 1986;78:417.

28   Immune-Complex Allergic Diseases

Abba I. Terr, MD

This chapter discusses allergic diseases mediated by immune complexes of allergen with IgG or IgM antibodies. Activation of complement by immune complexes generates chemotactic and vasoactive mediators that cause tissue damage by a combination of immune-complex deposition, alterations in vascular permeability and blood flow, and the action of toxic products from inflammatory cells. The pathology of immune complexes has been extensively studied in animals, and the process is detailed in Chapter 13. Tissue injury caused by immune complexes is believed to occur also in certain nonallergic diseases discussed elsewhere in this book. These include systemic lupus erythematosus (see Chapter 31), vasculitis (see Chapter 34), glomerulonephritis (see Chapter 36), rheumatoid arthritis (see Chapter 31), and acute allograft rejection (see Chapter 52).

The classic immune-complex allergic diseases are the cutaneous **Arthus reaction** and systemic **serum sickness.** In **allergic bronchopulmonary aspergillosis** a two-phase immunologic mechanism is involved in which immune complexes of *Aspergillus* antigens and IgG antibodies produce bronchial inflammation and bronchopulmonary tissue destruction in the presence of a concomitant IgE response to the allergen.

THE ARTHUS REACTION

In 1903, Nicholas-Maurice Arthus showed that the intradermal injection of a protein antigen into a hyperimmunized rabbit produced local inflammation that progressed to a hemorrhagic necrotic ulcerating skin lesion. Later investigations established that the Arthus phenomenon is a localized cutaneous inflammatory response to the deposition of immune complexes in dermal blood vessels. It therefore serves as a model system for all immune complex-mediated diseases.

The immunologic pathogenesis depends on antigen and antibody concentrations necessary to form immune complexes capable of initiating complement activation. Intermediate-size complexes activate complement most readily and therefore are the most damaging to tissues. Large insoluble complexes are rapidly cleared by the mononuclear phagocytes,

whereas small complexes fail to activate complement receptors. Immune complexes activate complement through fixation of the Fc portion of antibody to the Fc receptor on C1q. C3a and C5a anaphylatoxins are liberated. These molecules activate mast cells to release permeability factors, permitting localization of the immune complexes along the endothelial cell basement membrane. Chemotactic factors from various complement components attract neutrophils. Neutrophils, macrophages, lymphocytes, and other cells with membrane Fc receptors are activated. The activated neutrophils are especially important in the Arthus reaction. They release toxic chemicals such as oxygen-containing free radicals, generate proteolytic enzymes from cytoplasmic granules, and phagocytose the immune complexes.

Arthus reactions are rare in humans. Examples are shown in Table 28–1. Hemorrhagic necrosis at the site of injection of a drug or an insect bite or sting could suggest an Arthus reaction, but the distinction from a toxic reaction or secondary infection requires laboratory or immunohistochemical evidence of the presence of the relevant immune complexes. A limited form of the Arthus reaction occurs commonly at the site of allergy desensitization injections after sufficient doses of injected allergens have been given to generate IgG-"blocking" antibodies (see Chapter 51). Because the level of IgG antibodies achieved in allergy therapy is relatively low, the cutaneous and subcutaneous tissue inflammation produces only mild erythema and induration. This begins several hours after the injection and usually subsides in less than 24 hours.

Occasionally the condition can be traced to an unusual antigenic source. Lymphocytes from uninfected donors infused into their HIV-infected identical twin siblings produced mild Arthus reactions caused by antibodies to trace amounts of fetal calf serum used in the in vitro lymphocyte culture medium.

The reaction might accompany a toxigenic bacterial infection. The B-cell superantigen staphylococcal protein A has been shown to initiate a passive reverse Arthus reaction by its ability to bind nonspecifically to the Fab portion of human IgG (different from the complement-binding region) and to certain variable regions of heavy and light chains of circulating antibodies.

Table 28–1. Causes of Arthus reactions.

Class of Agent	Example
Nonprotein drugs	Beta-lactams
Protein drugs	LMW heparin Incidental foreign protein (fetal calf serum)[a]
Vaccines	Tetanus toxoid Diphtheria toxoid Allergens
Microbial antigens	Superantigens (Staph protein A)[a]
Insect sites and stings	Mosquitoes Spiders

[a] See text.

Table 28–2. Causes of serum sickness.

Class of Agent	Example
Nonprotein drug	Antibiotics Penicillin Sulfonamides Minocycline Cefaclor Others
Protein drugs	Heterologous antiserum Polyclonal (*horse, rabbit*) Antivenin (*snake, spider, scorpion*) Other antitoxin (*Botulinum*) Antirabies serum Antilymphocyte globulin (ALG) Antithymocyte globulin (ATG) Intravenous human gamma globulin Vaccines
Murine monoclonal antibody (Mab)	Antitumor necrosis factor
Insect sites, stings	Mosquito bites Hymenoptera insect stings

SERUM SICKNESS

Major Immunologic Features

- Systemic immune-complex complement-dependent inflammatory reaction to an extrinsic antigen
- Severity antigen dose-dependent
- Typical reaction produced by heterologous serum can occur in milder forms from other drugs

General Considerations

Serum sickness was first recognized in the preantibiotic era when heterologous antiserum was used as passive immunization for treatment of a number of infectious and toxic illnesses. Today, specific "serum therapy" with heterologous (usually equine) serum or gamma globulin is restricted to passive immunization for a very few toxic diseases and the use of antilymphocyte (ALG) or antithymocyte (ATG) globulin for immunosuppressive therapy.

Murine monoclonal antibodies to cytokines and similar agents are being used for treatment of cancer, sepsis, and so on. Serum sickness occurs infrequently and often in a mild form to the administration of other protein and nonprotein drugs, vaccines, and even to insect stings and bites (Table 28–2).

A. Definition: Serum sickness is an acute, self-limited allergic disease caused by immune complex-activated complement-generated inflammation after injection of a protein or haptenic drug. The cardinal features are fever, dermatitis, lymphadenopathy, and joint pains.

B. Epidemiology: Serum sickness is caused by the therapeutic injection of foreign material that is potentially antigenic, so the prevalence of this disease depends on the prevalence of certain forms of medical treatment. Therapeutic injections of large quantities of heterologous serum produce serum sickness in proportion to the dose. The attack rate was approximately 90% when a 200-mL dose of horse serum was given. The gamma globulin fraction of foreign serum containing the therapeutic antibodies is only marginally less antigenic with attack rates of the disease from ALG or ATG generally 50% or higher. The reason that certain drugs (eg, minocycline, cefaclor) are more likely to cause this reaction than are others within their class (tetracyclines, cephalosporins) is unknown. No prevalence statistics are available today, but reports of serum sickness are now uncommon.

C. Immunologic Pathogenesis: The pathogenesis of human serum sickness is believed to be similar to the mechanism of "one-shot" serum sickness produced experimentally in immunized rabbits (Figure 28–1). Following a single large dose of injected antigen a brief period of equilibration occurs between blood and tissues followed by slow degradation of antigen over several days as the primary antibody response is initiated. Antibody synthesis leads to its release into the circulation, where antigen-antibody complexes gradually form under conditions of moderate antigen excess. Intermediate-size complexes deposit in small blood vessels in various organs, triggering the events previously described for the Arthus reaction. This gives rise to the clinical and pathologic manifestations of disease. Free antigen is removed more rapidly from the circulation as antibody production and immune-complex formation increases. The circulating complexes then shift to antibody excess, thereby decreasing in size and clearing more rapidly. Finally, free antibody circulates, no further lesions appear, and healing takes place.

The optimal conditions for serum sickness occur during the initial antibody response of the previously immunized host. With subsequent exposures to the same antigen, the anamnestic antibody response facilitates rapid antigen clearance and greatly reduces the amount and persistence of immune complexes in the circulation.

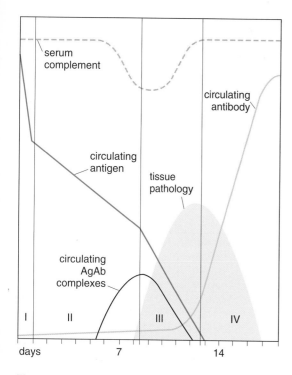

Figure 28–1. Immunologic events in experimental "one-shot" serum sickness in rabbits. The pathogenesis of human serum sickness is similar. A single high dose of antigen is given intravenously on day 0. Phase I: Equilibration of antigen between blood and tissues. Phase II: Primary antibody response. Near the end of this phase, antibody combines with antigen to form circulating immune complexes. Phase III: Tissue pathology and progression of clinical disease. Circulating complexes activate complement and deposit in tissues. The serum complement level falls transiently, and residual antigen is rapidly cleared from the blood. Phase IV: Remission. Antigen is no longer available, and the level of circulating antibody rises. No further immune complexes form, complement levels return to normal, pathologic lesions repair, and symptoms subside.

Clinical Features

A. Symptoms and Signs: Primary serum sickness begins 4–21 days (usually 7–10 days) after initial exposure to the causative antigen. The first sign is often a pruritic **rash,** which may be urticarial, maculopapular, or erythematous. There may be angioedema, particularly of the face, and the injection site usually becomes inflamed. **Fever, lymphadenopathy, arthralgias,** and **myalgias** complete the clinical presentation. Joint swelling and redness may occur, and occasionally the patient experiences headache, nausea, and vomiting. Recovery takes 7–30 days. Clinically significant cardiac or renal involvement is unusual. Neurologic manifestations may take place, usually in the form of mononeuritis involving especially the brachial plexus, and rarely polyneuritis, Guillain-Barré syndrome, or even meningoencephalitis.

Secondary serum sickness occurs in patients previously sensitized to the antigen. The latent period is short, only 2–4 days, and the clinical course of the disease may be brief but the manifestations can be severe. Repeated use of the same drug, such as ALG or ATG may cause repeated bouts of the disease with decreasing severity and latency, but therapeutic efficacy is usually maintained.

Recently, "despeciated" antivenin has been prepared by enzymatic digestion of the immunoglobulin Fc fragment leaving a functional F(ab')$_2$ fragment that causes serum sickness in only 1% or less of patients.

B. Laboratory Findings: Slight leukocytosis occurs. Plasma cells in the bone marrow are increased in number and may appear in the blood. Eosinophilia may be present, but this is not characteristic. The erythrocyte sedimentation rate is increased. Circulating immune complexes and reduced levels of serum complement components are often detected in disease caused by heterologous serum, but they are not usually detected in drug-induced serum sickness (for detection methods, see Chapter 15). Mild proteinuria, hematuria, and casts; transient electrocardiographic abnormalities; and pleocytosis are not unusual.

Immunologic Diagnosis

No specific test is diagnostic. The diagnosis is made on the basis of a compatible history of typical symptoms at an appropriate interval after drug administration, along with the physical and laboratory evidence. The disease is almost always benign and self-limited, with good prospects for complete recovery, so invasive tests such as tissue biopsy are not indicated.

Serum IgG and IgE antibodies specific to the relevant antigen may be detected in the time course illustrated in Figure 28–1 if confirmation of the diagnosis is required.

Treatment

Treatment should be conservative and symptomatic. Aspirin and antihistamines are effective. A short high-dose course of oral corticosteroids is warranted if symptoms are severe.

Complications & Prognosis

Complications are rare. Occasionally laryngeal edema may cause respiratory obstruction. The neuritis rarely is permanent.

ALLERGIC BRONCHOPULMONARY ASPERGILLOSIS

Major Immunologic Features

- Both IgE and IgG antibodies to *Aspergillus* involved in the pathogenesis of pulmonary disease
- IgE antibodies directed to spore allergens
- IgG antibodies directed to mycelial allergens

- Nonspecific elevation of serum IgE level during acute exacerbations of disease

General Considerations

Allergic bronchopulmonary aspergillosis (ABPA) is an unusual but not rare illness that affects young atopic adults with allergic asthma. It is caused by a concomitant IgE and IgG antibody response to the ubiquitous fungus *Aspergillus fumigatus.* Airborne spores of this organism prevail both indoors and outdoors year-round in many geographic areas, and it is a common saprophyte in the normal upper respiratory tract. The disease may occur in infants and children. It causes bronchiectasis and other destructive lung changes, but tissue damage can be prevented if the condition is diagnosed and treated properly.

A. Epidemiology: It is estimated that ABPA occurs in 1–2% of patients with asthma. Most cases have been reported in the United States and United Kingdom, but the disease probably occurs throughout the world. With rare exceptions, it is a disease of persons with atopic asthma, but it also occurs in 10% of children with cystic fibrosis. It has not been reported as an occupational disease. There is no known genetic predilection other than that related to atopy, and no human leukocyte antigen (HLA) association has yet been confirmed.

B. Immunologic Pathogenesis: *A fumigatus* is ubiquitous in the air and soil, and it may be found indoors where moisture and organic matter favor mold growth. Occasional cases are caused by *A ochraceus* or *A terreus.* Exposure to *Aspergillus* is universal, but there is no evidence that excessive environmental exposure causes the disease. High-dose exposure, however, may trigger acute attacks in the sensitized subject.

The **pathogenesis** of the disease is not entirely clear. The consensus is that ABPA is an allergic disease that requires both IgE and IgG antibodies to *Aspergillus* and that their corresponding immunologic effector mechanisms of inflammation result in the observed tissue damage (see Chapter 13). Inhalation of *Aspergillus* spores causes an immediate IgE-mediated bronchospastic reaction to an allergen in the spore, thereby trapping the organisms in the intraluminal mucus of the larger proximal bronchi. When the spores germinate and produce mycelia, the reaction of IgG antibodies to a different mycelial antigen produces tissue damage and inflammation, probably from immune complex-activated complement-derived products. Repeated episodes weaken the bronchial wall, leading to focal bronchiectasis. The significance of pathologic evidence of T-cell-mediated inflammation in disease pathogenesis is unknown. The inflammatory process extends to the peribronchial lung parenchyma, causing acute inflammatory infiltrates and ultimately chronic parenchymal destruction and fibrosis.

C. Pathology: The disease is confined to the lungs, where pathologic effects are twofold: those of the underlying asthma, and those associated with the acute inflammatory episodes and its sequelae. *Aspergillus* hyphae and inflammatory cells can be found in mucus plugs. The adjacent bronchial wall is infiltrated with mononuclear cells and eosinophils. A similar infiltrate affects peribronchial tissues, producing areas of interstitial pneumonia. Granulocytic inflammation and vasculitis are notably absent. Immunofluorescence studies have generally not shown immune-complex deposits in the lung, although these have been demonstrated in the late-onset skin test site in this disease (see later discussion). The reason for this discrepancy is unclear, but it may reflect the timing of the biopsy studies. Areas of chronic inflammation show noncaseating granulomas. Bronchiectasis and pulmonary fibrosis are late effects in the disease. The pathology, like the clinical manifestations, is variable.

Clinical Features

A. Symptoms and Signs: The clinical picture of ABPA is that of **asthma** with superimposed acute episodes of **fever, cough** productive of **mucus plugs, chest pains,** and **malaise.** Hemoptysis may occur. Other nonspecific symptoms include headache, arthralgias, and myalgias. Some patients present with chronic lung damage, which suggests that the acute inflammatory episodes may be asymptomatic. Physical findings are those of asthma, as well as rales in the presence of pulmonary infiltration.

B. Laboratory Findings: The diagnosis of ABPA is readily confirmed by objective evidence for the appropriate immune responses. Intradermal skin testing elicits an initial IgE antibody-mediated wheal-and-flare reaction to *A fumigatus* extract, followed by an Arthus reaction. Immunofluorescence at the height of the late response 6–12 hours after the intradermal injection reveals deposition of immunoglobulins and C3, distinguishing this response from a late-phase IgE reaction. Prick testing may not be sensitive enough to elicit the IgG antibody Arthus response, but it is usually sufficient for detecting the immediate IgE wheal and flare.

Serum precipitins to *Aspergillus* are found in about 70% of cases, and most of the remainder are positive if their sera are concentrated fivefold. IgG and IgE antibodies in serum can also be detected by radioallergosorbent test (RAST) or enzyme-linked immunosorbent assay (ELISA), but the high sensitivities of these techniques result in low specificity for diagnosis of disease.

The **total serum IgE level** is characteristically high in ABPA, and the level varies directly with disease activity. The mechanism for this is unknown, but IgE levels have important diagnostic and prognostic significance. The majority of the excess IgE cannot be accounted for by *Aspergillus*-specific antibody. Eosinophilia is present in blood and sputum, as it is in any case of asthma. Smear and culture of mucus plugs or sputum may yield the *Aspergillus* organism.

Pulmonary function testing reveals reversible airway obstruction, but the acute inflammatory episodes can be distinguished from simple asthma by reduction in diffusing capacity. In chronic disease, obstruction may be only partially reversible and a restrictive component may be prominent. **Bronchial provocation testing** with *Aspergillus* extract produces a dual immediate bronchospastic component followed by a late-phase obstructive-restrictive component accompanied by fever and leukocytosis.

The **chest roentgenogram** may show a variety of abnormalities, but it may also be normal. No radiologic finding is pathognomonic in this disease. Abnormalities that do occur may be found in many other lung diseases. During the acute phase, mucus plugs may produce focal areas of atelectasis or even segmental or lobar collapse. The peribronchial inflammation appears as migratory infiltrates, especially in the upper lobes and hilar areas. Chronic disease from repeated acute insults can cause volume loss, particularly in the upper lobes. Bronchiectasis revealed by bronchography or tomography is saccular and proximal, less commonly cylindrical.

Clinical Diagnosis

The diagnosis of ABPA is made on the basis of certain clinical and laboratory findings listed in Table 28–3. No single test is diagnostic. The diagnosis is definite when all seven major criteria are met and probable when six are met. All major and minor criteria can be found in other illnesses, but the critical importance of a definitive diagnosis is that it alerts the clinician to the need for corticosteroid therapy to prevent irreversible pulmonary damage. Any patient with a history of asthma and recurrent pulmonary infiltrates not otherwise explained should be given a diagnostic skin test with *Aspergillus*. Absence of the immediate reaction virtually rules out ABPA, but if the test is positive, a search for serum precipitins and radiographic evidence of bronchiectasis is indicated.

Differential Diagnosis

A fumigatus can cause other respiratory diseases. **Invasive aspergillosis** is an opportunistic infection that may complicate immunosuppression caused by drugs or disease. **Aspergilloma** is a localized growth of the organism invading a lung cavity or cyst. It typically induces a very marked precipitating antibody response, with a negative Arthus skin test, probably because of antibody excess at the skin site. *Aspergillus* hypersensitivity pneumonitis is a rare cause of farmer's lung. Finally, the organism is an atopic allergen in some cases of **allergic asthma.**

The variable clinical and radiologic features of the disease mimic **other pulmonary diseases,** including asthma with periodic mucus plugging or intercurrent viral infections, tuberculosis, hypersensitivity pneumonitis, pulmonary infiltration with eosinophilia

(PIE syndrome), mucoid impaction, and bronchocentric granulomatosis.

ABPA in Cystic Fibrosis

By using the criteria of Table 28–3, the diagnosis of ABPA is made more frequently in children with cystic fibrosis than in the atopic asthmatic population. It is difficult to be sure whether this reflects a fundamental predisposition or a secondary opportunistic effect. Both atopy and *Aspergillus* infections are prevalent in children with cystic fibrosis, setting the stage for the necessary immune response involved in the pathogenesis of ABPA. Markedly elevated and fluctuating serum IgE levels, eosinophilia, and dramatic roentgenographic resolution of infiltrates with corticosteroid treatment are important diagnostic clues that ABPA is present in this disease.

Treatment

A definitive diagnosis is important, because **high-dose systemic corticosteroid therapy** promptly resolves the acute allergic inflammatory episode and prevents the occurrence of long-term irreversible bronchial and parenchymal lung damage. The mechanism of the therapeutic effect can only be surmised, but it is probably antiinflammatory rather than immunosuppressive. An initial dose of 60 mg of prednisone daily in divided doses should be maintained until clinical and radiologic cure of the episode is evident, after which a slowly tapering dose with maintenance at 20–30 mg once on alternate days should prevent relapses. It is useful to monitor total serum IgE levels, which fall during remissions and rise again with recurrences. There is some evidence that the serum IgE rise might precede the clinical exacerbation. Serial chest roentgenograms should also be part of the monitoring process.

The concurrent asthma is treated in the standard fashion, including desensitization if indicated. Injections of *Aspergillus* extract, however, should probably be avoided because this might theoretically enhance the IgG antibody response and hence worsen

---

Table 28–3. Diagnostic criteria for ABPA.

Major criteria
1. Episodic bronchial obstruction.
2. Peripheral blood eosinophilia.
3. Positive immediate skin reactivity.
4. Serum precipitating antibodies.
5. Elevated serum IgE.
6. History of pulmonary infiltrates.
7. Central bronchiectasis.

Minor criteria
1. *A fumigatus*-positive sputum culture.
2. History of expectorating brown plugs or flecks.
3. Arthus' (late) skin reactivity.

Source: Reproduced, with permission, from Slavin RG: Allergic-bronchopulmonary aspergillosis. *Clin Rev Allergy* 1985; **3:**167.

the disease. Inhaled corticosteroids are not indicated for acute attacks, but they can be used to control the asthma between attacks. Chest physiotherapy and inhaled bronchodilators are helpful adjuncts to improve expectoration of mucus plugs, but antifungal drugs are of unproven benefit.

Complications & Prognosis

Table 28–4 is a scheme for staging untreated disease. The course is variable and unpredictable and may depend on factors of environmental exposure, so that not all patients proceed through all stages. Nevertheless, early recognition and adequate treatment prevent deterioration in pulmonary function and subsequent development of chronic airway obstruction and restrictive disease with pulmonary fibrosis. Occasionally, aspergilloma develops in a bronchiectatic or emphysematous cyst in ABPA. Cor pulmonale is likely to occur in stage V disease.

Table 28–4. Proposed stages of increasing severity and chronicity in ABPA.

Stage	Description
I	Acute episode responsive to systemic corticosteroids
II	Remission
III	Recurrent exacerbations
IV	Recurrent exacerbations with steroid-dependent severe asthma
V	Pulmonary fibrosis, irreversible obstruction, advanced radiographic changes, cavitation and upper lobe contraction, severe bronchiectasis, emphysema

Source: Reproduced, with permission, from Patterson, R et al: Allergic bronchopulmonary aspergillosis: Staging as an aid to management. *Ann Intern Med* 1982;**96**:286.

REFERENCES

ARTHUS REACTION

Selvaggi TA et al: Development of antibodies to fetal calf serum with Arthus-like reactions in human immunodeficiency virus-infected patients given syngeneic lymphocyte infusions. *Blood* 1997;89:776.

Sylvestre DL, Ravetch JV: Fc receptors initiate the Arthus reaction: Redefining the inflammatory cascade. *Science* 1994;265:1095.

SERUM SICKNESS

Bielory L et al: Human serum sickness: A prospective analysis of 35 patients treated with equine antithymocyte globulin for bone marrow failure. *Medicine* 1988;67:40.

Erffmeyer JE: Serum sickness. *Ann Allergy* 1986;56:105.

Heard K et al: Antivenom therapy in the Americas. *Drugs* 1999;58:5.

Naguwa SM, Nelson BL: Human serum sickness. *Clin Rev Allergy* 1985;3:117.

ALLERGIC BRONCHOPULMONARY ASPERGILLOSIS

Cockrill BA, Hales CA. Allergic bronchopulmonary aspergillosis. *Annu Rev Med* 1999;50:303.

Greenberger PA: Diagnosis and management of allergic bronchopulmonary aspergillosis. *Allergy Proc* 1994; 15:335.

Knutsen AP, Slavin RG: Allergic bronchopulmonary aspergillosis in patients with cystic fibrosis. *Clin Rev Allergy* 1991;9:103.

Patterson R et al: Allergic bronchopulmonary aspergillosis: Staging as an aid to management. *Ann Intern Med* 1982; 96:286.

29

Cell-Mediated Hypersensitivity Diseases

Abba I. Terr, MD

Certain allergic diseases are mediated by specifically sensitized effector T lymphocytes (T_{DH} cells) and not by specifically sensitized antibodies. The immunologic mechanism is often called **delayed hypersensitivity.** It is called cell-mediated immunity in response to infection by certain microorganisms, especially those that cause intracellular infections. This chapter discusses two very different T-cell-mediated allergic diseases: allergic contact dermatitis, which is very common, and hypersensitivity pneumonitis, which is quite uncommon but not rare.

Allergic contact dermatitis in its usual form is a pure form of T-cell hypersensitivity. (Occasionally, allergens that contact the skin or mucous membranes may elicit an IgE antibody response, especially urticaria but rarely systemic anaphylaxis.) **Hypersensitivity pneumonitis** is a clinically heterogenous disease that may assume several forms involving antibodies, T cells, or both, depending on factors of allergen dose and the form and duration of allergen exposure. It is included in this chapter because T-cell mechanisms are predominant in most clinically recognized cases.

ALLERGIC CONTACT DERMATITIS

Major Immunologic Features
- Mediated by specifically sensitized T cells
- Caused most often by contact with haptenic chemicals
- Patch testing efficient and accurate in diagnosis

General Considerations
A. Definition: Allergic contact dermatitis (also known as eczematous contact allergy) is an eczematous skin disease caused by cell-mediated hypersensitivity to an environmental allergen. Both sensitization and elicitation of the reaction involve contact of the allergen with the skin. Allergens causing the disease are numerous and include both natural and synthetic chemicals.

B. Epidemiology: The disease occurs worldwide and affects both sexes and all age groups. The most common allergen, pentadecylcatechol, found in poison ivy and poison oak, affects 50% of the US population clinically and another 35% subclinically.

C. Immunologic Pathogenesis: Allergic contact dermatitis is mediated by cutaneous T-cell hypersensitivity. The dose of allergen necessary for sensitization varies widely. Once sensitization occurs, it lasts for years, if not for life, and is generalized. Reactions can be elicited anywhere on the skin. In some instances systemic reactions have been provoked when the allergen enters the body by ingestion or injection.

Many important sensitizing allergens are organic chemicals, and some are metals. It is assumed that they function as haptens and that their binding to a carrier protein is an essential step in their subsequent recognition by T cells. The source and nature of the carrier protein in the skin are unknown. Some sensitizers, such as urushiol, the allergen in poison ivy, have intrinsic proinflammatory properties, which may explain their particularly virulent clinical expression.

In the sensitization stage of contact dermatitis, allergen penetrates the skin and is taken up by resident epidermal dendritic cells, also known as Langerhans' cells. Following capture of allergen, the dendritic cells differentiate into potent antigen-presenting cells and migrate to regional lymph nodes. There they encounter naive CD4 T cells, triggering the activation of those T cells whose antigen receptors are specific for the allergen in the form of processed antigen bound to the class II major histocompatibility class (MHC) molecules displayed on the surface of the dendritic cell. The activated allergen-specific T cells proliferate in the lymph node and differentiate into effector and memory cells, usually of the T_H1 type. Importantly, they acquire receptors, such as cutaneous lymphocyte-associated antigen (CLA), that allow them to home in on inflamed skin after exiting the lymph node. Allergen-specific memory T cells persist long after sensitization and retain the ability to migrate preferentially to the skin. When allergen again penetrates the skin, these memory cells rapidly evolve into effectors that mediate a delayed-type hypersensitivity reaction at the site of penetration.

D. Pathology: The inflammatory response in allergic contact dermatitis is characterized by perivenular cuffing with lymphocytes, epidermal cell vesiculation and necrosis, infiltration with basophils and eosinophils, interstitial fibrin deposition, and dermal and epidermal edema.

Clinical Features

A. Symptoms and Signs: The skin eruption appears acutely as erythema, swelling, and vesiculation. In severe cases, extensive blistering, scaling, and weeping may occur. In chronic milder disease, papules and scaling are more prominent. The lesion is pruritic or frankly painful if severe. The rapidity of onset after contact is directly proportional to the degree of sensitivity and may range from 6 hours to several days.

The location of the eruption on the skin is helpful in diagnosing the cause. Certain areas of skin, particularly the eyelids, react more easily than others, such as the palms. Metal dermatitis, usually caused by sensitivity to nickel, appears in discrete patches corresponding to the area of contact with jewelry, watches, or metal objects on clothing. A variety of allergens, such as dyes and fabric finishes, are found in clothing, causing a skin eruption on areas of skin covered by the apparel. Volatile allergens affect exposed areas, usually the face and arms. *Rhus* dermatitis from poison oak or poison ivy produces an especially severe disease with prominent vesicles and bullae and characteristic streaks of vesicles corresponding to brushing of the skin by the plant leaves.

B. Laboratory Findings: There are none.

Allergens

The list of known allergens is enormous and theoretically unlimited. All types of chemicals can produce this disease, but metallic inorganic compounds and organic chemicals are the most likely, in contrast to the protein allergens that dominate as the cause of other types of allergic conditions. The reason for this is unknown but is probably associated with the unique handling of foreign materials by the skin. The most common contact allergens are listed in Table 29–1. Nickel sensitivity is the most common of these, as evidenced by a positive patch test in 15–20% of the population. Allergic contact dermatitis of the hands caused primarily by rubber accelerators in natural latex gloves is becoming increasingly prevalent in health care workers.

Clinical Diagnosis

The diagnosis of allergic contact dermatitis is suggested by the physical appearance of the eruption and distribution of lesions. By history, reactions may appear suddenly, or they may present as a chronic, low-grade, smoldering dermatitis. The history must then be directed to exposures in the home, work, and recreational environment for possible allergens.

Immunologic Diagnosis

The diagnosis is confirmed by **patch testing,** a time-honored, well-standardized procedure that is

Table 29–1. Common contact allergens and concentrations.

Benzocaine 5%
Mercaptobenzothiazole 1%
Colophony 20%
p-Phenylenediamine 1%
Imidazolidinyl urea 2%
Cinnamic aldehyde 1%
Lanolin alcohol 30%
Carba mix 3%
Neomycin sulfate 20%
Thiuram mix 1%
Formaldehyde 1%
Ethylenediamine dihydrochloride 1%
Epoxy resin 1%
Quaternium 15 2%
p-tert-Butylphenol formaldehyde resin 1%
Mercapto mix 1%
Black rubber mix 0.6%
Potassium dichromate 0.25%
Balsam of Peru 25%
Nickel sulfate 2.5%

both an immunologic skin test and a provocation test that reproduces the disease "in miniature." Standard patch test allergens in concentrations that elicit allergic but not irritant reactions are available commercially for a number of the common contact sensitizers (see Table 29–1). Reactions are read in 48 hours for localized eczema at the patch test site (Table 29–2). Patch testing to the common allergens used in routine screening has an overall sensitivity of 77% and a specificity of 71%, which is acceptable for a bioassay. Weak (1+) reactions have poorer reproducibility than stronger ones.

Differential Diagnosis

Eczema refers to a general pattern of response of the skin to a variety of injurious stimuli. Scratching of the skin from any pruritic dermatosis can cause eczematization. The most common causes are atopic dermatitis; localized or generalized neurodermatitis; skin infection by bacteria or fungi; primary contact irritation by chemicals, foods, saliva, sweat, or urine; and dyshidrosis.

Table 29–2. Patch test interpretation.[a]

Result	Interpretation
1	Weak (nonvesicular) reaction: erythema, infiltration, papules (+)
2	Strong (edematous or vesicular) reaction (++)
3	Extreme (spreading, bullous, ulcerative) reaction (+++)
4	Doubtful reaction, macular erythema only
5	Irritant reaction (IR)
6	Negative reaction (–)
7	Excited skin
8	Not tested

[a] Reporting of results as recommended by the North American Contact Dermatitis Group.

Treatment

The disease responds to systemic **corticosteroids,** which should be given as early as possible. Small localized areas of involvement can be treated with a topical steroid cream. Applications of cool, wet dressings containing Burow's solution (aluminum acetate) are helpful for treating acute lesions. Chronic lichenified dermatitis requires a potent fluorinated steroid ointment with an occlusive dressing. Extensive areas of involvement or severe bullous lesions should be treated with a brief oral burst of high-dose prednisone or with intramuscular triamcinolone or methylprednisolone. An antibiotic may be indicated for secondary infection. Antihistamines are generally not effective for controlling the pruritus.

Prognosis

A cure is to be expected in the case of acute allergic contact dermatitis if the allergen is identified correctly and avoided. Exposure to the same or to a cross-reacting allergenic chemical, however, may cause a recurrence. Chromate allergy tends to be chronic, despite avoidance.

Prevention

The only means of prevention of the dermatitis in a sensitized patient is avoidance. Tolerance to contact sensitivity by prior oral ingestion of allergen has no practical application in humans, although it may be effective in animal models of the disease. Some patients with mild nickel sensitivity can tolerate jewelry that is treated with a protective coating. *Rhus* dermatitis can probably be lessened, if not prevented, if the skin is thoroughly washed with water immediately after contact.

Desensitization with oral or injected *Rhus* extract or pentadecylcatechol has advocates in clinical practice, but there is, as yet, no sound evidence of effectiveness. Some patients appear to lose sensitivity after repeated natural exposure, a phenomenon known as "hardening," but this also remains to be documented.

PHOTOALLERGIC CONTACT DERMATITIS

Major Immunologic Features
* Allergen requires activation by ultraviolet light
* Immunologic mechanism identical to that of allergic contact dermatitis

General Considerations

A. Definition: Photoallergic contact dermatitis is an uncommon eczematous skin disease caused by cell-mediated hypersensitivity to certain environmental chemicals that require sunlight activation to render them allergenic. The skin eruption appears on sun-exposed areas of the skin only.

B. Epidemiology: The disease has been associated primarily with drugs or chemical constituents of topical products, such as soaps, cosmetics, and topical drugs. It therefore appears from time to time in epidemic form when a new product is introduced. The epidemic subsides when the product is withdrawn from the market once the photosensitivity potential is discovered.

C. Immunologic Pathogenesis: The mechanism is identical to ordinary allergic contact dermatitis, except that the causative chemical agent must be activated by ultraviolet light to become allergenic. The mechanism of allergen activation is unknown. Two theories have been proposed. Ultraviolet radiation may cause an alteration in tertiary structure to generate the necessary allergen epitope, or, alternatively, free radicals generated by ultraviolet light may be necessary for binding of the hapten chemical to a skin carrier protein.

D. Pathology: The pathology is indistinguishable from that of allergic contact dermatitis.

Clinical Features

The dermatitis varies in its clinical appearance from an exaggerated sunburn to typical eczema to a severe vesiculobullous dermatosis. The distribution corresponds to sunlight exposure, but severe reactions may involve partially covered areas of skin as well. The eruption caused by a topically applied sensitizer is limited to the area of application.

Clinical Diagnosis

The disease is diagnosed by the combination of dermatitis in a sun-exposed distribution and a history of concurrent exposure to a known or suspected photoallergic sensitizer. A high index of suspicion facilitates diagnosis.

Immunologic Diagnosis

Photopatch testing is a modification of the standard patch test. The suspected agent is applied in the standard fashion for patch testing, and then the site is exposed to artificial ultraviolet light or sunlight. A test site not exposed to light is used as a control. The appearance of an eczematous eruption at the light-exposed site only is a positive test.

Differential Diagnosis

Certain chemicals and drugs produce dermatitis in sun-exposed areas of skin in all individuals, provided that sufficient amounts of the compound accumulate in the skin and that there is exposure to a particular wavelength of ultraviolet light. These are called phototoxic reactions and are not mediated immunologically. Differential diagnosis also includes ordinary contact dermatitis, sunburn, and other causes of photosensitivity.

Allergens

Some of the important drugs and chemicals that cause photoallergic and phototoxic contact dermatitis are listed in Table 29–3. Some drugs taken systemically produce photodermatitis.

Treatment

Avoidance of the sensitizing agent and sunlight and treatment with topical corticosteroids are usually sufficient. Systemic corticosteroids may be required in severe cases.

Prognosis

Occasionally the dermatitis persists despite avoidance measures. The reason for this is unknown.

HYPERSENSITIVITY PNEUMONITIS

Major Immunologic Features

- Complex immunopathogenesis with primary role of effector T cells
- Antibody precipitins useful in establishing exposure to the allergen
- Allergens usually airborne components of biologic organisms or their products

General Considerations

Hypersensitivity pneumonitis (also known as **extrinsic allergic alveolitis**) has been known as an occupational disease for well over two centuries, but more recently has been recognized as an allergic disease. It was first thought to be a pulmonary Arthus reaction caused by immune complexes of inhaled allergen and precipitating IgG antibodies, but persuasive evidence from clinical, pathologic, epidemiologic, and experimental studies has shown that the disease is mediated predominantly by T-lymphocyte (cellular) effector mechanisms. It shares some pathologic features with sarcoidosis and the pneumoconioses, but it differs from the former disease by having a recognized environmental cause and from the latter group of diseases by its immune responses to inhaled material. Hypersensitivity pneumonitis, like

allergic asthma, is produced by inhaled allergens, and in fact allergens can cause either disease. IgE antibodies, however, play no known role in the pathogenesis of hypersensitivity pneumonitis.

A. Definition: Hypersensitivity pneumonitis is an allergic disease of the lung parenchyma with inflammation in the alveoli and interstitial spaces induced immunologically by acute or chronic inhalation of a wide variety of inhaled materials. The disease may present in an acute, subacute, or chronic form. It is not currently possible to ascribe all features of the illness to a single immunologic mechanism. Several different immune pathways appear to operate separately or concurrently in this condition, but the most compelling evidence favors allergen-specific cell-mediated hypersensitivity as the mechanism of pathogenesis. Interstitial pneumonitis is the primary clinical manifestation for all forms of the disease.

B. Epidemiology: Cases have been reported worldwide. Disease prevalence depends on case definition, exposure, and host factors. It is frequently caused by occupational allergens, which further influence the prevalence and geographic, age, and sex distribution. Males aged 30–50 years are therefore usually affected. Farmer's lung, the prototype and most widely reported form of hypersensitivity pneumonitis, is caused by thermophilic actinomycetes, usually from warm, moist, moldy hay, and therefore the disease predominates in wet regions and especially among dairy farmers. Surveys suggest that 0.04–4% of farmers are affected. Bird handler's disease (also known as bird fancier's lung, pigeon breeder's disease, and bird breeder's disease) has been diagnosed in 15–21% of exposed individuals. Humidifier lung disease occurs in 23–71% of those exposed to contaminated humidifiers. Many published reports identify a single case or a small epidemic in a workplace. Once recognized, elimination of the environmental source of the allergen eliminates the disease.

C. Allergens: Hundreds of sources of allergens have been reported to cause hypersensitivity pneumonitis, usually in single cases. Some of the more common ones are shown in Table 29–4. The exact allergenic molecule has been isolated only infrequently, but these include a variety of heterologous proteins and organic or inorganic compounds. In many cases the chemical identification has been made by serologic or skin testing in the affected patient. As explained later, precipitins and skin tests may be epiphenomena, so definitive identification of the allergen requires bronchial provocation testing. (See the section on Immunologic Diagnosis.)

The allergens come from many environmental sources. The most common ones are microorganisms, especially bacteria and fungal spores, and animal products, such as feathers and particles of dried excreta. The few industrial chemicals so far identified with this disease have been highly reactive ones, such

Table 29–3. Some topical agents causing photoallergic and phototoxic reactions.

Photoallergic	Phototoxic
Drugs	Drugs
Sulfonamides	Sulfonamides
Phenothiazines	Phenothiazines
Soaps containing halogenated salicylanilides	Plant oils
	Psoralens
Sunscreen agents	Coal tar and its derivatives in
p-Aminobenzoate esters	dyes, perfumes, and
Benzophenones	other synthetics
Fragrances	Acridine
	Anthracene
	Phenothrene

Table 29–4. Allergens causing hypersensitivity pneumonitis.

Allergen	Source	Disease
Bacteria		
Thermophilic actinomycetes	Contaminated hay or grains	Farmer's lung
	Contaminated bagasse	Bagassosis
	Mushroom compost	Mushroom worker's lung
Bacillus subtilis	Contaminated walls	Domestic hypersensitivity pneumonitis
Streptomyces albus	Contaminated fertilizer	*Streptomyces* hypersensitivity pneumonitis
Fungi		
Aspergillus spp	Moldy barley	Malt worker's lung
	Moldy tobacco	Tobacco worker's lung
	Compost	Compost lung
Aureobasidium, Graphium spp	Redwood bark, sawdust	Sequoiosis
	Contaminated sauna water	Sauna worker's lung
	Contaminated humidifier	Humidifier lung
Cryptostroma corticale	Maple bark	Maple bark disease
Penicillium casei	Moldy cheese	Cheese worker's lung
Saccharomonospora viridis	Dried grass	Thatched roof disease
Various undetermined puffball spores	Moldy dwellings	Domestic hypersensitivity pneumonitis
	Mold in cork dust	Suberosis
	Lycoperdon puffballs	Lycoperdonosis
Alternaria, Penicillium spp	Wood pulp, dust	Woodworker's lung
Trichosporon cutaneum	House dust (reported in Japan)	Summer-type hypersensitivity pneumonitis
Insects		
Sitophilus granarius (wheat weevil)	Infested flour	Wheat miller's lung
Organic chemicals		
Isocyanates	Various industries	Chemical worker's lung
Miscellaneous		
Pituitary snuff	Medication	Pituitary snuff taker's lung
Coffee bean protein	Coffee bean dust	Coffee worker's lung
Rat urine protein	Laboratory rats	Laboratory worker's lung
Animal fur protein	Animal pelts	Furrier's lung
Unknown	Contaminated tap water	Tap water hypersensitivity pneumonitis

as isocyanates and acid anhydrides. Many cases have been associated with inhalation of a product such as dust from a food or droplets of contaminated water without identification of the source, although microbial contamination is usually suspected.

To date most reported cases have been **occupational** because these are more likely to be acute illnesses from high-dose exposure easily traced to the workplace by a history of an epidemic in a particular occupational site. The relatively few instances of disease caused by **domestic** exposure have been traced to thermophilic actinomycetes, fungi, mites, amebae, pet birds, and unknown organisms in contaminated water of home or automobile air conditioners, heaters, vaporizers, and evaporative air coolers. These tend to cause chronic and insidious pulmonary impairment. Physicians should be aware of these potential causes of "idiopathic" pulmonary fibrosis.

The allergen must be inhaled as an aerosol or particle that is capable of reaching the alveoli during normal respiration. Particulates, whether in the form of an organic dust or microorganism, must be less than 3 μm in diameter.

Many of the allergens associated with hypersensitivity pneumonitis have biologic properties, in addition to allergenicity, that may be important in causing disease. The thermophilic actinomycetes, which are classified in the same order as *Mycobacterium tuberculosis,* contain immunologic adjuvants for both antibody synthesis and cell-mediated immunity. Many of

the allergens can activate alveolar macrophages and the alternative complement pathway nonimmunologically.

D. Pathology: The histopathology of hypersensitivity pneumonitis depends on the stage of disease. During the acute phase immediately after exposure, the centrilobular respiratory bronchioles, alveoli, and blood vessels are intensely infiltrated by granulocytes, monocytes, and plasma cells. There is Arthus-like vasculitis of alveolar capillaries. Some studies show bronchiolar destruction. Alveolar wall thickening occurs but without necrosis. Immunofluorescence studies show deposition of immunoglobulins, C3, and fibrin in and around affected blood vessels. Thus, any role of precipitating antibodies causing immune complex deposition and complement-mediated Arthus-like vasculitis, alveolitis, and terminal bronchiolitis would be restricted to the early acute illness after allergen exposure.

The subacute phase, beginning within 3 weeks of exposure, is characterized by noncaseating granulomas in the interstitial spaces accompanied by lymphocytes and plasma cells with only occasional eosinophils and no vasculitis. Mild bronchiolitis obliterans is seen in 50% of cases.

Chronic disease is characterized by persistence of the subacute pathology. Lymphocytes are present in alveolar walls, and interstitial fibrosis accompanies the granulomatous and mononuclear interstitial and alveolar inflammation. No eosinophilia occurs, and immunofluorescence shows no immunoglobulin or complement deposits. Monoclonal antibody reagents reveal the presence of activated macrophages and T lymphocytes, predominantly CD8 cells.

The histopathology of hypersensitivity pneumonitis is not pathognomonic, with the possible exception of histiocytes with foamy cytoplasm surrounded by lymphocytes, which are seen in the chronic phase.

E. Pathogenesis: The allergic pathogenesis of hypersensitivity pneumonitis was first suspected in farmer's lung because of the granulomatous interstitial inflammation, a hallmark of T-cell-mediated immunity. The discovery of precipitating antibodies to extracts of thermophilic actinomycetes in these patients' sera, however, led to a persisting concept that this is an immune-complex disease, even after many studies showed that precipitins correlated with exposure to allergens and not necessarily to the presence of pulmonary disease. As explained earlier, an Arthus mechanism could be operative in the acute form of hypersensitivity pneumonitis. However, a complex mechanism of disease induction and resolution emerges from studies of bronchoalveolar lavage, serology, and pathology, as well as from experimental disease in rats and mice. Antigen-specific T-cell responses generate both T_H1 and T_H2 profiles of cytokine production and release. Tumor necrosis factor (TNF) and interleukin (IL) -1 activation of macrophages produce monokines, including macrophage-activating factor (MAF), migration inhibitory factor (MIF), and macrophage chemotactic factor (MCF). These monokines recruit and activate immature monocytes forming the interstitial granuloma, which is composed of epithelioid and mononucleated giant cells. CD8 T cells predominate in bronchoalveolar lavage fluid during active disease, but CD4 T cells predominate when the allergen exposure ceases. B-cell involvement is also evident by the presence of specific IgG and IgA antibodies, although their role in disease pathogenesis is less clear than is the role of pulmonary mucosal cellular immunity.

Immunogenetic and other immunoregulatory factors presumably are important in patient susceptibility to the disease and its various manifestations. Many of the inhaled allergens identified with this disease have intrinsic biologic properties that may have an adjuvant effect causing nonspecific immune stimulation, activation of macrophages, and nonimmunologic activation of the alternative complement pathway.

Unlike IgE-mediated diseases, allergen exposure by inhalation must be either intensive and massive or prolonged. It has been calculated that a farmer working with moldy hay may inhale 750,000 fungal spores per minute.

In experimental disease in animals, inhalation of soluble antigens produces a very mild disease or an acute hemorrhagic Arthus alveolitis analogous to human illness in workers exposed occupationally to high doses of trimellitic anhydride or isocyanate who develop high-titer circulating and alveolar-fluid antibodies and a restrictive infiltrative pulmonary disease with hemoptysis and anemia. On the other hand, the typical human hypersensitivity pneumonitis is best reproduced in animals by inhalation of particulate antigens that elicit alveolitis and interstitial granulomas, specific local and systemic cell-mediated hypersensitivity, activation of alveolar macrophages, local lymphokine production in alveolar fluid, and precipitins. Allergen inhalation challenge responses can be passively transferred by sensitized lymphocytes, and the disease can be inhibited with corticosteroids, with antimacrophage serum, and by neonatal thymectomy, all of which are consistent with cellular hypersensitivity.

Experiments in mice shed some light on the development and variability of the human disease. By using high- and low-responder strains, it has been shown that the disease is associated with a deficiency in allergen-specific suppressor T lymphocytes in the lung. The deficiency is determined by a dominant gene or genes linked to the immunoglobulin V_H haplotype but not to H-2 (analogous to human HLA) genes. Repeated exposure to the allergen causes a phenomenon of desensitization, with disappearance of infiltrates, refractoriness to disease by other, unrelated allergens, and cell-mediated anergy in some animals but not others. The anergic state is caused by an allergen-nonspecific suppressor macrophage, whose presence is controlled by a single recessive gene. Animals lacking this gene have sustained granulomatous disease and have failed to develop anergy. These intriguing experiments stress the role of genetic factors of immunoregulation that probably also control susceptibility to and expressions of the disease in humans.

Clinical Features

A. Symptoms: Clinical patterns are wide-ranging, but they may be classified into acute, subacute, and chronic forms. Acute reactions are characterized by single or multiple episodes of dyspnea, cough, malaise, fever, chills, and chest pain. Each episode begins 4–8 hours after a high-dose allergen exposure and clears within 24 hours. Weight loss and hemoptysis are rare. Subacute disease begins insidiously over a period of weeks, resulting in cough, dyspnea, and weight loss. The cough is initially dry and later productive. Dyspnea may become progressively profound, and cyanosis may be evident. Chronic disease occurs from low-dose continuous exposure, as in the case of hypersensitivity to a single bird in the home. Fatigue and weight loss may be the first indication of illness. Gradual progressive dyspnea may be overlooked or denied until it is noticed at rest.

B. Signs: During acute reactions, the temperature is elevated to as high as 39.5°C. The patient appears acutely ill, with tachypnea and tachycardia. Bilateral crackling rales can be heard, especially at the lung bases, as well as occasional rhonchi and wheezes, but the lungs may be clear. In chronic disease, breath sounds are diminished, and the expiratory phase may be prolonged if an obstructive component is present.

C. Laboratory Findings: In acute disease slight leukocytosis without eosinophilia usually occurs. The erythrocyte sedimentation rate is normal or mildly elevated. In chronic disease, serum immunoglobulin levels may be slightly increased, and low-titer rheumatoid factor and antinuclear antibody may be present.

Pulmonary function tests performed during the acute phase of the disease reveal a reversible restrictive pattern with reduced lung compliance and reduced diffusing capacity. Arterial blood gases show hypoxemia. The spirometric findings in chronic disease are those of irreversible restriction with or without an accompanying obstructive component due to bronchiolitis obliterans. In some patients an additional element of bronchial hyperirritability may occur.

Chest radiographic findings are highly variable. During an acute episode, the presence of multiple bilateral small nodules sparing the apices and bases is the typical pattern. This indicates the presence of interstitial inflammation and an alveolus-filling infiltrate. Less common findings are patchy pneumonia or a normal radiograph. In chronic disease a fibrotic linear pattern with or without nodules increases in intensity toward the periphery. A loss of volume that is most marked in upper lobes, honeycombing, and cor pulmonale-induced cardiac enlargement may occur. The disease does not cause pleural effusion or thickening, hilar adenopathy, calcification, cavitation, atelectasis, or coin lesions.

The classification just described should not obscure the fact that hypersensitivity pneumonitis is highly variable and that individual cases can be "atypical." Clinical manifestations depend on the chemical and physical properties of the allergen and the frequency and intensity of exposure, as well as on host factors. Clinical descriptions have been dominated by occupational syndromes such as farmer's lung, bagassosis, and bird handler's disease. Many unique case reports have been published with quaint names and unusual allergen sources, such as New Guinea thatched roof lung (contaminated thatch), paprika slicer's lung *(Mucor stalonifer),* Bible printer's lung (contaminated ink), and coptic lung (mummy cloth wrappings).

Clinical Diagnosis

The clinical diagnosis requires a high index of suspicion and information from an exposure history, compatible symptomatology, physical examination of the lungs, pulmonary function testing, chest radiography, serum antibodies, and, in some instances, bronchial provocation testing.

Any history of recurrent pneumonia of uncertain etiology, "idiopathic" restrictive or fibrotic lung disease, or unexplained pulmonary abnormality on chest radiograph is a prime suspect. The environmental, especially occupational, history is essential for providing clues for possible causative allergens.

No signs from physical examination, routine laboratory tests, or chest films are pathognomonic. Even pulmonary function testing may not show evidence of the restrictive abnormality during asymptomatic periods between acute attacks of early disease. Lung biopsy is likewise not pathognomonic because histopathology is similar to that of other interstitial diseases, but it is useful mainly to rule out other diagnoses.

Immunologic Diagnosis

Serum antibodies are not usually involved in disease pathogenesis, but their presence establishes the fact of exposure. Large quantities of **precipitating antibodies** are usually present, especially in early or acute disease, but they may disappear after a prolonged period of allergen avoidance. Ouchterlony analysis usually detects precipitins (see Chapter 15). The more sensitive radioimmunoassay, radioallergosorbent test (RAST), enzyme-linked immunosorbent assay (ELISA), and complement fixation test procedures lack specificity for diagnostic purposes. Serum complement component levels are normal or occasionally increased with acute allergen exposure.

When precipitating antibodies are present in serum, an intradermal skin test elicits a cutaneous Arthus reaction, characterized by localized diffuse edema and mild inflammation and erythema appearing at 4–6 hours and subsiding completely by 24 hours. Commercial test antigens are available for extracts of fungi and diluted avian serum. Many crude extracts of allergens known to cause this disease, such as thermophilic actinomycetes, are too irritating for skin testing. The Arthus skin test, like the precipitin test, is an indication of exposure and is not by itself diagnostic of the disease.

Bronchial provocation testing with allergen extract currently has the highest sensitivity and specificity for diagnosis, but it is an experimental procedure because of technical limitations and danger. It should be done in a hospital with 24-hour monitoring. A reversible restrictive lung defect begins at 4–6 hours, peaks at 8 hours, and resolves by 24 hours. Although the timing of response is similar to a late-phase asthmatic response, the abnormality in pulmonary function is different.

A simpler alternative to bronchial provocation is "on-site" challenge to observe changes in symptoms, lung auscultation, pulmonary functions, and chest radiograph by trial exposure of the patient to the suspected environment (eg, home or work) after an adequate period of avoidance. If an acute reaction is provoked, the site must be investigated to uncover the causative allergen. Environmental assessment might require the specialized services of engineers, microbiologists, or others.

Brochoalveolar lavage fluid contains large numbers of CD8 lymphocytes. This is characterisitic of active disease, and following removal from exposure to the allergen, the pattern returns to the normal CD4-predominant pattern. Activated macrophages, natural killer cells, and mast cells are also present during disease activity. Specific antibodies can also be recovered, but their diagnostic significance is unknown.

Differential Diagnosis

Pulmonary mycotoxicosis (atypical farmer's lung) is a disorder caused by acute massive exposure to moldy silage. The disease presents with fever, chills, and coughing that last for several days to a week. Diffuse infiltrations are apparent on chest x-ray radiograph, and fungal organisms are evident in alveoli and bronchioles, but no serum precipitins occur. The cause is unknown, but the illness is probably a toxic pneumonitis from a fungal product. Recurrent infectious pneumonias, other causes of interstitial lung disease, asthma, allergic bronchopulmonary aspergillosis, and pneumoconioses must also be differentiated from hypersensitivity pneumonitis.

Treatment

Avoidance of the allergen is the accepted form of treatment and prevention, although this may require a change in work that can seriously affect the patient and his or her family. Systemic corticosteroid therapy is indicated for resolution of acute reactions and for terminating and reversing severe or progressive disease. The drug should not be used as an alternative to avoidance of the allergen, but it may be necessary to protect the patient by suppressing inflammation if the allergen source has not been identified. Inhaled corticosteroids are not indicated.

Complications

Respiratory failure and cor pulmonale may result from chronic disease. Bronchiolitis obliterans may lead to irreversible obstructive pulmonary disease. Death from respiratory failure is possible during any phase of the disease.

Prognosis

Prognosis for recovery is good in the acute or subacute stages once the cause has been identified and avoided. Some patients with bird handler's disease, however, have progressive pulmonary insufficiency even with complete avoidance of birds. On the other hand, farmers can continue to have some exposure to thermophilic actinomycetes without progressive illness as long as the acute febrile symptomatic attacks are avoided.

Prevention

Avoidance is the only means of preventing this disease. Effective treatment therefore requires a specific immunologic diagnosis whenever possible because the same allergen may be found in different environments (see Table 29–4). The purpose of avoidance is prevention of irreversible lung disease.

Occupational preventive measures are obvious for the currently recognized causes. Proper workplace hygiene, filters and masks where appropriate, and other measures should be employed. Diseases caused by allergens in homes, automobiles, and offices are best prevented by physician awareness of the disease.

REFERENCES

ALLERGIC CONTACT DERMATITIS

Adams RM: *Occupational Skin Disease,* 3rd ed. WB Saunders, 1999.

Belsito DV: The rise and fall of allergic contact dermatitis. *Am J Contact Derm* 1997;8:193.

Beltrani VS (editor): Contact dermatitis: Irritant and allergic. *Immunol Allergy Clin North Am* 1997;17:345 (entire issue).

Huntley AC (editor): Allergic contact dermatitis. *Clin Rev Allergy* 1989;7:345 (entire issue).

Kalish RS, Askenase PW: Molecular mechanisms of CD8+ T cell-mediated delayed hypersensitivity: Implications for allergies, asthma, and autoimmunity. *J Allergy Clin Immunol* 1999;103:192.

Nethercott J: The positive predictive accuracy of patch tests. *Immun Allergy Clin North Am* 1989;9:549.

Rietschel RL, Fowler JF, Jr: *Fisher's Contact Dermatitis,* 4th ed. Lea & Febiger, 1995.

HYPERSENSITIVITY PNEUMONITIS

Ando M, Suga M: Hypersensitivity pneumonitis. *Curr Opin Pulm Med* 1997;3:391.

Calvert JE et al: Pigeon fanciers lung. *Clin Exp Allergy* 1999;29:166.

Craig TJ, Richerson HB: Update on hypersensitivity pneumonitis. *Compr Ther* 1996;22:559.

Salvaggio JE: Extrinsic allergic alveolitis (hypersensitiviy pneumonitis): Past, present, and future. *Clin Exp Allergy* 1997;27: Suppl 11;18.

Sharma OP, Fujimura N: Hypersensitivity pneumonitis: A noninfectious granulomatosis. *Semin Respir Infect* 1995; 10:96.

30

Drug Allergy

Jeffrey L. Kishiyama, MD, Allyson T. Tevrizian, MD, & Pedro C. Avila, MD

Introduction

Adverse reactions to drugs are common, affecting an estimated 2–30% of hospitalized inpatients. Undesired and unintended reactions may be **immunologic,** the subject of this chapter, or **nonimmunologic.** The latter include **side effects, intolerance, drug toxicity,** and **idiosyncratic** reactions.

Immunologic Basis of Drug Hypersensitivity

Immunologically mediated drug reactions result from the specific interaction of a drug or one of its metabolites with circulating IgG or IgM antibody, IgE antibody bound to mast cells or basophils, or sensitized lymphocytes. The ensuing allergic reaction represents the clinical manifestations of the inflammatory response. Immunogenicity of a drug is related to both genetic factors and physical characteristics of the antigen (drug) itself. High-molecular-weight drugs (eg, insulin, heparin, and heterologous or animal proteins) are immunogenic without modification, but most drugs (eg, penicillin, sulfonamides, and phenytoin) are low-molecular-weight compounds that are not antigenic unless modified through a process called **haptenation** (Figure 30–1). In this case a drug or its metabolite forms acyl-, amide- or disulfide-bonds (or rarely noncovalent bonds) with the patient's cell surfaces, soluble proteins, and other molecules with free amino or sulfhydryl groups. The resulting complex or haptenated drug is then recognized as foreign by the immune system and capable of inducing an immunologic response. Because many drugs are not chemically reactive in their native state, biotransformation or hydrolysis during metabolism is responsible for generating reactive compounds, that is, haptens. A full understanding of the **immunochemistry** of a low-molecular-weight drug is necessary to develop diagnostic allergy testing.

Drug-related **risk factors** for allergy are reflected in the prevalence of clinical hypersensitivity. Penicillin and other β-lactam antibiotics cause hypersensitivity in approximately 2–3% of the population by several different pathogenetic mechanisms. Therapeutic heterologous serum, such as antivenin and antithymocyte globulin, carry a high prevalence of immunopathologic reactions. The **route of administration** and pattern of exposure can also influence sensitization, which is more likely to occur after topical exposure. High-dose intravenous therapy is more immunogenic than oral or brief courses of treatment. Antihistamines, for example, rarely cause allergic reactions when taken systemically, but frequently sensitize for allergic contact dermatitis when used topically, probably because of the highly proficient antigen-presenting Langerhans' cells in the skin.

Patient-related risk factors are both genetic and acquired. Surprisingly, atopic status does not increase the risk of immediate hypersensitivity to drugs, but a familial propensity to develop drug allergies has been reported. Genetic factors determine drug metabolism, and certain human leukocyte antigen (HLA) phenotypes have been linked to increased reactivity. Genetic or acquired differences in N-acetylation rate (acetylation phenotype) or N-oxidation rate affect the risk for reaction to sulfonamides, hydralazine, and procainamide. Concurrent disease or concomitant drug administration also affects the risk of reaction. Epstein-Barr virus and human immunodeficiency virus (HIV) infection significantly increase the risk of cutaneous reactions to ampicillin and sulfonamides, respectively. Despite the lack of CD4 helper lymphocytes in acquired immunodeficiency disease, there is evidence that immunoreactive CD8 cytotoxic cells can produce the cytokines that enhance IgE production, eosinophilia, or cell-mediated drug-induced immunopathology. The spectrum of frequent drug-induced reactions in HIV infection includes fever, rash, anaphylaxis, Stevens-Johnson syndrome, toxic epidermal necrolysis, and hematologic and hepatic reactions.

Immunopathologic Classification

The clinical manifestations and their temporal relationship to drug exposure are important clinical clues in diagnosis. The **Gell and Coombs** classification of clinical hypersensitivity is especially useful for allergic drug reactions (Table 30–1).

Type I immediate hypersensitivity reactions are IgE-mediated and include acute urticaria, allergic bronchospasm, angioedema, or anaphylaxis (see Chapter 26). In the previously sensitized patient, symp-

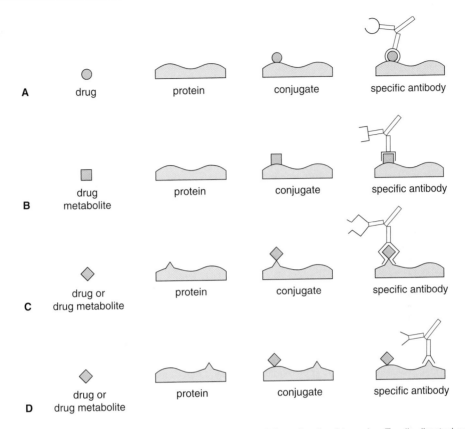

Figure 30–1. The interaction of a drug with tissue protein may result in antibodies (shown) or T cells directed against various determinants. **A:** The specific antibodies are directed against the native molecule. **B:** The antibodies are directed against a hydrolysis or biotransformation product of the drug. **C:** The antibodies are directed against a new determinant formed by the interaction of the drug or drug metabolite and the protein. **D:** Conjugation of the drug or its metabolites results in a conformational change in the tissue protein, which is then recognized as foreign by the immune system.

toms develop within minutes after drug exposure. If IgE antibodies are synthesized de novo during the course of drug treatment, the onset of clinical symptoms is delayed by days to weeks. Approximately 90% of systemic **anaphylactic** reactions include cutaneous features, such as generalized flushing, pruritus, urticaria, or angioedema. These findings alone may occur during parenteral therapy in the absence of immediate hypersensitivity.

Type II cytotoxic reactions are mediated by IgG or IgM antibodies and complement. A circulating or bone marrow cell (erythrocyte, leukocyte, megakaryocyte) is affected as an "innocent bystander" because the drug or drug-immune complex adheres to it, so that immune activation of complement results in lysis through the action of the "membrane attack complex" (C5-9). In theory, a similar drug-induced immune complex-complement-mediated pathway could damage a solid organ, such as the liver, kidney, or lung.

Table 30–1. Gell and Coombs 1963 classification of immunopathology.

Class	Specific Immune Reactant	Mediators	Diseases
I	IgE antibodies	Mast cell and basophil-derived	Atopy Anaphylaxis Urticaria/angioedema
II	IgG, IgM antibodies	Complement	Immune hemolytic anemia, neutropenia, thrombocytopenia
III	IgG, IgM antibodies	Complement	Serum sickness
IV	T lymphocytes	T-cell cytokines	Allergic contact dermatitis

Classic **serum-sickness** disorders are **type III** hypersensitivity reactions, e.g., serum sickness, and arise from the generation of circulating **immune complexes** (soluble antigen–antibody complexes). Pathologic lesions develop from the deposition of soluble immune-complexes in tissues such as elastic lamina of arteries, glomeruli, articular cartilage, and skin basement membranes. **Products resulting from complement activation** are strongly chemotactic for polymorphonuclear leukocytes, which activate and produce reactive oxygen metabolites and proteolytic lysosomal enzymes. These inflammatory mediators cause vascular and tissue damage, which can be magnified if the clotting system is also activated. Fever, arthralgias, lymphadenopathy, glomerulonephritis, and vasculitis are the **clinical manifestations,** which typically appear 10–21 days after administration of the offending medication. The time course of disease development reflects the generation of specific antibody, formation of immune complexes, and a relative state of soluble antigen excess. The appearance of symptoms can be more rapid, in a matter of 2–4 days, when antibody is preexisting because of previous sensitization. In the days before the introduction of antibiotics, the use of foreign animal serum was used as a treatment for infection, and approximately 50% of treated patients developed clinical serum sickness. Heterologous serum is still used as antivenin for treatment of snake and toxic spider bites and can cause type III reactions, but even low-molecular-weight drugs can trigger immune complex-mediated disease after haptenation with soluble proteins. Penicillin may be the most common drug causing type III reactions in clinical practice. Many other drugs have been reported to cause similar reactions, including sulfonamides, NSAIDs, hydantoins, metronidazole, thiouracils, and cephalosporins. The current use of foreign monoclonal antibody therapy for a wide variety of disorders has brought a resurgence of immune complex-mediated illness.

Type IV reactions are cell-mediated, delayed hypersensitivity **reactions involving sensitized lymphocytes. Allergic contact dermatitis (ACD)** is a classic type IV immunopathologic reaction. In cutaneous reactions, antigen (hapten–protein conjugate) is processed by antigen-presenting (Langerhans') cells, which interact with antigen-specific T helper cells, stimulating interleukin-1 (IL-1) production, upregulating Langerhans' cell function and T lymphocyte synthesis of interleukin-2 (IL-2) and interferon gamma (IFN-γ). These cytokines orchestrate the dermal inflammatory infiltration by cytotoxic T cells and mononuclear phagocytes, epidermal edema, and intraepidermal vesicles. Acute lesions are characterized by erythema, pruritus, papules, and vesicles. Chronic or subacute lesions may be difficult to distinguish from other dermatoses, with lichenification, scaling, and excoriation being the more predominant features. The typical interval between exposure and clinical symptoms is 12–48 hours in sensitized patients, but the actual process of sensitization may take days to years, depending on the intensity of exposure and the nature of the allergen. Drugs causing allergic contact dermatitis include topical neomycin, anesthetic agents, *para*-amino (PABA) compounds, penicillin, sulfonamides, bacitracin, and chloramphenicol. ACD has also been reported to transdermally administered medications such as clonidine, nitroglycerin, estradiol, and scopolamine. An additive such as ethylene diamine or fragrance, rather than the drug itself, is commonly the allergen. Ironically, topical corticosteroids used to treat ACD, are occasionally contact allergens as well.

Drug-induced **photosensitivity** can be either phototoxic (direct thermal injury) or photoallergic. Phototoxic reactions are not immunologic. Instead, a drug or its metabolite is transformed in vivo into a toxic compound by sunlight exposure, producing tissue injury that clinically resembles sunburn. In photoallergic reactions, the solar radiation alters the drug or its metabolites in vivo forming a reactive compound or complete hapten that elicits an immune response. The rash is a type IV eczematous lesion like allergic contact dermatitis. Drugs causing photoallergic reactions include sulfonamides, sulfonylurea, chlorpromazine, hexachlorophene, furosemide, isoniazid, naproxen, and amiodarone.

Some immunologic drug reactions do not easily fit the Gell and Coombs classification. **Drug fever** can be caused through a variety of immunologic and nonimmunologic mechanisms. Jarisch–Herxheimer reactions are febrile responses to pyrogens or endotoxin released by dying organisms. Fever may be caused by bacteremia or a Jarisch–Herxheimer reaction in patients receiving antibiotics, but fever accompanied by eosinophilia and a rash with rapid defervescence after discontinuation of the drug suggests an immunologic etiology. **Acute interstitial nephritis** (AIN) has been reported during therapy with methicillin and many other antibiotics that are not intrinsically nephrotoxic. NSAIDs, captopril, allopurinol, sulfonamides, rifampin, and phenytoin have also been implicated in AIN, which may present 10–20 days after initiation of therapy and lead to acute renal failure but may also be more occult and insidious in onset. **Autoimmune diseases** can be initiated by a drug. Drug-induced lupus has been associated with procainamide, hydralazine, isoniazid, methyldopa, and quinidine therapy. The majority of patients taking procainamide develop antinuclear antibodies, but fortunately a smaller proportion actually develops clinical symptoms. Cytotoxic antibody responses and immune complex-mediated mechanisms are likely to be involved, but T-cell functions can also be abnormal and potentially contribute to the disease.

The diagnosis of drug allergy is outlined in Table 30–2. The ability to confirm immunologic drug hypersensitivity is important in the diagnosis of a cur-

Table 30–2. Diagnostic procedure in drug allergy.

1. Obtain history of reaction, including
   A. Time course
   B. Temporal relation to suspected drug(s)
2. List all current medications by
   A. Known propensity for allergy
   B. History of prior reaction in the patient
3. Classify the reaction as most likely
   A. Immunologic
   B. Pharmacologic
   C. Toxic
   D. Drug–drug interaction
   E. Idiosyncratic or intolerance
4. If most likely immunologic, classify by suspected Immunopathologic mechanism
5. Perform testing appropriate to the suspected mechanism
   A. Skin or in vitro test, if available. If not
   B. Test-dose challenge

rent suspected reaction and in the selection of a drug for future treatment. The appropriate in vivo and in vitro methods are available (Table 30–3). In the case of IgE-mediated reactions, their use for suspect drugs that are macromolecules, especially proteins such as insulin, streptokinase, chymopapain, and heterologous polyclonal or monoclonal antibodies, are diagnostically dependable. In the case of low-molecular-weight organic drugs, which constitute the vast majority of the current armamentarium, allergy tests are limited by the need to know the immunochemistry of the drug and its metabolites (as well as cross-reacting drugs and their metabolites) in order to engineer the proper test reagent and by the need for extensive prospective trials to establish the positive and negative predictive values of the test results on a heterogeneous population of persons with and without a history of reaction to each drug being tested. Currently, these criteria are met only in the case of penicillin and other β-lactam drugs.

Patch testing is appropriate for drug reactions that present as allergic contact dermatitis from topically applied substances. The utility of patch testing in the evaluation of maculopapular rashes from orally or parenterally administered drugs is controversial.

The tests are read approximately 48 hours after ap-

Table 30–3. Drug allergy testing methods.

Immunologic Reaction	In Vivo	In Vitro
Type I	Immediate skin prick and intradermal	RAST, ELISA
Type II	None	Coombs[a]
Type III	Intradermal Arthus test	Precipitin test, RAST, ELISA
Type IV	Patch test	Lymphocyte proliferation[a]

[a] Requires specialized research laboratory.
Abbreviations: RAST = radioallergosorbent assay, ELISA = enzyme-linked immunosorbent assay.

plication and assessed for erythema, induration, and vesicle formation. The presence of these features suggests a type IV allergic response. Because many of the components of any topical medications can cause sensitization, from the active agent to components of the vehicle or the preservatives, broad panels of test substances are commonly applied. Frequently, these panels include nickel sulfate, thimerosal, formaldehyde, quaternium-15, thirams, ethylenediamine, and phenylenediamine, in addition to the active medication. Positive test reactions must be correlated with the history and physical examination findings to assess their clinical relevance.

Provocative or incremental challenge, also known as **"test-dose challenge"** can be useful when an allergic reaction to a drug is of low probability and diagnostic testing is not feasible. The test-dose challenge is below the dose that would likely cause a serious reaction. If tolerated, the dosing progresses at large incremental increases until a reaction occurs or full dose therapy is reached.

The initial dose is generally 0.1–1% of the desired treatment dose, and approximately threefold dose escalations are given until the desired dose is reached. For IgE-mediated reactions, a reaction is expected within 30 minutes of the test dose, so doses are given at this interval. For a late reaction such as macular-papular eruptions, the intervals between dosing increase should be 24–48 hours. Test dosing is contraindicated if a history of Stevens-Johnson syndrome or toxic epidermal necrolysis is elicited. Premedication with antihistamine and steroids is not advised because it can mask early symptoms and allow dosing to proceed further than advisable.

The **radioallergosorbent test (RAST)** and **enzyme-linked immunosorbent assay (ELISA)** are quantitative immunoassays for detection of IgE antibodies to specific antigens. These tests apply when the antigenic determinant of a drug is known. Currently, RAST and ELISA tests are available for protein drugs such as insulin, chymopapain, streptokinase, and for the major determinant of penicillin allergy. The sensitivity and specificity of these tests are not well characterized, so skin testing may be preferred. Detecting serum IgG and IgM antibodies to drug antigens is theoretically diagnostic for serum sickness, but their sensitivity and specificity for the disease are currently unknown. Late-onset reactions (eg, morbilliform rash) to nonprotein drugs are thought to be mediated by sensitized lymphocytes, but various in vitro drug-specific lymphocyte proliferation assays have generated inconsistent results. Although highly desirable clinically, these assays require knowledge of the immunochemistry and clinically relevant antigenic epitopes of many drugs, and they are expensive and time-consuming.

Acute rapid drug desensitization may be indicated in patients with a confirmed drug allergy, for which no satisfactory alternative treatment is possible or if no diagnostic testing is available. The disease should be serious enough to warrant the risk of possible anaphylaxis from the treatment. In theory, desensitization provides univalent haptens, which bind surface-bound IgE without cross-linking. Once the cell-bound specific IgE antibodies are saturated with hapten, the mast cell is refractory to further drug exposure and will not degranulate. Desensitization is an active but reversible process dependent on continuous presence of drug. Repeat desensitization is required for subsequent treatment courses with the same drug.

Desensitization is achieved by administering progressive doubling doses of drug at regular intervals (eg, every 15 minutes) at a starting dose typically 10^{-4}–10^{-5} of the full dose, until a therapeutic dose is tolerated. Oral administration carries a lower risk of life-threatening reactions, but parenteral administration may be necessary for certain drugs. Premedication with antihistamines or steroids may mask early signs of anaphylaxis and allow dosing to proceed further than advisable. Complications of penicillin desensitization are pruritus, urticaria, wheezing, inflammation at the infusion site, and, less commonly, serum sickness, hemolytic anemia, and glomerulonephritis. Desensitization dosing protocols have been published for penicillin, insulin, and sulfonamides, but these can be adapted for other medications. Slower "desensitization" (eg, daily) for non-IgE-mediated reactions is often effective although the mechanism of action is unknown.

The incidence of non-IgE-mediated late-onset morbilliform eruption from trimethoprim–sulfamethoxazole (TMP-SMZ) is increased tenfold in patients infected with HIV. **Slow oral TMP-SMZ "desensitization"** is safe and effective but should not be attempted in patients with Stevens–Johnson syndrome, multiple mucous membrane involvement, hepatitis, or hemolytic anemia.

Allergy to Specific Drugs

Beta-lactam antibiotics (penicillins and cephalosporins) are the most common drugs causing hypersensitivity, with an incidence of 0.7–8% (Figure 30–2). Less than 10% of patients who are history-positive for an adverse reaction to **penicillin,** however, have penicillin-specific IgE antibodies confirmed by testing. There is a time-dependent decline in the rate of positive skin tests in patients with confirmed immediate hypersensitivity. Patient-related historical accounts are not always accurate, but suspected hypersensitivity should be taken seriously. Anaphylactic reactions to penicillin are life-threatening in 1–5/10,000 courses of treatment. Benzylpenicillin (Penicillin G) is one of the few drugs whose metabolites and antigenic determinants have been identified immunochemically. The β-lactam ring structure is shared by all semisynthetic penicillins and is responsible for significant immunogenic cross-

Figure 30–2. Core structures of the five groups of β-lactam antibiotics. R1, R2, R3, sidechains. X stands for the oxygen atom or CH_2 in penems.

reactivity. (Figure 30–3) The primary metabolite is benzylpenicilloyl, referred to as the **"major determinant"** because 95% of tissue-bound penicillin is in this form. The metabolites comprising the other 5% are termed collectively the **"minor determinants."** Other antigenic sites exist on unique sidechains of various semisynthetic penicillins, but virtually all patients with immediate hypersensitivity possess IgE antibodies against the major or minor determinants. The major determinant is available commercially as a

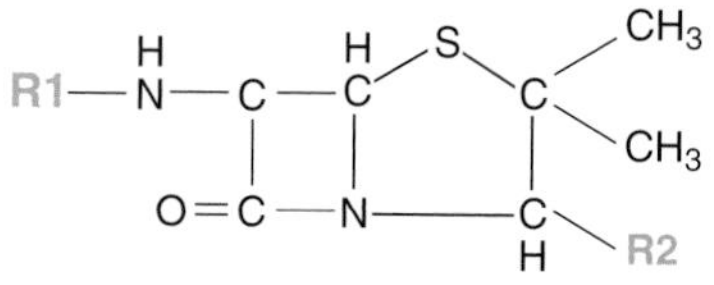

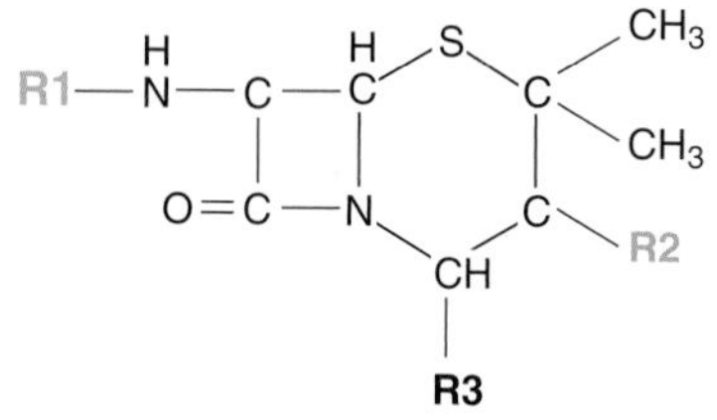

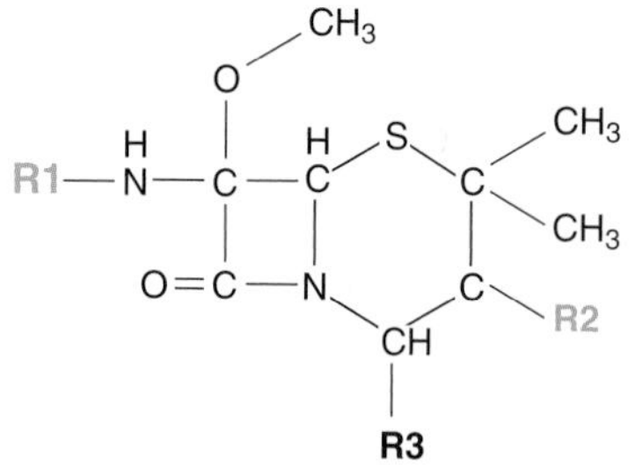

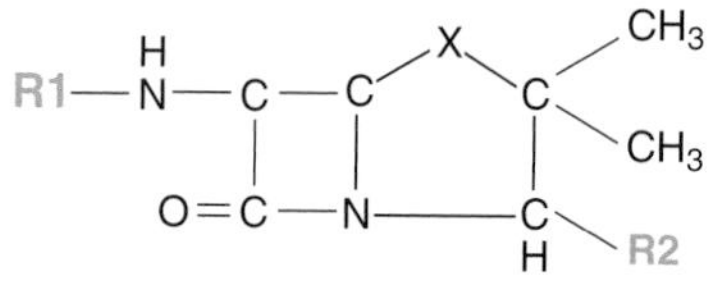

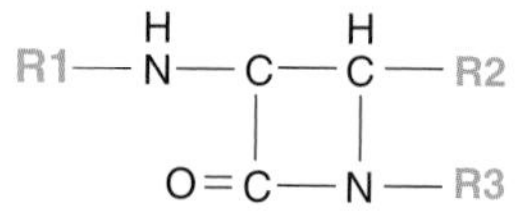

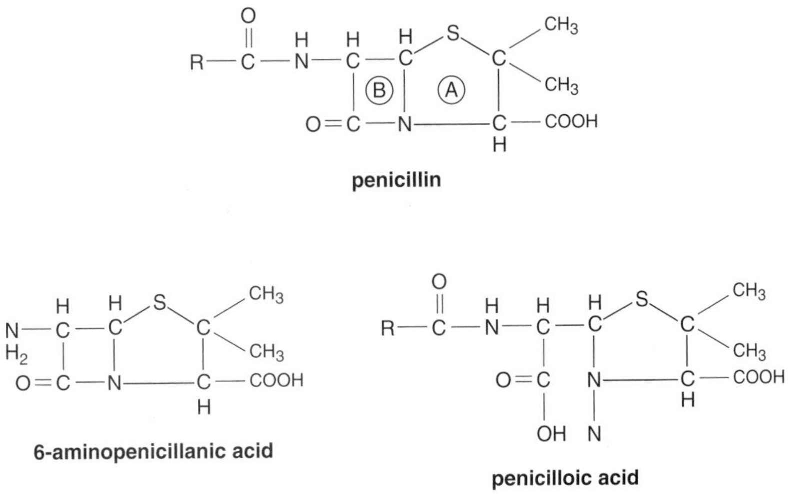

Figure 30–3. Penicillin and two allergenic biotransformation products. **A:** Thiazolidine ring. **B:** β-Lactam ring.

polylysine conjugate for skin testing, and the minor determinants are available only at selected allergy/immunology centers. Allergy testing with native penicillin and the major determinant identify only 85–90% of patients at risk for immediate hypersensitivity reactions, but the most severe reactions may occur in patients allergic to the minor determinants. Testing with both the major and minor determinants raises the sensitivity above 95%. Life-threatening reactions in history-positive, skin test-negative patients are extraordinarily rare.

Positive skin tests to either the major or minor determinants suggest that the patient is at significant (67%) risk of a hypersensitivity reaction and should undergo acute rapid desensitization if the drug must be used.

The value of penicillin allergy skin testing in patients suspected of **cephalosporine** allergy is uncertain. In vitro immunologic cross-reactivity between the penicillins and cephalosporins is substantial, but the incidence of in vivo cross-reactivity for first-generation cephalosporins is probably less than 10%, and much lower with second- and third-generation cephalosporins. Significant immunologic cross-reactivity occurs between penicillin and imipenem, but none with aztreonam, a monobactam.

The majority of adverse reactions to drugs used during **general anesthesia** are immediate reactions, involving either IgE- or non-IgE-mediated mechanisms. The distinction is important. Non-IgE-mediated release of histamine from mast cells and basophils can be triggered by drug-induced osmotic changes, complement activation, stimulation of the kinin–kallikrein system, and direct cellular activation. True IgE-mediated **anaphylactic reactions** require previous sensitization with synthesis of drug-specific

IgE antibodies, whereas these **pseudoallergic reactions,** also known as "anaphylactoid" reactions (ie, anaphylactic-like but not mediated by IgE antibodies) can occur on first exposure (See Table 30–1). Furthermore, the distinction between IgE-mediated anaphylaxis and pseudoallergic reactions is not merely a semantic one, but carries clinical importance. Some pseudoallergic reactions can be prevented with premedication (antihistamines and glucocorticoids), but this is not reliable for true systemic IgE-mediated anaphylaxis. Immunologic (ie, allergen) cross-reactivity depends on similarities in chemical structure, whereas pseudoallergic reactions depend on the biologic function of the drug.

The prevalence of anaphylaxis and anaphylactoid reactions during anesthesia administration is approximately 1 in 3500 procedures. About 50–60% are allergic (IgE-mediated). In one study, 50% of IgE-mediated anaphylactic reactions from anesthesia agents were caused by **muscle relaxants,** particularly the quaternary ammonium compound succinylcholine (suxamethonium) but also alcuronium, vecuronium, gallamine, and, less frequently, pancuronium. Cross-reactive quaternary ammonium ionic compounds in many consumer products and cosmetics are the suspected sensitizer because 90% of reacting patients are female. **Other drugs** implicated in anaphylactic shock during anesthesia are thiopental, *d*-tubocurarine, latex, sedative–hypnotics, plasma substitutes, opioids, benzodiazepines, propofol, and antibiotics. Some of these can cause mast cell degranulation both by IgE- and non-IgE-mediated mechanisms.

Local anesthetics are extremely rare causes of IgE-mediated hypersensitivity. Most adverse reactions are pharmacologic; toxic; vasovagal; or caused by hyperventilation, anxiety, rapid absorption, or inadvertent intravascular administration. These compounds, however, can cause allergic contact dermatitis, especially as an occupational disease in health care workers from frequent handling (eg, dentists). The diagnosis is confirmed by patch testing, which shows that the allergenic drug contains the *para*-aminophenyl group in its chemical structure (eg, procaine, tetracaine, benoxinate, benzocaine, or butamben). Those that do not (eg, lidocaine, mepivacaine, dibucaine, bupivacaine, proparacaine, dimethisoquin, cyclomethycaine, pramoxine, and cocaine) can be used safely.

Several distinct allergic and pseudoallergic reactions are associated with **aspirin (ASA)** and **nonsteroidal antiinflammatory drugs (NSAIDs).** Type I IgE-mediated **immediate hypersensitivity,** to ASA or NSAIDs may account for 1–3% of patients presenting with anaphylaxis or acute urticaria. Cross-reactivity is absent because these drugs are chemically different. **ASA sensitivity with asthma, nasal polyposis,** and **aspirin-induced bronchospasm and rhinosinusitis** is pseudoallergic and occurs with all of these drugs in each patient. The suspected mechanism is the pharmacologic inhibition of cyclooxygenase-1 (COX-1) enzymes and an aberrant generation of vasoactive and bronchospastic leukotrienes via the 5-lipoxygenase (5-LO) pathway. Weak COX-1 inhibitors (eg, acetaminophen) may cause symptoms when given in very high doses. Nonacetylated salicylates, such as choline magnesium trisalicylate and COX-2⁻ inhibitor NSAID drugs, do not cause the reaction. Some cases of chronic urticaria and angioedema may be due to a similar mechanism without the association with asthma and nasal polyps. Very rare cases of NSAID-induced aseptic meningitis and hypersensitivity pneumonitis are suspected to be due to cellular reactivity (type IV reactions).

Oral ASA desensitization is universally effective in the prevention of aspirin-induced asthma in patients with asthma, rhinosinusitis, and nasal polyposis. It requires continuous low-dose administration of daily ASA, and high-dose daily aspirin appears to improve the rhinosinusitis but not the asthma. Desensitization is not effective for ASA/NSAID urticarial angioedema.

REFERENCES

GENERAL

Adkinson NF: Drug allergy. In *Allergy Principles & Practice,* 5th edition. Middleton E et al (editors). Mosby-Year Book, 1998.

Levenson D et al: Cutaneous manifestations of adverse drug reactions. *Immunol Allergy Clin North Am* 1991; 11:443.

Patterson R et al: Drug allergy and protocols for management of drug allergies. *Allergy Proc* 1994;15:238.

Storrs F: Contact dermatitis caused by drugs. *Immunol Allergy Clin North Am* 1991;11:509.

ASPIRIN SENSITIVITY

Stevenson DD et al: Long term ASA desensitization-treatment of aspirin sensitive asthmatic patients: Clinical outcome studies. *J Allergy Clin Immunol* 1996;98:751.

PENICILLIN ALLERGY

Kishiyama JL, Adelman DC: The cross-reactivity and immunology of β-lactam antibiotics. *Drug Safety* 1994; 10:318.

Sullivan TJ: Antigen-specific desensitization of patients allergic to penicillin. *J Allergy Clin Immunol* 1982;69:500.

REACTIONS DURING GENERAL ANESTHESIA

Gall H et al: Adverse reactions to local anesthetics: Analysis of 197 cases. *J Allergy Clin Immuno* 1996;97:933.

Gueant JL et al: Diagnosis and pathogenesis of the anaphylactic reactions to anaesthetics. *Clin Exp Allergy* 1998; 28 (Suppl 4):65.

Thacker MA, Davis FM. Subsequent general anaesthesia in patients with a history of previous anaphylactoid/anaphylactic reaction to muscle relaxant. Annaesth Intensive Care 1999;27:190.

DESENSITIZATION

Caumes E et al: Efficacy, safety of desensitization with sulfamethoxazole & trimethoprim in 48 previously hypersensitive patients infected with human immunodeficiency virus. *Arch Dermatol* 1997;133:465.

Sark B et al: Acute and chronic desensitization of penicillin allergic patients using oral penicillin. *J Allergy Clin Immunol* 1987;79:523.

Rheumatic Diseases

31

Kenneth E. Sack, MD, & Kenneth H. Fye, MD

Many of the major rheumatologic disorders are autoimmune in nature. A thorough understanding of the mechanisms of the immune response is therefore essential to an understanding of these diseases. This chapter discusses the rheumatologic diseases with proved or hypothesized immunologic pathogenesis.

SYSTEMIC LUPUS ERYTHEMATOSUS

Major Immunologic Features

- Autoantibodies to multiple nuclear antigens, including double-stranded DNA
- Numerous other autoantibodies present as well
- Depression of serum complement levels occurs during flares of disease activity
- Immunoglobulins and complement deposit in the kidney and at the dermal–epidermal junction
- Genetic risk factors include deficiencies of early components of the classical complement cascade

General Considerations

Systemic lupus erythematosus (SLE) is a chronic systemic inflammatory disease that follows a course of alternating exacerbations and remissions. Involvement of multiple organ systems occurs during periods of disease activity. The cause of SLE is unknown. The disease affects predominantly females (4:1 over males) of childbearing age; however, the age at onset ranges from 2 to 90 years. It is more prevalent among nonwhites (particularly blacks) than whites.

Immunologic Pathogenesis

The hallmark of SLE is the production of autoantibodies directed against nuclear components, including single-stranded and double-stranded DNA, histones, small nuclear ribonucleoproteins (snRNPs), and the Ro (SS-A) ribonucleoprotein particle. Although cell-mediated immunity contributes to certain manifestations of SLE, autoantibodies appear to play the key role in pathogenesis. Complexes of these antibodies and their antigens can damage tissues by activating

complement and by engaging Fc receptors on macrophages and other inflammatory cells. DNA-anti-DNA immune complexes are of particular importance in the causation of lupus glomerulonephritis. SLE patients also can make antibodies to organ-specific, cell surface antigens, such as autoantibodies to platelets and erythrocytes leading to thrombocytopenia and hemolytic anemia, respectively.

The concordance rate for SLE is five to tenfold greater in monozygotic than in dizygotic twins but still is less than 50%. Thus, both genetic and environmental factors likely contribute to the development of SLE. The identification of susceptibility genes is an area of active investigation. HLA-DR2 and HLA-DR3 confer a modest increased risk of SLE. Human leukocyte antigen (HLA) class II alleles also are associated with the development of antibodies to particular autoantigens, with the strongest link between certain HLA-DQ alleles and antibodies to the Ro particle. The most common known susceptibility gene is a null allele at the C4A locus, which is located in the HLA class III region and carries a relative risk of SLE of 6 to 10. Even homozygous C4A deficiency does not result in lack of C4 protein because C4B alleles also encode for C4. The prevalence of SLE is high in those rare individuals who have complete deficiencies of C4 protein or of other early components (C1q, C1r, or C2) of the classical complement pathway. Impaired clearing of immune complexes may explain the association of SLE with these complement deficiencies. Alternatively, the association may reflect impaired clearance of apoptotic bodies in the absence of early complement components. Nuclear autoantigens (eg, nucleosomal DNA, snRNPs, Ro) concentrate in blebs found on the surface of keratinocytes undergoing programmed cell death. Thus, impaired clearance of apoptotic bodies may enhance exposure to the target antigens of the antinuclear antibodies seen in SLE. Ultraviolet light, which exacerbates disease activity in the majority of SLE patients, can induce apoptosis of keratinocytes.

Tolerance to many self-components fails in SLE, but the precise mechanisms are unknown. A wide range of abnormalities of T and B cells occurs in SLE. In general, B cells from SLE patients appear to be hyperactive, with increases in the numbers of B cells that spontaneously produce immunoglobulins in vitro. Whether this B-cell hyperactivity reflects intrinsic abnormalities of B cells or is due to aberrant T-cell regulation is unknown. In mouse models of lupus, however, the development of autoantibodies and disease depends on T cells.

SLE, like many rheumatic disorders, occurs predominantly in women. Estrogens enhance anti-DNA antibody formation and increase the severity of renal disease in animal models. Androgens have the opposite effect on both anti-DNA antibody production and renal disease.

Pathology

Numerous pathologic changes are characteristic of SLE:

1. The verrucous endocarditis of Libman-Sacks consists of ovoid vegetations, 1–4 mm in diameter, which form along the base of the valve.
2. A peculiar periarterial concentric fibrosis results in the so-called onion skin lesion seen in the spleen.
3. A pathognomonic finding in SLE, the **hematoxylin body,** consists of a homogeneous globular mass of nuclear material that stains bluish purple with hematoxylin. Hematoxylin bodies occur in the heart, kidneys, lungs, spleen, lymph nodes, and serous and synovial membranes.

It should be emphasized that patients with fulminant SLE involving the central nervous system, skin, muscles, joints, and kidneys may not have any distinctive pathologic abnormalities at autopsy.

Clinical Features

A. Symptoms and Signs: The onset of SLE can be acute or insidious. Constitutional symptoms include fever, weight loss, malaise, and lethargy. Every organ system may become involved.

1. Joints and muscles—Polyarthralgia or arthritis is the most common manifestation of SLE. The arthritis is symmetric and can involve almost any joint. It resembles rheumatoid arthritis, but bony erosions and severe deformity are unusual.

Avascular necrosis of bone is common in SLE. The femoral head is most frequently affected. Corticosteroids, which are major therapeutic agents in SLE, may play a role in the pathogenesis of this problem. Myalgias, with or without frank myositis, are common.

2. Skin—The most common skin lesion is an erythematous rash involving areas of the body chronically exposed to ultraviolet light. A few patients with SLE develop the classic "butterfly" rash. Sometimes lesions typical of discoid lupus erythematosus occur. This rash may resolve without sequelae, but it can result in scar formation, atrophy, and hypopigmenta-

tion or hyperpigmentation. A nonscarring skin lesion termed subacute cutaneous lupus erythematosus occurs predominantly in patients with anti-SS-A (Ro)antibodies. In addition, bullae, purpura, urticaria, angioneurotic edema, patches of vitiligo, subcutaneous nodules, and thickening of the skin may be seen. Vasculitic lesions, ranging from palpable purpura to digital infarction, are common. Alopecia, which may be diffuse, patchy, or circumscribed, is usually seen in active disease. Mucosal ulcerations, involving both oral and genital mucosa, occur in about 15% of cases.

3. Polyserositis—Pleurisy, with chest pain and dyspnea, is a frequent complication of SLE. Although one third of cases have pleural fluid, massive effusion is rare. Pericarditis is the commonest form of cardiac involvement and can be the first manifestation of SLE. The pericarditis is usually benign, leading only to mild chest discomfort and a pericardial friction rub, but severe pericarditis with tamponade can occur. Isolated peritonitis is extremely rare, although 5–10% of patients with pleuritis and pericarditis have concomitant peritonitis.

4. Kidneys—Renal involvement is a frequent and serious feature of SLE. Seventy-five percent of patients have nephritis at autopsy. The study of renal tissue by light microscopy, immunofluorescence, and electron microscopy may show five distinct histologic lesions, each associated with rather distinctive clinical features. (1) Mesangial glomerulonephritis manifests as hypercellularity and the deposition of immune complexes in the mesangium. This is a benign form of lupus nephritis. (2) In focal glomerulonephritis, segmental proliferation occurs in less than 50% of glomeruli. Immune complexes are found in the mesangium and in the subendothelium of the glomerular capillary. Focal glomerulonephritis is often a benign process, but it may progress to a diffuse proliferative lesion. (3) Diffuse proliferative glomerulonephritis is characterized by extensive cellular proliferation in more than 50% of glomeruli. Immunofluorescence reveals subendothelial deposits of immune complexes. This process frequently leads to renal failure. (4) In membranous glomerulonephritis, glomerular cellularity is normal, but the capillary basement membrane is thickened. Immune complexes occur mainly in subepithelial and intramembranous areas. This lesion may be associated with the development of the nephrotic syndrome. (5) Sclerosing glomerulonephritis is defined by an increase in mesangial matrix, glomerulosclerosis, capsular adhesions, fibrous crescents, interstitial fibrosis with tubular atrophy, and vascular sclerosis. This lesion portends a poor prognosis and is unresponsive to drugs.

It should be emphasized that a benign renal lesion may evolve into a more serious one.

Systemic hypertension is a common finding in acute or chronic lupus nephritis and may contribute to renal dysfunction.

5. Lungs—Pleuritic chest pain occurs in about 50% of patients with SLE. Pleural effusions are less common, are typically unilateral, and resolve quickly with treatment. Clinically apparent lupus pneumonitis is unusual. When a pulmonary infiltrate develops in a patient with SLE, particularly one being treated with corticosteroids or immunosuppressive drugs, infection must be the first diagnostic consideration. Alveolar hemorrhage is also a well-recognized complication of SLE, particularly in patients with anti-Sm antibodies. Restrictive interstitial lung disease is the commonest form of parenchymal involvement. It may be asymptomatic and detectable only by pulmonary function tests. The chest radiograph is usually normal but may show "plate-like" atelectasis or interstitial fibrosis with "honeycombing." Other pulmonary manifestations include pulmonary hypertension, pneumothorax, hemothorax, and vasculitis.

6. Heart—Clinically apparent myocarditis occurs rarely in SLE but when present may result in arrythmia or congestive heart failure. The verrucous endocarditis of SLE, with the characteristic Libman–Sacks vegetations, is usually asymptomatic and diagnosed only by echocardiography or at autopsy. Thickening of the aortic valve cusps with resultant aortic insufficiency can occur. Coronary artery disease, possibly related to corticosteroid therapy, is common.

7. Nervous system—Disturbances of mentation and aberrant behavior, such as psychosis or depression, are the commonest manifestations of central nervous system involvement. Convulsions, cranial nerve palsies, aseptic meningitis, migraine headache, transverse myelitis, peripheral neuritis, and cerebrovascular accidents may also occur.

8. Eyes—Ocular involvement is present in 20–25% of patients. The characteristic retinal finding (the cytoid body) is a fluffy white exudative lesion caused by focal degeneration of the nerve fiber layer of the retina secondary to retinal vasculitis. Scleritis is also a manifestation of ocular vasculitis. Corneal ulceration occurs in conjunction with Sjögren's syndrome (see item 12).

9. Gastrointestinal system—Gastrointestinal vasculitis can occur in SLE. Manifestations include abdominal pain, diarrhea, and hemorrhage. Pancreatitis, cholecystitis, acute and chronic hepatitis, bowel infarction, and protein-losing enteropathy may be seen.

10. Hematopoietic system—See (section B) Laboratory Findings.

11. Vascular system—Small-vessel vasculitis commonly occurs in active SLE. Cutaneous manifestations of small-vessel disease include splinter hemorrhages, periungual occlusions, finger pulp infarctions, and atrophic ulcers. Small-vessel vasculitis may also cause a "stocking-glove" peripheral neuropathy. Medium-vessel arteritis, involving arteries 0.5–1 mm in diameter, also occurs in SLE. Manifestations range from bowel infarction to mononeuritis multiplex to cerebrovascular accidents. Hypercoagulation leading to arterial and venous occlusive disease is seen in patients with antiphospholipid antibodies. Raynaud's phenomenon occurs in 15% of patients with SLE.

12. Sjögren's syndrome—Up to 30% of patients with SLE develop the sicca complex (keratoconjunctivitis sicca, xerostomia).

13. Drug-induced lupus-like syndrome—Certain drugs may provoke a lupus-like picture in susceptible individuals. The most commonly implicated drugs are hydralazine and procainamide, but minocycline, quinidine, chlorpromazine, methyldopa, isoniazid, and phenytoin are also known to produce this syndrome. Typical manifestations of drug-induced lupus are arthralgias, arthritis, rash, fever, and pleurisy. Nephritis and central nervous system involvement are rare. The disease usually remits when the offending drug is discontinued. Antihistone and antisingle-stranded DNA antibodies are typical of drug-induced lupus.

B. Laboratory Findings: Anemia is the most common hematologic finding in SLE. Eighty percent of patients present with a normochromic, normocytic anemia due to marrow suppression. A few develop Coombs-positive hemolytic anemia. Leukopenia and thrombocytopenia are common. Urinalysis may show hematuria, proteinuria, and erythrocyte and leukocyte casts. The sedimentation rate is typically high in active SLE. In central nervous system lupus, the cerebrospinal fluid protein concentration is sometimes elevated, and occasionally a mild lymphocytic pleocytosis occurs.

Immunologic Diagnosis

A. Complement: The serum complement is frequently reduced in active disease because of increased use by immune complexes together with reduced liver synthesis of complement components. Individual complement components, including C3 and C4, and total hemolytic complement activity may be decreased during disease activity. The serum of patients with active SLE occasionally contains circulating cryoglobulin consisting of IgM/IgG aggregates and complement.

B. Autoantibodies:

1. Antinuclear antibodies—Immunoglobulins of all classes may form antinuclear antibodies (ANA). Six different morphologic patterns of immunofluorescent staining have been described, five of which have clinical significance (Table 31–1).

a. The "homogeneous" ("diffuse," or "solid") pattern is the morphologic expression of antihistone antibodies and occurs in patients with systemic or drug-induced lupus erythmatosus. In this pattern, the nucleus shows diffuse uniform staining.

b. The "peripheral" ("shaggy," or "outline") pattern denotes the presence of anti-ds-DNA antibodies. The outline pattern is best seen when human leukocytes

Table 31–1. Antinuclear antibodies.

Pattern	Antigen	Associated Diseases
Peripheral	Double-stranded DNA	SLE
Homogeneous	DNA–histone complex	SLE, drug-induced lupus, occasionally other connective tissue disease
Speckled	Sm (Smith antigen)	SLE
	RNP (ribonucleo-protein)	Mixed connective tissue disease, SLE, Sjögren's syndrome, scleroderma, polymyositis
	SS-A (Ro)	Sjögren's syndrome, SLE
	SS-B (La)	Sjögren's syndrome, SLE
	Jo-1	Polydermatomyositis
	Mi-2	Dermatomyositis
	Scl-70	Scleroderma
	Centromere	Limited scleroderma
Nucleolar	Nucleolus-specific RNA	Scleroderma
	PM-Scl	Polymyositis

Abbreviations: SLE = systemic lupus erythematosus.

are used as substrate. It is characteristic of active SLE.

c. The "speckled" pattern reflects the presence of antibodies directed against non-DNA nuclear constituents. The anti-ENA (extractable nuclear antigen) assay detects antibodies against two saline-extractable nuclear antigens: the Sm (Smith) antigen and RNP (ribonucleoprotein) antigen. Antibodies against the Sm antigen are characteristic of SLE. High titers of anti-RNP antibodies are the hallmark of mixed connective tissue disease, but low-titer anti-RNP antibodies may occur in SLE.

d. The "nucleolar" pattern is caused by the homogeneous staining of the nucleolus. It has been suggested that this antigen may be the ribosomal precursor of ribonucleoprotein. This pattern is rare in SLE and is most often associated with scleroderma or polymyositis-dermatomyositis.

e. The "centromere" pattern is caused by anticentromere antibodies and is typically seen in patients with limited scleroderma.

The pattern of a positive ANA test must be interpreted with caution because (1) the serum of a patient with any rheumatic disease may contain many autoantibodies to different nuclear constituents, so that a ho-

mogeneous pattern may obscure a speckled or nucleolar pattern; (2) different antibodies in the serum can be present in different titers, so that by diluting the serum one can change the pattern observed; (3) the stability of the different antigens is different and can be changed by fixation or denaturation; and (4) the pattern observed appears to be influenced by the types of tissues or cells used as substrate for the test.

The ANA test is occasionally positive in normal individuals, in patients with various chronic diseases, and in the aged. Absence of ANA is strong evidence against a diagnosis of SLE.

2. Anti-DNA antibodies and immune complexes—Three major types of anti-DNA antibodies can be found in the sera of lupus patients: (1) anti-single-stranded or, "denatured," DNA (ss-DNA); (2) anti-double-stranded, or "native," DNA (ds-DNA); and (3) antibodies that react to both ss-DNA and ds-DNA. These antibodies may be either IgG or IgM classes. High titers of anti-ds-DNA antibodies are characteristic of SLE. In contrast, anti-ss-DNA antibodies are not specific and can be found in other autoimmune diseases, such as rheumatoid arthritis, chronic active hepatitis, primary biliary cirrhosis, and drug-induced lupus. Complement-fixing and high-avidity anti-ds-DNA antibodies may be associated with the development of renal disease. The amount of antibody usually correlates with disease activity, and the antibody titer frequently decreases when patients enter remission.

Circulating immune complexes are present in the sera of patients with active disease. Different assay techniques, however, are required to detect complexes of different sizes, and there is controversy about how closely the level of soluble circulating immune complexes correlates with disease activity.

3. Antierythrocyte antibodies—These antibodies belong to the IgG, IgA, and IgM classes and can be detected by the direct Coombs' test. The prevalence of these antibodies among SLE patients ranges from 10% to 65%. Hemolytic anemia does occasionally occur and, when present, is associated with a complement-fixing warm antierythrocyte antibody.

4. Circulating anticoagulants, antiphospholipids, and antiplatelet antibodies—Antiphospholipid antibodies develop in 10–15% of patients with SLE. These antibodies often are associated with a false-positive Venereal Disease Research Laboratory (VDRL) test for syphilis and can possess anticoagulant activity in vitro ("lupus anticoagulant"), leading to prolongation of the partial thromboplastin and Russell viper venom times. Paradoxic thrombotic states may develop owing to actions of antiphospholipid antibodies on platelets, vascular endothelial cells, or erythrocytes. Patients with antiphospholipid antibodies are at increased risk for thrombotic events, and women with these antibodies are subject to recurrent spontaneous abortions. Specific antifactor

VIII antibodies have also been described. These antibodies are potent anticoagulants and may be associated with bleeding. Antiplatelet antibodies are found in 75–80% of patients with SLE and can induce thrombocytopenia.

5. Rheumatoid factors—Almost 30% of patients with SLE have a positive latex fixation test for rheumatoid factors.

6. Anticytoplasmic antibodies—Numerous anticytoplasmic antibodies (antimitochondrial, antiribosomal, antilysosomal) have been found in patients with SLE. These antibodies are not organ- or species-specific. Antiribosomal antibodies are found in the sera of 25–50% of patients. The major antigenic determinant is ribosomal RNA. Antimitochondrial antibodies are more common in other diseases (eg, primary biliary cirrhosis) than in SLE.

C. Tissue Immunofluorescence

1. Kidneys—Irregular or granular accumulation of immunoglobulin and complement occurs along the glomerular basement membrane and in the mesangium in patients with lupus nephritis. On electron microscopy, these deposits are seen in subepithelial, subendothelial, and mesangial sites.

2. Skin—Almost 90% of patients with SLE have immunoglobulin and complement deposition in the dermal-epidermal junction of sun-exposed skin that is *not* involved with an active lupus rash. The immunoglobulins are IgG or IgM and appear as a brightly staining homogeneous or granular band. Patients with discoid lupus erythematosus show deposition of immunoglobulin and complement only in involved skin.

Differential Diagnosis

The diagnosis of SLE in patients with classic multisystem involvement and a positive ANA test is not difficult. The polyarthritis of SLE, however, is often similar to that seen in viral infections, infective endocarditis, mixed connective tissue disease, rheumatoid arthritis, and rheumatic fever. When Raynaud's phenomenon is the predominant complaint, progressive systemic sclerosis should be considered. SLE can present with a myositis similar to that of polymyositis-dermatomyositis. The clinical constellation of arthritis, alopecia, and a positive VDRL may denote secondary syphilis. Felty's syndrome (thrombocytopenia, leukopenia, splenomegaly in patients with rheumatoid arthritis) can simulate SLE. Takayasu's disease should be considered in a young woman who presents with arthralgias, fever, and asymmetric pulses. Some patients with discoid lupus erythematosus may develop leukopenia, thrombocytopenia, hypergammaglobulinemia, a positive ANA, and an elevated sedimentation rate. Ten percent of patients with discoid lupus erythematosus have mild systemic symptoms. The frequent presence of anti-ds-DNA in discoid lupus erythemato-

sus suggests that SLE and discoid lupus erythematosus are part of a single disease spectrum.

Treatment

The efficacy of the drugs used in the treatment of SLE is difficult to evaluate because spontaneous remissions do occur. Few controlled studies have been conducted because it is difficult to withhold therapy in the face of the life-threatening disease that can develop in fulminant SLE. Depending on the severity of the disease, no treatment, minimal treatment (nonsteroidal antiinflammatory drugs, antimalarials), or intensive treatment (corticosteroids, cytotoxic drugs) may be required.

When arthritis is the predominant symptom and other organ systems are not significantly involved, high-dose aspirin or another fast-acting nonsteroidal antiinflammatory drug may suffice to relieve symptoms. When the skin or mucosa is predominantly involved, antimalarials (hydroxychloroquine or chloroquine) and topical corticosteroids are very beneficial. Antimalarials also may be effective in the treatment of systemic disease.

Systemic corticosteroids are used to treat severe SLE and can suppress disease activity and prolong life. The mode of action is unknown, but the immunosuppressive and antiinflammatory properties of these agents presumably play a significant role in their therapeutic efficacy. High-dose corticosteroid treatment is recommended in acute fulminant lupus, acute lupus nephritis, acute central nervous system lupus, acute autoimmune hemolytic anemia, and thrombocytopenic purpura. One or more courses of "pulse" therapy may be effective in patients with recalcitrant disease. The course of corticosteroid therapy should be monitored by the clinical response and meticulous follow-up of laboratory and immunologic parameters.

If the clinical and immunologic status of the patient fails to improve or if serious side effects of corticosteroid therapy develop, immunosuppressive therapy with cytotoxic agents, such as cyclophosphamide, azathioprine, or methotrexate is indicated. Intravenous pulse therapy with cyclophosphamide is a practical and effective means of treating lupus nephritis or CNS lupus (see Chapter 53).

Complications & Prognosis

SLE may run a very mild course confined to one or a few organs, or it may be a fulminant fatal disease. Renal failure and central nervous system lupus were the leading causes of death until the corticosteroids and cytotoxic agents came into widespread use. Since then, the complications of therapy, including atherosclerosis, infection, and cancer, have become common causes of death. The 5-year survival rate of patients with SLE has markedly improved over the past decade and now approaches 80–90%.

RHEUMATOID ARTHRITIS

Major Immunologic Features

- Presence of rheumatoid factors (autoantibodies directed against the Fc portion of IgG) in serum and synovial fluid
- Infiltration of lymphocytes and activated macrophages into involved synovium
- Local production of tumor necrosis factor-α and other proinflammatory cytokines in inflamed synovium

General Considerations

Rheumatoid arthritis is a chronic, recurrent, systemic inflammatory disease primarily involving the joints. It affects 1–3% of people in the United States, with a female-to-male ratio of 3:1. The disease characteristically begins in the small joints of the hands and feet and progresses in a centripetal and symmetric fashion. Elderly patients may present with more proximal large-joint involvement. Deformities are common. Extraarticular manifestations include vasculitis, atrophy of the skin and muscle, subcutaneous nodules, serositis, pneumonitis, lymphadenopathy, splenomegaly, and leukopenia.

Immunologic Pathogenesis

The cause of rheumatoid arthritis is unknown. Current paradigms generally propose that the disease results from an autoimmune response triggered in a genetically susceptible individual by an environmental event, such as an infection. There is no consensus as to the identity of potential initiating infections or other environmental events. Inheritance of certain HLA-DRB1 alleles—DRB1*0101, DRB1*0401, DRB1*0404, DRB1*0405, DRB1*0408, DRB1*1001, and DRB1*1402—increases the relative risk of rheumatoid arthritis in many, but not all, populations studied. The protein product of the HLA-DRB1 allele, the β chain, is one of the two chains of HLA-DR, a class II major histocompatibility (MHC) molecule that presents peptides to CD4 T cells (Chapter 6). The disease-associated alleles share a similar sequence in the β chain (amino acids 70–74) that could influence peptide binding and interactions with T-cell receptors.

The link with HLA-DRB1 polymorphisms provides circumstantial evidence that T-cell recognition of antigen plays an important role in the pathogenesis of rheumatoid arthritis. T cells are a prominent component of the inflammatory infiltrate in the rheumatoid synovium. These synovial T cells have a memory phenotype and appear to be polyclonal; their antigen specificities are unknown. Although there are reports of a bias toward T_H1-like cytokine production by these cells, the more striking observation is the general paucity of T-cell-derived cytokines in synovial tissue. In contrast, there is a wide range of readily detectable macrophage-derived products, including proinflammatory cytokines such as tumor necrosis factor-α and interleukin-1, that can activate synovial fibroblasts and other cells to produce matrix metalloproteinases involved in the degradation of cartilage. According to one hypothesis, macrophages direct much of the ongoing synovial inflammation in rheumatoid arthritis, with T cells playing a critical role in the initiation of the synovitis but not in its propagation. The synovial infiltrate also contains activated B cells, and the synovium is a site for production of rheumatoid factors (antibodies specific for the Fc region of IgG). Immune complexes formed by IgG and rheumatoid factor can fix complement and may amplify the inflammatory process. In contrast to the mononuclear cell predominance in rheumatoid synovial tissues, polymorphonuclear neutrophilic leukocytes predominate in the synovial fluid. Neutrophils contribute to joint inflammation through the production of prostaglandins and the release of proteolytic enzymes and reactive oxygen species.

Rheumatoid factors may play a role in the causation of extraarticular disease. Patients with rheumatoid vasculitis have high titers of monomeric and pentameric IgM, IgA, and IgG rheumatoid factors. Antigen–antibody complexes infused into experimental animals in the presence of IgM rheumatoid factor induce necrotizing vasculitis. Theoretically, immune complexes initiate vascular inflammation by the activation of complement. Pulmonary involvement is associated with the deposition of 11S and 15S protein complexes containing aggregates of IgG in the walls of pulmonary vessels and alveoli. 19S IgM rheumatoid factor has also been detected in arterioles and alveolar walls adjacent to cavitary nodules.

Clinical Features

A. Symptoms and Signs:

1. Onset—The usual age at onset is 20–40 years. In most cases the disease presents with joint manifestations.

2. Articular manifestations—Patients experience stiffness and joint pain, which are generally worse in the morning and improve throughout the day. These symptoms are accompanied by signs of articular inflammation, including swelling, warmth, erythema, and tenderness on palpation. The arthritis is symmetric, involving the small joints of the hands and feet. Large joints (knees, hips, elbows, ankles, shoulders) commonly become involved later in the course of the disease, although in some patients large-joint involvement predominates. The cervical spine may be involved; the thoracic and lumbosacral spine is usually spared.

The most characteristic deformities in the hand are ulnar deviation of the fingers, the "boutonnière" deformity (flexion of the proximal interphalangeal joints and hyperextension of the distal interphalangeal joints resulting from volar slippage of the lateral bands of the superficial extensor tendons), and the "swan neck" deformity (hyperextension of the proximal interphalangeal joints and flexion of the distal interphalangeal joints resulting from contactures of intrinsic muscles of the hand).

3. Extraarticular manifestations—From 20% to 25% of patients (particularly those with severe disease) have subcutaneous or subperiosteal nodules, so-called rheumatoid nodules. Rheumatoid nodules consist of an irregularly shaped central zone of fibrinoid necrosis surrounded by a margin of large mononuclear cells with an outer zone of granulation tissue containing plasma cells and lymphocytes. They are thought to be a late stage in the evolution of a vasculitic process. Mature nodules are firm, nontender, round or oval masses that can be movable or fixed. They frequently develop over bony prominences, most commonly the olecranon process and proximal ulna, but can occur in visceral sites as well. Rheumatoid nodules may also be found in the myocardium, pericardium, heart valves, pleura, lungs, sclera, dura mater, spleen, larynx, and synovial tissues.

Lung involvement includes pleurisy, interstitial lymphocytic pneumonitis or fibrosis, pulmonary nodulosis, bronchiolitis obliterans, and pulmonary hypertension. The manifestations of rheumatoid cardiac disease include pericarditis, myocarditis, valvular insufficiency, and conduction disturbances.

Several types of vasculitis occur in rheumatoid arthritis. The most common is a small-vessel obliterative vasculitis that leads to periungual infarctions, splinter hemorrhages, and peripheral neuropathy. Less common is a subacute cutaneous arteriolitis associated with ischemic ulceration of the skin. The rarest form of rheumatoid vasculitis is a necrotizing vasculitis of medium and large vessels indistinguishable from polyarteritis nodosa. The major neurologic abnormalities in rheumatoid arthritis involve peripheral nerves. In addition to the peripheral neuropathy associated with vasculitis, a number of entrapment syndromes occur due to impingement by periarticular inflammatory tissue or amyloid on nerves passing through tight fascial planes. The carpal tunnel syndrome is a well-known complication of wrist disease; however, entrapment can also occur at the elbow, knee, and ankle. Destruction of the transverse ligament of the odontoid can result in atlantoaxial subluxation with cord or nerve root impingement.

Sjögren's syndrome (keratoconjunctivitis sicca and xerostomia) occurs in up to 30% of patients. Myositis with lymphocytic infiltration of involved muscle is rare. Ocular involvement ranges from benign inflammation of the surface of the sclera (episcleritis) to severe inflammation of the sclera, with nodule formation. Scleronodular disease can lead to weakening and thinning of the sclera (scleromalacia). A catastrophic but rare complication of scleromalacia is perforation of the eye with extrusion of vitreous (scleromalacia perforans).

4. Felty's syndrome—Felty's syndrome is the association of rheumatoid arthritis, splenomegaly, and neutropenia. Possible mechanisms of the hematologic abnormalities seen in these patients include antistem cell antibodies, antigranulocyte antibodies, and splenic sequestration of immune complex-coated polymorphonuclear leukocytes. The syndrome almost always develops in patients with high rheumatoid factor titers and rheumatoid nodules, although the arthritis itself is frequently inactive. Other features of hypersplenism and lymphadenopathy may also be present. These patients are at increased risk of developing bacterial infections.

B. Laboratory Findings: A normochromic, normocytic anemia and thrombocytosis are common among patients with active disease. The sedimentation rate is elevated, and the degree of elevation correlates roughly with disease activity.

The synovial fluid is more inflammatory than that seen in degenerative osteoarthritis or SLE. The leukocyte count is usually 5000–20,000/μL (occasionally higher than 50,000/μL) with a predominance of neutrophils.

The rheumatoid pleural effusion is an exudate containing fewer than 5000 mononuclear or polymorphonuclear leukocytes per microliter. Protein exceeds 3 g/dL, and glucose is often reduced below 20 mg/dL. Rheumatoid factors can be detected, and complement levels are usually low.

C. Radiographic Findings: The first detectable radiographic abnormalities are soft tissue swelling and juxtaarticular demineralization. The destruction of articular cartilage leads to joint space narrowing. Bony erosions develop first at the junction of the synovial membrane and the bone just adjacent to articular cartilage. Destruction of the cartilage and laxity of ligaments lead to maladjustment and subluxation of articular surfaces. Spondylitis is usually limited to the cervical spine and may lead to osteoporosis, joint space narrowing, erosions, and, finally, subluxation of the involved articulations.

Immunologic Diagnosis

The most important serologic abnormality is the presence of rheumatoid factor, which is found in 80% of patients, including virtually all cases complicated by rheumatoid nodules or other manifestations of extraarticular disease. Despite its name, rheumatoid factor is not specific for rheumatoid arthritis. Elevated titers can be seen in other autoimmune diseases (eg, SLE, Sjögren's syndrome, polymyositis), in chronic infections (eg, hepatitis C, subacute bacterial endocarditis), in malignancy, and in otherwise normal individuals, particularly the elderly.

Many patients have antinuclear antibodies. Serum complement levels are usually normal but may be low in the presence of active vasculitis. Cryoglobulins are often seen in patients with rheumatoid vasculitis (Chapter 15).

Differential Diagnosis

In the patient with classic articular changes, bony erosions of the small joints of the hands and feet, and positive rheumatoid factors, the diagnosis of rheumatoid arthritis is not difficult. Early in the disease, or when extraarticular manifestations dominate the clinical picture, other rheumatic diseases (including SLE, Reiter's syndrome, gout, psoriatic arthritis, degenerative osteoarthritis, and the peripheral arthritis of chronic inflammatory bowel disease) or infectious processes may mimic rheumatoid arthritis. Patients with SLE can be distinguished by their characteristic skin lesions, renal disease, and diagnostic serologic abnormalities. Reiter's syndrome occurs predominantly in young men, generally affects joints of the lower extremity in an asymmetric fashion, and is often associated with urethritis and conjunctivitis. Gouty arthritis is usually an acute monarthritis with negatively birefringent sodium urate crystals present within the white cells of inflammatory synovial fluid. Psoriatic arthritis is usually asymmetric and often involves distal interphalangeal joints. Degenerative arthritis is characterized by Heberden's nodes, lack of symmetric joint involvement, and involvement of the distal interphalangeal joints. The peripheral arthritis of bowel disease usually occurs in large weight-bearing joints and is often associated with bowel symptoms. The polyarthritis associated with rubella vaccination, parvovirus infection, viral hepatitis, sarcoidosis, and infectious mononucleosis can mimic early rheumatoid arthritis.

Treatment

A. Physical Therapy: A rational program of physical therapy is vital in the treatment of patients with rheumatoid arthritis. Such a program should consist of an appropriate balance of rest and exercise and the judicious use of heat or cold therapy.

B. Drug Treatment: A major goal of drug treatment is to reduce synovial inflammation in order to improve symptoms and to preserve joint function. Most therapeutic regimens employ one or more of the so-called disease-modifying antirheumatic drugs (DMARDs), such as methotrexate, sulfasalazine, leflunomide, and hydroxychloroquine (see Chapter 53). Approximately 70% of patients respond to methotrexate, the most widely used DMARD in the United States. However, sustained, complete remissions are uncommon with methotrexate or any other DMARD. Several studies suggest that combinations of DMARDs (eg, methotrexate + sulfasalazine + hydroxychloroquine) may be more efficacious than treatment with single agents. The immunosuppressive agents azathioprine and cyclosporine are sometimes used for recalcitrant disease. Gold and penicillamine, once used extensively in the treatment of rheumatoid arthritis, are now prescribed infrequently.

A promising new therapeutic approach to the treatment of rheumatoid arthritis is neutralization of tumor necrosis factor with etanercept (see Chapter 53). Etanercept is effective when used alone or in combination with methotrexate for recalcitrant disease. Ongoing studies are examining the role of etanercept in early rheumatoid disease and the ability of etanercept to slow the progression of joint erosions.

Nonsteroidal antiinflammatory drugs (NSAIDs; see Chapter 53) are useful adjuncts to DMARD treatment but rarely control disease activity when used alone. NSAIDs provide some symptomatic relief and can reduce inflammation but probably do not prevent joint destruction.

Low-dose oral corticosteroids are often used as adjunctive therapy in patients with suboptimal responses to DMARDs. They may slow the progression of erosions in early disease. Because corticosteroids lead to rapid responses, they are sometimes used as bridge therapy to provide symptomatic relief when starting DMARDs, which take weeks or even months to work. Intermittent intraarticular injection of corticosteroid is useful for patients with only a few symptomatic joints. Relief may last for months.

C. Orthopedic Surgery: Surgery to correct or compensate for joint damage is often an essential part of the general management of rheumatoid arthritis. Arthroplasty is employed to relieve pain and to maintain or improve joint motion. Arthrodesis can be used to correct deformity and alleviate pain, but it results in loss of motion. Early synovectomy might prevent joint damage or tendon rupture and decreases pain and inflammation in a given joint, but the synovium often grows back and symptoms may return.

Complications & Prognosis

Several clinical patterns of rheumatoid arthritis are apparent. Spontaneous remission rarely occurs. Some patients have brief episodes of acute arthritis with longer periods of low-grade activity or remission. Rare patients have sustained progression of active disease resulting in deformity and death. Involvement of more than 20 joints during the first 6 months of disease, the presence of rheumatoid nodules, and high titers of rheumatoid factor are unfavorable prognostic factors.

Follow-up of patients after 10–15 years shows that 50% are stationary or improved, 70% are capable of full-time employment, and 10% are completely incapacitated. Death from vasculitis or atlantoaxial subluxation is rare. Fatalities are more often associated with sepsis or the complications of therapy.

JUVENILE ARTHRITIS

Major Immunologic Features

- Overt or "hidden" rheumatoid factors
- Antinuclear antibodies in some patients

General Considerations

Juvenile arthritis consists of a group of disorders that occur in individuals younger than 16 years of age. The incidence of the disease peaks in boys at age 2 and again at age 9, whereas in girls it peaks between 1 and 3 years of age. Juvenile arthritis may present as a systemic illness (Still's disease), as a seronegative pauci- or polyarthritis, or as a seropositive polyarthritis identical to adult rheumatoid arthritis. The outlook for girls with pauciarticular disease is excellent, whereas boys with pauciarticular disease are at risk for the development of ankylosing spondylitis. Although upper respiratory infections and trauma have both been implicated as precipitating factors, the roles of infection, trauma, and heredity in the pathogenesis of the disease are unclear.

Immunologic Pathogenesis

The basic immunopathogenic mechanisms in juvenile arthritis are unknown. Both humoral and cellular defects occur in these patients, however. Diffuse hypergammaglobulinemia, involving IgG, IgA, and IgM, is present. Rheumatoid factors of all immunoglobulin classes have been detected. Approximately 10% of children with juvenile arthritis have a positive test for IgM rheumatoid factor. The sera from some patients with negative tests may actually contain IgM rheumatoid factors. Two major theories have been offered in an attempt to explain the presence of these "hidden" rheumatoid factors in juvenile arthritis. First, IgM rheumatoid factor may bind avidly to native IgG in the patient's serum and therefore may not be able to bind IgG coating the latex particles. Second, an abnormal IgG may be present that preferentially binds IgM, thereby blocking latex fixation. Cold-reacting (4°C) pentameric IgM rheumatoid factors (cryoglobulins) are associated with severe disease.

Serum components of both the classic and alternative (properdin) complement systems are elevated, although this elevation is less in patients who have rheumatoid factors or severe disease. Elevation of serum complement may reflect a secondary overcompensation in response to increased consumption, or a general increase in protein synthesis. Studies of the metabolism of complement actually demonstrate hypercatabolism. The depression of complement in synovial fluid is probably secondary to complement activation by immune complexes, similar to that seen in rheumatoid arthritis.

Studies suggest that patients with juvenile arthritis possess certain HLA tissue types with greater than expected frequencies. Thus, patients with early-onset pauciarticular disease tend to be HLA-DR5- or HLA-DR8-positive, whereas those with late-onset pauciarticular disease tend to be HLA-B27-positive. Patients with rheumatoid factor-positive polyarticular disease tend to be HLA-D4-positive, and those with systemic disease tend to be HLA-DR5-positive.

Clinical Features

A. Symptoms and Signs:

1. Onset—

a. Twenty percent of children, usually younger than age 4, present with high, spiking fever, an evanescent rash, polyserositis, hepatosplenomegaly, and lymphadenopathy (Still's disease).

b. Forty percent of patients present with polyarthritis (more than four joints involved during the first 6 months of illness), sometimes accompanied by low-grade fever and malaise. In 25% of this group, the onset is in late childhood and is associated with rheumatoid factor.

c. Forty percent of patients present with pauciarticular (involvement of four or fewer joints) disease and few systemic manifestations. Slightly more than 50% of these patients are young girls.

2. Joint manifestations—Even in the presence of severe arthritis, young children may not complain of pain but may instead limit the use of a joint. The knees, wrists, ankles, and neck are common sites of initial involvement. Older children occasionally develop symmetric involvement in the small joints of the hands (metacarpophalangeal, proximal interphalangeal, and distal interphalangeal) similar to that seen in adults. In seronegative patients, the metacarpophalangeal joints may be spared. With severe hand involvement, children are more likely to develop radial rather than ulnar deviation. Involvement of the feet may lead to hallux valgus or to "hammer toe" deformity. Achillobursitis and achillotendinitis may cause tender, swollen heels.

3. Systemic manifestations—Fever, often with a high evening spike, is characteristic of Still's disease. Anorexia, weight loss, and malaise are common. Most children with Still's disease develop an evanescent, salmon-colored maculopapular rash that coincides with periods of high fever. Occasional patients manifest cardiac involvement. Pericarditis occurs commonly but rarely leads to dysfunction or constriction. Myocarditis is an unusual manifestation of the cardiac disease, but, when present, can lead to heart failure. Acute pneumonitis or pleuritis sometimes occur, but chronic lung disease is rare.

Iridocyclitis occurs most commonly in young girls with pauciarticular disease and a positive ANA and can precede articular involvement. It typically runs an insidious course and often persists even when joint disease becomes quiescent. Iridocyclitis is best monitored by frequent slit lamp examinations, at least through puberty.

Lymphadenopathy and hepatosplenomegaly are associated with severe systemic disease and are uncommon in patients with chiefly articular manifestations.

Subcutaneous nodules occur in children with polyarticular disease, usually in association with a positive test for rheumatoid factors.

Rarely, Still's disease occurs in adults. Characteristic manifestations include high spiking fevers, evanescent rash, arthritis, and elevated leukocyte count and hepatic enzyme levels.

4. Complications—The major complication of juvenile arthritis is impairment of growth and development secondary to early epiphyseal closure. This is particularly common in the mandible, causing micrognathia, and in the metacarpals and metatarsals, leading to abnormally small fingers and toes. The extent of growth impairment usually correlates positively with the severity and duration of disease but may also reflect the growth-inhibiting effects of steroids. Children in whom arthritis begins before age 5 occasionally undergo increased growth of an affected extremity. Vasculitis and encephalitis are sometimes observed in patients with juvenile arthritis. Secondary amyloidosis occurs rarely.

B. Laboratory Findings: Mild leukocytosis (15,000–20,000/μL) is the rule, but some patients develop leukopenia. A normochromic microcytic anemia, an elevated erythrocyte sedimentation rate, and an abnormal C-reactive protein occur commonly. Elevations of serum ferritin, sometimes to very high levels, are seen in active Still's disease. Positive tests for rheumatoid factors occur in older children with polyarticular disease, whereas antinuclear antibodies are found both in patients with polyarticular disease and in young patients with pauciarticular disease. A positive ANA almost never occurs in Still's disease. Serum protein electrophoresis shows an increase in acute-phase reactants (α-globulins) and a polyclonal increase of γ-globulin. The synovial fluid in active juvenile rheumatoid arthritis is exudative, with a leukocyte count of 5000–20,000/μL (mostly neutrophils). Mononuclear cells may predominate in the synovial fluid of patients with pauciarticular disease.

C. Radiographic Findings: Radiographic changes early in the disease include juxtaarticular demineralization, periosteal bone accretion, premature closure of the epiphyses, cervical zygapophyseal fusion (particularly at C2-3), osseous overgrowth of the interphalangeal joints, and erosion and narrowing of the joint space. Carpal arthritis with ankylosis is seen as a late manifestation of Still's disease.

Immunologic Diagnosis

Currently, the diagnosis of juvenile arthritis is based on clinical criteria. Although certain abnormalities of immunoglobulins, complement, and cellular immunity are compatible with the diagnosis of juvenile arthritis, no specific immunologic test is diagnostic.

Differential Diagnosis

The diagnosis of juvenile arthritis is extremely difficult because the disease can present with nonspecific constitutional signs and symptoms in the absence of arthritis. Other causes of fever, particularly infections and cancer, must be considered. Leukemia can present in childhood with fever, lymphadenopa-

thy, and joint pains. Rheumatic fever closely resembles juvenile arthritis, particularly early in the disease, but the patient with juvenile arthritis tends to have higher spiking fevers, lymphadenopathy and hepatosplenomegaly in the absence of carditis, and a more refractory, long-lasting arthritis. Patients with rheumatic fever are more likely to have evidence of recent streptococcal infection, including elevated titers of antihyaluronidase, antistreptokinase, and antistreptodornase antibodies. In addition, patients with rheumatic fever tend to have a less intense leukocytosis and respond more dramatically to low doses of aspirin. An expanding skin lesion followed in weeks or months by arthritis suggests the diagnosis of Lyme disease, an inflammatory arthropathy caused by the spirochete *Borrelia burgdorferi*. Rheumatic diseases that may begin in childhood, such as SLE or dermatomyositis, can be differentiated by their different clinical course, different organ system involvement, and characteristic serologic abnormalities.

When juvenile arthritis presents as a monoarticular arthritis, examination of synovial fluid is of paramount importance to exclude infection.

Treatment

The major goals of therapy are to relieve pain, prevent contractures and deformities, and promote normal physical and emotional development. These goals are best achieved by a comprehensive program of physical, medical, and, when necessary, surgical therapy.

A. Physical Therapy: Exercise promotes muscle strength, encourages growth, and helps to prevent deformity. The goal in children is to maintain mobility.

B. Drug Treatment:

1. Aspirin—The disease often responds to antiinflammatory doses of aspirin or to many of the NSAIDs (Chapter 53). Because the clinical signs of aspirin toxicity are subtle in children, it is essential to monitor serum salicylate levels during aspirin therapy.

2. Remittive agents—Children with refractory arthritis may benefit from gold, antimalarials, sulfasalazine, or methotrexate.

3. Corticosteroids—Intraarticular corticosteroid injections are useful in pauciarticular disease. Systemic corticosteroids are reserved for patients with myocarditis, vasculitis, refractory iridocyclitis, or Still's disease that is unresponsive to aspirin therapy. Patients with iridocyclitis may require prolonged corticosteroid therapy. In children, the major toxic effects of corticosteroid therapy include subcapsular cataract formation, vertebral osteoporosis and collapse, infection, premature skeletal maturation with diminished growth, and pseudotumor cerebri with intracranial hypertension.

C. Surgical Treatment: The aims of surgery in juvenile arthritis are to relieve pain and maintain or improve joint function. Synovectomy may diminish pain due to chronic synovitis, but long-term effectiveness is questionable. Synovectomy for severe extensor tenosynovitis of the hand may prevent tendon rupture. Tendon release procedures help relieve joint contractures. Hip replacement is of benefit in selected cases but should be delayed as long as possible because in some children hip cartilage may regenerate with continued weight-bearing.

Complications & Prognosis

Seventy percent of patients experience a spontaneous and permanent remission by adulthood. Patients with Still's disease tend to have several recurrences per year. Patients presenting with oligoarthritic disease, particularly if they are female, tend to remain oligoarthritic, and those presenting with polyarthritis remain polyarthritic. Rarely, the disease persists into adulthood. This usually occurs in children with symmetric polyarthritis similar to that seen in adults. Sometimes a patient with juvenile arthritis in apparent remission develops rheumatoid arthritis as an adult. In an occasional unfortunate case, the disease is relentless and crippling. Small-joint involvement, positive serum rheumatoid factor, and onset in later childhood all portend a poor prognosis.

SJÖGREN'S SYNDROME

Major Immunologic Features

- Infiltration of salivary and lacrimal glands by CD4 T cells and B cells
- Autoantibodies to the ribonucleoproteins Ro (SS-A) and La (SS-B)
- Genetic predisposition linked to HLA region

General Considerations

Sjögren's syndrome is a chronic inflammatory disease of unknown cause characterized by diminished lacrimal and salivary gland secretion resulting in keratoconjunctivitis sicca and xerostomia. There is dryness of the eyes, mouth, nose, trachea, bronchi, vagina, and skin. In half of patients, the disease occurs as a primary pathologic entity (primary Sjögren's syndrome). In the other half, it occurs in association with rheumatoid arthritis or other connective tissue disorders. Ninety percent of patients with Sjögren's syndrome are female. Although the mean age at onset is 50 years, the disease does occur in children. Sjögren's syndrome may carry an increased risk for the development of B-cell lymphomas.

Immunologic Pathogenesis

Cell-mediated immune mechanisms likely play a central role in the inflammation that leads to tissue damage in Sjögren's syndrome. CD4 T cells predominate in the focal lymphocytic infiltrates that characterize involved salivary and lacrimal glands. These appear to be activated T_H1-type cells, based on the presence of interleukin-2 and interferon-γ and absence of interleukin-4. Epithelial cells in the salivary glands of Sjögren's patients, but not in control subjects, express HLA class II molecules and B7 molecules, suggesting that they might present antigens to CD4 T cells. The antigen specificities of lesional T cells, however, are unknown.

Considerable evidence suggests B-cell abnormalities. Although somewhat less prominent than T cells, B cells and plasma cells also are present in glandular infiltrates. Patients with Sjögren's syndrome frequently have hypergammaglobulinemia, elevated levels of rheumatoid factor, and autoantibodies to the ribonucleoproteins Ro (or SS-A) and La (or SS-B). The Ro and La particles can physically associate, and the majority of patients with primary Sjögren's syndrome develop autoantibodies to both. In selected ethnic groups, certain DRB1 extended haplotypes are associated with an increased risk of Sjögren's and with the development of antibodies to Ro and La. The tissue expression of Ro and La is ubiquitous. Whether anti-Ro and anti-La antibodies contribute to organ-specific (ie, salivary and lacrimal gland) inflammation in Sjögren's syndrome or how they might do so is unknown. These antibodies are not specific for Sjögren's syndrome. Antibodies to Ro occur in up to 50% of patients with SLE, and transplacental transfer of anti-Ro and anti-La appear to play a direct role in the pathogenesis of neonatal lupus.

Pathology

Histologically, lymphocytic infiltration occurs in the exocrine glands of the respiratory, gastrointestinal, and vaginal tracts, as well as in the glands of the ocular and oral mucosa. Histologic demonstration of lymphocytic infiltration in a biopsy specimen taken from the minor labial salivary glands is the most specific and sensitive single diagnostic test for Sjögren's syndrome.

Clinical Features

A. Symptoms and Signs:

1. Oral—Dryness of the mouth is usually the most distressing symptom and is often associated with burning discomfort and difficulty in chewing and swallowing dry foods. Parotid salivary flow is less than the normal 5 mL/10 minutes/gland. Polyuria and nocturia develop as the patient drinks increasing amounts of water in an effort to relieve oral symptoms. The oral mucous membranes are dry and erythematous, and the tongue becomes fissured and ulcerated. Severe dental caries is often present. Half of patients have intermittent parotid gland enlargement. The parotid gland in Sjögren's syndrome is firm, in contrast to the soft parotid enlargement characteristic of diabetes mellitus or alcohol abuse. Glossitis and angular cheilitis are manifestations of oral candidiasis in Sjögren's syndrome.

2. Ocular—The major ocular finding is keratoconjunctivitis sicca. Symptoms include burning, itching, decreased tearing, ocular accumulation of thick mucoid material during the night, photophobia, pain, and a "gritty" or "sandy" sensation in the eyes. Decreased tearing is demonstrated by diminished flow of tears down a strip of filter paper inserted into the lower palpebral fissure (Schirmer's test). Rose bengal or fluorescein reveals punctate staining of the conjunctiva and cornea. Tear break-up time is shortened. Severe ocular involvement may lead to ulceration, vascularization with opacification, or perforation of the cornea.

3. Miscellaneous—Dryness of the nose, posterior oropharynx, larynx, and respiratory tract may lead to epistaxis, dysphonia, recurrent otitis media, tracheobronchitis, or pneumonia. Dryness of the vagina may cause dyspareunia. Active synovitis is a common finding, particularly in patients who also have rheumatoid arthritis. Twenty percent of patients with primary Sjögren's syndrome complain of Raynaud's phenomenon. Ten percent of patients have extraglandular lymphocytic infiltrates, particularly in the kidneys, lungs, lymph nodes, and muscles. A few such patients develop lymphoma.

B. Laboratory Findings: Anemia, leukopenia, and an elevated erythrocyte sedimentation rate are common features. Secretory sialography with radiopaque dye demonstrates glandular disorganization. Salivary scintigraphy with technetium ^{99m}Tc pertechnetate reveals decreased parotid secretory function.

Immunologic Diagnosis

No immunologic test is diagnostic for Sjögren's syndrome; however, a myriad of nonspecific immunologic abnormalities occur in these patients. Hypergammaglobulinemia is seen in half of patients. Although serum protein electrophoresis usually shows a polyclonal hypergammaglobulinemia, occasional patients develop a monoclonal IgM paraproteinemia, usually of the kappa type. Patients who develop lymphoma sometimes become severely hypogammaglobulinemic and show disappearance of autoantibodies. Rheumatoid factors can be detected in 90% of patients with Sjögren's syndrome. ANA in a speckled or homogeneous pattern is present in 70% of patients. Antibodies against La or SS-B are relatively specific for patients with primary Sjögren's syndrome. Antibodies to Ro (SS-A) may be found in Sjögren's syndrome alone or in Sjögren's syndrome associated with SLE. Patients with Sjögren's syndrome and rheumatoid arthritis have neither anti-SS-A nor anti-SS-B antibodies.

Differential Diagnosis

The diagnosis of Sjögren's syndrome can be made on the basis of two of the three classic manifestations of xerostomia, keratoconjunctivitis sicca, and a connective tissue disease. The varied and multisystemic nature of the disease, however, may obscure the diagnosis. Other causes of bilateral parotid swelling include nutritional deficiencies, endocrine disorders, sarcoidosis, drug reactions, infections (including human immunodeficiency virus [HIV] and hepatitis C), amyloid, and obesity. Parotid gland cancer must always be considered in a patient with unilateral parotid swelling.

Treatment

A. Symptomatic Measures:

1. Oral—Patients must be urged to maintain fastidious oral hygiene, with regular use of fluoride toothpaste and mouthwashes and with regular dental examinations. Frequent sips of water and the use of sugarless gum or candy to stimulate salivary secretion are sometimes helpful in relieving xerostomia. Pilocarpine is sometimes useful in cases that do not respond to conservative measures. Many patients find aerosolized preparations of artificial saliva helpful. A bedroom humidifier helps decrease nocturnal xerostomia and nasal dryness.

2. Ocular—Artificial tears alleviate ocular signs and symptoms. Shielded glasses offer protection against the drying effects of wind. Therapy for refractory ocular complications includes mucolytic agents, punctal occlusion, soft contact lenses, and partial tarsorrhaphy.

3. Other—Dryness of the skin can be treated with moisturizing skin creams or oils. Vaginal and nasal dryness is often relieved with sterile, water-miscible lubricants.

B. Systemic Measures: Sjögren's syndrome can usually be controlled with symptomatic therapy. Nonsteroidal antiinflammatory drugs are useful in the treatment of the nonerosive arthritis of Sjögren's syndrome. Corticosteroids or immunosuppressive agents may be required in treating patients with severe or life-threatening disease, such as lymphoma, Waldenström's macroglobulinemia, or massive lymphocytic infiltration of vital organs.

Complications & Prognosis

In the vast majority of patients, significant lymphoproliferation is confined to salivary, lacrimal, and other mucosal glandular tissue, resulting in a benign chronic course of xerostomia and xerophthalmia. Rarely, patients develop significant extraglandular lymphoid infiltration or neoplasia.

Splenomegaly, leukopenia, and vasculitis with leg ulcers may occur. Hypergammaglobulinemic purpura, often associated with renal tubular acidosis, has been described and may be a presenting complaint. Five percent of patients with Sjögren's syndrome develop chronic autoimmune thyroiditis. Other associations include primary biliary cirrhosis, chronic active hepatitis, gastric achlorhydria, pancreatitis, renal and pulmonary lymphocytic infiltration, cryoglobulinemia with glomerulonephritis, hyperviscosity syndrome, and adult celiac disease. Neuromuscular complications include polymyositis, peripheral or cranial (particularly trigeminal) neuropathy, and cerebral vasculitis. Rarely, patients with Sjögren's syndrome develop lymphoma, immunoblastic sarcoma, or Waldenström's macroglobulinemia.

PROGRESSIVE SYSTEMIC SCLEROSIS (SCLERODERMA)

Major Immunologic Features

- Frequent occurrence of antinuclear antibodies with a speckled or nucleolar pattern
- Anticentromere antibodies, particularly in limited scleroderma
- Antibodies against topoisomerase 1 (Scl-70), particularly in generalized disease

General Considerations

Scleroderma is a disease of unknown cause characterized by abnormally increased collagen deposition in the skin. The course is usually slowly progressive and chronically disabling, but it can be rapidly progressive and fatal because of involvement of internal organs. It commonly begins in the third or fourth decade of life, but children are occasionally affected. The prevalence of the disease is one case per 100,000 in the population. Women are affected twice as often as men. There is no racial predisposition.

Scleroderma has been categorized based on the nature and extent of end-organ involvement. Patients with extensive visceral involvement often have widespread skin involvement (progressive systemic sclerosis). In limited scleroderma, skin thickening usually involves the distal extremities and, sometimes, the face and neck. CREST syndrome, which is defined by the presence of soft-tissue calcinosis, Raynaud's phenomenon, esophageal dysmotility, and telangiectasias, is the major form of limited scleroderma. Morphea is a scleroderma-like cutaneous lesion without visceral involvement.

Immunologic Pathogenesis

Little is definitively known about the pathogenesis of scleroderma. Any pathogenetic scheme must explain the vasomotor instability, microvasculature abnormalities, and accumulation of extracellular matrix that are prominent features of scleroderma. The association of scleroderma with several autoimmune disorders (primary biliary cirrhosis, Sjögren's syndrome, and thyroiditis), the existence of overlap syndromes that have features of both scleroderma and SLE, and the clinical similarities between scleroderma and graft-versus-host disease provide circumstantial evidence for a role for immune mechanisms in the pathogenesis of scleroderma. Similarly, the presence of autoantibodies to nuclear components in the great majority of patients with scleroderma suggests an abnormality of the immune system. Cell-mediated immune mechanisms, antibodies, and immune complexes have the potential to injure vascular endothelium, and cytokines produced by T cells and macrophages can activate fibroblasts to produce collagen and other matrix components. At present, however, there is little hard evidence that these events are critical in the pathogenesis of scleroderma.

Pathology

Biopsy of clinically involved skin reveals thinning of the epidermis with loss of the rete pegs, atrophy of the dermal appendages, hyalinization and fibrosis of arterioles, and a striking increase of compact collagen fibers in the reticular dermis.

Synovial findings range from an acute lymphocytic infiltration to diffuse fibrosis with relatively little inflammation.

The histologic changes in muscles include interstitial and perivascular inflammatory infiltration followed by fibrosis and myofibrillar necrosis, atrophy, and degeneration.

In patients with renal involvement, the histologic appearance of the kidney is similar to that of malignant hypertensive nephropathy, with intimal proliferation of the interlobular arteries and fibrinoid changes in the intima and media of more distal interlobular arteries and of afferent arterioles.

Collagen deposition is increased in the lamina propria, submucosa, and muscularis of the gastrointestinal tract. Small-vessel changes similar to those that occur in the skin may also result. With loss of normal smooth muscle, the large bowel is subject to development of the characteristic wide-mouthed diverticula and to infiltration of air into the wall of the intestine (pneumatosis cystoides intestinalis).

Clinical Features

A. Symptoms and Signs:

1. Onset—Raynaud's phenomenon heralds the onset of the disease in at least 90% of patients. It may precede the other manifestations by many years. Scleroderma frequently begins with skin changes, but in one third of patients polyarthralgias and polyarthritis are the first manifestations. Initial visceral involvement without skin changes occurs rarely.

2. Skin abnormalities— The clinical evolution of scleroderma occurs in three stages. In the edematous phase, symmetric nonpitting edema is present in the hands and, rarely, in the feet. The edema can progress to the forearms, arms, upper anterior chest, abdomen, back, and face. In the sclerotic phase, the skin is tight, smooth, and waxy and seems bound down to underlying structures. Skin folds and wrinkles disappear. The hands are involved in most patients, with painful, slowly healing ulcerations of the fingertips in half of those cases. The face appears stretched and mask-like, with thin lips and a "pinched" nose. Pigmentary changes and telangiectases are frequent at this stage.

The skin changes may stabilize for prolonged periods and then either progress to the third (atrophic) stage or soften and return to normal. It should be emphasized that not all patients pass through all the stages. Subcutaneous calcifications, usually in the fingertips (calcinosis circumscripta), occur more often in women than in men. The calcifications vary in size from tiny deposits to large masses and may develop over bony prominences throughout the body.

3. Joints and muscles—Articular complaints are very common and may begin at any time during the course of the disease. The arthralgias, stiffness, and frank arthritis seen in progressive systemic sclerosis may be difficult to distinguish from those of rheumatoid arthritis, particularly in the early stages of the disease. Involved joints include the metacarpophalangeals, proximal interphalangeals, wrists, elbows, knees, ankles, and small joints of the feet. Flexion contractures caused by changes in the skin or joints are common. Muscle involvement is usually mild but may be clinically indistinguishable from that of polymyositis, with muscle weakness, tenderness, and pain of proximal muscles of the upper and lower extremities.

4. Lungs—The lungs are frequently involved in progressive systemic sclerosis, either clinically or at autopsy. Interstitial fibrosis is the major pulmonary manifestation and may occur early in patients with truncal involvement. Pulmonary hypertension, which can best be detected by echocardiography, is more likely to be seen in limited scleroderma. Patients with diffuse pulmonary involvement have intimal proliferation of small and medium-size pulmonary arteries and arterioles and may have an intense bronchiolar epithelial proliferation.

5. Heart—Because of the frequency of pulmonary fibrosis, cor pulmonale is the most common cardiac finding. Myocardial fibrosis, leading to resistant left-sided heart failure, carries a poor prognosis. Cardiac arrhythmias and conduction disturbances are common manifestations of myocardial fibrosis. Pericarditis is usually asymptomatic and is found incidentally at autopsy. Although 40% of patients have pericardial effusion, tamponade is extremely rare.

6. Kidneys—Renal involvement is an uncommon but life-threatening development in patients with diffuse disease. Although renal insufficiency may follow an indolent course, it frequently presents as rapidly progressive oliguric renal failure with or without malignant hypertension. Marked changes are seen on renal arteriography in patients with scleroderma kidney. Irregular arterial narrowing, tortuosity of the interlobular arterioles, persistence of the arterial phase, and absence of a nephrogram phase are typical findings.

7. Gastrointestinal tract—The gastrointestinal tract is commonly affected. The esophagus is the most frequent site of involvement, with dysphagia or symptoms of reflux esophagitis occurring in 80% of patients. Gastric and small-bowel involvement presents with cramping, bloating, and diarrhea alternating with constipation. Hypomotility of the gastrointestinal tract with bacterial overgrowth may result in malabsorption. Colonic scleroderma is associated with chronic constipation. The barium enema may reveal large, wide-mouthed diverticula along the antimesenteric border of the colon.

8. Sjögren's syndrome—Sicca syndrome is seen in 5–7% of patients.

B. Laboratory Findings: The normochromic normocytic anemia of chronic inflammatory disease is occasionally seen in progressive systemic sclerosis. Microangiopathic anemia can also occur. An elevated erythrocyte sedimentation rate and polyclonal hypergammaglobulinemia are common.

Immunologic Diagnosis

Polyclonal hypergammaglobulinemia is a frequent serologic abnormality in progressive systemic sclerosis. The fluorescent ANA test shows a speckled or nucleolar pattern in 90% of cases. Anticentromere antibodies occur commonly in patients with limited scleroderma. Antibodies to topoisomerase 1 (Scl-70) typically are seen in patients with diffuse disease.

Differential Diagnosis

When classic skin changes and Raynaud's phenomenon are associated with characteristic visceral complaints, the diagnosis is obvious. In patients presenting with visceral or arthritic complaints and no skin changes, the diagnosis is difficult. Mixed connective tissue disease is a syndrome with features of scleroderma, rheumatoid arthritis, SLE, and polymyositis–dermatomyositis. The manifestations of the disease include arthritis, Raynaud's phenomenon, scleroderma of the fingers, muscle weakness and tenderness, interstitial lung disease, and a skin rash resembling either dermatomyositis or SLE. These patients have a high-titer speckled pattern of ANA and antibody to the ribonuclease-sensitive component of extractable nuclear antigen (eg, RNP). Renal disease is unusual in these patients. Patients with eosinophilic fasciitis present with marked thickening of the skin similar to that seen in the edematous phase of scleroderma. In eosinophilic fasciitis, however, Raynaud's phenomenon and visceral involvement are rare and fibrosis and inflammatory cell infiltration are seen in the deep facial layers, whereas in scleroderma the fibrosis occurs predominantly in the dermis. The differential diagnosis also includes scleromyxedema, polyvinyl chloride toxicity, L-tryptophan-induced eosinophilia myalgia syndrome, toxic oil syndrome, carcinoid syndrome, phenylketonuria, porphyria cutanea tarda, amyloidosis, Werner's syndrome, and progeria.

Treatment

There is no cure for scleroderma. Most manifestations of the disease are discouragingly refractory to antiinflammatory and immunosuppressive agents. Corticosteroids are beneficial for the myositis of scleroderma but not for other visceral manifestations of the disease. Uncontrolled studies suggest that monthly intravenous pulses of cyclophosphamide may be of modest benefit for the treatment of interstitial lung disease. Much of the care in scleroderma is supportive (eg, use of proton pump inhibitors for esophageal reflux, antibiotics for bacterial overgrowth of the small bowel, skin lubricants to alleviate dryness and cracking).

Vasodilatory agents, particularly calcium channel blockers and angiotensin-converting enzyme (ACE) inhibitors provide relief for some patients with severe Raynaud's phenomenon. These patients also should avoid exposure to cold and tobacco.

Hypertensive crisis in renal disease associated with progressive systemic sclerosis is very difficult to control even with potent hypotensive agents. ACE inhibitors can be of benefit in treating the renal disease associated with scleroderma.

Complications & Prognosis

Spontaneous remissions occur, but the usual course of the disease is one of relentless progression from dermal to visceral involvement. Involvement of the heart, lungs, or kidneys is associated with a high mortality rate. Aspiration pneumonia resulting from esophageal dysfunction is a complication in advanced disease.

Although the prognosis for any given patient is extremely variable, the overall 5-year survival rate for progressive systemic sclerosis is approximately 40%.

POLYMYOSITIS-DERMATOMYOSITIS

Major Immunologic Features

- Autoantibodies to aminoacyl-tRNA synthetases, signal recognition particle, and nuclear antigens
- Increased expression of class I and class II HLA molecules on myocytes
- CD8 T-cell infiltration of muscle in polymyositis
- Perivascular infiltrates of B cells and CD4 T cells in muscle in dermatomyositis
- Deposition of immunoglobulin and membrane attack complex (C5-C9) in microvasculature in dermatomyositis

General Considerations

Polymyositis-dermatomyositis is an acute and chronic inflammatory disease of muscle and skin that may occur at any age. Women are affected twice as commonly as men. There is no racial preponderance. The prevalence of the disease is one per 200,000 population.

Polymyositis-dermatomyositis can be subclassified into six categories: (1) idiopathic polymyositis, (2) idiopathic dermatomyositis, (3) polymyositis-dermatomyositis associated with cancer, (4) childhood polymyositis-dermatomyositis, (5) polymyositis-dermatomyositis associated with other rheumatic diseases (Sjögren's syndrome, SLE, progressive systemic sclerosis, mixed connective tissue disease), and (6) inclusion body myositis.

Immunologic Pathogenesis

The inflammatory myopathies appear to result from an immune response directed against muscle and instigated by as yet unidentified environmental events. As is the case with many putative immune-mediated diseases, polymyositis and dermatomyositis are associated with particular HLA class II alleles. Inheritance of the HLA haplotype containing the linked alleles DRB1*301 and DQA1*0501 is important risk factor for the development of inflammatory myopathies in some (white, Hispanic, and African-American) but not other (Korean) ethnic populations. Genetic susceptibility for the development of antisynthetase antibodies and other myositis-specific autoantibodies maps to the HLA DQA1 locus.

Muscle damage in polymyositis and inclusion body myositis appears to be the result of a cell-mediated immune response. Mononuclear infiltrates composed of CD8 T cells, CD4 T cells and macrophages surround and invade nonnecrotic muscle fibers. Several lines of evidence implicate perforin-dependent cytotoxicity by CD8 T cells as the major cause of muscle damage. Infiltrating CD8 cells in polymyositis, and probably in inclusion body myositis as well, display restricted use of T-cell receptor gene segments, consistent with an antigen-driven response. Muscle fibers in myositis express increased levels of HLA class I molecules and, therefore, can present antigens to CD8 T cells (which are class I restricted). The CD8 T cells that are in direct contact with muscle fibers orient their perforin vectorially toward the fiber, as occurs during an antigen-driven response. The identity of the antigen(s) presented by muscle is unknown. Extensive searches for an underlying viral infection have yielded negative results, suggesting that the T cells may be responding to an endogenous muscle antigen and that the response is an autoimmune one.

Humoral immunity likely has a large role in mediating tissue damage in dermatomyositis. Compared with polymyositis, mononuclear infiltrates in muscle in dermatomyositis are more perivascular, have more CD4 T cells, and have fewer CD8 T cells. The membrane attack complex of complement (C5b-C9) deposits in endomyseal capillaries in dermatomyositis and may induce perivascular inflammation and subsequent tissue damage. The membrane attack complex also deposits in the small vessels of the cutaneous lesions of dermatomyositis.

Pathology

Biopsy of involved muscles is diagnostic in only 50–80% of cases. A normal muscle biopsy, therefore, does not rule out the diagnosis of polymyositis-dermatomyositis in a patient with a characteristic clinical picture, muscle enzyme elevations, and an abnormal electromyogram. The histologic findings in acute and subacute polymyositis–dermatomyositis include (1) focal or extensive primary degeneration of muscle fibers, (2) signs of muscle regeneration (fiber basophilia, central nuclei), (3) necrosis of muscle fibers, (4) a focal or diffuse lymphocytic infiltration, and (5) perivascular inflammation. Chronic myositis leads to a marked variation in the cross-sectional diameter of muscle fibers and a variable degree of interstitial fibrosis. Patients with inclusion body myositis have evidence of nuclear inclusion bodies on light and electron micrography.

Clinical Features

A. Symptoms and Signs:

1. Onset—Although the symptoms may begin abruptly, the onset of the disease is usually insidious.

2. Muscle involvement—The commonest manifestation is weakness of involved striated muscle. The proximal muscles of the extremities are most often affected, usually progressing from the lower to the upper limbs. The distal musculature is involved in only 25% of patients. Weakness of the cervical muscles with inability to raise the head and weakness of the posterior pharyngeal muscles with dysphagia and dysphonia are also seen. Facial and extraocular muscle involvement is unusual. Muscle pain, tenderness, and edema also occur.

3. Skin involvement—The characteristic rash of dermatomyositis, present in approximately 40% of patients, consists of raised, smooth or scaling, dusky red plaques over bony prominences of the hands, elbows, knees, and ankles. An erythematous telangiectatic rash may appear over the face and sun-exposed areas. Less commonly seen is the characteristic "heliotrope" rash (a dusky, lilac suffusion of the upper eyelids). One fourth of patients have various dermatologic manifestations ranging from skin thickening to scaling eruptions to erythroderma.

4. Cancer—Some patients with polymyositis-dermatomyositis are found to have a concomitant malignant tumor. In middle-aged patients the association between polymyositis-dermatomyositis and cancer appears to be more common. Removal of the tumor can result in a dramatic improvement in the polymyositis-dermatomyositis.

5. Miscellaneous features—A mild transitory arthritis is not unusual. Sjögren's syndrome occurs in 5–7% of cases. In children, vasculitis may result in gastrointestinal ulceration with abdominal pain, hematemesis, and melena. Patients with severe muscle disease are particularly susceptible to the development of interstitial pneumonia and pulmonary fibrosis. Raynaud's phenomenon occurs occasionally.

B. Laboratory Findings: An elevated erythrocyte sedimentation rate and a mild anemia are very common. Half of patients have elevated α_2- and γ-globulins on serum protein electrophoresis. Myoglobinemia and myoglobinuria are often seen. Up to 20% of patients with acute polymyositis have nonspecific T-wave abnormalities on the ECG.

1. Muscle enzymes—When muscle cells are injured, a number of muscle enzymes, including glutamic–oxaloacetic transaminase, creatine phosphokinase, and aldolase, are released into the blood. The serum enzyme elevation reflects the severity of muscle damage as well as the amount of muscle mass involved.

2. Electromyography—When involved muscles are examined, 70–80% of patients demonstrate myopathic changes on electromyography. These changes are nonspecific but can point to the diagnosis of myositis. They include (1) spontaneous "sawtooth" fibrillatory potentials and irritability on insertion of the test needle; (2) complex polyphasic potentials, often of short duration and low amplitude; and (3) salvos of repetitive high-frequency action potentials (pseudomyotonia).

Immunologic Diagnosis

Antibodies to the histidyl-sRNA synthetase (Jo-1) occur in a substantial number of patients with polymyositis, particularly those with steroid-resistant disease and those with pulmonary involvement. Patients with dermatomyositis have antibodies to the nuclear antigen Mi-2. Those with acute-onset polymyositis may have antibodies to a cytoplasmic antigen, signal recognition particle (SRP). Antibodies to PM-Scl (a nucleolar antigen) are more common in patients with polymyositis and scleroderma. Anti-RNP antibodies occur most frequently in patients with myositis as a component of mixed connective tissue disease.

Differential Diagnosis

At least three of the following criteria must be present for a definite diagnosis of polymyositis: (1) weakness of the shoulder or pelvic girdle musculature, (2) biopsy evidence of myositis, (3) elevation of muscle enzymes, and (4) electromyographic findings of myopathy. Typical skin changes reflect a definite diagnosis of dermatomyositis. A number of diseases can affect muscles and lead to clinical and laboratory abnormalities that are identical to those seen in polymyositis–dermatomyositis. The diagnostic criteria outlined previously cannot be strictly applied in patients with infection (including HIV), sarcoidosis, muscular dystrophy, SLE, progressive systemic sclerosis, mixed connective tissue disease, drug-induced myopathy (alcohol, clofibrate), rhabdomyolysis, and various metabolic and endocrine disorders (McArdle's syndrome, hyperthyroidism, myxedema, acid maltase deficiency, carnitine palmityl transferase deficiency, and adenosine monophosphate [AMP] deaminase deficiency). In addition, various neuropathies and muscular dystrophies can mimic inflammatory myopathy. A diligent search for occult cancers should be made in any adult patient who develops polymyositis-dermatomyositis.

Treatment

A. Corticosteroids: Prednisone, 60–80 mg orally daily, usually decreases muscle inflammation and improves strength. The dose is tapered slowly, with clinical and laboratory monitoring. Assessment of muscle strength and determination of serum enzyme levels are helpful indicators of disease activity. Some patients require chronic prednisone therapy (5–20 mg daily) to control the disease.

B. Other Agents: Methotrexate and azathioprine have each been used with success in patients who do not respond to corticosteroids or who develop severe complications of corticosteroid therapy. Cyclosporine or intravenous gamma globulin may be beneficial in refractory cases.

Complications & Prognosis

Polymyositis–dermatomyositis is a chronic disease characterized by spontaneous remissions and exacerbations. Most patients respond to corticosteroid therapy. Patients with severe muscle atrophy show little response to either corticosteroid or other immunosuppressive therapy. When the disease is associated with cancer, the prognosis depends on the response to tumor therapy.

BEHÇET'S DISEASE

Behçet's disease is a chronic recurrent inflammatory disease affecting adults of both sexes. The major manifestations of the disease are aphthous stomatitis, iritis, and genital ulcers. Other findings include vasculitis (particularly of the skin), pulmonary artery aneurysms, arthritis, meningomyelitis, enterocolitis, erythema nodosum, thrombophlebitis, and epididymitis. Pathergy (a pustular lesion appearing after needle puncture of the skin) is highly suggestive of Behçet's disease.

Genetic and environmental factors probably play a role in pathogenesis. Some studies show an increased prevalence of HLA-B5 and HLA-B51 in Behçet's disease. There is also evidence suggesting that a virus may play a role in disease causation. Antibodies against various human mucosal antigens have been detected, and indirect immunofluorescence has demonstrated vascular deposition of immunoglobulins as well as circulating anticytoplasmic antibodies. Lymphocytes and plasma cells are prominent in the perivascular infiltrate of Behçet's vasculitis. Amyloidosis may develop in some patients.

Local corticosteroids are useful in the treatment of mild ocular and oral disease. Systemic corticosteroids are helpful in the treatment of systemic manifestations, but chlorambucil is thought to be the most useful agent for treating severe ocular or central nervous system disease. Unproved remedies include levamisole, colchicine, cyclosporine, and thalidomide.

SPONDYLOARTHROPATHIES

The spondyloarthopathies include ankylosing spondylitis, Reiter's syndrome, psoriatic arthritis, and the arthritis of inflammatory bowel disease. These distinct clinical entities share certain features: seronegativity (the absence of rheumatoid factor); a predilection for axial skeletal involvement, particularly the sacroiliac joints; an asymmetric pattern of peripheral joint involvement; tenosynovitis producing dactylitis ("sausage digits"); and an association with HLA-B27.

ANKYLOSING SPONDYLITIS

Ankylosing spondylitis is a chronic progressive inflammatory disorder involving the sacroiliac joints, spine, and large peripheral joints. Ninety percent of cases occur in males, with the usual age at onset being the second or third decade of life.

The disease begins with the insidious onset of low back pain and stiffness, usually worse in the morning. Manifestations include pain on compression of the sacroiliac joints and spasm of the paravertebral muscles. Findings in advanced disease include ankylosis of the sacroiliac joints and spine, with loss of lumbar lordosis, marked dorsocervical kyphosis, and decreased chest expansion. Peripheral arthritis, when present, usually involves the shoulder or hips. Twenty-five percent of patients also have iritis or iridocyclitis. Carditis with or without aortitis occurs in 10% of patients, and a few patients develop insufficiency of the aortic valves. Pericarditis and pulmonary fibrosis are rare complications of ankylosing spondylitis.

Patients with ankylosing spondylitis are seronegative for rheumatoid factors and ANA, but an elevated erythrocyte sedimentation rate and a mild anemia are common during active disease. Electrocardiographic abnormalities, such as atrioventricular block, left or right bundle branch block, and left ventricular hypertrophy reflect cardiac involvement. Radiographs of the sacroiliac joints reveal osteoporosis and erosions early in the disease and sclerosis with fusion in advanced disease. Calcification of the anterior longitudinal ligament of the spine and squaring of the vertebrae are seen on lateral radiographs of the spine. Ossification of the outer margins of the intervertebral disk (syndesmophyte formation) may lead to fusion of the spine.

The proliferative synovitis in these patients is similar pathologically to that of rheumatoid arthritis. In advanced disease the characteristic skeletal change is ossification of the sacroiliac joints and interspinous and capsular ligaments. Pathologic cardiac findings include focal inflammation and fibrous thickening of the aortic wall and the base of the valve cusps.

The pathogenesis of ankylosing spondylitis is poorly understood. Family and twin studies suggest that ankylosing spondylitis is largely a genetic disease that develops in response to ubiquitous environmental trigger(s). Although multiple genes may be involved, only one has been identified: HLA-B27 (a group of closely related MHC class I alleles; see Chapter 6). Inheritance of HLA-B27 increases the relative risk of ankylosing spondylitis approximately 100 fold but, according to recent genetic modeling, probably contributes only about 15–20% of the total genetic risk. In the United States, approximately 90% of white patients with ankylosing spondylitis have HLA-B27 compared with 8% of the healthy white population. It is unknown whether HLA-B27 predisposes to the development of disease by presenting an "arthritogenic" peptide to T lymphocytes, by acting as an autoantigen, or by some other mechanism.

Rodents that express human HLA-B27 transgenes develop disease with features of the human spondyloarthropathies. A germ-free environment prevents disease in HLA-B27-transgenic rats, and exposure to normal bacterial bowel flora, particularly Bacteroides species, triggers full expression of spondyloarthropathy. Inflammatory bowel disease is a prominent, early feature of disease in these transgenic rats, suggesting an important role for bowel inflammation in pathogenesis. Humans with ankylosing spondylitis do not have clinically apparent bowel involvement but, despite the absence of symptoms, frequently have microscopic changes consistent with inflammatory bowel disease. Moreover, patients with either Crohn's disease or ulcerative colitis can develop sacroiliitis and spondylitis indistinguishable from ankylosing spondylitis, again suggesting a link between bowel inflammation and the development of ankylosing spondylitis.

The treatment of ankylosing spondylitis consists of giving antiinflammatory agents to decrease acute inflammation and relieve pain and of instituting physical therapy to maintain muscle strength and flexibility. Therapy is designed to maintain a position of function even if ossification and ankylosis progress. Posturing exercises (lying flat for periods during the day, sleeping without a pillow, breathing exercises), the judicious use of local heat, and job modification are all part of a rational physical therapy program. Total hip replacement may offer considerable relief to patients with ankylosis of the hips, although recurrent ankylosis is sometimes a problem.

REITER'S SYNDROME

Reiter's syndrome is clinically defined as a triad consisting of arthritis, urethritis, and conjunctivitis.

The arthritis, however, is frequently accompanied by only one of the other characteristic manifestations or may occur isolation. Although Reiter's syndrome usually affects men, it may also occur in women and children. The arthritis tends to be asymmetric, and oligoarticular, involving primarily joints of the lower extremity. Fever, malaise, and weight loss occur commonly with episodes of acute arthritis. Frequently the urethritis is asymptomatic. The conjunctivitis is mild, but 20–50% of patients develop iritis. Balanitis circinata, painless oral ulcerations, and keratoderma blennorrhagicum (thick keratotic lesions of the palms and soles) are mucocutaneus manifestations. Complications include spondylitis and carditis. The manifestations of Reiter's syndrome appear to be more severe in patients with AIDS.

Most patients have a mild leukocytosis. The urethral discharge is purulent, but smear and culture are negative for *Neisseria gonorrhoeae*. Synovial fluid is sterile, with a leukocyte count of 2000–50,000/μL, mostly polymorphonuclear neutrophils (PMNs). The classic radiographic finding is fluffy periosteal proliferation of the heels, ankles, metatarsals, phalanges, knees, and elbows. Bony erosions may be seen in severe cases but rarely, if ever, occur in upper extremities. Approximately 80% of patients with Reiter's syndrome have HLA-B27.

Many, but not all, cases of Reiter's syndrome follow a clinically apparent bacterial infection. Well-defined initiating events include enteric infections with shigellae, salmonellae, yersiniae, and campylobacters and genitourinary infection with chlamydiae. The arthritis usually follows within 1 to 3 weeks of the infection. Because cultures of fluid and synovia from involved joints are sterile, viable organisms probably are not present, and the disease likely reflects an autoimmune response triggered by the infection. Consistent with this notion, antibiotics are ineffective in the treatment of postenteric Reiter's syndrome. Prolonged treatment with a tetracycline appears to be of some benefit for postchlamydial Reiter's disease. Tetracyclines, however, have substantial antiinflammatory effects, and it is unclear whether the observed benefit is due to the antimicrobial or the antiinflammatory properties of the drug.

NSAIDs or slow-acting antirheumatic drugs like sulfasalazine may be used to control acute inflammation. Immunosuppressive drugs, such as methotrexate or azathioprine, may be necessary in treatment of patients with recalcitrant disease. Although the acute attack usually subsides in a few months, recurrences are common and some patients develop a chronic deforming arthritis.

PSORIATIC ARTHRITIS

Psoriatic arthritis is a chronic, recurrent, asymmetric, erosive polyarthritis that occurs in about 25% of patients with psoriasis. The onset of the arthritis may be acute or insidious and is usually preceded by skin disease. It characteristically involves the distal interphalangeal joints of the fingers and toes and may involve the hips, sacroiliac joints, and spine. Distal interphalangeal joint disease is frequently accompanied by nail pitting or onycholysis secondary to psoriasis of the nail matrix or nail bed. Constitutional signs and symptoms, such as fever and fatigue, may occur. Severe erosive disease may lead to marked deformity of the hands and feet (arthritis mutilans), and marked vertebral involvement can result in ankylosis of the spine.

An elevated erythrocyte sedimentation rate and a mild anemia are common. Hyperuricemia is occasionally seen in patients with severe skin disease. Serum immunoglobulin levels are normal, and rheumatoid factor is absent. Synovial fluid examination reveals a leukocyte count of 5000–40,000/μL, mostly PMN. Characteristic radiographic findings include "pencil cup" erosions, fluffy periosteal proliferation, and bony ankylosis of peripheral joints. Sacroiliac changes, including erosions, sclerosis, and ankylosis similar to that in Reiter's syndrome, occur in 10–30% of patients.

The cause of psoriasis and psoriatic arthritis is unknown. Genetic factors appear to play a role in disease causation. Psoriasis and rheumatic diseases are found in family members of approximately 15% of patients. Patients with psoriasis and peripheral arthritis have an increased prevalence of HLA Cw*0602. Forty-five percent of patients with psoriasis and spondylitis have HLA-B27. Evidence for an immunopathogenesis in psoriatic arthritis includes the presence of antibodies directed against skin antigens and of activated T cells in skin and synovium.

Skin and arthritic manifestations require therapy. Topical corticosteroids, coal tar and ultraviolet light, or immunosuppressive drugs can be used to treat the skin disease. Treatment of arthritis is similar to that of rheumatoid arthritis.

RELAPSING POLYCHONDRITIS

Relapsing polychondritis is a rare disease characterized by recurrent episodes of inflammatory necrosis involving cartilaginous tissues of the ears, nose, upper respiratory tract, and peripheral joints. It may occur alone or in association with other diseases such as rheumatoid arthritis, SLE, systemic vasculitis, or malignancy. Relapsing polychondritis begins abruptly with swollen, painful, erythematous lesions of the nose or ears, usually associated with fever. Destruction of supporting cartilaginous tissues leaves patients with characteristic "floppy ear" and "saddle nose" deformities and can lead to collapse of the trachea. The commonest cause of death in these patients is airway obstruction. Recurrent episcleritis, anterior

inflammatory ocular disease, auditory and vestibular defects, systemic vasculitis, necrotizing glomerulitis, vasculitis, and arthritis are other manifestations of relapsing polychondritis. Aortic insufficiency due to destruction and dilatation of the aortic valve ring occurs rarely.

Laboratory abnormalities include an elevated erythrocyte sedimentation rate, increased serum immunoglobulins, a false-positive VDRL, and mild anemia. Pathologic examination reveals infiltration of the cartilage–connective tissue interface with lymphocytes, plasma cells, and PMNs. As the lesion evolves, the cartilage loses its basophilic stippling and becomes acidophilic. Eventually, the cartilage becomes completely replaced by fibrous tissue.

The pathogenesis of this disease is unknown; however, some evidence suggests that autoimmune phenomena play a role. Immune complexes are present at the fibrocartilaginous junction. Antibodies to human type II collagen occur but are also seen in other rheumatic diseases. Cell-mediated immune responses may be important: CD4 T cells are present in inflammatory infiltrates, and T cells from patients can respond to cartilage-derived antigens in vitro.

Corticosteroids, dapsone, colchicine, nonsteroidal antiinflammatory drugs, and cytotoxic agents have been used with success in the treatment of relapsing polychondritis.

RELAPSING PANNICULITIS
(Weber-Christian Disease)

Relapsing panniculitis is a rare syndrome characterized by recurrent episodes of discrete nodular inflammation and nonsuppurative necrosis of subcutaneous fat. Most patients are women. Painful, erythematous nodules usually appear over the lower extremities but may involve the face, trunk, and upper limbs. Lesions often progress to local atrophy and fibrosis. Occasionally, they may undergo necrosis, with the discharge of a fatty fluid. Constitutional signs, including fever, usually accompany an acute episode. Histologically, one sees edema, mononuclear cell infiltration, fat necrosis, perivascular inflammatory cuffing, and endothelial proliferation. The differential diagnosis includes superficial thrombophlebitis, polyarteritis nodosa, necrotizing vasculitis, erythema induratum, erythema nodosum, and factitious disease.

The cause of relapsing panniculitis is unknown, and, in fact, the syndrome may be simply a nonspecific response to any one of a number of inciting factors, including trauma, cold, exposure to toxic chemicals, and infection. It has been seen in patients with SLE, rheumatoid arthritis, diabetes mellitus, sarcoidosis, tuberculosis, withdrawal from corticosteroid therapy, acute and chronic pancreatitis, pancreatic carcinoma, and α_1-antitrypsin deficiency. An autoimmune mechanism is suggested by the presence of hypocomplementemia, circulating immune complexes, and the association of relapsing panniculitis with several autoimmune diseases. The only autoantibodies demonstrated to date are circulating leukoagglutinins.

Acute episodes respond to corticosteroid therapy. NSAIDs, antimalarial drugs, and immunosuppressive agents have been used to treat severe disease.

HYPOGAMMAGLOBULINEMIA & ARTHRITIS

Hypogammaglobulinemia is an acquired or congenital disorder that may involve all or any one of the specific classes of immunoglobulin (see Chapter 21). Hypogammaglobulinemia is associated with infections, chronic inflammatory bowel disease, sarcoidosis, SLE, scleroderma, Sjögren's syndrome, polymyositis–dermatomyositis, and cancer. Patients with classic adult and juvenile rheumatoid arthritis may develop hypogammaglobulinemia.

Patients with severe hypogammaglobulinemia may develop a seronegative, symmetric arthritis, with morning stiffness, occasional nodule formation, and radiographic evidence of demineralization and joint space narrowing. Bony erosions are rarely seen. Biopsy of the synovium reveals chronic inflammatory changes without plasma cells. Despite the reduction of serum immunoglobulins, immunoglobulin may be detected in the inflammatory synovial fluid. Total hemolytic complement is commonly depressed in the synovial fluid, suggesting immune complex formation.

The mono- or pauciarticular arthritis seen in hypogammaglobulinemia may be caused by mycoplasma, ureaplasma, or enterovirus infection.

Hypogammaglobulinemic arthritis may improve after the administration of gamma globulin.

REFERENCES

SYSTEMIC LUPUS ERYTHEMATOSUS

Bansal VK, Beto JA: Treatment of lupus nephritis: a meta-analysis of clinical trials. *Am J Kidney Dis* 1997;29:193.

Cabral AR, Alarcón-Segovia D: Autoantibodies in systemic lupus erythematosus. *Curr Opin Rheum* 1998;10:409

Cervera R et al: Systemic lupus erythematosus: Clinical and immunologic patterns of disease expression in a cohort of 1,000 patients. *Medicine* 1993;72:113.

Cervera R et al: Morbidity and mortality in systemic lupus erythematosus during a 5-year period: A multi-center prospective study of 1,000 patients. *Medicine* 1999;78: 167.

Huong DLT et al: The pulmonary manifestations of systemic lupus erythematosus. *Semin Arth Reum* 1999;78: 148.

McCarty DJ et al: Incidence of systemic lupus erythematosus: Race and gender differences. *Arth Rheum* 1995;38: 1260.

Petri M: Systemic lupus erythematosus and pregnancy. *Rheum Dis Clin North Am* 1994;20:87.

Segal AM et al: The pulmonary manifestations of systemic lupus erythematosus. *Semin Arth Rheum* 1985;14:202.

West S: Lupus and the central nervous system. *Curr Opin Rheum* 1996;8:408.

RHEUMATOID ARTHRITIS

Alarcón GS: Epidemiology of rheumatoid arthritis. *Rheum Dis Clin North Am* 1995;21:589.

Arnett FC et al: The American Rheumatism Association 1987 revised criteria for the classification of rheumatoid arthritis. *Arth Rheum* 1988;31:315.

Hurd ER: Extra-articular manifestations of rheumatoid arthritis. *Semin Arthritis Rheum* 1979;8:151.

Pincus T et al: Quantitative analysis of hand radiographs in rheumatoid Arthritis: Time course of radiographic changes, relation to joint examination measures, and comparison of DiFerrante scoring methods. *J Rheumatol* 1995;22:1983.

Seldin MF et al: The genetics revolution and the assault on rheumatoid arthritis. *Arth Rheum* 1999;42:1071.

JUVENILE ARTHRITIS

Cassidy JT et al: The development of classification criteria for children with juvenile rheumatoid arthritis. *Bull Rheum Dis* 1989;38:1.

De Inocencio J et al: Can genetic markers contribute to the classification of juvenile rheumatoid arthritis? *J Rheumatol* 1993;20:12.

Giannini EH et al: Comparative efficacy and safety of advanced drug therapy in children with juvenile rheumatoid arthritis. *Semin Arthritis Rheum* 1993;23:34.

Lawrence JM: Autoantibody studies in juvenile rheumatoid arthritis. *Semin Arthritis Rheum* 1993;22:265.

Woo P, Wedderburn LR: Juvenile chronic arthritis. *Lancet* 1998;351:969.

SJÖGRENS SYNDROME

Daniels TE, Fox PC: Salivary and oral components of Sjögren's Syndrome. *Rheum Dis Clin North Am* 1992; 18:571.

Daniels TE, Whitcher JP: Association of patterns of labial salivary gland inflammation with keratoconjunctivitis sicca: Analysis of 618 patients with suspected Sjögren's Syndrome. *Arth Rheum* 1994;37:869.

Fox RI, Saito I: Criteria for diagnosis of Sjögren's syndrome. *Semin Arth Rheum* 1995;25:117.

Fox RI: Evolving concepts of diagnosis, pathogenesis, and therapy of Sjögren's syndrome. *Curr Opin Rheum* 1998; 10:446.

PROGRESSIVE SYSTEMIC SCLEROSIS

Barnett A et al: A survival study of patients with scleroderma over 30 years (1953–1983): The value of a simple cutaneous classification in the early stages of disease. *J Rheumatol* 1988;15:276.

Black CM et al: Systemic sclerosis: current pathogenetic concepts and future prospects for targeted therapy. *Lancet* 1998;347:145.

Okano Y: Antinuclear antibody in systemic sclerosis (scleroderma). *Rheum Dis Clin North Am* 1990;22:709.

Rocco V, Hurd E: Scleroderma and scleroderma-like disorders. *Semin Arthritis Rheum* 1986;16:22.

Steen VD: Systemic sclerosis. *Rheum Dis Clin North Am* 1990;16:641.

Subcommittee for Scleroderma Criteria of the American Rheumatism Association Diagnostic and Therapeutic Criteria Committee: Preliminary criteria for the classification of systemic sclerosis (scleroderma). *Arth Rheum* 1980;23:581.

POLYMYOSITIS-DERMATOMYOSITIS

Plotz PH et al: Myositis: Immunologic contributions to understanding cause, pathogenesis, and therapy. *Ann Int Med* 1995;122:715.

Targoff IN et al: Classification criteria for the idiopathic inflammatory myopathics. *Curr Opin Rheum* 1997;9:527.

BEHÇETS DISEASE

Kaklamani VG et al: Behçets disease. *Semin Arth Rheum* 1998;27:197.

ANKYLOSING SPONDYLITIS

Gram JT, Husby G: Clinical, epidemiologic, and therapeutic aspects of ankylosing spondylitis. *Curr Opin Rheum* 1998;10:292.

Khan MA: An overview of clinical spectrum and heterogeneity of spondyloarthropathies. *Rheum Dis Clin North Am* 1992;18:1.

van der Linden S, van der Heijde D: Ankylosing spondylitis: Clinical features. *Rheum Dis Clin North Am* 1998; 24:663.

REITER'S SYNDROME

Amor B: Reiter's syndrome: Diagnosis and clinical features. *Rheum Dis Clin North Am* 1998;24:677.

Calin A, Fries J: An "experimental" epidemic of Reiter's syndrome revisited: Follow-up evidence on genetic and environmental factors. *Ann Intern Med* 1976;84:564.

Schumacher, HR: Reactive arthritis. *Rheum Dis Clin North Am* 1998;24:261.

PSORIATIC ARTHRITIS

Aladman, D: Psoriatic arthritis. *Rheum Dis Clin North Am* 1998;24:829.

RELAPSING POLYCHONDRITIS

Trentham DE, Le CH: Relapsing polychondritis. *Ann Intern Med* 1998;129:114.

Zeuner M et al: Relapsing polychondritis: Clinical and Immunogenetic analysis of 62 patients. *J Rheumatol* 1997; 24:96.

PANNICULITIS

Panush R et al: Weber-Christian disease: Analysis of 15 cases and review of the literature. *Medicine* 1985;64: 181.

HYPOGAMMAGLOBULINEMIA & ARTHRITIS

Lee AH et al: Hypogammaglobulinemia and rheumatic disease. *Semin Arthritis Rheum* 1993;22:252.

James R. Baker, Jr., MD

In the more than 40 years since the first demonstration of the immune basis for thyroiditis, autoimmune disease has been identified as a major cause of dysfunction of all endocrine organs. It is now apparent that such diverse disorders as idiopathic Addison's disease, insulin-dependent diabetes mellitus (IDDM), and the polyglandular endocrinopathy syndromes share an autoimmune pathogenesis.

MECHANISM OF DEVELOPMENT OF AUTOIMMUNE ENDOCRINE DISEASE

Endocrine disease has become a favored model for the study of autoimmune pathogenesis. It is postulated that autoimmunity begins with an inflammatory process, possibly of infectious origin, in the endocrine organ. The inflammatory cells in the gland produce interferon gamma and other cytokines, which induce the aberrant de novo expression of class II human leukocyte antigen (HLA) molecules on endocrine cell membranes and enhance the function of localized antigen-presenting cells (Figure 32–1). Class II HLA-expressing endocrine cells may function as antigen-presenting cells for their own cellular proteins, which are recognized by autoreactive T and B cells. This leads to destruction of endocrine cells through apoptosis (programmed cell death), which releases additional cellular proteins for processing by antigen-presenting cells, propagating the autoimmune response.

Cross-reactivity between autoantigens and environmental or dietary antigens may be important in initiating autoimmune responses. The mechanism by which an immune response to a pathogen or an environmental or dietary protein might lead to a loss of tolerance to an autoantigen is not understood. Several examples are now documented for Graves' disease and IDDM, however, and it is apparent that this cross-reactivity may occur at either the T- or B-cell level.

ORGAN-SPECIFIC AUTOANTIBODIES

The presence of organ-specific autoantibodies is often used as an adjunct to the diagnosis and occasionally the management of some autoimmune disorders. Table 32–1 presents the relative sensitivity and specificity of autoantibodies in different diseases and should be referred to during study of this chapter.

Organ-specific antibodies are defined by several methods, including their binding to tissue as determined by immunohistologic staining and the binding of specific proteins, lipids, carbohydrates, and hormones in immunoassays. In addition, autoantibody activity is characterized by the inhibition of hormone binding to receptor or through physiologic alterations of organ and cells in vitro. Difficulties arise, however, in the use of these autoantibodies in diagnosis and evaluation of autoimmune diseases. Inconsistencies often occur in the way many of the bioassays are conducted, leading to variability in sensitivity of autoantibody results. Also, in immunoassays for antibodies to ill-defined antigens, differences in the antigen preparation can vary the results.

Often, even well-characterized autoantibodies are not specific for an associated autoimmune disorder, which raises concern about the pathogenic role of the autoantibody in the autoimmune disorder. For example, antithyroglobulin antibodies can develop in healthy relatives of patients with autoimmune thyroid disease and in some healthy elderly individuals. In contrast, some antibodies found in only a small proportion of patients with autoimmune disease, such as insulin receptor antibodies, correlate well with disease activity in those patients (see Table 32–1). Thus, it is always important to evaluate autoantibody findings in the context of the patient's clinical situation.

THYROID AUTOIMMUNE DISEASES

HASHIMOTO'S THYROIDITIS

Major Immunologic Features
- Lymphocytic infiltration of the thyroid gland
- Antibodies to thyroid antigens
- Cellular sensitization to thyroid antigens
- Increased apoptosis of thyroid cells

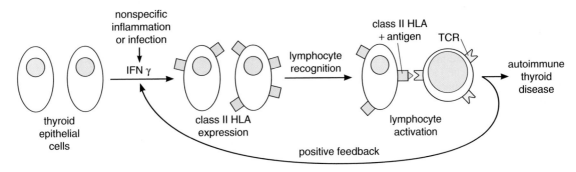

Figure 32–1. Initiation of autoimmunity through class II HLA expression. The expression of class II HLA results in prsentation of antigens to T cells, leading to T-cell activation, and the production of more lymphokines. These cause feedback stimulation of HLA expression and produce cytotoxic cells, which can destroy epithelial cells. *Abbreviations:* IFNγ = interferon gamma; HLA = human lymphocyte antigen; TCR = T-cell receptor.

General Considerations

Hashimoto's thyroiditis (also called chronic thyroiditis) is an inflammatory disorder of unknown cause, which results in progressive destruction of the thyroid gland. Found most commonly in the middle-aged and elderly, it also occurs in other age groups, including children in whom it may cause goiter. Females make up the vast majority, about 85%, of patients. Although it is distributed throughout the world without racial or ethnic restriction, it occurs more commonly in families in which another member has an autoimmune thyroid disease. It is observed in conjunction with Graves' disease in a form of autoimmune-overlap syndrome. In addition, it is associated with other autoimmune disorders, such as systemic lupus erythematosus (SLE), chronic active hepatitis, dermatitis herpetiformis, and scleroderma. Although no formal mode of inheritance is recognized, associations have been reported with several class II HLA antigens, including DR4 and DR5. These associations, however, are not consistent among different ethnic populations.

Table 32–1. Antigens implicated in autoimmune endocrine diseases.

Disorder	Antigen	Antigen Function	Disease Specificity
Hashimoto's disease	Thyroglobulin	Hormone precursor	High
	Thyroid peroxidase	Enzyme	High
	TSH receptor	Hormone receptor	Moderate
Graves' disease	TSH receptor	Hormone receptor	High
	Thyroid peroxidase	Enzyme	Moderate
	Thyroglobulin	Hormone precursor	Low-moderate
	64-kd antigen	Unknown	Unknown
	70-kd heat shock protein	Stress response protein	Unknown
Type I diabetes	Insulin/proinsulin	Hormone	High
	Insulin receptor	Hormone receptor	High
	Glutamic acid		
	Decarboxylase	Enzyme	High
	β-cell granule	Transport protein	High
	Pancreatic cytokeratin	Cellular matrix	
		protein	Unknown
	64-kd antigen	Unknown	Unknown
	Glucagon	Hormone	Unknown
	65-kd heat shock protein	Stress response protein	Unknown
Addison's disease	21-Hydroxylase	Enzyme	High
	P450 sidechain cleavage enzyme	Enzyme	High
	17-Hydroxylase	Enzyme	High
Idiopathic hypoparathyroidism	200-kd and 130-kd	Unknown	Unknown
	Endothelial antigen	Unknown	Unknown
	Mitochondrial antigen	Unknown	Low

Abbreviation: TSH = thyroid-stimulating hormone.

Pathology

The hallmark of Hashimoto's thyroiditis is lymphocytic infiltration that almost completely replaces the normal glandular architecture of the thyroid (Figure 32–2). Plasma cells and macrophages abound, and dying thyroid cells with acidophilic granules called Askanazy cells are scattered through this infiltrate. Formations of germinal centers often give the impression that the thyroid gland is being converted into a lymph node. Lymphocytes infiltrating the thyroid are mainly B cells and CD4 T cells, although CD8 cytotoxic T cells have been cloned from Hashimoto's glands.

Clinical Features

Hashimoto's thyroiditis is primarily associated with symptoms of altered thyroid function. Early in the course of the disease euthyroidism is usually the case, but clinical hyperthyroidism may arise due to the inflammatory breakdown of thyroid follicles with release of thyroid hormones. In contrast, late in the disease hypothyroidism often occurs because of progressive destruction of the thyroid gland. The most common eventual outcome of Hashimoto's disease is hypothyroidism.

A consistent physical sign seen in Hashimoto's disease is an enlarged thyroid gland. The goiter is often large and "rubbery" and may feel nodular, similar to its condition in other goitrous diseases. Often, lymph nodes surrounding the gland become enlarged. Rarely, patients show evidence of generalized vasculitis with urticaria and nephritis, and these findings have been associated with the presence of circulating immune complexes.

General laboratory findings are not helpful in making the diagnosis and relate primarily to the thyroid status of the patient. Patients with hyperthyroidism are differentiated from those with Graves' disease by the demonstration of patchy or decreased uptake on a radioiodine scan of the thyroid.

Immunologic Diagnosis

The hallmark of the diagnosis of Hashimoto's disease is the presence of circulating autoantibodies to thyroglobulin and thyroid microsomal antigen (now known to be the enzyme thyroid peroxidase). These antibodies were first detected by immunofluorescence (Figure 32–3), but they are now measured by agglutination assays or enzyme-linked immunosorbent assay (ELISA) (see Chapter 15). They are present in the serum of more than 90% of patients with Hashimoto's disease, with thyroid peroxidase antibodies being more common and of higher titer than antithyroglobulin antibodies. In patients without serum antibodies, autoantibody production may be localized to the intrathyroidal lymphocytes and plasma cells. Interestingly, the immune responses to both thyroglobulin and thyroid peroxidase are heterogeneous, with several areas of each molecule conferring immunogenicity.

Other thyroid antibodies are often present in Hashimoto's disease patients, including antibodies

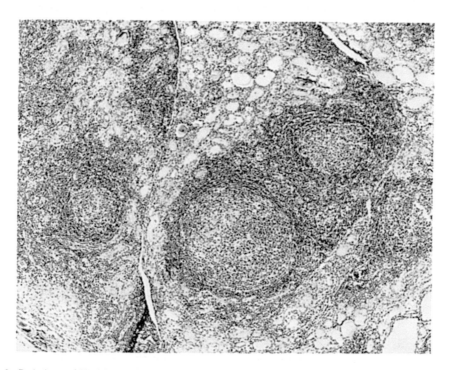

Figure 32–2. Pathology of Hashimoto's thyroiditis. Note the germinal centers that disrupt normal thyroid architecture. (Original magnification ×100.)

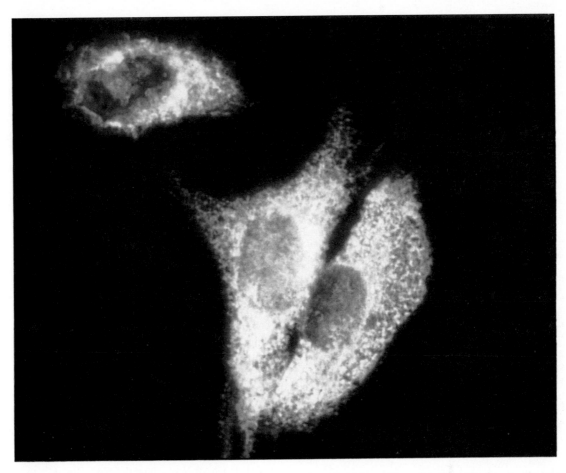

Figure 32–3. Immunofluorescent staining of a cultured human thyroid cell by antithyroglobulin antibodies showing the distribution of the antigen. (Original magnification ×400.) (Courtesy of Donald Sellitti.)

that displace thyroid-stimulating hormone (TSH) from its receptor on thyroid cells and others that stimulate thyroid cells to produce hormones. Other important thyroid antigens stimulate the production of autoantibodies because multiple unidentified protein bands are recognized by sera from patients with Hashimoto's thyroiditis in Western blots of thyroid membranes. In addition, lymphocytes of these patients proliferate in response to thyroid antigens.

Differential Diagnosis

Clinical criteria and antithyroid antibody titers help differentiate Hashimoto's disease from other forms of goiter. On occasion, the rapid enlargement of one lobe of the thyroid gland is confused with thyroid cancer or thyroid lymphoma, which are observed with an increased incidence in Hashimoto's glands. In these cases, needle biopsy of the nodule may be helpful, whereas computed tomograms or magnetic resonance images of the neck can be used to evaluate cervical adenopathy.

Treatment

Treatment of Hashimoto's disease usually consists of thyroid hormone replacement for hypothyroidism. If the patient has a symptomatic goiter, doses of thyroid hormone that suppress TSH secretion can often decrease the size of the gland. Rarely, thyroidectomy is necessary for an unusually large or painful gland.

Prognosis

The prognosis of Hashimoto's disease is excellent, but serial thyroid function tests, especially TSH levels, are necessary to monitor the requirement for thyroid hormone replacement.

TRANSIENT THYROIDITIS SYNDROMES

Major Immunologic Features

- Giant-cell infiltration of the thyroid
- Transient production of antithyroid antibodies

General Considerations

Several heterogeneous, self-limited thyroiditis syndromes have transient immune activity against the thyroid. The two most often encountered are subacute (de Quervain's) thyroiditis and postpartum thyroiditis. Subacute thyroiditis is possibly caused by a viral infection of the thyroid gland. It has a seasonal and geographic distribution common to infections with mumps virus, coxsackievirus, and echovirus. Patients with this disorder usually have an acute phase of thyroiditis in which the gland may be painful and antithyroid antibodies may be present. At this time, patients are thyrotoxic, with an elevated serum T4 and decreased radioiodine uptake. Progressive euthyroid and hypothyroid periods of 4–8 weeks may follow before thyroid functions finally normalize.

Similar in clinical course, postpartum thyroiditis is a common disorder that usually presents within 3 months of delivery. Patients may experience either hypothyroidism or hyperthyroidism, and a significant percentage develop chronic thyroid dysfunction. Interestingly, patients who have this disorder often have recurrent courses with subsequent pregnancies.

Postpartum thyroiditis occurs in about 5–8% of pregnant women and, unlike subacute thyroiditis, is thought to be unrelated to a viral infection of the thyroid. Supporting this contention are the presence of thyroid peroxidase antibodies preceding the onset of clinical disease and an association with HLA-DR3 and -DR5 haplotypes.

Pathology

Although the lymphocytic infiltrate seen in subacute thyroiditis is similar to that in Hashimoto's disease, two findings in subacute thyroiditis are distinctive. First, giant cells with a small center of thyroid colloid can be seen (this is known as colloidophagy), and the follicular infiltration tends to progress to form granulomas. These findings are not seen in postpartum thyroiditis, however.

Clinical Features

Subacute thyroiditis and postpartum disease have in common the clinical presentation of rapidly enlarging thyroid gland and signs of thyroid dysfunction. Subacute thyroiditis has a much more acute course than postpartum disease and is more commonly associated with pain and tenderness in the area of the gland. Postpartum thyroiditis and other types of transient thyroiditis without pain or other symptoms are sometimes termed "silent" thyroiditis.

Subacute thyroiditis is also accompanied by an elevated erythrocyte sedimentation rate. Both syndromes can cause "low-uptake" toxicosis; that is, they can produce elevated serum levels of thyroid hormones in the face of low to normal levels of radioactive iodine uptake.

Immunologic Diagnosis

Antibodies to thyroid peroxidase occur in both syndromes, but they tend to be transient and of low titer in subacute thyroiditis. Thyroid-stimulating antibodies develop in a few patients with postpartum disease.

Treatment & Prognosis

In most cases thyroid function returns to normal within several months in both disorders. Patients with subacute thyroiditis who have especially painful glands may be treated with antiinflammatory drugs. Postpartum patients who are clinically hypothyroid can benefit from thyroid hormone replacement. This finding offers a means for monitoring patients for eventual therapy with thyroid hormone or antithyroid drugs.

GRAVES' DISEASE

Major Immunologic Features

- Antibodies against thyroid antigens stimulate thyroid cell function and displace TSH binding
- Increased growth and proliferation of thyroid cells
- Associated autoimmune ophthalmopathy and dermopathy

General Considerations

Graves' disease is an autoimmune disorder of unknown cause, which presents as thyrotoxicosis with a diffuse goiter. It is unique among autoimmune disorders because it is probably mediated by autoantibodies that actually stimulate thyroid cellular activity. Patients with Graves' disease often have associated phenomena of ophthalmopathy and a proliferative dermopathy, which appear to be autoimmune in nature. The endocrine, skin, and eye disorders are most commonly seen in combination. They can exist separately, however, and often have different clinical courses even when they coexist in the same patient.

Graves' disease is most common in the third and fourth decades of life and has a marked female predominance of 7:1. Unlike Hashimoto's disease, it rarely occurs in children but is often seen in individuals past the fifth decade of life. It is a relatively common disorder, occurring in 0.1–0.5% of the general population.

Graves' disease was among the first autoimmune disorders noted to have an association with HLA haplotypes. There is a strong association with DR3 and several DQβ and a DQα genotype in whites and with Bw35 and Bw46 in Asians. Also, the disease tends to occur in families and is linked with HLA and Gm haplotypes in affected kindred. The disease seems to be associated with a type of generalized "autoimmune susceptibility" in some families because other family members often have autoimmune disorders such as Hashimoto's disease and antibodies to gastric parietal cells and intrinsic factor.

Pathology

Thyroid glands from patients with Graves' disease present as uniformly enlarged and diffuse goiters. Microscopic analysis reveals small thyroid follicles with hyperplastic epithelium, but little colloid. Although a lymphocytic and plasma cell infiltrate often occurs, it is much less intense and does not have the associated destruction of normal tissue seen in Hashimoto's disease. These findings resolve in patients treated with antithyroid drugs.

Immunofluorescence analysis indicates that a high proportion of thyroid cells express HLA-DR antigens on their surface. In addition, analysis of the lymphocyte subsets in the gland reveals both CD4 and CD8 T and B cells.

Clinical Features

Graves' disease typically presents with diffuse goiter and thyrotoxicosis. The signs of hyperthyroidism are heat intolerance, hand tremor, nervousness, irritability, warm moist skin, weight loss, muscle reflex changes, hyperdynamic cardiovascular status with tachycardia, hyperdefecation, and changes in mental status. The exception to these symptoms occurs in the elderly, in whom apathetic hyperthyroidism may present with tachycardia as the sole clinical manifestation. Patients with accompanying ophthalmopathy may have proptosis, lid lag, and a characteristic "stare." Dermopathy usually presents as a swelling in the pretibial area (myxedema), and in the feet, face, or hands.

Laboratory findings are those of hyperthyroidism, with elevated levels of total and free T3 and T4. TSH levels in this disease are low or undetectable because the stimulation of the thyroid gland is exogenous rather than from the pituitary axis and the elevated levels of the thyroid hormones cause a feedback inhibition of pituitary TSH secretion.

The thyroid gland in patients with Graves' disease always shows an increased uptake of radioactive iodine. A diffuse homogeneous uptake on a radioisotopic scan of the thyroid is almost pathognomonic of Graves' disease.

Immunologic Diagnosis

The immunologic diagnosis of Graves' disease rests on the identification of antithyroid antibodies with the ability to alter thyroid cell function. These antibodies tend to fall into three categories (Figure 32–4): (1) antibodies that stimulate the production of cyclic adenosine monophosphate (cAMP) (thyroid-stimulating immunoglobulins [TSI]), (2) antibodies causing proliferation of thyroid cells as measured by the incorporation of [³H]thymidine into their DNA (thyroid growth-stimulating immunoglobulins [TGSI]), and (3) antibodies that displace the binding of TSH from its receptor (thyroid-binding inhibitory immunoglobulins [TBI]). Although these antibodies have been found in several other disorders, especially

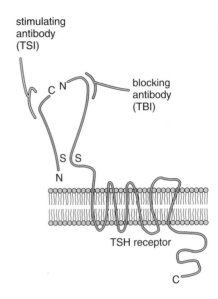

Figure 32–4. TSH receptor structure and antibody-binding sites. The TSH receptor is a major antigen in autoimmune thyroid disease. Autoantibodies bind to different sites on the external domain of the receptor and mediate stimulation of the receptor (in Graves' disease) or inhibition of receptor activation by TSH (atrophic thyroiditis). *Abbreviations:* TSH = thyroid-stimulating hormone; TBI = thyroid-binding inhibitory immunoglobulins; TSI = thyroid-stimulating immunoglobulins.

Hashimoto's thyroiditis, their presence in the appropriate clinical setting is virtually pathognomonic of Graves' disease. In addition, monitoring the function of these antibodies may, in some cases, correlate with the clinical course of the disease and its response to antithyroid drugs.

Initial efforts to measure the activity of TSI involved injecting IgG fractions from patients with Graves' disease into animals and measuring thyroid activity. This test has been replaced by the Fisher rat thyroid line 5 (FRTL-5) or cells transfected with, and expressing, recombinant TSH receptor. These cells are grown in culture with IgG from patients with Graves' disease, and the effect on cell function (either the production of cAMP or the incorporation of [³H]thymidine) is measured. The ability of the IgG to displace TSH from its receptor is still measured as described more than 15 years ago. The test involves the incubation of IgG with porcine thyroid membranes and radiolabeled TSH. The amount of TSH bound to the membrane is then calculated and compared with the amount bound in the presence of control IgG or unlabeled TSH. This results in a "percent displacement" of radiolabeled TSH, which gives a relative activity of the IgG.

Recently, studies with recombinant TSH receptor protein have tried to identify specific sites in the receptor bound by autoantibodies. These studies are inconclusive but suggest that several sites exist in the external domain of the receptor to which autoantibodies bind. It appears from these studies that antibodies that stimulate or block the TSH receptor bind to different sites on the receptor. This suggests that the autoantibody response to the TSH receptor in Graves' disease is complex and heterogeneous.

Differential Diagnosis

The differential diagnosis of Graves' disease involves exclusion of other thyroid disorders manifesting hyperthyroidism, such as Hashimoto's disease, pituitary tumors, or thyroid adenomas. Most of these can be ruled out by determining that the thyroid gland has a diffuse increase in iodine uptake. The presence of ophthalmopathy and dermopathy also supports the diagnosis of Graves' disease.

Treatment

The initial treatment of Graves' disease involves the inhibition of symptomatic β-adrenergic hyperstimulation with β-adrenergic blocking agents. Therapy with drugs to inhibit thyroid cell function is also given soon after diagnosis. These drugs, propylthiouracil and methimazole, offer several advantages in the treatment of Graves' disease. They not only inhibit the production of thyroid hormones, relieving hyperthyroidism, but also decrease the size and vascularity of the goiter, making it more amenable to definitive therapy with surgery or radioactive iodine. Of interest, these drugs may also interrupt the perpetuation of the underlying autoimmune process, possibly through the resolution of the hyperthyroidism because thyroid hormones appear to have nonspecific immunostimulatory activities in vitro.

Recently, it has been shown that administering suppressive doses of thyroid hormone in conjunction with antithyroid drugs may lead to long-term remission of Graves' disease. The mechanism of this effect is unknown but may be the result of suppression of thyrocyte autoantigen expression.

Definitive therapy for Graves' disease involves the destruction of the thyroid gland, either by ^{131}I or by complete surgical removal of the gland. Although personal preference and experience often dictate which therapy is used, surgery has been the therapy of choice in women of childbearing age because of the potential risks of radiation to the gonads and fetus. Recent studies do not show risk to the ovaries, however, and radioiodine is becoming increasingly popular in premenopausal women once pregnancy is ruled out.

Prognosis & Complications

The prognosis for most patients is very good once their thyroid function is controlled. The most serious problems in Graves' disease often come from the associated ophthalmopathy and dermopathy, which in some cases do not respond to treatments that normalize thyroid function. Treatment with corticosteroids provides relief in some cases, but occasionally the ophthalmopathy progresses to a point that vision is threatened. At that point, radiotherapy or surgical decompression of the orbit is often required. More aggressive treatment protocols with immunosuppressive drugs such as cyclosporine have shown some success in reversing the autoimmune process in these patients.

PRIMARY HYPOTHYROIDISM

Major Immunologic Features
- Lymphocytic infiltration of the thyroid gland
- Antithyroid antibodies can be present

General Considerations

Primary hypothyroidism, or thyroid atrophy, is the most common cause of hypothyroidism (other than iatrogenic ablation) in adults. Much like the other autoimmune thyroid diseases, it is more common in women than men and occurs most often from age 40 to 60 years. The atrophy probably results from asymptomatic or unrecognized thyroiditis with resulting progressive destruction of the gland. Data suggest, however, that some cases are related to antibodies that block TSH binding to its receptor, thereby inhibiting the trophic effect of the hormone. Thyroid atrophy also occurs as part of the polyglandular syndromes (see Autoimmune Polyglandular Syndromes).

Pathology

The thyroid is markedly atrophic and often fibrotic. In some cases residual lymphocytic infiltration occurs.

Clinical Features

Although most patients demonstrate the usual findings of hypothyroidism and a small, impalpable thyroid gland, some present with palpable fibrosis in the area of the thyroid gland. Laboratory findings include elevated TSH levels with low (or low normal) levels of circulating thyroid hormones. TSH response to thyrotropin-releasing hormone (TRH) administration is often exaggerated, indicating an increased state of activation of the pituitary axis.

Immunologic Diagnosis

Antithyroid antibodies are found in a high proportion of patients (>80%), but they are not necessary for the diagnosis. No other specific immunologic tests are available. However, studies may identify the sites in the TSH receptor where blocking antibodies bind. This information could lead to the development of specific assays.

Treatment

Treatment consists of lifelong thyroid hormone replacement.

DISORDERS OF THE ENDOCRINE PANCREAS

INSULIN-DEPENDENT DIABETES MELLITUS

Major Immunologic Features
- Monocytic and lymphocytic infiltration of the islets of Langerhans
- Antibodies against multiple antigens of islet β cells
- HLA-DR expression on the β cells
- Increased apoptosis of the β cells

General Considerations

Insulin-dependent diabetes mellitus (IDDM or Type I Diabetes) is a disorder in which the destruction of the insulin-producing β cells of the pancreatic islets of Langerhans results in a deficiency of insulin. This destruction is in contrast to the defect in type II diabetes mellitus, in which resistance of target organs to the effects of insulin is present. IDDM is an autoimmune disease. The postulated sequence of events leading to islet cell destruction is similar to the scheme outlined for autoimmune thyroid disease in Figure 32–1. After an initiating event such as a viral infection, an inflammatory response to the β cells of the islets results. This inflammation is characterized by HLA-DR expression on the β cells and lymphocytic infiltration of the islets. Subsequently, either a persistent stimulation of the immune system or a defect in immune regulation allows the propagation of the autoimmune response in a genetically predisposed individual. This causes destruction of the β cells and leads to insulin deficiency.

The hypothesis that a viral infection is the initial insult leading to the development of IDDM in humans is unproved. Considerable circumstantial evidence, however, favors this hypothesis, including reports of the development of IDDM following infections with viruses, such as mumps virus, cytomegalovirus, influenza virus, and rubella virus, and direct evidence links viral infection and diabetes in experimental animals. Mumps virus, coxsackievirus types B3 and B4, and reovirus type 3 can infect and destroy human islet cells in vitro. In addition, amino acid sequence similarities exist between coxsackievirus proteins and the islet cell autoantigen, glutamic acid decarboxylase. As yet, however, no direct causal link exists between the common occurrence of infections with these viruses and the rare event of developing autoimmune diabetes mellitus. The heterogeneous genetic susceptibility to development of autoimmunity may make identification of a specific environmental cause difficult.

Epidemiologic studies support the concept of a genetic susceptibility to developing IDDM. Seen almost entirely in individuals under the age of 30 years, IDDM has a peak age of onset between 10 and 14 years. It occurs predominantly in whites and has a prevalence of approximately 0.25% in both the United States and Europe. Unlike most other autoimmune disorders, males are more commonly affected than females by a small margin. The incidence of this disorder has increased slightly over the past 50 years. Seasonal fluctuations also occur.

The genetics of type I diabetes mellitus have come under intense study recently. More than 90% of patients have HLA-DR3, -DR4, or both, and there is a negative association with HLA-DR2. An additive risk occurs when both HLA-DR3 and -DR4 are present. Few individuals who have the HLA-DR3 and -DR4 haplotypes develop IDDM, however. This paradox may be partially explained by the association of these HLA antigens with particular DQβ genotypes. Unique substitutions of amino acids at critical positions in the DQβ chain may be related to susceptibility to diabetes. One substitution (an uncharged amino acid for Asp at position 57) was also noted in animals genetically susceptible to diabetes. Although this substitution does not perfectly identify humans at risk for this disease, it underscores the potential importance of HLA antigens in diabetes. Studies in animals with spontaneous autoimmune diabetes (NOD mice) indicate that many genetic elements may be involved in this disorder.

Pathology

Patients show evidence of lymphocytic infiltration in the pancreatic islets even before evidence of glucose intolerance is noted. This inflammatory lesion progresses to cause apoptosis of the β cells with atrophy and scarring of the islets. The other endocrine cells in the islets usually remain functional.

Immunofluorescence staining of the islet inflammation reveals several interesting findings. First, there is HLA-DR expression on the β cells, as well as on the infiltrating lymphocytes. The majority of these lymphocytes stain positively with monoclonal antibodies for CD8, indicating a cytotoxic phenotype. Antibody-producing cells are also seen, and antibody and complement components are present on the surface of the β cells.

Clinical Features

The signs and symptoms are well known and are beyond the scope of this chapter. Unlike type II disease, a true insulin deficiency occurs in type I diabetes mellitus, which leaves the patient prone to greater fluctuations in blood glucose concentration and to subsequent ketosis.

The laboratory diagnosis still rests on the documentation of elevated blood glucose concentrations. A fasting blood glucose level greater than 140 mg/dL in the appropriate clinical setting is diagnostic for diabetes. If the fasting glucose concentration is normal, the use of a glucose tolerance test may be helpful, but this is controversial. The level of hemoglobin A1c is helpful primarily in monitoring the ongoing control of blood glucose concentrations in patients on therapy.

Immunologic Diagnosis

Presently, no immunologic test is useful clinically. Antibodies to specific islet cell antigens such as glutamic acid decarboxylase (GAD) or insulin can be helpful in determining whether a susceptible individual will develop the disease.

Treatment

Treatment of diabetes requires normalization of blood glucose concentrations by using oral hypoglycemic drugs or insulin injections. Most patients with IDDM require insulin, and the availability of human insulin may allow better therapy for some patients with insulin antibodies. Segmental pancreas or islet cell transplantation may offer a more physiologic form of insulin replacement in the future.

Many trials of immunosuppressive therapy have attempted to reverse the inflammatory process that causes islet cell destruction. Although most of these trials were started a short time after the development of glucose intolerance, some have shown successful increases in insulin-connecting peptide (C peptide) levels and clinical improvement in blood glucose control, obviating a need for insulin injections in a very few subjects. All of these drugs have potentially severe toxicity, which has prevented their use in most diabetics.

ADDISON'S DISEASE

Major Immunologic Features
- Circulating antibodies against specific antigens from adrenal cells
- Complement fixed on the surface of adrenal cells
- Associated with other autoimmune diseases

General Considerations

Since the decline of tuberculosis, idiopathic Addison's disease is the most common form of adrenal insufficiency, accounting for 70–80% of all cases. The prevalence is relatively low, only 40–50 cases per million, and it tends to affect young individuals in their third or fourth decade. The female-to-male ratio is lower than that seen in other autoimmune disorders, only 1.8:1. It can present as an isolated disorder or in combination with other autoimmune diseases. It is most commonly seen as part of a polyglandular syndrome (see Autoimmune Polyglandular Syndromes), which accounts for up to 40% of the cases of this disease. The disease is associated with HLA-DR 3/4 in a manner similar to type I diabetes mellitus, except when part of a polyglandular syndrome.

Pathology

Grossly, adrenal glands from patients with idiopathic Addison's disease show progressive scarring and atrophy. Microscopic examination often reveals a lymphocytic infiltrate early in the course of the disease, and immunofluorescence shows antibody and complement fixed to cortical cells.

Clinical Features

Idiopathic Addison's disease is usually slowly progressive, with the development of clinical manifestations such as salt wasting, hypotension, anorexia, malaise, and hyperpigmentation occurring so gradually that they can easily go undetected. Serum levels of adrenocorticotropic hormone (ACTH) are often elevated long before clinical disease develops. The finding of small, noncalcified adrenal glands on computed tomography of the abdomen helps to differentiate this disorder from adrenal insufficiency secondary to carcinoma (primary or metastatic) and tuberculosis. The laboratory diagnosis rests on the lack of a cortisol (and possibly aldosterone) response to ACTH administration.

Immunologic Diagnosis

Serum antibodies against adrenal cortical cells are demonstrable by immunofluorescence in up to 80% of cases. Antibodies against specific antigens can now be detected by immunoassay.

Treatment

Treatment consists of corticosteroid hormone replacement and, when needed, replacement of mineralocorticoid hormones. No trials of immunosuppressive therapy have been published.

LYMPHOCYTIC ADENOHYPOPHYSITIS

Lymphocytic adenohypophysitis is a rare disorder characterized by the rapid development of hypopituitarism without evidence of pituitary adenoma. It occurs most often in women during or after pregnancy. Although the incidence of this disorder is unknown, the finding of antibodies against pituitary cells in 18% of patients with Sheehan's syndrome suggests that at least some of these patients may have had an autoimmune basis for their hypopituitarism. It also occurs as part of a polyglandular syndrome (see Autoimmune Polyglandular Syndromes), in which it has been associated with isolated deficiencies of gonadotropic hormones.

PREMATURE OVARIAN FAILURE

Evidence is accumulating that some individuals may have an autoimmune basis for premature gonadal failure. In several cases autoimmune oophoritis has been associated with other autoimmune endocrine diseases, especially adrenal insufficiency.

IDIOPATHIC HYPOPARATHYROIDISM

This is an uncommon disorder seen primarily in polyglandular autoimmune syndromes. Although antibodies against parathyroid tissue commonly occur in the polyglandular syndromes, their presence does not correlate with overt hypoparathyroidism. Antibodies from patients with this disorder have been reported to cause complement-mediated cytolysis of parathyroid cells, suggesting that a subset of antibodies may have pathogenic significance.

AUTOIMMUNE POLYGLANDULAR SYNDROMES

Major Immunologic Features
- Circulating antibodies against multiple endocrine organs
- Evidence of HLA-DR expression on affected cells
- Genetic susceptibility to autoimmunity

General Considerations
Polyglandular syndromes are groupings of multiple endocrine dysfunctions of autoimmune origin in a genetically susceptible individual. The recently developed classification scheme replaces the many eponymic versions of these disorders (Table 32–2).

A. Type I Syndrome: The type I syndrome occurs in childhood, usually before the age of 10 years, with a slight female predominance. It was previously known as mucocutaneous candidiasis endocrinopathy. The most common association is between candidiasis and hypoparathyroidism (>70% of cases), but 40–70% of patients also go on to develop adrenal insufficiency. With the exception of gonadal failure,

Table 32–2. Classification of polyglandular syndromes.

Syndrome	Major Criteria	Minor Criteria
Type I	Candidiasis Adrenal failure Hypoparathyroidism	Gonadal failure Alopecia Malabsorption Chronic hepatitis
Type II	Adrenal failure Thyroid disease IDDM	Gonadal failure Vitiligo Nonendocrine autoimmune disease
Type III[a]	Thyroid disease	a. IDDM b. Gastric disease c. Nonendocrine autoimmune disease

Abbreviation: IDDM = insulin-dependent diabetes mellitus.
[a] Type III is composed of thyroid disease plus only one of a, b, or c.

which occurs in approximately 40% of patients, the other autoimmune endocrine disorders are less common in the type I syndrome. An association exists, however, with chronic active hepatitis (10–15% of cases), alopecia areata, malabsorption, and pernicious anemia.

The pathogenesis of this disorder is unknown, but the problems with chronic fungal infection suggest a defect in cell-mediated immunity. Autoantibodies against cells from most affected organs are also seen in a large percentage of patients.

Although type I polyglandular syndrome occurs sporadically, it is more commonly seen as a familial disorder with inheritance suggestive of an autosomal-recessive trait. It has not been associated with a particular HLA haplotype.

B. Type II Syndrome: Type II polyglandular syndrome was originally known as Schmidt's syndrome. It tends to occur most often between the ages of 20 and 30 years and has a 2:1 female predominance. It is a rare disorder, with a prevalence of 20 per million. It is characterized by the presence of a second, autoimmune disorder (usually diabetes or thyroid disease or both) with idiopathic Addison's disease. Gonadal failure occurs in a smaller percentage of cases, and nonendocrine autoimmune disorders have been occasionally noted.

Although at least half the cases of type II polyglandular syndrome are familial, the mode of inheritance is unknown. Both autosomal-dominant and -recessive patterns have been suggested, and the frequency of HLA-DR3 in these patients is also high. Autoantibodies against cells of the affected organs are present in the majority of patients, and there have also been reports of alterations in cell-mediated immunity.

C. Type III Syndrome: Type III polyglandular syndrome is the least well characterized but probably the most common of the disorders. It is defined by the presence of autoimmune thyroid disease with another autoimmune disorder. This syndrome comprises at least three clinical entities. The first is the association of diabetes mellitus with autoimmune thyroid disease. The second is the association of autoimmunity against gastric components such as parietal cells or intrinsic factor in association with autoimmune thyroid disease. The association of any other organ-specific autoimmune disorder, such as myasthenia gravis, with autoimmune thyroid disease constitutes the third component. Patients with type III polyglandular syndrome, by definition, do not have Addison's disease.

The cause of type III polyglandular syndrome is unclear, but it tends to primarily involve female patients (7:1 female predominance) who have HLA-DR3-associated autoimmune disease. Again, organ-specific autoantibodies are present in the sera of patients with this disorder.

D. Other Considerations: The pathology, symptoms, and treatment of patients with the polyglandular syndromes are the same as for the individual autoimmune disorders, with a few important exceptions. Patients with type I polyglandular syndrome should have their candidiasis treated with ketoconazole, which not only provides symptomatic relief but also may help resolve some of the defects in cell-mediated immunity. In addition, all patients with the polyglandular syndromes should be monitored for the development of other autoimmune disorders associated with their syndrome. This minimizes the possibility of missing disorders such as Addison's disease, which may develop later in the course of the syndrome.

REFERENCES

GENERAL

Baker JR Jr: Autoimmune endocrine disease. *JAMA* 1997; 278:1931.

Caillat-Zucman S: Genetic predisposition to autoimmune endocrine diseases. *Ann Med Inter* 1999;15:221.

Lernmark A: Immune surveillance: Paraneoplastic or environmental triggers of autoimmunity. *Crit Rev Immunol* 1997;17:437.

Lorini R et al: IDDM and autoimmune thyroid disease in the pediatric age group. *J Pediatr Endocrinol Metab* 1996; 9:89.

Tomer Y, Davies TF: Infections and autoimmune endocrine diseases. *Baillieres Clin Endocrinol Metab* 1995;9:47.

Zouali M et al: Autoimmune diseases—At the molecular level. *Immunol Today* 1993;14:473.

THYROID DISEASES

Ajjan RA et al: Cytokines and thyroid function. *Adv Neuroimmunol* 1996;6:359.

Arscott PL, Baker JR, Jr: Apoptosis and thyroiditis. *Clin Immunol Immunopathol* 1998;87:207.

Baker JR Jr et al: Seronegative Hashimoto thyroiditis with thyroid autoantibody production localized to the thyroid. *Ann Intern Med* 1988;108:26.

McIntosh RS et al: The antibody response in human autoimmune thyroid disease. *Clin Sci* 1997;92:529.

Paschke R, Ludgate M: The thyrotropin receptor in thyroid diseases. *N Engl J Med* 1997;337:1675.

Perros P, Kendall-Taylor P: Thyroid-associated ophthalmopathy: Pathogenesis and clinical management. *Baillieres Clin Endocrinol Metab* 1999;9:115.

Prabhakar BS et al: Thyrotropin-receptor-mediated diseases: A paradigm for receptor autoimmunity. *Immunol Today* 1997;18:437.

Spitzweg C, Heufelder AE: Update on the thyroid sodium iodide symporter: A novel thyroid antigen emerging on the horizon. *Eur J Endocrinol* 1997;137:22.

DIABETES

Atkinson MA, Maclaren NK: The pathogenesis of insulin-dependent diabetes mellitus. *N Engl J Med* 1994; 331: 1428.

Azar ST et al: Type I (insulin-dependent) diabetes is a T_H1- and T_H2-mediated autoimmune disease. *Clin Diagn Lab Immunol* 1999;6:306.

Baekkeskov S et al: Identification of the 64K autoantigen in insulin-dependent diabetes as the GABA-synthesizing enzyme glutamic acid decarboxylase. *Nature* 1990;347: 151.

Baekkeskov S et al: The glutamate decarboxylase and 38 kd autoantigens in type 1 diabetes: Aspects of structure and epitope recognition. *Autoimmunity* 1993;15(Suppl): 24.

Baisch JM et al: Analysis of HLA-DQ genotypes and susceptibility in insulin-dependent diabetes mellitus. *N Engl J Med* 1990;322:1836.

Becker KG. Comparative genetics of type 1 diabetes and autoimmune disease: Common loci, common pathways? *Diabetes* 1999;48:1353.

Bonifacio E et al: Islet autoantibody markers in IDDM: Risk assessment strategies yielding high sensitivity. *Diabetologia* 1995;38:816.

Gottsater A et al: Glutamate decarboxylase antibody levels predict rate of beta-cell decline in adult-onset diabetes. *Diabetes Res Clin Pract* 1995;27:133.

Lernmark A: Type 1 diabetes. *Clin Chem* 1999;45:1331.

Lernmark A: Molecular biology of IDDM. *Diabetologia* 1994;37(suppl 2):S73.

Muntoni S, Muntoni S: New insights into the epidemiology of type 1 diabetes in Mediterranean countries. *Diabetes Metab Res Rev* 1999;15:133.

Riley WJ et al: A prospective study of the development of diabetes in relatives of patients with insulin-dependent diabetes. *N Engl J Med* 1990;323:1167.

Slavin S et al: New approaches for control of anti-self reactivity in type 1 diabetes mellitus and transplantation of pancreatic islets. *J Mol Med* 1999;77:223.

ADDISON'S DISEASE

Chen S et al: Autoantibodies to steroidogenic enzymes in autoimmune polyglandular syndrome, Addison's disease, and premature ovarian failure. *J Clin Endocrinol Metab* 1996;81:1871.

Falorni A et al: High diagnostic accuracy for idiopathic Addison's disease with a sensitive radiobinding assay for autoantibodies against recombinant human 21-hydroxylase. *J Clin Endocrinol Metab* 1995;80:2752.

Falorni A et al: 21-Hydroxylase autoantibodies in adult patients with endocrine autoimmune diseases are highly specific for Addison's disease. Belgian Diabetes Registry. *Clin Exper Immunol* 1997;107:341.

Seissler J et al: Autoantibodies to adrenal cytochrome P450 antigens in isolated Addison's disease and autoimmune polyendocrine syndrome type II. *Exper Clin Endocrinol Diabetes* 1999;107:208.

Weetman AP et al: HLA associations with autoimmune Addison's disease. *Tissue Antigens* 1991;38:31.

Winqvist O et al: 21-Hydroxylase, a major autoantigen in idiopathic Addison's disease. *Lancet* 1992;339:1559.

Winqvist O. Soderbergh A. Kampe O. The autoimmune basis of adrenocortical destruction in Addison's disease. *Mol Med Today* 1996;2:282.

LYMPHOCYTIC ADENOHYPOPHYSITIS & HYPOPARATHYROIDISM

Brandi ML et al: Antibodies cytotoxic to bovine parathyroid cells in autoimmune hypoparathyroidism. *Proc Natl Acad Sci U S A* 1986;83:8366.

Guay AT et al: Lymphocytic hypophysitis in a man. *J Clin Endocrinol Metab* 1987;64:631.

Homberg JC: Hypoparathyroidism, ovarian insufficiency, and adrenal insufficiency of autoimmune origin. *Rev Prat* 1986;36:3505.

McDermott MW et al: Lymphocytic adenohypophysitis. *Can J Neurol Sci* 1988;15:38.

AUTOIMMUNE OVARIAN FAILURE

Moncayo R, Moncayo HE: The association of autoantibodies directed against ovarian antigens in human disease: A clinical review. *J Intern Med* 1993;234:371.

POLYGLANDULAR AUTOIMMUNE DISEASE

Ahonen P: Autoimmune polyendocrinopathy candidosis ectodermal dystrophy (APECED): Autosomal recessive inheritance. *Clin Genet* 1985;27:535.

Appleboom TM, Flowers FP: Ketoconazole in the treatment of chronic mucocutaneous candidiasis secondary to autoimmune polyendocrinopathy candidiasis syndrome. *Cutis* 1982;30:71.

Betterle C et al: Clinical review 93: Autoimmune polyglandular syndrome type 1. *J Clin Endocrinol Metab* 1998;83:1049.

Betterle C et al: Type 2 polyglandular autoimmune disease (Schmidt's syndrome). *J Pediatr Endocrinol Metab* 1996;9(Suppl 1):113.

Chung AD, English JC 3rd: Cutaneous hyperpigmentation and polyglandular autoimmune syndrome type II. *Cutis* 1997;59:77.

Leshin M: Polyglandular autoimmune syndromes. *Am J Med Sci* 1985;290:77.

Obermayer-Straub P, Manns MP: Autoimmune polyglandular syndromes. *Baillieres Clin Gastroenterol* 1998;12:293.

Perheentupa J. Autoimmune polyendocrinopathy-candidiasis-ectodermal dystrophy (APECED). *Horm Metab Res* 1996;28:353.

Presotto F, Betterle C: Insulin-dependent diabetes mellitus: A constellation of autoimmune diseases. *J Pediatr Endocrinol Metab* 1997;10:455.

33

Hematologic Diseases

J. Vivian Wells, MD, FRACP, FRCPA, & James P. Isbister, FRACP, FRCPA

Many areas in hematology are significantly affected by immunologic processes. An important group of disorders—the autoimmune hemolytic anemias, autoimmune neutropenias, and immune thrombocytopenias—are characterized by immunologic destruction of circulating blood cells. Even hematopoietic precursor cells in the bone marrow may be affected by immunologic mechanisms, as seen in pure erythrocyte aplasia and some cases of aplastic anemia. Another large group of hematologic disorders—the plasma cell dyscrasias, lymphatic leukemias, and lymphomas—represent abnormal proliferations of primary cells of the immune system (see Chapter 43).

This chapter is devoted primarily to hematologic disorders in which immunologic cells or mechanisms play a major role. The chapter discusses immunologic disorders of leukocytes, erythrocytes, and hemostasis.

LEUKOCYTE DISORDERS

LEUKOPENIA

Leukopenia is defined as a reduction in the number of circulating leukocytes below 4000/μL. Granulocytopenia may be caused either by decreased granulocyte production by the bone marrow or by increased granulocyte utilization or destruction. Decreased granulocyte production occurs in aplastic anemia, leukemia, and other diseases marked by bone marrow infiltration; many drugs also cause leukopenia by this mechanism. Increased granulocyte use or destruction occurs in hypersplenism, autoimmune neutropenia, and some forms of drug-induced leukopenia. The major causes of leukopenia are listed in Table 33–1.

1. AUTOIMMUNE NEUTROPENIA

Autoimmune neutropenia may occur as an isolated disorder or secondary to an autoimmune disease. These patients may be asymptomatic or may have recurrent infections. Antigranulocyte antibodies have been detected by a variety of procedures, including fluorescence or antiglobulin consumption techniques that use antiimmunoglobulin antisera, functional assays, and cytotoxicity assays. The presence of leukoagglutinins does not correlate well with leukopenia. Bone marrow function is relatively normal in autoimmune neutropenia, with myeloid hyperplasia and a shift to the left in maturation, or maturation arrest, presumably in response to increased peripheral granulocyte destruction. The autoantibody may also suppress bone marrow myeloid cell growth in vitro and in vivo.

Autoimmune neutropenia may also be seen in systemic lupus erythematosus (SLE), Felty's syndrome (rheumatoid arthritis, splenomegaly, and severe neutropenia), and other autoimmune disorders. Immune neutropenia in these disorders may be caused by adsorption of immune complexes onto the neutrophil membrane with premature cell destruction rather than by an antibody directed at specific neutrophil antigens. Some patients with Felty's syndrome also appear to have depressed granulocyte production by the bone marrow, probably also on an immunologic basis.

2. CYCLIC NEUTROPENIA

These patients have a 3- to 6-week cycle, which includes a period of neutropenia lasting 4–10 days. Patients may be asymptomatic, but many show a pattern of recurrent fever, pharyngitis, recurrent aphthous stomatitis, lymphadenopathy, and infections during the period of neutropenia. The treatment of choice for symptomatic patients is granulocyte colony-stimulating factor (G-CSF; see section on management of neutropenia).

3. DRUG-INDUCED IMMUNE NEUTROPENIA

Although most drugs produce neutropenia by bone marrow suppression, some may cause neutropenia by the attachment of drug-antibody immune complexes

Table 33–1. The major causes of leukopenia.

Infections
  Viral—rubella
  Bacterial—typhoid fever, miliary tuberculosis, brucellosis
  Rickettsial
Therapy
  Ionizing radiation
  Cytotoxic drugs
  Drugs
    Selective neutropenia
    Agranulocytosis
    Aplastic anemia
Hematologic diseases
  Megaloblastic anemia
  Acute leukemia
  Myelodysplasia
  Aplastic anemia
  Multiple myeloma
  Paroxysmal nocturnal hemoglobinuria
  Leukoerythroblastic anemia
    Metastatic carcinoma
Autoimmune neutropenia
  Hypersplenism
  SLE
  Felty's syndrome
Chronic idiopathic neutropenia
Cyclic neutropenia
Miscellaneous
  Anaphylaxis
  Hypopituitarism

Abbreviations: SLE = systemic lupus erythematosus.

to the surface of the granulocytes, with premature cell destruction. This "innocent-bystander" mechanism is known to occur in drug-induced immune hemolytic anemia and thrombocytopenia. Cephalothin causes granulocytopenia in approximately 0.1% of patients given the drug, probably by this mechanism.

4. AGRANULOCYTOSIS

Agranulocytosis is characterized by the total absence of granulocytes and granulocyte precursors from the peripheral blood and bone marrow. This most often results from exposure of the patient to certain drugs, such as aminopyrine, dipyrone, and phenylbutazone. Patients with agranulocytosis usually present with infections—often serious, life-threatening ones. Prior to the antibiotic era, agranulocytosis was almost invariably fatal. Patients now usually recover with intensive antibiotic treatment, G-CSF, and granulocyte transfusions when necessary. Unlike drug-induced aplastic anemia, agranulocytosis usually resolves spontaneously within a few days to a few weeks after discontinuing the offending drug.

Although antigranulocyte antibodies or leukocyte drug-dependent antibodies generally have not been demonstrated in agranulocytosis, there is circumstantial evidence that immunologic damage to peripheral blood and bone marrow granulocytic cells is the mechanism of cell destruction, at least in some cases.

Such patients often develop agranulocytosis after taking the responsible drug for weeks or months. If they recover from the agranulocytosis after the drug is discontinued and later are rechallenged with a small test dose of the same drug, acute agranulocytosis occurs immediately, associated with the acute onset of fever, chills, and hypocomplementemia.

5. MANAGEMENT OF NEUTROPENIA

The first step in the management of neutropenia is identification of any underlying disease or drugs that may be responsible for the neutropenia.

The offending drug should be withdrawn, unless it is "essential" treatment, such as antitumor cytotoxic chemotherapy, antiretroviral therapy in human immunodeficiency virus (HIV) treatment, or recombinant interferon alfa therapy. Underlying diseases such as SLE should be treated appropriately, and generally no specific treatment is required for the neutropenia, which tends to resolve as the underlying disease goes into remission or is controlled. On occasion, patients with autoimmune neutropenia have required treatment with corticosteroids, immunosuppressive drugs, or splenectomy.

The major advance in the management of cytopenias has been the therapeutic use of hemopoietic growth factors.

Cytokines are bioactive cell secretions, which function as hormones for immune and other cells. The growth factors function as growth regulators, and more than 20 such factors have been identified and their genes cloned, including erythropoietin, the colony-stimulating factors, and the interleukins (IL). A few are now used in clinical practice (see Chapter 10), but their use is still restricted in many ways. Many ongoing clinical trials are assessing the role of cytokines in treating various diseases. Table 33–2 lists the major cytokines currently in clinical use or suggested for further studies.

For the management of neutropenia, cytokine therapy has been used in the following clinical settings:

1. Chronic Neutropenia/Cyclic Neutropenia: G-CSF is now the treatment of choice.

2. Autoimmune Neutropenia: G-CSF is considered for symptomatic patients not responding to corticosteroid therapy.

3. Drug-Associated Neutropenia: GM-CSF has been used in HIV infections significant neutropenia has developed after treatment with the antiretroviral agent zidovudine. Its role in this setting is still unproven.

4. Neutropenia Associated with Hairy Cell Leukemia: G-CSF is effective in this setting.

5. Cytotoxic Chemotherapy: Neutropenia is virtually inevitable following full-dose multidrug cytotoxic therapy. Several trials have studied G-CSF and GM-CSF to determine whether they prevent or

Table 33–2. Cytokines/hemolymphopoietic growth factors with clinical applications.

Cytokine	Major Biologic Effects	Clinical Applications[a]
Erythropoietin	Erythrocyte production	Anemia of end-stage renal disease Zidovudine anemia in AIDS patients
Granulocyte colony-stimulating factor (G-CSF)	Granulocyte lineage and differentiation Early myeloid stem cell action Neutrophil phagocytosis increase. Release of neutrophils from bone marrow	Neutropenia Aplastic anemia Transplantation
Granulocyte–monocyte colony-stimulating factor (GM-CSF)	Granulocyte, macrophage, and megakaryocyte proliferation and differentiation Enhancement of neutrophil functions	Neutropenia Aplastic anemia Transplantation
Colony-stimulating factor-1 (CSF-1)	Macrophage–monocyte proliferation and differentiation (lesser for granulocytes) Stimulation of macrophage activities	Neutropenia (Cancer)
Interleukin-2 (IL-2)	Growth induction for T cells Activation of cytotoxic T cells Enhancement of NK function	(AIDS) (Cancer)
Interleukin-3 (IL-3)	Stimulatin of proliferation and differentiation of granulocyte, macrophage, mast cell, megakaryocyte, early myeloid stem cell, and T- and B-cell lineages	Neutropenia Aplastic anemia Transplantation
Interleukin-6 (IL-6)	Stimulation of B-cell differentiation and IgG secretion Synergy with IL-3 for stimulation of early myeloid stem cells Stimulation of platelet production	(Aplastic anemia) (Transplantation)

Abbreviations: AIDS = acquired immunodeficiency syndrome; NK = natural killer.
[a] Items in parentheses indicate conditions that have been tested but not proven.

modify the severity of the neutropenia and permit complete treatment courses at full dosage. G-CSF is now widely used in cytotoxic chemotherapy-induced neutropenia.

6. Transplantation: Cytokine therapy has two possible uses in transplantation medicine. The first is to increase the neutrophil count in patients who have neutropenia after transplantation. The second is in nonneutropenic patients to mobilize stem cells from bone marrow to the periphery for collection, cryopreservation and, autografting.

7. Aplastic Anemia: GM-CSF, G-CSF, and interleukin-3 (IL-3) have all produced increases in neutrophil counts in such patients, but only while the drug is continued and with no effect on red cell and platelet counts. Their current use in this setting is therefore limited, mainly to supporting patients pending bone marrow transplantation for severe aplastic anemia.

8. Myelodysplasia: G-CSF is increasingly being used in patients with infections secondary to neutropenia or abnormal neutrophil function. The side effects of G-CSF are few, mainly axial bone pain during intravenous (but not subcutaneous) therapy and splenomegaly with long-term treatment. GM-CSF has a wider range of side effects, including fever and, at higher doses, capillary leak (fluid retention) syndrome, pericarditis, and pleuritis.

It is clear that cytokine/growth factor therapy will increase in the future, especially with the development of combination therapy for multilineage effects (eg, IL-3 and G-CSF or GM-CSF).

ERYTHROCYTE DISORDERS

The erythrocyte disorders in which immune processes play an important role are the immune hemolytic anemias, paroxysmal nocturnal hemoglobinuria, and aplastic anemia and related disorders.

IMMUNE HEMOLYTIC ANEMIAS

The immune hemolytic disorders are classified in Table 33–3. The classification is based on the behavioral characteristics of the antibodies involved and whether an underlying disease is demonstrable. The clinical picture may be one of an acute self-limiting hemolytic disorder but is more often chronic. Because identification of the type of antibody is essential to correct diagnosis in patients with suspected immune hemolytic anemia, the immunologic laboratory investigation is discussed before the individual diseases.

Immunologic Laboratory Investigations

Two groups of immunologic tests are used to investigate patients with suspected immune hemolytic anemias: (1) tests to detect and characterize antibod-

Table 33–3. Classification of immune hemolytic anemias.

Autoimmune hemolytic anemias
  A. Warm antibody types
    1. Idiopathic warm autoimmune hemolytic anemia (AIHA)
    2. Secondary warm autoimmune hemolytic anemias
      a. SLE and other autoimmune disorders
      b. Chronic lymphocytic leukemia, lymphomas, etc
      c. Hepatitis and other viral infections
  B. Cold antibody types
    1. Idiopathic cold agglutinin syndrome
    2. Secondary cold agglutinin syndrome
      a. *Mycoplasma pneumoniae* infection; infectious mononucleosis and other viral infections
      b. Chronic lymphocytic leukemia, lymphomas, etc
    3. Paroxysmal cold hemoglobinuria
      a. Idiopathic
      b. Syphilis, viral infections
Drug-induced immune hemolytic anemias
    1. Drug absorption mechanism
    2. Membrane modification mechanism
    3. Immune complex mechanism

  Partial list of drugs:

Aminosalicylic acid (PAS)	Methyldopa
Antihistamines	Penicillin
Carbromal	Phenacetin
Cephalothin	Pyramidon
Chlorinated hydrocarbons	Quinidine
Chlorpromazine	Quinine
Dipyrone	Rifampin
Insulin	Stibophen
Isoniazid	Sulfonamides
Levodopa	Sulfonylureas
Mefenamic acid	Tetracyclines
Melphalan	

Alloantibody-induced immune hemolytic anemias
  A. Hemolytic transfusion reactions
  B. Hemolytic disease of the newborn
  C. Allograft-associated anemias

ies involved in the hemolytic process and (2) tests to aid in diagnosis of possible underlying disease processes. Tests that define underlying disorders include detection of anti-DNA antibodies and antinuclear antibody (ANA) in SLE, rheumatoid factors in rheumatoid arthritis, and monoclonal B cells in chronic lymphocytic leukemia.

The serologic tests used to characterize antibodies in serum and on erythrocytes are basic blood-banking procedures, with the addition of monospecific antisera to identify specific proteins on erythrocytes and titration techniques to precisely quantitate antibody activity. Laboratory evaluation of such patients addresses a series of questions:

1. Are the erythrocytes of the patient coated with immunoglobulin, complement components, or both?
2. How heavily are the erythrocytes sensitized?
3. What antibodies are eluted from the erythrocytes?
4. What antibodies are present in the serum?

Routine screening is performed by means of the direct antiglobulin (Coombs') test by tube or slide agglutination (see Chapter 17) using antisera with broad specificity. Subsequent evaluation requires testing the red cells with dilutions of monospecific antisera, especially antisera to IgG and C3. The autoantibody is examined at different temperatures to see whether the temperature of maximal activity identifies it as a "warm" or "cold" antibody.

False-negative and false-positive results can be obtained in direct antiglobulin tests. Approximately 20% of all patients with immune hemolytic anemias have a negative or only weakly positive direct antiglobulin test unless the antiserum contains adequate titers of antibodies to complement components, especially C3. A positive direct antiglobulin test may be seen in situations other than autoantibodies on erythrocytes and does not necessarily mean autoimmune hemolytic anemia. Causes of such reactions include (1) antibody formation against drugs rather than intrinsic erythrocyte antigens (see section on drug-induced hemolytic anemia); (2) damage to the erythrocyte membrane due to infection or cephalosporins, leading to nonimmunologic binding of proteins; (3) in vitro complement sensitization of erythrocytes by low-titer cold antibodies (present in many normal individuals) in clotted blood samples stored at 4°C prior to separation; (4) delayed transfusion reactions; and (5) unknown mechanisms. The above-mentioned reactions are generally weak and can be differentiated by clinical and detailed serologic studies.

Serologic investigations of the patient's serum and erythrocyte eluates should answer these questions: (1) Are antibodies present? (2) Do they act as agglutinins, hemolysins, or incomplete antibodies? (3) What is their thermal range of activity? (4) What is their specificity?

The patient's serum is tested both undiluted and with fresh added complement against untreated and enzyme-treated pools of erythrocytes. The tests are run at both 37 and 20°C and examined after 1 hour for agglutination and lysis. Cold agglutinin titration at 4°C is also performed. Erythrocyte eluate is similarly tested.

Specialized tests may be performed to detect antibodies to drugs (eg, penicillin) in cases of drug-induced immune hemolytic anemia.

The specificity of the antibodies is tested at different temperatures with a panel of erythrocytes of different Rh genotypes and with cells of different types in the Ii blood group system.

The results of the serologic investigations are then correlated with clinical and other laboratory investigations to establish a definitive diagnosis.

1. WARM AUTOIMMUNE HEMOLYTIC ANEMIA

Major Immunologic Features

• Positive direct antiglobulin (Coombs') test

- Possible associated lymphoreticular cancer or autoimmune disease
- Splenomegaly common

General Considerations

Warm antibody autoimmune hemolytic anemia is the most common type of immune hemolytic anemia. It may be either idiopathic or secondary to chronic lymphocytic leukemia, lymphomas, SLE, or other autoimmune disorders or infections (see Table 33–3). The idiopathic form may follow overt or subclinical viral infection.

Clinical Features

A. Symptoms and Signs: Patients usually present with symptoms of anemia and hemolysis. Underlying disease, such as lymphadenopathy, hepatosplenomegaly, or manifestations of autoimmune disease may also be manifested.

B. Laboratory Findings: Normochromic normocytic or slightly macrocytic anemia is usually present; spherocytosis is common, and nucleated erythrocytes may occasionally be found in the peripheral blood. Leukocytosis and thrombocytosis are often present, but occasionally (especially in SLE) leukopenia and thrombocytopenia are seen. A moderate to marked reticulocytosis usually occurs. The bone marrow shows marked erythroid hyperplasia with plentiful iron stores. The serum level of unconjugated bilirubin increases. Stool and urinary urobilinogen may be greatly increased. Transfused blood has a shortened survival time.

Immunologic Diagnosis

The results of the serologic tests discussed earlier are summarized in Table 33–4. The most common pattern is IgG and complement on erythrocytes, with IgG in the eluate. The eluate generally has no activity if the erythrocytes are sensitized only with complement.

Warm hemolysins active against enzyme-treated erythrocytes occur in 24% of sera, but warm serum agglutinins or hemolysins against untreated erythrocytes are rare. The indirect antiglobulin test (see Chapter 17) is positive at 37°C in approximately 50–60% of patients' sera tested with untreated erythrocytes but in 90% of serum samples tested with enzyme-treated erythrocytes. This warm antibody is usually IgG but rarely may be IgM, IgA, or both.

The specificity of antibodies in warm antibody autoimmune hemolytic anemia is complex, but the main specificity is directed against determinants in the Rh complex.

Differential Diagnosis

Congenital nonspherocytic hemolytic anemia, hereditary spherocytosis, and hemoglobinopathies can usually be differentiated by the family history, routine hematologic tests, hemoglobin electrophoresis, and a negative direct antiglobulin test.

Treatment

A. General Measures: Treatment of the primary disease is necessary. Blood transfusions may be necessary for life-threatening anemia but should be avoided when possible, since the transfused cells are

Table 33–4. Summary of serologic findings in patients with autoimmune hemolytic anemia.

	Erythrocytes		Serum		
Disease Group	Direct Antiglobulin Test	Eluate	Immunoglobulin Type	Serologic Characteristics	Specificity
Warm antibody type	IgG 30% IgG + complement 50% Complement 20%	IgG IgG No activity	IgG (rarely also IgA or IgM)	Positive indirect antiglobulin test 50% Agglutination of enzyme-treated erythrocytes 90% Hemolysis of enzyme-treated erythrocytes 24% Agglutination of untreated erythrocytes (20 °C) 20% Agglutination or hemolysis of untreated erythrocytes (37 °C). Very rare	Rh system (often with a "nonspecific" component)
Cold agglutinin syndrome	Complement	No activity	IgM (rarely IgA)	High-titer cold agglutinin (usually 1:1000 at 4 °C) up to 32 °C; monoclonal IgM in chronic disease	Anti-I usually (can be anti-i or anti-Pr)
Paroxysmal cold hemoglobinuria (very rare)	Complement	No activity	IgG	Potent hemolysin also agglutinates normal cells. Biphasic (usually sensitizes cells in cold up to 15 °C and hemolyzes them at 37 °C)	Anti-P blood group

Source: Modified, with permission, from Petz LD, Garratty G: Laboratory correlations in immune hemolytic anemias. In: *Laboratory Diagnosis of Immunologic Disorders.* Vyas GN et al (editors). Grune & Stratton, 1975, p. 139.

rapidly destroyed. Careful serologic studies are needed to minimize the risks of serious hemolytic transfusion reactions, and successful crossmatching can be difficult or impossible in this situation. Alloantibodies are common and are difficult to detect.

B. Specific Measures: Hemolysis can be controlled with high doses of corticosteroids in most patients (40–120 mg of prednisone per day). The steroids are fairly rapidly tapered and then slowly reduced until the clinical state, hemoglobin level, and reticulocyte count indicate the appropriate maintenance dose. Occasionally it is possible to gradually withdraw steroids completely. Regular monitoring is necessary because relapses often occur.

Monitoring generally includes serologic studies, such as direct and indirect antiglobulin tests, and these may show improvement with reduced amounts of IgG and complement on erythrocytes and lower antibody titers or a negative antibody test. There is no consistent correlation between clinical response and serologic tests; however, prednisone often induces clinical remissions in patients with warm antibody autoimmune hemolytic anemia despite persistently positive direct antiglobulin tests.

If prednisone therapy fails or if unacceptable side effects occur, splenectomy is usually performed. Splenectomy is the treatment of choice if hemolysis persists after 2–3 months of corticosteroids and 60% respond to this procedure. ^{51}Cr-labeled erythrocyte survival studies can be used to identify abnormal splenic erythrocyte sequestration prior to splenectomy; however, clinical remissions may occur after splenectomy even when abnormal splenic sequestration cannot be documented. Continued significant hemolysis or late relapse sometimes occurs after splenectomy and requires therapy with steroids with or without other immunosuppressive agents.

Other immunosuppressive drugs include oral azathioprine, cyclophosphamide at low dosage, or cyclosporine.

Prognosis

The prognosis of idiopathic warm antibody autoimmune hemolytic anemia is fairly good; however, relapses are not infrequent, and death sometimes occurs. The prognosis of secondary warm autoimmune hemolytic anemia is determined by the underlying disease (eg, SLE or lymphoma).

2. COLD AGGLUTININ SYNDROMES

These diseases may be primary or secondary to infection or lymphoma (see Table 33–3). The infections include mycoplasmal pneumonia and infectious mononucleosis and other viral infections.

The clinical features are often those of the underlying disease. Cold-reactive symptoms such as Raynaud's phenomenon, livedo reticularis, or vascular purpura are seen in some patients. Hemolysis is generally mild but occasionally severe, especially in cases secondary to lymphoproliferative disease. The onset may be acute in cases secondary to infection. The idiopathic form is generally gradual in onset and runs a chronic and usually benign course in older patients.

These diseases usually are characterized by high serum titers of agglutinating IgM antibodies that react optimally in the cold. These patients have cold agglutinin titers in the thousands or millions, whereas normal individuals may have low-titer IgM cold agglutinins, and patients with chronic parasitic infections and most patients with *Ancylostoma* infection have titers up to 1:500. The presence of hemolysis is determined by the thermal range of the cold agglutinin. The high-titer, narrow-thermal-range antibodies cause acral ischemic symptoms. Some, however, may have a low titer but a thermal range reacting up to 37°C. The specificity of the IgM is generally anti-I in the Ii system, but occasionally it is anti-I or anti-Pr (see Table 33–4). In chronic idiopathic cases or cases associated with lymphoproliferative disease, the cold agglutinin is generally a monoclonal IgM-κ paraprotein. The direct antiglobulin test is always positive using antiserum to C3.

Treatment consists of keeping the patient warm and waiting for spontaneous resolution in acute cases. Chronic cases sometimes respond to chlorambucil or cyclophosphamide in low doses. Corticosteroids and splenectomy are probably not helpful, unless an underlying lymphoma is present.

The prognosis is generally good except for patients with severe underlying disease such as malignant lymphoma.

3. DRUG-INDUCED IMMUNE HEMOLYTIC ANEMIA

Many cases of immune hemolytic anemia have been reported in association with drug administration; the most common examples are included in Table 33–3. Investigating suspected drug-induced hemolytic anemia proceeds in three stages: (1) a history of intake of the drug, (2) confirmation of hemolysis, and (3) serologic tests. Detailed serologic tests are necessary because different drugs produce hemolysis by different mechanisms. The immunopathologic mechanisms and clinical and laboratory features are summarized in Table 33–5. The mechanisms are classified as immune complex formation, hapten adsorption, nonspecific adsorption, and other, unknown mechanisms.

1. Immune-Complex Formation: Circulating preformed immune complexes between the drug and antibody to the drug sensitize the erythrocyte ("innocent-bystander" phenomenon). Quinine in low doses

Table 33–5. Summary of immunopathologic mechanisms and clinical and laboratory features in drug-induced immune hemolytic disorders.

Mechanism	Drugs	Clinical Findings	Serologic Evaluation	
			Direct Antiglobulin Test	Antibody Characterization
Immune complex formation (drug + antidrug antibody)	Quinine, quinidine, phenacetin	History of small doses of drugs. Acute intravascular hemolysis and renal failure. Thrombocytopenia occasionally found	Complement (IgG) occasionally also present)	Drug + patient's serum + enzyme-treated erythrocytes → Hemolysis, agglutination, or sensitization Antibody often complement-fixing IgM Eluate generally nonreactive
Drug adsorption to erythrocyte membrane (combination with high-titer serum antibodies to drug)	Penicillins, cephalosporins	History of large doses of drugs Other allergic features may be absent Usually subacute extravascular hemolysis	IgG (strongly positive if hemolysis occurs) Rarely, weak complement sensitization also present	Drug-coated erythrocytes + serum → Agglutinaton or sensitization (rarely hemolysis) High-titer antibody Eluate reacts only with antibiotic-coated erythrocytes
Membrane modification (nonimmunologic adsorption of proteins to erythrocytes)	Cephalosporins	Hemolytic anemia rare	Positive with reagents with antibodies to a variety of serum proteins	Drug-coated erythrocytes + serum → Sensitization to antiglobulin antisera in low titer
Unknown	Methyldopa	Gradual onset of hemolytic anemia Common	IgG (strongly positive if hemolysis occurs)	Antibody sensitizes normal erythrocytes without drug Antibody in serum and eluate identical to warm antibody No in vitro tests demonstrate relationship to drug

Source: Adapted, with permission, from Garratty G, Petz LD: Drug-induced immune hemolytic anemia. *Am J Med* 1975;**58**:398.

is a typical example. Clinical features and serologic findings vary greatly.

2. Drug (Hapten) Adsorption: The drug acts as a hapten in that it is bound to the erythrocyte membrane and stimulates the production of a high titer of antidrug antibodies.

3. Nonspecific Adsorption: The drug affects the erythrocytes so that various nonimmunologic proteins are adsorbed onto erythrocytes and give a positive Coombs' test. This does not result generally in marked hemolysis.

4. Unknown Mechanisms: This type is exemplified by the positive Coombs' test that develops within 3 months in 20% of patients treated with methyldopa. The IgG that coats erythrocytes in these patients does not have antibody activity against the drug, and the drug is not required in in vitro tests.

The hemolysis may be acute and severe, but only rarely is blood transfusion required. The main treatment is to stop the offending drug and monitor the patient to be sure the hemolysis disappears. The prognosis is therefore excellent.

4. PAROXYSMAL COLD HEMOGLOBINURIA

This rare disease may be transient or chronic and constitutes 10% of the cold autoimmune hemolytic anemias. It may occur as a primary idiopathic disease or secondary to syphilis or viral infection. It is characterized clinically by signs of hemolysis and hemoglobinuria following local or general exposure to cold. Symptoms may include combinations of fatigue; pallor; aching and pain in the back, legs, or abdomen; chills and fever; and the passing of dark brown urine. The symptoms may appear from within a few minutes to a few hours after exposure to cold.

The disease is characterized by the presence of the classic biphasic Donath–Landsteiner antibody. This polyclonal IgG antibody sensitizes erythrocytes in the cold (usually below 15°C), so that complement components are detected on the erythrocytes by the direct antiglobulin test after rewarming. Heavily sensitized cells are hemolyzed when warmed to 37°C. The antibody has specificity for the P antigen.

Acute attacks are treated symptomatically, and

postinfectious cases generally resolve spontaneously, but transfusion is often necessary.

5. HEMOLYTIC DISEASE OF THE NEWBORN

See Chapter 17.

PAROXYSMAL NOCTURNAL HEMOGLOBINURIA

Paroxysmal nocturnal hemoglobinuria (PNH) is a rare acquired disease that can occur in adults as a chronic hemolytic anemia with acute exacerbations. It may follow other hematologic disorders such as idiopathic or drug-induced bone marrow aplasia and may terminate in acute myelogenous leukemia. The intravascular hemolysis causes intermittent hemoglobinemia and hemoglobinuria. This activity fluctuates throughout the day, but the classic nocturnal timing of hemoglobinuria is seen in only 25% of cases. Venous thrombosis is a recognized complication.

The diagnosis is suggested by the findings of intermittent or chronic intravascular hemolysis, iron deficiency, hemosiderinuria, a low leukocyte alkaline phosphatase value, and frequently pancytopenia. The diagnosis of PNH is confirmed by any of the following: the acid hemolysis (Ham) test, the sugar water test, and the inulin test. These tests detect the abnormal clones with the two presently known abnormalities in PNH: the exquisite sensitivity of PNH erythrocytes to complement lysis and the abnormally low acetylcholinesterase activity in the erythrocyte membrane. PNH is not an autoimmune-mediated disease, but instead represents failure to regulate the alternative pathway of complement activation.

In PNH the synthesis by hematopoietic cells of the glycosyl-phosphatidylinositol molecules that anchor proteins to the cell membrane is deficient. Complement-mediated hemolysis is a prominent feature of the disease due to deficient cell surface expression of decay-accelerating factor (DAF), CD55, and CD59, which protect blood cells from the action of complement. DAF operates at the level of C3/C5 activation. DAF does not have a central role in controlling hemolysis of erythrocytes, but it regulates the deposition of C3 on nucleated cells. PNH arises from a mutant hemopoietic clone, which explains the association with several other blood disorders such as aplastic anemia and leukemia.

The end result is that cells from such patients are more easily destroyed by complement than are normal cells. Patients' cells are lysed by approximately 4% of the amount of complement required to lyse normal erythrocytes.

Treatment is mainly symptomatic but otherwise unsatisfactory. Transfusions are often required, and reactions are not infrequent. Androgens may be useful if underlying bone marrow hypoplasia is present. Corticosteroids and splenectomy are probably not useful. Rarely, bone marrow transplantation may be possible.

APLASTIC ANEMIA & RELATED DISORDERS

Some cases of aplastic anemia and related disorders may be immunologic in origin.

Pure Erythrocyte Aplasia

This rare form of anemia is characterized by a marked reduction or absence of bone marrow erythroblasts and blood reticulocytes, with normal granulopoiesis and thrombopoiesis. It occurs as an acquired disorder in adults, either in an idiopathic form or associated with thymoma (in 30–50% of cases), lymphoma, other tumors, or certain drugs. In children red cell aplasia is usually associated with parvovirus infection. Patients usually present with progressive anemia requiring transfusion support. Bone marrow examination confirms the diagnosis. Thymoma is present in a small number of patients. Other immunologic abnormalities, such as hypogammaglobulinemia, monoclonal gammopathy, autoimmune hemolytic anemia, myasthenia gravis, and features of SLE may be seen in patients with pure erythrocyte aplasia.

Many patients with pure erythrocyte aplasia, with or without thymoma, have serum IgG antibodies that fix complement and are cytotoxic for bone marrow erythroblasts. This IgG antibody in plasma from patients with pure erythrocyte aplasia suppresses in vitro erythropoiesis by normal bone marrow.

Patients with pure erythrocyte aplasia usually require total erythrocyte transfusion support. Patients with thymomas should have these tumors removed, which produces a remission in about 30% of these patients. Patients with idiopathic pure erythrocyte aplasia and those who do not respond to thymectomy should be treated with intravenous gamma globulin (IVIG) if they do not have parvovirus infection. If not responsive to IVIG, the next step is immunosuppressive drugs. Corticosteroids are usually used first, but few patients respond, and most are subsequently treated with cyclophosphamide plus prednisone. This combination produces remissions in 30–50% of patients, but relapses may occur when drugs are discontinued. Splenectomy has also been advocated for refractory pure erythrocyte aplasia, as has plasma exchange.

Aplastic Anemia

Aplastic anemia is defined as pancytopenia due to bone marrow aplasia. Patients with severe aplastic anemia have no hematopoietic precursor cells present in their bone marrow and must be supported with erythrocyte and platelet transfusions and antibiotics.

In the past, aplastic anemia was usually associated with exposure to toxic drugs or chemicals (benzene, chloramphenicol, arsenicals, gold, anticonvulsants, etc). Hepatitis of unknown cause may be a precursor, as well. Recent series, however, indicate that most patients have no such exposure and no other associated illness, so that they are classified as having idiopathic aplastic anemia. Such patients should be tested for HIV infection.

Lymphocytes from the bone marrow of about one third of patients with aplastic anemia suppress the growth of or kill granulocyte colonies from normal bone marrow in vitro. When these abnormal suppressor lymphocytes are separated from the marrow granulocytic stem cells or killed with a specific cytotoxic antilymphocyte serum, increased granulocyte colony formation occurs. Other investigators found that peripheral blood lymphocytes from patients with aplastic anemia may suppress erythropoiesis of normal bone marrow when cultured in vitro.

Problems in management exist with continuing transfusion support; even with optimal supportive care, severe aplastic anemia rarely undergoes spontaneous remission, and the mortality rate is a 75–90%. Trials have confirmed the efficacy of antilymphocyte globulin (ALG) in selected patients, with response occurring in approximately 50%. Treatment with high doses of androgens may benefit some patients, but few patients with severe aplasia respond. Treatment with GM-CSF, G-CSF, IL-3, or CSF-1 is only a short-term measure. Bone marrow transplantation produces long-term remissions in 50–80% of patients with severe aplastic anemia, and early bone marrow transplantation is currently considered the treatment of choice for patients with a histocompatibly matched donor.

Aplastic anemia, therefore, may result from different defects involving the stem cells, the hematopoietic environment, cytokines/hemolymphopoietic growth factors, or suppressor cells. Characterization of the nature of the defects would permit more rational management of aplastic anemia because those cases with evidence of increased suppressor cell activity would be considered for treatment with immunosuppressive drugs or antithymocyte globulin (ATG) and those with obvious stem cell defects would be considered for early bone marrow transplantation.

PLATELET DISORDERS

Thrombocytopenia may be caused by decreased platelet production, increased platelet destruction, or abnormal platelet pooling. Immunologic thrombocytopenias, the subject of this section, are caused by increased platelet destruction, usually following platelet sensitization with antibody. Thrombocytopenias from decreased platelet production (aplastic anemia, leukemias, etc) have already been discussed with regard to immunologic features. Thrombocytopenia due to abnormal platelet pooling in an enlarged spleen (hypersplenism) is generally not associated with immunologic abnormalities.

Immunologic Mechanisms of Platelet Destruction

Several immunologic mechanisms of platelet damage leading to thrombocytopenia have been described. Platelet autoantibodies sensitize circulating platelets in idiopathic thrombocytopenic purpura and related disorders, leading to premature destruction of these cells in the spleen and generally involving Fc receptors on macrophages and other parts of the monocyte-machrophage system (see following section). Platelet alloantibodies may develop after multiple transfusions with blood products, or maternal sensitization can occur during pregnancies. Such platelet alloantibodies are becoming a major problem in long-term platelet support for patients with bone marrow failure. Alloantibodies may cause shortened platelet survival after transfusion or produce immediate platelet lysis with severe fever and chill reactions. Shortened platelet survival appears to be mediated by noncomplement-dependent IgG or IgM antibodies similar to autoantibodies seen in idiopathic thrombocytopenic purpura (ITP) and platelet lysis by complement-dependent cytotoxic antibodies. These alloantibodies are directed primarily at human leukocyte antigens (HLA), but non-HLA platelet antigens may also be involved. Alloantibody-dependent lymphocyte-mediated cytotoxicity has also been described in some patients.

The classification of platelet-specific antigens has continued to pose problems. The antigens of the five human platelet antigen (HPA) systems are inherited in an autosomal-codominant manner. The clinically relevant platelet alloantigens have their origins in single amino acid substitutions within the polypeptide chain of the glycoprotein (GP) that bears the alloantigenic epitope. The original platelet antigen system was based on the name of the patients, but this has resulted in major problems with nomenclature. The new classification system, based on internationally agreed-on platelet antigen numbers, has not been universally accepted.

Other immunologic mechanisms of platelet destruction include development of antibodies to drugs or other antigenic substances (haptens) absorbed to the platelet membrane and adsorption of preformed antigen-antibody complexes onto the platelet membrane, with rapid removal of these sensitized cells from the circulation (innocent-bystander phenomenon). The reactions are often complement-dependent. These mechanisms occur in drug-induced immune thrombocytopenia, in some infections, especially

Table 33–6. Classification of immune thrombocytopenias.

Idiopathic (autoimmune) thrombocytopenic purpura (ITP)

Secondary autoimmune thrombocytopenias
Systemic lupus erythematosus (SLE) and other autoimmune disorders
Chronic lymphocytic leukemia, lymphomas, some nonlymphoid malignancies
Human immunodeficiency virus (HIV) infection
Infectious mononucleosis and some other infections

Drug-induced immune thrombocytopenias (partial list of drugs)

Acetazolamide	Imipramine
Allymid	Meprobamate
Aminosalicylic acid (PAS)	Methyldopa
Antazoline	Novobiocin
Apronalide	Phenolphthalein
Aspirin	Phenytoin
Carbamazepine	Quinidine
Cephalothin	Quinine
Chlorthiazide	Rifampin
Digitoxin	Spironolactone
Factor VIII concentrate	Stibophen
Heparin	Sulfamethazine
Hydrochlorothiazide	Thioguanine

Posttransfusion purpura

Thrombotic thrombocytopenic purpura (TTP)

Neonatal immune thrombocytopenias
Due to autoantibodies (ITP)
Due to alloantibodies (maternal sensitization)

Due to alloantibodies (destruction of transfused platelets)
Sensitization from previous transfusions
Maternal sensitization during pregnancies

HIV, and in autoimmune disorders such as SLE. It has been suggested that cell-mediated immunity, that is, lymphocyte activation, may alone be able to cause platelet damage and thrombocytopenia. Lymphocyte activation has been observed in response to autologous platelets in some patients with ITP. Whether this represents a true cellular immune response or that the lymphocytes are reacting to immune complexes or otherwise altered platelets remains uncertain. Finally, it is known that bacterial endotoxin can cause thrombocytopenia directly, usually involving activation of the complement system. Antibodies are not required for this reaction.

Table 33–6 shows a classification of immunologic thrombocytopenias that are discussed in more detail in the following section.

IDIOPATHIC THROMBOCYTOPENIC PURPURA

Major Immunologic Features

- Antiplatelet antibodies demonstrable on platelets and in serum
- Shortened platelet survival
- Therapeutic response to prednisone, intravenous immunoglobulin, and splenectomy

General Considerations

Idiopathic thrombocytopenic purpura is an autoimmune disorder characterized by increased platelet destruction by antiplatelet autoantibody. IgG autoantibodies sensitize the circulating platelets, leading to accelerated removal of these cells by the macrophages of the spleen and at times of the liver and other components of the monocyte–macrophage system. Enhanced T helper cell/antigen-presenting interactions may have a role in IgG antiplatelet autoantibody production. Platelet autoantibodies are directed against a number of glycoprotein antigens on the platelet surface, usually anti-GPIIb/IIIa antibodies or, less commonly, against GPIb/IX. Although there is a compensatory increase in platelet production by the bone marrow (total platelet turnover may be 10–20 times the normal rate), thrombocytopenia occurs, and, depending on the severity, gives rise to the two typical clinical features of the disease: purpura and bleeding.

Idiopathic thrombocytopenic purpura most often occurs in otherwise healthy children and young adults. Childhood ITP often occurs within a few weeks following a viral infection, suggesting possible cross-immunization between viral and platelet antigens or adsorption of immune complexes or a hapten mechanism. Adult ITP is less often associated with a preceding infection. An identical form of autoimmune thrombocytopenia can also be associated with SLE, chronic lymphocytic leukemia, lymphomas, nonlymphoid cancers, infectious mononucleosis, and other viral and bacterial infections. Certain drugs can also cause immune thrombocytopenia, and these can produce a clinical picture that is indistinguishable from ITP.

Although adult and childhood ITP appear to have similar basic pathophysiologic features, they are significantly different in their course and therefore their treatment. The features of ITP in children and adults are compared in Table 33–7. Most children have spontaneous remissions within a few weeks to a few months, and splenectomy is rarely necessary. Adult patients, on the other hand, rarely have spontaneous remissions and usually require splenectomy within the first few months after diagnosis. HIV-associated immune thrombocytopenic purpura is recognized more frequently in patients with HIV who have not yet had an AIDS-defining disease.

Table 33–7. Idiopathic thrombocytopenic purpura in children and adults.

Parameter	Children	Adults
Peak age incidence (yr)	2–6	20–30
Sex incidence (M:F)	1:1	1:3
Clinical onset	Acute	Gradual
Antecedent infection	Common	Uncommon
Average duration of disease	1 mo	Months to years
Spontaneous remission	90%	10–20%
Presenting platelet count	$<20 \times 10^9$ L	$(30–50) \times 10^9$ L

Table 33–8. Tests for platelet autoantibodies in idiopathic thrombocytopenic purpura (ITP).

Method	Percent Positive
Standard immunologic tests (agglutination, complement fixation, etc)	0
Transfusion of plasma from patients with ITP into normal donors	63–75
Platelet factor 3 release	65–70
^{14}C-serotonin release	60
Lymphocyte activation by autologous platelets	70
Lymphocyte activation by platelet-antibody immune complexes	90+
Phagocytosis of platelet-antibody immune complexes by granulocytes	90+
Measurement of platelet-associated IgG by competitive binding assays	90+
Radiolabeled Coombs antiglobulin test	90+
Fluorescein-labeled Coombs antiglobulin	90+
Enzyme-linked immunosorbent assay (ELISA)	90+

Immunologic Diagnosis

W. Harrington and coworkers first showed in 1951 that the plasma from patients with ITP caused thrombocytopenia when transfused into normal human recipients. Their introduction of a clinically useful laboratory test for antiplatelet antibodies has been disappointing. Techniques to detect antiplatelet antibodies are shown in Table 33–8. Immunoinjury techniques (platelet factor 3 release, ^{14}C-serotonin release) detect antiplatelet antibodies in the serum of 60–70% of adult patients with ITP. Other methods to show positive results in almost all patients with ITP include methods to detect platelet–autoantibody complexes by lymphocyte activation or ingestion by granulocytes, or competitive binding assays or antiglobulin tests for the measurement of antiplatelet antibodies on the platelet surface. Methods using incubation of patient serum or plasma with intact platelets has resulted in greater sensitivity.

Platelet Kinetics

^{51}Cr-platelet kinetic studies show that all patients with ITP and other types of autoimmune thrombocytopenia have markedly shortened platelet survival times ($t_{1/2}$ 0.1–30 hours; normal $t_{1/2}$ 100–120 hours) and have normal or only slightly subnormal platelet recoveries at t_0 (40–80%; normal 60–80%). About 75% of patients have splenic platelet sequestration, and 25% have both splenic and hepatic sequestration. Patients with thrombocytopenia due to an enlarged splenic platelet pool can be easily distinguished from patients with autoimmune thrombocytopenia by these kinetic methods. Both groups had an 85–90% complete remission rate at 2 years' follow-up after splenectomy.

Clinical Features

A. Symptoms and Signs: The onset may be acute, with sudden development of petechiae; ecchymoses; epistaxis; and gingival, gastrointestinal, or genitourinary tract bleeding. More commonly, the disease is gradual in onset and chronic in course. Often, however, chronic ITP is slowly progressive or suddenly becomes acute.

B. Laboratory Findings: The platelet count is usually less than 20,000–30,000/mL in acute cases and 30,000–100,000/mL in chronic cases. Moderate anemia due to blood loss and iron deficiency may occur. The leukocyte count is normal or slightly increased but may be low in SLE. Platelets are often larger than normal on peripheral blood smear, and no immature leukocytes are present. The bone marrow shows normal or increased numbers of megakaryocytes and is otherwise normal. The megakaryocytes may be normal or immature in appearance but at times are larger than normal with increased numbers of nuclei.

Differential Diagnosis

All causes of thrombocytopenia must be considered when evaluating a patient with suspected ITP (Table 33–9). Patients with ITP characteristically feel and look well, and all physical and laboratory findings are normal except for thrombocytopenia and the associated purpura and possible bleeding. Patients with "consumptive" thrombocytopenias, on the other hand, tend to be acutely ill, often with fever and evidence of multisystem disease, especially renal disease. These patients generally have microangiopathic hemolytic anemia, the fragmented erythrocytes being a critical diagnostic finding on the peripheral blood smear. Abnormalities of clotting function are also often present. Patients with acute leukemia, aplastic

Table 33–9. Differential diagnosis of thrombocytopenic purpuras.

Thrombocytopenias due to increased platelet destruction
  Immune thrombocytopenias
    Idiopathic thrombocytopenic purpura
    Secondary autoimmune thrombocytopenias
    Drug-induced immune thrombocytopenias
    Posttransfusion purpura
    Neonatal immune thrombocytopenias
    Thrombocytopenia due to use of factor VIII concentrate
    HIV infection
  Consumptive thrombocytopenias
    Thrombotic thrombocytopenic purpura
    Hemolytic–uremic syndrome
    Disseminated intravascular coagulation
    Vasculitis
    Sepsis
  Hypersplenism
Thrombocytopenias due to decreased platelet production
  Bone marrow suppression by drugs, alcohol, toxins, infections
  Aplastic anemia
  Leukemias and other bone marrow cancers
  Megaloblastic anemia
  Refractory anemias, preleukemia, hematopoietic dysplasia

anemia, and other serious bone marrow disorders are also often acutely ill, and bone marrow examination is diagnostic. Patients with hypersplenism sufficient to cause thrombocytopenia usually have an easily palpable spleen; hypersplenism alone rarely causes a platelet count of less than 50,000/μL.

Secondary causes of autoimmune thrombocytopenia, such as HIV infection and SLE, must be ruled out by appropriate laboratory tests. If a patient with apparent ITP has been taking any suspicious drugs, the possibility of drug-induced thrombocytopenia must be considered. In some areas, HIV-associated disease is now the most common cause of thrombocytopenic purpura, especially in males between 20 and 50 years of age. Testing for antibodies to HIV is an essential part of the assessment of ITP.

Treatment

Treatment of patients with ITP is based mainly on clinical features and progress. If the patient is asymptomatic and the platelet count remains over 30,000/μL, observation is the preferred approach.

Children with mild or moderately severe ITP should be observed without therapy. In children who require active treatment, IVIG is the treatment of choice. A 5-day course of 400 mg/kg/d is given. Responses occur in 75% in 1–4 days, but many patients respond for only a short time, and repeat courses may be necessary.

Splenectomy is the treatment of choice for adult patients with ITP with persistent symptomatic thrombocytopenia. Corticosteroids (prednisone, 1–2 mg/kg/d) usually increase the platelet count temporarily but do not alter the course of the underlying disease, and most patients relapse when steroid use is tapered or discontinued. Adults rarely have spontaneous remissions, and splenectomy is therefore usually necessary within the first few months after diagnosis. Large doses of steroids over long periods should be avoided in these patients, since 75–90% will have prolonged complete remissions following splenectomy. Immunosuppressive therapy with cytotoxic drugs should generally not be used until the patient has had the benefit of splenectomy; this is particularly true for younger patients because these drugs may cause serious late adverse effects.

Vincristine seems to be a valuable agent in treating patients with autoimmune thrombocytopenia who do not respond to splenectomy, who relapse after an initial response to splenectomy, or in whom the risk of splenectomy is unacceptable. A significant increase in platelet count occurs in 70–80% of patients with refractory autoimmune thrombocytopenia treated with vincristine. Vincristine appears to be more effective, less toxic, and better tolerated than cyclophosphamide or other standard immunosuppressive drugs. Resistant cases may respond to cyclosporine. IVGG may be used as a short-term measure in adults prior to splenectomy, if corticosteroid therapy has failed to maintain a satisfactory platelet count at an acceptable dose. Response to IVIG is a good predictor of response to splenectomy. IVIG is also used in patients with HIV-associated immune thrombocytopenic purpura, prior to splenectomy, cases in which long-term immunosuppressive and cytotoxic therapy is contraindicated. Zidovudine (AZT) is effective in raising platelet counts in patients with HIV-associated immune thrombocytopenic purpura.

Corticosteroids may be given when severe thrombocytopenia and bleeding occur in children, although the platelet count does not respond as consistently to steroids in children as in adults. Splenectomy should be considered in children only when severe thrombocytopenia persists for 3–6 months because most children will have had a spontaneous remission by that time. The postsplenectomy state is much more likely to predispose young children to serious or overwhelming infection than in adults. Immunosuppressive drugs should generally not be used in children.

DRUG-INDUCED IMMUNE THROMBOCYTOPENIAS

The principal drugs that may cause immune thrombocytopenic purpura are listed in Table 33–6. The best studied example was the sedative apronalide (Sedormid) (no longer in use); the drugs most commonly used in clinical practice that can produce immune thrombocytopenic purpura are sulfonamides, thiazide diuretics, chlorpropamide, quinidine, heparin, and gold. A syndrome resembling acute drug-induced immune thrombocytopenia has also been observed in heroin addicts. Further reports have confirmed the increasing frequency of the heparin-induced thrombocytopenia syndrome (HIT). This unusual combination includes clinical features of hemorrhagic tendencies due to development of thrombocytopenia in patients treated with heparin for thrombosis. It appears that the heparin-dependent IgG-class antibody induces thromboxane synthesis and aggregation of the platelets.

The period of sensitization varies after initial exposure to the drug, but subsequent drug reexposure is rapidly followed by thrombocytopenia. Patients therefore usually give a history of having taken the drug in the recent past or at least several weeks ago if this is their first exposure. A very small plasma concentration of the drug and very small amounts of antibody may induce severe thrombocytopenia. The drug itself generally shows only weak and reversible binding to the platelet; the thrombocytopenia in most cases appears to be caused by antibody development to platelet factor 4 (PF4) and adsorption of the drug-antibody complexes to the platelet membrane with complement activation.

Treatment consists mainly of withdrawal of the offending drug (or all drugs) and monitoring for return of normal platelet counts, generally within 7–10 days. Thrombocytopenia may persist if the drug is excreted slowly. When a patient who is taking a number of suspicious drugs is first seen, it is often impossible to tell if the condition is drug-induced immune thrombocytopenia or ITP. In vitro tests can now be used in some centers to confirm drug-antibody reactions involving platelets. Because they are too hazardous, in vivo drug challenges of sensitized patients for confirmation of drug-induced immune thrombocytopenia should be avoided. In HIT it is important that alternative anticoagulation is used to prevent thrombosis. Heparinoid may be used as there is usually no cross reaction with the heparin antibody.

POSTTRANSFUSION PURPURA

There are two types of posttransfusion purpura. The first is due to dilution and occurs during massive blood replacement, as in the treatment of hemorrhage and shock. Further bleeding from the dilutional thrombocytopenia may complicate clinical management. The second type, which is due to alloantibodies, is an acute severe thrombocytopenic state appearing about 1 week after transfusion of a blood product. It occurs almost exclusively in women. It is mediated by an alloantibody, usually directed against the platelet Pl^{A1} antigen. Platelets both with and without the Pl^{A1} antigen are destroyed.

The diagnosis is suspected when acute thrombocytopenia occurs 7–10 days after blood transfusion. Coagulation studies are normal, and the bone marrow shows abundant megakaryocytes. The anti-Pl^{A1} antibody is detected in the plasma.

Gradual recovery from posttransfusion purpura usually occurs in 1–6 weeks. Corticosteroids do not appear to alter the course of the disease. Massive exchange transfusions have been associated with more rapid recovery, but severe transfusion reactions often occur. Aggressive plasma exchange or IVIG have also been shown to be effective without the risks of severe transfusion reactions.

NEONATAL ALLOIMMUNE THROMBOCYTOPENIA

Neonatal alloimmune thrombocytopenia (NAIT) is a rare syndrome, occurring in approximately 1 in 5000 newborn infants as a result of maternal alloimmunization against a platelet-specific antigen on fetal platelets for which the mother is antigen-negative. The syndrome is characterized by an isolated, transient, severe thrombocytopenia due to platelet destruction by maternal IgG alloantibody that has crossed the placenta. It may result in serious intrauterine, neonatal, or perinatal immune thrombocytopenia, which may cause extensive hemostatic failure, especially intracerebral hemorrhage. It is now possible to establish immune thrombocytopenia, allowing for the cause of appropriate treatment and eventually the care of future pregnancies. Treatment in utero of fetomaternal alloimmunization has altered the natural course of fetal thrombocytopenia, assisting in the management of pregnancies at risk.

NAIT should be suspected in neonates with otherwise unexplained isolated thrombocytopenia and confirmed with demonstration of a platelet antibody in the mother's serum. The typical presentation for an infant with NAIT is dramatic petechiae, purpura, and extreme thrombocytopenia in an otherwise healthy infant. There is significant risk of serious, life-threatening hemorrhage. The mother has no significant obstetric history, the maternal platelet count is normal, and there is no present or past history of ITP. If the mother or infant have other perinatal or hematologic problems, alternative diagnosis need to be considered to explain the thrombocytopenia, including maternal autoimmune or drug-induced, preeclampsia hemolysis-elevated liver enzymes low platelet count syndrome (HELLP), sepsis, congenital viral infections, congenital bone marrow hypoplasia, osteopetrosis, prematurity, and birth asphyxia. Babies of first pregnancies are affected in about half the cases.

Treatment is dictated by the presence of bleeding and the degree of thrombocytopenia. Infants who are bleeding or severely thrombocytopenic should receive a platelet transfusion compatible with the mother's serum. Washed and irradiated maternal platelets are suitable. A single platelet transfusion is usually adequate. High-dose IVIG can serve as an alternative form of treatment if compatible platelets cannot be procured. Pregnancies known to be at risk for NAIT should be monitored with ultrasound examinations from about the 20th week of gestation. Fetal blood sampling for platelet count and allotype should be considered around 20 weeks. This should be performed at a center experienced in percutaneous umbilical cord blood sampling (PUBS) and capable of preparing maternal platelets for transfusion. The importance of cooperative care among the obstetrician, hematologist, and neonatologist cannot be overemphasized. Accurate assessment of the past obstetric and transfusion history is important. Before the next pregnancy or early in subsequent pregnancies, the father's platelets should be phenotyped to determine if all subsequent infants will have the target antigen.

THROMBOTIC THROMBOCYTOPENIC PURPURA

Thrombotic thrombocytopenic purpura (TTP) is a rare potentially fulminant and life-threatening disorder characterized by platelet microthrombi in small vessels resulting in organ dysfunction and a microangiopathy. Coagulation activation is not a prominent feature. The clinical syndrome is manifested by the pentad of thrombocytopenia, microangiopathic hemolytic anemia, fever, renal dysfunction, and neurologic abnormalities. Abdominal symptoms, hepatic dysfunction, and pulmonary abnormalities may also occur. With the clinical features and a microangiopathic blood smear with thrombocytopenia the diagnosis is relatively easy. The acute form of the condition can be fulminant and life-threatening and in the past was rapidly fatal in the majority of patients.

The pathophysiology of this syndrome is enigmatic, and the mechanisms may not be the same in individual cases. There could be a final common pathway for a variety of initiating causes. Pathologically, an abnormal interaction appears to exist between the vascular endothelium and platelets. Recent evidence suggests TTP may be caused by an autoimmune-induced deficiency of metalloprotease involved in the proteolysis of von Willebrand factor (vWF). The high-molecular-weight vWF multimers are not cleaved under high shear stress conditions and thus predispose to thrombosis. The rare familial TTP has been identified as due to a congenital deficiency of metalloprotease. In some cases, circulating platelet-aggregating factors or abnormalities in high-molecular-weight vWF multimers may mediate the platelet aggregation.

The primary idiopathic form usually has an acute presentation and probably has an underlying autoimmune mechanism. This form may be associated with a variety of prodromal infections (viral—CMV, HIV, herpes—and bacterial) and typically may occur in the third trimester of pregnancy. Bacterial cytotoxins, produced by *Shigella dysenteriae* I and certain *Escherichia coli* serotypes, have been related to TTP and hemolytic–uremic syndrome (HUS) probably in initiating damage to vascular endothelial cells, possibly via cytokine mechanisms. TTP may be associated with various drugs (cytotoxic agents), toxins, and bites. Chemotherapy-associated TTP/HUS may be associated with a range of cytotoxic medications, especially mithramycin. Pathogenesis may be related to drug toxicity on endothelial cells in the kidney microvasculature or the formation of soluble circulating platelet aggregators, such as immune complexes, autoantibodies, or abnormal amounts of large-molecular-weight vWF multimers from stimulated endothelial cells. Severe microangiopathy resembling TTP has also been reported as a complication of acute graft-versus-host disease in patients receiving cyclosporine prophylaxis following allogeneic bone marrow transplantation. It is hypothesized that cytokines may induce the endothelial damage.

In the past, TTP was fatal in 90% of patients, but dramatic improvement in its outcome has occurred over the past two decades with the development of effective therapy. Plasma infusion or exchange have become the cornerstones of the treatment of TTP. Cryoprecipitate-poor plasma (depleted in vWF) may offer advantages over whole fresh-frozen plasma. It is now possible to achieve remissions in the majority of patients, and cures are now common, but unfortunately up to half the patients relapse. The clinical course at relapse is usually milder than the disease at presentation, and less aggressive therapy may be needed. Patients resistant to this approach may respond to alternative therapy, including high-dose intravenous immunoglobulin, dextran, platelet inhibitory drugs, corticosteroids, vincristine, or splenectomy.

HEMOLYTIC-UREMIC SYNDROME

This syndrome has many similarities to TTP, but renal involvement is the hallmark in association with microangiopathic hemolytic anemia and thrombocytopenia. It usually occurs in children and is related to bacterial or viral infections. It may rarely be seen in adults, in whom the disease is commonly drug-related and may take a more chronic and serious course. Quinine-associated hemolytic-uremic syndrome (HUS) has been recently described and probably occurs more often than is recognized. It is important to recognize this syndrome in order to avoid further quinine exposure. The prognosis and approach to management of HUS is similar to that for TTP.

QUININE-INDUCED IMMUNE THROMBOCYTOPENIA WITH HEMOLYTIC-UREMIC SYNDROME

Quinine-induced immune thrombocytopenia with HUS is a recently defined clinical entity. The disease is characterized by the onset of chills, sweating, nausea and vomiting, abdominal pain, oliguria, and petechial rash following quinine exposure. Anemia, severe thrombocytopenia, increased serum lactate dehydrogenase levels, and azotemia are noted. Quinine-dependent platelet-reactive antibodies can usually be identified. Patients are treated with plasma exchange (range 1–12 procedures), and may also require hemodialysis. All survive without residual abnormality. Adult patients presenting with HUS should routinely be asked about exposure to quinine in the form of medication or beverages. The mechanism of renal failure is unclear but may be due to drug-induced antibodies reactive with endothelial cells leading to margination of granulocytes in renal glomeruli. Quinine-induced HUS has a better prognosis than other forms of adult HUS.

CIRCULATING INHIBITORS OF COAGULATION

Abnormal bleeding is occasionally due to circulating inhibitors that block one or more plasma coagulation factors, have in most cases been shown to be IgG antibodies. Inhibitors against factor VIII and von Willebrand factor occur most often, but inhibitors directed against factors V, IX, XIII, and vWF have also been reported. There are rare reports of human monoclonal proteins (especially IgM) with antibody activity directed against clotting components, for example factor VIII, and phospholipid. Inhibitors may appear abruptly and be associated with life-threatening hemorrhage or may be chronic and associated with little or no bleeding.

Factor VIII inhibitors develop in 15% of patients with classic hemophilia after they have been transfused with factor VIII-containing blood products; genetic factors appear to determine which patients develop inhibitors. Factor VIII inhibitors also occasionally occur spontaneously in postpartum women, in patients with autoimmune disorders such as SLE, and in older patients without demonstrable underlying disease. Rarely, the paraprotein in a monoclonal gammopathy has specific inhibitor activity against factor VIII or other clotting factors.

High-titer factor VIII inhibitors (antibodies) often cause serious bleeding and require aggressive treatment. Patients with serious bleeding can be given several times the calculated amount of factor VIII to saturate the inhibitor, provided the inhibitor titer is not too high. When bleeding cannot be stopped, even after giving large amounts of factor VIII, activated prothrombin complex concentrates should be given because these often stop the bleeding by providing activated clotting factors that bypass the factor VIII step. If this is unsuccessful, aggressive large-volume plasma exchange can be used to remove the inhibitor.

Combination therapy with factor VIII, cyclophosphamide, vincristine, and prednisone (CVP) is highly effective in the eradication of factor VIII inhibitors in nonhemophiliacs, but not in hemophiliacs.

ANTIPHOSPHOLIPID SYNDROME

Major Immunologic Features
- Anticardiolipin antibodies (ACA)(IgG or IgM class) present
- Ninety percent of patients with lupus anticoagulants (LA) also have ACA
- Eleven percent of ACA cross-react with heparin and heparan sulfate
- Frequent association with SLE

General Considerations
Antiphospholipid syndrome (APS) comprises a clinical diagnosis of arterial or venous thrombosis, thrombocytopenia, or recurrent fetal loss, and laboratory results of positive tests for IgG-class or IgM-class ACA or lupus anticoagulants on at least two occasions 12 weeks apart.

The female-to-male ratio is 2:1, and smoking, hy-perlipidemia, and hypertension are additional risk factors.

The condition is primary if associated autoimmune disease (especially SLE) has been excluded. There are no clear differences in major features or treatment of primary or secondary anticardiolipin antibody syndrome.

Immunologic Pathogenesis
The cause of the production of these antibodies is unknown, but frequently an infection precedes the development and detection of the various antibodies. In some cases the antiphospholipid antibodies appear to follow the use of drugs, such as procainamide, hydralazine, chlorpromazine, quinidine, isoniazid, and methyldopa.

Many mechanisms of action of LA have been postulated, but none explains the coagulation abnormalities found in all cases. Binding of autoantibodies to protein phospholipid complexes provides the unifying model. Most antiphospholipid antibodies require the presence of anionic phospholipid binding proteins (eg β-2-glycoprotein I and prothrombin). Mechanisms proposed to explain the hypercoagulable state include antibody cross-linking of membrane-bound antigens altering kinetics of phospholipid-dependent reactions and antibody cross-linking of antigens bound to surface receptors triggering transduction and cellular activation.

Clinical Features
A. Symptoms and Signs:
1. Venous Thrombosis: This may occur in up to 50% of patients (especially younger patients) and included deep venous thrombosis, venous thromboembolism, and thrombosis at unusual sites.

2. Arterial Ischemic and Infarct Syndromes: These may take various forms and occur in up to 50% of patients and include stroke, transient ischemic attacks, multiinfarct dementia, migraine headaches; myocardial infarction; vasculitic rashes and arthralgias in 50%; digital infarcts or skin necrosis; pulmonary hypertension; retinal artery or venous occlusion; amaurosis fugax; splenic infarction or hyposplenism; adrenal infarction and hemorrhage; and livedo reticularis and multiple ischemic cerebrovascular lesions (Sneddon's syndrome).

3. Recurrent Fetal Loss: This may occur in up to 35% of pregnant patients. IgG or IgM anticardiolipin antibodies occur in 2% of women with one or two fetal losses, 9% of women with two losses and 10% of women with three or more. Anticardiolipin antibodies may occur with severe preeclampsia late in the second or early in the third trimester.

4. Cardiac Abnormalities: Valvular insufficiency or stenosis may result from verrucous endocardial lesions or Libman–Sacks endocarditis. There is a strong association with anticardiolipin antibodies in patients with SLE.

5. Autoimmune Hemolytic Anemia: Anticardiolipin antibodies may have a direct role in the production of hemolytic anemia in some patients with SLE by acting as autoantibodies to red blood cells.

6. Drug-Induced APS: This syndrome may appear following drug treatment, and many patients show features of SLE. The drugs include procainamide, hydralazine, chlorpromazine, quinidine, isoniazid, and methyldopa. More frequently, patients treated with drugs who develop autoantibodies are asymptomatic. These antibodies include anticardiolipin (especially IgM class), lupus anticoagulants, and ANA and DNA antibodies.

7. Association with Infections: It is uncommon to find the clinical features of APS although it is common for ACA and lupus anticoagulants to develop with an infection and disappear with resolution of the infection. Infections include syphilis; Lyme disease; and viral infections due to adenovirus, rubella, chickenpox, and HIV.

B. Laboratory Findings:

1. Thrombocytopenia: Thrombocytopenia occurs in 30–50%, especially in patients with SLE.

2. Anticardiolipin Antibody: Cofactor (b2-glycoprotein)-dependent ACA have been associated with autoimmune disease and the presence of clinical manifestations of the syndrome. This is in contrast to cofactor-independent ACA in which the association is with infectious diseases and drug-induced ACA.

Lupus anticoagulant activity is demonstrated on two occasions, 12 weeks apart, in 50% of patients.

Antiphospholipid antibodies prolong the phospholipid-dependent coagulation assays. Not all reagents in clotting assays are equally sensitive to lupus anticoagulant. The combination of anticardiolipin antibody and β_2-glycoprotein is essential for binding to cardiolipin and lupus anticoagulant activity. Low β_2-glycoprotein levels (<50 mg/L) may result in false-negative lupus anticoagulant tests.

3. Other Serology: ANA is present in 50% of cases in low titer 1/40–1/160. Antibodies to single-stranded DNA are frequent. Occasionally the Coombs' direct antiglobulin test is positive with associated autoimmune hemolytic anemia. Antibodies to double-stranded DNA and ENA are negative.

Treatment

Treatment of the clinical features of APS remains controversial and is often unsatisfactory. This is partly because of the multifactorial nature of the syndrome, partly because definition of the syndrome is still developing, and partly because of the marked clinical variability.

If SLE is associated with APS, then treatment of the underlying SLE is a priority (see Chapter 31). With mild thrombotic symptoms, aspirin is the most common first-line drug therapy. With more severe thrombotic features, more aggressive anticoagulant treatment is given, with varying claims for its efficacy. Corticosteroid therapy is often used now in women with the syndrome who experience recurrent early fetal loss to attempt to achieve a viable fetus.

REFERENCES

LEUKOPENIA

Dale DC: Immune and idiopathic neutropenia. *Curr Opin Hematol* 1998;5:33.

Stroncek DF: Neutrophil antibodies. *Curr Opin Hematol* 1997;4:455.

ERYTHROCYTE DISORDERS

Hashimoto C: Autoimmune hemolytic anemia. *Clin Rev Allergy Immunol* 1998;16:285.

Smith LA: Autoimmune hemolytic anemias: Characteristics and classification. *Clin Lab Sci* 1999;12:110.

PLATELET DISORDERS

Amiral J: Meyer D Heparin-induced thrombocytopenia: Diagnostic tests and biological mechanisms. *Baillieres Clin Haematol* 1998;11:447.

Aster R: Drug-induced immune thrombocytopenia: An overview of pathogenesis. *Semin Hematol* 1999;36:2.

Blanchette V et al: Management of chronic immune thrombocytopenic purpura in children and adults. *Semin Hematol* 1998;35(Suppl l):36.

Eldor A: Thrombotic thrombocytopenic purpura: Diagnosis, pathogenesis and modern therapy. *Baillieres Clin Haematol* 1998;11:475.

Esplin MS: Branch DW Diagnosis and management of thrombotic microangiopathies during pregnancy. *Clin Obstet Gynecol* 1999;42:360.

Gillis S, Eldor A: Immune thrombocytopenic purpura in adults: Clinical aspects. *Baillieres Clin Haematol* 1998;11:361.

Greinacher A: Heparin-induced thrombocytopenia: Pathophysiology and clinical concerns. *Baillieres Clin Haematol* 1998;11:461.

Harrington WL et al: Demonstration of thrombocytopenic factor in the blood patients with thrombocytopenic purpura. *J Lab Clin Med* 1951;38:1.

Imbach P, Kuhne T: Immune thrombocytopenic purpura ITP. *Vox Sang* 1998;74 Suppl 2:309.

Kaplan KL, Francis CW: Heparin-induced thrombocytopenia. *Blood Rev* 1999;13:1.

Moake JL: von Willebrand factor in the pathophysiology of thrombotic thrombocytopenic purpura. *Clin Lab Sci* 1998;11:362.

Porcefijn L, von dem Borne AE: Immune-mediated thrombocytopenias: Basic and immunological aspects. *Baillieres Clin Haematol* 1998;11:1.

Ruggenenti P, Remuzzi G: Pathophysiology and management of thrombotic microangiopathies. *J Nephrol* 1998; 11:300.

Sutor AH, Gaedicke G: Acute autoimmune thrombocytopenia. *Baillieres Clin Haematol* 1998;11:381.

Tarantino MD, Goldsmith G: Treatment of acute immune thrombocytopenic purpura. *Semin Hematol* 1998;35 (Suppl 1):28.

COAGULATION DISORDERS

Esmon NL et al: Lupus anticoagulants, thrombosis and the protein C system. *Haematologica* 1999;84:446.

Galli M, Barbui T: Antiprothrombin antibodies: detection and clinical significance in the antiphospholipid syndrome. *Blood* 1999;93:2149.

Harris EN et al: Diagnosis of the antiphospholipid syndrome: A proposal for use of laboratory tests. *Lupus* 1998;7(Suppl 2): S 144.

Kandiah DA et al: Current insights into the "antiphospholipid" syndrome: Clinical, immunological, and molecular aspects. *Adv Immunol* 1998;70:507.

Roubey RA: Mechanisms of autoantibody-mediated thrombosis. *Lupus* 1998;7(Suppl 2):S 114.

Thiagarajan P, Shapiro SS: Lupus anticoagulants and antiphospholipid antibodies. *Hematol Oncol Clin North Am* 1998;12:1167.

Inflammatory Vasculitides

34

Kenneth H. Fye, MD, FACP, FACR, & Kenneth E. Sack, MD, FACR

General Considerations

The vasculitides are a group of inflammatory disorders united by their common target organ, the vascular tree. They represent a spectrum of pathologic and clinical disease ranging from acute necrotizing vasculitis to chronic indolent vascular inflammation. Although extravascular granuloma formation may be observed in some of the vasculitides, the major pathologic finding is inflammation of blood vessels. The various vasculitides can be distinguished using a combination of findings: the type of involved vessels (eg, large arteries, small arteries, venules, etc), the pattern of vascular involvement (eg, extracranial circulation, etc), and the histology, and presence or absence of certain laboratory abnormalities. Nonetheless, the classification of the vasculitides has proved to be particularly difficult and is still evolving. This chapter will focus on the primary vasculitides and will not review vasculitis secondary to another disease process, such as systemic lupus or subacute bacterial endocarditis.

Immunologic processes likely play a critical pathogenic role in most of the primary vasculitides. Interest has focused on three general mechanisms: immune complex-mediated inflammation, autoantibodies [eg, antineutrophil cytoplasmic antibodies (ANCA) and antibodies to endothelial cells], and T-cell-mediated vascular damage. More than one mechanism may be operative in any particular form of vasculitis.

It has long been recognized that immune complexes can induce vascular damage. For example, injection of antigen in the form of horse serum or bovine albumin into rabbits results in an inflammatory arteritis coincident with the development of a host antibody response and the formation of immune complexes. The intravenous injection of preformed immune complexes, particularly in the presence of rheumatoid factors, induces vasculitis in rats. Vasculitis is a prominent component of serum sickness in humans. Complexes of antibodies and antigen can deposit in vessel walls where they induce inflammation by triggering the complement cascade and by recruiting and activating Fc receptor-bearing cells, such as macrophages and polymorphonuclear leukocytes.

Adhesion molecules play an important role in the pathogenesis of vasculitis by allowing the leukocytes to "roll" along the vascular endothelium, to adhere to the endothelium, and to extravasate into the perivascular tissues.

Antiendothelial cell antibodies are commonly seen in the vasculitides, and there is evidence to suggest that the levels of antiendothelial cell antibodies may correlate with activity of disease. These antibodies can induce antibody-dependent cell-mediated cytotoxicity, activate complement, stimulate intravascular thrombosis, and induce chemotaxis.

ANCA directed against either myeloperoxidase or serine protease 3 are seen in several of the small vessel vasculitides and may play a role in the pathogenesis of vascular inflammation. For example, activation of neutrophils leads to a translocation of serine protease 3 from the cytosol to the cell surface. Attachment of antiserine protease 3 antibodies to surface serine protease 3 may enhance cell activation and lead to degranulation, respiratory burst, and granulocyte adherence to endothelial cells.

Cell-mediated mechanisms also appear to play a pathogenetic role in some of the vasculitides. In these disorders CD4 and CD8 cells and T-cell-derived cytokines have been observed in vessel walls, raising the possibility that a T-cell response to a vascular antigen contributes to the vasculitis.

POLYARTERITIS NODOSA

Major Immunologic Features

- Immunoglobulin and complement deposits in the walls of involved vessels
- Circulating immune complexes in patients with hepatitis B related disease
- Vascular infiltrates composed largely of neutrophils with variable numbers of macrophages and lymphocytes

General Considerations

Polyarteritis nodosa (PAN) is a necrotizing vasculitis of medium-size muscular arteries (0.5–1 mm in diameter). The disease usually affects middle-aged men and, in many patients, is associated with hepatitis B infection. Although localized forms of PAN occur, the disorder is generally systemic, with protean manifestations reflecting multiple organ system involvement.

Immunologic Pathogenesis

Experimental immune complex disease can cause an arteritis in animals that resembles PAN. Immunofluorescent studies in humans have demonstrated immunoglobulin and complement in vessel walls during active disease, consistent with the possibility of immune complex-mediated inflammation. In patients with circulating hepatitis B antigen, the antigen, either alone or with antihepatitis B immunoglobulin or complement, may be deposited in the vessel walls. In these patients the levels of circulating immune complexes appear to correlate with disease activity. Evidence of hepatitis B infection varies with the population studied but can be seen in up to half of patients with PAN.

Immunohistochemical studies have demonstrated CD4 lymphocytes and macrophages in perivascular infiltrates. Activation markers, such as human leukocyte antigen (HLA)-DR and interleukin-2 receptor, can be seen on infiltrating T cells. Such observations suggest that cell-mediated immune mechanisms also may contribute to PAN.

Clinical Features

A. Symptoms and Signs: Constitutional manifestations, including fever, fatigue, lethargy, myalgias, arthralgias, and weight loss reflect the systemic nature of the disorder. Specific organ failure is usually due to multiple infarctions caused by vascular occlusions brought on by inflammation in involved vessels. Inflammation of the vessel wall can cause microaneurysms, which may rupture and bleed.

1. Renal—The kidneys are involved in 70% of patients, and renal failure is the commonest cause of death in PAN patients. Renin-dependent renovascular hypertension occurs in 50% of patients. Rupture of microaneurysms in the renal circulation is associated with renal or perirenal hematomas. Periureteral vasculitis may cause ureteral fibrosis and obstructive uropathy.

2. Cardiac—Sixty percent of patients have cardiac involvement. Congestive heart failure is the commonest manifestation of cardiac involvement, but atrioventricular heart block and coronary artery insufficiency with myocardial infarction can be seen.

3. Gastrointestinal—Half of the patients with PAN develop vasculitis of the gastrointestinal tract, manifested by pancreatitis, hepatitis, infarction of the liver, cholecystitis, bowel ischemia (sometimes with infarction or perforation), and gastrointestinal bleeding. Small-bowel ischemia, malabsorption, or pancreatitis indicate a poor prognosis. On occasion, a medium-vessel vasculitis histologically identical to

PAN may affect the appendix or gallbladder in the absence of systemic disease.

4. Pulmonary—The lungs are affected infrequently. Typical manifestations include asthma, bronchitis, pneumonitis, or, rarely, pleuritis.

5. Neurologic—Peripheral neuropathy, particularly affecting the lower extremities, occurs in 70% of patients. Although mononeuritis multiplex is characteristic of PAN, many patients present with just a sensory "stocking-glove" peripheral neuropathy. Cranial nerve involvement occurs uncommonly. Central nervous system vasculitis may cause strokes because of infarctions or rupture of microaneurysms with hemorrhage.

6. Cutaneous—Half of the patients develop skin manifestations, including livido reticularis, digital infarctions, palpable purpura, and subcutaneous nodules.

7. Musculoskeletal—Twenty percent of cases develop myositis, with muscle weakness, pain, and tenderness. The arthritis seen in PAN occurs early in the disease. It is an asymmetric, inflammatory, oligoarticular process affecting primarily weight bearing joints.

8. Ocular—Ocular manifestations include retinal vasculitis, retinal detachment, and scleritis.

9. Genitourinary—Although traditionally a favorite site for biopsy, less than 20% of patients have testicular involvement. Orchitis is more common, however, in PAN associated with hepatitis B infection.

B. Laboratory Findings: Most patients have a normochromic, normocytic anemia, a leukocytosis (occasionally with eosinophilia), an elevated erythrocyte sedimentation rate (ESR) and an elevated level of C-reactive protein. Patients with renal involvement may have hematuria or proteinuria, as well as elevated serum creatinine and blood urea nitrogen. Elevated alkaline phosphatase and serum transaminases are particularly likely in patients with serologic evidence of hepatitis B infection. Elevated serum amylase and lipase reflect pancreatitis. A positive ANCA, generally due to antimyeloperoxidase antibodies, is seen in about 10% of cases. Polyclonal hypergammaglobulinemia, cryoglobulinemia, a positive rheumatoid factor, and antiphospholipid antibodies can all be seen on occasion.

C. Diagnosis: Ultimately, the diagnosis of PAN rests on either biopsy or angiographic confirmation of medium-vessel vasculitis. Biopsies of involved skin, muscle, sural nerve, or testicle are particularly helpful. Visceral angiograms are positive in 70% of patients, whether or not there is clinical evidence of abdominal or renal involvement. The angiographic characteristics of PAN include loss of the fine arborialization of the visceral vasculature, "corkscrewing" and wall irregularities of involved vessels, and microaneurysms of medium-size arteries, 0.5–1.0 mm in diameter. Angiograms of the celiac axis, superior mesenteric artery, and renal arteries are most likely to reveal diagnostic changes. Angiographic abnormalities may resolve with therapy.

Treatment

Before the advent of modern therapy the 2-year survival rate of patients with PAN was only 10%. With the use of systemic corticosteroids the 5-year survival rate increased to 50%. The introduction of cytotoxic therapy raised the 5-year survival rate to 80%.

Oral corticosteroids are the cornerstone of therapy. The usual starting dose of 60–80 mg/day is tapered to maintenance levels after the disease process has been controlled. In life-threatening disease 1000 mg/day of methylprednisolone is administered intravenously on each of 3 consecutive days.

Several oral cytotoxic drugs are of likely benefit in the treatment of PAN. In life-threatening or recalcitrant disease, cyclophosphamide, an alkylating agent administered either in the form of monthly intravenous pulses or daily low oral doses, is often efficacious but carries considerable toxicity, particularly with the daily oral regimens. A second alkylating agent, chlorambucil, is an alternative to cyclophosphamide. Azathioprine, a purine antagonist, has an excellent safety profile. Methotrexate and cyclosporine are occasionally effective in the treatment of PAN. Plasmapheresis can sometimes be of benefit in patients who do not respond to pharmacologic therapy, particularly those with circulating immune complexes. Plasmapheresis must be used in conjunction with cytotoxic therapy to prevent "rebound" formation of immune complexes.

Prognosis

PAN is a potentially fatal disorder that must be treated aggressively before irreversible organ damage occurs. Involvement of the kidneys, nerves, muscles, and bowel portend a poor prognosis. Recurrences of PAN are unusual in patients who respond well to initial therapy, and the 10-year survival rate is similar to that after 5 years—(80%). Much of the late mortality seen in PAN is a consequence of the toxicities of long-term corticosteroid or cytotoxic therapy.

MICROSCOPIC POLYANGIITIS

Major Immunologic Features

• A positive ANCA due to antimyeloperoxidase antibodies
• Necrotizing inflammation of small vessels

General Considerations

Microscopic polyangiitis (MPA) is a systemic necrotizing vasculitis that affects small vessels (arterioles, venules, capillaries). The average age of onset is 50 years, and men are affected twice as often as women. The cause of the disease is unknown. The majority of patients have a positive ANCA. Although 80% of these patients have a pANCA due to antimyeloperoxidase antibodies, 20% will have a positive cANCA due to antiserine protease 3 antibodies. Some patients with MPA also have antiendothelial cell antibodies.

Clinical Features

A. Signs and Symptoms: Constitutional manifestations, including fever, weight loss, malaise, and lethargy, occur in 75% of patients, sometimes months before the diagnosis of vasculitis is apparent.

1. Renal—Rapidly progressive crescentic glomerulonephritis is the major clinical manifestation of MPA, affecting virtually 100% of patients. Without treatment, renal function deteriorates rapidly. There are typically no immune deposits in the kidney.

2. Pulmonary—The lungs are involved in half the patients. Pulmonary capillaritis results in diffuse alveolar damage with pulmonary infiltrates, hemorrhage, and hemoptysis. Interstitial fibrosis is a late complication.

3. Musculoskeletal—Myalgias, arthralgias, and a nondeforming arthritis are seen in 75% of patients.

4. Cutaneous—Palpable purpura is the commonest cutaneous manifestation of MPA. Splinter hemorrhages, periungual infarctions, and cutaneous ulcers also occur.

5. Gastrointestinal—The intestines are affected in approximately 50% of patients. Major manifestations include abdominal pain and diarrhea. Bowel infarctions are rare. Hepatosplenomegaly occurs in 20% of patients.

6. Other—Episcleritis occurs in a third of patients. Upper respiratory manifestations include oral ulcers, epistaxis, and sinusitis. Both the central and peripheral nervous system can be affected. The commonest cardiac manifestation is pericarditis.

B. Laboratory Findings: Patients typically have a normochromic, normocytic anemia, leukocytosis, thrombocytosis, and elevated ESR and C-reactive protein. Serum complement levels are normal or elevated. Renal involvement is characterized by hematuria, proteinuria, an active urinary sediment, and, in cases of renal failure, elevated serum creatinine and blood urea nitrogen. Eighty percent of patients have a positive ANCA, generally due to antimyeloperoxidase antibodies. The rheumatoid factor is positive in over half of patients, and a third have a positive ANA.

C. Diagnosis: A systemic inflammatory disorder with renal, pulmonary, musculoskeletal, and cutaneous involvement in the presence of a positive pANCA is suggestive of a necrotizing vasculitis, but the definitive diagnosis rests on histologic evidence of small-vessel vascular inflammation. Skin and lung are the most fruitful biopsy sites. Renal biopsy typically reveals a pauciimmune, crescentic, rapidly progressive glomerulonephritis. Pulmonary infiltrates seen on chest radiograph reflect the presence of pulmonary hemorrhage. Visceral angiograms are normal.

Treatment

MPA with clinically significant major organ involvement is treated with a combination of high-dose corticosteroids and cytotoxic agents (usually cyclophosphamide in the form of intravenous pulses or small daily doses). Azathioprine can be used to maintain remissions induced by cyclophosphamide.

Prognosis

The 5-year survival rate of patients with fulminant MPA is 65%. Age at onset of greater than 50 years and the development of renal failure are indicators of a poor prognosis. Relapses are common, particularly when treatment is discontinued, so chronic therapy with prednisone or low doses of cytotoxic drugs is often necessary.

WEGENER'S GRANULOMATOSIS

Major Immunologic Features

- A positive cANCA due to antiserine protease 3 antibodies
- Activated T cells with a T_H1-like cytokine profile in inflammatory infiltrates

General Considerations

Wegener's granulomatosis(WG) is a necrotizing granulomatous angiitis affecting small and medium-size arteries and veins. The three major areas of involvement are the upper respiratory tract, the lung parenchyma, and the kidneys. Men and women are affected equally. Before the advent of modern therapy, systemic WG was uniformly fatal, with a 12-month survival rate of only 18%. With the introduction of cyclophosphamide, remissions and long-term survival became possible. Some patients have a limited form of the disease that responds to less toxic therapies, such as trimethoprim–sulfamethoxazole or methotrexate.

The prominent involvement of the upper airways and lung in WG suggests that the disease may result from an inhaled antigen or pathogen, but there is little firm evidence to support this possibility. The presence of granulomas and activated T cells in involved tissues suggest that cell-mediated immune response are important. However, over 90% of patients with active systemic WG have a positive ANCA, generally due to antiserine protease 3 antibodies. As noted earlier, these antibodies may play a role in the pathogenesis of the disease. Antiendothelial cell autoantibodies are also seen in WG and may contribute to vascular inflammation.

Clinical Features

A. Signs and Symptoms: WG affects adults of both sexes equally. It can present as an acute, severe life-threatening disease or as a chronic, indolent inflammatory disorder. Most patients have upper respiratory, lower respiratory, and renal involvement, but some have only upper airway disease ("limited WG"). Unexplained fever and weight loss may precede the typical manifestations of the disease.

1. Upper Respiratory—Upper airway disease is the commonest manifestation of WG, occurring in over 90% of patients. Signs of nasal involvement include nasal ulcers, mucosal inflammation with nasal obstruction, septal perforation, and necrosis of nasal cartilage with "saddle nose" deformity. Acute and chronic sinusitis, often with secondary infection, occurs in over 80% of patients. Other manifestations include oral ulcers, chronic gingivitis, and subglottic stenosis. Manifestations of ear involvement include chondritis of the external ear, otitis externa, granulomata of the tympanic membrane, otitis media, vertigo, and hearing loss (either conductive or sensory).

2. Lower Respiratory—WG can cause pulmonary infiltrates, pulmonary nodules (which may cavitate), and pulmonary hemorrhage. Endobronchial inflammation can lead to obstructive lung disease, whereas interstitial involvement proceeds to restrictive lung disease with respiratory insufficiency. Hilar or mediastinal masses may occur.

3. Renal—Glomerulonephritis is seen in 80% of patients, half of whom develop renal insufficiency. Findings include fibrinoid necrosis, proliferative changes and epithelial crescents without immune complex deposition, and glomerulosclerosis. Vasculitis of medium-size arteries and granuloma formation occur less commonly in the kidney.

4. Musculoskeletal—About 70% of patients complain of myalgias and arthralgias, whereas a third develop a true nondeforming, nonerosive arthritis.

5. Cutaneous—Skin lesions are common and include palpable purpura, cutaneous ulcers, pyoderma gangrenosum, and Raynaud's phenomenon. Cutaneous manifestations of WG typically respond well to corticosteroid or immunosuppressive therapy.

6. Neurologic—WG affects both the peripheral and central nervous systems. Peripheral manifestations include mononeuritis multiplex and peripheral symmetric polyneuropathy. Central nervous system disease consists of cranial neuropathy, infarction, subdural or subarachnoid hemorrhage, seizures, or diffuse cerebritis.

7. Gastrointestinal—Common manifestations of gastrointestinal involvement are abdominal pain, diarrhea, and bleeding, reflecting the presence of small- or large-bowel ulceration. Involvement of medium-size vessels can cause bowel infarction with perforation.

8. Cardiac—Approximately 10% of WG patients have clinical evidence of cardiac disease. Manifestations include pericarditis, coronary arteritis, conduction defects, and cardiomyopathy.

9. Genitourinary—Genitourinary manifestations include ureteral obstruction, urethritis, orchitis, and epididymitis. Necrotizing vasculitis of the bladder wall can lead to hemorrhagic cystitis that is difficult to distinguish from the hemorrhagic cystitis caused by cyclophosphamide therapy.

B. Laboratory Findings: Patients generally present with a normochromic, normocytic anemia, leukocytosis, thrombocytosis, and an elevated ESR. An active urinary sediment with red cells and red cell casts typifies renal involvement, and a rising creatinine signifies renal failure. A positive rheumatoid factor is seen in 50% of patients. The ANCA is positive in over 90% of patients with active systemic disease and in about 40% of patients in remission. Although most patients have a cANCA due to the presence of antiserine protease 3 antibodies, some have a positive pANCA caused by antimyeloperoxidase antibodies.

C. Diagnosis: Signs and symptoms of upper and lower respiratory inflammation in a patient with glomerulonephritis and a positive ANCA is compatible with a clinical diagnosis of WG, but the final diagnosis depends on biopsy evidence of vasculitis, tissue necrosis, and granuloma formation. Small- and medium-size arteries, capillaries, and veins can all be affected in WG. Biopsies of upper airway tissues are rarely diagnostic; the most reliable diagnostic tissue is obtained by open lung biopsy. Renal biopsy findings, generally a pauciimmune crescentic glomerulonephritis with varying amounts of fibrinoid necrosis, are not specific for WG but are of considerable diagnostic value in the right clinical setting.

Treatment

Cyclophosphamide is the mainstay of treatment of severe WG and significantly increases survival. Systemic corticosteroids can temporarily ameliorate the inflammatory manifestations of the disease and are often used as initial therapy until the patient responds to the slower acting cyclophosphamide. Because of the toxicity of long-term oral cyclophosphamide, there is considerable interest in regimens with fewer complications. Monthly pulses of intravenous cyclophosphamide are less toxic but may not be as effective as the oral form of the agent. Methotrexate and azathioprine may be useful in maintaining remissions induced by cyclophosphamide and may allow for shorter courses of cyclophosphamide. Trimethoprim–sulfamethoxazole has been used with success as adjunct therapy in WG, particularly in the limited form of the disease. Its greatest value may be in maintaining remissions induced by more potent agents. Reduction in respiratory tract infections, which may trigger relapses, may explain the efficacy of this antibiotic.

Prognosis

Over 90% of WG patients respond to therapy, with 5-year survival rates greater than 80%. Unfortunately, relapses are common when treatment is discontinued, and 75% of patients have persistent morbidity, including chronic renal failure, nasal deformities, tracheal stenosis, chronic sinusitis, and hearing loss. In addition, many patients suffer significant morbidity related to chronic immunosuppressive therapy.

CHURG-STRAUSS SYNDROME

Major Immunologic Features

- Positive pANCA due to antimyeloperoxidase antibodies
- Elevated levels of IgE
- Granuloma formation

General Considerations

Churg-Strauss syndrome (CSS), also called allergic granulomatosis and angiitis, is a necrotizing, granulomatous, small-vessel vasculitis associated with asthma, sinusitis, and eosinophilia. It affects adults, and men twice as often as women. Pulmonary involvement is the cardinal feature of this vasculitis.

Immunologic Pathogenesis

The cause of the disease is unknown, but it may be partly an allergic phenomenon. Increased levels of IgE and peripheral eosinophilia are common in untreated patients, and asthma, sinusitis, and allergic rhinitis are major manifestations of the disease. The ANCA is positive in two thirds of patients, generally because of the presence of antimyeloperoxidase antibodies.

Clinical Features

A. Signs and Symptoms: Constitutional symptoms, such as weight loss, fever, myalgias, and arthralgias, are common. Patients generally have a long history of upper respiratory allergies, asthma, and eosinophilia before the onset of the full-blown syndrome.

1. Pulmonary—Adult-onset asthma is the most common manifestation of CSS, affecting nearly all patients. Other respiratory features include allergic rhinitis, sinusitis, and nasal polyposis. Patchy pulmonary infiltrates, seen in half the patients, are generally evanescent and may sometimes be associated with pleural effusions.

2. Neurologic—Peripheral neuropathy (either mononeuritis multiplex or symmetric polyneuropathy) occurs in 75% of patients. The commonest CNS manifestation is ischemic optic neuritis.

3. Cardiac—Myocardial granulomata and small-vessel coronary vasculitis are a major cause of morbidity and mortality in CSS patients. Manifestations of cardiac disease include congestive heart failure, restrictive cardiomyopathy, and pericarditis.

4. Renal—The typical renal lesion, seen in 50% of patients, is a focal segmental glomerulonephritis, sometimes with crescents and necrosis. Other renal lesions include vasculitis, granulomata, and eosinophilic interstitial infiltrates.

5. Gastrointestinal—Abdominal pain, diarrhea, or gastrointestinal bleeding due to bowel vasculitis is seen in up to 50% of patients. Bowel perforation occurs rarely.

6. Cutaneous—Cutaneous manifestations, including palpable purpura, subcutaneous nodules, skin infarction, and livido reticularis, are seen in over half the patients.

B. Laboratory Findings: Anemia, eosinophilia, elevated IgE levels, and an elevated ESR are common. An active urinary sediment with red cells, red cell casts, and proteinuria are manifestations of renal involvement. Increases in serum creatinine and blood urea nitrogen signify renal insufficiency. A positive pANCA is seen in 75% of patients.

C. Diagnosis: A diagnosis of CSS is likely in an adult with asthma, allergic rhinitis or sinusitis, transient pulmonary infiltrates, peripheral neuropathy, eosinophilia, and a positive ANCA. Biopsy confirmation of vasculitis is mandatory, however. The most fruitful biopsy sites are nerve, skin, lung, and kidney. Typical histologic findings include inflammation of arterioles and venules, extravascular granuloma formation, and perivascular eosinophilic infiltrates.

Treatment

Usually, the disease responds well to high-dose corticosteroids, and most patients require a low maintenance dose of prednisone. In patients who do not respond adequately to or who cannot tolerate corticosteroids, cytotoxic agents, such as cyclophosphamide, azathioprine, chlorambucil, and methotrexate are usually effective.

Prognosis

The long-term prognosis for patients with CSS is good, with a 5-year survival rate of greater than 75%. Mortality is most often related to myocardial infarction and congestive heart failure due to the disease or to the atherosclerotic complications of corticosteroid therapy. Renal failure, bowel infarction, and respiratory failure also increase mortality.

GIANT-CELL ARTERITIS

Major Immunologic Features

- T_H1 type CD4 cells and macrophages infiltrating the walls of involved vessels

General Considerations

Giant-cell arteritis (GCA), also called temporal ar-

teritis, cranial arteritis, and giant-cell arteritis of the aged, is an indolent vasculitis of large arteries, particularly in the extracranial circulation, that affects patients 50 years of age or older. Whites of northern European extraction are particularly susceptible. The major complications of this disorder are caused by occlusion of involved vessels. GCA is usually self-limited, with an average duration of disease activity of approximately 2 years. The cause is unknown.

Immunologic Pathogenesis

The inflammatory process appears to be T-cell mediated, with the vascular infiltrate consisting of T_H1 type CD4 lymphocytes and macrophages. Lesional macrophages produce interleukins 1 and 6 as well as other inflammatory cytokines.

Clinical Features

A. Signs and Symptoms: The disease occurs exclusively in patients older than 50 years of age and affects women twice as often as men. Constitutional manifestations are common and include fever, malaise, weight loss, myalgias, and proximal muscle stiffness (particularly in the morning).

1. Cranial Arteritis—Involvement of extracranial vessels can cause headache, temporal artery tenderness, glossitis, and jaw claudication. Without treatment, GCA can cause blindness due to infarction of the optic nerve or, less commonly, due to occlusion of the central retinal artery.

2. Aortitis—Aortitis, particularly of the thoracic aorta, is not uncommon. Although generally asymptomatic, dissection can occur in patients with active disease. Aortic aneurysm formation can also occur as a late complication of GCA.

3. Cerebrovascular Occlusion—Cerebrovascular occlusions, particularly in the posterior circulation, occur in GCA. The carotid and vertebral arteries, as well as intracranial vessels can be involved in these patients. Deafness and vertigo may occur in patients with vertebral artery involvement.

4. Musculoskeletal—Polymyalgia rheumatica (PMR) is characterized by stiffness and pain of the shoulder and pelvic girdle musculature. Like GCA, it targets patients older than 50 years of age and is seen twice as frequently in women as in men. Blind temporal artery biopsy reveals histologic evidence of GCA in 60% of patients with PMR. Nonspecific synovitis, particularly of the shoulders, can be demonstrated by bone scan or biopsy.

5. Hepatic—A mild lymphocytic portal triaditis is seen in 25% of patients. Although elevations in serum levels of transaminases may occur, an elevated serum alkaline phosphatase is more common.

B. Laboratory Findings: An elevated ESR is the most characteristic laboratory abnormality. The magnitude of the elevation reflects the activity of the disease and is a rough gauge of the patient's response to therapy.

C. Diagnosis: The diagnosis rests primarily on the presence of a typical history and physical examination, an elevated ESR, and a prompt and dramatic clinical response to corticosteroid therapy. Because the treatment of GCA involves the use of long-term corticosteroids, however, it is important to confirm the diagnosis by temporal artery biopsy. Histologic findings include mononuclear cell infiltration, giant-cell formation, intimal thickening, and fragmentation of the internal elastic lamina. Because vascular involvement is discontinuous, at least 2.5 cm of vessel should be examined. Sometimes a biopsy of both temporal arteries is necessary to confirm the diagnosis.

Treatment

Corticosteroids eliminate the acute symptoms and prevent the occlusive complications of GCA, including blindness. Oral prednisone is usually initiated at doses of 40–60 mg qd. The dose is tapered over the ensuing months to the lowest dose needed to control symptoms. Within a year most patients will be on maintenance doses of less than 10 mg qd. The ESR generally decreases with therapy and increases with a relapse of symptoms. Because occlusive complications of the disease can occur quickly and be irreversible, prednisone therapy should be initiated as soon as the diagnosis is entertained. If an appropriate diagnostic evaluation does not reveal GCA, the prednisone can be quickly discontinued. Temporal artery biopsy will yield positive findings for at least a week after the initiation of corticosteroid therapy. Methotrexate can serve as a steroid-sparing agent in patients with chronic, recalcitrant disease.

Prognosis

GCA typically remits after an average of 2 years, although some patients have persistent disease for longer than 4 years. Late clinical relapses occasionally occur after discontinuation of corticosteroids. Inadequate corticosteroid therapy is associated with an increased mortality due to myocardial infarction, stroke, and dissecting aortic aneurysm. The incidence of aortic aneurysm increases in patients who have a distant history of GCA. Fortunately, the long-term survival of patients with GCA who go into remission does not differ from that of a normal population.

TAKAYASU'S ARTERITIS

Takayasu's arteritis (TA) is an indolent inflammatory arteritis that is histologically indistinguishable from giant-cell arteritis. It characteristically affects women of childbearing years, particularly those of Asian ancestry. The immunopathogenesis remains uncertain, but there is evidence of dysfunctional cellular and humoral immunity including increased CD4 and decreased CD8 cells, enhanced expression of HLA antigens and ICAM-1, positive rheumatoid factors, increased levels of circulating immune complexes, and antiendothelial antibodies.

The major clinical manifestations are due to inflammation of large arteries, with stenosis, occlusion, or aneurysm formation. The aorta and its branches are particularly affected. Transient ischemic attacks, stroke, and carotidynia reflect cerebrovascular involvement. Inflammation in coronary arteries may result in angina, myocardial infarction, ischemic cardiomyopathy, or sudden death. Abdominal pain, intestinal claudication, and hypertension reflect visceral vessel involvement. Peripheral claudication occurs when major nutrient vessels of the extremities are affected. Dermatologic manifestations include erythema nodosum, pyoderma gangrenosum, and Raynaud's phenomenon. Retinal arteries are involved up to a third of patients. There are no laboratory abnormalities characteristic of TA, but the ESR is frequently elevated and may be a valuable guide to therapy. The diagnosis rests on the presence of typical angiographic findings, which include extensive irregular stenoses or occlusions of the aorta and its major branches, particularly the subclavian arteries. Eventually, the inflammation leads to loss of the integrity of the vessel wall with fusiform or saccular aneurysm formation.

Systemic corticosteroids are the mainstay of therapy. Some patients, however, will require cytotoxic agents, such as cyclophosphamide or methotrexate. Percutaneous angioplasty or bypass grafting may be necessary in patients with established occlusive disease and ischemia. Although TA is a chronic recurrent process, the 5-year survival rate approaches 90%.

BUERGER'S DISEASE

Buerger's disease (BD), or thromboangiitis obliterans, is an acute and chronic inflammatory process affecting small and medium-size arteries and veins. The cause is unknown, but BD primarily affects young males who smoke tobacco. It is associated with an increased prevalence of HLA-B5 and HLA-A9. Antiendothelial cell antibodies that react with both surface and intracellular epitopes have been identified in the majority of patients. The initial histologic manifestation of the disease is polymorphonuclear cell infiltration of the vessel wall with thrombus formation. Eventually, mononuclear cells, giant cells, and fibroblasts replace the polymorphonuclear cells, and the involved vessel undergoes fibrotic obliteration. Clinical manifestations include arthralgias, Raynaud's phenomenon, distal peripheral claudication, digital ischemia and gangrene, cutaneous ulcers, and superficial venous thrombophlebitis. Angiography reveals smooth tapered lesions in distal vessels in the absence of proximal atherosclerotic disease. Diagnosis requires histologic demonstration of typical vascular inflammation. Cessation of smoking is the mainstay of therapy. Surgery, including debridement, bypass grafting, and amputation, may be necessary in selected cases.

HENOCH-SCHÖNLEIN PURPURA

Henoch-Schönlein purpura (HSP) is the commonest form of childhood vasculitis. It is a small-vessel vasculitis that often follows upper respiratory infections or exposure to drugs. Immunologic abnormalities include elevated serum levels of IgA and circulating immune complexes containing IgA. Immune deposits containing IgA, complement, and fibrin can be found in the walls of affected vessels, and deposits of IgA can be seen in the mesangium of patients with glomerulonephritis. HSP typically affects male children, with the peak incidence at 4 years of age. Manifestations include purpura, urticaria, arthritis, abdominal pain, gastrointestinal bleeding, and glomerulonephritis. The severity of renal involvement varies from microscopic hematuria to nephritic syndrome with renal failure. Pulmonary vasculitis with pulmonary hemorrhage occurs rarely. Laboratory abnormalities include leukocytosis, thrombocytosis, an elevated ESR, and the previously described IgA abnormalities.

Treatment with nonsteroidal antiinflammatory agents will suffice in most children. Patients with rapidly progressive glomerulonephritis or gastrointestinal vasculitis, however, may require corticosteroid or cytotoxic therapy. The prognosis is generally excellent, but chronic renal failure may occur in 2–5% of patients.

KAWASAKI'S DISEASE

Kawasaki's disease (KD), also called mucocutaneous lymph node syndrome, is a systemic necrotizing vasculitis that affects children, generally boys, younger than age 5 years. The epidemiologic pattern suggests that KD is a result of an infection, but no specific agent has been identified. Immunologic factors play a major role in pathogenesis. Antiendothelial cell antibodies, ANCA, and circulating immune complexes are seen in patients with KD. Typical manifestations include fever, polymorphous rash, erythema and desquamation of the palms and soles, erythema of the lips and oral mucosa, conjunctival injection, cervical lymphadenopathy, and cardiovascular disease. Cardiac involvement, which occurs in a third of patients, can lead to pericarditis, coronary artery or ventricular aneurysm formation, myocardial infarction, or congestive heart failure. Less common are arthritis, gastrointestinal disease, proteinuria, and CNS involvement with cranial neuropathy or convulsions. Laboratory abnormalities, in addition to the immunologic findings, include anemia, leukocytosis, thrombocytosis, elevated ESR and C-reactive protein, proteinuria, and, in children with CNS involvement, CSF pleocytosis.

The treatment of choice is aspirin and high-dose intravenous gamma globulin. Treatment of the cardiac complications may include antiplatelet therapy, thrombolysis, or coronary revascularization surgery. Corticosteroids may increase the incidence of coronary artery involvement and should be avoided. The prognosis is excellent, although patients with cardiac involvement are vulnerable to premature coronary atherosclerosis.

HYPERSENSITIVITY ANGIITIS

Hypersensitivity angiitis (HA), also called hypersensitivity vasculitis is a small-vessel cutaneous vasculitis that occurs as a reaction to any of a number of foreign antigens, including drugs, vaccines, chemicals, or infectious agents. The vasculitis is limited to the skin, although patients may develop fever, arthralgias or arthritis, and constitutional symptoms, such as malaise, lethargy, and fatigue. Biopsy of early lesions typically reveals debris from a granulocytic infiltration (leukocytoclastic vasculitis). Biopsy of a subacute or chronic lesion reveals a lymphocytic vasculitis. Laboratory abnormalities include leukocytosis, thrombocytosis, an elevated ESR, low complement levels (especially in urticarial vasculitis), and circulating immune complexes. Immunofluorescent staining of involved vessels reveals the deposition of IgG, IgM, or IgA immunoglobulins, complement, and fibrin.

Removal of the offending agent generally results in resolution of the vasculitis, although the temporary use of systemic corticosteroids may be necessary in some cases.

REFERENCES

POLYARTERITIS NODOSA

Calabrese LH et al: Therapy of resistant systemic necrotizing vasculitis. Polyarteritis, Churg-Strauss syndrome, Wegener's granulomatosis, and hypersensitivity vasculitis group disorders. *Rheum Dis Clin North Am* 1995; 21:41.

Guillevin L et al: Polyarteritis nodosa related to hepatitis B virus. A prospective study with long-term observation of 41 patients. *Medicine* 1995;74:238.

Lie JT: Histopathologic specificity of systemic vasculitis. *Rheum Dis Clin North Am* 1995;21:883.

MICROSCOPIC POLYANGIITIS

Guillevin L et al: Microscopic polyangiitis. Clinical and laboratory findings in eighty-five patients. *Arth Rheum* 1999;42:421.

Jennette JC, Falk RJ: Small-vessel vasculitis. *New Engl J Med* 1997;337:1512.

WEGENER'S GRANULOMATOSIS

deGroot K et al: Therapy for the maintenance of remission in sixty-five patients with generalized Wegener's granulomatosis. *Arth Rheum* 1996;39:2052.

Guillevin L et al: A prospective, multicenter, randomized trial comparing steroids and pulse cyclophosphamide versus steroids and oral cyclophosphamide in the treatment of generalized Wegener's granulomastosis. *Arth Rheum* 1997;40:2187.

Rao JK et al: The role of antineutrophil cytoplasmic antibody (c-ANCA) testing in the diagnosis of Wegener granulomatosis. *Ann Int Med* 1995;123:925.

CHURG-STRAUSS SYNDROME

Guillevin L et al: Churg-Strauss syndrome. Clinical study and long-term follow-up of 96 patients. *Medicine* 1999;78:26.

Guillevin et al: Prognostic factors in polyarteritis nodosa and Churg-Strauss syndrome. *Medicine* 1996;75:17.

GIANT-CELL ARTERITIS

Brack A et al: Disease pattern in cranial and large-vessel giant cell arteritis. *Arth Rheum* 1999;42:311.

Salvarani Carlo, Hunder GG: Musculoskeletal manifestations in a population-based cohort of patients with giant cell arteritis. *Arth Rheum* 1999;42:1259.

Weyland CM, Goronzy JJ: Arterial wall injury in giant cell arteritis. *Arth Rheum* 1999;42:844.

TAKAYASU'S ARTERITIS

Hoffman GS et al: Treatment of glucocorticoid-resistant or relapsing Takayasu's arteritis with methotrexate. *Arth Rheum* 1994;37:578.

Kerr GS et al: Takayasu arteritis. *Ann Int Med* 1994; 120:919.

BUERGER'S DISEASE

Joyce JW: Buerger's disease (thromboangiitis obliterans). *Rheum Dis Clin North Am* 1990;16:463.

Szuba A, Cooke JP: Thromboangiitis obliterans. An update on Buerger's disease. *West J Med* 1998;168:255.

HENOCH-SCHÖNLEIN PURPURA

Garcia-Porrua C, Gonzalez-Gay MA: Comparative clinical and epidemiological study of hypersensitivity vasculitis versus Henoch-Schönlein purpura in adults. *Semin Arth Rheum* 1999;28:404.

Tancrede-Bohin E et al: Schönlein–Henoch purpura in adult patients. Predictive factors for IgA glomerulonephritis in a retrospective study of 57 cases. *Arch Derm* 1997;133: 438.

KAWASAKI'S DISEASE

Bradley DJ, Glode MP: Kawasaki disease. The mystery continues. *West J Med* 1998;168:23.

Leung DYM et al: The immunopathogenesis and management of Kawasaki syndrome. *Arth Rheum* 1998;41:1538.

HYPERSENSITIVITY ANGIITIS

Martinez-Taboada VM et al: Clinical features and outcome of 95 patients with hypersensitivity vasculitis. *Am J Med* 1997;102:186.

Michael BA et al: Hypersensitivity vasculitis and Henoch-Schönlein purpura: A comparison between the 2 disorders. *J Rheumatol* 1992;19:721.

Gastrointestinal, Hepatobiliary, & Orodental Diseases

Warren Strober, MD, Stephen P. James, MD, & John S. Greenspan, BDS, PhD, FRCPath

GASTROINTESTINAL DISEASES

Warren Strober, MD

The gastrointestinal tract, by virtue of its proximity to the myriad of potential antigens in the resident microflora and the foodstream, is a site of intense immunologic activity. In normal individuals, this activity does not usually give rise to immune effector responses capable of mediating inflammation. On the contrary, the immune system associated with the gastrointestinal tract, the mucosal immune system, is distinguished by its capacity to down-regulate responses to harmless floral and food antigens in a manner that does not preclude its capacity to mount effector response to pathogens (see Chapter 14). Unfortunately, this immune regulation sometimes suffers a breakdown owing either to the presence of certain untoward genetic factors or to adverse environmental conditions. When this occurs, immunologically related diseases of the gastrointestinal tract can develop.

GLUTEN-SENSITIVE ENTEROPATHY

Major Immunologic Features
- Hypersensitivity to cereal grain proteins (eg, wheat gliadin)
- Diagnostic IgA antigliadin and antiendomesial antibodies
- Small-intestinal mucosa villous atrophy accompanied by lymphocytic infiltration of the lamina propria and increased numbers of intraepithelial lymphocytes
- Strong association with HLA-B8, DR3, DQ2 (DQA1*0501, DBQ1*0201)
- T cells reactive to gliadin peptides presented by antigen-presenting cells in association with DQ2

General Considerations
Gluten-sensitive enteropathy (GSE) (celiac sprue or nontropical sprue) is a disease of the small intes-

tine characterized by villous atrophy and malabsorption. It is caused by a hypersensitivity to cereal grain storage proteins, most importantly, the gliadin fraction of gluten in wheat and similar storage proteins in barley and rye. It is either limited to the intestine or associated with a vesicular skin disease, dermatitis herpetiformis (GSE-DH).

Pathology
The inflammatory lesions of the gastrointestinal (GI) tract are found largely in the small intestine, the area of greatest contact with ingested gliadin. The earliest lesion is characterized by the presence of increased numbers of lamina propria mononuclear cells underlying normal intestinal crypts and villi. This progresses to "compensated" GSE marked by a further increase in the infiltrate and the development of hypertrophic crypts, which elaborate crypt epithelial cells at a rate that compensates for the loss of epithelial villous cells; in both of these lesions villous length remains relatively normal, and symptoms, if present, are mild. With further progression, the inflammation reaches a "destructive stage" of disease characterized by intense mononuclear infiltrate associated with crypt hyperplasia that can no longer keep pace with the loss of villous cells; as a result, the villi become shortened or even flattened, and the patients now develop the characteristic malabsorption of GSE (Figure 35–1).

If the GSE inflammation is prolonged, the mature lesion may progress to a fibrotic or burned out stage in which the destruction of villous architecture is permanent and the patient no longer fully recovers when placed on a gluten-free diet.

At the destructive stage of GSE, the lymphocyte infiltrate is composed of B cells, T cells, and macrophages. The B cells consist primarily of IgA B cells, although IgG cells are disproportionately increased; in contrast, few if any IgE B cells are present. The lamina propria (LP) T-cell population consists of $\alpha\beta$ T-cell receptor (TCR) -bearing T-cell populations (both CD4 and CD8) that more frequently bear surface markers indicative of cell maturation and activation than T cells in the normal LP T-cell population. In addition, the T cells consist of

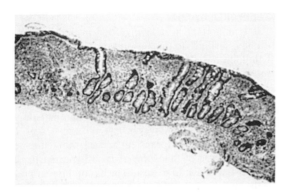

Figure 35–1. Gluten-sensitive enteropathy, destructive phase. Jejunal biopsy specimen showing complete loss of villi, elongation of crypts, and massive lymphocytic infiltrate.

increased numbers of intraepithelial (IEL) cells consisting primarily of CD8 T cells bearing either $\alpha\beta$ or $\gamma\delta$ TCR. The $\alpha\beta$TCR-bearing IEL also express markers of cell proliferation as well as markers of maturation that wax and wane according to exposure to ingested gliadin. In contrast, the $\gamma\delta$TCR-bearing population of T cells does not vary in relation to gliadin ingestion and thus may not be associated with disease pathogenesis. Finally, the macrophage and dendritic cell populations bear markers of activation and express human leukocyte antigen (HLA)-DQ, the major histocompatibility complex (MHC) restriction molecule implicated in the presentation of gliadin peptides to T cells.

Immunologic Pathogenesis

GSE is due to an immune reactivity to certain cereal storage protein peptides. The main pathologic component of this reactivity is the induction of T cells by antigen-presenting cells, which present gliadin peptides to T cells in the context of MHC antigens associated with GSE. The T cells thus induced are T_H1 cells producing IFNγ and TNFα, which then act on intestinal macrophages to produce proinflammatory cytokines such as IL-1β and TNFα. Recent evidence indicates that these cytokines induce fibroblasts to produce metalloproteinases that are the proximal cause of injury to the LP matrix supporting the villi. A second potential pathologic mechanism involving T cells in GSE is that $\alpha\beta$TCR-bearing IEL recognize and lyse epithelial cells expressing gliadin peptides presented in the context of nonclassical MHC antigens. This mechanism is most responsible for the loss of villous cells so characteristic of GSE.

B cells specific for gliadin also occur in lesions and give rise to characteristic IgA antigliadin antibodies. In addition, antibodies specific for complexes of gliadin and an endogenous enzyme that reacts with gliadin, a transglutaminase, also occur. These antibodies are the GSE-specific antiendomesial antibodies noted later on. Whether either of these antibodies contribute to tissue injury in the mature GSE lesion is still unknown although lesions contain deposits of activated complement proteins indicative of complement activation.

The underlying mechanism that sets these pathologic events in motion appears to be a genetically determined inability to induce oral tolerance to gliadin peptides. Thus, although patients become normally unresponsive to the vast array of ingested proteins in the foodstream, they form immunogenic effector T cells specific for gliadin. The basis for this antigen-specific defect in oral tolerance is still unknown. One possibility relates to the fact that the great majority of patients with GSE bear HLA antigens (particularly, DQA1*0501 and DQB1*0201), which shift the mucosal response from one of tolerance induction to one of immune effector cell induction. The HLA genes associated with GSE may have arisen in human prehistory as a means of responding vigorously to infectious agents, and it is only when the cultivation and ingestion of wheat became common that these genes became "disease genes." The HLA antigens found in GSE also occur in normal individuals; thus, other immunologic mechanisms must also come into play.

Clinical Features of GSE & GSE-DH

The clinical course of GSE is dominated by gastrointestinal tract symptoms relating to malabsorption, whereas that of GSE-DH it is dominated by a vesicular skin eruption and intestinal symptoms are usually absent or, when present, are mild. The intestinal symptoms of GSE are highly variable and usually consist of weight loss, diarrhea, symptoms due to nutritional deficiencies, and, in children, growth failure. The dermatologic manifestations of GSE-DH are marked by the presence of an intensely pruritic, vesicular eruption on extensor and exposed skin surfaces. Typical laboratory findings in GSE include evidence of malabsorption such as increased fecal fat, abnormal D-xylose absorption, vitamin deficiencies, anemia, and, in severe cases, biochemical evidence of osteomalacia and abnormal blood coagulation due to vitamin K deficiency. Intestinal contrast studies during active disease show dilation of the proximal small bowel and thickening of the bowel wall.

Immunologic Diagnosis

The diagnosis of GSE is established by the presence of characteristic circulating antibodies and by a small-bowel biopsy that demonstrates the presence of villous atrophy. The most important of the antibodies are IgA antigliadin and IgA antiendomesial antibodies because these are both specific to GSE and occur in the vast majority of patients. When these antibodies are present, the patient is assigned the presumptive diagnosis of GSE, which is then verified by small-bowel biopsy. Typically, these antibodies disappear when a patient is placed on a gluten-free diet, and the histologic abnormality resolves.

Differential Diagnosis

GSE must be distinguished from other causes of villous atrophy and malabsorption, including those due to other food hypersensitivities, certain allergic manifestations of the GI tract, and autoimmune diseases of the GI tract—such as those associated with common variable immunodeficiency (see discussion below). In addition, in underdeveloped countries it must be distinguished from tropical sprue, a villous atrophy due to exposure to an increased ambient microbial load.

Treatment

Treatment of GSE consists of lifelong elimination of gliadin-containing foods from the diet. Such treatment must be instituted even in patients with mild disease because a major complication of GSE is increased prevalence of small-bowel carcinoma and lymphoma in untreated or poorly treated cases. Nutritional supplements should be instituted in patients with active disease or recovering from the disease. Very severe disease, particularly that associated with severe villous atrophy and small-bowel ulceration may require treatment with corticosteroids. GSE-DH also responds to a gliadin-free diet, but although the GI lesions are highly responsive to the latter, skin lesions require prolonged and strict gliadin exclusion. For this reason, patients are usually treated with diaminodiphenyl sulfone (dapsone), an antiinflammatory drug that brings about rapid resolution of the skin lesions with relatively few side effects.

Complications & Prognosis

Unrecognized and untreated GSE may lead to severe debility and death, whereas treated GSE is compatible with normal health and a normal life expectancy. As noted earlier, the likelihood of intestinal carcinoma and lymphoma is increased in GSE, but this problem is obviated by the early institution of a gliadin-free diet. Patients with long-standing intestinal changes may be relatively unresponsive to a gliadin-free diet and may require corticosteroid therapy.

VILLOUS ATROPHY NOT DUE TO GLUTEN SENSITIVITY

Major Immunologic Features

- Food hypersensitivity due to exposure to food substances prior to development of oral tolerance; mimics GSE, but not associated with GSE antibodies
- A spectrum of diseases broadly related to allergy of the GI tract
- Autoimmune gastroenteropathies mediated for the most part by T-cell-mediated tissue injury

General Overview

It is important to recognize that intestinal villous atrophy leading to malabsorption can result from pathologic processes other than a genetically determined sensitivity to gliadin (GSE). The most frequent of such conditions is a hypersensitivity to one of several proteins, most commonly cow milk protein, that mimics GSE both clinically and pathologically. In this case, however, the disease occurs in young children and is transient and self-limited in nature. The basis of this form of food hypersensitivity is most likely due to exposure to a food protein prior to the maturation of the capacity to develop oral tolerance to that protein. Thus, unlike GSE, the cause of the hypersensitivity is mainly environmental rather than genetic, and the condition is not associated with particular HLA markers. This form of food hypersensitivity is also distinguished from GSE by the fact that patients do not develop high-titer IgA antigliadin or antiendomesial antibodies and have more normal IEL levels on small-bowel biopsy. They do, however, develop IgA antibodies to the food components inducing the disease, such as antimilk protein. Treatment consists of elimination of the offending foods from the diet, usually for several years.

A second category of nongluten-sensitive villous atrophy includes cases of enteropathy that fall broadly into the category of allergy to food substances. This is a somewhat complex spectrum of disorders, some of which are still poorly understood. One form consists of IgE-mediated GI allergy associated with other non-GI allergic symptoms or a chronic IgE-mediated eosinophilic gastroenteritis marked by some degree of villous atrophy and protein-losing enteropathy. Yet another disease in this category is a non-IgE-mediated enteropathy, also marked by eosinophilic infiltration of the small intestine or the antral area of the stomach. In some cases, these various forms of allergy can be related to a single offending food substance, whereas in other cases, they cannot, even if the change is associated with a high IgE level. In the latter regard, an allergic GI diathesis can "spread" to become an allergic hypersensitivity to food protein in general. Treatment of these conditions involves removal of the offending food from the diet or, when this does not lead to disease amelioration, to administration of corticosteroids.

Finally, non-GSE-associated villous atrophy can occur in the somewhat ill-defined group of gastroenteropathies resulting from autoimmunity of the GI tract. This form of villous atrophy overlaps non-IgE-associated gastroenteropathy as described earlier and may be part of a more general autoimmune condition because it frequently occurs along with autoimmunity involving other organs. In some cases it occurs in association with the presence of antiepithelial cell antibodies; however, this is likely to be an epiphenomenon because the real cause of the disease is probably T-cell-mediated intestinal injury as in GSE. Such "autoimmune gastroenteropathy" is occasionally a feature of common variable immunodeficiency (CVI) or IgA deficiency, in which case it is associated with a distinctive histopathologic change characterized by the presence of intestinal lymphoid nodules. Treatment of autoimmune gastroenteropathy is mainly the administration of corticosteroids; however, this may lead to severe and sometimes fatal infections if an underlying immunodeficiency is present.

WHIPPLE'S DISEASE

Major Immunologic Features
- Massive infiltration of the lamina propria with macrophages containing PAS-positive bacteria or bacterial remnants
- Infection with *Tropheryma whippelii*
- Macrophages manifesting a defect in the capacity to produce IL-12

General Overview
Whipple's disease is a rare infectious disease caused by the bacterium *Tropheryma whippelii*. The infection is usually centered in the GI tract, and thus the disease is marked by weight loss, malabsorption, and diarrhea. The infection may involve multiple organs, however, and may thus give rise to CNS symptoms of various types, as well as joint, cardiac, and lung manifestations. In the GI tract, one sees a massive infiltration with macrophages containing periodic acid-Schiff (PAS)-positive bacteria or bacterial breakdown products as well as free-lying PAS-positive bacteria. This pathologic picture, coupled with identification of the organism by 16S RNA typing, is the means of diagnosis. The massive infiltration leads to clubbed villi and lymphatic obstruction, the former causing malabsorption and the latter causing protein-losing enteropathy and a low albumin level. In most cases, the disease responds to various antibiotic regimens.

The basis of susceptibility of patients with Whipple's disease to *T whippelii* infection is unclear. However, recently it has been shown that macrophages from patients produce reduced amounts of IL-12 which, in turn, leads to reduced T-cell production of IFN-γ, a major macrophage activation factor. Evidence that this defect is an etiologic factor comes from the observation that several patients with antibiotic-resistant Whipple's disease have been successfully treated with IFN-γ. Although the IL-12 defect may be necessary for the pathogenesis of Whipple's disease, it cannot be the sole abnormality because it does not explain why patients with infection due to a low-grade pathogen, *T whippelii*, do not have a more general immunodeficiency.

INTESTINAL LYMPHANGECTASIA & OTHER PROTEIN-LOSING ENTEROPATHIES

Major Immunologic Features
- Protein-losing enteropathy leading to hypoalbuminemia and hypogammaglobulinemia
- Immunodeficiency due to loss of lymphocytes into the GI tract

General Overview
Protein-losing enteropathy (PLE) is a syndrome occurring in many GI diseases that is marked by bulk loss of circulating protein into the GI tract. These include diseases associated with mediator release such as allergic gastroenteropathy, diseases marked by autoimmunity or inflammation such as inflammatory bowel diseases, GSE, and CVI, and finally, disorders of the intestinal lymphatics, such as intestinal lymphangiectasia. This last disease is usually the cause of the most severe PLE and thus is the "prototype" protein-losing disease.

Intestinal lymphangiectasia can result from as a primary defect of the intestinal lymphatics that leads to lymphatic obstruction and loss of lymph fluid into the GI tract; in this case, it is frequently associated with abnormalities of the peripheral lymphatics as well, producing a characteristic asymmetric peripheral edema. Alternatively, intestinal lymphangiectasia can be a secondary syndrome in which an underlying cardiac abnormality (eg, constructive pericarditis), GI abnormality (eg, Whipple's disease or Crohn's disease), or neoplastic disease leads to physical obstruction of the lymphatics or a lupus-like inflammation causing functional obstruction of the lymphatics. Although these secondary forms of intestinal lymphangiectasia lead to loss of lymph into the GI tract, they are not associated with peripheral lymphatic abnormalities (and asymmetric edema).

The loss of lymphatic fluid into the GI tract in intestinal lymphangiectasia results in hypoalbuminemia and hypogammaglobulinemia; however, the latter is not as severe as in primary hypogammaglobulinemias such as CVI and does not itself require therapy with intravenous immunoglobulin. In addition, the loss of lymphatic fluid leads to depletion of lymphocytes contained in the lymph fluid, particularly in the recirculating CD4+/CD45RA+ T cells most at risk for such loss. As a result, patients may develop profound lymphocytopenia and secondary T-cell-mediated immunodeficiency. Intestinal lymphangiectasia is therefore a unique immunodeficiency disease in which loss of immune elements, rather than their abnormal products, is the cause of the immunodeficiency. In evaluating patients with intestinal lymphangiectasia it is important to distinguish between primary and secondary forms of the disease because the latter can be cured.

IMMUNOPROLIFERATIVE SMALL-INTESTINAL DISEASE (IPSID), MEDITERRANEAN LYMPHOMA, ALPHA HEAVY-CHAIN DISEASE

Major Immunologic Features

- Infiltration of the GI tract lamina propria with pre-malignant or malignant B cells
- B cells producing α heavy chains and other aberrant immunoglobulins

General Overview

The immunoproliferative small-intestine diseases (IPSIDs) consist of a rare group of premalignant or malignant lymphomas that are limited primarily to the small bowel and its draining lymph nodes. The pathognomonic feature is infiltration of the lamina propria with aberrant B cells (plasma cells) that frequently produce Ig α heavy chains (α chains) unassociated with light chains. These α chains result from the occurrence of cells manifesting heavy-chain deletions that include the heavy chain-/light chain-binding sites. The cellular infiltrate leads first to villous effacement and malabsorption and then to intestinal obstruction.

Cases of IPSID are rare and are usually found in underdeveloped countries, especially those in the Middle East, and in countries surrounding the Mediterranean Sea. Characteristically, it occurs in young patients with malnutrition. It has been suggested that the disease has its origin in excessive antigenic response to environmental mucosal antigens associated with various bacterial agents. This would explain its responsiveness at an early stage to antibiotic therapy. In this sense, IPSID is similar in its pathogenesis to mucosa-associated lymphoid tissue (MALT) lymphoma, which is etiologically linked to *Helicobacter pylori* infection (see later discussion). Diagnosis is made by identification of α heavy chains in the serum or by in situ tissue staining; in addition, the involved tissues have a characteristic histology. Treatment consists of prolonged antibiotics in early cases and chemotherapy in late cases. Patients can also be treated with chemotherapy followed by autologous bone marrow transplantation because the marrow is not involved in this disease.

PERNICIOUS ANEMIA

Major Immunologic Features

- Antiparietal cell and antiintrinsic factor antibodies
- Infiltrating CD4 T cells mediate tissue injury

General Considerations

Pernicious anemia (PA) is an organ-specific autoimmune disease characterized by chronic inflammation of the fundus and body of the stomach, and loss of gastric parietal cells. As a result, patients with PA develop achlorhydria, decreased production of pepsinogen 1, and decreased production of intrinsic factor. The decrease in intrinsic factor, in combination with antibodies that block intrinsic factor function, leads to vitamin B_{12} (cobalamin) malabsorption and its consequences—megaloblastic anemia and neuropathy.

The chronic gastritis associated with PA has been called type A gastritis, which is distinguished by the fact that the inflammation spares the antrum of the stomach and thus is associated with gastric gland hyperplasia (due to lack of negative feedback by gastric acid) and elevated serum gastrin levels. Type A gastritis differs from type B gastritis in that the latter involves the entire stomach and is associated with low serum gastrin levels. As discussed in the following section, this form of gastritis is due to chronic infection with *H pylori*.

PA usually occurs in older individuals (usually women) and may be part of a polyendocrine autoimmune state involving the thyroid gland (Hashimoto's thyroiditis), the adrenal gland (Addison's disease), or the islet cells (juvenile diabetes melitis). In addition, it has been associated with other organ-specific autoimmunities manifested by ovarian failure, vitiligo, and myasthenia. Finally, it is associated with an increased incidence of carcinoid cancer and gastric carcinomas. It is important to note that PA is only one of several causes of cobalamin deficiencies; other causes include the aforementioned type B gastritis that results from chronic *H pylori* infection, terminal ileal disease or resection, and intestinal bacterial overgrowth or infection with the fish tapeworm *Diphyllobothrium latum.*

Immunologic Pathogenesis

It has been known for quite some time that PA is associated with the presence of antibodies to parietal cells, and it was assumed that such antibodies were the cause of the inflammation. Recently, however, it has been shown that these antibodies target H^+/K^+-ATPase, an intracellular enzyme not readily accessible to antibodies. It is unlikely, therefore, that these antibodies are the initial cause of tissue injury. Another hypothesis concerning the pathogenesis of PA comes from studies of mouse models of gastritis in which it can be shown that CD4 T cells (also specific for H^+/K^+-ATPase) can transfer gastritis to naive recipients. Thus, it appears that CD4 T cells are the chief effectors of gastritis in mice, and, by extension, in human gastritis and PA. Of interest, T cells causing autoimmune gastritis in mice occur after the mice are subject to neonatal thymectomy. This has led to the view that normal mice develop suppressor cells in the thymus that prevent autoimmune gastritis, as well as associated autoimmune states. Thus, the real cause of autoimmune gastritis (and PA) in humans may be the loss of a normally occurring counterregulatory cell.

Although the pathogenesis of type A gastritis may be largely due to T cells, the pathogenesis of PA is due to both T cells and B cells. T cells take part by causing gastric cell loss and thus reduced intrinsic factor synthesis. B cells take part by producing anti-intrinsic factor antibody, which interferes with the formation of the intrinsic factor cobalamin complexes necessary for intrinsic factor uptake in the ileum.

Pathology

The gastric lesion in PA is characterized by the infiltration of mononuclear cells between gastric glands and in the submucosa. The infiltrate is a mixed one, consisting of T cells, B cells, and macrophages. As the disease progresses, the infiltrate is accompanied by loss of parietal and zymogen cells, giving rise ultimately to gastric atrophy and thinning of the gastric mucosa. As indicated earlier, this lesion results in achlorhydria associated with hypergastrinemia due to antral sparing and hypertrophy of gastrin-producing cells (G cells).

The hematologic findings of PA consist of myeloblastic anemia associated with macrocytes and hypersegmented polymorphonuclear leukocytes. Patients manifest low serum vitamin B_{12} and low levels of serum transcobalamin-2, the protein that carries vitamin B_{12} to cells.

Diagnosis

The diagnosis of PA is made on the basis of the histologic picture described here and the presence of an abnormal Schilling's test for the detection of vitamin B_{12} malabsorption. The latter consists of the administration of radiolabeled vitamin B_{12} by mouth, followed by measurement of the uptake of the label and its appearance in the stool. Reduced uptake and increased excretion of the labeled vitamin B_{12} indicates the presence of PA. Characteristically, the Schilling's test "corrects" if labeled vitamin B_{12} is coadministered with exogenous intrinsic factor. Serologic tests are also used in diagnosis and consist of determination of the presence of autoantibodies to gastric parietal cells that are detected by immunofluorescence and of antibodies to intrinsic factor that are detected by enzyme-linked immunosorbent (ELISA) assays.

Treatment

Treatment of PA consists of parenteral vitamin B_{12} injection. Although this treatment reverses the hematologic abnormalities, it may have little effect on preexisting neurologic abnormalities. Because such treatment does not affect the underlying gastric atrophy and inflammation, patients must continue to be followed for the possible development of gastric carcinoma.

HELICOBACTER PYLORI-ASSOCIATED CHRONIC GASTRITIS & MUCOSA-ASSOCIATED LYMPHOID TISSUE LYMPHOMA

Major Immunologic Features

- Chronic *H pylori* infection of the stomach leading to chronic gastritis, gastric and duodenal ulcers, and gastric cancer
- Chronic *H pylori* infection leading to B-cell lymphoma (MALT lymphomas)

General Overview

In recent years it has become apparent that *H pylori* infection of the gastric lining occurs in the majority of individuals. Although such infection most commonly causes chronic gastritis that has no pathologic consequences, it is an important risk factor for the occurrence of gastric and duodenal ulcers and the development of upper GI tumors, including both adenocarcinoma and MALT lymphomas.

H pylori infection is initiated by adherence of the organism to the gastric epithelial cells, followed by the initiation of a complex immune response. This response includes a B-cell component resulting in the production of antibodies, which may either control infection or cause inflammation via cross-reactivity with endogenous mucosal antigens. In addition, it includes a T-cell component that leads to the production of proinflammatory cytokines such as IFNγ and TNFα. This immune response leads to an inflammatory response that ultimately causes chronic gastritis. Finally, the tissue injury caused by the immunologic response to the organism may be augmented by the organism itself via the production of a cytotoxin (AcG A protein), which plays a role in the formation of ulcers. Diagnosis of *H pylori* infection is made by histologic examination of the stomach mucosa, presence of anti-*H pylori* antibodies, and a breath test to detect the presence of various enzymes produced by the organism. Treatment consists of antibiotic therapy coupled with antisecretory therapy to decrease acid secretion.

An important complication of chronic *H pylori* infection is the occurrence of MALT lymphomas arising from neoplastic transformation of the B cells that are stimulated in response to the infection. Once these occur, they are further induced by T cells specific for *H pylori* antigens. Thus, a situation arises that is similar to the nonspecific induction of lymphoma in IPSIDs (see earlier section). Early MALT lymphomas respond to eradication of the *H pylori* infection, but most cases require chemotherapy.

INFLAMMATORY BOWEL DISEASES

General Overview

The inflammatory bowel diseases (IBDs) can be broadly defined as chronic inflammations of the GI tract, most likely due to an abnormal immune response to antigenic constituents in the gastrointestinal lumen. They actually comprise two usually distinct diseases: Crohn's disease and ulcerative colitis (UC) (see description in following sections). The IBDs are grouped under a single name because they frequently occur together in members of the same family, and are sometimes indistinguishable when disease is limited to the large bowel.

Both Crohn's disease and UC have complex genetic bases. Evidence of genetic factors initially consisted of the occurrence of disease in families and later in the association of disease with various genetic markers (most importantly HLA and TNFα types); recently, however, the occurrence of disease has been linked to defined genetic areas on several chromosomes. Thus far, Crohn's disease and UC appear to be multigenic and, therefore, have no clear-cut pattern of inheritance. There is also evidence of environmental factors. IBD is a disease of urbanization, and its highest incidence occurs in European and North American populations. Paradoxically, this may relate to improvements in public hygiene in these areas and to the consequent lack of exposure to a large array of organisms that formerly accompanied human habitation. Through the years, organisms have been said to cause IBDs, particularly Crohn's disease. Recently, for instance, an atypical *Mycobacterium (M paratuberculosis)* has been put forward as an infectious agent in Crohn's disease; however, in no instance has such an infectious cause been proved, and in the case of *M paratuberculosis,* it has been clearly disproved. On the other hand, data supporting the concept that IBDs are due to an immune dysregulation have steadily gained stature.

In the 1990s, the understanding of IBD took a great leap forward with the discovery of numerous mouse models of chronic intestinal inflammation resembling Crohn's disease or UC. These mouse models are of several types, including: (1) particular strains of mice subjected to various antigenic stresses such as SJL/J mice given the haptenating agent trinitrobenzene sulfonic acid per rectum; (2) mice with particular gene defects such as complete deficiencies of IL-2, IL-10, or TCRα chain or overexpression of TNFα; and (3) mice with severe combined immunodeficiency (SCID) that have been adaptively repleted with naive T cells from normal mice of a slightly different MHC type. Several broad conclusions emerge from the studies of such models. First, they show that chronic mucosal inflammation requires the presence of a normal bacterial flora because it is not seen in a strictly germ-free environment. This suggests that the immune dysregulation leads to abnormal immune responses to antigens in the normal flora. Second, the chronic mucosal inflammation occurs in states of immune dysregulation rather than immune deficiency. Third, regardless of the underlying defect or the mode of induction of im-

mune deficiency, the inflammation results from a final common pathway of an immune dysfunction, either an excessive T_H1-mediated response (which pathologically resembles Crohn's disease) or an excessive T_H2-mediated response (which pathologically resembles ulcerative colitis). The models show that excessive inflammation can occur as a result of excessive T_H1 drive (ie, IL-12/IFNγ production) or T_H2 drive (ie, IL-4 production) or, contrariwise, inadequate counterregulation of T_H1/T_H2 response by suppressor cytokines such as TGFβ or IL-10. Applying these principles to human IBD, we can say that although Crohn's disease and UC can conceivably have multiple specific defects, in each case these defects lead to the final common pathway of an exaggerated and inflammatory T_H1 or T_H2 cell response which is driven by antigens present in the normal flora. The T_H1 cell response is indicative of Crohn's disease because Crohn's disease is characterized by increased IL-12/IFNγ production, and the T_H2 cell response is indicative of UC, because UC is associated with elevated IL-5 production and autoantibodies.

CROHN'S DISEASE

Major Immunologic Features
- Transmural granulomatous inflammation of the bowel wall
- Excessive T_H1 cell response with overproduction of IL-12 and IFNγ

General Considerations
Crohn's disease (regional ileitis, granulomatous ileitis, or colitis) is characterized by transmural inflammation of any portion of the bowel wall. Its prevalence ranges from 10 to 70 per 100,000, and it is much more common in urbanized countries. The disorder most typically begins between the ages of 15 and 30 years but can begin at any age. There is familial aggregation of cases but no clear-cut mode of inheritance.

Immunopathologic Findings
Crohn's disease may involve any part of the alimentary tract from the mouth to the anus, although most patients exhibit the typical pattern of the disease characterized by predominant involvement of the ileocolic, small-intestinal, and colonic–anorectal regions. The gross pathology of Crohn's disease is characterized by transmural inflammation of the bowel wall, often in a discontinuous fashion, with ulceration, strictures, and fistulae being frequent features. The histopathologic findings are those of a granulomatous inflammatory process (true granulomas are found in about 60% of surgically resected specimens) (Figure 35–2), associated with crypt abscesses, fissures, and aphthous ulcers. The inflammatory infiltrate is mixed, consisting of lymphocytes

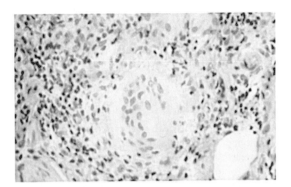

Figure 35–2. Crohn's disease. Rectal biopsy specimen with mucosal granuloma.

(both T and B cells), plasma cells, and macrophages. Plasma cells of all isotypes are increased, with IgM- and IgG-secreting plasma cells increased relative to IgA-secreting plasma cells. The number of T cells is increased, but a normal CD4/CD8 ratio is maintained.

Recent studies have shown that lamina propria macrophages from patients with active Crohn's disease produce increased amounts of IL-12. This is associated with increased activation of the signal transducer and activator of transcription (STAT)4 T-cell-signaling pathway and, as a result, with increased IFNγ secretion. Lamina propria macrophages also elaborate increased amounts of TNFα and other inflammatory cytokines. This mirrors the situation seen in mouse models of transmural ileitis and colitis, such as is seen in mice with IL-12-dependent TNFα overproduction. Finally, lamina propria T cells from patients with Crohn's disease manifest proliferative and cytokine responses to their own bowel flora, whereas normal individuals do not. This suggests that the disease is due to an altered response to constituents in the bowel flora as indicated previously in the discussion of animal models of the disease.

Clinical Features

Typical symptoms of Crohn's disease include abdominal pain; anorexia; weight loss; fever; diarrhea; perianal discomfort and discharge; and extraintestinal symptoms involving the skin, eyes, and joints. The manifestations vary somewhat according to the predominant pattern of intestinal involvement: involvement of the small bowel typically leads to symptoms of intestinal obstruction, or fistula or abscess formation; involvement of the large bowel results in bleeding and perianal problems. Extraintestinal manifestations are not unusual and include arthritis, erythema nodosum, pyoderma gangrenosum, aphthous mouth ulcers, uveitis, anemia, urinary calculi, and sclerosing cholangitis. Typical laboratory abnormalities in-

clude anemia (due to chronic disease, iron deficiency, vitamin B_{12} deficiency, or folate deficiency), leukocytosis, thrombocytosis, elevation of the erythrocyte sedimentation rate, hypoalbuminemia, electrolyte abnormalities (in cases with severe diarrhea), and the presence of occult blood in the stool. Many radiographic abnormalities may be present in small-bowel and colon contrast studies; these include aphthous ulcerations, linear ulcerations, edema, and thickening of the bowel wall (Figure 35–3), as well as strictures, fissures, fistulae, and mass lesions (inflammatory masses or abscesses); the chronic inflammation also may lead to a characteristic "cobblestone" pattern of the mucosal surface. When the areas involved are accessible, endoscopy provides a direct method of evaluating disease activity and permits collection of biopsy material for pathologic confirmation as well as screening for colon carcinoma.

Immunologic Diagnosis

Multiple abnormalities of immune function have been described, but none has diagnostic specificity (see previous discussion).

Differential Diagnosis

Diseases sometimes having an appearance similar to Crohn's disease are appendicitis, diverticulitis, intestinal neoplasia, and intestinal infections (*M tuberculosis, Chlamydia, Yersinia enterocolitica, Campylobacter jejuni, Entamoeba histolytica, Cryptosporidium,* herpes simplex virus, cytomegalovirus, *Salmonella,* and *Shigella* infections). A combination of stool cultures, intestinal

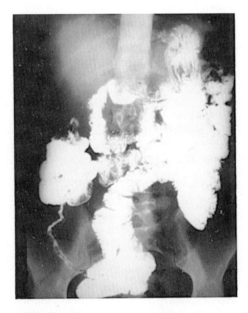

Figure 35–3. Crohn's disease. Small-bowel barium contrast radiograph showing marked narrowing of the terminal ileum as a result of transmural inflammation.

biopsies, and clinical follow-up are usually sufficient to exclude these possibilities.

Treatment

The antiinflammatory drug sulfasalazine and newer 5-aminosalicylic acid (5-ASA) agents are useful in treating mild colonic Crohn's disease and are commonly used in an attempt to maintain remissions. Metronidazole is similar in efficacy to sulfasalazine and appears to be particularly useful for treating perianal disease. In more severe active disease, corticosteroids at high doses are effective both in treating acute exacerbations and at low doses in maintaining remission. Azathioprine and 6-mercaptopurine are used as steroid-sparing drugs in patients who require high doses of corticosteroids for long periods and who are not amenable to surgical therapy; in addition, these drugs have been shown to have a role in long-term prophylaxis. It has been shown that agents that block TNFα activity (infliximab or etanercept; see Chapter 53) ameliorate inflammation in a substantial number of patients who fail other forms of therapy. This is particularly true of Crohn's disease patients who also have fistulae. The long-term efficacy of these agents, or indeed other anticytokine agents such as anti-IL-12, warrants further clinical study.

Other approaches to the treatment of Crohn's disease include dietary management with elemental diets or total parenteral nutrition. Although these have proved useful in repairing the nutritional status of patients and in inducing symptomatic improvement of acute disease, they do not lead to sustained clinical remissions. Antibiotics are used in treating secondary small bacterial overgrowth and in treating pyogenic infections. Finally, surgical treatment is necessary when the disease is not controlled medically and when various complications occur (see following paragraph).

Complications & Prognosis

Patients typically have recurrent episodes of active disease with periods of intervening quiescence. Often, however, they have low-grade symptoms even during periods of apparent disease inactivity. Approximately two thirds of patients require surgery at some time during their life for disease not treatable with tolerable doses of steroids or for complications such as obstruction, abscess, fistula, hemorrhage, or megacolon. Nevertheless, the disease is clearly not curable by surgical resection because it recurs at a rate approaching 90% when patients are followed long term. The mortality rate from Crohn's disease is approximately twice that in the general age-matched population although most deaths occur early in the course of the disease. The incidence of intestinal carcinoma in Crohn's disease is increased, but the frequency is much lower that that associated with ulcerative colitis, possibly because chronic disease usually requires resection.

ULCERATIVE COLITIS

Major Immunologic Features

- Chronically inflamed and ulcerated colonic mucosa
- Frequent occurrence of anticolon antibodies such as ANCA

General Considerations

Idiopathic ulcerative colitis (UC) is a chronic inflammation of the mucosa limited to the colon. As with Crohn's disease, UC is found primarily in urbanized areas, although it does occur worldwide. The prevalence ranges from 37 to 80 per 100,000 and is increased in Ashkenazi Jewish populations. There are two peaks of incidence: one in the third and one in the fifth decade. There is a significant familial association but no clear-cut pattern of inheritance.

Immunopathologic Findings

UC, in contrast to Crohn's disease, is limited to the colon and involves mainly the superficial layers of the bowel. In addition, the inflammation is continuous and is not associated with granulomas. Typically, the disease is found in the distal colon and rectosigmoid area, but it extends proximally to involve the entire colon in more severe cases. Gross pathologic findings include edema, increased mucosal friability, and frank ulceration. Histologic features are crypt abscesses consisting of accumulations of polymorphonuclear cells adjacent to and within crypts, necrosis of the epithelium, and surrounding accumulations of chronic inflammatory cells (Figure 35–4); over time, this leads to distortion of the crypt architecture. Finally, in long-standing disease, epithelial cell dysplasia and colonic carcinomas can be found.

As with Crohn's disease, the pathogenesis of UC is thought to be related to an abnormal response to normal mucosal constituents. However, UC differs from Crohn's disease both in its anatomic distribution and in its relatively superficial pattern of inflammation. It

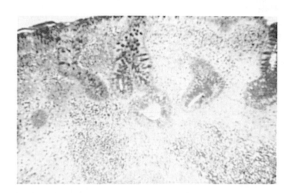

Figure 35–4. Ulcerative colitis. Rectal biopsy specimen showing distortion of crypts and lymphoid aggregates.

also differs from Crohn's disease immunologically in that the controlling response is not a T_H1 cell (IFNγ)-driven immune response. Evidence of the reciprocal hypothesis that UC is a T_H2 T-cell-driven response is supported by several pieces of evidence. First, murine models of inflammation that most clearly resemble UC (TCRα chain-deficient mice and SJL/J mice with induced colitis due to intrarectal administration of oxazolone) are dominated by T_H2 responses. Second, although IL-4 production is not elevated in UC, IL-5 production, another T_H2 cytokine, is elevated. Third and finally, UC is associated with the production of autoantibodies, a pathologic response usually seen in T_H2-cell-driven inflammations. The fact that IL-4 production is not elevated in UC as it is in other T_H2 T-cell responses does raise some question as to whether the inflammatory response is not a T_H2 response, but rather a unique response that is neither T_H1 or T_H2 in origin. Further work will be necessary to settle this question.

The prevalence of autoantibodies is higher in UC than in Crohn's disease. These include antibodies to colonic epithelial cell components that in some cases cross-react with colonic organisms. Most prominent are antineutrophil cytoplasmic antibodies (ANCA) with specificities for catalase, α-enolase and lactoferrin but not proteinase 3, as occurs in Wegener's granulomatosis. These antibodies are found in a large number of cases of UC as well as in small number of cases of Crohn's disease; thus the ability of ANCA testing to differentiate between the two diseases is poor. Early studies demonstrated that lymphocytes from patients with UC can be cytotoxic for colonic epithelial cells in vitro, probably due to "arming" of Fc-receptor-bearing killer cells (NK cells) with antiepithelial antibodies. It is highly questionable, however, that this mechanism plays a pathologic role in vivo.

Clinical Features

The clinical features of UC are highly variable. The onset may be insidious or abrupt. Symptoms include diarrhea, tenesmus, and relapsing rectal bleeding. With fulminant involvement of the entire colon, toxic megacolon, a life-threatening emergency may occur. Extraintestinal manifestations include arthritis, pyoderma gangrenosum, uveitis, and erythema nodosum. Colonic dysplasia and carcinoma may ensue in long-standing disease. Typical laboratory abnormalities include anemia (chronic disease, iron deficiency), leukocytosis, thrombocytosis, elevation of the erythrocyte sedimentation rate, electrolyte abnormalities (in severe diarrhea), and the presence of occult blood in stool. A barium enema study may demonstrate ulcerations and, in more severe disease, pseudopolyps. In chronic disease the colon may be shortened, narrowed, and tubular. Colonoscopy is useful for direct assessment of the degree and extent of inflammation, for biopsy confirmation of the diagnosis, and for screening for dysplasia and carcinoma.

Immunologic Diagnosis

No immunologic test is specific for the disease. Anticolon epithelial cell antibodies have been identified in research laboratories, but they have not been proven to have significant diagnostic utility. ANCA have been identified in subgroups of patients, but their presence does not correlate with disease activity and is not specific for ulcerative colitis.

Differential Diagnosis

The differential diagnosis is similar to that of Crohn's disease, with the addition of ischemic colitis, radiation-induced enteritis, and pseudomembranous colitis. UC may be difficult to distinguish from Crohn's disease when the latter is limited to the large bowel or when the large-bowel inflammation has features of Crohn's disease such as transmural inflammation. The distinction is not critical, however, because treatment is the same in both cases.

Treatment

As is true for Crohn's disease, sulfasalazine and related salicylate-containing drugs are effective in mild cases and corticosteroid drugs are effective in severe cases of UC. Topical administration of either salicylates or corticosteroids is effective in some patients, particularly those with disease limited to distal bowel, and is associated with decreased side effects compared with systemic use. Supportive measures such as administration of iron and antidiarrheal agents are sometimes indicated. Azathioprine, 6-mercaptopurine, and methotrexate are sometimes used in refractory corticosteroid-dependent cases. Newer anticytokine medication have yet to be tested in UC; however, it is not likely that anticytokines directed against T_H1 cytokines will be useful in UC because this is a non-T_H1 disease.

Complications & Prognosis

Patients with UC usually respond to medical therapy and enjoy a reasonable quality of life without surgical intervention. Patients with severe intractable disease or with megacolon, however, may require colectomy. In contrast to Crohn's disease, surgical treatment (colectomy) completely eliminates the disease. In patients who have the disease for longer than two decades, the incidence of colon carcinoma increases significantly, mandating periodic screening examinations. Whether the presence of colonic dysplasia is an indication for prophylactic colectomy is controversial.

HEPATOBILIARY DISEASES

Stephen P. James, MD

Hepatobiliary diseases, no less than gastrointestinal diseases, may have their origin in a disorder of the immune system. Whether these diseases are also due to an abnormality of mucosal immune regulatory mechanisms (as in the case of the inflammatory bowel diseases) remains to be seen.

AUTOIMMUNE CHRONIC ACTIVE HEPATITIS

Major Immunologic Features
- Type 1: Antinuclear antibodies, antismooth muscle antibodies; association with DRB1*03, DRB1*04
- Type 2: Antinuclear antibody negative, antiliver/kidney microsome antibody type-1 positive
- Destruction of hepatocytes associated with portal infiltration of lymphocytes
- Multiple overlap syndromes

General Considerations

Autoimmune hepatitis comprises a group of uncommon diseases characterized by a chronic hepatitis that frequently progresses to cirrhosis and by the presence of a variety of autoimmune phenomena. The diseases typically affect women and are more common in individuals of northern European descent. There are two major subtypes. The most common form, type 1, is characterized by chronic hepatitis, particularly in younger or middle-age women in association with high-titer antinuclear antibodies (originally described as "lupoid" hepatitis). Type 1 has a significant association with HLA-DR3 and -DR4. Type 2 is defined by absence of antinuclear antibodies and the presence of liver or kidney microsome type 1 autoantibodies. This form is rare or nonexistent in North America, affects women at a much younger age, and typically has an aggressive clinical course. Autoimmune hepatitis is also a component of clinical overlap syndromes, including primary biliary cirrhosis without antibodies to mitochondria (autoimmune cholangiopathy). Cryptogenic cirrhosis may represent an end-stage of autoimmune hepatitis.

Immunopathology Findings

The major histologic findings in the liver of patients with autoimmune hepatitis are not specific and consist of necrosis of hepatocytes in the periportal region (piecemeal necrosis), disruption of the limiting plate of the portal tract, and local infiltration of lymphoid cells. The degree of necrosis is variable, but in some patients is associated with bridging fibrosis or cirrhosis. The lymphoid cells infiltrating lesions of autoimmune hepatitis consist predominantly of plasma cells and CD4 T cells. The histologic findings may be indistinguishable from chronic viral hepatitis or drug-induced hepatitis.

The mechanism of liver damage in autoimmune hepatitis is unknown. Although autoantibodies against liver have been shown to be present and are sus-pected to mediate hepatocyte injury, this has not yet been proven. Lymphocyte-mediated killing of autologous hepatocytes has also been demonstrated in vitro; however, the specificity and mechanism of this killing are also uncertain. On a deeper level, it is unknown why either B-cell or T-cell elements that mediate autoimmunity directed at hepatocytes develop in autoimmune hepatitis patients, other than the fact that the disease has a genetic basis, suggesting that the inflammation does not represent a response to a cryptic infection. In this regard, it should be noted that autoimmune hepatitis is associated with a set of HLA genes that commonly occur in a number of autoimmune diseases, and it is likely that genes associated with HLA genes play an important role in disease pathogenesis.

Clinical Features

Typical symptoms of autoimmune hepatitis result from nonspecific features of chronic liver disease and include easy fatigability, jaundice, dark urine, abdominal discomfort, anorexia, myalgia, delayed menarche, and amenorrhea. These features are superseded late in the disease by nonspecific symptoms attributable to progressive liver disease. Abnormal physical findings include hepatomegaly, jaundice, splenomegaly, spider nevi, and Cushingoid features. Common laboratory findings include elevation of serum aminotransferase levels and hypergammaglobulinemia.

Immunologic Diagnosis

Autoimmune hepatitis has no pathognomonic laboratory diagnosis features. Polyclonal hypergammaglobulinemia is typically found, and autoantibodies are present, by definition. Type 1 disease is characterized by the presence of antinuclear antibodies and, frequently, other autoantibodies such as antismooth muscle antibodies. Type 2 disease is defined by the presence of antiliver-microsomal type 1 autoantibodies, which have cytochrome monooxygenase P450 IID6 as its target. Patients with autoimmune hepatitis have an increased frequency of false-positive antibodies against hepatitis C using early immunoassays but do not have hepatitis C antibodies using more current, more specific immunoassays.

Differential Diagnosis

The most important conditions in the differential diagnosis of autoimmune hepatitis are chronic viral hepatitis and drug-induced hepatitis, which are the most common chronic liver diseases. The diseases can be confused with hepatitis C in rare patients who are antibody- and PCR-negative for the viral antigen. Drug-induced hepatitis can closely mimic autoimmune hepatitis and must be excluded by thorough drug histories and drug elimination. Sclerosing cholangitis may also resemble autoimmune hepatitis but is associated with typical biliary imaging findings that are absent in autoimmune hepatitis. Uncommon metabolic liver disease, such as Wilson's disease or α_1-antitrypsin deficiency, may mimic autoimmune hepatitis clinically and histologically but are marked by characteristic metabolic abnormalities and the absence of autoantibodies.

Treatment

Patients with autoimmune hepatitis typically display good responses to treatment with corticosteroids, with or without addition of azathioprine. In patients with severe disease, treatment appears to retard disease progress and prolong survival. Ursodeoxycholic acid administration does not appear to be helpful. Other immunosuppressive drugs are undergoing evaluation for possible efficacy. Patients with complications of end-stage liver disease are good candidates for liver transplantation.

PRIMARY BILIARY CIRRHOSIS

Major Immunological Features

- Lymphocytic infiltration and destruction of intrahepatic bile ducts
- Associated autoimmune syndromes
- Presence of antimitochondrial antibodies

General Considerations

Primary biliary cirrhosis (PBC) is a chronic disease of unknown cause, primarily affecting middle-age women. It is characterized by chronic intrahepatic cholestasis due to chronic inflammation and necrosis of intrahepatic bile ducts and progresses insidiously to biliary cirrhosis. Although syndromes resembling PBC may follow ingestion of drugs such as chlorpromazine or contraceptive steroids, no toxic or infectious agent has been identified. It has been suggested that PBC is an autoimmune disease because of the frequent association of other autoimmune syndromes, the presence of autoantibodies, and histologic features of the disease. Its prevalence has been estimated to be 2.3–14.4 per 100,000. The distribution of the disease is worldwide, without predilection for any racial or ethnic group.

The usual age of diagnosis of PBC is in the fifth and sixth decades, but age at onset varies widely from the third to the eighth decade. Ninety percent of patients are female. Familial aggregation has been reported but is rare; however, the prevalence of immunologic abnormalities has been reported to be increased in family members. There are no known HLA associations.

Immunopathology

The histopathologic abnormalities occurring in the liver of PBC patients have been divided into four stages; however, these often overlap and more than one stage may be found in biopsy specimens from the same patient. The earliest changes (stage I) are most specific and consist of localized areas of infiltration of intrahepatic bile ducts with lymphocytes and necrosis of biliary epithelial cells; these lesions may have granulomas in close proximity (Figure 35–5). Stage II is marked by proliferation of bile ductules, prominent infiltration of portal areas with lymphoid cells, and early portal fibrosis. Stage III is characterized by reduction of the inflammatory changes, paucity of bile ducts in the portal triads, and increased portal fibrosis. Finally, stage IV, is associated with biliary cirrhosis and a marked increase in hepatic copper. Overall, then, the pathologic process of PBC is characterized by slowly progressive, spotty destruction of bile ducts, with associated inflammation and fibrosis, and, ultimately, cirrhosis. Hepatocellular necrosis is not a prominent feature, although occasional cases of primary biliary cirrhosis/chronic active hepatitis overlap syndromes occur with piecemeal necrosis. Studies of hepatic tissue in PBC, using immunofluorescence, show that the plasma cells in portal triads are predominantly of the IgM class and are associated with deposition of IgM. CD4 T cells predominate in portal triads, but CD8 T cells have been observed in close proximity to damaged epithelial cells. HLA-DR antigen expression is increased on biliary epithelial cells, a finding associated with other forms of autoimmunity.

Although the mechanisms of liver injury in this disease are unknown, the association of PBC with autoimmune syndromes and autoantibodies suggests that PBC is an autoimmune disease. Patients frequently have circulating immune complex-like substances, abnormalities of the complement cascade, and, in almost all cases, antimitochondrial antibodies. These antibodies display several different specificities, the most prevalent being the E2 component of pyruvate dehydrogenase, which is present on the inner mitochondria membrane. A molecule that cross-

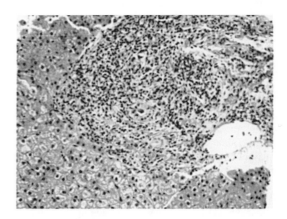

Figure 35–5. Primary biliary cirrhosis. Percutaneous liver biopsy specimen showing bile duct surrounded by a dense lymphoid infiltrate typical of stage I disease.

reacts with the E2 component is expressed on biliary epithelium and as such may be a target of cytotoxic T cells. The underlying factors leading to the autoimmunity of PBC are still poorly understood. One important possibility is that patients with PBC have defects in the immunoregulatory systems that ordinarily suppress the autoimmune reactions characteristic of the disease.

Clinical Features

The onset of symptoms in PBC is typically insidious and as many as half of all patients are asymptomatic at diagnosis. Typical symptoms include pruritus, fatigue, increased skin pigmentation, arthralgias, and dryness of the mouth and eyes. Jaundice and gastrointestinal bleeding from varices are uncommon presentations. There may be no abnormalities on physical examination. With disease progression, patients manifest hepatomegaly, splenomegaly, skin hyperpigmentation, excoriations, xanthelasma, spider telangiectasia, and, late in the disease, deep jaundice, petechiae, purpura, and signs of hepatic decompensation. PBC is also characterized by symptoms or signs relating to autoimmunity involving organs other than the liver. These include keratoconjunctivitis sicca, arthritis, hypothyroidism, scleroderma (CREST variant), Raynaud's phenomenon, and pulmonary alveolitis.

Common laboratory abnormalities include elevation of serum alkaline phosphatase and γ-glutamyl transpeptidase. Total bilirubin is normal early in the disease but increases progressively as the disease advances. Hypercholesterolemia is also frequently present. Nonspecific laboratory changes of hepatic decompensation are found late in the disease. Cholangiography is normal early in the disease but may reveal distortion of bile ducts due to cirrhosis late in the disease.

Immunologic Diagnosis

The nearly pathognomonic immunologic feature of primary biliary cirrhosis is the presence in high titer of nonspecies-specific, nonorgan-specific antibodies against the inner-membrane components of mitochondria. Antimitochondrial antibodies are found in other autoimmune syndromes but only in low titer. Less than 10% of PBC patients lack these antibodies. Many other autoantibodies are commonly found in patients but are not useful in diagnosis. Other immunologic abnormalities, such as circulating immune complex-like materials, complement abnormalities, and abnormalities of lymphocyte function, are not useful in diagnosis.

Differential Diagnosis

Chronic cholestasis may follow the administration of drugs such as chlorpromazine, but this does not lead to progressive loss of bile ducts, and it resolves following withdrawal of the drug. Hepatic sarcoidosis may closely mimic PBC, but antimitochondrial antibodies are absent. Graft-versus-host disease and liver allograft rejection have clinical abnormalities that may resemble PBC, but these can be distinguished on the basis of clinical and liver biopsy features. Hepatic allograft rejection may also be associated with nonsuppurative destructive cholangitis.

Treatment

Medical treatments includes supportive treatment, such as anion exchange resins to relieve pruritus and administration of lipid-soluble vitamins for nutritional deficiencies. Attempts to suppress the primary inflammatory process of PBC have been disappointing. Corticosteroids are considered to be contraindicated because of their tendency in uncontrolled studies to exacerbate the metabolic bone disease that complicates the disease. Azathioprine and colchicine may improve survival marginally. D-Penicillamine has been used, but does not increase survival and is associated with severe side effects. Cyclosporine has been used on an investigational basis, but has not yet proved to be efficacious. Treatment of PBC with ursodeoxycholic acid has been associated with improved clinical findings and chance of survival in some patients. The only treatment for end-stage disease is hepatic transplantation.

Complications & Prognosis

Progressive disease is often associated with metabolic bone disease and may lead to chronic hepatic decompensation. Survival from the time of diagnosis varies greatly; asymptomatic patients may have a normal life span. For symptomatic patients, survival from diagnosis is about 12 years from the time of diagnosis. Patients with end-stage disease may be excellent candidates for transplantation, and the long-term prognosis in patients who survive the procedure is good.

PRIMARY SCLEROSING CHOLANGITIS

Major Immunologic Features

- Chronic inflammation and fibrosis of intrahepatic and extrahepatic bile ducts
- Frequent association with inflammatory bowel disease
- Autoimmune features of inflammatory bowel disease, particularly p-ANCA

General Considerations

Primary sclerosing cholangitis (PSC) is a disease of unknown cause characterized by inflammation, fibrosis, and stricture formation of both intrahepatic and extrahepatic bile ducts. Unlike many autoimmune diseases, it has a male predominance. It is usually associated with inflammatory bowel disease, typically ulcerative colitis but occasionally Crohn's disease, which may be mild or asymptomatic. The liver disease is usually progressive and leads to biliary cirrhosis, independent of the severity or treatment response of the associated inflammatory bowel disease. There is a significant risk of cholangiocarcinoma.

The symptoms are similar to those of chronic cholestatic liver disease and include fatigue, pruritus, hyperpigmentation, xanthelasma, and jaundice. Patients may have recurrent fever and abdominal pain due to superimposed acute bacterial cholangitis due to biliary strictures. Symptoms of underlying inflammatory bowel disease may be present. Extrahepatic manifestations other than inflammatory bowel disease are uncommon. Routine clinical laboratory findings may be similar to those in PBC.

Pathology & Immunopathogenesis

The characteristic features of PSC are an inflammatory, fibrous, obliterative process that occurs in a segmental fashion in intrahepatic and extrahepatic bile ducts. The cellular infiltrate in PSC is mixed, but activated CD8 T cells predominate. B cells are not a prominent feature in contrast to autoimmune hepatitis and PBC. There is aberrant expression of HLA class II molecules on biliary epithelium. Antibodies cross-reactive with colonic and biliary epithelium have been identified; however, the specific antigens involved and their role in pathogenesis is uncertain. Patients with ulcerative colitis have a high frequency of perinuclear (p)-ANCA, which is not a tissue-specific autoantigen.

Immunologic Diagnosis

The diagnosis of PSC is based on typical clinical features and characteristic findings on cholangiography. It is not yet known whether magnetic resonance cholangiography is useful for diagnosis of this condition. Immunologic testing is not helpful for diagnosis other than for exclusion of other conditions, such as viral hepatitis, autoimmune hepatitis, and PBC.

Treatment & Prognosis

Clinically apparent PSC is usually progressive and leads to death from liver failure or cholangiocarcinoma. It is uncertain whether mild liver abnormalities commonly found in patients with inflammatory bowel disease, which is often not progressive, represent a mild form of PSC. Treatment is largely palliative, consisting of dilation of dominant structures by biliary endoscopy and antibiotic therapy for superimposed bacterial cholangitis. Antiinflammatory and immunosuppressive therapies have not been shown to improve prognosis. Patients with end-stage liver disease may be excellent candidates for liver transplantation, although the disease may recur in the allograft.

ORODENTAL DISEASES

John S. Greenspan, BDS, PhD, FRCPath

The mouth is the portal of entry for a variety of antigens, including numerous microorganisms, into the alimentary and respiratory systems. Normally, these antigens do not cause disease and are flushed away with swallowed saliva into the distal parts of the alimentary tract. The mucosal barrier, continual desquamation of oral epithelium, toothbrushing, and other forms of mouth cleansing mechanically protect the mouth. Immunologic defense mechanisms, particularly secretory IgA antibodies, probably prevent adherence of microorganisms to mucosal and tooth surfaces by aggregating them and possibly rendering them more susceptible to phagocytosis.

Several of the most important oral diseases, including caries, the common forms of gingival and periodontal disease, oral herpes simplex virus infections, candidal infections, and the oral manifestations of primary and secondary immunodeficiency (especially AIDS), are due to an imbalance between oral organisms and the host response. This imbalance results from hypersensitivity, immunologic deficiency, or direct tissue damage regardless of the status of the host response, as in the case of dental caries and chronic inflammatory periodontal disease.

Another group of oral diseases in which immunologic factors have been implicated are those in which oral tissues are a target for autoimmune reactions. Manifestations may be confined to the mouth or may involve other systemic organs. Many are mucocutaneous diseases, several are rheumatoid diseases, and others involve mainly the gastrointestinal tract. The role of tumor immune mechanisms in oral homeostasis and the part that defects in these mechanisms play in the cause and pathogenesis of oral precancerous lesions and mucosal malignancy constitute a growing field of interest. Tumor immune mechanisms are probably important but must be considered in the context of other factors, including oncogenic viruses and chemical carcinogens.

LOCAL ORAL DISEASES INVOLVING IMMUNOLOGIC MECHANISMS

1. INFLAMMATORY PERIODONTAL DISEASES: GINGIVITIS & PERIODONTITIS

Major Immunologic Features
- Bacterial dental plaque-induced inflammation of tissues immediately surrounding the teeth
- Local responses of the host ineffective in eliminating the bacteria, which continue to adhere to the tooth surfaces

- Local responses include complement activation, infiltration of leukocytes, release of lysosomal enzymes and cytokines, and production of a serious gingival crevicular exudate
- Inflammatory agents from bacteria and immunopathologic reactions of host result in gingivitis and periodontitis

General Considerations

Inflammation of the supporting tissues of the teeth produces one of the most common forms of human diseases. Depending on its severity, the destructive process may involve both the gingiva (gingivitis) and the periodontal ligament and alveolar bone surrounding and supporting the teeth (periodontitis). Periodontitis may involve both the direct cytotoxic and proteolytic effects of dental plaque and the indirect pathologic consequences of the host immune response to the continued presence of bacterial plaque microorganisms (Figure 35–6).

Dental plaque consists of a mass of bacteria that adheres tenaciously to the tooth surfaces. In gingivitis, the plaque generates inflammation of the gingival tissue without affecting the underlying periodontal ligament and bone. In periodontitis, attachment between the gingiva and the involved teeth is lost, subgingival bacterial plaque forms on the root surfaces, and bone loss is clinically apparent (Figures 35–7 and 35–8). Elimination of the plaque usually stops the inflammatory process. In children with poor oral hygiene, gingivitis is common, but periodontitis is rare.

The microflora of the dental plaque is complex, comprising many different strains of bacteria, including gram-positive rods and cocci and gram-negative rods, cocci, and filamentous forms. In general, the healthy gingival crevice contains only a few gram-positive streptococcal and facultative *Actinomyces* species. As gingivitis develops, many more gram-negative organisms are found, including *Fusobacterium nucleatum, Prevotella intermedia,* and *Haemophilus* species. Many motile rods and spirochetes are also seen. In advanced adult periodontitis, the organisms usually cultured are predominantly gram-negative anaerobic rods, such as *P intermedia, Porphyromonas gingivalis,* and *F nucleatum.* Furthermore, phase-contract examination shows that as many as 50% of organisms from such lesions are motile rods and spirochetes. There is some indirect evidence for a relationship between particular forms of periodontal disease and specific microorganisms. Thus, elevated levels and increased frequency of serum antibodies to *Actinobacillus actinomycetemcomitans, Capnocytophaga* spp., and *Eikenella corrodens* are found in localized juvenile periodontitis (rapidly progressive periodontitis) (see Section II: Juvenile Periodontitis).

Immunologic Pathogenesis

A delicate balance exists between dental plaque organisms and the host response. In healthy individuals, the immunologic response provides a well-regulated specific defense against infiltration by plaque substances. The tissue-destructive mechanisms thought to be involved in periodontal diseases include direct effects of plaque bacteria, polymorphonuclear-induced damage, complement-mediated damage initiated by both antibody and the alternative pathway, and cell-mediated damage.

Clinically apparent gingivitis is probably the result of an exaggerated response to bacterial plaque. Individuals with mild gingivitis have, in addition to a continued polymorphonuclear infiltration, a gingival influx of a few T lymphocytes. Those with prolonged severe gingivitis and severe periodontitis, however, have an influx composed mainly of B lymphocytes and plasma cells, with resulting IgG antibody production. Most noteworthy in severe periodontal disease is the extremely low proportion of gingival plasma cells committed to IgG2 production, whereas serum levels of the other IgG subclasses are normal. The proportions of antibodies of IgG3, IgG1, or IgG4 subclass with specific antibody activity for plaque antigens in the gingival tissues are unknown. This unusual local IgG subclass response may indicate a degree of nonspecific activation of B lymphocytes arriving in the inflamed area, possibly caused by a variety of mechanisms involving bacterial mitogens and proteinases. The bacteria may also activate the alternative complement pathway. Associated with gingivitis is the generation of a serum exudate known as crevicular fluid, which flows from around the teeth and contacts the dental plaque. This exudate, like serum, contains functional complement components as well as low levels of specific antibodies to the various plaque antigens.

The onset of flow of crevicular fluid is an important stage in the progression of periodontal disease. Crevicular fluid complement is rapidly activated by a combination of effects. These include activation of the classical pathway by IgG and IgM antibodies to subgingival plaque antigens; activation of the alternative complement pathway by endotoxins and peptidoglycan from gram-negative and gram-positive microorganisms, respectively; and activation of complement components by host and bacterial proteolytic enzymes. Complement activation results first in the release of C3a and C5a, which cause additional edema and increase crevicular fluid flow, and subsequently in the chemotactic attraction of polymorphonuclear leukocytes. Other chemotactic factors are produced directly by the plaque microorganisms. The release of proteolytic enzymes with collagenase and trypsin-like activities by host cells is believed to damage tissue and activate additional complement components and subsequent release of prostaglandin E. In vitro, prostaglandin E can induce bone resorption through its effects on osteoclasts.

Cell-mediated immunity may also play a role in the progression of periodontal disease. In some studies, individuals with periodontal disease generally

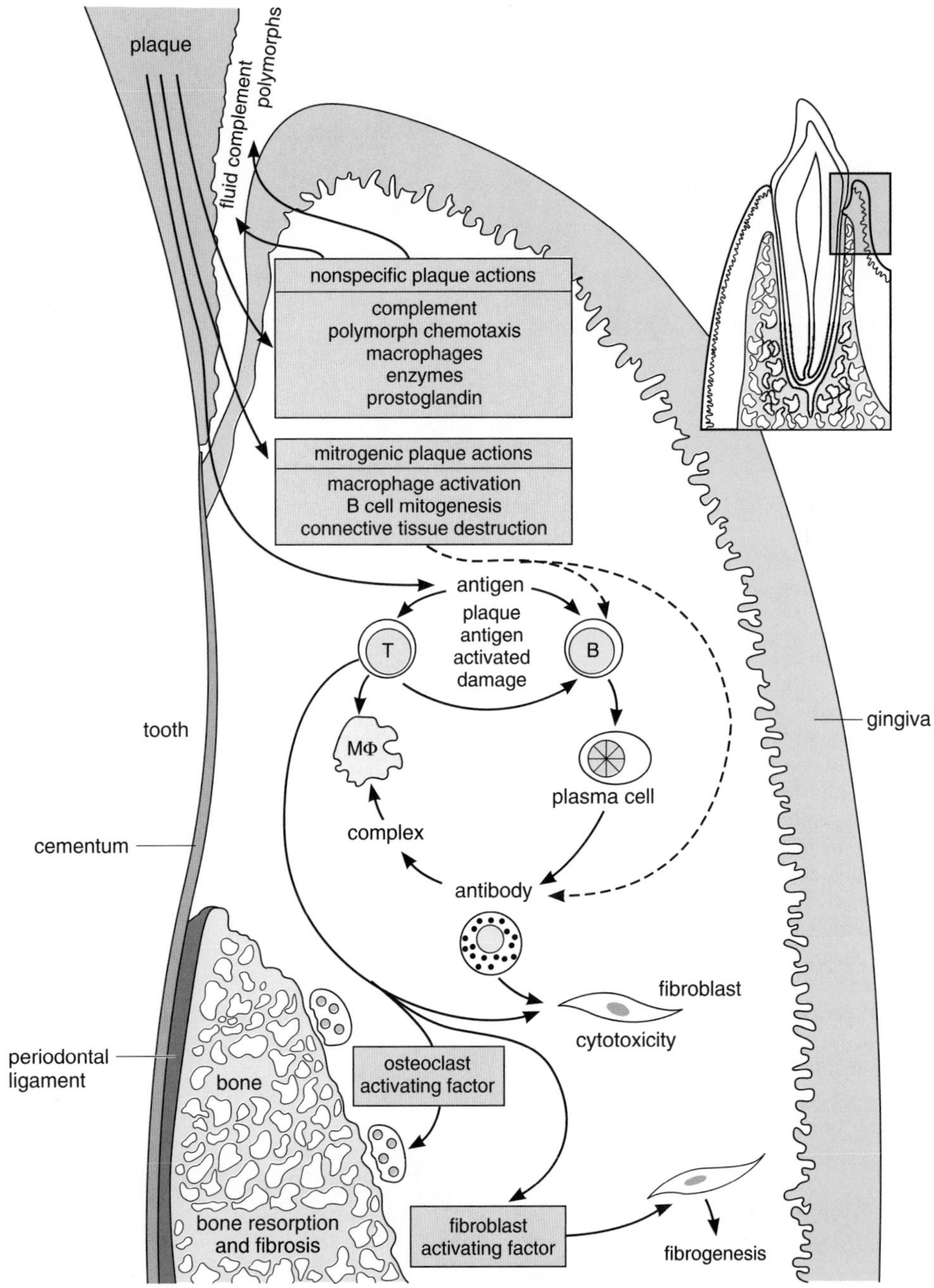

Figure 35–6. The pathogenesis of periodontal disease.

exhibit increased peripheral blood T-lymphocyte reactivity to plaque antigens. Yet, for reasons unknown, in severe gingivitis and severe periodontitis the local T-cell response to the plaque is conspicuously small. Bone destruction in periodontal disease may be mediated by lymphokines, including osteoclast-activating factor, as well as by parathyroid hormone and prostaglandins. Individuals with reduced immunologic capacity, notably primary immunodeficiency and immunodeficiency secondary to treatment associated with kidney transplantation, do not have more gingival and periodontal disease than do normal

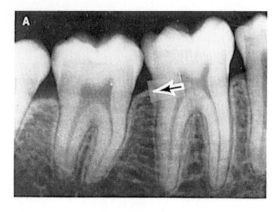
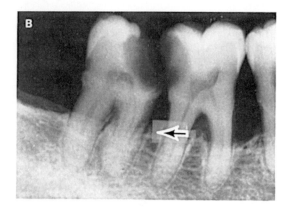

Figure 35–7. Radiographs of the lower molars of **A:** a 25-year-old man with normal periodontium and **B:** a 45-year-old man with severe dental caries and advanced periodontitis. Arrows denote supporting alveolar bone, half of which has been destroyed in the patient with periodontitis. (Courtesy of GC Armitage.)

controls. Severe periodontal disease is seen in association with HIV infection, however.

Treatment

Although gingivitis and periodontitis are apparently caused by dental bacterial plaque, there is a reluctance to treat this disease with antibiotics because elimination of one group of organisms by antibiotics may lead to the emergence of antibiotic-resistant strains. Some clinicians, however, use local application of tetracycline depending on the severity of the periodontal disease. Treatment may range from simply good routine oral hygiene to periodontal surgery. Reduction of plaque accumulation to an absolute minimum is essential for the arrest of gingivitis or the reduction of periodontal ligament destruction and bone loss. Topical antibacterial agents, notably chlorhexidine, are valuable for this purpose.

2. JUVENILE PERIODONTITIS

In a small percentage of the population, periodontal bone loss occurs very rapidly, sometimes within 2–5 years. In juvenile periodontitis, formerly known simply as periodontosis, conventional periodontal treatment is ineffective. Characteristic gram-negative anaerobic flora are present, different from those in the more slowly progressive form of periodontitis. Short-term antibiotics are probably useful in these cases, but there is no evidence that the results of such treatment are permanent. Several reports suggest that defects in granulocyte or monocyte function may be involved.

RECURRENT APTHOUS ULCERATION

Major Immunologic Features

- Lymphocyte infiltration present at the earliest stage of the lesion

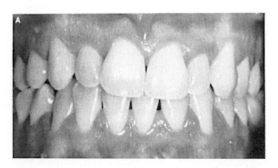
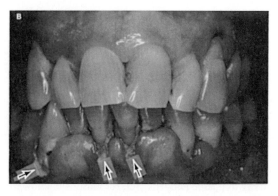

Figure 35–8. Clinical appearance of the anterior teeth and periodontal tissues of **A:** a 22-year-old man with healthy gingiva and **B:** a 48-year-old man with advanced periodontitis. Note the heavy deposits of plaque and calculus (*arrows*). Gingival inflammation is particularly marked around the lower anterior teeth, and most teeth have either pocket formation or extensive gingival recession. (Courtesy of GC Armitage.)

- Circulating antibodies to oral mucous membranes present in some patients may cross-react with oral organisms
- Cellular immunity to the same antigens
- Possibly abnormal levels of circulating cytokine
- Circulating immune complexes found in some patients
- Association with HLA-B12
- Favorable response to topical or systemic corticosteroids

General Considerations

After caries and chronic periodontal disease, oral ulceration probably represents the most common lesion of the mouth. Although oral ulcers can be due to a large number of diseases, the most common form is recurrent aphthous ulceration (RAU) (aphthous stomatitis) (Figure 35–9). Recurrent oral ulcers usually occur alone but may be a local manifestation of Behçet's disease when accompanied by uveitis, genital ulcers, and perhaps lesions of other systems. Estimates of the prevalence of recurrent oral ulceration vary, but probably 20% of the population experiences it. The condition may recur only once or twice a year or may be so frequent that a new set of ulcers overlaps a previous group. There is slight evidence of a familial incidence. Severe RAU can be seen in association with HIV infection. Emotional, hematologic, and nutritional factors may play a causative role, and an association has been suggested with changes in the hormone status during the menstrual cycle. Extensive searches for specific bacterial or viral causes have been unsuccessful. A possible role for herpes simplex virus type I has again been raised by the observation that part of the herpes simplex virus genome is present and transcribed in peripheral blood mononuclear cells of patients with recurrent aphthae and Behçet's disease. Similarly, some studies implicate varicella-zoster virus, *Helicobacter,* and human herpesvirus 8 (HHV8), the etiologic agent of Kaposi's sarcoma. Additional evidence indicates a possible role for *Streptococcus sanguis* because this organism has been cultured from the ulcers and patients exhibit delayed hypersensitivity reactions to the organism and significant inhibition of leukocyte migration by antigens of this organism in vitro. The organism is a common commensal, however. One study has shown reduced lymphocyte transformation to *S sanguis* in patients compared with controls. A likely role for bacterial or viral agents in this disease is that of cross-reacting antigens, which elicit host responses to autologous oral mucosal membrane antigens.

Immunologic Pathogenesis

Patients have a raised level of circulating antibody to a saline extract of fetal oral mucous membrane. Slightly raised levels of the same antibody have been found in other ulcerative conditions but in lower titers. The antibodies are of the agglutinating and complement-fusing type, suggesting that antibody cytotoxicity might be involved in the tissue destruction. Some studies, however, show poor correlation between the level of antimucous membrane antibody and clinical features of the disease. In addition, two other mechanisms could explain the presence of circulating autoantibodies of this type. The antibodies may cross-react with antigens of an organism present in the mouth, such as *S sanguis* or a virus, and oral mucous membrane epithelial cells. Alternatively, the antibodies may be a response to exposed tissue antigens from chronic ulcerations that had previously been protected from the immune system. Attempts to show that patient serum containing significant titers of this antibody has a direct cytotoxic effect against oral epithelial cells have been unsuccessful. Thus, it is unlikely that a cytotoxic antioral mucosal antibody is directly involved in the pathogenesis.

The earliest histologic changes in RAU involve an infiltrate of lymphocytes; other cells do not appear until a later stage. Patients with RAU have peripheral blood lymphocytes that are sensitized to oral mucous membrane antigen. These two observations support the hypothesis that a cell-mediated hypersensitivity mechanism might be involved in the pathogenesis of RAU. Lymphocytes from some patients with RAU are cytotoxic to oral epithelial cells. The antigen eliciting the cytotoxic reaction has not been identified. Increased antibody-dependent cell-mediated cytotoxicity has been found, but the identity of the population of lymphocytes involved in these reactions is also unknown. Increased production of tumor necrosis factor (TNF) and other cytokines by peripheral blood lymphocytes of patients with RAU has been observed. At present no acceptable hypothesis links oral mucous membrane autoantigens and effector mechanisms, although transient defects in immunoregulation have been postulated.

Patients with Behçet's disease and recurrent oral ulceration show elevated levels of serum C9 and cir-

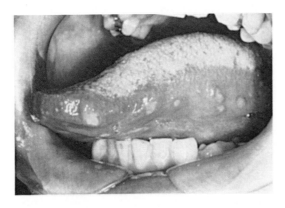

Figure 35–9. Recurrent aphthous ulcers.

culating soluble immune complexes. IgG and C3 have also been demonstrated in the basement membrane zone of the lesions. It is unclear whether these observations are clues to the immunologic pathogenesis of the disease or represent epiphenomena. There is also some evidence for an increased incidence of HLA-B12 in recurrent oral ulceration.

Treatment & Prognosis

Effective treatment depends on identification of any underlying systemic disease. In such cases, treatment of the systemic condition usually leads to cure of the oral ulceration. For the remaining group, uncomplicated by known systemic disease, several treatment forms are available, including the use of topical corticosteroids, antibiotics, and immunostimulants. Some cases of major aphthous ulceration are sufficiently severe to warrant the use of systemic prednisone. Furthermore, thalidomide has been effective in treating severe, intractable aphthous ulcers in HIV-infected patients. Tetracycline mouth rinses have been used with some success in the herpetiform variety of RAU.

ACQUIRED IMMUNODEFICIENCY SYNDROME

The oral mucosa is particularly hospitable to opportunistic pathogens. Thus, primary and recurrent herpes simplex virus, varicella-zoster virus, and several fungi, notably *Candida* species, are frequent features of primary cellular immunodeficiency syndromes (see Chapters 22 and 46). The same conditions, as well as a number of others, are seen in patients whose immune systems are compromised by chemotherapy, are receiving bone marrow transplants, have leukemia or lymphoma, and have clinical expressions of HIV-induced immunosuppression.

The oral features of acquired immunodeficiency syndrome (AIDS) include Kaposi's sarcoma, non-Hodgkin's lymphoma, and severe oral candidiasis (Figure 35–10), as well as persistent herpesvirus lesions (herpes simplex virus and varicella-zoster virus). Other conditions seen in AIDS and other HIV diseases include severe periodontal disease, oral warts, and the recently described lesion known as oral hairy leukoplakia.

Hairy leukoplakia (Figure 35–11) is seen on the tongue in HIV-immunosuppressed patients. Clear evidence for the presence of Epstein–Barr virus (EBV) in lesions comes from immunocytochemistry with monoclonal antibodies, from electron microscopic morphology, and from DNA studies with EBV probes. Southern blot hybridization provides evidence for the presence of EBV DNA in complete linear virion form and in very high copy number.

Oral hairy leukoplakia is a significant indicator of HIV-induced immunosuppression and is highly pre-

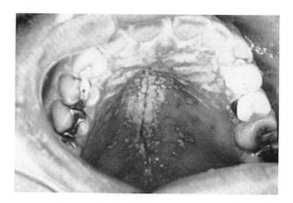

Figure 35–10. Pseudomembranous candidiasis in an HIV-positive man.

dictive of the subsequent development of AIDS, although rare cases are seen in HIV-negative people, primarily in association with other forms of secondary immunodeficiency. It appears to be one of only two oral lesions specifically associated with HIV infection. It is the first form of oral leukoplakia consistently associated with a virus or viruses. The mechanism whereby HIV favors oral opportunistic infection presumably involves viral elimination of helper T cells and thus the loss of cell-mediated immunity to herpesviruses and fungi as well as to other organisms. Other mechanisms may also mediate the immune defect, however, including loss of Langerhans' cells or their functions as well as polymorphonuclear cell and macrophage aberrations.

ORAL CANDIDIASIS

Major Immunologic Features
- Many associated immunologic defects
- Most significant oral indication of an underlying immunodeficiency

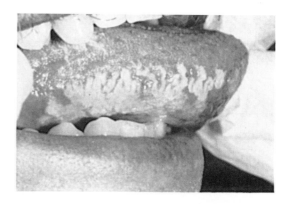

Figure 35–11. Hairy leukoplakia in an HIV-positive man.

- Prominent feature of HIV-induced immunodeficiency

General Considerations

Oral candidiasis is the most common oral fungal disease. It may occur in acute or chronic form at any age. The disease may be a sign of life-threatening systemic disease or may be confined to a small part of the oral mucous membrane and have no general significance. *Candida* species are frequent oral commensals, and it has not yet been established whether candidiasis is predominantly of endogenous or exogenous origin.

Immunologic Pathogenesis

The immunologic features of generalized candidiasis are discussed in Chapters 22 and 47. A wide range of immunologic defects have been found, including defects in cytotoxicity to *Candida,* reduced lymphokine production, failure of anticandidal antibody response of one or more classes, generalized cytotoxicity defects, failure of lymphocyte activation to candidal antigen, absence of the delayed hypersensitivity skin test to *Candida* or to many antigens, and presence of an abnormal suppressor T-cell population.

Immunologic defects alone do not explain the pathogenesis of candidiasis, however. High glucose levels in diabetics and low levels of serum iron transferrin and blood folate are also important factors. Granulocyte defects have been shown in some patients, as have defects in leukocyte myeloperoxidase. A few patients have been described in whom antibody production to *Candida* and other antigens was enhanced while cellular immune function was depressed.

Diagnosis

The diagnosis of pseudomembranous candidiasis (thrush) is based on the clinical appearance and history (see Figure 35–10). Differentiating candidal leukoplakia from other white oral lesions involves smear, culture, and biopsy.

Treatment & Prognosis

Treatment of localized oral candidiasis consists of elimination of predisposing factors, when known, and administration of topical antifungal therapy. This may be prolonged in the treatment of chronic oral candidiasis. Systemic therapy is used in cases that are resistant to local measures and in generalized mucocutaneous candidiasis.

REFERENCES

GENERAL

Strober W, Neurath MF: Immunologic diseases of the gastrointestinal tract In: *Clinical Immunology, Principles and Practice.* Rich RR et al (editors). Mosby, 1996.

GASTROINTESTINAL DISEASES

Gluten-Sensitive Enteropathy

Strober W, Fuss IJ: Gluten-sensitive enteropathy and other immunologically mediated enteropathies In: *Mucosal Immunity,* 2nd ed. Ogra PL et al (editors). Academic Press, 1999.

Fry L: Dermatitis herpetiformis. *Baillieres Clin Gastroenterol* 1995;9:371.

Villous Atrophy Not Due to Gluten Sensitivity

Catassi C et al: Severe and protracted diarrhea: Results of 3-year SIGEP multicenter survey. *J Pediatr Gastroenterol Nutr* 1999;29:63.

Savilahti E: Food-induced malabsorption syndromes. *J Pediatr Gastroenterol Nutr* 2000;30(Suppl):S61.

Whipple's Disease

Marth T et al: Defects in monocyte interleukin-12 production and humoral immunity in Whipple's disease. *Gastroenterology* 1997;13:442.

Marth T, Strober W: Whipple's disease. *Semin Gastroenterol Dis* 1996;7:41.

Intestinal Lymphangiectasia

Strober W, Fuss IJ: Protein-losing enteropathies. In: *Mucosal Immunity,* 2nd ed. Ogra PL et al (editors). Academic Press, 1999.

IPSID

Fine KD, Stone MJ: Alpha-heavy chain disease, Mediterranean lymphoma and immunoproliferative small intestinal disease: A review of clinicopathological features, pathogenesis, and differential diagnosis. *Am J Gastroenterol* 1999;94:1139.

Pernicious Anemia

Toh BH et al: Pernicious anemia. *New Engl J Med* 1997; 337:1441.

Helicobacter Infection

Isaacson PG: Gastrointestinal lymphoma of T- and B-cell types. *Mod Pathol* 1999;12:151.

Inflammatory Bowel Disease

Strober W et al: Mucosal immunoregulation and inflammatory bowel disease: New insights from murine models of inflammation. *Scand J Immunol* 1998;48:453.

Peppercorn MA: Inflammatory bowel disease. *Gastroenterol Clin North Am* 1995;24:1.

LIVER DISEASES

Autoimmune Hepatitis

McFarlane IG: Pathogenesis of autoimmune hepatitis. *Biomed Pharmacother* 1999;58:255.

Czaja AJ: The variant forms of autoimmune hepatitis. *Ann Intern Med* 1996;125:588.

Czaja AJ: Drug therapy in the management of type 1 autoimmune hepatitis. *Drugs* 1999;57:49.

Primary Biliary Cirrhosis

Laurin JM, Lindor KD: Primary biliary cirrhosis. *Dig Dis* 1994;12:331.

Primary Sclerosing Cholangitis

Lee YM, Kaplan MM: Primary sclerosing cholangitis. *N Engl J Med* 1995;332:924.

ORODENTAL DISEASES

Periodontal Disease

Graves DT: The potential role of chemokines and inflammatory cytokines in periodontal disease progression. *Clin Infect Dis* 1999;28:482.

Ranney RR: Immunologic mechanisms of pathogenesis in periodontal disease: An assessment. *J Periodontal Res* 1991;26:243.

Williams RC: Periodontal disease. *N Engl J Med* 1990;332:373.

AIDS & Candidiasis

Agabian N: Candidiasis and HIV infection. In: *Oral Manifestations of HIV Infection.* Greenspan JS, Greenspan D (editors). Quintessence, 1995.

Greenspan D, Greenspan JS: HIV-related oral disease. *Lancet* 1996;348:729.

Renal Disease

36

Jean L. Olson, MD

INTRODUCTION

Immune-mediated renal disease is the most common cause of end-stage renal disease worldwide. There are several distinct mechanisms by which the immune system can damage the kidney (Table 36–1): the deposition of circulating immune complexes, the formation of immune complexes in situ, and T-cell-mediated injury. Circumstantial evidence also suggests that antineutrophil cytoplasmic antibodies (ANCA) play a direct role in the pathogenesis of the glomerulonephritis seen in the ANCA-associated diseases. These mechanisms will be discussed in turn in the following section. Once these have initiated injury, secondary mediators of inflammation continue the process. Such mediators known to be involved in renal disease will be briefly cataloged. Finally, specific immune-mediated renal diseases will be described with respect to clinical features, pathology with correlation to pathogenesis, and therapy.

IMMUNOLOGIC MECHANISMS OF RENAL INJURY

ANTIBODY-MEDIATED MECHANISMS

CIRCULATING IMMUNE COMPLEXES

The deposition of immune complexes from the circulation on various structures within the kidney was the first recognized immune-mediated mechanism of renal injury. Longcope noted the similarity between serum sickness and glomerulonephritis. Using a model of bovine serum albumin (BSA)-induced serum sickness, Germuth and associates studied the temporal relationship between the elimination of the antigen (BSA), the formation of anti-BSA antibodies, and the occurrence of glomerulonephritis. They found that BSA was eliminated from the serum by binding to specific anti-BSA antibodies. Furthermore, the development of glomerulonephritis began concurrently with the formation of these complexes, peaked after the disappearance of the complexes from the serum, and then slowly declined in severity over several weeks. Dixon and coworkers were able to produce various forms of glomerulonephritis by changing the timing, concentration, and nature of antigen injected.

The properties of immune complexes that influence deposition in the kidney include charge, size, and duration of persistence within the circulation. Cationic complexes are able to deposit in the subepithelial space secondary to the intrinsic anionic charge of the glomerular basement membrane (GBM). When preformed immune complexes are injected into experimental animals, larger complexes tend to deposit in the subendothelial space or in the mesangium. Persistence of the immune complexes in the circulation is now thought to be the most important of the factors that determine the occurrence of renal disease in the setting of circulating immune complexes. Large lattice structure (the number of antigen and antibody molecules) causes complexes to persist for longer periods in the circulation. The Kupffer cells in the liver usually remove these larger complexes, but this clearance mechanism can become saturated, allowing deposition within the kidney.

Examples of human renal diseases that are considered to be secondary to the deposition of circulating immune complexes include serum sickness nephritis, cryoglobulinemic glomerulonephritis, postinfectious glomerulonephritis, and lupus nephritis. Serum sickness nephritis is rare now, but it is the prototype for immune complex deposition. Mixed cryoglobulins (types II and III) are themselves circulating immune complexes. The membranoproliferative glomerulonephritis associated with cryoglobulinemia shows large deposits chiefly located in the subendothelial space with fewer deposits in the mesangium. Although this location supports the idea that they have come largely from the circulation, there is no direct correlation between the quantitative amount of circulating cryoglobulins and the presence or severity of glomerular disease. Postinfectious glomerulonephritis bears simi-

Table 36–1. Immune mechanisms in renal diseases.

Mechanisms	Renal Diseases
Circulating immune complexes	Serum sickness Postinfectious glomerulonephritis Lupus nephritis Membranoproliferative glomeru- lonephritis with cryoglobulinemia
In situ immune complex formation	Membranous glomerulonephritis Anti-GBM disease IgA nephropathy Henoch–Schönlein nephritis
Antineutrophil cytoplasmic antibody	Wegener's granulomatosis Microscopic polyangiitis Churg–Strauss vasculitis
T-lymphocyte-mediated	Tubulointerstitial nephritis

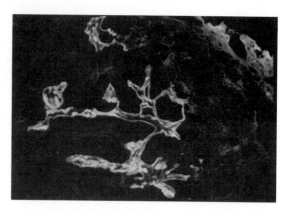

Figure 36–1. Immunofluorescence photomicrograph of a glomerulus from a patient with anti-GBM disease. Note the smooth linear staining for IgG along the glomerular basement membrane (×100).

larities to serum sickness nephritis with respect to the temporal relationship between the infection and the appearance of glomerulonephritis and also in the nature of the large subepithelial deposits. The particular antigen has not been identified, however, nor is it known if this antigen is actually present in the circulating complexes or the deposits. The severity of lupus nephritis does correspond to the level of circulating immune complexes and to depression of serum complement; however, at least some of the deposits in this disease are now thought to be due to in situ deposition. Current thinking is that circulating immune complexes play a role in each of these conditions, but that in situ formation is more important in most immune-complex-mediated renal diseases.

IN SITU IMMUNE COMPLEX FORMATION

In situ formation of immune complexes occurs when antibodies from the circulation bind to antigens within the kidney. These antigens may be intrinsic constituents of the kidney (eg, type IV collagen of the GBM) or may have become planted in the kidney (eg, charge-dependent binding of cationic proteins to the anionic portions of the GBM or epithelial cells). In the case of intrinsic components two patterns of immune deposition are noted by immunofluorescence microscopy. Linear staining of the GBM or tubular basement membrane (TBM) is indicative of antibody binding to a component of the GBM or TBM, respectively (Figure 36–1). Granular staining suggests the presence of a discontinuous antigen (Figure 36–2) and may reflect antibody binding to either intrinsic cellular antigens or to deposited antigens.

Anti-GBM Deposition

The only example of this form of deposition in humans is anti-GBM disease (see later discussion). It has been studied extensively in two experimental models: nephrotoxic nephritis (Masugi nephritis) and

autoimmune glomerulonephritis (Steblay nephritis). In the nephrotoxic nephritis model, anti-GBM antibodies produced in one animal species (usually sheep) are injected into a different animal species (eg, rabbit, mouse or rat). These heterologous antibodies bind to the GBM, and proteinuria results. This heterologous phase of renal injury is followed by an autologous phase in which the host immune response generates antibodies to the heterologous anti-GBM. These autologous antibodies engage the GBM-bound heterologous antibodies, further accentuating renal injury through the recruitment and activation of neutrophils, macrophages, and other inflammatory cells. Crescent formation (proliferation of parietal epithelial cells, infiltration of mononuclear cells, and deposition of fibrin within Bowman's space) frequently results. The second model of anti-GBM disease—autoimmune glomerulonephritis—is produced by immunizing sheep with heterologous GBM in Freund's

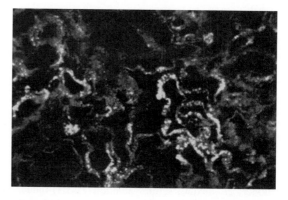

Figure 36–2. Immunofluorescence photomicrograph of a glomerulus from a patient with membranous glomerulonephritis. Note the granular staining for IgG along the capillary loops. Compare with the linear staining seen in Figure 36–1 (×125).

adjuvant. This produces a glomerulonephritis mediated by antibodies directed against the noncollagenous (NC1) domain of type IV collagen found in the GBM. This model is similar to the human disease, which also is caused by host anti-GBM antibodies directed against the NC1 domain of type IV collagen.

Anti-TBM nephritis also exists as an experimental model and as a form of human disease. Immunizing guinea pigs with rabbit TBM emulsified in complete Freund's adjuvant produces the experimental model. This results in linear staining of the TBM on immunofluorescent study and by the induction of severe tubulointerstitial nephritis with tubulitis. This nephritis can be transferred to another animal by antibodies but not by cells, demonstrating that it is due to humoral-mediated immunity. In humans anti-TBM tubulointerstitial nephritis is rare. It can be seen as a result of exposure to several drugs, such as methicillin and allopurinol. In those cases it is believed that a drug-derived hapten binds to the TBM. Anti-TBM tubulointerstitial nephritis may also be seen in association with a variety of glomerulonephritides, most commonly anti-GBM disease.

Antibodies to Cellular Components

Some experimental models of nephritis are induced by antibodies to each of the three cell types of the glomerulus (ie, the epithelial cell, the endothelial cell, and the mesangial cell). Heymann's nephritis is the oldest and best known of these models. This antiepithelial cell nephritis was originally described in 1959 and was induced in rats by the intraperitoneal injection of a suspension of renal cortex in adjuvant. Nephrotic-range proteinuria ensued weeks later accompanied by microscopic changes characteristic of membranous glomerulonephritis with granular capillary loop immunofluorescence for IgG and C3 and subepithelial deposits when viewed with electron microscopy. It is now known that the antigen is a complex of a glycoprotein, megalin, and a receptor-associated protein. This complex is present both on the brush border of the proximal tubule and on the pedicel of the glomerular epithelial cell. The antibodies to megalin bind to the antigen on the foot of the pedicels, and the immune complexes are then shed to the subepithelial space where they form immune deposits. Heymann's nephritis is accepted as a valid model for human membranous glomerulonephritis although it is not yet known if the nephritogenic antigen is identical. It seems likely that several different antigens may be capable of producing the same pathologic picture. In humans both primary and secondary forms of membranous glomerulonephritis occur. In the secondary forms, putative antigens or at least sources for antigens have been identified. We will return to this point in the discussion of membranous glomerulonephritis.

Experimental models with antibodies against components of both mesangial and endothelial cells have been developed but their relevance to human glomerulonephritis is not yet well established. Rat mesangial cells contain a surface glycoprotein known as Thy 1.1, which was originally found expressed on thymocytes. Administration of anti-Thy 1.1 sera to rats results in acute mesangiolysis secondary to the in situ deposition of complement-fixing immune complexes in the mesangium. Mesangial proliferation and complete resolution of the lesion follow unless multiple doses of the antiserum are given. The model has been used chiefly to study the processes involved in glomerulosclerosis. Mesangiolysis is an unusual lesion that has been observed in a number of disparate glomerular diseases, often without any clear relationship to immune complexes. On the other hand, antimesangial antibodies have been reported to occur in IgA nephropathy and Henoch-Schönlein purpura. These glomerular diseases are characterized pathologically by mesangial proliferation. A single model with antiendothelial antibodies has been developed. It was induced by the administration of antiangiotensin-converting enzyme antibodies to rabbits. A transient mild glomerulonephritis was noted to be associated with deposits of IgG and C3 in the capillary wall and with endothelial cell swelling. Circulating antiendothelial antibodies have been identified in a number of different glomerular lesions, but their pathogenetic significance is unknown.

Planted Antigens

Several experimental models suggested the possibility that foreign antigens, particularly those that are cationic, might become planted in the glomerular filter by charge interactions. In the models, investigators perfused the kidney with a cationic protein such as lysozyme followed by antibodies to lysozyme. In situ formation of immune complexes was demonstrated by the finding of subepithelial deposits. It is unknown whether any human glomerular disease occurs due to this mechanism. Some workers have evidence to suggest that trapped bacterial antigen may play a role in the pathogenesis of poststreptococcal glomerulonephritis. It is possible that trapped cationic tumor antigens could be responsible for the membranous glomerulonephritis sometimes found in association with certain solid tumors.

ANTINEUTROPHIL CYTOPLASMIC AUTOANTIBODIES

A possible role for antineutrophil cytoplasmic autoantibodies (ANCA) in the pathogenesis of vasculitis and glomerulonephritis was first recognized in 1985. ANCAs are specific for proteins in the granules of neutrophils and lysosomes of monocytes. The two target antigens are myeloperoxidase (MPO), which produces the perinuclear (p)-ANCA pattern and pro-teinase-3 (PR3), which shows the cytoplasmic (c)-ANCA pattern, in indirect immunofluorescence assays. A possible sequence of events in ANCA-mediated vasculitis follows. All neutrophils contain ANCA antigens within their granules. Stimulation by cytokines triggers expression of these ANCA antigens on the surface of the neutrophils where they are ex-posed to circulating ANCAs. This interaction results in adhesion of the neutrophils to endothelial cells. ANCAs may also form complexes in situ with ANCA antigens adsorbed to endothelial cells. These interac-tions also lead to apoptosis and necrosis.

The systemic vasculitides associated with ANCAs include Wegener's granulomatosis, microscopic poly-angiitis, and Churg–Strauss syndrome. Occasional pa-tients have renal-limited disease. Several arguments provide evidence supporting a possible pathogenic role for ANCAs in these diseases. First, 80-90% of pa-tients with these diseases have circulating ANCAs. The specificity of ANCAs in these diseases is sup-ported by the lack of ANCAs in patients with other acute or chronic inflammatory conditions. Second, there is a general correlation between ANCA titer and disease activity. Third, ANCAs have been detected in certain drug-induced vasculitides; in particular those associated with propylthiouracil. In this case with-drawal of drug causes disappearance of both ANCA and the vasculitis. Fourth, there is in vitro demonstra-tion of activation of cytokine-primed neutrophils by ANCAs. Neutrophils primed with tumor necrosis fac-tor alpha (TNFα) degranulate and produce oxygen metabolites on exposure to IgG from ANCA-positive serum. This degranulation does not occur in the pres-ence of IgG from controls or from patients with other renal disease. Fifth, several animal models support a possible role for ANCAs in these diseases. In one of these models human neutrophil granules were injected into rats that had been immunized with human MPO. The rats developed a glomerulonephritis without evi-dence of significant immune complex deposition—similar to the pauciimmune glomerulonephritis ob-served in human ANCA-associated disease. Other investigators, however, using a similar model showed a more typical immune complex glomerulonephritis. Other models have shown that anti-MPO antibodies worsen the expression of anti-GBM disease. None of the models to date provide incontrovertible evidence for a pathogenic role for ANCAs.

T-LYMPHOCYTE-MEDIATED RENAL INJURY

T-lymphocytes are required for both cell- and anti-body-mediated immune responses. In the kidney they are important both as inducers and as secondary me-diators of disease. They can be involved directly in local cell-mediated immunity but may also regulate some of the antibody-dependent processes discussed earlier.

T LYMPHOCYTES & ACUTE TUBULOINTERSTITIAL NEPHRITIS

Several animal models of tubulointerstitial nephri-tis (TIN) are useful for our understanding of the role of T lymphocytes in these diseases. Most notably, ge-netically susceptible strains of mice develop a cell-mediated form of TIN 6–7 weeks after being immu-nized with rabbit TBM. These mice produce both anti-TBM antibodies and anti-TBM T lymphocytes. Transfer of the disease is accomplished by immune cells, however, and not by transfer of serum to non-immunized animals. Effector T lymphocytes recov-ered from affected kidneys can induce disease in less than a week when injected into kidney of nonimmu-nized animals.

The evidence for a possible role of cell-mediated immunity in human TIN comes chiefly from exami-nation of the nature of the inflammatory infiltrates in these diseases. The pathologic features of TIN include infiltrates composed largely of activated lymphocytes and macrophages, sometimes with granulomatous features. Such injury is usually encountered in the set-ting of drug-induced injury, allograft rejection, my-cobacterial and fungal infections, and sarcoidosis. Thus, the target of the immune response may be a drug-induced hapten, an alloantigen, an antigen from an organism or an autoantigen, respectively. The TIN that accompanies glomerulonephritis may also have activated lymphocytes and macrophages as the pri-mary effector cells. It is not certain whether this is caused by specific antigen recognition by the T cell or by a nonspecific reaction to the cytokines spilling out of the damaged glomeruli.

T LYMPHOCYTES & ACUTE GLOMERULONEPHRITIS

T-cell dysregulation may play a role in acute glomerulonephritis. It is thought that loss of T-cell tolerance to type IV collagen is important in deter-mining susceptibility to human anti-GBM disease. In the experimental models discussed earlier, adjuvants are required to interfere with the natural self-toler-ance. T-cell-dependent polyclonal B-cell activation may play a role in lupus nephritis and in the model of repeated injections of mercuric chloride. In the latter, an initial anti-GBM-like disease characterized by the production of multiple autoantibodies is followed by membranous glomerulonephritis. The autoimmunity can be transferred to normal rats by injection of T cells as long as the suppressor cells are depleted. Currently, however, little evidence supports the theory of a primarily T-cell-mediated glomerulonephritis. Experimental studies have provided some evidence that such a disease could exist. For example, mice lacking the mu immunoglobulin gene develop crescentic glomerulonephritis when injected with heterologous globulin despite their inability to produce antibody.

SECONDARY MEDIATORS OF ACUTE INFLAMMATION

CELLS

The neutrophil is a major agent of injury in postinfectious glomerulonephritis. Macrophages play a crucial role in most other forms of proliferative glomerulonephritis. Macrophages accumulate in glomeruli secondary to the production of cytokines, chemokines, complement, and enhanced expression of adhesion molecules. They can cause glomerular injury by producing oxygen metabolites, cytokines, plasminogen activator, eicosanoids, and nitric oxide and may affect glomerular hemodynamics. They also play a role in the induction of apoptosis and in the formation of crescents. Finally, they are a potential source of growth factors that induce mesangial proliferation and increased mesangial matrix. Conversely, macrophages also may help to resolve glomerulonephritis by phagocytosing immune complexes. Intrinsic cells of the glomerulus are another source of inflammatory mediators. The mesangial cells are best studied because they are easiest to maintain in vitro. Table 36–2 indicates some of the sources of the important cytokines and other mediators.

Table 36–2. Molecular mediators in glomerulonephritis.

Mediators	Cellular Source
Cytokines	
Interleukin-1	Macrophage
	Mesangial cell
Tumor necrosis factor α	Macrophage
	Mesangial cell
Interleukin-4	T cells
Interleukin-6	Mesangial cells
	Macrophages
Adhesion molecules	
Selectins	Endothelial cells
β_2-Integrins	Macrophages
β_1-Integrins	Macrophages
	T cells
	Epithelial cells
	Mesangial cells
Immunoglobulin-like molecules	Endothelial cells
	Mesangial cells

MOLECULAR MEDIATORS

Proinflammatory cytokines are important in the pathogenesis of glomerular injury. Interleukin (IL)-1β and TNFα are two of the many cytokines involved in this process. Administration of these cytokines can induce or worsen experimental glomerulonephritis. Glomerular synthesis of these two cytokines precedes the expression of the glomerulonephritis, and use of antibodies or specific antagonists nullifies their effects. These cytokines are present in several different proliferative forms of human glomerulonephritis. Other cytokines shown to have a role in glomerulonephritis are shown in Table 36–2. The adhesion molecules are responsible for leukocyte adhesion to the area of injury. Furthermore, they facilitate leukocyte migration out of the capillaries and into the mesangium or interstitium. The chemokines listed in Table 36–3 also attract effector cells to the area of injury. Use of antibodies to these substances markedly ameliorates experimental glomerulonephritis. Reactive oxygen metabolites may be the triggering mechanism for these chemokines and for the adhesion molecules in the setting of glomerulonephritis.

The importance of the complement cascade in glomerular injury has been known for a long time. Complement may become fixed to the tissue in the immune complexes. However, glomerular epithelial, endothelial, and mesangial cells can also synthesize complement. Complement components C3 and C5 are chemoattractant for leukocytes. Complement depletion prevents glomerulonephritis in some models and species. The terminal complement components C5b-9, membrane attack complex (MAC), causes cell lysis. MAC also induces reactive oxygen metabolites and certain prostaglandins. Complement inhibitory proteins such as CD59 and decay-accelerating factor closely regulate the complement system. Inhibition of these molecules in experimental models leads to more severe injury. The complement system also aids in the clearance of immune complexes. Patients with inherited deficiencies of the early components of the classical complement cascade often develop immune complex renal disease (Chapter 25).

Table 36–3. Chemokines in renal disease.

Chemokines	Target Cells
CXC Family	Neutrophils
MIP-1α	
IL-8	
CC Family	Monocytes
MCP-1	
RANTES	
MIP-1β	

[1] Chemokine acronyms are defined in Table 11-1

Reactive oxygen metabolites are known to be direct mediators of glomerular injury. Renal infusion of phorbol myristate acetate, which stimulates the respiratory burst, induces glomerular injury. However, when this is accompanied by catalase, which degrades hydrogen peroxide, the injury is prevented. Scavengers of reactive oxygen metabolites nullify glomerular injury in a variety of models. Reactive oxygen metabolites are produced by neutrophils and may be produced by macrophages and mesangial cells. Proteases may also directly mediate renal injury. In particular proteases may damage glomerular basement membrane or mesangial matrix by degrading their protein components. Proteases may be derived from neutrophils, macrophages and mesangial cells.

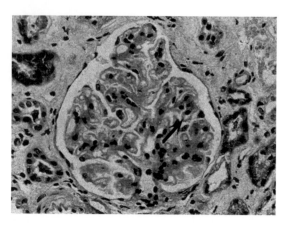

Figure 36–3. Light micrograph of a glomerulus from a patient with membranous glomerulonephritis. Note the thickened capillary walls (*arrow*) with mild mesangial prominence. The cellularity is within normal limits (H&E, ×125).

SPECIFIC IMMUNE-MEDIATED RENAL DISEASES

PRIMARY GLOMERULONEPHRITIS

MEMBRANOUS GLOMERULONEPHRITIS

Clinical Features & Course

Membranous glomerulonephritis is a disease principally of adults. The most common presentation is the nephrotic syndrome, but as many as half of the patients in one study had only asymptomatic proteinuria or an abnormal urinalysis. It is the most common cause of nephrotic syndrome in white adults. Half of the patients have increased serum creatinine level and hypertension at presentation. A few patients have hematuria at presentation but most develop this sign during the course of their disease. The natural history of the disease is usually indolent with spontaneous remission occurring in approximately 25% of patients after many years. After 8–10 years another 25% develop end-stage disease or die. The remaining patients progress to mild chronic renal insufficiency.

Pathology & Immunopathology

By light microscopy the glomeruli show uniform thickening of capillary loops with at most mild mesangial hypercellularity (Figure 36–3). Silver stain shows typical "spikes," and trichrome stain demonstrates the deposits on the epithelial side of the GBM. The presence of segmental sclerosis, many obsolete glomeruli, tubular atrophy and interstitial fibrosis, or hyaline arteriolosclerosis suggests a greater likelihood of progressive renal insufficiency. Immunofluorescence reveals granular capillary loop staining for IgG and C3. Electron microscopy shows numerous subepithelial deposits with extensive effacement of foot processes. The presence of immunoglobulin and

complement within deposits is typical of an immune complex-mediated disease. As discussed earlier, Heymann's nephritis is believed to be a good model of this disease, suggesting that membranous glomerulonephritis results from in situ formation of complexes. In the idiopathic forms, the exact antigen(s) is unknown. It seems likely that the exact antigen may vary from case to case.

The occurrence of mesangial deposits suggests the possibility of a secondary form of the disease. Approximately 25% of patients have membranous glomerulonephritis secondary to infections (hepatitis B, syphilis, etc), drugs (gold, penicillamine, etc), neoplasms (lung, stomach, etc), and autoimmune disease (lupus, mixed connective tissue disease, etc). In most of these examples the antigen is known, and in some has been identified within the immune deposits. Some may be planted antigens. For example, in the membranous glomerulonephritis associated with hepatitis B infection, HBeAg is often found in the deposits. HBeAg is small enough to pass to the epithelial slit diaphragm, where it can become planted. This protein produces cationic antigens, which pass to the slit as a result of their positive charge. The likelihood of the in situ formation of such complexes is increased by the persistent nature of hepatitis infection, which allows continuous seeding of the GBM by both antigen and antibody.

Another interesting characteristic of membranous glomerulonephritis is the paucity of infiltrating inflammatory cells. The most likely explanation is that the injury in this disease is complement-mediated but independent of inflammatory cells. MAC has been found in the deposits of membranous glomerulonephritis and is thought to be responsible for the renal injury.

Treatment

Treatment for membranous glomerulonephritis has always been problematic. The possibility of spontaneous remissions confounds interpretation of small or uncontrolled studies. Steroids were the original drugs of choice, but more recent studies have failed to demonstrate efficacy. Encouraging results have been reported with alkylating agents (cyclophosphamide or chlorambucil) and cyclosporine, but definitive studies have not yet been published.

POSTINFECTIOUS GLOMERULONEPHRITIS

Clinical Features & Course

Postinfectious glomerulonephritis is most commonly associated with infection with group A *Streptococcus*. In those cases, it occurs 1–4 weeks (on average 10–11 days) following an episode of pharyngitis in children or young adults. The classic presentation is the abrupt onset of dark or smoky-colored urine accompanied by periorbital edema. Laboratory data reveal elevated serum creatinine, low serum complement, low-grade proteinuria, and hematuria with red blood cell casts. Clinical recovery is expected in most cases in children although it may take as long as 10 years for complete resolution of the changes. Approximately two thirds of adults show complete recovery.

Other agents that have been implicated in infection-related glomerulonephritis include *Staphylococcus, Pneumococcus, Klebsiella, Mycoplasma,* and many viruses. These organisms can be involved in glomerulonephritis associated with endocarditis, deep-seated abscesses, shunt nephritis, pneumonia, and certain skin infections. These cases of glomerulonephritis occur in the setting of ongoing infection, and, in contrast to poststreptococcal glomerulonephritis, recovery usually depends on eradication of the seat of primary infection.

Pathology & Immunopathology

The light microscopic hallmark of postinfectious glomerulonephritis is diffuse cellular proliferation chiefly within capillary lumina (Figure 36–4). The neutrophil is the predominant cell at early stages, but the numbers of monocytes increase during the course of the disease. The site of proliferation shifts to the mesangial compartment. Crescents are frequently present and have been associated with poorer prognosis in some studies but not in others. On occasion, the glomerular changes are associated with a nonspecific interstitial nephritis. The most common immunofluorescence finding is coarsely granular staining for IgG and C3 along capillary loops and sometimes in the mesangium. IgM and properdin may also be seen. The latter in combination with the lack of staining for C1q

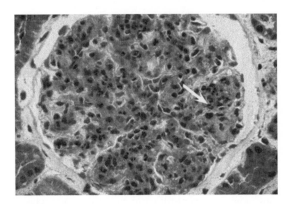

Figure 36–4. Light micrograph of a glomerulus from a patient with postinfectious glomerulonephritis. Note the increased mesangial and endocapillary cellularity. In particular, neutrophils (*arrow*) may be seen (H&E, ×150).

suggests that the alternative pathway is involved. On electron microscopy large subepithelial deposits, the so-called humps, are typically scattered on most capillary loops (Figure 36–5). Mesangial deposits are not uncommon. Rarely, one may find subendothelial deposits. Although the nonstreptococcal variants may be identical to the picture described earlier, other morphologic appearances also occur. For example, in the variant associated with endocarditis, a focal segmental proliferative lesion may be present sometimes associated with fibrinoid necrosis. In the case of either shunt nephritis or deep-seated abscess, the pattern of

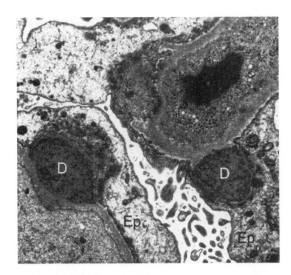

Figure 36–5. Electron micrograph of a portion of a glomerulus from a patient with postinfectious glomerulonephritis. Note the hump-like subepithelial deposits (D) with a variegated appearance. Epithelial cells (Ep) show extensive effacement of foot processes (Uranyl acetate and lead citrate, ×7500).

glomerular injury is more often akin to membranopro-liferative glomerulonephritis (see following section).

It is well accepted that postinfectious glomeru-lonephritis is immune complex-mediated. As dis-cussed earlier, it fits well with the serum sickness model. The exact mechanism of immune complex deposition is still unclear, however, and the antigen has not been defined. Investigators have variously implicated circulating immune complexes or in situ formation of such complexes with either a "planted" antigen or cross-reaction to an autoantigen. It is not even known whether the antigen is a component of the infectious agent itself or a modification of en-dogenous protein resulting in an autoimmune type of reaction. As stated earlier, it is believed that the alter-native pathway is important in the activation of com-plement in this disease and the resulting renal injury. Cell-mediated immunity may play an ancillary role.

Treatment

No particular treatment is instituted in most cases of poststreptococcal glomerulonephritis except to treat acute or chronic renal failure that may ensue. In the cases of glomerulonephritis that are related to some sort of chronic or subacute infection such as endocarditis or abscess, treatment of the primary in-fection with antibiotics has been reported to result in resolution of the renal disease in the long-term for most patients.

IGA NEPHROPATHY

Clinical Features & Course

IgA nephropathy is the most prevalent form of glomerulonephritis worldwide and a major contribu-tor to end-stage renal disease. The overall frequency varies by geographic region due to differences in the rate of renal biopsy as well as to differences in risk within different populations. It is more frequent in Asia than in North America. Certain Native American groups have an increased risk for developing the dis-ease. It begins predominantly in the second and third decades of life although it has been reported to occur in the very young and in the elderly. Males are more frequently affected than females in a ratio of 2:1.

Three typical clinical presentations have been de-scribed. The first is the classical presentation of episodic macroscopic hematuria occurring at the time of pharyngitis or other viral illness. This presentation is the most common, is seen predominantly in young males, and has the best prognosis. The second is characterized by persistent or intermittent micro-scopic hematuria. These patients are more likely to have proteinuria, to be older than 30 years of age, and to progress to end-stage renal failure. The final group is generally older than 50 years of age when they present with chronic renal failure and hyperten-sion. Although 10% of patients with IgA nephropa-thy have been reported to have a spontaneous remis-sion, few maintain it. Overall 60–70 % of patients progress to chronic renal insufficiency, with 20–30% developing end-stage disease.

Pathology & Immunopathology

IgA nephropathy may have any appearance by light microscopy, but the most common pattern is that of mesangioproliferative glomerulonephritis. The mesangial areas show increased matrix and cells usually of glomerular origin. The capillary loops are unremarkable. In other cases one may see focal pro-liferative glomerulonephritis in association with endocapillary proliferation and either necrotizing le-sions or crescents. The presence of crescents in greater than 70% of glomeruli or of significant global glomerulosclerosis portends a poor prognosis. The disease is defined by the immunofluorescence find-ings. Mesangial staining for IgA must predominate. IgA is the only immunoglobulin in about 25% of cases and may be accompanied by IgG, IgM, or a combination of both. C3 is almost always present without other complement components, suggesting probable alternative pathway activation. Electron mi-croscopic examination reveals the presence of large mesangial deposits with smaller paramesangial de-posits. Subendothelial and subepithelial deposits may also occur, but chiefly in those patients with endo-capillary proliferation by light microscopy.

IgA nephropathy is an immune complex-mediated disease. Circulating immune complexes containing IgA are regularly found. Recent evidence suggests that the IgA in this disease is abnormally glycosy-lated. This alteration leads to prolonged survival in the circulation, more rapid glomerular deposition, and increased capacity of IgA to activate comple-ment. The temporal relationship between pharyngitis or gastroenteritis and the episodes of hematuria and nephritis suggest that a viral antigen may be impor-tant, but no specific antigen has been identified yet. Another possible pathogenetic factor is reduced clearance of immune complexes due to alteration in the complement system or to reduced phagocytic up-take. Defects in immunoregulation may also play a role in the pathogenesis of this disease. The exact role has not been determined, however, nor is it known if these defects are acquired or genetic. Fa-milial clusters of IgA nephropathy are widely re-ported.

Treatment

The treatment of IgA nephropathy is controversial. The most common regimens have included the use of fish oil high in ϖ-3 fatty acids or antiplatelet agents such as dipyridamole. Various immunosuppressive agents, such as steroids, azathioprine, and cyclophos-phamide, have had only mixed results. Plasmaphere-sis is rarely used and only in cases of severe acute re-nal failure.

MEMBRANOPROLIFERATIVE GLOMERULONEPHRITIS

Clinical Features & Course

The idiopathic forms of membranoproliferative glomerulonephritis (MPGN), types I and II, affect children and young adults although they can appear in older adults as well. Some patients present with an acute nephritic picture with hematuria, hypertension, renal insufficiency, and oliguria. Most also have proteinuria; many with the nephrotic syndrome. The two types of MPGN have similar clinical features. Both are characterized by low serum complement, particularly C3. Each also may show elevated levels of C3 nephritic factor (C3NeF), although type II MPGN shows that abnormality more consistently. The clinical course is generally progressive over years to end-stage renal disease for both types. In some patients persistent proteinuria occurs, whereas others have a remitting and relapsing course. Secondary forms of type I MPGN are well known. They are associated with a variety of infections, most notably hepatitis C virus; neoplasms; hereditary complement deficiencies; mixed cryoglobulinemia (most of these are related to hepatitis C); and a host of miscellaneous conditions such as Castleman's disease, sickle cell anemia, and Gaucher's disease.

Pathology & Immunopathology

All forms of MPGN show the same light microscopic appearance. The glomeruli have a lobular architecture with accentuation of the mesangial areas by increased matrix and hypercellularity. In addition, the capillary walls are thickened with "double contours" visible on the silver stain, representing two layers of basement membrane with subendothelial deposits between them. Two features may help to distinguish the cryoglobulinemic form of MPGN from all other types. The cryoglobulins may form "coagula", PAS-positive globules, within the capillary loops. Furthermore, these cases have increased numbers of monocytes within the capillary lumina. In fact, the proliferation in these cases is chiefly endocapillary. Immunofluorescence findings are quite characteristic. In both types C3 is the predominant deposit. In type I MPGN it is typically in a broken linear pattern with mesangial staining. In type II the pattern is described as peripheral lobular but the mesangium may also stain. Immunoglobulins may also be present, but they generally show less intense staining. Electron microscopy is necessary to distinguish with certainty between the two types. Type I MPGN has mesangial and subendothelial deposits accompanied by mesangial cell interposition. Type II MPGN shows a pathognomonic dense ribbon-like transformation of the glomerular basement membrane. Of the secondary forms, cryoglobulinemic forms can be suggested on the basis of finding the typical "ring and cylinder" substructure within the deposits.

The evidence suggests that MPGN is immune complex-mediated. It bears some similarities to membranous glomerulonephritis inasmuch as many secondary forms occur. The presence of these secondary forms supports the idea that a chronic antigenemia exists, which is sometimes related to chronic infection or to tumor or an autoimmune condition. In most cases, however, the precise causative agent is unknown. The difference between the two diseases lies in the pattern of immune complex deposition. The prominence and severity of the hypocomplementemia as well as the presence of C3NeF has led to the idea that complement activation is important in the pathogenesis of MPGN. C3NeF is an IgG that stabilizes the alternative pathway C3 convertase (see Chapter 12). This stabilization is not reversible by factor H, and thus C3Nef allows continuous activation of the alternative complement pathway. The resulting hypocomplementemia may make the patient susceptible to various infections resulting in MPGN. The association of MPGN with various complement deficiencies lends further credence to the role of defects in complement regulation in the pathogenesis of MPGN. An animal model in Yorkshire pigs further supports this idea. These pigs have a deficiency of factor H that leads to an accumulation of C3 convertase and depletion of complement. They develop type II MPGN. Hypocomplementemia may also lead to a decrease in the solubilization and clearance of immune complex deposits.

Treatment

No specific therapy has been proven effective in any form of this disease. Some authors believe that steroids or cyclophosphamide (or both) may slow its progression. Other authors have advocated the use of platelet inhibitors, but their efficacy has not been demonstrated. These diseases are rare so that it is difficult to mount the sort of trial that would be necessary to determine effectiveness of a new drug therapy.

GLOMERULONEPHRITIS ASSOCIATED WITH SYSTEMIC DISEASE

LUPUS NEPHRITIS

Clinical Features & Course

The renal manifestations of systemic lupus erythematosus (SLE) are a major cause of both morbidity and mortality within this disease. Fifty percent of patients with SLE develop lupus nephritis, usually within the first year after presentation. On occasion the lupus nephritis precedes the other clinical and even serologic manifestations of SLE. A wide range of presentations is possible accompanied by a similarly broad spectrum of pathologic changes (Table 36–4). Patients may present with asymptomatic hematuria or proteinuria. Other patients develop nephrotic syndrome. Some patients present with rapid onset of acute renal failure. Lupus nephritis is characterized by a remitting and relapsing course with changes of the morphologic type from one class to another. The renal biopsy in these cases helps to determine therapy and prognosis. The course of the disease is as variable as the clinical presentation. Currently the survival rate at 10 years is about 88% for all types of lupus nephritis.

Pathology & Immunopathology

As stated earlier lupus nephritis comes in many forms (see Table 36–4). Class I shows no alterations. Class II is characterized by cellular proliferation limited to the mesangium accompanied by varying degrees of mesangial matrix increase. Capillary loops are thin and delicate. Class III is typified by involvement of some glomeruli in a segmental pattern with increased mesangial cellularity that extends into the capillary lumen. Class IV shows a diffuse pattern of involvement exemplified by global hypercellularity, increased matrix, and thickened capillary loops often described as "wire loops." Silver stain often delineates subendothelial deposits. Classes Va and Vb are manifest by thickened capillary loops with "spikes" on silver stain. On occasion, mesangial matrix is increased, but only mild increases occur in cellularity. Classes Vc and Vd demonstrate a combination of classes III or IV with class Va. Additional changes that may be seen are crescents, necrotizing lesions, hyaline thrombi, and hematoxylin bodies. These forms may transform from one class into another. Any class may be accompanied by interstitial nephritis (see later discussion). Immunofluorescence studies commonly show a "full house"—three immunoglobulins (IgG, IgA, and IgM) and two complement components (C3 and C1q). The pattern of deposition (mesangial vs loop) is determined by the location of deposits. Electron microscopy confirms the diagnosis by determining the deposits' site with greater sensitivity. Class I has no deposits. Class II shows only mesangial deposits. Classes III and IV contain mesangial and subendothelial deposits (Figure 36–6). The subendothelial

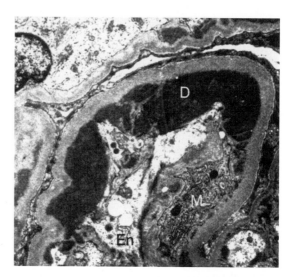

Figure 36–6. Electron micrograph of a portion of a glomerulus from a patient with diffuse proliferative lupus nephritis. Note the large subendothelial deposit (D). The endothelial cell (En) is swollen, and the mesangial cell (M) has interposed itself into the subendothelial space (Uranyl acetate and lead citrate, ×5000).

deposits in class III are smaller and fewer than those seen in class IV. Class Va shows only subepithelial deposits. Class Vb contains both mesangial and subepithelial deposits. Classes Vc and Vd demonstrate deposits in all three locations: subepithelial, subendothelial, and mesangial. Other ultrastructural features include tubuloreticular inclusions in endothelial cells, fingerprints in the deposits, and other substructure suggestive of cryoglobulins.

Lupus nephritis is another prototype of immune complex-mediated renal disease. In this case many candidate autoantibodies and antigens are present. Autoantibodies to dsDNA, histones, and ribonucleoprotein have been detected in the glomerular deposits and eluted from the kidney. These antiDNA antibodies may cross-react with a number of different glomerular constituents. Thus, in situ formation of complexes is one mechanism operating in lupus nephritis. There is also evidence for "planting" of autoantigens such as histone that have affinity for glomerular constituents.

Table 36–4. Pathologic classification of lupus nephritis.

Class	Pathologic Description	Clinical Presentation
I	Normal	Asymptomatic
II	Mesangial	Hematuria; normal renal function
III	Focal proliferative	Hematuria; proteinuria; normal or mild renal insufficiency
IV	Diffuse proliferative	Hematuria; proteinuria; acute renal insufficiency
Va or Vb	Membranous	Nephrotic syndrome
Vc or Vd	Mixed membranous and proliferative	Hematuria, nephrotic syndrome; often renal insufficiency

Once bound to the glomerulus they can interact with circulating autoantibodies to form immune complexes. The role of deposition of preformed circulating immune complexes is thought to be less important in lupus nephritis. (See Chapter 31 for further discussion of the immunopathogenesis of SLE.)

Treatment

As stated earlier, the renal biopsy helps to direct therapy in lupus nephritis. Class II lupus requires only that the extrarenal manifestations be treated. Class III nephritis with low activity can be treated with steroids alone. The therapy for class III nephritis with high activity or for class IV lupus must be individualized but usually includes a combination of steroids and cyclophosphamide. The treatment of class V lupus nephritis is similar to that of idiopathic membranous glomerulonephritis with the use of cyclosporine or alkylating agents the current agents of choice.

HENOCH-SCHÖNLEIN PURPURA

Clinical Features & Course

Henoch-Schönlein purpura (HSP) is a small-vessel vasculitis that is manifest by purpura, abdominal pain, arthralgias, and nephritis. Nephritis occurs in approximately 40% of patients and may be the presenting sign. Microscopic or macroscopic hematuria is present in nearly all patients. Other common clinical features include proteinuria, hypertension, and acute renal failure. The purpuric rash typically begins on the extensor surfaces of the legs and buttocks. Abdominal pain is nonspecific and may be accompanied by other gastrointestinal symptoms. The arthralgias generally affect the larger joints. Outcome depends on the extent of renal involvement. Sixty percent of patients enjoy a complete recovery within 6 months. Only 10% of all patients with HSP (25% of those with renal disease) progress to end-stage renal disease. IgA nephropathy is considered a kidney-limited form of HSP by some authors.

Pathology & Immunopathology

The changes are similar to those of IgA nephropathy. In fact these two entities are indistinguishable on pathologic grounds alone. Light microscopy is characterized by a predominantly mesangial proliferative picture although there is a slight tendency to increased endocapillary proliferation in HSP compared with IgA nephropathy. Necrotizing lesions and crescents may be present. The prognosis is worse in that group of patients who have crescents in more than 50% of glomeruli. IgA is the predominant immunoglobulin by definition. It may be accompanied by other immunoglobulin or by C3. IgA may also be seen in tubular basement membrane. This finding may distinguish HSP from IgA nephropathy. Both of these diseases may show IgA in the skin around post-

capillary venules. As many as 20% of the normal population also have this finding, however, rendering it nonspecific. Electron microscopy shows mesangial deposits in most cases. As many as half of the patients have subendothelial deposits, and one third have occasional subepithelial deposits. In some patients, the GBM is split with lamination reminiscent of the changes seen in hereditary nephritis.

HSP is considered an immune-mediated renal disease. Infection seems a likely precipitating factor as HSP shows seasonal variation and is often accompanied by a viral prodrome. The pathogenesis may be similar to IgA nephropathy. Both IgA nephropathy and HSP are thought to result from activation of the alternative pathway. The fact that the acute glomerular injury is more severe, as well as the occurrence of systemic involvement, speaks to some important differences, however. These differences may be due to the nature of the inciting agent. For example, experimental injection of bacterial cell wall antigens from different strains of *Streptococcus pneumoniae* into mice resulted into two distinct patterns of involvement similar to the differences between IgA nephropathy and HSP.

Treatment

No specific treatments are recommended for HSP. Over the years, steroids, azathioprine, and cyclophosphamide have been tried with uneven results. In severe crescentic cases with a rapidly progressive picture, plasmapheresis is sometimes instituted. The high percentage of cases with spontaneous resolution confounds efforts to conduct and interpret therapeutic trials.

VASCULITIS-ASSOCIATED GLOMERULAR LESIONS

ANTIGLOMERULAR BASEMENT MEMBRANE DISEASE

Clinical Features & Course

Antiglomerular basement membrane (anti-GBM) disease is characterized by rapidly progressive glomerulonephritis and pulmonary hemorrhage (Goodpasture's syndrome). Approximately half of the patients develop both pulmonary and renal disease, and the remaining patients have renal-limited anti-GBM disease. Young men tend to present with the full-blown syndrome, and older women tend to manifest the renal-limited form. A flu-like illness often precedes the onset of hematuria. Occasionally one may elicit a history of hydrocarbon exposure. Serology shows the presence of anti-GBM antibodies. Antineutrophil cytoplasmic antibodies (ANCA) may also be present in as many as one third of patients with anti-GBM antibody. The presence of ANCA in addition to anti-GBM antibody gives a better prognosis than anti-GBM antibody alone. The mortality rate is currently about 10%, and half of the patients progress to end-stage renal disease.

Pathology & Immunopathology

The characteristic light microscopic findings in anti-GBM disease are segmental necrotizing lesions and crescents. Silver stain demonstrates local destruction of the GBM. The unaffected glomeruli and noninvolved portions of glomerular tufts usually show normal cellularity and capillary loops. Multinucleated giant cells are commonly seen in the crescents. Bowman's capsule is also frequently disrupted with spillage of the inflammation into the adjacent renal parenchyma. This change is seen more frequently in either anti-GBM disease and ANCA-associated lesions than in immune-complex mediated crescentic glomerulonephritis. Linear staining of GBM by IgG is characteristically bright on immunofluorescent study. It is important to always examine a control such as albumin as patients with diabetes may show linear staining of both GBM and TBM for IgG and albumin. Electron microscopy confirms the light microscopic findings. No deposits are identified.

The target antigen of circulating anti-GBM antibodies in human disease is the C-terminal noncollagenous (NC1) portion of the α3 chain of type IV collagen. 90 to 100% of patients with anti-GBM antibodies have reactivity with α3(IV) NC1, with 15% having an additional reactivity with α1(IV) NC1 and 3% with α4(IV) NC1. The triggering event for the induction of the formation of the anti-GBM antibodies is unknown although several potential factors are recognized. A genetic association has been made between anti-GBM disease and HLA DR2 (DRB1-1501 and DQB1-0602 alleles). Exposure to hydrocarbons or infection with influenza A2 has also been temporally associated with onset of this disease. Cigarette smoking has also been implicated. In a study of patients with anti-GBM disease, all smokers had both pulmonary and renal manifestations, but only 20% of the nonsmokers had pulmonary hemorrhage.

Treatment

High-dose corticosteroids, other immunosuppressive drugs, and plasmapheresis are the mainstays in the treatment of anti-GBM disease. Plasmapheresis in conjunction with immunosuppressive agents hastens the disappearance of the anti-GBM antibodies. The outcome is better if the serum creatinine is less than 6 mg/dL at the time of institution of therapy.

ANTINEUTROPHIL CYTOPLASMIC AUTOANTIBODIES-ASSOCIATED DISEASE

Clinical Features & Course

The ANCA-associated diseases that manifest as small-vessel vasculitis include Churg-Strauss syndrome (CSS), Wegener's granulomatosis (WG), and microscopic polyangiitis (MPA). WG is usually associated with cANCA directed against proteinase3, whereas both MPA and CSS usually have detectable pANCA directed against myeloperoxidase (Table 36–5). Patients with any of these diseases may present with fever, arthralgias, myalgias, purpura, and peripheral neuropathy. CSS is defined by the presence of asthma and eosinophilia. WG typically includes more frequent involvement of upper airways and lungs. MPA has considerable overlap with WG with respect to organ involvement. Renal-limited variants of WG and MPA may occur. The exact presentation and course depend on the pattern of organ involvement. Clinical evidence of crescentic pauci-immune glomerulonephritis occurs in 45% of patients with CSS, 80% of patients with WG, and 90% of patients with MPA. These patients may have a very explosive picture with rapidly progressive glomerulonephritis in which the renal function deteriorates from normal to severe renal insufficiency within weeks. Other patients have a slower course to renal failure over several months.

Table 36–5. Differential diagnosis of crescentic glomerulonephritis.

Disease	Immunologic Mechanism	Immunofluorescent Pattern
Wegener's granulomatosis	cANCA	Pauciimmune
Microscopic polyangiitis	pANCA	Pauciimmune
Churg–Strauss syndrome	pANCA	Pauciimmune
Anti-GBM disease	Anti-GBM antibodies	Linear GBM staining with IgG
Proliferative lupus nephritis	Immune complexes	Full-house granular and mesangial staining
IgA nephropathy/HSP	Immune complexes	Mesangial IgA and C3
Postinfectious glomerulonephritis	Immune complexes	Granular IgG and C3

Abbreviations: cANCA = cytoplasmic antineutrophil cytoplasmic antibodies; pANCA = perinuclear antineutrophil cytoplasmic antibodies; GBM = glomerular basement membrane; HSP = Henoch–Schönlein purpura; Ig = immunoglobulin.

Pathology & Immunopathology

It is not possible to distinguish among these diseases based on the pathology of the kidney. The characteristic light microscopic alteration is the segmental necrotizing lesion with crescent formation similar to that change seen in anti-GBM disease. This is frequently accompanied by interstitial nephritis. One may find an interstitial capillaritis in as many as half of the cases of WG. Rarely, one will find necrotizing granulomatous inflammation in the interstitium in WG, but such changes may also be seen in MPA. Frank vasculitis is seldom found in renal biopsies although one may consider the fibrinoid necrosis of the glomerular tuft a form of vasculitis. Immunofluorescence studies are generally negative although occasional nonspecific segmental staining may be seen with IgG and C3, thus the name pauciimmune glomerulonephritis. Electron microscopy does not contribute to the diagnosis.

These diseases often begin with a viral prodrome. Such an illness may be accompanied by circulating cytokines, which, in turn, could prime neutrophils and monocytes to express ANCA antigens on their cytoplasmic surfaces. The question then arises as to why such a flu-like illness is followed by small-vessel vasculitis in only a small proportion of people who suffer a viral illness. This is an important consideration that needs to be answered before the precise role of ANCAs in the pathogenesis of these fascinating diseases can be determined with certainty.

Treatment

Severe disease usually is treated initially with cyclophosphamide, often in combination with high-dose corticosteroids (see Chapters 31 and 53).

TUBULOINTERSTITIAL DISEASES

LUPUS-ASSOCIATED TUBULOINTERSTITIAL NEPHRITIS

Clinical Features & Course

The most common form of immune complex-associated tubulointerstitial nephritis (TIN) is that seen in the setting of SLE. Half of all patients with lupus glomerulonephritis have an accompanying TIN. This is most often seen in the proliferative forms of lupus nephritis (WHO classes III and IV). Interstitial inflammation is one of the features of the activity index, which can contribute to a poorer prognosis. On rare occasion TIN may occur in the absence of significant glomerular disease in SLE. Such patients present with acute renal failure and urinalysis typical of TIN rather than glomerulonephritis.

Pathology & Immunopathology

The light microscopy of the TIN of lupus nephritis is often indistinguishable from other forms of TIN and is characterized by tubular epithelial cell injury, a mixed chronic inflammatory infiltrate with macrophages, lymphocytes, and plasma cells, and interstitial edema. On occasion, apoptosis is quite prominent unlike in other forms of TIN. These lesions evolve with time to a chronic TIN characterized by tubular atrophy and loss and interstitial fibrosis. Immunofluorescence studies show the presence of IgG, C3, and C1q in a granular pattern along the tubular basement membrane (TBM) or in the interstitium. Electron microscopy demonstrates dense deposits along the outer aspects of the TBM or surrounding intertubular capillaries.

These lesions seem to be mediated by immune complex deposition. Most of the infiltrating cells are T lymphocytes with fewer macrophages, B lymphocytes, and natural killer (NK) cells. A greater proportion of CD8 cells is found relative to other forms of TIN. The predominance of T cells in the infiltrate suggests that cellular immunity may be involved in these lesions. Furthermore, the presence of NK cells suggests that antibody-dependent cellular cytotoxicity may also play a role in the injury.

Treatment

The treatment is the same as described for lupus nephritis. The addition of severe TIN in lupus worsens the activity index, potentially requiring the more cytotoxic drugs. But individual tailoring of therapy is always required in this disease.

ANTITUBULAR BASEMENT MEMBRANE NEPHRITIS

Primary antitubular basement membrane (anti-TBM) nephritis is exceedingly rare, with fewer than 10 well-documented cases appearing in the world's literature. Secondary forms are most often associated with anti-GBM nephritis. Anti-TBM antibodies may be found in as many as 50–70% of such patients. The light microscopic changes are nonspecific but show tubular epithelial injury with a mixed chronic inflammatory infiltrate. Linear immunofluorescent staining of the TBM with antisera to IgG is pathognomonic.

T-LYMPHOCYTE-MEDIATED TIN

Clinical Features & Course

TIN induced by T cells occurs in many different settings, including drug-induced injury, allograft rejection, reaction to infectious agents, and sarcoidosis. The clinical features vary with the disease, but in most cases acute renal failure is a common compo-

Table 36–6. Pathology of T-cell mediated TIN.

Disease	Characteristic Pathologic Feature(s)	Treatment
Drug-induced injury	Eosinophils, granulomatous inflammation	Withdrawal of drug; ? steroids
Allograft rejection	Tubulitis, endothelialitis	Increased immunosuppression
Infection	Bacterial – neutrophils Virus – typical inclusions Fungal/mycobacterial – granulomas Special stains to identify organisms	Appropriate antibiotic
Sarcoidosis	Noncaseating granulomas	Steroids

nent. The course also differs according to the disease and the chronicity of the injury at the time of diagnosis.

Pathology & Immunopathology

The pathology of the different types of T-cell-mediated injury is briefly summarized in Table 36–6. In general, tubular epithelial injury must be present accompanied by an interstitial inflammatory infiltrate. The nature of the infiltrate may aid in determining the diagnosis. Neither immunofluorescence nor electron microscopy is helpful; however, special stains for organisms including immunoperoxidase stains may be useful.

As discussed earlier, the evidence for the existence of T-cell-mediated TIN has come chiefly from animal models. Delayed-type hypersensitivity is likely important in drug reactions and sarcoidosis. The mechanisms of allograft rejection are complex and are discussed elsewhere (Chapter 52).

Treatment

Appropriate therapy depends on the cause of the TIN and is shown briefly in Table 36–6.

REFERENCES

GENERAL

Jennette JC et al: *Heptinstall's Pathology of the Kidney,* 5 ed. Philadelphia: Lippincott-Raven, 1998.

Neilson EG, Couser WG: *Immunologic Renal Diseases.* Lippincott-Raven, 1997.

IMMUNOLOGIC MECHANISMS OF RENAL INJURY

Dixon FJ: Pathogenesis of immunologic disease. *J Immunol* 1972;109:187.

Germuth FG Jr et al: Immune complex disease. I. Experimental acute and chronic glomerulonephritis. *Johns Hopkins Med J* 1967;120:225.

Heeringa P et al: Animal models of anti-neutrophil cytoplasmic antibody associated vasculitis. *Kidney Int* 1998; 53:253.

Hellmark T et al: Characterization of anti-GBM antibodies involved in Goodpasture's syndrome. *Kidney Int* 1994; 46:823.

Jansen JH et al: In situ complement activation in porcine membranoproliferative glomerulonephritis type II. *Kidney Int* 1998;53:331.

Longcope WT: Some observations on the course and outcome of hemorrhagic nephritis. *Trans Am Clin Climatol Assoc* 1937;53:153.

Salant DJ: ANCA: Fuel for the fire or the spark that ignites the flame? *Kidney Int* 1999;55:1125.

Segerer S et al: Chemokines, chemokine receptors, and renal disease: From basic science to pathophysiologic and therapeutic studies. *J Am Soc Nephrol* 2000;11:152.

Sheerin NS et al: Altered distribution of intraglomerular immune complexes in C3-deficient mice. *Immunology* 1999;97:393.

Yamazaki H et al.: All four putative ligand-binding domains in megalin contain pathogenic epitopes capable of inducing passive Heymann nephritis. *J Am Soc Nephrol* 1998;9:1638.

SPECIFIC IMMUNE-MEDIATED RENAL DISEASE

Bolton WK et al: Goodpasture's syndrome. *Kidney Int* 1996; 50:1753.

Foster MH, Kelley VR: Lupus nephritis: Update on pathogenesis and disease mechanisms. *Semin Nephrol* 1999; 19:173.

Guillevin L et al.: Microscopic polyangiitis—Clinical and laboratory findings in eighty-five patients. *Arthritis Rheum* 1999;42:421.

Johnson RJ et al.: Renal manifestations of hepatitis C virus infection. *Kidney Int* 1994;46:1255.

Montseny JJ et al: The current spectrum of infectious glomerulonephritis: Experience with 76 patients and review of the literature. *Medicine* 1995;74:63.

Dermatologic Diseases

37

Neil J. Korman, PhD, MD

A large and growing number of autoimmune skin diseases are characterized by **skin blisters.** They are among the most intriguing, well-characterized and potentially serious skin diseases known. The clinical presentation, morphology, and lesion distribution of blistering diseases are important in developing a working diagnosis. Absolute diagnosis requires histologic, immunopathologic, immunochemical, and ultrastructural studies. It has become increasingly clear that the associated **autoantibodies** bind to specific structures within the skin (Figures 37–1 and 37–2) and their discovery has revolutionized the understanding and classification of these diseases. Furthermore, these autoantibodies, which may also be found circulating in the blood, serve as important diagnostic markers, and they have been used to identify and characterize several cell adhesion proteins in the skin.

The most accurate diagnostic features for routine histology are obtained from skin biopsies that sample early lesions including inflamed skin or small vesicles. **Direct immunofluorescence,** which detects antibodies bound to the skin, should be performed on perilesional, unaffected skin. **Indirect immunofluorescence** detects the presence of circulating antibodies that are directed against molecules found in the skin.

BULLOUS PEMPHIGOID

Major Immunologic Features
- Linear deposition of IgG and C3 at the dermal-epidermal junction
- Circulating IgG binds to bullous pemphigoid antigens in the lamina lucida of the dermal-epidermal junction

General Considerations
A. Definition: Bullous pemphigoid is characterized by tense, often pruritic blisters on the flexor surfaces of the extremities, axilla, groin, and lower abdomen. Characteristic deposition of IgG or C3 or both occurs at the dermal–epidermal junction, without which the diagnosis is in question.

B. Etiology: In vivo and in vitro models suggest that the binding of IgG to bullous pemphigoid antigens (named for the disease) at the lamina lucida of the dermal–epidermal junction is an initiating event in the disease. **Autoantibodies** in bullous pemphigoid recognize two distinct keratinocyte hemidesmosomal proteins named BP 230 (BPAG1) and BP 180 (BPAG2). BP 230 is a cytoplasmic protein, whereas BP 180 is a transmembrane protein, whose clinically relevant epitopes map to a short region between an extracellular collagenous domain and the transmembrane domain. The genes for BP 230 and BP 180 are located on chromosomes 6 and 10, respectively. The primary stimulus for production of the autoantibody is unknown. The disease has been passively transferred to animals by the injection of antibody from patients. Immunohistochemical studies also demonstrate activation of both the classical and alternative complement pathways. Antibody, complement, and mast cell activation in situ cause influx of inflammatory cells, including eosinophils, into the area. The release of mediators from inflammatory cells, including proteolytic enzymes, may contribute to characteristic separation of the epidermis from the dermis. The typical distribution of lesions on the body surface may correlate with the regional distribution and concentration of the bullous pemphigoid antigen.

C. Prevalence: Bullous pemphigoid is an uncommon but not rare disease. There is no sex or race predominance. Although occasionally identified in children, it is primarily a disease of individuals 60 years of age or older. There are no known patterns of inheritance or HLA associations.

Pathology
Biopsy specimens (3–4 mm in diameter) obtained from the edge of a fresh blister containing perilesional skin reveal a subepidermal bulla with inflammatory infiltrate that may be eosinophil-rich (Figure 37–3). The epidermis is intact and not necrotic. Biopsy of older lesions may give the false appearance of an intraepidermal blister if the epidermis has begun to regenerate. The dermal infiltrate will vary depending on whether the base of the clinical lesion is grossly inflamed or normal, the former being char-

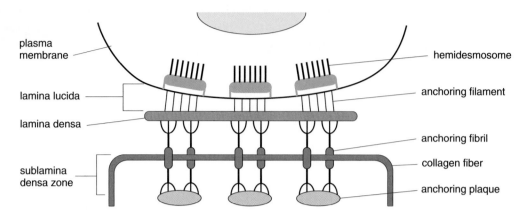

Figure 37–1. Schematic of epithelial basement membrane zone indicates major regions and structures. The lamina lucida is the electron-lucent region just below the keratinocyte plasma membrane and just above the electron-dense lamina densa. Skin incubated in 1 mol/L NaCl splits through the lamina lucida. (Reproduced and modified, with permission, from Gammon WR et al: Immunofluorescence on split skin for the detection and differentiation of basement membrane zone autoantibodies. *J Am Acad Dermatol* 1992;27:79.)

acterized by an infiltrate in the papillary dermis similar to that seen in the blister cavity.

Clinical Features

A. Signs and Symptoms: The classic lesion of bullous pemphigoid is a tense blister of 1 cm or more diameter on a normal or erythematous base (Figure 37–4). The tenseness of the blisters usually correlates with the thickness of the blister roof, which in bullous pemphigoid is full-thickness epidermis (see Figure 37–3). The lesions may be very pruritic, but this varies. Bullae are distributed over the extremities and trunk and may rupture and then heal. Smaller blisters

(vesicles) are sometimes seen (vesicular pemphigoid). Blisters may remain localized to areas such as the lower legs (localized pemphigoid). Elderly patients frequently present with urticarial lesions preceding the eruption of blisters (urticarial pemphigoid). Recognizing these clinical variants suggests the appropriate skin biopsy specimens for routine stains and direct immunofluorescence. Blisters may occur in the oral cavity in up to one third of patients and, rarely, on other mucous membranes, including the esophagus, vagina, and anus.

B. Laboratory Findings: Peripheral eosinophilia and elevated serum IgE have been found in 50% and

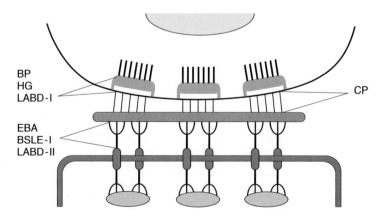

Figure 37–2. Schematic of the epithelial basement membrane zone shows ultrastructural binding sites of basement membrane zone (BMZ) autoantibodies. BP = bullous pemphigoid; BSLE-I = bullous systemic lupus erythematosus type I; CP = cicatricial pemphigoid; EBA = epidermolysis bullosa acquisita; LABD = linear IgA bullous disease. (Reproduced and modified, with permission, from Gammon WR et al: Immunofluorescence on split skin for the detection and differentiation of basement membrane zone autoantibodies. *J Am Acad Dermatol* 1992;27:79.)

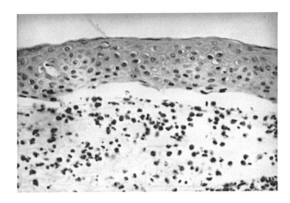

Figure 37–3. Histopathology of bullous pemphigoid. Note the full thickness of epidermis that makes up the blister roof. (Courtesy of Philip LeBoit.)

70% of patients, respectively, and may correlate with disease activity.

Immunologic Diagnosis

Direct immunofluorescence studies of normal-appearing or erythematous nonbullous perilesional skin reveal linear basement membrane zone (BMZ) deposits of IgG (Figure 37–5) and C3 in the majority of patients, as well as in epidermolysis bullosa acquisita, mucous membrane pemphigoid, herpes gestationis, and bullous eruption of systemic lupus erythematosus. Approximately 70% of patients have circulating IgG antibodies that bind to the basement membrane. Similar findings may also be observed in patients with epidermolysis bullosa acquisita so that distinction between the two disease requires special studies, such as indirect immunofluorescence utilizing **salt-split skin,** in which normal human skin is treated with 1.0 M NaCl solution for three days. This causes a split within the epidermal basement membrane so that most bullous pemphigoid antibodies will bind to the epidermal side only, whereas all epidermolysis bullosa acquisita antibodies will bind solely to the dermal side. Approximately 85–95% of

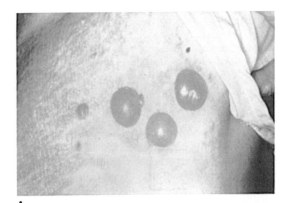

A

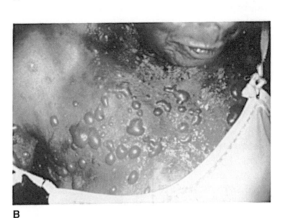

B

Figure 37–4. A: Tense blisters on a red base on the back of a patient with bullous pemphigoid. **B:** Multiple blisters on the chest of a patient. (Courtesy of Richard Odom.)

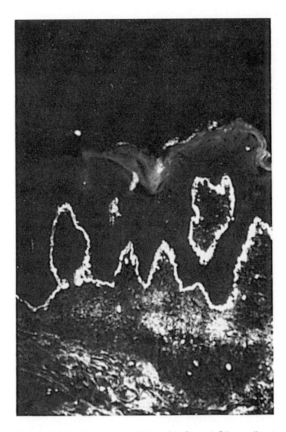

Figure 37–5. Linear deposition of IgG and C3 on direct immunofluorescence of lesional skin. (Courtesy of Richard Odom.)

patients with bullous pemphigoid have circulating IgG autoantibodies by this method.

Differential Diagnosis

Several diseases are characterized by blistering and may more often be distinguished from bullous pemphigoid by immunofluorescence and histopathology than by clinical features and natural course. In elderly patients with tense blisters, a subepidermal blister on light microscopy and the linear BMZ deposition of IgG or C3 or both on direct immunofluorescence is very suggestive of the diagnosis. However, indirect immunofluorescence studies demonstrating circulating IgG antibody binding to the roof or to both the roof and base of salt-split skin are required to absolutely confirm the diagnosis of bullous pemphigoid. The same clinical, histologic, and immunologic features in a young woman who is pregnant or taking oral contraceptive drugs, however, strongly suggests the diagnosis of herpes gestationis. A bullous drug eruption may be similar histologically but has negative immunofluorescence studies. Bullous erythema multiforme often has a few target, or bull's eye, lesions with central blisters but distinct histologic and usually negative or nonspecific immunofluorescence findings. Mucous membrane pemphigoid, dermatitis herpetiformis, pemphigus vulgaris, epidermolysis bullosa acquisita, and porphyria cutanea tarda are distinguished from bullous pemphigoid on clinical grounds and laboratory findings.

Treatment

Localized disease can often be treated successfully with low-dose steroids. Mild generalized disease is usually treated successfully with low-dose prednisone (approximately 0.5 mg/kg/day, in a single morning dose). More severe disease requires moderate dose prednisone (0.75–1.25 mg/kg/day), in a single morning dose, tapering to an alternate-day regimen as the disease comes under control. Patients with contraindications to systemic therapy may be treated with dapsone, a combination of tetracycline and nicotinamide, or immunosuppressive drugs, particularly azathioprine (1.0–1.5 mg/kg/day). Older patients with severe disease can often be successfully treated with moderate-dose prednisone and azathioprine. Mycophenolate mofetil has also been used successfully. Progressive uncontrollable disease may require moderate- to high-dose prednisone with cyclophosphamide or chlorambucil, pulse steroids, and plasmapheresis.

Prognosis

Bullous pemphigoid is usually a self-limited disease with a benign, if sometimes prolonged, course. Factors predictive of prognosis have been difficult to identify; however, recent studies demonstrated a correlation between the amount of anti-BP180 antibodies and disease severity. Fatal complications may arise in the oldest and most debilitated patients. The key to successful management is adequate control of the disease while avoiding the complications of systemic corticosteroids. Patients with bullous pemphigoid were in the past thought to have an increased prevalence of age-associated cancers, but recent data have refuted this impression.

MUCOUS MEMBRANE PEMPHIGOID

Major Immunologic Feature
- Linear deposits of IgG and C3 and sometimes IgA at the submucosal–epithelial junction

Cicatricial pemphigoid (**mucous membrane pemphigoid**) refers to a group of subepithelial blistering diseases involving primarily mucosal surfaces and, occasionally, the skin. The lesions frequently, but not always, heal with scarring, which often is responsible for the major morbidity. Involved mucosae include oral, ocular, nasopharyngeal, laryngeal, anogenital, and esophageal. The histology of mucous membrane pemphigoid consists of a subepidermal blister with an inflammatory cell infiltrate. Direct immunofluorescence may reveal linear deposits of IgG, IgA, and C3 at the epidermal basement membrane. Indirect immunofluorescence may reveal circulating IgG or IgA antibodies (or both) depending on the type and number of substrates used and the clinical phenotype. The majority of patients have antibodies that bind to the epidermal side of split skin. Recent sophisticated immunopathologic and immunochemical studies have uncovered several distinct **subgroups.** Patients with antibodies directed against laminin have circulating IgG autoantibodies that bind to the dermal side of salt-split skin and recognize epiligrin, now known as laminin-5, and occasionally laminin-6. Patients with pure ocular disease in the absence of skin, oral, or other mucous membrane disease rarely have circulating IgG antibodies, have no antibody to any defined BMZ antigens, but many have IgG antibodies directed against the β_4-integrin. Patients with both mucosal disease and skin lesions tend to have circulating IgG antibodies to bullous pemphigoid antigens. Finally, a heterogeneous group of patients have oral mucosal disease with or without ocular or other mucosal disease but no skin disease.

Mucous membrane pemphigoid is a chronic disease, and treatment should be directed to the involved organs. Disease limited to the nasopharynx or oropharynx may be treated with topical or intralesional steroids, short bursts of oral corticosteroids, or dapsone. If the eyes, esophagus, or larynx become involved, morbidity can be severe, including blindness and asphyxiation; therefore, aggressive therapy with systemic corticosteroids and immunosuppressive drugs is warranted. Cyclophosphamide has been most effective in the treatment of patients with severe involvement, and the majority go into clinical remission after an 18–24-month course.

HERPES GESTATIONIS

Major Immunologic Features
- The third component of complement is always, and IgG is occasionally, deposited linearly along the dermal-epidermal junction of a perilesional skin biopsy.
- Frequently, circulating IgG antibodies avidly bind complement

General Considerations
A. Definition: Herpes gestationis is characterized by extremely pruritic vesicles and bullae appearing during pregnancy. *Herpes* is the Greek word meaning "to creep," but this disease has no association with herpes simplex virus or varicella-zoster virus. Because it shares several features in common with bullous pemphigoid, it is sometimes called pemphigoid gestationis.

B. Etiology: The primary stimulus for antibody production is unknown, but the antigen is the same BP 180 (BPAG2) epidermal basement membrane hemidesmosomal protein that is one of the target antigens in bullous pemphigoid. The onset of herpes gestationis appears to require placental tissue, choriocarcinoma, or hydatidiform moles; recurrences may be caused by exogenous estrogen alone. Antibodies to placental tissue in these patients do not cross-react with those to the skin, but they do react with the amnion epithelial basement membrane of second-trimester and full-term placentas, although the significance of this finding is unclear. Activation of the classical complement pathway may be involved in the blistering.

C. Prevalence: Herpes gestationis is rare, ranging from 1:3000–1:10,000 births in early studies to 1:50,000 births in recent studies. There have been few reports in blacks, which may reflect their lower frequency of HLA-DR4. Between 61% and 83% of patients have the HLA-DR3 haplotype, and 45% have both HLA-DR3 and DR4, compared with 3% of women in the general population. However, the HLA type does not correlate with duration, severity, or recurrence of disease or with antibody titer. Abnormal regulation of anti-HLA idiotype antibodies during pregnancy was demonstrated in one patient, but the prevalence and significance of this defect is unknown.

Pathology
The "classic" light microscopy of a subepidermal bulla with eosinophils in the blister cavity is seen in only a minority of cases. The papillary dermis shows edema and a mixed perivascular lymphohistiocytic infiltrate with eosinophils. Spongiosis (edema be-

tween epidermal cells), with or without eosinophils, liquefactive degeneration, or necrosis in the epidermis may be present. Eosinophils are an important histologic feature when present (Figure 37-6A).

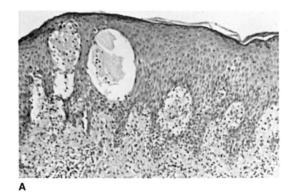

A

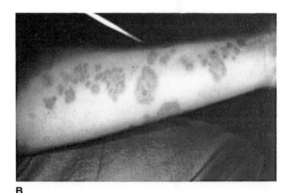

B

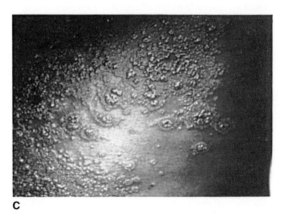

C

Figure 37–6. A: Histopathology of herpes gestationis showing early subepidermal blister formation. The tear-drop-shaped vesicle at the left is characteristic of early herpes gestationis. (Courtesy of Philip LeBoit.) **B:** Hive-like and ringed lesions with vesicular edges on the arm of a patient with herpes gestationis. (Courtesy of Richard Odom.) **C:** Rings of vesicles at the edges of plaques in herpes gestationis. (Courtesy of Richard Odom.)

Clinical Features

A. Signs and Symptoms: The onset is usually in the second or third trimester; in 20% of cases it occurs in the first few days postpartum. **Intense pruritus** accompanies and at times precedes the eruption, which often begins around the umbilicus or on the extremities as hive-like plaques, blisters, or rings of vesicles at the edges of hive-like plaques (see Figures 37–6B and 37–6C). The disease may worsen at delivery. It tends to recur with subsequent pregnancies and lasts for weeks to months postpartum, occasionally flaring with ovulation, menstruation, or use of oral contraceptives. Lactation may shorten the natural course of untreated postpartum skin disease. Barring secondary bacterial infection, the blisters heal without scarring.

B. Laboratory Findings: Routine investigations are not clinically useful. Peripheral eosinophilia may occur, with an elevated erythrocyte sedimentation rate. Serum complement concentrations are usually normal.

Immunologic Diagnosis

A skin biopsy specimen obtained at the edge of a fresh blister for direct immunofluorescence testing reveals linear deposition of C3 at the epidermal BMZ in virtually all cases. IgG is also found in 25%. Routine indirect immunofluorescence studies are usually negative, but when positive, the pattern is identical to that seen in bullous pemphigoid. The complement fixation assay is positive in about 50% of cases.

Differential Diagnosis

The onset of pruritic, hive-like plaques with tense blisters in a pregnant woman requires punch biopsy specimens for light and immunofluorescence microscopy to confirm the diagnosis. Diseases causing pruritus and hive-like rashes must be ruled out by histology and immunofluorescence in cases of herpes gestationis prior to the appearance of blisters. These include atopic dermatitis, scabies, and dry skin. A large number of poorly defined pruritic cutaneous syndromes are reported in pregnant women. Hive-like or edematous plaques may be caused by pruritic urticarial papules and plaques of pregnancy (which, unlike herpes gestationis, typically spares the umbilicus), urticaria, and erythema multiforme.

Treatment & Prognosis

Treatment should be undertaken in collaboration with the patient's obstetrician. Prednisone at 40–60 mg/day controls the disease in most cases within a week. If not, higher or divided doses may be necessary. The dose is then slowly tapered over several weeks to a maintenance dose. Some patients improve spontaneously in the third trimester, but the condition flares at delivery. Cytotoxic immunosuppressive drugs should be avoided during pregnancy. Antihistamines have little, if any, effect.

Herpes gestationis often recurs in subsequent pregnancies, and then it may appear earlier. Skin lesions in infants are uncommon and usually transient, requiring no therapy. Early studies suggested an increased fetal mortality rate, but subsequent studies have not supported this. There is an increased probability of low birth weight and premature infants, so delivery should be performed in a facility that has a neonatal intensive care unit.

EPIDEMOLYSIS BULLOSA ACQUISITA

Major Immunologic Feature

- IgG and, less frequently, IgA, IgM, and C3 linearly deposited at the BMZ in the sublamina densa zone

General Considerations

Epidermolysis bullosa acquisita is a blistering disease marked by skin fragility. It occurs on noninflamed skin over the distal extremities and heals with scarring. Immunoelectron microscopy detects linear immunoglobulin deposits in the sublamina densa zone of the dermal-epidermal junction. These may also be seen by salt-split skin immunofluorescence microscopy on the dermal side of the dermal-epidermal junction.

The cause is unknown. The epidermolysis bullosa acquisita antigen is the globular carboxy terminus of type VII procollagen, which is also synthesized by epidermal cells and fibroblasts in culture. Aggregates of type VII collagen form the anchoring fibrils that bind the epidermis and dermis together. In vitro organ culture models of the disease indicate that epidermolysis bullosa acquisita antibody fixes complement and directs an influx of leukocytes into the skin, resulting in epidermal-dermal separation.

Pathology

A subepidermal blister is present. Other features, especially the dermal infiltrate, are variable and correlate with clinical characteristics.

Clinical Features

A. Signs and Symptoms: Epidermolysis bullosa acquisita is a disease of adult onset with two distinct presentations. The classic presentation involves acral skin fragility and blisters, which heal with scarring and milia. Alternatively, almost half of all patients have widespread vesicles and bullae on red or inflamed bases; these are associated with pruritus, erosion, and erythematous plaques. The lesions may be accentuated in skin folds and flexural areas. This second presentation resembles bullous pemphigoid. Both presentations may occur during the evolution of the disease. Some patients also have nail changes, oral lesions, or scarring in the scalp, leading to hair loss. Epidermolysis bullosa acquisita may be significantly associated with inflammatory bowel disease, particularly Crohn's disease.

B. Laboratory Findings: Routine tests and urine porphyrin levels are normal.

Immunologic Diagnosis

Direct immunofluorescence examination of perilesional skin demonstrates a broad linear band of IgG, C3, and, occasionally, other immune deposits at the dermal-epidermal junction, but these are not pathognomonic. However, 25–50% of patients have positive indirect immunofluorescence of the BMZ below stratified squamous epithelium; the autoantibodies do not cross-react with the lungs and kidneys. Salt-split skin indirect immunofluorescence shows characteristic staining on the dermal side, which helps define epidermolysis bullosa acquisita. In the absence of positive indirect immunofluorescence, immunoelectron microscopy localizes the immune deposits to the sublamina densa fibrillar zone.

Differential Diagnosis

Family history and immunofluorescence testing help rule out the hereditary form of epidermolysis bullosa. Noninflammatory lesions may clinically and histologically be confused with those of porphyria cutanea tarda, which can be diagnosed by 24-hour urinary porphyrin excretion and the finding of immune deposits in dermal vessels. Bullous pemphigoid may be similar clinically and histologically to one presentation of epidermolysis bullosa acquisita. However, immunoelectron microscopy, indirect immunofluorescence on split-skin substrates, the presence or absence of scarring and milia, and the response to treatment aid in distinguishing between the two diseases. The bullous eruption of systemic lupus erythematosus (SLE) may be very difficult to distinguish from epidermolysis bullosa acquisita by clinical and histologic features, immunofluorescence testing, and Western immunoblot analysis of patient sera against epidermolysis bullosa acquisita antigen. However, bullous SLE responds more readily to dapsone, has less skin fragility, heals without scars and milia, and tends to have a more granular staining pattern at the dermal-epidermal junction on direct immunofluorescence.

Treatment

Management is difficult because patients respond poorly to topical and systemic corticosteroid therapy, even with the addition of dapsone, colchicine, and various immunosuppressive drugs. Treatment with cyclosporin A has shown promising results but must be undertaken with great caution because of its nephrotoxicity. Extracorporeal photopheresis has recently been found of value in a few patients and has few side effects. Local measures to promote cleanliness, control infections, and minimize trauma are important.

Prognosis

Epidermolysis bullosa acquisita is a chronic, nonremitting disease with morbidity from painful erosions of blisters that heal with scarring.

DERMATITIS HERPETIFORMIS

Major Immunologic Features

- Granular deposits of IgA and complement components at the dermal-epidermal junction in dermal papillae in lesional and normal-appearing skin
- Critical sensitivity to dietary gluten

General Considerations

Dermatitis herpetiformis is characterized by pruritic grouped papules, papulovesicles, and vesicles and the granular deposition of IgA in dermal papillae at the dermal-epidermal junction. The stimuli that produce IgA antibodies found on the skin, the antigen(s) to which they are bound, and cellular and biochemical causes of the disease remain to be determined. The IgA antibody does not react with gluten or gliadin and may be found in clinically normal-appearing skin. It is presumed that the primary stimulus for the disease occurs in the gastrointestinal tract.

Prevalence estimates are 10–37 persons/100,000 in Scandinavia, but much lower in Japan. Between 80% and 95% of patients with granular deposits of IgA in normal skin have the HLA-B8 haplotype, and up to 95% have HLA-DR3. More than 90% of patients may express the HLA antigen DQw2. The strongest HLA associations on a molecular level are with HLA-DQB1*0201 and HLA-DQA1*0501 and HLA-DRB1*0301, as seen with gluten-sensitive enteropathy. The association with HLA-DP antigens is weaker than with HLA-DQw2 or HLA-DR3. HLA-DB8 is also associated with "ordinary" gluten-sensitive enteropathy without skin lesions (see Chapter 35).

Pathology

Light microscopy of early papules or fresh, unbroken vesicles reveals neutrophils at the dermal papillary tips in early lesions that may evolve into subepidermal blisters. Eosinophils and a mild perivascular lymphohistiocytic infiltrate may be seen. Older vesicles and crusted lesions may yield nondiagnostic findings.

Clinical Features

Grouped red papules, hive-like plaques, and vesicles symmetrically distributed on the elbows and knees, upper back, buttocks, and posterior neck and scalp (Figure 37–7) are helpful in making the diagnosis. The lesions are **extremely pruritic** or may burn or sting. It is uncommon for patients to present with intact vesicles because the extreme pruritus leads to severe scratching and erosions.

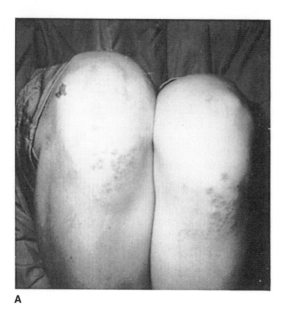
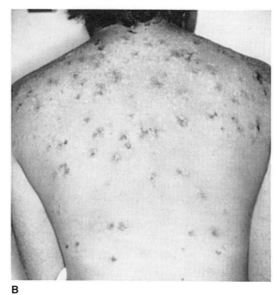

A

B

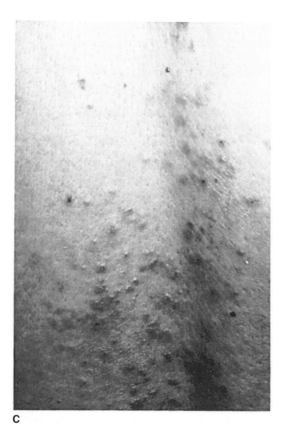
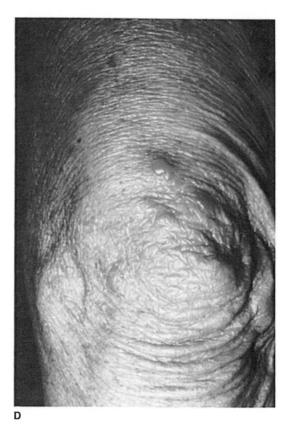

C

D

Figure 37–7. Dermatitis herpetiformis. **A** and **B:** Typical distribution of lesions on knees and upper back. (Courtesy of Richard Odom.) **C:** Papular lesions on the middle of the back. (Courtesy of John Reeves.) **D:** Close-up view of papulovesicular lesions on elbow. (Courtesy of John Reeves.)

There are no diagnostic laboratory findings. Endoscopy with biopsy or radiographic studies may detect signs of gluten-sensitive enteropathy, but this is neither clinically useful nor necessary for diagnosis or management. Both hyperthyroidism and hypothyroidism occur more frequently in patients with dermatitis herpetiformis.

Immunologic Diagnosis

Direct immunofluorescence of normal-appearing perilesional skin reveals granular deposits of polyclonal IgA along dermal papillae in all patients, and this defines the disease (Figure 37–8). IgA may not always be found in lesional skin. C3 may also be found.

Differential Diagnosis

Other vesicular diseases include varicella, herpes simplex, and herpes zoster. Cytologic smears and cultures, as well as the nongrouped or asymmetric distribution of lesions in these diseases, distinguish them from dermatitis herpetiformis. A clinically similar disease with different HLA associations, called linear IgA disease, is characterized by linear deposits of IgA in or below the lamina lucida of the BMZ. Direct immunofluorescence can also rule out diseases such as bullous pemphigoid and herpes gestationis, although they are usually distinguishable clinically as well.

Treatment

Although difficult to achieve, strict **avoidance of dietary gluten** may control the disease entirely after 1–4 years, lower the dosage of sulfones required, and clear skin IgA deposits after more than a decade. Dapsone, 100–200 mg/day can completely control the skin disease in most patients. Erythrocyte G6PD deficiency must be ruled out prior to therapy with dapsone. Patients on dapsone must be monitored for hemolysis (which may occur at high doses even in patients with normal G6PD levels) and methemoglobinemia, as well as for hepatic, renal, and neurologic complications of therapy.

Prognosis & Associated Diseases

Dermatitis herpetiformis is a chronic disease unless dietary avoidance of gluten is maintained. Even after lesions have cleared, reintroduction of gluten results rapidly in disease exacerbation. Lesions heal without scarring, although pigmentary changes may remain. There are reported associations of dermatitis herpetiformis with antigastric parietal cell antibodies, gastric hypochlorhydria or achlorhydria, antithyroid antibodies, IgA nephropathy, and, possibly, gastrointestinal lymphoma.

LINEAR IGA BULLOUS DERMATOSIS

Major Immunologic Feature
• Linear BMZ deposits of IgA

Linear IgA bullous dermatosis is an acquired autoimmune blistering skin disease that in the past was considered a variant type of dermatitis herpetiformis. It may resemble dermatitis herpetiformis or bullous pemphigoid. It occurs with increased frequency in patients older than 60 years of age, but it may also be seen throughout adulthood. A blistering disease known as chronic bullous disease of childhood is the childhood counterpart of linear IgA bullous disease. Lesions consist of papulovesicles or blisters along with urticarial plaques. Some patients have an arcuate pattern with a "cluster of jewels" grouping of blisters. Patients with linear IgA bullous disease do not have any gastrointestinal disease, an increased frequency of the HLA-B8/DRW3 phenotype, or benefit from a gluten-free diet. The lesions are more generalized than are those in dermatitis herpetiformis and are not usually symmetric. Oral mucous membrane lesions are frequent. Occasional ocular involvement with subsequent scarring may occur that is very similar to that found in mucous membrane pemphigoid.

The histology of subepidermal vesicles with eosinophil or neutrophil predominance is very similar to that of bullous pemphigoid and dermatitis herpetiformis. Neutrophilic microabscesses may also be seen. Direct immunofluorescence studies reveal a predominance of linear IgA deposits at the BMZ in all patients. Some may also have less intense linear BMZ deposits of IgG, C, and IgM. Indirect immunofluorescence studies demonstrate the presence of IgA anti-BMZ antibodies in 30–50% when monkey esophagus or human skin is used as the substrate. When salt-split human skin is used as the substrate, circulating IgA anti-BMZ antibodies usually bind to the epidermal side in 80–90% of patients. Sera from patients with linear IgA bullous dermatosis contain IgA

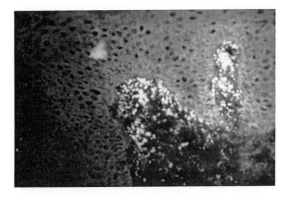

Figure 37–8. Direct immunofluorescence of perilesional skin demonstrates IgA deposition in dermal papillae in dermatitis herpetiformis. (Courtesy of Richard Odom.)

antibodies that recognize a molecule originally called LAD-1, now known to be a portion of the 180-kd BPAG2.

Treatment of linear IgA bullous disease depends on the severity of disease and the areas of involvement. Most patients with disease limited to the skin respond very well to dapsone. Sometimes a partial response to dapsone will improve with the addition of prednisone. Interferon alfa has been used to manage severe disease that only partially responded to prednisone and dapsone. Conjunctival involvement, which may be indistinguishable from mucous membrane pemphigoid, requires aggressive therapy with both prednisone and cyclophosphamide to prevent ocular scarring.

PEMPHIGUS VULGARIS & PEMPHIGUS FOLIACEOUS

Major Immunologic Features
- IgG deposited on the epidermal cell surface
- Circulating IgG antibody binds to the cell surface of stratified squamous epithelium

General Considerations

Pemphigus vulgaris and pemphigus foliaceous are described together because they are blistering diseases characterized by acantholysis and the deposition of cell surface autoantibodies. They may be distinguished clinically, histologically, and immunologically.

Pemphigus vulgaris and pemphigus foliaceous are characterized by widespread **blistering** and **denudation** of skin and mucous membranes. They have a distinctive histopathology of **acantholysis** (loss of cohesion) of epidermal cells and a typical direct immunofluorescence pattern. The lesion is superficial in pemphigus foliaceous and deeper in pemphigus vulgaris.

A. Etiology: A large body of clinical and experimental evidence demonstrates that pemphigus autoantibodies are pathogenic. Circulating antibody titers correlate with disease activity in many patients, and treatment with plasmapheresis has induced short-term remissions in some. Neonatal pemphigus vulgaris, which resolves spontaneously by several months of age is consistent with transplacental maternal pemphigus IgG antibody as the cause. Treatment of skin in organ culture with pemphigus vulgaris or pemphigus foliaceous IgG (without complement or inflammatory cells) leads to epidermal acantholysis (in the suprabasilar and granular layer, respectively). In this system, acantholysis is mediated by the release of a protease thought to be plasminogen activator. Finally, neonatal mice injected with either pemphigus foliaceous or pemphigus vulgaris IgG antibodies develop the clinical, histologic, and immunopathologic features of the corresponding subtype of pemphigus.

The specificity of antibodies for keratinocyte cell surface molecules has been studied and found to involve molecular complexes that contain adhering junction molecules. Patients with pemphigus vulgaris have circulating autoantibodies directed against a 130-kd cadherin, desmoglein III, a desmosomal protein that is bound to plakoglobin, an 85-kd molecule of desmosomes and adherens junctions. Patients with pemphigus foliaceous have circulating autoantibodies directed against desmoglein I, a 160-kd desmosomal protein, which is also bound to plakoglobin. Although the exact sequence of events after pemphigus antibody binds to the epidermal cell surface is unknown, there is evidence to support a role for proteolytic enzymes and complement activation. Thus, pemphigus autoantibodies probably interfere directly with assembly or function of cell adhesion junctions and, thereby, lead to blister formation.

B. Epidemiology: Pemphigus vulgaris occurs predominantly but not exclusively in persons of Jewish or Mediterranean ancestry. It may occur in all age groups, with an incidence of 0.5–3.2 cases/100,000/year but is more common in the fourth and fifth decades and is rare after age 60. The familial occurrence of pemphigus has been reported in 25 families.

C. Genetics: HLA-A10 was first identified as being more commonly represented among patients with pemphigus vulgaris than in the general population. More recently it has been shown that 95% of pemphigus vulgaris patients are HLA-DR4/DQw3 or HLA-DRw6/DQw1, and it is thought that pemphigus may segregate with DQ alleles. In a series of 13 DQw1-positive patients with pemphigus vulgaris, all were identified as positive for an allele designated PV6 allele in codon 57, where asparagine replaces valine or serine.

Pathology

Skin biopsy shows a suprabasal intraepidermal blister with loss of cohesion of keratinocytes (acantholysis) in pemphigus vulgaris (Figure 37–9) and a superficial subcorneal or subgranular acantholytic blister in pemphigus foliaceous.

Clinical Features

Pemphigus vulgaris is characterized by blisters that most commonly affect the scalp, chest, umbilicus, and body folds (Figure 37–10). In contrast to the lesions of bullous pemphigoid, these blisters are flaccid and fragile because the epidermal split occurs within the epidermis, resulting in a thinner roof (see Figure 37–9). Lesions may easily rupture, and in some cases only crusts and no blisters are seen. Oral lesions may be initial or, uncommonly, the only presentation of the disease. Nikolsky's sign (sloughing of the epidermis after lateral pressure with a cotton applicator or tongue blade) is positive in involved skin. Pemphigus foliaceous, with its more superficial

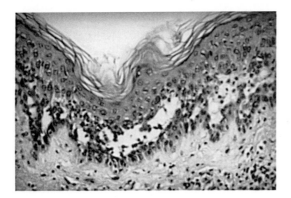

Figure 37–9. Histopathology of pemphigus vulgaris demonstrates intraepidermal blister formation with loss of cohesion of keratinocytes (acantholysis). (Courtesy of Philip LeBoit.)

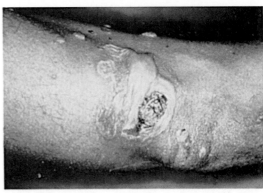

A

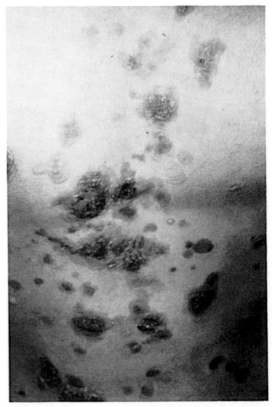

B

histologic process of blistering, may show only scaly, crusted, and superficial erosions without frank blisters. Oral lesions are rare in pemphigus foliaceous. Routine laboratory tests are not helpful in diagnosis or management.

Immunologic Diagnosis

Direct immunofluorescence reveals the deposition of IgG in virtually all patients and complement components (mostly C3) on the epidermal cell surface forming a honeycomb pattern (Figure 37–11) in 50% of all patients. Between 80 and 90% of patients also have circulating IgG that stains the cell surface of stratified squamous epithelium of monkey esophagus. Monkey esophagus gives the best results for the diagnosis of pemphigus vulgaris; guinea pig esophagus for pemphigus foliaceous.

Differential Diagnosis

Pemphigus vulgaris is suspected in a disease featuring blisters, crusting, and appropriate immunofluorescence studies. Oral lesions may be confused with aphthous ulcers or oral erythema multiforme. Scalp lesions may appear similar to impetigo. Pemphigus vulgaris resembles other pemphigus variants, including pemphigus foliaceous and pemphigus erythematosus, but light microscopy is helpful in this situation. Other blistering eruptions (see earlier discussion) are readily distinguished by clinical appearance (size, grouping, distribution, and tenseness of blisters), histopathology, and immunofluorescence pattern. Because pemphigus vulgaris and pemphigus foliaceous may be sometimes confused with widespread dermatitis or impetigo, persistent empirical treatment without a biopsy often delays the correct diagnosis.

Figure 37–10. A: Flaccid blister on the elbow of a patient with pemphigus vulgaris (compare with the tense blister in bullous pemphigoid in Figure 37–4). **B:** Crusted and bullous lesions on the chest of a patient with pemphigus vulgaris. (Courtesy of Richard Odom.)

Treatment

All patients with pemphigus vulgaris require systemic therapy with glucocorticosteroids, generally prednisone at 1–2 mg/kg/day in a single morning

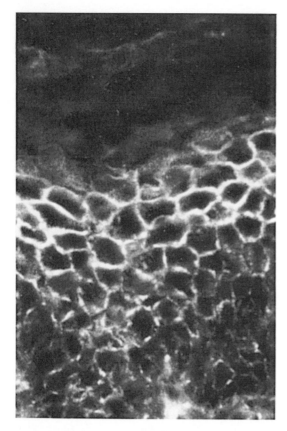

Figure 37–11. Direct immunofluorescence pattern of IgG deposition in pemphigus vulgaris. The immunoglobulins and complement components are deposited in intercellular regions in the epidermis forming a honeycomb pattern. (Courtesy of Denny Tuffanelli.)

dosage, depending on disease severity, then tapering toward an alternate day dosage within 1–3 months as the disease allows. Pemphigus foliaceous patients tend to have a more benign course, can often be treated with lower dosages of glucocorticosteroids, and occasionally respond to topical steroid therapy alone.

Immunosuppressive drugs, most commonly cyclophosphamide and azathioprine, are used, particularly in pemphigus vulgaris, for their steroid-sparing effects. Cyclophosphamide appears to be the more effective, and both have significant toxicities. Mycophenolate mofetil may have less morbidity than cyclophosphamide and azathioprine and has recently been used successfully in pemphigus vulgaris. Other, less effective, steroid-sparing drugs used in pemphigus include dapsone, the combination of tetracycline and niacinamide, hydroxychloroquine sulfate, gold, and cyclosporine. Patients with the most severe disease may be treated with the combinations of systemic glucocorticosteroids, immunosuppressive drugs, and plasmapheresis.

Prognosis & Associated Diseases

Age, extent of disease activity, and duration of disease before treatment all predict the clinical outcome of pemphigus. Elderly patients have a worse prognosis. One large study found that the average age of death within 3 months of the initiation of therapy was 75 years compared with 55 for those surviving the first 3 months of therapy. Patients with generalized disease have a higher mortality rate. Patients with minimal disease activity for prolonged periods do better than patients whose disease rapidly progresses before beginning therapy. Several studies show that the majority of patients who die from pemphigus do so within the first few years of diagnosis.

Although the dose of glucocorticosteroids necessary to control disease has been cited as an important prognostic factor, complications of systemic steroid therapy make it difficult to separate disease-related from treatment-related morbidity and mortality. Systemic glucocorticoid and immunosuppressive therapy has reduced the mortality rate from 60–90% to 5–10%.

Pemphigus may occur in association with myasthenia gravis or thymoma or rarely with other autoimmune diseases. Certain medication, including penicillamine and captopril, may occasionally lead to a drug-related pemphigus.

PARANEOPLASTIC PEMPHIGUS

Major Immunologic Features

- Cell surface deposits of IgG and C3 along with occasional granular basement membrane deposits of C3 on direct immunofluorescence
- Circulating IgG antibodies that bind to cell surface of skin and mucosa in typical pemphigus pattern but in addition bind to simple, columnar and transitional epithelia

Paraneoplastic pemphigus is an autoimmune syndrome that has features reminiscent of both pemphigus vulgaris and erythema multiforme. Patients with this disease have an underlying malignancy, usually **lymphoreticular.** The disease is characterized by ocular and oral blisters and erosions along with generalized skin lesions that may resemble erythema multiforme, toxic epidermal necrolysis, lichen planus, or bullous pemphigoid. There are histologic features of both pemphigus vulgaris and erythema multiforme. Immunofluorescence studies show circulating and tissue bound IgG antibodies that bind to the cell surface of stratified squamous epithelia in a pattern indistinguishable from that of pemphigus antibodies. These circulating IgG antibodies also recognize the cell surface of simple columnar and transitional epithelia such as colon, small bowel, liver, lung, and bladder, in contrast to pemphigus IgG antibodies, which recognize only the cell surface of stratified squamous epithelia. In addition, IgG antibodies that bind to the basement membrane may occur. The circulating antibodies in paraneoplastic pemphigus react with a complex of five proteins of 250, 230, 210, 190, and 170 kd. The 250-kd molecule is desmoplakin I, the 230-kd molecule is bullous pemphigoid antigen I, the 210 band is a doublet consisting of envoplakin and desmoplakin II, the 190-kd molecule is periplakin, and the 170-kd molecule is uncharacterized. Recent studies also demonstrate that some patients have circulating IgG antibodies that also recognize desmoglein I and desmoglein III, the autoantigens found in pemphigus foliaceous, respectively. Although the cause of this severe mucocutaneous disease is poorly understood, it may result from the combination of both a cellular and humoral immune response to tumor antigens that also have overlapping reactivity to normal components of skin and other epithelia.

Paraneoplastic pemphigus must be considered in patients with severe mucocutaneous disease reminiscent of pemphigus who present with atypical features. The patient may not have a known neoplasm at the time of presentation. If paraneoplastic pemphigus is suspected, then a search for an occult neoplasm is warranted. Investigation may be extensive because associated tumors include rare entities such as retroperitoneal sarcoma, thymoma, Waldenström's macroglobulinemia, as well as more commonly recognized ones such as Hodgkin's lymphoma and chronic lymphocytic leukemia.

The prognosis of paraneoplastic pemphigus is related to the type of associated neoplasm. Patients with a benign tumor tend to have remission after the first tumor is resected, whereas those with malignant tumors have a poorer prognosis. The best treatment is removal of the tumor, but, unfortunately in most cases it is malignant. Aggressive regimens that include systemic corticosteroids, cyclophosphamide, azathioprine, cyclosporine, plasmapheresis, and intravenous immunoglobulins have all been used with limited success in the treatment of paraneoplastic pemphigus associated with a malignant neoplasm. This very aggressive therapy has numerous potential complications and should not be undertaken without the collaboration of experienced oncologists. A potentially promising new therapy is immunoablative high-dose cyclophosphamide without stem cell rescue for lymphoma associated paraneoplastic pemphigus.

REFERENCES

BULLOUS PEMPHIGOID

Ahmed AR et al: Bullous pemphigoid: Clinical and immunologic follow-up after successful therapy. *Arch Dermatol* 1977;113:1043.

Berk MA, Lorincz AL: The treatment of bullous pemphigoid with tetracycline and niacinamide. *Arch Dermatol* 1986;122:670.

Bernard P et al: Anti-BP180 autoantibodies as a marker of poor prognosis in bullous pemphigoid: A cohort analysis of 94 elderly patients. *Br J Dermatol* 1997;136:694.

Dubertret L et al. Cellular events leading to blister formation in bullous pemphigoid. *Br J Dermatol* 1980;104:615.

Giudice GJ et al: Cloning and primary structural analysis of the bullous pemphigoid autoantigen BP180. *J Invest Dermatol* 1992;99:243.

Hadi SM et al: Clinical, histological, and immunological studies in 50 patients with bullous pemphigoid. *Dermatologica* 1988;176:6.

Jordon RE et al: Basement membrane zone antibodies in bullous pemphigoid. *JAMA* 1967;200:751.

Korman NJ: Bullous pemphigoid: The latest in diagnosis, prognosis and therapy. *Arch Dermatol* 1998;134:1137.

Meuller S et al: A 230 kd basic protein is the major bullous pemphigoid antigen. *J Invest Dermatol* 1989;92:33.

Nousari HC et al: Successful therapy for bullous pemphigoid with mycophenolate mofetil. *J Am Acad Dermatol* 1998;37:497.

Stanley JR: A specific antigen–antibody interaction triggers the cellular pathophysiology of bullous pemphigoid. *Br J Dermatol* 1985;113(suppl 28):67.

Tanaka M et al: Clinical manifestation in 100 Japanese bullous pemphigoid cases in relation to autoantigen profiles. *Clin Exp Dermatol* 1996;21:23.

Venecie PY et al: Bullous pemphigoid and malignancy: Relationship to indirect immunofluorescence findings. *Acta Dermatol Venereol* (Stockh) 1984;64:316.

Venning VA, Wojnarowska F: Lack of predictive factor for the clinical course of bullous pemphigoid. *J Am Acad Dermatol* 1992;26:585.

Wintroub BU et al: Morphologic and functional evidence for release of mast cell products in bullous pemphigoid. *N Engl J Med* 1978;298:417.

MUCOUS MEMBRANE PEMPHIGOID

Chan LS et al: Immune-mediated subepithelial blistering diseases of mucous membranes. Pure ocular cicatricial pemphigoid is a unique clinical and immunopathological entity distinct form bullous pemphigoid and other subsets identified by antigenic specificities of autoantibodies. *Arch Dermatol* 1993;129:448.

Chan LS et al: Laminin-6 and laminin-5 are recognized by autoantibodies in a subset of cicatricial pemphigoid. *J Invest Dermatol* 1997;108:848.

Domloge-Hultsch N et al: Anti-epiligrin cicatricial pemphigoid. A subepithelial bullous disorder. *Arch Dermatol* 1994;130:1521.

Foster CS: Cicatricial pemphigoid. *Trans Am Ophthalmol Soc* 1986;84:527.

Mutasim DF et al: Cicatricial pemphigoid. *Dermatol Clin* 1993;11:499.

Tyagi S et al: Ocular cicatricial pemphigoid antigen: Partial sequence and biochemical characterization. *Proc Natl Acad Sci U S A* 1996;93:14714.

HERPES GESTATIONIS

Holmes RC, Black MM: The specific dermatoses of pregnancy. *J Am Acad Dermatol* 1983;8:405.

Jordon RE et al: The immunopathology of herpes gestationis: Immunofluorescence studies and characterization of "HG factor." *J Clin Invest* 1976;57:1426.

Katz SI et al: Herpes gestationis: Immunopathology and characterization of the HG factor. *J Clin Ivest* 1976; 57:1434.

Lawley TJ et al: Pruritic urticarial papules and plaques of pregnancy. *JAMA* 1979;241:1696.

Morrison LH et al: Herpes gestationis autoantibodies recognize a 180 kd human epidermal antigen. *J Clin Invest* 1988;81:2023.

Shornick JK et al: Herpes gestationis: Clinical and histologic features of twenty-eight cases. *J Am Acad Dermatol* 1983;8:214.

EPIDERMOLYSIS BULLOSA ACQUISITA

Briggaman RA et al: Epidermolysis bullosa acquisita of the immunopathological type (dermolytic pemphigoid). *J Invest Dermatol* 1985;85(suppl);79.

Crow LL et al: Clearing of epidermolysis bullosa acquisita on cyclosporine. *J Am Acad Dermatol* 1988;19:937.

Gammon WR et al: Epidermolysis bullosa acquisita—A pemphigoid-like disease. *J Am Acad Dermatol* 1984;11: 820.

Gammon WR et al: Direct immunofluorescence studies of sodium chloride-separated skin in the differential diagnosis of bullous pemphigoid and epidermolysis bullosa acquisita. *J Am Acad Dermatol* 1990;22:664.

Gordon KB et al: Treatment of refractory epidermolysis bullosa acquisita with extracorporeal photochemotherapy. *Br J Dermatol* 1997;136:415.

Woodley DT et al: Review and update of epidermolysis bullosa. *Semin Dermatol* 1988;7:111.

DERMATITIS HERPETIFORMIS

Fronek Z et al: Molecular analysis of HLA-DP and DQ genes associated with dermatitis herpetiformis. *J Invest Dermatol* 1991;97:799.

Fry L: Fine points in the management of dermatitis herpetiformis: Recent advances. *J Am Acad Dermatol* 1987;16: 1129.

Kadunce DP et al: The effect of an essential diet with and without gluten on disease activity in dermatitis herpetiformis. *J Invest Dermatol* 1991;97:175.

Katz SI et al: HLA-B8 and dermatitis herpetiformis in patients with IgA deposits in skin. *Arch Dermatol* 1977; 113:155.

Mazzola G et al: Immunoglobulin and HLA-DP genes contribute to the susceptibility to juvenile dermatitis herpetiformis. *Eur J Immunogenet* 1992;19:129.

Otley CC et al: DNA sequence analysis and restriction fragment length polymorphism typing of the HLA-Dqw2 alleles associated with dermatitis herpetiformis. *J Invest Dermatol* 1991;97:318.

LINEAR IgA DISEASE

Chan LS, Cooper KD: Interferon alpha for linear IgA bullous dermatosis. *Lancet* 1992;340:425.

Chorzelski TP et al: Linear IgA bullous dermatosis of adults. *Clin Dermatol* 1992;9:383.

Webster GF et al: Cicatrizing conjunctivitis as a predominant manifestation of linear IgA bullous dermatosis. *J Am Acad Dermatol* 1994;30:355.

Wojnarowska F et al: Chronic bullous disease of childhood, childhood cicatricial pemphigoid, and linear IgA disease of adults. *J Am Acad Dermatol* 1988;19:792.

Zone JJ et al: The 97 kd linear IgA disease antigen is identical to a portion of the extracellular domain of the 180 KD bullous pemphigoid antigen. *J Invest Dermatol* 1998;110:207.

PEMPHIGUS

Ahmed AR et al: Pemphigus-current concepts. *Ann Intern Med* 1980;92:376.

Amagai M et al: Autoantibodies against a novel epithelial cadherin in pemphigus vulgaris, a disease of cell adhesion. *Cell* 1991;67:869.

Anhalt GJ et al: Induction of pemphigus in neonatal mice by passive transfer of IgG from patients with the disease. *N Engl J Med* 1982;306:1189.

Beutner EH, Jordon RE: Demonstration of skin antibodies in sera of pemphigus vulgaris patients by indirect immunofluorescent staining. *Proc Soc Exp Bio Med* 1964;117: 505.

Bystryn JC: Adjuvant therapy of pemphigus. *Arch Dermatol* 1984;120:941.

Enk AH, Knop J: Mycophenolate is effective in the treatment of pemphigus vulgaris. *Arch Dermatol* 1999;135: 54.

Fellner MJ et al: Successful use of cyclophosphamide and prednisone for initial treatment of pemphigus vulgaris. *Arch Dermatol* 1978;114:889.

Judd KP, Lever WF: Correlation of antibodies in skin and serum with disease severity in pemphigus. *Arch Dermatol* 1979;115:428.

Korman NJ: Pemphigus vulgaris, pemphigus foliaceus and paraneoplastic pemphigus. *J Geriatric Dermatol* 1996;4: 53.

Korman NJ et al: Demonstration of an adhering-junction molecule (plakoglobin) in the autoantigens of pemphigus foliaceus and pemphigus vulgaris. *N Engl J Med* 1989; 321:631.

Krain LS: Pemphigus. Epidemiologic and survival characteristics of 59 patients, 1955–1973. *Arch Dermatol* 1974; 110:862.

Lever WF: Pemphigus. *Medicine* 1953;32:1.

Lever WF, Schaumberg-Lever G: Immunosuppressants and prednisone in pemphigus vulgaris. Therapeutic results obtained in 63 patients between 1961 and 1975. *Arch Dermatol* 1977;113:1236.

Lever WF, White H: Treatment of pemphigus with corticosteroids. Results obtained in 46 patients over a period of 11 years. *Arch Dermatol* 1963;87:12.

PARANEOPLASTIC PEMPHIGUS

Anhalt GJ et al: Paraneoplastic pemphigus. *N Engl J Med* 1990;323:1729.

Camisa C et al: Paraneoplastic pemphigus: A report of three cases including one long-term survivor. *J Am Acad Dermatol* 1992;27:547.

Fullerton SH et al: Paraneoplastic pemphigus with autoantibody deposition in bronchial epithelium after autologous bone marrow transplantation. *JAMA* 1992;267:1500.

Joly P et al: Overlapping distribution of autoantibody specificities in paraneoplastic pemphigus and pemphigus vulgaris. *J Invest Dermatol* 1994;103:65.

Kiyokawa C et al: Envoplakin and periplakin are components of the paraneoplastic pemphigus antigen complex. *J Invest Dermatol* 1998;111:1236.

Korman NJ: Paraneoplastic pemphigus: A distinctive autoimmune syndrome. *Med Surg Dermatol* 1995;2:3.

Mehregan DR et al: Paraneoplastic pemphigus: A subset of patients with pemphigus and neoplasia. *J Cut Pathol* 1993;20:203.

Nousari HC et al: Immunoablative high-dose cyclophosphamide without stem cell rescue in paraneoplastic pemphigus: Report of a case and review of this new therapy for severe autoimmune disease. *J Am Acad Dermatol* 1999;49:750.

Rybojad M et al: Paraneoplastic pemphigus in a child with a T-cell lymphoblastic lymphoma. *Br J Dermatol* 1993;128:418.

Su WPD et al: Paraneoplastic pemphigus: A case with high titer of circulating anti-basement zone antibodies. *J Am Acad Dermatol* 1994;30:841.

38

Neurologic Diseases

Olaf Stüve, MD, & Scott S. Zamvil, MD, PhD

In recent years, major advances have been made in understanding how cellular and humoral immune responses contribute to the pathogenesis of many neurologic diseases. Autoimmune mechanisms in which tolerance to self-antigens is compromised are now considered important in the initiation and perpetuation of several of these disorders. One such mechanism is **molecular mimicry,** a process in which the host response to an infectious pathogen elicits immune responses to determinants shared with self antigens. This mechanism is thought to contribute to the pathogenesis of multiple sclerosis and acute disseminated encephalomyelitis, two central nervous system demyelinating diseases, and to Guillain-Barré syndrome, a demyelinating disease of the peripheral nervous system. Traditionally, the brain has been considered an immunologically privileged site separated by the blood-brain barrier. It is now clear, however, that lymphocytes do enter the central nervous system in some disease states and interact with accessory cells in producing pathologic immune responses. Although a majority of studies have emphasized the importance of cellular immune responses in central nervous system demyelinating conditions, recent work has indicated that antibodies to specific myelin antigens may also participate in these conditions. Humoral autoimmunity has a key role in the weakness characteristic of myasthenia gravis, a disease in which autoantibodies to the acetylcholine receptor inhibit neuromuscular transmission. Antibodies to self nervous system tissue antigens are observed in other diseases, including the paraneoplastic syndromes, amyotrophic lateral sclerosis, and some chronic neuropathies, although their significance is uncertain. It is now realized that autoimmune features may also be important in certain forms of stroke and epilepsy, two conditions not previously associated with immune abnormalities. Secondary immune responses may occur in neurodegenerative diseases, such as Alzheimer's disease, although their role in pathogenesis of these conditions is conjectural.

DEMYELINATING DISEASES

Demyelinating diseases are some of the clinically most important neurologic disorders. The pathologic hallmark of demyelinating diseases is their destruction of myelin sheaths surrounding nerve fibers with relative sparing of neurons and axons. Perivascular infiltration of mononuclear cells within demyelinating lesions, T-cell reactivity to myelin proteins, the association of susceptibility with genes within the major histocompatibility complex (MHC), and the favorable clinical response to immune suppression suggest that primary or secondary immune mechanisms participate in the pathogenesis of multiple sclerosis (MS).

MULTIPLE SCLEROSIS

Major Immunologic Features
- Inflammatory demyelination in the central nervous system (CNS) white matter with perivascular infiltration of mononuclear cells
- Cellular and humoral immune responses to myelin antigens
- Association with HLA-DR2
- Response to immunosuppressive and immunomodulatory therapy

General Considerations
MS is a chronic inflammatory demyelinating disease of the central nervous system (CNS), causing relapsing and progressive neurologic disabilities. It is the most common and clinically important demyelinating disease in humans. Approximately 300,000 (0.1%) individuals in the United States have MS. Women are affected twice as often as men. The peak age of onset is between 20 and 40, although less commonly, MS may develop in children and in older individuals. MS susceptibility involves both genetic and environmental factors. Caucasians are more fre-

quently diagnosed with MS than other ethnic groups. The prevalence varies between 50–100 per 100,000 in high-risk areas such as the Scandinavian countries or the northern United States, to less than 5 per 100,000 in Africa and Japan. Individuals that migrate from high-risk to low-risk regions, or vice versa, after age 15 carry their native risk for contracting MS, suggesting that exposure to an environmental factor, possibly one of several different viruses, during adolescence is critical in determining MS susceptibility. Reports regarding localized clusters of MS cases, most notably the outbreak many years ago on the Faroe Islands, have suggested that a transmissible agent may contribute to this illness. Genetic studies have shown that the risk of MS is 10–20 times higher for first-degree relatives of individuals with MS than in the general population. The concordance rate among monozygotic (identical) twins is 30–35% and only 2–5% for a dizygotic (fraternal) twins and other siblings. Studies of multiplex MS families (more than one family member affected) indicate that 15–20 loci may contribute to MS susceptibility. However, linkage to the class II human leukocyte antigen (HLA-D) region of the MHC located on chromosome 6p21 is the most consistently identified factor in genetic studies of MS. The strongest association is with HLA-DR2 (DRB*1501, DQB*0602).

It is thought that activated myelin-reactive CD4 T_H1 cells have a central role in MS pathogenesis. Myelin basic protein, proteolipoprotein, and myelin oligodendrocyte glycoprotein are the three candidate autoantigens most commonly examined. The frequency of activated CD4 T cells that recognize these autoantigens is increased in MS patients. A disproportionate number of activated CD4 T cells occur within MS lesions, especially at the leading (active) edges, although it is unclear if the T cells identified in these lesions have specificity for myelin antigens. Substantial evidence for the role of myelin-specific T cells in CNS demyelinating diseases has been derived from investigations of experimental autoimmune ("allergic") encephalomyelitis (EAE), the archetypal model for MS. Activated CD4 T_H1 cells that recognize one of the candidate myelin antigens mediate EAE, causing relapsing paralysis and CNS demyelination. Concepts regarding the pathogenesis of MS and other organ-specific autoimmune diseases have emerged from EAE studies. For example, it has been observed that induction of EAE by immunization with a major (dominant) determinant of one of these autoantigens, is often followed by recruitment of CD4 T cells that recognize secondary (subdominant or cryptic) determinants of the same autoantigen or a determinant(s) of one of the other encephalitogenic autoantigens. This observation led to development of the concepts of intramolecular and intermolecular determinant spreading, respectively. Evidence indicates that determinant spreading, also known as **repertoire broadening,** is important in the development of relapses in

EAE and may have similar importance in the development and progression of MS and other diseases.

Several immunoregulatory defects occur in MS. Clinical MS exacerbations are associated with relative deficiency in activity of regulatory (suppressor) T_H2 cells that secrete IL-4 and IL-10. Not surprisingly, myelin-reactive T cells from MS patients and CD4 T cells that mediate EAE secrete increased amounts of T_H1 cytokines, interferon-γ, and IL-2. Interferon-γ is required for induction of class II MHC molecules on nonprofessional antigen-presenting cells (APC), including astrocytes and microglia, resident APCs in the CNS that are thought to present myelin antigens to pathogenic T cells. Interferon-γ also causes these APCs to up-regulate expression of B7 (B7-1 and B7-2) molecules, which are required for CD28 T cell costimulation. Convincing evidence for the key role of interferon-γ in this disease emerged from a clinical trial involving patients with relapsing-remitting (RRMS) when it was learned that systemic administration of interferon-γ provoked clinical exacerbations remitting MS. Myelin-specific CD4 T cells in individuals with MS and CD4 T_H1 cells that induce EAE also secrete other important proinflammatory cytokines, such as tumor necrosis factor (TNF), and proinflammatory chemokines. CD4 T cells from MS patients express CD40 ligand, which binds CD40, a costimulatory molecule expressed on some APCs and causes them to produce IL-12, a cytokine that induces secretion of interferon-γ and promotes T_H1 differentiation. Several immunosuppressive medications used in the treatment of MS interfere with the production of these proinflammatory cytokines and down-regulate MHC class II expression on APC.

Whether T cells have a primary role in the initial events leading to myelin destruction is unknown. It is also unclear whether the inciting events occur within or outside the CNS. CD4 T cells recognize antigen in association with MHC class II molecules. The normal CNS is almost devoid of MHC class II molecules, however. Furthermore, the normal brain contains an intact blood-brain barrier (BBB), which is composed of cerebrovascular endothelial cells connected by tight junctions. It is now known that activated, but not resting, lymphocytes can penetrate the BBB and enter the CNS parenchyma. Thus, it is currently thought that through the secretion of interferon-γ and other proinflammatory cytokines, activated myelin-specific T cells that enter the CNS cause up-regulation of MHC class II molecules and costimulatory molecules, which are often detected on astrocytes and microglia within demyelinating MS lesions. What then initiates T-cell activation? In one model, molecular mimicry, infection with a pathogen(s) that contains a protein(s) with amino acid homology or structural similarity to myelin protein antigens may activate these cells, which then enter the CNS (Figure 38–1). Although no one virus has proven to cause MS, several different viruses, including human T-cell lymphotropic virus (HTLV)-1

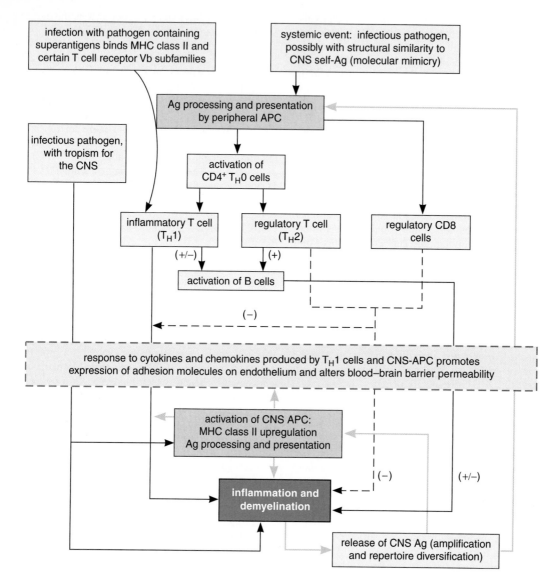

Figure 38–1. Potential mechanisms for induction and progression of inflammation and demyelination in multiple sclerosis. (1) Infectious pathogens, possibly with tropism for the central nervous system (CNS), may participate directly in CNS initial inflammation and demyelination. (2) During systemic infection antigenic components of a pathogen may be presented to CD4 and CD8 T cells by antigen-presenting cells (APC) and infected cells, respectively. If the CNS antigen (Ag) and pathogen share structural similarity or amino acid sequence homology, T cells that recognize myelin (self) antigens may be activated (molecular mimicry). (3) Systemic infection with a pathogen containing superantigen(s) may contact major histocompatibility complex (MHC) class II and T-cell receptor Vβ subfamily utilized by myelin (self) antigen-specific T cells causing their activation. Activated T cells secrete proinflammatory cytokines, penetrate the blood-brain barrier, and activate CNS APC (endothelial cells, astrocytes, microglia, and infiltrating macrophages) to up-regulate MHC class II molecules and present CNS antigens to T cells. Release of myelin antigens during the inflammatory cascade may lead to recruitment of T cells that recognize other myelin antigens (repertoire diversification). Activation of regulatory CD4 (T$_H$2) and CD8 cells that counteract inflammatory immune responses may occur. Inflammatory CD4 T$_H$1 and regulatory CD4 T$_H$2 cells may also activate B cells. It is thought that antibodies secreted by plasma cells could also participate in alteration or damage of myelin sheaths. Black lines and arrows represent immune pathways originating in the systemic circulation, and blue lines and arrows represent immune responses within the CNS. Dotted lines and arrows represent potential regulatory mechanisms.

and other retroviruses, herpesvirus-6, and Epstein-Barr virus have been implicated in MS pathogenesis. In support of molecular mimicry, myelin-specific CD4 T-cell clones from some MS patients react to with proteins derived from some of these viruses, and immunization with specific viral peptides that share homology with myelin proteins can induce EAE. Viruses, possibly with tropism for the CNS, may also cause direct injury to the CNS or disruption of the BBB, facilitating release of CNS autoantigen(s), not normally exposed, in an immunogenic manner, which may lead to expansion of myelin-specific T cells. In this regard, evidence for prior infection has been demonstrated for different viruses by the detection of virus-specific antibodies within the cerebrospinal fluid (CSF) of MS patients and the detection of viral DNA or RNA within their brain tissue or mononuclear cells. The difficulty in establishing an association with one specific virus may reflect the possibility that multiple viruses may be involved in the etiology of MS.

Superantigens (SAgs), proteins produced by certain viruses and bacteria, are potential stimuli that may also participate in the activation of T cells that cause demyelination (Figure 38–2). These proteins

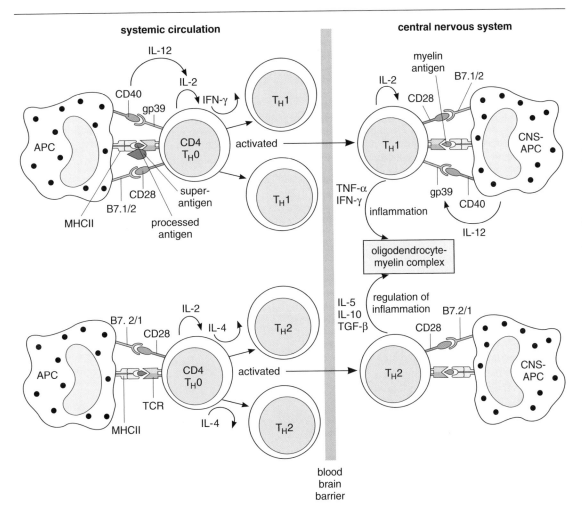

Figure 38–2. Model for activation of encephalitogenic CD4 T_H1 and regulatory CD4 T_H2 cells in central nervous system (CNS) demyelinating disease. First, an antigen (Ag) with amino acid homology or structural similarity to a self-myelin antigen is internalized and processed by peripheral antigen-presenting cells (APC) that express major histocompatibility complex (MHC) class II molecules and costimulatory signals (B7-1, B7-2, CD40). These APC present antigen to CD4 T_H0 cells that differentiate into proinflammatory T_H1 cells or regulatory T_H2 cells. Alternatively, superantigens that contain specificity for the appropriate T-cell receptor V_β subfamily used by encephalitogenic T cells may lead to their activation. After activation, CD4 cells can enter the CNS. On recognition of CNS self-antigen presented by CNS APC, T_H1 cells mediate effector function and secrete inflammatory cytokines. APC may present myelin Ag to T_H2 cells, which in turn secrete regulatory cytokines that counterbalance inflammatory responses. Abbreviations: TCR = T-cell receptor; TNF = tumor necrosis factor; IFN = interferon; IL = interleukin

bind and bridge the MHC class II molecules on APCs with specific T-cell receptor β chains expressed on T cells, leading to T-cell activation in an antigen-non-specific manner. Specific SAgs that bind the subfamily of T-cell receptor Vβ chains used by some encephalitogenic T cells have been shown to induce relapses in EAE. T-cell activation by viral SAgs is also one potential mechanism thought to be involved in MS exacerbations, which commonly occur in association with viral infection.

Although a majority of studies in MS and EAE have emphasized the role of T cells, investigators have examined the role of B cells in these conditions. The presence of elevated intrathecal levels of IgG and oligoclonal bands in approximately 80% of MS patients has suggested a intrinsic CNS humoral immune response. The target antigens for these lymphocytes have never been clearly identified, however. It has also been observed that B-less (μ-knockout) mice are susceptible to EAE and develop CNS demyelinating lesions, indicating that B cells are not obligatory for induction of CNS demyelinating disease. Nevertheless, in recent studies, autoantibodies specific for myelin oligodendrocyte glycoprotein have been detected in acute MS lesions. Furthermore, in certain EAE models, transfer of myelin oligodendrocyte glycoprotein-specific autoantibodies has facilitated demyelination and caused clinical exacerbations. Thus, there is considerable interest in characterizing the role of myelin-specific antibodies in MS.

Pathology

MS lesions are confined to the CNS white matter and are found most frequently in the periventricular region of the cerebrum, the cerebellum, brain stem, optic nerves, and spinal cord. Located primarily in the perivascular zones within these structures, lesions can vary in size from a few millimeters to several centimeters. Nineteenth-century French neurologists, credited with the original description correlating clinical and pathologic features of MS, observed that these lesions were sharply demarcated and referred to them as *plaques,* the French word meaning "scars" or "patches." In early stages of lesion development, infiltration with CD4 T cells, CD8 T cells, B cells, plasma cells, and macrophages is usually observed. Reactive astrocytes and phagocytic macrophages are the predominant cell types in older demyelinating lesions. Although oligodendrocytes are usually lost in older lesions, there is also sometimes evidence of remyelination. Plasma cells within demyelinating lesions are thought to be responsible for increased intrathecal levels of IgG and the presence of oligoclonal IgG. In general, lesions at different ages are found at the same time and are thought to account for the appearance of clinical signs and symptoms at separate times. Axonal loss and cerebral atrophy can occur later in MS.

Clinical Features

Inflammatory demyelinating lesions in MS can occur throughout the CNS, accounting for the variety of symptoms that may develop in individual patients. Common presenting symptoms of MS include focal sensory deficits (eg, facial or extremity numbness), imbalance, unilateral or bilateral visual loss (optic and retrobulbar neuritis), double vision (diplopia), fatigue, and weakness. With recurrent episodes (exacerbations) and progression, individuals often develop permanent neurologic impairments. Urinary and bowel dysfunction, as well as sexual impairment, symptoms usually attributed to spinal cord involvement, may develop. Moderate cognitive impairment, and sometimes psychiatric symptoms, can develop later. Several disease patterns are possible. A relapsing-remitting (RR) course with frequent early exacerbations, incomplete remissions, and accumulation of some disability affects 65% of all patients (Figure 38–3A). Exacerbations often last from days to weeks. Approximately 10–15% of patients with RRMS have a milder form, sometimes called "benign" MS, which is characterized by fewer exacerbations that are associated with complete or near-complete resolution and little or no accumulation of detectable disability (Figure 38–3B). It is estimated that 25% patients have

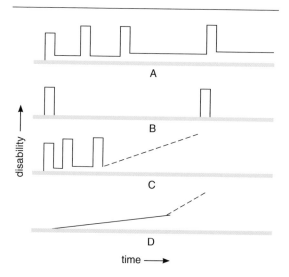

Figure 38–3. Different disease patterns in multiple sclerosis. **A:** Relapsing–remitting, a course with frequent early exacerbations, periods of stability, and little accumulation of permanent disability. **B:** Benign, a course with fewer exacerbations, complete or nearly complete resolution of neurologic symptoms, and minimal permanent disability. **C:** Secondary progressive, characterized by an initial relapsing–remitting course followed by a progressive phase with accelerated accumulation of permanent neurologic disability. **D:** Primary progressive, a disease pattern with insidious onset, no remissions, and steady progression of neurologic disability.

secondary progressive (SP) MS, a course characterized initially by relapses and remissions (RRMS) followed by a progressive phase associated with accumulation of permanent dysfunction (Figure 38–3C). Approximately 10% patients have primary progressive (PP) MS, a form associated with gradual progression from onset without remissions (Figure 38–3 D). Interestingly, in Asia, where the incidence is lower, MS is manifested by bilateral visual loss and paralysis of the extremities due to localization of demyelinating lesions to the optic nerves and spinal cord, respectively. Unlike disseminated (western) MS which is associated with HLA-DR2 (DRB*1501), Asian MS appears to have a different genetic predisposition.

Diagnosis

Recurrent episodes of neurologic impairment representing dysfunction in different anatomic locations within the CNS are clinical features that support the diagnosis of MS. Magnetic resonance imaging (MRI) is the most useful test for diagnosis of MS. Using T_2- and fluid-attenuated inversion recovery (FLAIR) weighted MRI, white matter lesions can be detected in 95% MS patients (Figure 38–4). CSF examination from MS patients often reveals a mild pleocytosis.

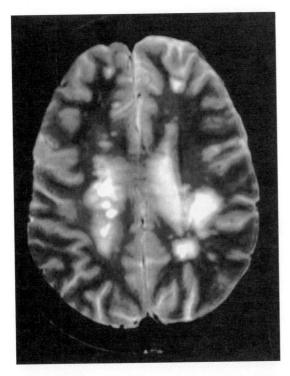

Figure 38–4. T_2-weighted magnetic resonance image (MRI) obtained during a multiple sclerosis exacerbation reveals numerous areas of increased signal intensity in areas of inflammation surrounding the lateral ventricles (courtesy of Dr. James Bowen).

An elevated IgG index (ratio of CSF to serum IgG corrected for albumin concentration in each compartment) indicates that intrathecal IgG synthesis is taking place. Two or more oligoclonal IgG bands within the CSF, presumably secondary to stimulation of discrete clones of B cells and plasma cells, are detected by electrophoresis in approximately 80% of MS patients. Electrophysiologic tests [visual evoked potentials (VEP), brain stem auditory evoked responses (BAER), and somatosensory evoked potentials (SSEP)] can also be used to identify regions of white matter dysfunction not detectable by imaging. Although tests used for diagnosis of MS are highly sensitive, they are not specific for this diagnosis.

Differential Diagnosis

A number of infectious, inflammatory, and autoimmune conditions can sometimes produce signs, symptoms, spinal fluid, and even MRI abnormalities that mimic MS. These illnesses include sarcoidosis, neurosyphilis, Lyme disease, systemic lupus erythematosus (SLE), CNS vasculitis, Behçet's disease, and Sjögren's syndrome. HTLV-1-associated myelopathy, also known as tropical spastic paraparesis (TSP), is considered when patients present with slowly progressive paraparesis. Certain metabolic disorders, including vitamin B_{12} deficiency and hypothyroidism, may be considered in the initial diagnostic evaluation. Diagnostic tests specific for many of these other conditions permit the clinician to eliminate them from the differential diagnosis. Although relapsing symptoms are not characteristic features of strokes, brain tumors, and arteriovenous malformations, these structural lesions are sometimes considered in the differential diagnosis. Some spinocerebellar degenerative diseases, such as Friedereich's ataxia, produce cerebellar signs and symptoms that occur in MS patients. As these conditions tend to be familial and are associated with normal spinal fluid, they can be distinguished from MS.

Treatment

After the publication of a multicenter, double-blind, placebo-controlled investigation in 1993, which demonstrated that subcutaneous injections of recombinant interferon-β 1b (IFNβ-1b; Betaseron) every other day reduced the frequency of exacerbations and the appearance of new or enlarging lesions on MRI, IFNβ-1b became the first medication approved for the treatment of RRMS. In 1996, a slightly different molecule, recombinant interferon-β 1a (IFNβ-1a; Avonex), was also shown to be effective in early RRMS. IFNβ-1a also had a modest effect in slowing progression of disability. Shortly thereafter, it was reported that copolymer-1 (glatiramer acetate; Copaxone), a synthetic polypeptide composed of a random mixture of four amino acids (alanine, glutamic acid, lysine, and tyrosine) that was previously found to be effective in prevention and treatment of EAE, reduced exacerbation frequency and accumulation of disability in RRMS. These three agents, commonly referred to as the "ABC" (Avonex, Betaseron, and Copaxone) medications, appear to have similar efficacy, reducing the relapse rate by 30%. The IFNβs and Copaxone may have several different mechanisms of action. Treatment with IFNβ-1a is associated with increased IL-10 levels. IFNβ also prevents interferon-γ-induced up-regulation of MHC class II molecules on various APCs. Because it has been shown that IFNβ suppresses lymphocyte production of matrix metalloproteases and inhibits their capability to penetrate extracellular matrix, IFNβ may reduce lymphocyte traffic into the CNS. Copaxone may act as an altered peptide ligand (APL), interfering with MHC class II binding of myelin antigens or with the binding of myelin antigen-specific T-cell receptors. In fact, evidence indicates that Copaxone inhibits the binding of myelin basic protein to HLA-DR molecules. In contrast, some data indicate that Copaxone may act as a mimic, and induce myelin-reactive T_H2 cells. Because Copaxone and IFNβ have separate mechanisms of action, they may have synergistically beneficial effects when given in combination, a possibility that is being investigated.

High-dose intravenous steroids (eg, methylprednisolone) are the most widely used medication to treat acute MS exacerbations. Steroids suppress acute MS symptoms and appear to shorten attack duration. Although useful in acute exacerbations, there are no data substantiating that steroids alter the natural course of MS. Hyperglycemia (glucose intolerance), hypertension, and osteopenia are some of the potential side effects that limit prolonged steroid use.

Treatment of PPMS and SPMS has been more challenging. In 1999, however, results reported from a large trial revealed a highly significant delay in progression in patients with SPMS who were treated with IFNβ-1b. The IFNβ medications and Copaxone are currently being evaluated in the treatment of PPMS. Other immunosuppressive medications, including azathioprine, cyclophosphamide, and cyclosporine, have been used in the treatment of progressive MS, although with mixed results. Serious side effects from these medications have also restricted their clinical use. Despite the possibility that autoantibodies may participate in MS pathogenesis, studies have failed to show clear benefit from plasmapheresis or intravenous immunoglobulin in progressive and RRMS.

Several experimental immunomodulatory agents have been evaluated in MS treatment. Targeted therapy with anti-CD4 monoclonal antibodies, which was effective in both prevention and treatment of EAE, did not appear to be beneficial in MS. Oral administration of myelin induces tolerance to myelin antigens and prevents EAE. The results from a trial evaluating oral tolerance with bovine myelin in RRMS was disappointing, however. Although EAE has been invaluable for studies of pathogenesis and evaluation of potential treatments, favorable results in EAE have not necessarily translated into clinical efficacy in MS. Other promising approaches are being tested. APLs that interfere with MHC class II binding of myelin antigens are being investigated in RRMS. Autologous hematopoietic stem cell transplantation, which may eliminate pathogenic myelin autoantigen-specific T-cell clones, is being evaluated in advanced MS.

Complications & Prognosis

MS is one of the leading causes of significant disability in patients between the ages of 20 and 50 in the United States. The prognosis for disability varies and depends mainly on the form of MS. Favorable prognostic factors in adults include early onset, female sex, a remitting–relapsing course, and minimal disability 5 years after onset of symptoms. A population-based study showed that 10 years after onset of symptoms, a third of all patients require unilateral assistance to ambulate. After 30 years, this number increases to 80% of all patients. After diagnosis, the 25-year expected survival rate is 74% compared with an expected rate of 82% in the general population.

ACUTE DISSEMINATED ENCEPHALOMYELITIS

Major Immunologic Features

- Often preceded by an infectious illness or a vaccination
- Cellular and humoral responses to myelin antigens
- Response to immunosuppressive therapy

General Considerations

Acute disseminated encephalomyelitis (ADEM) is considered a monophasic demyelinating disease of the CNS that occurs most often following an infection or vaccination. Although ADEM is uncommon, it is an important illness because of the widespread use of vaccinations for prevention of infectious diseases and because ADEM often causes severe permanent neurologic disabilities. Clinical illness usually occurs several days to weeks following vaccination. In cases due to natural viral infection, neurologic symptoms can begin during (parainfectious) or after (postinfectious) the acute viral illness. A number of viral pathogens have been associated with ADEM, including the measles, rubella, and varicella zoster viruses. Less commonly, ADEM has been reported following infection with the influenza, mumps, coxsackie B, Epstein–Barr, herpes simplex, human immunodeficiency, and human herpesvirus-6. With measles virus, ADEM occurs in approximately 1 out of 1000 infections. The incidences of ADEM after varicella and rubella virus infections are <1:10,000 and <1:20,000, respectively. In addition to viruses, ADEM subsequent to infection with *Mycoplasma pneumoniae* and *Legionella cincinnatiensis* have also been reported.

Postimmunization encephalomyelitis is most commonly associated with measles, mumps, and rubella vaccinations. The incidence is 1–2 per 10^6 for live measles vaccine immunizations, significantly lower than that for postinfection encephalomyelitis from measles itself. In fact, in comparison with the rate of developing ADEM after a natural virus infection, the risk of developing ADEM after a vaccination is nearly 20 times lower.

Experimental models indicate that both infectious mechanisms and a secondary autoimmune responses contribute to CNS demyelination in ADEM. Infection of susceptible mice with Theiler's murine encephalomyelitis virus (TMEV) causes acute encephalitis and CNS demyelination associated with activation of CD4 and CD8 T cells. A fulminant monophasic form of EAE with quadriparesis and variable degrees of CNS demyelination occurs following immunization with myelin extract or purified myelin antigens in complete Freund's adjuvant. As for MS, myelin-specific T cells are thought to have a central role in ADEM pathogenesis. Humoral immune responses to CNS autoantigens (eg, gangliosides) may also be involved in the pathogenesis of ADEM.

Pathology

ADEM lesions are observed throughout the brain and spinal cord. Large areas of inflammation and demyelination with perivenous cuffs containing mononuclear cells, occasional neutrophils, and lipid-laden macrophages are usually observed. As the disease progresses, astrocytic hyperplasia and gliosis are found.

Clinical Features

ADEM usually affects infants and young children, although infrequently it has been reported in middle-age and elderly individuals. In postimmunization and postinfectious ADEM, patients initially develop fever and nonspecific respiratory illness. Neurologic symptoms usually follow after 1–20 days. Common clinical features of ADEM include headaches, meningismus, seizures, weakness, spasticity, obtundation, and sometimes coma associated with respiratory distress. After a period of stabilization, patients frequently improve. It has been reported that some patients may develop recurrent symptoms, however, it is difficult to distinguish these exacerbations from the attacks of RRMS. Thus, when recurrent symptoms do occur, the diagnosis of RRMS is pursued, and use of a disease modifying agent approved for the treatment of MS is considered.

Immunologic Diagnosis

The CSF often shows a mild lymphocytic pleocytosis and protein elevation. Elevated CSF IgG and the presence of oligoclonal bands on electrophoresis, which are found in MS and other CNS inflammatory conditions, are often detected. As in other conditions causing acute injury to CNS myelin, myelin basic protein may be detected in the CSF in ADEM. Increased cellular immune responses to myelin basic protein have also been demonstrated. In cases of postinfectious ADEM it is sometimes possible to detect individual pathogens by culture or gene expression in CSF; however, it is often difficult to establish a causal effect in ADEM.

Differential Diagnosis

The diagnosis of ADEM is strongly suggested when the onset of the characteristic neurologic symptoms follow soon after a viral exanthem or immunization. This diagnosis is supported when neuroimaging demonstrates extensive white matter disease and analysis of CSF reveals a pleocytosis and elevated IgG. ADEM may be difficult to distinguish from acute fulminant MS, however. In both of these illnesses, MRI imaging demonstrates multiple patchy areas of increased T2 signal intensity in the periventricular and subcortical white matter. In general, the lesions of ADEM are symmetric and more widespread than in MS. Vasculitis in systemic lupus erythematosus can affect the CNS, but the symptoms in that condition are usually more focal than in ADEM. Encephalitis caused by herpes simplex virus and the arboviruses can cause seizures, obtundation, and coma, but tend to involve both gray matter and white matter. In contrast with ADEM, herpes simplex virus encephalitis causes predominantly unilateral or bilateral temporal lobe lesions that are often associated with hemorrhage. Neurosarcoidosis, the leukodystrophies, and the subacute encephalitis of acquired immunodeficiency syndrome (AIDS) are sometimes considered in the differential diagnosis, although these illnesses often develop more slowly.

Treatment

High-dose intravenous corticosteroids are commonly used as a first-line treatment because they are believed to shorten the duration of neurologic symptoms. Some case studies have reported that plasmapheresis or intravenous gamma globulins are sometimes beneficial. Thus, when patients do not respond to steroids, neurologists often administer these immunomodulatory therapies.

Complications & Prognosis

The mortality rate of postimmunization ADEM is approximately 5%. In postinfectious ADEM secondary to measles virus infection the estimated mortality rate is nearly 25%, and 30–35% of these survivors have persistent neurologic sequelae. Poor prognosis has been correlated with abrupt onset and greater severity of symptoms. In contrast, the incidence of major neurologic sequelae from ADEM from rubella and varicella virus infections is lower. Relapses of ADEM are rare, and when the do occur, the diagnosis of MS should be considered.

ACUTE INFLAMMATORY DEMYELINATING POLYNEUROPATHY

- An acute viral infection or an enteric infection with *Campylobacter jejuni* often precedes neurologic symptoms
- Cellular and humoral immune responses to peripheral nerve and cranial nerve antigens
- Immunomodulatory treatments shorten recovery

General Considerations

The Guillain-Barré syndrome (GBS), or acute inflammatory demyelinating neuropathy (AIDP), is the most common acquired peripheral demyelinating disease. The incidence is approximately 0.6–1.9 per 100,000, with equal sex predilection. A viral upper respiratory tract or gastrointestinal tract infection may precede the neurologic symptoms by several days or weeks. Gastrointestinal infection with *Campylobacter jejuni* triggers 10–30% of all cases of the GBS. Viral pathogens that have been associated with the GBS include human immunodeficiency virus (HIV), Epstein-Barr virus, and cytomegalovirus. There has been a small, but definable, increased risk of developing GBS after immunization, which became most apparent after the 1976 swine-flu vaccine program. Recent surgical procedures have also been associated with GBS, and in some studies, have accounted for up to 5% of all cases.

Immunization of susceptible animals with galactocerebrosides or peripheral nerve myelin protein, P2, induces experimental autoimmune neuritis (EAN), causing clinical symptoms and histopathologic changes found in GBS. Molecular mimicry is considered an important pathogenic mechanism when GBS follows infection or immunization.

Pathologic Findings

Lesions of the peripheral and cranial nerves are characterized histologically by segmental regions of infiltration with mononuclear cells (T cells, B cells, and macrophages) and demyelination. After a prolonged disease course, there may be evidence of axonal loss and wallerian degeneration. In GBS due to *Campylobacter* infection, axonal degeneration and less demyelination occur.

Clinical Presentation

The characteristic feature of GBS is an acute, rapidly progressive, ascending, and symmetric weakness with loss of deep tendon reflexes. The majority of patients initially experience tingling (paraesthesias) in their feet and hands and muscle aches (myalgia). Facial, oculomotor, oropharyngeal, and respiratory muscles may become involved, and some patients then require respiratory support. When the autonomic nerves are involved, individuals can develop hemodynamic instability and cardiac arrhythmias. The sever-

ity of clinical deficits typically peaks within the first 2 weeks of onset, but some will progress for 3–4 weeks. Most patients will improve and return to normal function within 6–9 months; however, relapses and a prolonged disease course with residual neurologic deficits have been reported. In a variant of the GBS syndrome, the Miller-Fisher syndrome, patients present with paresis of their extraocular muscles (ophthalmoplegia), unsteadiness (ataxia), and loss of their deep tendon reflexes (areflexia).

Electrophysiologic studies provide important diagnostic information. Within a week of onset of clinical symptoms, nerve conduction studies usually show prolonged distal motor latencies and prolonged or absent F waves. Electromyography may show evidence of muscle denervation by 4–6 weeks.

Immunologic Diagnosis

Within several days from onset in most patients the CSF will reveal elevated protein, a key feature for diagnosis. Typically the CSF is acellular, although occasionally the numbers of mononuclear cells may be slightly elevated. Other diagnoses should be considered if the number of mononuclear cells exceeds 25 cells/μL. Increased IgG and IgA antibody titers to GM1 ganglioside can be found in the axonal variant of GBS, whereas antibodies to GQ1b are associated with the Miller-Fisher syndrome.

Differential Diagnosis

It is not difficult to diagnosis GBS when patients present with rapidly progressive ascending weakness and loss of deep tendon reflexes. An evolving acute transverse myelitis is one of the most common early diagnostic errors because it can present similarly to GBS, with muscle weakness and areflexia. In this disorder, however, deep tendon reflexes typically increase and muscle tone becomes spastic after several days or weeks. Other differential diagnoses include acute intermittent porphyria, diphtheric neuropathy, and botulism.

GBS has been observed in patients infected with HIV. The clinical and electrophysiologic presentation in these patients is often identical to that of non-HIV-infected patients, and the presence of pleocytosis in the CSF (usually greater than 25 cells per microliter) may be the only distinguishable feature. Cases of HIV-associated GBS often occur early in the clinical course of this infection and may herald the onset of other HIV-associated clinical complications.

Treatment

Early plasmapheresis and intravenous immunoglobulin therapy have been shown to be equally effective in accelerating recovery in GBS. The role of other immunosuppressive drugs, such as high-dose steroids, is currently unsettled. In the acute phase it is necessary to monitor respiratory function and treat mechanical respiratory failure. Because autonomic dysfunction can occur, hemodynamic monitoring is required. Hypertension is treated with antihypertensive medications and hypotension with volume and vasopressor agents.

Complications & Prognosis

The overall prognosis of the GBS is quite good, with full recovery of neurologic function occurring in about two thirds of patients. The remaining cases have a prolonged or incomplete recovery with residual limb weakness, bulbar weakness, or muscular atrophy. In about 10% of these patients, the residual disability is severe. Widespread axonal damage is associated with poor outcome. About 10% of patients experience a relapse during their recovery, and 2% experience a recurrence of the disease after complete recovery. The most dangerous complications of the GBS are respiratory complications secondary to aspiration and pulmonary embolism, as well as autonomic dysfunction, such as hypotension, hypertension, and cardiac arrhythmias. The mortality rate of GBS is 3–5%.

CHRONIC INFLAMMATORY NEUROPATHIES

Chronic inflammatory demyelinating polyradiculoneuropathy (CIDP) is a disorder of presumed autoimmune cause, which accounts for one third of all initially undiagnosed acquired neuropathies. In approximately 10% of cases, CIDP is preceded by an infection. Similar to GBS, patients can present with extremity, truncal, and facial musculature weakness. CIDP begins insidiously, however, and progresses slowly. Patients present with a relapsing-remitting (one third of cases), stepwise progressive (one third of cases), chronic progressive, or monophasic disease pattern (together one third of cases). There is evidence of mononuclear cell infiltration with focal demyelination, and hypertrophic changes of the proximal peripheral nerve, spinal ganglia, and spinal roots are observed. CSF examination typically reveals normal or increased protein with a mononuclear pleocytosis. In contrast to GBS, CIDP is considered highly responsive to corticosteroids. The response to plasmapheresis and intravenous immunoglobulins varies.

In a number of other chronic demyelinating diseases, humoral immune responses have also been postulated to play a key role in pathogenesis. Approximately 50% of patients with osteosclerotic multiple myeloma and 15% of patients with osteolytic multiple myeloma and IgG and IgA monoclonal gammopathies develop a predominantly motor segmental demyelinating polyneuropathy. Painful dysesthesias and muscle weakness in the distal limbs are frequent clinical manifestations. A subgroup of patients have Crow-Fukase syndrome (hyperpigmentation of skin, edema, excessive hair growth, papilledema, hepatosplenomegaly, hypogonadism, hypothyroidism,

and elevated protein in the CSF) or POEMS syndrome (polyneuropathy, organomegaly, endocrinopathy, myeloma, and skin changes). A similar polyneuropathy is associated with monoclonal gammopathy of undetermined significance (MGUS). The IgG or IgA light chain type is typically lambda. A causal role of these antibodies in demyelination has yet to be proven. Many patients show significant clinical improvement after plasma exchange or corticosteroid treatment.

Multifocal motor neuropathy (MMN) with conduction block is another form of chronic peripheral neuropathy. MMN is characterized by the subacute onset of muscle weakness involving one or more nerves in the upper or lower limbs. Electrophysiologic studies show focal motor conduction block that can be proximal or intermediate. There may be multiple areas of block in an individual nerve, which do not occur at the usual sites of nerve entrapment. MMN with conduction block is associated with high titers of GM1 ganglioside antibodies. Myelin-associated glycoprotein (MAG) antibody has been detected in patients with benign monoclonal gammopathy and peripheral neuropathy. The latter two diseases are successfully treated with immunosuppressive agents, plasmapheresis, or intravenous immunoglobulins.

Lupus erythematosus and systemic vasculitis are autoimmune diseases associated with neuropathy. The vasculitis may be confined exclusively to the peripheral nerves or associated with systemic disease. Biopsy specimens show inflammatory cell infiltrates, necrosis of blood vessel walls, and axonal degeneration. The treatment of choice is immunosuppressive agents.

Chronic neuropathies have also been observed in sarcoidosis, systemic amyloidosis, and rheumatoid arthritis. The underlying disease mechanisms are not fully understood.

DISORDERS OF NEUROMUSCULAR TRANSMISSION

Myasthenia gravis and the paraneoplastic Lambert-Eaton myasthenic syndrome are disorders of transmission at the neuromuscular junction characterized by fluctuating weakness and fatigability of skeletal muscles. Humoral autoimmune mechanisms have been established in these conditions.

MYASTHENIA GRAVIS

Major Immunologic Features
• A humoral immune response against the acetylcholine receptor on the postsynaptic membrane

- Reproduction of symptoms with passive transfer of antiacetylcholine receptor antibody
- Increased incidence of other autoimmune diseases in myasthenia gravis patients
- Response to immunosuppressive therapy and thymectomy

General Considerations

Myasthenia gravis (MG) is the most common disorder of the neuromuscular junction. The estimated prevalence in the United States is 3 per 100,000 (or about 9000 cases). MG is characterized by variable weakness of limb muscles, extraocular muscles, and pharyngeal muscles. There are two peak disease incidences: The first occurs within the second and third decades and a second peak occurs within the seventh and eighth decades. Before age 40, women are three times more commonly affected, whereas in the older age group males predominate. Family members of patients with MG are approximately 1000 times more likely to develop this disease than the general population. In young women, MG is associated with HLA B-8 and DR3 haplotypes. In the older age group, MG patients without evidence of thymoma have an association with HLA-A3, -B7, and DR2. In addition, MG has frequently been reported in association with other autoimmune diseases, including insulin-dependent diabetes mellitus and autoimmune thyroiditis.

Immune mechanisms participate directly in the pathogenesis of MG. Autoantibodies directed against the nicotinic acetylcholine receptor (AChR) block these receptors on the postsynaptic membrane and interrupt electrical transmission. Passive transfer of anti-AChR antibodies from MG patients into naive animals results in clinical, electrophysiologic, and pathologic features of MG. In the animal model of MG, experimental autoimmune myasthenia gravis (EAMG), immunization with purified AchR protein induces AChR-specific T-cell and B-cell responses that are responsible for muscle weakness.

Pathology

In healthy individuals, the postsynaptic membrane of the neuromuscular junction is characterized by a folded pattern with abundant AChR on the tip of each fold (Figure 38–5A). In muscle biopsy specimens from MG patients, antibodies are attached to the postsynaptic membrane, receptors are lost, and postsynaptic folds are sparse and shallow (Figure 38–5B). In 70-90% of biopsy specimens, the thymus is "hyperplastic," with the presence of active germinal centers in the medulla. Ten percent of MG patients have a locally invasive thymoma. Because thymic myoid cells within thymoma and thymic hyperplasia can express AChR, and both AChR-specific CD4 T cells and antibody-secreting B cells have been detected in thymoma and hyperplastic thymic tissue

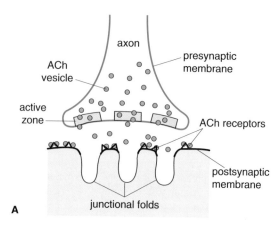

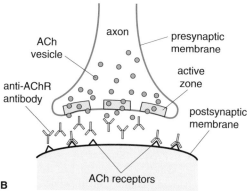

Figure 38–5. Electrical transmission at the neuromuscular junction in **A:** healthy state and in **B:** myasthenia gravis. When an electrical signal propagates along an axon and reaches the synapse, acetylcholine (ACh) is released from the presynaptic membrane. In healthy individuals, the postsynaptic membrane of the neuromuscular junction is characterized by a folded pattern with abundant ACh receptors (AChR) on the tip of the folds. ACh crosses the synaptic cleft and binds to AChR, which leads to transmission of the electric signal to the muscle cell. In patients with myasthenia gravis, AChR antibodies block the AChR, and eventually lead to a decreased number of AChR on the postsynaptic membrane. The postsynaptic folds are sparse and shallow. The degree of reduction of AChR correlates with the severity of myasthenia gravis.

in MG, it has been postulated that the thymus may be a primary site of autosensitization.

Clinical Features

The prominent clinical feature of MG is variable weakness of selected muscle groups. More than half of all patients present initially with symptoms caused by impairment of extraocular eye muscles, such as drooping of an eyelid (ptosis) or double vision (diplopia). Other common presenting symptoms are hoarseness, nasal speech, slurred speech, difficulties with chewing, and swallowing. Limb and neck flexor weakness typically occur later in the disease. Symptoms from MG usually worsen over the course of the day, and are often brought on by activities that stress the affected muscle group.

Immunologic Diagnosis

Anti-AChR IgG can be found in 90% of MG patients. IgG_2 and IgG_4 are the predominant subclasses. The presence of anti-AChR antibody in the appropriate clinical setting confirms the diagnosis. Anti-AchR antibodies, however, are not specific for clinical MG. These antibodies can be found in asymptomatic relatives of MG patients as well as in patients with other autoimmune diseases. Edrophonium (Tensilon) is used in diagnosis of MG. Intravenous injection of this acetylcholinesterase inhibitor relieves muscle weakness instantaneously by increasing the availability of ACh in the synaptic cleft.

Approximately 10% of patients who test negative for anti-AChR antibody have other factors that interfere with the turnover of acetylcholine at the neuromuscular junction. A number of nonreceptor muscle antibodies have been identified in MG patients. An anti-AchR-directed CD4 T-cell immune response may contribute significantly to disease activity in AchR antibody-negative MG patients. In fact, the predominant anti-AchR T-cell response in MG and EAMG is directed against the main immunogenic region on the AchR alpha chain, which contains the myasthenogenic determinant in EAMG.

Differential Diagnosis

Fluctuating weakness of the ocular, oropharyngeal, and limb muscles differentiates MG from some of the other diseases with weakness, including the Miller–Fisher syndrome or progressive bulbar palsy. Periodic paralysis, which is a group of disorders, known as channelopathies, caused by mutations in potassium, sodium, and calcium channel proteins does not respond to acetylcholinesterase inhibitors. Other disorders of the neuromuscular junction, such as botulinum and organophosphate intoxication, Lambert-Eaton syndrome, or snake bites, can respond somewhat to acetylcholinesterase inhibitors, but are usually easily distinguished on the basis of the clinical history and repetitive stimulation in EMG. Patients with rheumatoid arthritis, scleroderma, or Wilson's disease, who are being treated with penicillamine, may experience symptoms similar to MG. Discontinuation of penicillamine usually results in full resolution of muscle weakness.

Treatment

Acetylcholinesterase inhibitors, surgical thymectomy, and immunosuppressive medications are used to treat MG. Acetylcholinesterase inhibitors are the first line of treatment. Long-term immunosuppression with corticosteroids, azathioprine, or cyclosporine are often used. Plasmapheresis and intravenous IgG (IVIG) are beneficial, but frequently need to be repeated at variable intervals. Plasmapheresis removes IgG including anti-AChR IgG, and IVIG may act as a competitive inhibitor. Surgical thymectomy is recommended for patients with generalized myasthenia from puberty until the age of 60. Eighty percent of MG patients with thymomas become asymptomatic after thymectomy.

Complications & Prognosis

Before the introduction of intensive care therapy and the different treatment options listed earlier, a third of the patients died as a direct consequence of their disease, a third of the patients remained clinically stable, and another third showed significant symptomatic improvement. When treatment is delayed, respiratory complications may occur. Respiratory complications can also occur from excessive use of acetylcholinesterase inhibitors, causing a "cholinergic crisis." Aminoglycoside antibiotics and procainamide can lead to exacerbation of weakness in MG. Overall the mortality rate from MG is quite low.

LAMBERT-EATON MYASTHENIC SYNDROME

Patients with an underlying malignancy, most commonly small-cell carcinoma of the lung, can sometimes develop clinical features that resemble MG. This syndrome, which causes proximal muscle weakness, mainly of the lower extremities, has been termed Lambert-Eaton myasthenic syndrome (LEMS). LEMS can be distinguished from MG by the presence of muscle stiffness, autonomic changes, and absence of deep tendon reflexes. In contrast with the exertional fatigue of MG, in LEMS muscle strength typically increases with repetitive muscle contractions. Neurologic signs and symptoms may precede the diagnosis of the underlying neoplasm. Electrodiagnostic testing shows an incremental response on repetitive nerve stimulation. IgG antibodies to presynaptic voltage-gated calcium channels have been demonstrated in the serum of patients with LEMS (Table 38–1). These antibodies interfere with the release of acetylcholine at nerve terminals and conduction of the electrical signal from the neuron to the muscle cell. This disease has successfully been transferred from humans to mice by passive transfer of these antibodies. Treatment of LEMS aims to reduce the titers of anticalcium channel antibodies. The clinical efficacy of IVIG has been shown in two controlled trials. Plasmapheresis, steroids, and other immunosuppressive agents have also been shown to be efficacious. Improvement with acetylcholinesterase inhibitors occurs only in two thirds of patients with LEMS and is less pronounced than in MG patients.

Table 38–1. Paraneoplastic disorders associated with antineuronal antibodies.

Antibody	Neuronal Antigen	Onconeural Antigen[a]	Syndrome	Associated Malignancy
Anti-Yo	Purkinje cell cytoplasm, 34 and 62 kd	CDR34, CDR62-1, CDR62-2	Cerebellar degeneration	Gynecologic, breast
Anti-Ri	Neuronal nuclei in the central nervous system, 55 and 80 kd	NOVA1, NOVA2	Cerebellar ataxia, opsoclonus	Gynecologic, breast, small-cell lung cancer
Anti-Ma	Neuronal nuclei and cytoplasm, 40 kd	Ma1, Ma2	Cerebellar, brain stem dysfunction	Multiple neoplasms
Anti-Tr	Neuronal cytoplasm, Purkinje cells, spiny dendrites	Unidentified	Cerebellar degeneration	Hodgkin's lymphoma
Anti-CV-2	Glia, 66 kd	POP66	Encephalomyelitis, cerebellar degeneration	Small-cell lung cancer and other
Anti-Hu	All neuronal nuclei, 35–40 kd	HuD, HuC, Hel-N1	Limbic encephalitis, sensory neuropathy	Small-cell lung cancer, neuroblastoma
Anti-Ta	Neuronal nuclei and cytoplasm	Ma2	Limbic encephalitis, brain stem dysfunction	Testicular cancer
Anti-Vgcc	Presynaptic voltage-gated calcium channels	α_1-Subunit of voltage-gated calcium channels	Lambert–Eaton myasthenic syndrome	Small-cell lung cancer
Anti-MysB	Presynaptic voltage-gated calcium channels	β-Subunit of voltage-gated calcium channels	Lambert–Eaton myasthenic syndrome	Small-cell lung cancer
Anti-Car	Retinal photoreceptor, 23 kd	Recoverin	Photoreceptor degeneration	Small-cell lung cancer and others
Antiamphiphysin	Synaptic vesicle, 128 kd	Amphiphysin	Stiff-person syndrome, encephalomyelitis	Breast cancer

[a] Onconeural antigens are normally only present in neurons. Paraneoplastic antibodies have been used to probe complementary DNA expression libraries to clone the antigen(s) identified by these antibodies.

IMMUNOLOGIC ABNORMALITIES IN OTHER NEUROLOGIC DISEASES

It has become clear that several different neurologic conditions result from secondary immune abnormalities in response to other disease states. Whereas a primary role for autoantibodies in MG has been established, nervous system autoantibodies that occur in response to certain malignancies are responsible for the nervous system dysfunction in specific paraneoplastic syndromes. Secondary immune responses may also contribute to the pathology of primary neurologic diseases. In fact, some data suggest that humoral immune responses may be involved in certain stage(s) in the pathogenesis of Alzheimer's disease. Immune abnormalities are associated with atypical stroke syndromes that occur in young individuals.

PARANEOPLASTIC SYNDROMES

In these conditions, immune responses are directed against "onconeural" antigens, normal self nervous system antigens that are expressed ectopically by tumors outside the nervous system. This form of molecular mimicry is thought to be responsible for several conditions, including paraneoplastic cerebellar degeneration and limbic encephalitis. Although these conditions have been defined and characterized by humoral antigen-specific responses, recent studies suggest that cellular immune responses, mediated by tumor-specific cytotoxic CD8 T cells, may also participate in the pathogenesis of some paraneoplastic nervous system syndromes. Often patients develop neurologic symptoms long before their primary tumor is discovered. When another cause cannot account for the neurologic symptoms, an extensive diagnostic evaluation is often pursued to identify an occult neoplasm.

Patients with paraneoplastic cerebellar degeneration can present with slurred speech, gait instability, and tremor. Paraneoplastic cerebellar degeneration is associated with ovarian cancer, breast cancer, small-cell lung cancer, and Hodgkin's disease. Characteristic histologic features of paraneoplastic cerebellar degeneration include extensive loss of Purkinje cells, the predominant neuron responsible for cerebellar output, and microglial proliferation. Patchy cerebellar lymphocytic infiltrates may also be observed. Five different antibodies have been identified thus far in patients with this disorder (see Table 38–1).

Limbic encephalitis is a paraneoplastic syndrome characterized by memory impairment, psychiatric changes, and seizures. Pathologic changes occur in the limbic system, which includes the hippocampus, amygdala, hypothalamus, and insular and cingulate cortices. Small-cell lung cancer is the primary malignancy diagnosed in approximately 80% of patients with paraneoplastic limbic encephalitis. Neuroblastoma is also associated with limbic encephalitis. Antibodies (see Table 38–1) targeted against the family of HU antigens, RNA-binding proteins found in the nuclei of some neurons and small-cell lung cancer cells, are identified in patients with limbic encephalitis. Limbic encephalitis has also been associated with testicular cancer. In these men, antitesticular antigen (anti-TA) antibodies targeted to one of the five Ma proteins found in both neurons and spermatogenic testicular cells have been identified.

Although appreciation for the paraneoplastic syndromes has increased dramatically in recent years, treatments are considered unsatisfactory. Immunosuppressive medications are sometimes considered to treat the "autoimmune" neurologic dysfunction. Because immune suppression may potentiate growth of the primary malignancy, these medications may not be used. Interestingly, it has been observed that tumor growth can be more indolent in individuals with paraneoplastic antibodies than in individuals with the same type of tumor without a paraneoplastic syndrome or without paraneoplastic antibodies.

AMYOTROPHIC LATERAL SCLEROSIS

Amyotrophic lateral sclerosis (ALS), commonly known as Lou Gehrig's disease or motor neuron disease, is a degenerative condition characterized by premature death of upper- and lower motor neurons. Subtypes of this disorder include the sporadic, familial, and western Pacific forms. Approximately 20% of patients with the familial form of ALS have one of 55 different mutations of the gene encoding for the cytosolic enzyme copper/zinc superoxide dismutase (SOD1). Depending on the clinical variant, either lower motor neurons innervating the bulbar muscles and the limb muscles, or the upper motor neurons are initially involved. Approximately 50% of patients with ALS die within 3 years from onset of clinical symptoms, usually from respiratory failure.

Although controversial, the results of several studies indicate that immune mechanisms may participate in the pathogenesis of ALS. Inhibitory antibodies to voltage-gated calcium channels have been identified in ALS patients and passive transfer of these antibodies into mice produced muscle weakness and motor neuron apoptosis. Antibodies to motor neuron neuro-

filament proteins have been found in 25% of patients with the sporadic form of ALS, compared with 13 % of controls. An autoimmune murine model caused by immunization with spinal cord gray matter results in inflammatory foci within the spinal cord accompanied by loss of upper and lower motor neurons, accumulation of IgG, and clinical weakness. Despite the evidence for humoral and cellular immunologic mechanisms ALS, thus far, immunomodulatory therapies have not altered the course of this fatal disease.

ALZHEIMER'S DISEASE

Alzheimer's disease (AD) accounts for more than 50% of all dementia in Europe and North America. It is a very heterogeneous disorder that is diagnosed clinically when other causes of dementia have been excluded. Typically, there is a progressive decline of cognitive function with mild plateaus. The average survival is 8–10 years after onset of symptoms. Characteristic clinical features include progressive short-term memory loss and language impairment. Behavioral symptoms, such as paranoid delusions and visual hallucinations, are also associated with AD. Some familial cases of AD have been associated with mutations in the amyloid precursor protein (chromosome 21), presenilin-1 (chromosome 14), and presenilin-2 (chromosome 1) genes. AD has been associated with decreased choline-acetyltransferase in the hippocampus and neocortex and with defects in amyloid precursor protein and tau protein.

Neuritic "senile" plaques, argyrophilic fibrous material with a central amyloid core, and neurofibrillary tangles composed of paired helical filaments, can be found in the frontal lobe and temporal lobe poles. The number of senile plaques correlates best with the severity of dementia. AD tissue shows small numbers of mononuclear infiltrates.

Secondary immune responses may contribute to the pathogenesis of AD. Activated microglia express high levels of MHC molecules and complement receptors. In plaques, amyloid-beta peptide is colocalized with proteins of the classical complement pathway, and it has been observed in vitro that amyloid-beta can bind C1q and initiate the complement cascade. Transgenic mice that overexpress mutant human amyloid precursor protein show clinical and pathologic features of AD. Recently, it was shown that amyloid-beta peptide-specific antibodies generated in response to immunization with amyloid-beta peptide could prevent the development of beta-amyloid plaques, neuritic dystrophy, and astrogliosis in these transgenic mice.

Use of nonsteroidal antiinflammatory drugs such as aspirin or ibuprofen has been associated with a decreased risk of developing AD. This observation is sometimes quoted in support for an inflammatory component to the neurodegenerative process in AD.

OTHER CENTRAL NERVOUS SYSTEM DISEASES WITH AUTOIMMUNE FEATURES

Autoimmune mechanisms are considered in the pathophysiology of two rare neurologic disorders, Rasmussen's encephalitis and stiff-person syndrome. Rasmussen's encephalitis is a syndrome of unilateral cerebral dysfunction that begins in childhood and is manifested by intractable unilateral focal seizures (epilepsia partialis continua), hemiparesis, and variable intellectual impairment. Both cellular and humoral immune responses may be involved in this disorder, which is characterized histologically by unilateral focal brain inflammation containing large numbers of T cells and cells that express increased MHC class I and class II molecules. Analysis of T-cell receptor gene expression by infiltrating T cells within these lesions revealed use of a limited repertoire of V genes and complementarity-determining region (CDR3) nucleotide motifs, suggesting that oligoclonal expansion of T cells recognizes a local brain tissue-specific antigen. One candidate autoantigen is the neuronal membrane receptor for the excitatory amino acid neurotransmitter glutamate. IgG antibodies to one subunit of this receptor, GluR3, are observed in patients with Rasmussen's encephalitis and immunization of animals with GluR3 induces a clinicopathologic syndrome similar to Rasmussen's encephalitis, including inflammatory infiltration of mononuclear cells in the CNS and the production of anti-GluR3 IgG antibodies. It has been observed that these IgG antibodies, as well as the anti-GluR antibodies found in some patients with Rasmussen's encephalitis, can induce hyperexcitability of cultured neurons. Medical management of Rasmussen's encephalitis is challenging. Treatment often includes anticonvulsant medications, corticosteroids, and plasmapheresis. Hemispherectomy is used when seizures are refractory to these medications.

Stiff-person syndrome is a condition characterized by excessive muscular contraction that results in spontaneous spasms, progressive rigidity, and the development of dystonic postures. These symptoms result from hyperactivity of spinal motor neurons similar to that seen in clinical tetanus. Although originally described as stiff-man syndrome, it is now known that it has no sex predilection. Stiff-person syndrome is considered to have an autoimmune basis for several reasons. It often occurs in association with other autoimmune diseases, including insulin-dependent diabetes mellitus, thyroiditis, myasthenia gravis, and pernicious anemia. In fact, as many as 37% of individuals with stiff-person syndrome have type I (insulin-dependent) diabetes. In 60–90% of individuals with stiff-person syndrome antibodies to glutamic acid decarboxylase (GAD), the major autoantigen in this condition, can be detected in both serum and cerebrospinal fluid. GAD is the enzyme responsible for synthesis of the inhibitory neurotransmitter, γ-aminobutyric acid (GABA). Some data indicate that the GAD-specific autoantibodies detected in individuals with stiff-person syndrome functionally inhibit synthesis of GABA. Most interestingly, GAD is considered a key autoantigen in the pathogenesis of type I diabetes and GAD-specific autoantibodies are detected in 50–80% of patients with this autoimmune disease. Despite the association of stiff-person syndrome with type I diabetes and the recognition of a common autoantigen, it appears that distinct epitopes of GAD are recognized in these two different conditions. Other (systemic) autoantibodies such as anti-smooth muscle, antinuclear, and antimitochondrial antibodies are common in stiff-person patients. Anti-amphiphysin antibodies, sometimes detected in the serum of patients with breast cancer, are also associated with stiff-person syndrome (see Table 38–1). Variable success has been obtained with high-dose corticosteroids, azathioprine, intravenous immunoglobulin, and plasmapheresis.

IMMUNOLOGIC FEATURES OF STROKE

An atypical pathophysiology often accounts for stroke in young individuals. Common risk factors for stroke in older individuals (ie, hypertension, diabetes mellitus, tobacco use, elevated cholesterol, and family history of vascular disease) are often absent. Young individuals (<40) with stroke may have circulating antibodies to phospholipids, major constituents of all cell membranes, which predispose them to thrombotic strokes. The lupus anticoagulant was the first antibody implicated in stroke conditions. It is not a true anticoagulant and is not always associated with systemic lupus erythematosus. The most common antiphospholipid antibodies accounting for these "hypercoagulable" strokes are anticardiolipin antibodies, which are responsible for the positive (and false-positive) serologic tests for syphilis. Antiphospholipid antibodies are usually of the IgG isotype. Patients with stroke associated with antiphospholipid antibodies are commonly women with a history of deep venous thrombosis, thrombocytopenia, or spontaneous abortions. In Sneddon's syndrome, antiphospholipid antibodies have been associated with skin rash (livedo reticularis), high blood pressure, and cerebrovascular ischemic infarcts. It has been postulated that antiphospholipid antibodies cause a coagulopathy by activation of clotting factors, inhibition of anticoagulants such as protein C and S, as well as endothelial cell activation. The treatment of choice remains anticoagulation, as immunosuppressive therapy, plasmapheresis, and IVIG have been proven unsuccessful.

After acute ischemic stroke, adhesion molecules

are up-regulated on cerebrovascular endothelial cells, a number of proinflammatory cytokines are secreted, and leukocytic infiltration occurs. Although neutrophils predominate, T cells and NK cells are also observed within 24 hours of ischemic stroke. It has been postulated that exposure of CNS antigens to systemic immunocompetent cells could potentiate inflammation in stroke. Based on this concept, one group recently investigated whether induction of tolerance to the CNS autoantigen by oral administration of myelin basic protein could alter the outcome of ischemic stroke. In their experimental model they observed that oral tolerance to myelin basic protein, in contrast to control antigen, reduced stroke size. Although highly speculative, these results raise the possibility that antigen-specific immune modulation may be a beneficial adjunctive therapy in certain types of ischemic stroke.

REFERENCES

MULTIPLE SCLEROSIS

European Study Group on interferon beta-1b in secondary progressive MS: Placebo-controlled multicentre randomised trial of interferon beta-1b in treatment of secondary progressive multiple sclerosis. *Lancet* 1998;352:1491.

Genain CP et al: Identification of autoantibodies associated with myelin damage in multiple sclerosis. *Nat Med* 1999;5:170.

The IFNB multiple sclerosis study group: Interferon beta-1b is effective in relapsing-remitting multiple sclerosis. I. Clinical results of a multicenter, randomized, double-blind, placebo-controlled trial. *Neurology* 1993;43:661.

Johnson KP et al: Copolymer 1 reduces relapse rate and improves disability in relapsing-remitting multiple sclerosis: Result of a phase III multicenter, double-blind placebo-controlled trial. The Copolymer 1 Multiple Sclerosis Study Group. *Neurology* 1995;45:1268.

Stüve O et al: Interferon beta-1b decreases the migration of T lymphocytes in vitro: Effects on matrix metalloproteinase-9. *Ann Neurol* 1996;40:853.

Weinshenker BG et al: The natural history of multiple sclerosis: A geographically based study. 4. Applications to planning and interpretation of clinical therapeutic trials. *Brain* 1991;114:1057.

Zamvil SS, Steinman L. The T lymphocyte in experimental allergic encephalomyelitis. Annu Rev Immunol 1990; 8:579.

ACUTE DISSEMINATED ENCEPHALOMYELITIS

Kesselring J et al: Acute disseminating encephalomyelitis. *Brain* 1990;113:291.

Murray PD et al: CD4+ and CD8+ T cells make discrete contributions to demyelination and neurologic disease in a viral model of multiple sclerosis. *J Virol* 1998;72:7320.

Stüve O, Zamvil SS: Pathogenesis, diagnosis, and treatment of acute disseminated encephalomyelitis. *Curr Opin Neurol* 1999;12:395.

ACUTE & CHRONIC INFLAMMATORY DEMYELINATING POLYNEUROPATHIES

Hahn AF. Guillain-Barré syndrome. *Lancet* 1998;352:635.

Hartung HP et al: Guillain-Barré syndrome, CIDP and other chronic immune-mediated neuropathies. *Curr Opin Neurol* 1998;11:497.

MYASTHENIA GRAVIS & MYASTHENIC SYNDROME

Bril V et al: The long-term clinical outcome of myasthenia gravis in patients with thymoma. *Neurology* 1998;51:1198.

Drachman DB: Myasthenia gravis. *New Engl J Med* 1994; 330:1797.

Takamori M: An autoimmune channelopathy associated with cancer: Lambert-Eaton myasthenic syndrome. *Intern Med* 1999;38:86.

PARANEOPLASTIC SYNDROMES

Dalmau JO, Posner JB: Paraneoplastic syndromes. *Arch Neurol* 1999;56:405.

Darnell RB: The importance of defining the paraneoplastic neurologic disorders. *N Engl J Med* 1999;340:1831.

AMYOTROPHIC LATERAL SCLEROSIS

Jackson CE, Bryan WW: Amyotrophic lateral sclerosis. *Semin Neurol* 1998;18:27.

Morrison BM, Morrison JH: Amyotrophic lateral sclerosis associated with mutations in superoxide dismutase: A putative mechanism of degeneration. *Brain Res Brain Res Rev* 1999;29:121.

Smith RG et al: Autoimmunity and ALS. *Neurology* 1996; 47:45.

ALZHEIMER'S DISEASE

Schenk D et al: Immunization with amyloid-β attenuates Alzheimer-disease-like pathology in the PDAPP mouse. *Nature* 1999;400:173.

St George-Hyslop PH, Westaway DA: Antibody clears senile plaques. *Nature* 1999;400:116.

Stewart WF et al: Risk of Alzheimer's disease and duration of NSAIDS use. *Neurology* 1997;48:626.

OTHER DISEASES OF THE CENTRAL NERVOUS SYSTEM WITH AUTOIMMUNE FEATURES

Antel JP, Rasmussen T: Rasmussen's encephalitis and the new hat. *Neurology* 1996;46:9.

Becker KJ: Inflammation and acute stroke. *Curr Opin Neurol* 1998;11:45.

Feldman E, Levine SR: Cerebrovascular disease with antiphospholipid antibodies: Immune mechanisms, significance, and therapeutic options. *Ann Neurol* 1995;37:114.

Levy LM et al: The stiff-person syndrome: An autoimmune disorder affecting neurotransmission of gamma-aminobutyric acid. *Ann Intern Med* 1999;131:522.

Li Y et al: Local-clonal expansion of infiltrating T lymphocytes in chronic encephalitis of Rasmussen. *J Immunol* 1997;158:1428.

Eye Diseases

39

Mitchell H. Friedlaender, MD, & G. Richard O'Connor, MD

The eye is frequently considered to be a special target of immunologic disease processes, but proof of the causative role of these processes is lacking for all but a few disorders. In this sense, the immunopathology of the eye is much less clearly delineated than that of the kidney, the testis, or the thyroid gland. Because the eye is a **highly vascularized organ** and because the rather labile vessels of the conjunctiva are embedded in a nearly transparent medium, inflammatory eye disorders are more obvious (and often more painful) than those of such other organs as the thyroid or the kidney. The iris, ciliary body, and choroid are the most highly vascularized tissues of the eye. The similarity of the vascular supply of the uvea to that of the kidney and the choroid plexus of the brain has given rise to justified speculation concerning the selection of these three tissues, among others, as targets of immune complex diseases (eg, serum sickness).

Immunologic diseases of the eye can be grossly divided into two major categories: antibody-mediated and cell-mediated diseases. As is the case in other organs, there is ample opportunity for the interaction of these two systems in the eye.

ANTIBODY-MEDIATED DISEASES

Before it can be concluded that a disease of the eye is antibody-dependent, the following criteria must be satisfied: (1) There must be evidence of specific antibody in the patient's serum or plasma cells. (2) The antigen must be identified and, if feasible, characterized. (3) The same antigen must be shown to produce an immunologic response in the eye of an experimental animal, and the pathologic changes produced in the experimental animal must be similar to those observed in the human disease. (4) It must be possible to produce similar lesions in animals passively sensitized with serum from an affected animal on challenge with the specific antigen.

Unless all of the preceding criteria are satisfied, the disease may be thought of as *possibly* antibody-dependent. In such circumstances, the disease can be regarded as antibody-mediated if only one of the following criteria is met: (1) antibody to an antigen is present in higher quantities in the ocular fluids than in the serum (after adjustments have been made for the total amounts of immunoglobulins in each fluid); (2) abnormal accumulations of plasma cells are present in the ocular lesion; (3) abnormal accumulations of immunoglobulins are present at the site of the disease; (4) complement is fixed by immunoglobulins at the site of the disease; (5) an accumulation of eosinophils is present at the site of the disease; or (6) the ocular disease is associated with an inflammatory disease elsewhere in the body for which antibody dependency has been proved or strongly suggested.

VERNAL CONJUNCTIVITIS & ATOPIC KERATOCONJUNCTIVITIS

These two diseases belong to the group of atopic-like disorders. Both are characterized by itching and lacrimation of the eyes but are more chronic than is hay fever conjunctivitis. Furthermore, both ultimately result in structural modifications of the lids and conjunctiva. The immunologic basis for these diseases is not delineated.

Vernal conjunctivitis characteristically affects children and adolescents; the incidence decreases sharply after the second decade of life. Like hay fever conjunctivitis, vernal conjunctivitis occurs only in the warm months of the year. Most of its victims live in hot, dry climates. The disease characteristically produces giant ("cobblestone") papillae of the tarsal conjunctiva (Figure 39–1).

Atopic keratoconjunctivitis affects individuals of all ages and has no specific seasonal incidence. The skin of the lids has a characteristic dry, scaly appearance. The conjunctiva is pale and boggy. Both the conjunctiva and the cornea may develop scarring in the later stages of the disease. Atopic cataract has also been described. Staphylococcal blepharitis, manifested by scales and crusts on the lids, commonly complicates this disease.

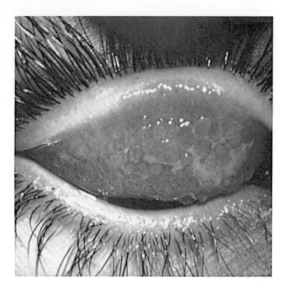

Figure 39–1. Giant papillae ("cobblestone") in the tarsal conjunctiva of a patient with vernal conjunctivitis.

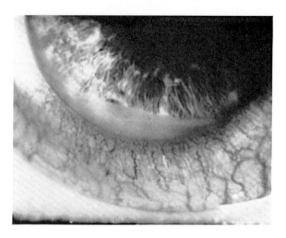

Figure 39–2. Acute iridocyclitis in a patient with ankylosing spondylitis. Note the fibrin clot in the anterior chamber.

RHEUMATOID DISEASES AFFECTING THE EYE

The diseases in this category vary greatly in their clinical manifestations depending on the specific disease entity and the age of the patient. Uveitis and scleritis are the principal ocular manifestations of the rheumatoid diseases. **Juvenile rheumatoid arthritis** affects females more frequently than males and is commonly accompanied by iridocyclitis of one or both eyes. The onset is often insidious, the patient having few or no complaints and the eye remaining white. Extensive synechia formation, cataract, and secondary glaucoma may be far advanced before the parents notice that anything is wrong. The arthritis generally affects only one joint (eg, a knee) in cases with ocular involvement.

Ankylosing spondylitis affects males more frequently than females, and the onset is in the second to sixth decades. It may be accompanied by iridocyclitis of acute onset, often with fibrin in the anterior chamber (Figure 39–2). Pain, redness, and photophobia are the initial complaints, and synechia formation is common. Over 90% of patients with ankylosing spondylitis and over 50% of all iridocyclitis patients express the human leukocyte antigen (HLA)-B27 allele.

Rheumatoid arthritis of adult onset may be accompanied by acute scleritis or episcleritis (Figure 39–3). The ciliary body and choroid, lying adjacent to the sclera, are often involved secondarily with the inflammation. Rarely, serous detachment of the retina results. The onset is usually in the third to fifth decade, and women are affected more frequently than men. The sclera may become thin and may even perforate.

Reiter's disease affects men more frequently than women. The first attack of ocular inflammation usually consists of a self-limited papillary conjunctivitis. It follows, at a highly variable interval, the onset of nonspecific urethritis and the appearance of inflammation in one or more of the weight-bearing joints. Subsequent attacks of ocular inflammation may consist of acute iridocyclitis of one or both eyes, occasionally with hypopyon (Figure 39–4). Over 90% of patients with Reiter's disease carry the HLA-B27 allele.

Immunologic Pathogenesis

Rheumatoid factor, an IgM autoantibody directed against the patient's own IgG, probably plays a major role in the pathogenesis of certain clinical manifestations of rheumatoid arthritis. The union of IgM antibody with IgG is followed by fixation of complement

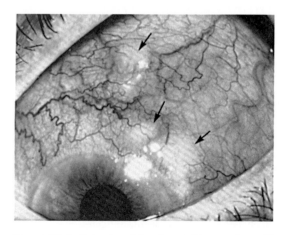

Figure 39–3. Scleral nodules *(arrows)* in a patient with rheumatoid arthritis. (Courtesy of S Kimura.)

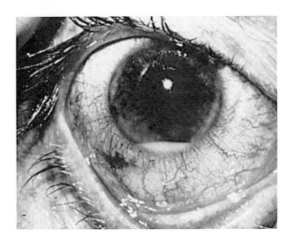

Figure 39–4. Acute iridocyclitis with hypopyon in a patient with Reiter's disease.

at the tissue site and the attraction of leukocytes and platelets to this area. An occlusive vasculitis resulting from this train of events is thought to form the rheumatoid nodule in the sclera and elsewhere in the body. The occlusion of vessels supplying nutrients to the sclera is thought to be responsible for the "melting away" of the scleral collagen that is so characteristic of rheumatoid arthritis (Figure 39–5).

Although this explanation may suffice for rheumatoid arthritis, patients with the ocular complications of juvenile rheumatoid arthritis, ankylosing spondylitis, and Reiter's syndrome usually have negative tests for rheumatoid factor, so other explanations must be sought.

Outside the eyeball itself, the **lacrimal gland** has been shown to be under attack by circulating antibodies. Destruction of acinar cells within the gland and invasion of the lacrimal gland (as well as the salivary glands) by mononuclear cells result in decreased tear secretion. The combination of dry eyes (keratoconjunc-

tivitis sicca), dry mouth (xerostomia), and rheumatoid arthritis (or other connective tissue disease) is known as Sjögren's syndrome (see Chapter 33).

A growing body of evidence indicates that the immunogenetic background of certain patients accounts for the expression of their ocular inflammatory disease in specific ways. Analysis of the HLA antigen system shows HLA-B27 is significantly more common in patients with ankylosing spondylitis and Reiter's syndrome than could be expected by chance alone. How this molecule controls specific inflammatory responses is unknown.

Immunologic Diagnosis

Rheumatoid factor can be detected in the serum by a number of standard tests involving the agglutination of IgG-coated erythrocytes or latex particles. Unfortunately, the test for rheumatoid factor is not positive in the majority of isolated rheumatoid afflictions of the eye.

The HLA types of individuals suspected of having ankylosing spondylitis and related diseases can be determined by standard cytotoxicity tests with specific antisera. These tests are generally done in tissue-typing centers where HLA typing for organ transplantation necessitates such studies. Radiography of the sacroiliac area is a valuable screening procedure that may show evidence of spondylitis prior to the onset of low back pain in patients with the characteristic form of iridocyclitis.

Treatment

Patients with uveitis associated with rheumatoid disease respond well to local instillations of corticosteroid drops (eg, dexamethasone 0.1%) or ointments. Orally administered corticosteroids must occasionally be resorted to for brief periods. Aspirin given orally in divided doses with meals is thought to reduce the frequency and blunt the severity of recurrent attacks. Atropine drops 1% are useful for the relief of photophobia during the acute attacks. Shorter acting mydriatics such as phenylephrine 2.5% should be used in the subacute stages to prevent synechia formation. Corticosteroid-resistant cases, especially those causing progressive erosion of the sclera, have been treated successfully with immunosuppressive drugs such as chlorambucil. Hydroxychloroquine, an antimalarial drug, has been useful in the treatment of Sjögren's syndrome and other collagen-vascular diseases. Eye examinations at 6- to 12-month intervals are recommended because deposits in the cornea and retina have been reported with high-dose hydroxychloroquine therapy.

OTHER ANTIBODY-MEDIATED DISEASES

The following antibody-mediated diseases are infrequently seen by the practicing ophthalmologist.

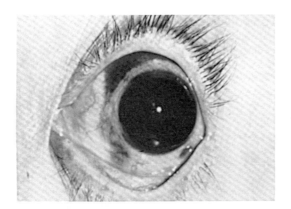

Figure 39–5. Scleral thinning in a patient with rheumatoid arthritis. Note the dark color of the underlying uvea.

Systemic lupus erythematosus (SLE), associated with the presence of circulating antibodies to DNA, produces an occlusive vasculitis of the nerve fiber layer of the retina. Such infarcts result in cytoid bodies, or "cotton-wool" spots, in the retina (Figure 39–6).

Pemphigus vulgaris produces painful intraepithelial bullae of the conjunctiva. It is associated with the presence of circulating antibodies to an intercellular antigen located between the deeper cells of the conjunctival epithelium.

Cicatricial pemphigoid is characterized by subepithelial bullae of the conjunctiva. In the chronic stages of this disease, cicatricial contraction of the conjunctiva may result in severe scarring of the cornea, dryness of the eyes, and, ultimately, blindness. Pemphigoid is associated with local deposits of tissue antibodies directed against one or more antigens located in the basement membrane of the epithelium.

Lens-induced uveitis is a rare condition that may be associated with circulating antibodies to lens proteins. It is seen in individuals whose lens capsules have become permeable to these proteins as a result of trauma or other disease. Interest in this field dates back to 1903, when P. Uhlenhuth first demonstrated the organ-specific nature of antibodies to the lens. R. Witmer showed in 1962 that antibody to lens tissue may be produced by lymphoid cells of the ciliary body.

CELL-MEDIATED DISEASES

This group of diseases appears to be associated with T-cell-mediated immunity (delayed hypersensi-

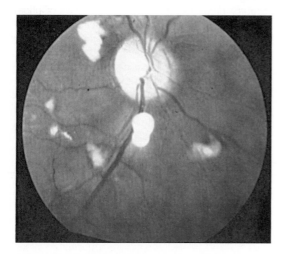

Figure 39–6. Cotton-wool spots in the retina of a patient with systemic lupus erythematosus.

tivity). Various structures of the eye are invaded by mononuclear cells, principally lymphocytes and macrophages, in response to one or more chronic antigenic stimuli. In chronic infections, such as tuberculosis, leprosy, toxoplasmosis, and herpes simplex, the antigenic stimulus has clearly been identified as an infectious agent in the ocular tissue. Such infections are often associated with delayed skin test reactivity following the intradermal injection of an extract of the organism.

More intriguing but less well understood are the granulomatous diseases of the eye for which no infectious cause has been found. Such diseases are thought to represent cell-mediated, possibly autoimmune processes, but their origin remains obscure.

OCULAR SARCOIDOSIS

Ocular sarcoidosis is characterized by a panuveitis with occasional inflammatory involvement of the optic nerve and retinal blood vessels. It often presents as iridocyclitis of insidious onset. Less frequently, it occurs as acute iridocyclitis, with pain, photophobia, and redness of the eye. Large precipitates resembling drops of solidified mutton fat are seen on the corneal endothelium. The anterior chamber contains a good deal of protein and numerous cells, mostly lymphocytes. Nodules are often seen on the iris, both at the pupillary margin and in the substance of the iris stroma. The latter are often vascularized. Synechiae are commonly encountered, particularly in patients with dark skin. Severe cases ultimately involve the posterior segment of the eye. Coarse clumps of cells ("snowballs") are seen in the vitreous, and exudates resembling candle drippings may be seen along the course of the retinal vessels. Patchy infiltrations of the choroid or optic nerve may also be seen.

Infiltrations of the lacrimal gland and of the conjunctiva have been noted on occasion. When the latter are present, the diagnosis can easily be confirmed by biopsy of the small opaque nodules.

Immunologic Pathogenesis

Although many infectious or allergic causes of sarcoidosis have been suggested, none has been confirmed. **Noncaseating granulomas** are seen in the uvea, optic nerve, and adnexal structures of the eye as well as elsewhere in the body. The presence of macrophages and giant cells suggests that particulate matter is being phagocytized, but this material has not been identified.

Patients with sarcoidosis are usually **anergic** to extracts of the common microbial antigens such as those of mumps, *Trichophyton, Candida,* and *Mycobacterium tuberculosis.* As in other lymphoproliferative disorders, such as Hodgkin's disease and chronic lymphocytic leukemia, suppression of T-cell immunity impairs normal delayed hypersensitivity responses to common antigens. Meanwhile, circulating immunoglobulins are usually detectable in the serum at higher than normal levels.

Immunologic Diagnosis

The diagnosis is largely inferential. Negative skin tests to a battery of antigens to which the patient is known to have been exposed are highly suggestive, and the same is true of the elevation of serum immunoglobulins. Biopsy of a conjunctival nodule or scalene lymph node may provide positive histologic evidence of the disease. Radiographs of the chest reveal hilar adenopathy in many cases. Elevated levels of serum lysozyme or serum angiotensin-converting enzyme may be detected. A gallium scan, using gallium-67, may be useful in detecting clinically inapparent lesions.

Treatment

Sarcoid lesions of the eye respond well to corticosteroid therapy. Frequent instillations of prednisolone acetate 1% eye drops generally bring the anterior uveitis under control. Atropine drops should be prescribed in the acute phase of the disease for the relief of pain and photophobia; short-acting pupillary dilators such as phenylephrine should be given later to prevent synechia formation. Systemic corticosteroids are sometimes necessary to control severe attacks of anterior uveitis and are always necessary for the control of retinal vasculitis and optic neuritis. The latter condition often accompanies cerebral involvement and carries a grave prognosis.

SYMPATHETIC OPHTHALMIA & VOGT-KOYANAGI-HARADA SYNDROME

These two disorders are discussed together because they have certain common clinical features. Both are thought to represent autoimmune phenomena affecting pigmented structures of the eye and skin, and both may give rise to meningeal symptoms.

Clinical Features

Sympathetic ophthalmia is an inflammation in the second eye after the other has been damaged by penetrating injury. In most cases, some portion of the uvea of the injured eye has been exposed to the atmosphere for at least 1 hour. The uninjured, or "sympathizing," eye develops minor signs of anterior uveitis after a period ranging from 2 weeks to several years. Floating spots and loss of the power of accommodation are among the earliest symptoms. The disease may progress to severe iridocyclitis with pain and photophobia. Usually, however, the eye remains relatively quiet and painless while the inflammatory disease spreads around the entire uvea. Despite the presence of panuveitis, the retina usually remains un-

involved except for perivascular cuffing of the retinal vessels with inflammatory cells. Papilledema and secondary glaucoma may occur. The disease may be accompanied by vitiligo (patchy depigmentation of the skin) and poliosis (whitening) of the eyelashes.

Vogt-Koyanagi-Harada syndrome consists of inflammation of the uvea of one or both eyes characterized by acute iridocyclitis, patchy choroiditis, and serous detachment of the retina. It usually begins with an acute febrile episode with headaches, dysacusis, and occasionally vertigo. Patchy loss or whitening of the scalp hair is described in the first few months of the disease. Vitiligo and poliosis are commonly present but are not essential for the diagnosis. Although the initial iridocyclitis may subside quickly, the course of the posterior disease is often indolent, with long-standing serous detachment of the retina and significant visual impairment.

Immunologic Pathogenesis

In both sympathetic ophthalmia and Vogt-Koyanagi-Harada syndrome, delayed hypersensitivity to melanin-containing structures is thought to occur. Although a viral cause has been suggested for both disorders, there is no convincing evidence of an infectious origin. It is postulated that some insult, infectious or otherwise, alters the pigmented structures of the eye, skin, and hair in such a way as to provoke delayed hypersensitivity responses to them. Soluble materials from the outer segments of the photoreceptor layer of the retina have recently been incriminated as possible autoantigens. Patients with Vogt-Koyanagi-Harada syndrome are usually of Asian ancestry, which suggests an immunogenetic predisposition to the disease.

Histologic sections of the traumatized eye from a patient with sympathetic ophthalmia may show uniform infiltration of most of the uvea by lymphocytes, epithelioid cells, and giant cells. The overlying retina is characteristically intact, but nests of epithelioid cells may protrude through the pigment epithelium of the retina, giving rise to **Dalen-Fuchs nodules.** The inflammation may destroy the architecture of the entire uvea, leaving an atrophic, shrunken globe.

Immunologic Diagnosis

Skin tests with soluble extracts of human or bovine uveal tissue are said to elicit delayed hypersensitivity responses in these patients. Several investigators have recently shown that cultured lymphocytes from patients with these two diseases undergo transformation to lymphoblasts in vitro when extracts of uvea or rod outer segments are added to the culture medium. Circulating antibodies to uveal antigens have been found in patients with these diseases, but such antibodies are to be found in any patient with long-standing uveitis, including those suffering from several infectious entities. The spinal fluid of patients with Vogt-Koyanagi-Harada syndrome may show increased numbers of mononuclear cells and elevated protein in the early stages.

Treatment

Mild cases of sympathetic ophthalmia may be treated satisfactorily with locally applied corticosteroid drops and pupillary dilators. The more severe or progressive cases require systemic corticosteroids, often in high doses, for months or years. An alternate-day regimen of oral corticosteroids is recommended for such patients to minimize adrenal suppression. The same applies to the treatment of patients with Vogt-Koyanagi-Harada syndrome. Occasionally, patients with long-standing progressive disease become resistant to corticosteroids or cannot take additional corticosteroid medication because of pathologic fractures, mental changes, or other reasons. Such patients may become candidates for immunosuppressive therapy. Chlorambucil and cyclophosphamide have used successfully for both conditions. More recently, cyclosporine has shown promise in the treatment of corticosteroid-resistant uveitis.

OTHER CELL-MEDIATED DISEASES

Giant-cell arteritis (temporal arteritis) (see Chapter 34) may have disastrous effects on the eyes, particularly in elderly individuals. The condition is manifested by pain in the temples and orbit, blurred vision, and scotomas. Examination of the fundus may reveal extensive occlusive retinal vasculitis and choroidal infarcts. Atrophy of the optic nerve head is a frequent complication. Such patients have an elevated erythrocyte sedimentation rate. Biopsy of the temporal artery reveals extensive infiltration of the vessel wall with giant cells and mononuclear cells.

Polyarteritis nodosa (see Chapter 34) can affect both the anterior and posterior segments of the eye. The corneas of such patients may show peripheral thinning and cellular infiltration. The retinal vessels reveal extensive necrotizing inflammation characterized by eosinophil, plasma cell, and lymphocyte infiltration.

Behçet's disease (see Chapters 31 and 34) has an uncertain place in the classification of immunologic disorders. It is characterized by recurrent iridocyclitis with hypopyon and occlusive vasculitis of the retinal vessels. Although it has many of the features of a delayed hypersensitivity disease, dramatic alterations of serum complement levels at the very beginning of an attack suggest an immune complex disorder. Furthermore, high levels of circulating immune complexes have recently been detected in patients with this disease. Most patients with eye symptoms are positive for HLA-B5 (subtype B51).

Contact dermatitis (see Chapter 29) of the eyelids represents a significant though minor disease caused by delayed hypersensitivity. Atropine, perfumed cosmetics, materials contained in plastic spectacle frames, and other locally applied agents may act as the sensitizing hapten. The lower lid is more extensively involved than the upper lid when the sensitizing agent is applied in drop form. Periorbital involvement with erythematous, vesicular, pruritic lesions of the skin is characteristic.

Phlyctenular keratoconjunctivitis (Figure 39–7) represents a delayed hypersensitivity response to certain microbial antigens, principally those of *M tuberculosis*. It is characterized by acute pain and photophobia in the affected eye, and perforation of the peripheral cornea has been known to result. The disease responds rapidly to locally applied corticosteroids. Phlyctenulosis is much less of a problem than it was before the advent of chemotherapy for pulmonary tuberculosis. It is still encountered occasionally, however, particularly among Native Americans and Inuit peoples. Rarely, other pathogens such as *Staphylococcus aureus* and *Coccidioides immitis* have been implicated in phlyctenular disease.

Acquired immunodeficiency syndrome (AIDS) (see Chapter 46) is commonly associated with ocular disorders. Cotton-wool exudates are the most common ocular sign. They have the same appearance as those seen in SLE (see Figure 39–6), but it is not known whether the cotton-wool spots of AIDS have the same pathogenesis. As is the case with SLE, patients suffering from AIDS may have elevated levels of serum immune complexes.

In addition to cotton-wool spots, AIDS patients may develop Kaposi's sarcoma of the conjunctiva or lids as well as chorioretinitis associated with any one of a number of different opportunistic pathogens such as cytomegalovirus, *Cryptococcus, Toxoplasma,* or *Candida.* These patients have a fundamental disor-

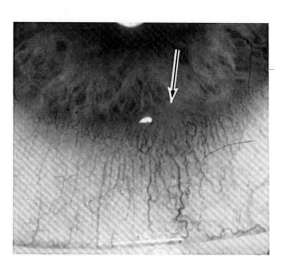

Figure 39–7. Phlyctenule (*arrow*) at the margin of the cornea. (Courtesy of P Thygeson.)

der of cell-mediated immunity reflected in reduced levels of CD4 cells and chronic infection by human immunodeficiency virus (HIV). These patients often die of systemic opportunistic infections such as *Pneumocystis carinii* pneumonia or toxoplasmal encephalitis. Because cotton-wool spots are an early sign of AIDS, the ophthalmologist may be the first physician to alert the patient to the existence of this serious disorder.

CORNEAL GRAFT REACTIONS

General Considerations

Blindness due to opacity or distortion of the central portion of the cornea is a remediable disease (Figure 39–8). If all other structures of the eye are intact, a patient whose vision is impaired solely by corneal opacity can expect great improvement from a graft of clear cornea into the stroma and a single-layered endothelium. Although the surface epithelium may be sloughed and later replaced by the recipient's epithelium, certain elements of the stroma and all of the donor's endothelium remain in place for the rest of the patient's life. This has been firmly established by sex chromosome markers in corneal cells when donor and recipient were of opposite sexes. The endothelium must remain healthy for the cornea to remain transparent, and an energy-dependent pump mechanism is required to keep the cornea from swelling with water. Because the recipient's endothelium is in most cases diseased, the central corneal endothelium must be replaced by healthy donor tissue.

A number of foreign elements exist in corneal grafts that might stimulate the immune system of the host to reject this tissue. In addition to those already mentioned, the corneal stroma is regularly perfused with IgG and serum albumin from the donor, although none—or only small amounts—of the other blood proteins are present. Although these serum proteins of donor origin rapidly diffuse into the recipient stroma, these substances are theoretically immunogenic.

Although the ABO blood group antigens have been shown to have no relationship to corneal graft rejection, the HLA antigen system probably plays a significant role in graft reactions. HLA incompatibility between donor and recipient has been shown by several investigators to be significant in determining graft survival, particularly when the corneal bed is vascularized. It is known that most cells of the body possess these HLA antigens, including the endothelial cells of the corneal graft as well as certain stromal cells (keratocytes). The epithelium has been shown to possess a non-HLA antigen that diffuses into the anterior third of the stroma. Thus, although much foreign antigen may be eliminated by purposeful removal of the epithelium at the time of grafting, the amount of antigen that has already diffused into the stroma is automatically carried over into the recipient. Such antigens may be leached out by soaking the donor cornea in tissue culture for several weeks prior to engraftment.

Immunologic Pathogenesis

Both antibody and cellular mechanisms have been implicated in corneal graft reactions. It is likely that **early graft rejections** (within 2 weeks) are cell-mediated reactions. Cytotoxic lymphocytes have been found in the limbal area and stroma of affected individuals, and phase microscopy in vivo has revealed an actual attack on the grafted endothelial cells by these lymphocytes. Such lymphocytes generally move inward from the periphery of the cornea, making what is known as a "rejection line" as they move centrally. The donor cornea becomes edematous as the endothelium becomes compromised by an accumulation of lymphoid cells.

Late rejection of a corneal graft may occur several weeks to many months after implantation of donor tissue into the recipient eye. Such reactions may be antibody-mediated because cytotoxic antibodies have been isolated from the serum of patients with a history of disease in this area. Trauma, including chemical burns, is one of the most common causes of central corneal opacity. Others include scars from herpetic keratitis, endothelial cell dysfunction with chronic corneal edema (Fuchs' dystrophy), keratoconus, and opacities from previous graft failures. All of these conditions represent indications for penetrating corneal grafts, provided the patient's eye is no longer inflamed and the opacity has been allowed maximal time to undergo spontaneous resolution (usually 6–12 months). It is estimated that ap-

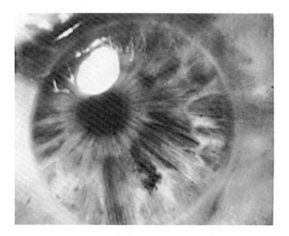

Figure 39–8. A cornea severely scarred by chronic atopic keratoconjunctivitis into which a central graft of clear cornea has been placed. Note how distinctly the iris landmarks are seen through the transparent graft.

proximately 10,000 corneal grafts are performed in the United States annually. Of these, about 90% can be expected to produce a beneficial result.

The cornea was one of the first human tissues to be successfully grafted. The fact that recipients of corneal grafts generally tolerate them well can be attributed to (1) the absence of blood vessels or lymphatics in the normal cornea and (2) the lack of presensitization to tissue-specific antigens in most recipients. Reactions to corneal grafts do occur, however, particularly in individuals whose own corneas have been damaged by previous inflammatory disease. Such corneas may have developed both lymphatics and blood vessels, providing afferent and efferent channels for immunologic reactions in the engrafted cornea.

Although attempts have been made to transplant corneas from other species into human eyes (xenografts), particularly in countries where human material is not available for religious reasons, most corneal grafts have been taken from human eyes (allografts). Except in the case of identical twins, such grafts always represent the implantation of foreign tissue into a donor site; thus, the chance for a graft rejection due to an immune response to foreign antigens is virtually always present.

The cornea is a three-layered structure composed of a surface epithelium, an oligocellular stroma, and a single endothelial layer of cells. Each layer can undergo single or multiple graft reactions in vascularized corneal beds. Graft reactions can be cell-mediated or antibody-mediated. These antibody reactions are complement-dependent and attract polymorphonuclear leukocytes, which may form dense rings in the cornea at the sites of maximum deposition of immune complexes. In experimental animals, similar reactions have been produced by corneal xenografts, but the intensity of the reaction can be markedly reduced either by decomplementing the animal or by reducing its leukocyte population through mechlorethamine therapy.

Treatment

The mainstay of the treatment of corneal graft reactions is corticosteroid therapy. This medication is generally given in the form of frequently applied eye drops (eg, prednisolone acetate 1%, hourly) until the clinical signs abate. These clinical signs consist of conjunctival hyperemia in the perilimbal region, a cloudy cornea, cells and protein in the anterior chamber, and keratic precipitates on the corneal endothelium. The earlier that treatment is applied, the more effective it is likely to be. Neglected cases may require systemic or periocular corticosteroids in addition to local eye drop therapy. Occasionally, vascularization and opacification of the cornea occur so rapidly that corticosteroid therapy is useless, but even the most hopeless-appearing graft reactions have occasionally been reversed by corticosteroid therapy. Topical corticosteroids are often used once or twice a day as prophylaxis against transplant rejection. More recently, topical cyclosporine eye drops have been used.

Patients known to have rejected many previous corneal grafts are treated somewhat differently, particularly if disease affects their only remaining eye. An attempt is made to find a close HLA match between donor and recipient. Pretreatment of the recipient with immunosuppressive agents such as azathioprine has also been resorted to in some cases. Although HLA testing of the recipient and the potential donor is indicated in cases of repeated corneal graft failure or in cases of severe corneal vascularization, such testing is not necessary or practicable in most cases requiring keratoplasty.

REFERENCES

Bielory L (editor): Ocular allergy. *Immunol Clin North Am* 1997;17:1. Entire issue.

Dugel PU, Rao NA: Ocular infections in acquired immunodeficiency syndrome. *Int Ophthalmol Clin* 1993; 33:103.

Friedlaender MH (editor): Ocular allergy. *Int Ophthalmol Clin* 1988;28:261.

Friedlaender MH: *Allergy and Immunology of the Eye,* 2nd ed. Raven, 1993.

Friedlaender MH: New and evolving ocular infections. *Int Ophthalmol Clin* 1993;33:1. Entire issue.

Gold DH: Systemic associations of ocular disease. *Int Ophthalmol Clin* 1991;31:1. Entire issue.

Mannis MJ et al: *Eye and Skin Disease.* Lippincott-Raven, 1996.

Michelson JB, Nozik RA: *Surgical Treatment of Ocular Inflammatory Disease.* Lippincott, 1988.

O'Connor GR, Chandler JW (editors): *Advances in Immunology and Immunopathology of the Eye.* Masson, 1985.

Smith R, Nozik R: *Uveitis: A Clinical Approach to Diagnosis and Management.* Williams & Wilkins, 1983.

Smolin G (editor): Infectious and immunologic diseases of the cornea. *Inl Opthalmol Clin* 1998;38:1. Entire issue.

Smolin G, O'Connor GR: *Ocular Immunology.* Little, Brown, 1986.

Tabbara KF: Posterior uveitis. Part 1. *Int Ophthalmol Clin* 1995;35:1. Entire issue.

Tabbara KF: Posterior uveitis. Part 2. *Int Ophthalmol Clin* 1995;35:1. Entire issue.

Tabbara KF, Hyndiuk RA: *Infections of the Eye.* Little Brown, 1996.

Respiratory Diseases

40

John F. Fieselmann, MD, & Hal B. Richerson, MD

Respiratory diseases of putative disordered immune regulation include those caused by a hypersensitivity (allergy) to an exogenous antigen, autoantibody, or immunodeficiency. **Hypersensitivity responses** to known antigens include hypersensitivity pneumonitis, allergic asthma (atopic and occupational), some examples of eosinophilic pneumonias (parasitic, drug-induced, and allergic bronchopulmonary aspergillosis), and other drug-induced lung diseases. These are covered in Chapters 26, 28, 29, and 30. Most respiratory diseases attributed to disordered immune regulation are of unknown cause, but their pathology appears to involve immunologic mechanisms. Examples include collagen-vascular diseases, granulomatous diseases, vasculitis syndromes, and idiopathic interstitial fibrosis. Respiratory diseases in patients with **primary** or **secondary immunodeficiency** are caused by infectious agents: viral, bacterial, fungal, or parasitic.

The lung must cope with antigens, including infectious organisms, that reach it by way of inspired air, aspiration, and the circulation. The pulmonary immune system normally mounts a protective effector response against harmful agents and ignores those that are harmless. Clearance mechanisms involving alveolar macrophages, ciliary action, secretions, cough, and a combination of innate (nonspecific) and acquired (specific) immunologic mechanisms protect the lung very well in general. Why the system fails and how it leads to disease in some individuals is not well understood for many of the conditions included in this chapter.

DRUG-INDUCED RESPIRATORY DISEASES

Drugs cause adverse pulmonary effects by several different mechanisms, although details of pathogenesis are lacking in most instances. Potential mechanisms include hypersensitivity, direct toxicity, production of free oxygen radicals, stimulation of collagen synthesis, and lipidosis induction. This section primarily considers reactions involving proven or suspected immunologic mechanisms. Lists of common drugs are provided in Table 40–1.

Immunologic Mechanisms

Drug-induced hypersensitivity reactions involving the lungs may be associated with one or more types of immunologic response that damage host tissue. In the Gell and Coombs classification system, hypersensitivity responses may involve IgE antibodies (type I), cellular cytotoxicity (type II), antigen–antibody complexes (type III), or T-cell-mediated hypersensitivity (type IV). Except for wheal-and-flare (immediate-type) skin tests in type I hypersensitivity, documentation of drug allergy by in vivo or in vitro testing has not been clinically useful. In the following section, selected drugs are discussed to illustrate prototypic manifestations of adverse pulmonary reactions.

Airway Involvement

Bronchospasm and cough are the most common symptoms of airway dysfunction. Asthma may be caused by drugs capable of IgE immunogenesis and subsequent IgE-mediated systemic or local anaphylaxis. This is seen in response to β-lactam antibiotics, foreign proteins, and exogenous hormones. **Latex** from surgical gloves or catheters is an increasing problem. Inhalation of **psyllium** (eg, Metamucil) dusts may induce asthma in a sensitized individual administering or otherwise handling the drug.

Aspirin and other nonsteroidal antiinflammatory drugs can cause sudden, severe bronchospasm. No evidence exists that IgE antibodies play a role; rather, shunting of the arachidonic pathway toward lipoxygenase products (leukotrienes C_4, D_4, and E_4) has been suggested as the probable mechanism. Asthma can also be provoked by the direct pharmacologic effects of β-adrenergic blockers or an idiosyncratic effect of angiotensin-converting enzyme (ACE) inhibitors.

Parenchymal Involvement

Parenchymal involvement induced by drugs includes diffuse, discrete, or interstitial infiltrates that may be associated with eosinophilia or with fibrosis. Chest computed tomography (CT) may help in the diagnosis and monitoring of pulmonary damage in patients receiving potentially toxic drugs. **Nitrofurantoin** may cause acute or, less commonly, chronic pulmonary disease. The acute form usually has a sud-

Table 40–1. Drug-induced respiratory diseases that may involve immunologic mechanisms.

Structure Affected or Disease Induced	Drug	Major Pulmonary Manifestations
Airways	ACE inhibitors Aspirin and other NSAIDs Sulfites Cisplatin, L-asparaginase D-Penicillamine Psyllium (inhaled)	Cough, asthma (rare) Asthma Bronchospasm Bronchospasm Bronchiolitis obliterans Asthma

Parenchyma	Anti-infectious agents
	  Isoniazid
	  Nitrofurantoin
	  p-Aminosalicylic acid
	  Penicillin
	  Sulfonamides
		Pulmonary infiltrates

	Chemotherapeutic agents
	  Azathioprine
	  Methotrexate
	  Procarbazine
		Pulmonary infiltrates

	Chemotherapeutic agents
	  Azathioprine
	  Bleomycin
	  Busulfan
	  Chlorambucil
	  Cyclophosphamide
	  Melphalan
	  Mitomycin
	  Nitrosureas
		Pulmonary fibrosis/pneumonitis

	Miscellaneous agents
	  Carbamazepine
	  Cromolyn
	  Gold salts
	  NSAIDs
		Pulmonary infiltrates

	Miscellaneous agents
	  Amiodarone
	  Diphenylhydantoin
	  D-Penicillamine
	  Fluoxetine
	  Methysergide
	  Nitrofurantoin
		Pulmonary fibrosis/pneumonitis

Pleura	Chemotherapeutic agents
	  Bleomycin, busulfan, methotrexate
	    mitomicin, procarbazine
	  Methysergide, ergonovine
	  Bromocryptine
	  Nitrofurantoin
		Pleurisy and effusion

Mediastinum	Diphenylhydantoin	Pseudolymphoma with adenopathy
Lupus syndrome	Diphenylhydantoin Hydralazine Isoniazid Procainamide	Infiltrates, pleuritis, effusion
Pseudo-Goodpasture's syndrome	D-Penicillamine	Pulmonary hemorrhage

Abbreviations: ACE = angiotensin-converting enzyme; NSAID = nonsteroidal antiinflammatory drug.

den onset of fever, cough, dyspnea, and occasionally pleurisy within 7–10 days of beginning medication. Crackles and wheezes may be heard, and eosinophilia is found in 20–30% of patients. Chest radiographs show an interstitial, alveolar, or mixed pattern most prominent at the bases (Figure 40–1). Patients usually improve rapidly after the drug is withdrawn. The un-common chronic form begins after months to years of nitrofurantoin use and is manifested by an insidious onset of dyspnea on exertion, bibasilar crackles, and diffuse interstitial pneumonitis or fibrosis. Some resolution typically occurs on discontinuation of the drug, but the fibrosis may progress. Studies suggest an immunologic pathogenesis in the acute form and cumu-

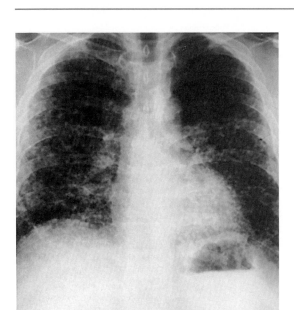

Figure 40–1. Chest radiograph of a patient with drug-induced lung disease secondary to nitrofurantoin showing nodular and linear interstitial infiltrates in the periphery and at the bases.

lative toxicity, perhaps from oxygen radicals, in the chronic form. **Amiodarone** pneumonitis occurs in 4–6% of patients taking this antiarrhythmic drug and results in death in about 25% of those affected. The risk of this complication is dose- and duration-related and is manifested by dyspnea and cough with radiographic findings of interstitial and alveolar infiltrates. Although hypersensitivity may play a role, the condition is associated with lipid accumulation in lung cells (lipidosis), which may be the cause of the inflammatory response. Withdrawing the drug early in the course of pulmonary involvement results in resolution in most patients. **Chemotherapeutic agents,** especially methotrexate, carmustine (*N,N′*-bis(2-chloroethyl)-*N*-nitrosourea [BCNU], and bleomycin, are well known to cause adverse pulmonary responses. Methotrexate generates pulmonary complications in about 8% of patients, but there appears to be a threshold dose requirement of 20 mg/week. The time interval before onset of symptoms may vary from days to years. The acute syndrome of fever, cough, dyspnea, and bilateral pulmonary infiltrates progresses over 1–2 weeks and then regresses whether or not methotrexate therapy is stopped. Acute lymphocytic leukemia of childhood seems to be a specific risk factor for the acute syndrome, and it results in death in 10% of those affected. BCNU, especially in higher doses, has been reported to cause pulmonary fibrosis in 20–30% of patients. The mechanism of injury is probably oxidant toxicity rather than an immunologic one. Bleomycin produces both acute and chronic pulmonary injury with inflammatory infiltrates and fibrosis. The chronic, but not the acute, form is dose-dependent, occurring in about 15% of patients receiving total doses that exceed 450 mg. Older age, previous irradiation, and oxygen therapy increase the risk. The chest x-ray film most commonly shows lower lobe linear or nodular densities.

Gold salts produce pneumonitis in fewer than 1% of patients; this condition occurs 1–26 months after institution of therapy. Eosinophilia and lymphokine production provide evidence favoring types I and IV hypersensitivity responses. **Sulfasalazine** has been reported to cause pulmonary infiltrates, eosinophilia, fibrosis, and bronchiolitis obliterans after months or years of therapy. Hypersensitivity is the most likely mechanism.

Pleura

Drugs causing inflammation of the pleura with or without other lung structures are listed in Table 40–1. Pleuritis may also occur as a part of a drug-induced lupus syndrome.

Mediastinum

Diphenylhydantoin may cause a pseudolymphoma affecting mediastinal as well as peripheral lymph nodes.

Lupus Syndrome

Procainamide and **hydralazine** are the most common agents that cause drug-induced systemic lupus erythematosus with pulmonary manifestations of pneumonitis or pleural effusions. **Isoniazid, D-penicillamine,** and **diphenylhydantoin** are less frequent lupus inducers. Features of the syndrome suggest hypersensitivity mechanisms that may involve an adjuvant effect or alteration of DNA nucleoproteins and subsequent autoantibody production.

Pseudo-Goodpasture's Syndrome

D-Penicillamine in high doses occasionally causes pseudo-Goodpasture's syndrome with abrupt onset of dyspnea, cough, hemoptysis, and hematuria, followed by increasing respiratory distress and renal failure. Intraalveolar hemorrhage and fibrosis are seen histologically. In contrast to Goodpasture's syndrome, antibasement membrane antibodies are not found.

EOSINOPHILIC PNEUMONIAS

Peripheral blood eosinophilia is commonly associated with atopic diseases, parasitic infestations, and some allergic drug reactions. There are many less common causes. When eosinophilia is present together with pulmonary infiltrates, however, the diagnostic possibilities are more limited and constitute the eosinophilic pneumonias or pulmonary infiltrates with eosinophilia (PIE) syndromes (Table 40–2). Although

Table 40–2. Eosinophilic pneumonias.

Disease Entity	Association with Asthma	Comments
Allergic bronchopulmonary aspergillosis	Essentially always (extrinsic asthma)	Complication of atopic asthma with evidence of IgE and IgG antibodies to *Aspergillus fumigatus*
Chronic idiopathic eosinophilic pneumonia (Carrington's)	Frequent (intrinsic asthma)	Subacute to chronic symptoms of cough, fever, dyspnea, sweats, and weight loss; classically peripheral infiltrates on radiogram
Allergic granulomatosis (Churg-Strauss syndrome)	Essentially always	Multisystem vasculitis with fever, malaise, weight loss, pulmonary infiltrates, peripheral neuropathy, arthralgias, myalgias
Acute simple idiopathic pulmonary eosinophilia (Löffler's syndrome)	Occasional	Migratory or transient infiltrates on chest x-ray and minimal or no symptoms
Acute eosinophilic pneumonia	None	Recently described noninfectious eosinophilic pneumonia with rapid progressive respiratory failure
Eosinophilia–myalgia syndrome	None	Caused by dietary supplements of tryptophan (L-tryptophan); sometimes associated with pulmonary infiltrates
Drug-induced eosinophilic pneumonia	None	Penicillins, sulfonamides, nitrofurantoin, isoniazid, and many others (see Table 40–3)
Parasite-induced eosinophilic pneumonia (including visceral larva migrans and tropical pulmonary eosinophilia)	Occasional	*Ascaris, Trichinella, Strongyloides, Dirofilaria, Wuchereria, Toxocara,* and others (see Table 40–3)
Hypereosinophilic syndrome	None	Eosinophilia >1500/mm^3 for 6 months or more; characteristic organ involvement; absence of secondary cause

the cause is usually unknown, hypersensitivity is suspected because similar syndromes result from hypersensitivity to known agents. Affected patients usually have peripheral blood eosinophilia over 10%, or 500 eosinophils/mm^3, but some have eosinophilic pulmonary infiltrates without peripheral eosinophilia.

Many eosinophilic pneumonias are associated with asthma, and the presence or absence of asthma is useful in the differential diagnosis (see Table 40–2).

Asthma essentially always occurs in and usually predates the onset of allergic bronchopulmonary aspergillosus (ABPA) and allergic granulomatosis of Churg and Strauss, and it is often associated with Carrington's chronic eosinophilic pneumonia. The patient is always atopic in ABPA (with demonstrable IgE antibodies to *Aspergillus fumigatus*), often atopic in Churg–Strauss allergic granulomatosis, but not atopic in Carrington's chronic eosinophilic pneumonia.

ABPA is fully discussed in Chapter 30.

Chronic Idiopathic Eosinophilic Pneumonia

This disease is often called Carrington's chronic eosinophilic pneumonia. Clinical manifestations include fever, night sweats, weight loss, and progressive dyspnea. Most patients are white women with a history of recent-onset nonatopic asthma. The classic radiograph shows widespread shadows in a peripheral distribution (Figures 40–2 and 40–3), described

as the "photographic negative" of that produced by pulmonary edema, although localized nonsegmental transient or migratory infiltrates are also found. Chest CT may reveal predominant peripheral airspace consolidation even when the radiograph does not. Glucocorticoid therapy produces prompt remission of this potentially fatal disease, but relapses are common after discontinuation of treatment.

Allergic Granulomatosis of Churg & Strauss

This disease typically begins with upper respiratory symptoms of rhinitis and sinusitis followed by asthma and marked peripheral blood eosinophilia, with concurrent or subsequent pulmonary infiltrates. This is followed by evidence of a systemic vasculitis that may involve the heart, skin, and peripheral nerves. The kidneys are spared or only mildly involved. Mononeuritis multiplex is common, but polyneuropathy also occurs. Treatment requires glucocorticoids in this previously fatal disease; in resistant cases, immunosuppressants such as cyclophosphamide or azathioprine are needed.

Simple Idiopathic Pulmonary Eosinophilia

This is a self-limited, relatively mild illness with transient or migratory pulmonary infiltrates and peripheral eosinophilia regardless of etiology. Also called Löffler's syndrome, this disease usually refers

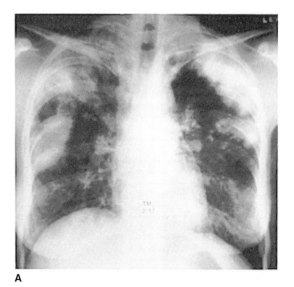

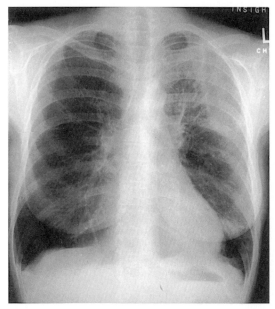

A

B

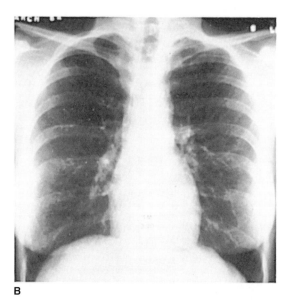

B

Figure 40–2. Chest radiograph of a patient with chronic idiopathic (Carrington's) eosinophilic pneumonia, **A:** showing peripheral distribution of infiltrates during the active phase of the disease and **B:** resolution of the lesions within days of starting glucocorticoid therapy.

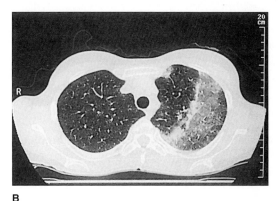

B

Figure 40–3. A: Chest radiograph of a 52-year-old woman during third exacerbation of chronic eosinophilic pneumonia, interpreted as showing a vague opacity overlying the peripheral margin of the left upper hemithorax and stranded opacities radiating out from the left heart border. **B:** High-resolution chest computed tomography taken on patient shown in **A** on the same day, with demonstration of confluent "ground-glass" densities in the left upper lobe. Note the rather distinct demarcation of the involved peripheral portion of the left upper lobe in this axial slice. Scattered areas of abnormal ground-glass density throughout both lungs were also seen.

to simple pulmonary eosinophilia of unknown cause; similar manifestations due to drugs or parasites are better classified under specific cause.

The condition is expected to resolve within a month, so the patient with minimal symptoms does not require treatment.

Acute Eosinophilic Pneumonia

This is an acute form of eosinophilic lung disease first reported in 1989 as distinct from previously de-

scribed syndromes. Specific features include (1) acute febrile illness, (2) severe hypoxemia, (3) diffuse infiltrates on the chest film, (4) over 25% eosinophils in bronchoalveolar lavage fluid, (5) no pulmonary or systemic infection, (6) no history of asthma or atopic illness, (7) prompt response to glucocorticoid therapy, and (8) complete resolution with no sequelae. Distinctive features are the rapid development of severe dyspnea and hypoxemia (PO_2 46–58 mm Hg) within a few days of onset of an acute febrile illness in a previously healthy subject. Lung biopsy has shown diffuse alveolar edema, intraalveolar and interstitial eosinophils, and no vasculitis.

The cause is unknown. Suggested inciting agents in individual patients have included drugs and parasites. Prognosis is excellent with early diagnosis and therapy. No recurrences have been reported to date.

Eosinophilia-Myalgia Syndrome

This syndrome is included here because it may present with pulmonary infiltrates and peripheral blood eosinophilia. The most notable clinical features are severe disabling myalgias, muscle weakness, skin rash, and soft tissue induration resembling scleroderma. It occurs from ingestion of L-tryptophan (containing one or more contaminants) used in large doses as a dietary supplement.

Drug-Induced Eosinophilic Pneumonias

Pulmonary diseases induced by drugs and involving suspected immunologic mechanisms were described earlier. Drugs most commonly incriminated in eosinophilic pneumonia are listed in Table 40–3. Nitrofurantoin may produce acute or chronic eosinophilic pneumonia, whereas most incriminated drugs produce acute syndromes beginning within a month of the institution of therapy. Treatment involves withdrawal of the drug with or without glucocorticoid therapy.

Parasite-Induced Eosinophilic Pneumonias

Eosinophilia is characteristic of all invasive **helminthic** infestations. Those that remain localized to the intestinal tract and cause minimal inflammatory lesions produce little if any eosinophilia; examples include oxyuriasis (pinworm) and trichuriasis (whipworm). Encystment of larval forms may be followed by disappearance of eosinophilia. Protozoan infestations (malaria, amebiasis, giardiasis, toxoplasmosis, leishmaniasis, trypanosomiasis) are not usually accompanied by eosinophilia. Thus, parasite-induced eosinophilic pneumonias are limited to tissue-invasive stages of helminthic parasites trafficking through the lung. Documented examples are listed in Table 40–3.

Visceral larva migrans most commonly affects young children and is caused by infection with the dog and cat ascarids, *Toxocara canis* and *T cati,* respectively; the raccoon ascarid *Baylisascaris procyonis,* hookworm, and *Strongyloides stercoralis* are occasionally responsible. Clinical manifestations are due to free migration of larvae in the liver, lungs, brain, eyes, heart, and skeletal muscles, causing inflammation, eosinophilia, and, eventually, granuloma formation. Patients are often asymptomatic but may present with fever, hepatomegaly, splenomegaly, skin rash, and recurrent pneumonia.

Table 40–3. Eosinophilic pneumonias secondary to drugs and parasites.

Drugs	
Ampicillin	Minocycline
Aspirin	Naproxen
Arsenicals	Nickel
Beclomethasone	Nitrofurantoin
Bleomycin	Aminosalicylic acid
Carbamazepine	Penicillamine
Chlorpromazine	Penicillin
Chlorpropamide	Phenothiazine
Clofibrate	Propylthiourasil
Crack cocaine	Phenylbutazone
Cromolyn	Piroxicam
Diclofenac	Streptomycin
Dilantin	Sulfasalazine
Gold salts	Sulfonamide
Hydralazine	Tetracycline
Imipramine	Thiazide
Mephenesin	Tolazamide
Methotrexate	Tricyclic antidepressants
Methylphenidate	

Parasites
Ancylostoma brasiliense (hookworm)
Ancylostoma duodenale (hookworm)
Ascaris species (roundworm)
Brugia malayi
Dirofilaria immitis (dog heartworm)
Fasciola hepatica (liver fluke)
Necator americanus (hookworm)
Schistosoma species (blood flukes)
Strongyloides stercoralis
Taenia saginata (beef tapeworm)
Toxocara canis (dog roundworm)
Toxocara cati (cat heartworm)
Trichinella spiralis
Trichuris trichiura (whipworm)
Wuchereria bancrofti

Tropical pulmonary eosinophilia is associated with microfilarial infection (*Wuchereria bancrofti* and *Brugia malayi*) and is characterized by fever, weight loss, fatigue, dyspnea, wheezing, and cough, which are usually worse at night. The disease is seen mainly in India, Southeast Asia, and South Pacific islands. Treatment with diethylcarbamazine is usually successful, but progressive fibrosis has been reported following inadequate eradication of the organisms.

Hypereosinophilic Syndrome

Diagnostic criteria for this idiopathic condition include (1) persistent eosinophilia greater than 1500 eosinophils/mm^3 for longer than 6 months; (2) lack of another known causes of eosinophilia; and (3) systemic involvement of the heart, liver, spleen, central nervous system, or lungs. Fever, weight loss, and anemia are common. The heart is frequently involved, with tricuspid valve abnormalities and biventricular restrictive and obliterative cardiomyopathy. Treatment is aimed at lowering the eosinophil count. Some patients progress with morphologic, cytologic, and karyotypic features of eosinophilic leukemia.

OCCUPATIONAL & ENVIRONMENTAL LUNG DISEASES

Indoor air quality has become an increasingly important issue for workplace and home environments. For the most part, immune-mediated occupational and environmental diseases involving the lung are either asthma (Chapter 26) or hypersensitivity pneumonitis (Chapter 29). The environmental antigens associated with these disorders make up long and growing lists.

In addition to asthma and hypersensitivity pneumonitis, environmental exposures may result in **nonimmunologic disorders,** such as the organic dust toxic syndrome (eg, grain fever caused by inhalation of endotoxin, mycotoxins, and other toxins) or the sick building syndrome, which has symptoms of cough, irritation of the nose or throat, headache, fatigue, and difficulty concentrating. Investigations of outbreaks of these and other symptoms reported by workers in modern office buildings determine a specific cause, such as accumulation of toxic gases or contaminated humidification systems, in only about 25% of cases. Inadequate ventilation with outdoor air has also been reported.

SARCOIDOSIS

Major Immunologic Features

- Accumulation of T cells and monocyte-macrophage populations through cell redistribution and in situ proliferation.
- Pattern of cytokines produced by activated CD4 T cells determines nature of immune response
- Granuloma formation through T_H1-associated cell-mediated immune response and macrophage release of mediators
- Polyclonal gammopathy
- Depression of cutaneous delayed-type hypersensitivity (anergy)

General Considerations

Sarcoidosis is a multisystem granulomatous disease of unknown origin that occurs most commonly in young adults. There appears to be a higher prevalence in the black population. It is characterized by a lymphocytic alveolitis or noncaseating granulomas (or both). Pulmonary manifestations occur in more than 90% of patients. Cutaneous, ocular, or hepatic manifestations are also common.

Immunologic Pathogenesis

The assumed inciting antigen of this disorder is unknown. Accumulation of T cells and monocyte–macrophage populations through cell redistribution and in situ proliferation is the earliest step in sarcoid inflammatory reactions. Activated CD4 T cells spontaneously release interferon γ, interleukin-2, and other cytokines. Interleukin-2 release produces a large number of T cells at the site of disease through two mechanisms: (1) chemotaxis of T cells from the circulation to sites of granuloma formation and (2) mitogenesis (the stimulation of T-cell proliferation at sites of granuloma formation). This compartmentalization of inflammatory cells in disease sites results in peripheral blood lymphocytopenia and a CD4 lymphocyte-rich alveolitis. Recent information suggests that the pattern of cytokines produced by CD4 T cells determines the nature of the immune response. Differentiated T_H1 cells cause lymphocyte proliferation and macrophage activation. Activated macrophages release cytokines and chemokines, enhance the proliferation and differentiation of T_H1 cells, and thus facilitate granuloma formation. Most components of the granuloma (macrophages, epithelioid cells, and multinucleated giant cells) are derived from blood monocytes.

Activated T cells at sites of granuloma formation are probably responsible for the polyclonal gammopathy sometimes found in sarcoid. T-cell/B-cell interactions release B-cell growth factor and B-cell differentiation factor, which nonspecifically activate B cells to differentiate into immunoglobulin-secreting plasma cells.

Clinical Features

Textbook descriptions of acute sarcoidosis include fever, erythema nodosum, iritis, and polyarthritis. More often, however, patients note the insidious onset of fatigue, weight loss, malaise, weakness, anorexia, fever, sweats, nonproductive cough, and progressive exertional dyspnea. They may also be asymptomatic, diagnosed only by the presence of an abnormality on a routine chest film. (Figure 40–4; Table 40–4). Pulmonary function studies may be normal or show restrictive lung disease characterized by loss of lung volume, decreased diffusing capacity,

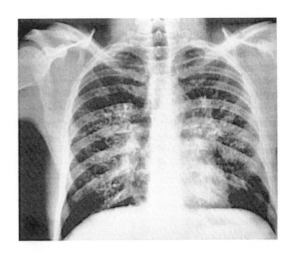

Figure 40–4. Chest radiograph of a patient with sarcoidosis (type II) showing bilateral hilar and parenchymal fibronodular infiltrates.

Table 40–4. Chest radiography in sarcoidosis.

Type	Description
0	Normal
I	Bilateral hilar adenopathy alone
II	Hilar adenopathy and parenchymal abnormalities
III	Parenchymal abnormalities without hilar adenopathy

and exercise-induced hypoxemia. Up to 40% of patients have airway involvement with an obstructive ventilatory defect.

Diagnosis

The diagnosis can be established by the following criteria: (1) a compatible clinical picture; (2) histologic evidence of a systemic granulomatous disease compatible with sarcoidosis; and (3) no evidence of exposure to an agent that is known to cause granulomatous disease. The disorder is also frequently associated with a peripheral blood T lymphocytopenia, anergy to a panel of skin tests for cellular immunity, hypergammaglobulinemia, circulating immune complexes, increased serum ACE activity, increased numbers of macrophages and a CD4/CD8 T-cell ratio greater than 3.5 in the bronchoalveolar lavage. These findings suggest but are not specific for sarcoidosis. The Kveim test, a cutaneous hypersensitivity test formerly used to diagnose sarcoidosis, is largely of historical interest because the antigen is unavailable and other tests are better.

Differential Diagnosis

Other granulomatous diseases include infections (particularly tuberculosis, nontuberculous mycobacterial infection, fungal infection), hypersensitivity pneumonitis, berylliosis, drug reactions, and neoplasms such as lymphomas. Type III sarcoidosis must also be distinguished from the large number of other interstitial lung disorders.

Treatment & Prognosis

The overall prognosis is favorable, with the likelihood of spontaneous remission somewhat linked to the stage of the disease. Patients with a type 0 or I chest film have a very good prognosis with a greater than 80% chance of spontaneous remission, whereas those with type II or III chest film have a less favorable prognosis. Treatment with corticosteroids is normally reserved for symptomatic pulmonary disease; systemic involvement of the eyes, myocardium, and central nervous system; disfiguring skin lesions; and hypercalcemia.

IDIOPATHIC PULMONARY FIBROSIS

Major Immunologic Features

- Possible immune complexes in the blood and lungs
- Alveolar and interstitial macrophages pivotal in

pathogenesis of lung fibrosis by release of neutrophilic chemoattractants, oxidants, and growth signals for mesenchymal cells

General Considerations

Except for a rare familial form, idiopathic pulmonary fibrosis is an interstitial lung disease of unknown origin. Therefore, known causes, including environmental inorganic dusts or toxic fumes; sarcoidosis; eosinophilic granuloma; collagen vascular disease; and pulmonary fibrosis secondary to lung infections, chronic aspiration, and drugs, must be excluded prior to making this diagnosis. Although some patients respond to treatment with corticosteroid or cytotoxic drug therapy, the prognosis, in general, is poor.

Immunologic Pathogenesis

Idiopathic pulmonary fibrosis (IPF) is a suspected cellular immune-mediated disorder. An influx of inflammatory cells results in injury to type I epithelial cells. Subsequent release of fibrogenic cytokines and growth factors results in fibroblast proliferation, type II cell hyperplasia, and deposition of extracellular matrix proteins. Recent data suggest a complex relationship among cellular components (macrophages, lymphocytes, neutrophils), their release of potent inflammatory mediators, and the cellular receptors that mediate or modify these responses. Alveolar and interstitial macrophages play an important role in the pathogenesis of lung fibrosis through the release of oxidants that injure pulmonary epithelium and chemotactic factors that attract neutrophils and eosinophils. Lung macrophages also secrete fibrogenic cytokines and growth factors, which lead to fibroblast proliferation and augmentation of collagen synthesis.

These cellular relationships may determine the pathologic features of IPF, including increased numbers of polymorphonuclear leukocytes and generalized fibrosis of the lung parenchyma. The pathogenic role of immune complexes in the circulation and lungs during the early, active phase of the disease is unclear.

Clinical Features

Although patients at any age can be affected by this disease, the average age at diagnosis is 60 years. The disease has an insidious onset, with patients often noting symptoms for weeks to months before seeking medical attention. The usual presenting symptoms are progressive dyspnea on exertion and a nonproductive cough. Constitutional symptoms such as fatigue, weight loss, malaise, and arthralgias are not uncommon. Physical examination reveals dry bibasilar crackles ("Velcro rales"). In advanced cases, one may find clubbing, cyanosis, and evidence of cor pulmonale. The chest radiograph shows interstitial fibrosis predominantly in the basilar areas of the lungs. Honeycombing may occur in later stages. A chest CT may show focal or diffuse "ground glass" infiltrates or increased interstitial markings that are more prominent in the bases and periphery. A peripheral honeycomb pattern is frequently observed (Figure 40–5). Pulmonary function testing shows a restrictive defect with decreases in lung volumes and diffusing capacity. Arterial blood gases show normal or decreased oxygen tension, which may fall significantly with exertion.

Diagnosis

Because this is a diagnosis of exclusion, no definitive or specific confirmatory tests exist. Serologic abnormalities may include positive tests for antinuclear antibodies or rheumatoid factor, increased amounts of immunoglobulins, and circulating immune complexes. Various immunologic tests are used primarily to exclude the presence of other interstitial lung disorders. Pathologic abnormalities often reveal wide variability among patients. Even when several biopsy specimens are taken from an individual patient, pathologic heterogeneity is not uncommon, suggesting that lung injury occurs at different rates. The histologic pattern varies from an acute alveolitis to an acellular stage with marked distortion of lung architecture and

fibrosis. Bronchoscopy with biopsy and lavage is often used to exclude other causes of chronic interstitial lung disease. Bronchoalveolar lavage reveals increased numbers of alveolar macrophages and polymorphonuclear leukocytes; the most characteristic feature is an increased percentage of both neutrophils and eosinophils. Because the histology of bronchoscopically obtained specimens is often nonspecific, an open or transthoracic thoracoscopic lung biopsy is usually necessary to exclude other disorders (eg, granulomatous infections, sarcoidosis, or bronchiolitis with obstructive pneumonia) and to select the patients most likely to respond to treatment.

Differential Diagnosis

The differential diagnosis includes a large number of interstitial lung diseases of both known and unknown origin (Table 40–5). The principal considerations, however, are sarcoidosis, hypersensitivity pneumonitis, collagen-vascular diseases, and certain inorganic dust exposures.

Treatment & Prognosis

Therapy is directed at suppressing active inflammation (alveolitis) and thus preventing further loss of

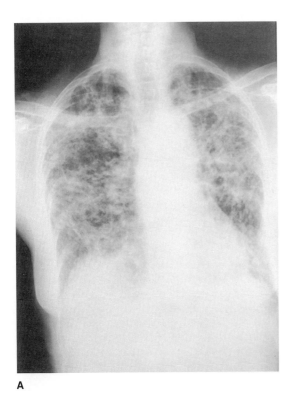

A

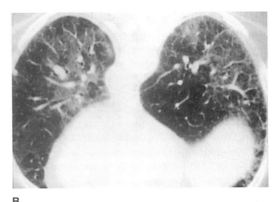

B

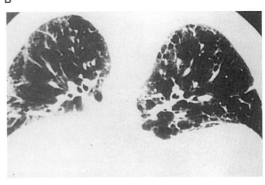

C

Figure 40–5. Radiographic evaluation of patients with idiopathic pulmonary fibrosis. **A:** Chest film shows diffuse, bilateral interstitial infiltrates. Chest CT examples show the spectrum and heterogeneity of this process. **B:** An alveolar filling process is noted, and **C:** a more chronic, fibrotic process with honeycombing.

Table 40–5. Differential diagnosis of idiopathic
pulmonary fibrosis.

Aspiration pneumonia
Collagen vascular diseases
Drugs (antibiotics and chemotherapy)
Eosinophilic lung syndromes
Histiocytosis X
Hypersensitivity pneumonitis
Infections (mycobacterial, viral, or fungal)
Lymphocytic interstitial diseases
Noxious gases (eg, oxides of nitrogen)
Pneumoconioses
Radiation
Sarcoidosis

function. High doses of corticosteroids may result in
improvement and stabilization of pulmonary functions
in approximately 20% of patients. Cytotoxic
drugs have also been reported to benefit some patients.
Unfortunately, despite treatment with corticosteroids
or cytotoxic drugs, the survival rate at 5 years
is only 50%. This high mortality is secondary to progressive
respiratory failure, infections related to treatment,
pulmonary emboli, lung cancer, right heart
failure, and the complications of prolonged immunosuppressive
therapy. Most recently, there has been
some enthusiasm for single-lung transplantation in
patients who respond poorly to medical trials.

ANTIGLOMERULAR BASEMENT MEMBRANE DISEASE (GOODPASTURE'S SYNDROME)

Major Immunologic Features

- Circulating antiglomerular basement membrane (anti-GBM) antibodies characteristically present early
- Anti-GBM antibodies primarily to the noncollagenous domain of the α3 chain of type IV collagen
- Linear deposits of immunoglobulin (typically IgG) and complement (C3) along the basement membrane of renal glomeruli and tubules, and pulmonary alveoli
- Pathogenesis probably antibody-mediated cytotoxicity

General Considerations

Antiglomerular basement membrane (anti-GBM) disease, also called **Goodpasture's syndrome,** is a disease of unknown origin with the triad of pulmonary hemorrhage, glomerulonephritis, and circulating antibody to basement membrane antigens. Intrapulmonary hemorrhage varies from insignificant to severe and life-threatening, often preceding renal involvement by 1–12 months. Rapidly progressive renal disease is common, with oliguric renal failure occurring within weeks to months of the clinical onset of the disease. Without early treatment, renal failure is permanent.

Immunologic Pathogenesis

In more than 90% of cases, circulating **anti-GBM antibodies** appear early in the course of the disease. These antibodies are directed against the noncollagenous domain of the α3 chain of type IV collagen in renal tubular, renal glomerular, and pulmonary alveolar basement membranes. Immunofluorescence techniques demonstrate antibody deposited in a characteristic linear pattern, often accompanied by C3 deposition. Antibody bound to basement membrane activates the complement cascade, resulting in the generation of chemotactic factors for various inflammatory cells, which subsequently destroy the renal tubular, renal glomerular, and pulmonary alveolar basement membranes via the release of various reactive oxygen species and proteolytic enzymes. This constitutes a type II hypersensitivity (cytotoxic) reaction. In addition, a host of other noncomplement mediators of inflammation are also activated.

Clinical Features

Goodpasture's syndrome occurs predominantly in young males, often following a viral infection. Pulmonary manifestations include pulmonary hemorrhage with or without hemoptysis, dyspnea, weakness, fatigue, and cough. Recurrent hemorrhage may result in iron deficiency anemia. The chest radiograph typically reveals bilateral opacities that radiate from the hilum predominantly in the middle and lower lobes in a confluent or acinar pattern. The pattern may change in intensity depending on the degree of interalveolar hemorrhage (Figure 40–6). Bronchoalveolar lavage produces hemosiderin-laden macrophages with or without erythrocytes. Renal involvement causes gross or microscopic hematuria and variable amounts of proteinuria, a decreased 24-

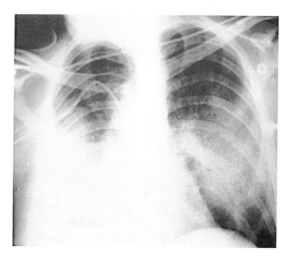

Figure 40–6. Chest radiograph of a patient with Goodpasture's
syndrome, showing extensive bilateral pulmonary
infiltrates typical of intraalveolar hemorrhage.

hour urine creatinine clearance, and an increase in blood urea and serum creatinine levels.

Differential Diagnosis

Pulmonary hemorrhage with renal failure may be seen in Wegener's granulomatosis, systemic lupus erythematosus, polyarteritis nodosa, and renal vein thrombosis with pulmonary embolism. These disorders lack the constellation of clinical, pathologic, and immunologic features on which the diagnosis of Goodpasture's syndrome is based.

Treatment & Prognosis

Because the disorder may be rapidly fatal, it is imperative that it be diagnosed and treated promptly. Treatment is directed at removal of circulating anti-GBM antibody, modulation of the inflammatory response, and suppression of new antibody synthesis. This has been effectively orchestrated with plasma exchange to remove anti-GBM antibodies and immunosuppressive drugs (corticosteroids and cytotoxic drugs) to suppress inflammation and new antibody formation. If instituted early in the course of the disease, this type of therapy may halt the progression of the disease and maintain renal function. A number of factors influence the response to treatment. The prognosis for recovery is poor when the initial serum creatinine level is >5 mg/dL and when crescents are present in >50% of glomeruli in the original renal biopsy. Bacterial infections during the recovery period are often associated with relapse. For patients with end-stage renal disease, renal transplantation has been successful after the disappearance of the circulating anti-GBM antibodies. Unfortunately, the transplanted kidney occasionally develops the disease. Mortality results from respiratory failure secondary to pulmonary hemorrhage, complications of renal failure, and infection.

PULMONARY VASCULITIS SYNDROMES

Granulomatous and nongranulomatous vasculitides of unknown cause affecting the lung are listed in Table 40–6, along with conditions presenting as pulmonary–renal syndromes. Although of unknown cause, histopathology suggests involvement of immunologic mechanisms. Wegener's granulomatosis, small-vessel vasculitis, and collagen–vascular diseases are discussed in Chapters 31 and 34.

Lymphomatoid Granulomatosis

Lymphomatoid granulomatosis, involving primarily the lungs, and **polymorphic reticulosis** (or lethal midline granuloma), involving primarily the nose and paranasal sinuses, are histopathologic entities. Recent studies have suggested that these conditions are Epstein–Barr virus-driven lymphoproliferative disor-

Table 40–6. Granulomatous and nongranulomatous vasculitis syndromes affecting the lung.

Granulomatosis–angiitis syndromes
Wegener's granulomatosis
Lymphomatoid granulomatosis
Necrotizing sarcoid granulomatosis
Bronctiocentric grancolomatosis
Allergic granulomatosis of Churg and Strauss
Sarcoidal vasculitis
Small-vessel vasculitis
Leukocytoclastic angiitis
Henoch–Schönlein purpura
Behçet's disease
Collagen-vascular disease
Pulmonary–renal syndromes
Goodpasture's syndrome
Wegener's granulomatosis
Lymphomatoid granulomatosis
Allergic granulomatosis of Churg and Strauss
Systemic lupus erythematosus
Progressive systemic sclerosis (scleroderma)

ders. Both diseases can involve other tissues, including the skin, central nervous system, and abdominal organs, and both may result in malignant lymphoma. Radiation therapy is successful in localized disease.

Clinical manifestations of lymphomatoid granulomatosis include cough, fever, and dyspnea. Most patients are in early middle age, and men predominate. Pulmonary lesions are commonly in the lower lung fields bilaterally in a peripheral location without hilar adenopathy, and they tend to wax and wane. Skin lesions occur in one half of the patients. Glomerulonephritis is absent, but nodular renal lesions occur. Nervous system involvement is common and may include central nervous system dysfunction and peripheral neuropathies. Treatment with cyclophosphamide and prednisone has been somewhat successful. From 12 to 47% of patients with lymphomatoid granulomatosis develop malignant lymphoma.

Necrotizing Sarcoid Granulomatosis

This relatively benign entity may be a variant of sarcoidosis with infrequent extrapulmonary manifestations, decreased prevalence of mediastinal or hilar lymphadenopathy, and a tendency for cavitation of lung nodules. Cough is the most common symptom, and dyspnea, chest pain, and constitutional symptoms may occur. Radiographs typically show multiple bilateral nodules in subpleural and peribronchovascular locations. Glucocorticoid therapy alone may be adequate treatment.

BRONCHOCENTRIC GRANULOMATOSIS

This condition consists of granulomas preferentially involving the bronchi and bronchioles. A prolonged course is usual, with symptoms of cough, dyspnea, pleuritic chest pain, and fever. The overall prognosis is favorable. Treatment generally involves glucocorticoids, especially in patients with asthma in whom bronchocentric granulomatosis may simulate or accompany allergic bronchopulmonary mycoses.

ALLERGIC ANGIITIS & GRANULOMATOSIS OF CHURG & STRAUSS

See section titled Eosinophilic Pneumonias.

PULMONARY MANIFESTATIONS OF IMMUNODEFICIENCY

Immunodeficiency diseases and disorders, including AIDS, are covered elsewhere in this volume (Chapters 21–25 and 46). These diseases increase the risk of specific pulmonary infections, depending largely on the type of defect in the immunocompromised host. Impaired antibody formation or complement deficiency predisposes patients to pneumonia caused by pyogenic organisms, chiefly *Streptococcus pneumoniae* and *Haemophilus influenzae*. Compromise of cellular immunity leads to increased risks for infections with mycobacteria and *Nocardia;* fungi such as *Pneumocystis carinii* (formerly classified as a protozoan), *Candida,* and agents of systemic mycoses; herpes viruses, vaccinia virus, and measles virus; and parasites including *Toxoplasma gondii* and *Strongyloides stercoralis.* Defects in granulocytes commonly result in staphylococcal abscesses that may involve the lung.

ADULT RESPIRATORY DISTRESS SYNDROME

General Considerations

The adult respiratory distress syndrome (ARDS) is a form of acute lung injury characterized by noncardiogenic pulmonary edema from increased vascular permeability. It can occur in the setting of a wide variety of clinical conditions, including sepsis, gastric acid aspiration, pancreatitis, trauma, fat emboli syndrome, and central nervous system insult.

Immunologic Pathogenesis

A putative pathogenetic mechanism is the activation of the complement system with recruitment and sequestration of neutrophils in pulmonary interstitial capillaries. A number of cytokines released from macrophages may play a significant role in the recruitment of neutrophils. **Tumor necrosis factor alpha (TNFα)** is probably the most important cytokine generated in response to endotoxin. The actual amount of TNFα released is modulated by the metabolites of arachidonic acid (PGE_2). In the capillaries, neutrophils responding to these signals accumulate and release a number of toxic products including oxygen free radicals and proteases, which cause endothelial cell damage, interstitial and intraalveolar edema, hemorrhage, and fibrin deposition.

Diagnosis

In the proper clinical setting, a diagnosis of ARDS is made when diffuse, bilateral infiltrates are evident on chest film (consistent with pulmonary edema), there is no evidence of increased pulmonary capillary hydrostatic pressure (this usually requires placement of a pulmonary artery catheter), and refractory hypoxemia occurs that cannot be corrected by high concentrations of oxygen. In the last decade, mortality rates have fallen in most studies to 40–50%. Mortality relates to the underlying cause of ARDS and to the development of multiple organ failure.

Treatment

At present, treatment of patients with ARDS is supportive. Clinical trials of receptor antagonists and monoclonal antibodies to specific mediators are in progress.

REFERENCES

DRUG-INDUCED RESPIRATORY DISEASES
Cooper JAD Jr: Drug-Induced Lung Disease. *Adv Int Med* 1997;42:231.
Rosenow EC III et al: Drug-induced pulmonary disease. *Chest* 1992;102:239.

EOSINOPHILIC PNEUMONIAS
Pope-Harmon AL, et al: Acute eosinophilic pneumonia: A summary of 15 cases and review of the literature. *Medicine* 1996;75:334.
Umeki S: Reevaluation of eosinophilic pneumonia and its diagnostic criteria. *Arch Int Med* 1992;152:1913.
Walker C et al: Activated T cells and cytokines in bronchoalveolar lavages from patients with various lung diseases associated with eosinophilia. *Am J Respir Crit Care Med* 1994;150:1038.

OCCUPATIONAL & ENVIRONMENTAL LUNG DISEASES
Grammer LC, Patterson R: Occupational immunologic lung disease. *Ann Allergy* 1987;58:151.
Reed CR: Hypersensitivity pneumonitis and occupational lung diseases from inhaled endotoxin. *Immunol Allergy Clin North Am* 1992;12:819.
Schwartz DA, Peterson MW: Occupational Lung Disease. *Adv Intern Med* 1997;42:269.

SARCOIDOSIS

Agostini C, Semenzato G: Cytokines in sarcoidosis. *Semin Respir Infect* 1998;13:184.

Hunninghake GW et al: American Thoracic Society Statement on Sarcoidosis. *Am J Respir Crit Care Med* 1999; 160:736.

Müller-Quernheim J: Sarcoidosis: Immunopathogenetic concepts and their application. *Eur Respir J* 1998;12: 716.

IDIOPATHIC PULMONARY FIBROSIS

Hunninghake GW, Kalica AR: Approaches to the treatment of pulmonary fibrosis. *Am J Resp Crit Care Med* 1995; 151:915.

Katzenstein AA, Myers JL: Idiopathic pulmonary fibrosis: Clinical relevance of pathologic classification. *Am J Respir Crit Care Med* 1998;157:1301.

GOODPASTURE'S SYNDROME

Ball JA, Young KR Jr.: Pulmonary manifestations of Goodpasture's syndrome: Antiglomerular basement membrane disease and related disorders. *Clin Chest Med* 1998; 19:777.

Hellmark T et al. Identification of a clinically relevant immunodominant region of collagen IV in Goodpasture disease. *Kidney Int* 1999;55:936.

Kelly PT, Haponik EF: Goodpasture's syndrome: Molecular and clinical advances. *Medicine* 1994;73:171.

GRANULOMATOSIS-VASCULITIS SYNDROMES

Davenport A et al: Clinical relevance of testing for antineutrophil cytoplasm antibodies (ANCA) with a standard indirect immunofluorescence ANCA test in patients with upper or lower respiratory tract symptoms. *Thorax* 1994; 49:213.

Frazier AA et el. Pulmonary angiitis and granulomatosis: Radiologic-pathologic correlation. *RadioGraphics* 1998;18: 687.

Strickler JG et al: Polymorphic reticulosis: A reappraisal. *Hum Pathol* 1994;25:659.

ADULT RESPIRATORY DISTRESS SYNDROME

Artigas A et al: Ventilatory, pharmacologic, supportive therapy, study design strategies, and issues related to recovery and remodeling. Acute respiratory distress syndrome. *Am J Resp Crit Care Med* 1998;157:1332.

Kollef MH, Schuster DP: The acute respiratory distress syndrome. *N Engl J Med* 1995;332:27.

Pittet J-F et al: Biological markers of acute lung injury: Prognostic and pathogenetic significance. *Am J Respir Crit Care Med* 1997;155:1187.

41

Reproduction & the Immune System

Karen Palmore Beckerman, MD, & Donald J. Dudley, MD

Perhaps, then, the zoologist is right to think of placentation as one of the more easily understood innovations of vertebrate phylogeny. But as it happens, not all the problems of viviparity have been satisfactorily solved. The relationship between mother and foetus is still in some degree teleologically inept, and it will be argued that certain trends in the evolution of viviparity raise special immunological difficulties for the foetus. (PB Medawar, 1953)

The purpose of this chapter is to acquaint the reader with basic principles of the immune response relevant to reproductive processes. Although many issues discussed here relate directly to contemporary cellular immunology, most of the questions are far from new, and, in fact, have remained essentially unanswered since they were first articulated by Medawar and his predecessors in the first half of this century.

The reader is introduced to the field of reproductive biology with a brief overview of the anatomy and histology of the male and female genital tracts. Recent findings regarding genital mucosal immunity are presented, followed by examination of the immune status of ovarian and testicular tissues and, of course, the remarkable immune privilege enjoyed by tissues of the fetus. Topics such as immune causes of infertility and abortion are discussed critically, receiving significant attention in scientific and lay journals.

Two areas of maternal-fetal medicine are presented in some detail because of their clinical relevance and their importance to contemporary immunologic understanding of cellular interactions during gestation and parturition. First is the perinatal transmission of HIV infection, which, although less completely understood, effectively illuminates neglected areas of investigation that have become indispensable to our understanding of the dynamics of maternal and fetal immune interactions. Second, we discuss the immunologic aberrations that characterize common obstetric problems, including preterm labor and preeclampsia.

REPRODUCTIVE TRACT ANATOMY & IMMUNITY

ANATOMY

Female

The mucosa of the vagina and outer portion of the uterine cervix (or **ectocervix**) is made up of a highly vascularized submucosa and a superficial, nonkeratinized, stratified squamous epithelium (Figure 41–1). This squamous epithelium abruptly changes to simple stratified columnar epithelium at the **transitional zone,** which marks the beginning of the inner portion of the cervix (or **endocervix**). This is the site of hormonally regulated secretion of specialized mucus that facilitates sperm transport. The endocervix ends in the uterine cavity, the lining of which is referred to as either **endometrium** in the nonpregnant state or **decidua** during pregnancy. Depending on the hormonal stimulation, the endometrium varies from 1 to 6 mm in thickness and is made of several glandular layers. The innermost layer, the **stratum functionale,** grows and thickens prior to and after ovulation. If pregnancy and implantation occur, it hypertrophies further to become the nutrient-rich, intensely glandular decidua; if pregnancy does not occur, this layer is shed at the time of menses.

The site of fertilization is the fallopian tube, a muscular membranous structure lined by a highly vascular mucosa **(endosalpinx),** consisting of ciliated and secretory cells. The endosalpinx is thrown into numerous, branched, slender longitudinal folds and is ideally suited to the maintenance, nutrition, and transport of the conceptus during its 5-day journey to the uterus.

Male

The character of the penile urethral epithelium varies in different places. The most distal portion of the urethra lies in the glans penis and is termed the

fossa navicularis. The urethral mucosa in this section is lined by stratified squamous epithelium. The remainder of the penile urethra **(pars cavernosa)** is composed of pseudostratified columnar epithelium. Both sections are surrounded by a highly vascular submucosa. Penile periurethral tissue contains many small, branched, tubular glands lined by columnar mucus-secreting cells **(glands of Littré),** which can become chronically infected after urethritis. Nearer to the bladder, the urethra is lined by transitional epithelium characteristic of the bladder itself.

MUCOSAL IMMUNITY

The mucosa of the female genital tract (see Figure 41–1) is an anatomic and immunologic barrier of critical importance to host defenses against the spread of sexually transmitted diseases, including HIV infection. It is composed of immunologically reactive tissues capable of mounting local responses to foreign antigens in a manner similar to other immunologically active surfaces such as the respiratory and gastrointestinal tracts. Inductive sites for mucosal immunity of the reproductive tract consist of the cervix; vagina; large intestine and rectum; and the obturator, iliac, and inguinal lymph nodes that drain these structures. Immunoglobulin A (IgA)-containing plasma cells have been demonstrated in the lamina propria of the fallopian tube, endometrium, endocervix, and vagina, supporting an immune effector role for these structures. Unique distributions of Langerhans' cells, dendritic cells, CD4 and CD8 T lymphocytes, and plasma cells have been described in surgical specimens of normal fallopian tube, cervix, vagina, and vulva.

The greatest number of intraepithelial and subepithelial lymphocytes is seen in the cervical transitional zone, suggesting that this site is an area of enhanced immune activity similar to other mucosal surfaces exposed to the external environment. As in the ileum, it appears that intraepithelial T cells of the fallopian tube and cervix are predominantly CD8, whereas subepithelial populations are CD4. The functional result of this tissue distribution is not entirely clear. Taken together, however, these findings support an important inductive role for cervical and fallopian tube lymphoid tissues in host mucosal defenses.

Vaginal immunization results in the appearance of specific IgA and IgG in vaginal secretions and IgG in the uterine cavity. Nasopharyngeal and intramuscular immunization induces low-level secretion of IgG (but not IgA) in the vagina and uterus coincident with increasing serum IgG titers. There is general agreement that cervical IgG is serum-derived, whereas cervical IgA is locally produced. Along with the cyclical hormonal effects on mucosal integrity and mucous production, immunoglobulin levels in the cervix apparently vary markedly during the menstrual cycle.

To date, although mucosal immunity has been well studied in the lower gastrointestinal tract, immune responses in the male genital mucosa have been less thoroughly characterized. It may be reasonable to assume that as the spread of sexually transmitted diseases is studied in further detail, similar mechanisms of mucosal immune defenses in the male will be described.

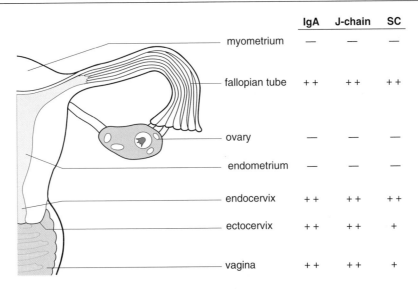

	IgA	J-chain	SC
myometrium	—	—	—
fallopian tube	+ +	+ +	+ +
ovary	—	—	—
endometrium	—	—	—
endocervix	+ +	+ +	+ +
ectocervix	+ +	+ +	+
vagina	+ +	+ +	+

Figure 41–1. The secretory immune system of the female genital tract. Immunofluorescence was used to analyze tissue from the uterus, fallopian tube, ovary, endocervix, ectocervix, and vagina. Note that fallopian tube and endocervix are the only sites strongly positive for the presence of IgA, J-chain, and secretory component (SC). Key: – = negative; + = weakly positive; ++ = strongly positive. (Reproduced, with permission, from Kutteh WH et al: *Mol Androl* 1993;4:183.)

DEFENSE AGAINST PATHOGENS VERSUS TOLERANCE OF SPERM "INVASION"

Covering, as it does, more than 400 m² of mucosa, the mucosal immune system is the largest component of a host's immune apparatus and contains the majority of the body's antibody-producing plasma cells. Much as in gut-associated lymphatic tissues, resident populations of macrophages, Langerhans' cells, dendritic cells, and T cells have been characterized in the superficial submucosa of the female genital tract. Antigen that reaches the cervical or vaginal submucosa is thought to be phagocytosed by antigen-presenting cells (presumably the resident macrophages and Langerhans' cells), which migrate to regional lymph nodes where processed antigen is presented. Once activated, T cells and B cells migrate to mucosal effector sites by specific binding to local postcapillary venule adhesion molecules. After arriving at mucosal tissues, B cells undergo clonal expansion as a result of activation by antigen, antigen-presenting cells, T cells, and cytokines to become IgA plasma cells. These cells contain J chains, and the IgA produced is largely polymeric. In addition, vaginal and cervical epithelium produces secretory component for transport of immunoglobulin into reproductive tract secretions. Despite the regular, repetitive inoculation of millions of foreign spermatozoa into sexually active women, the immune system of the female reproductive tract is typically unresponsive to sperm antigens. Several factors are postulated to account for this. First, the ejaculate contains factors that inhibit immune responses. It is also thought that characteristics unique to female genital mucosal immunity must play an essential role in tolerance to sperm antigens. Different studies have reported a 1–12% incidence of antisperm antibodies in fertile women, whereas sperm-reactive antibodies are formed in 75% of men engaged in oral–genital intercourse, suggesting that in the case of antisperm antibodies at least, the inductive arm of mucosal immunity in the cervix and the vagina is uniquely tolerant to sperm antigens.

Although the maternal immunologic response to sperm antigens is not dramatic or exuberant, a male factor clearly plays a role in female reproductive pathology. For example, women with less sperm antigen exposure appear to be more predisposed to the development of preeclampsia, and the risk for preeclampsia changes with different paternity (see later discussion). Also, some women have no reproductive problems with a certain partner but then encounter problems with recurrent pregnancy loss with a different partner. Although the pathophysiology for these problems is not elucidated, these observations suggest that different and specific responses to sperm antigens depend on the female host and male partner.

THE OVARY & TESTIS

The Testis

The observations that germ cell antigens can behave more as foreign than as self and that in the male, haploid germ cells do not develop until puberty, long after the fetal or neonatal period when self tolerance is established, led to the development of the theory that sperm autoantigens are sequestered behind a strong blood–testis barrier. Although tight junctional barriers between the supporting Sertoli cells that surround cells involved in spermatogenesis can be demonstrated, the immune privilege that must be enjoyed by male germ cells in the testis is not complete. The normal testis contains numerous class II-negative resident macrophages in the interstitial spaces between the seminiferous tubules. In the mouse, these cells can be induced to up-regulate their class II expression, and early germ cells, which lie outside the blood–testis barrier, can be immunogenic to their host, as discussed later in the section on infertility.

The Ovary

Unlike the testis, the ovary is clearly not a site of immune privilege. First, meiosis is not complete until just after sperm penetration of the egg, so that haploid female gamete antigens have little opportunity to be expressed. Still, ovarian antigens can produce autoimmune disease, as discussed later. Within the ovary, resident macrophages are a major component of the interstitial ovarian compartment, there is an influx of leukocytes around the time of ovulation, and numerous macrophages are observed in the corpus luteum after follicular rupture. Macrophage-secretory products have been shown to influence ovarian cells in vitro: tumor necrosis factor alpha (TNFα) inhibits steroid secretion by ovarian granulosa cells, whereas interleukin 1β (IL-1β) is cytotoxic to ovarian cell dispersates. Gonadotropin-dependent IL-1β gene expression has been identified in the human ovary prior to ovulation, along with expression of IL-1 receptor and IL-1 receptor antagonist. These and other observations have led some investigators to describe ovulation as an inflammatory-like reaction, with IL-1β as its centerpiece.

FERTILIZATION, IMPLANTATION, & THE IMMUNE RESPONSE TO FETAL TISSUES

SPERM-EGG FUSION

Fertilization is achieved following the successful completion of a complex sequence of events involving a spermatozoon and an egg. Although much of the cell biology of this process is well beyond the scope of this chapter, certain aspects of sperm–egg interactions deserve consideration. Fusion of gametes must require mutual, species-specific recognition of surface antigen and an initial adhesion step. Contact of gametes signals the **acrosome reaction,** whereby the covering of the head of the sperm is dissolved, activating enzyme systems that make it possible for the sperm to penetrate the cell mass **(cumulus oophorus)** and the thick, acellular mucopolysaccharide layer **(zona pellucida)** that surround the egg.

Complementary adhesion molecules have been characterized on the surface of mouse gametes. An 83,000-dalton glycoprotein, murine zona pellucida 3 (mZP3), appears to act as a primary sperm receptor. Adhesion is carbohydrate-mediated via serine–threonine–O-linked oligosaccharides and results in initiation of the acrosome reaction. Another glycoprotein, mZP2, is involved in maintaining sperm binding to the ovum. On the acrosomal membrane of the head of the sperm, a putative 56,000-dalton egg-binding protein has been identified as sp-56. It is assumed that homologous molecules regulate the early phases of fertilization in other mammals.

IMPLANTATION

After fertilization is completed and mitotic division is successfully initiated, it takes 6 days for the conceptus, surrounded by the zona pellucida, to traverse the fallopian tube and reach the uterus as an autonomous, cystic, embryonic cell mass known as the preimplantation **blastocyst.** Implantation of the blastocyst is regulated by complex interactions between peptide and steroid hormones that synchronize the preparation of the endometrium with development of the embryo. Progesterone secretion by the corpus luteum of the ovary is a critical component of these interactions and is necessary for decidual maintenance and development. Human chorionic gonadotropin (HCG) is secreted by embryonic tissues by the first day after implantation and is responsible for the conversion of the corpus luteum of the menstrual cycle to the corpus luteum of pregnancy. Thus, the early conceptus is responsible for supporting the ovarian progesterone secretion that is necessary for its own survival. Besides maintaining the endometrium of pregnancy, commonly called the **decidua,** progesterone, first of ovarian origin and later produced by the developing placenta itself, may also play a significant immunosuppressive role at the maternal-fetal interface. One mechanism by which progesterone may support pregnancy may be via its regulatory properties on cytokine production (see later discussion).

At the time of implantation, the decidua contains numerous leukocytes, including T cells and macrophages. Classic T-cell biology has focused on the highly adaptive αβ T cell. Although they are in the maternal decidua, T cells are low in numbers and tend to migrate from the uterus at the time of early pregnancy. Notably, there is an influx of a relatively new class of T cells in the maternal decidua. These γδ T cells can be found in relatively large numbers in the maternal decidua. γδ T cells tend to be less capable of adaptive immune responses than αβ T cells and are thought to be a more primitive lineage than αβ T cells. The function of these T cells is unknown, but some investigators speculate that they may act to prevent the adverse effects of viral infection in the maternal decidua. Their role in maintaining or supporting pregnancy is unclear.

Cytokine products are thought to be mediators of many of these interactions. For example, estrogen-dependent expression of epidermal growth factor (EGF) and its receptor have been identified in the mouse uterus, where they may regulate uterine angiogenesis and growth. The EGF receptor has been identified on the preimplantation blastocyst and in in vitro embryo cultures; EGF stimulates blastocyst development, suggesting a functional ligand-receptor interaction for EGF during preimplantation events. The colony-stimulating factor family of cytokines [granulocyte-macrophage colony-stimulating factor (GM-CSF), colony-stimulating factor-1 (CSF-1), and interleukin-3 (IL-3)] along with the c-*fms* receptor for CSF-1 have been identified in murine placenta and decidua and in human placental cell lines. Recent data suggest that these cytokines modify blastocyst membrane properties in preparation for implantation. Indeed, the homozygous female CSF-1-deficient osteopetrotic mouse is infertile in matings with homozygous-deficient males but can produce offspring in matings with heterozygotes.

Before implantation, the zona pellucida must be shed. Although it is unclear whether the source of enzymes needed for degradation of the zona pellucida is endometrial or embryonic, it does appear that a burst of uterine expression of the cytokine leukemia inhibitory factor (LIF) is required for adhesion and implantation of the blastocyst into the endometrium. Female mice lacking a functional LIF gene are fertile, but their blastocysts fail to implant and develop. These concepti are quite viable, however, and can be transferred to pseudopregnant wild-type controls, in which they implant and develop normally.

Other cytokines secreted by decidual T cells and macrophages can either facilitate or impede implantation events. In vitro studies show that IL-1β inhibits murine blastocyst attachment but enhances trophoblast outgrowth. Interferon gamma (IFNγ) inhibits trophoblast outgrowth and causes degenerative changes in these cells, suggesting that implantation events may be regulated by the types of cytokines present and the timing of their secretion and their relative abundance to embryonic development.

TROPHOBLAST INVASION
OF MATERNAL TISSUES

Human embryonic development requires rapid access to the maternal circulation. Once attached to the endometrium, a distinct subset of **cytotrophoblast** cells (which now surround the embryonic tissues of the blastocyst and are destined to differentiate into the placenta and the outer layer of the fetal membranes) quickly differentiate into the highly invasive **trophoblast.**

The invasive trophoblast first erodes into endometrial stroma and then invades endometrial arterioles by day 12 of human gestation; it then replaces maternal endothelium and vascular smooth muscle, establishing the maximally dilated, fetal trophoblast-lined, **uteroplacental circulation** (Figure 41–2). Despite the fact that maternal leukocytes are in continuous contact with these fetal tissues now lining maternal vessels of the decidua and placenta, all of these structures continue to transport nutrients and eliminate waste from the fetus for the remainder of the pregnancy without rejection or attack by the immune system of either the fetus or the mother.

THE PLACENTA AS AN
IMMUNE ORGAN

The placenta is a unique, short-lived organ. Along with producing protein and steroid hormones that regulate physiologic activities of pregnancy, it also acts as the fetal lung, kidneys, intestine, and liver. Its function as a complex tissue of immunologic significance has received considerable attention in recent years.

Trophoblast

The multinuclear **syncytiotrophoblast** layer of the placenta (see Figure 41–2) was traditionally thought to act as a sort of "shield" for the fetus by serving as a barrier to maternal immune effector mechanisms. This model alone, however, has not been sufficient to explain maternal tolerance of fetal tissues. The trophoblast secretes cytokines that have been primarily associated with mononuclear phagocytes, such as CSF-1 and its receptor c-*fms,* IL-3, and GM-CSF. Like macrophages, trophoblast expresses high levels of the LIF receptor (see earlier discussion), is capable of phagocytosis and syncytialization, and expresses FcR, CD4, and CD14. The one preliminary reporting of trophoblast expression of IL-10 indicates that the trophoblast is responsive to TNFα, IL-1, transforming growth factor beta (TGFβ), and IL-6. Taken together, these findings have led to speculation that the trophoblast could represent part of a network of macrophage-like tissues distributed throughout the body that share common cytokine pathways and other characteristics. Such a model may or may not

yield meaningful clinical information in the near future; however, the introduction of concepts such as cytokine signaling and other dynamic interactions between maternal and fetal tissues will be critical to further advances in our understanding of trophoblast development and survival.

The Hofbauer Cell

The Hofbauer cell is a macrophage-like cell found within the fetal portion of the placenta (chorionic villus) in the stromal tissue that surrounds the fetal vessels of the villous core (Figure 41–3). It is present early in gestation and is probably of fetal origin. Early in pregnancy this cell may play a significant role in flow dynamics within the fetal villus and later it is actively phagocytic; however, its function in placental development, physiology, and immunity has not been completely characterized.

Placental HLA Expression

It has become quite clear that the trophoblast is distinct from all other cell types in its ability to express human leukocyte antigen (HLA) molecules. The trophoblast does not express class I or class II HLA either constitutively or in response to IFNγ, despite the presence of abundant receptors for IFNγ in placental tissues and despite demonstrable enhancement of RNA synthesis, production of renin, and transferrin receptor expression by first-trimester trophoblast culture in response to the cytokine. The trophoblast does, however, constitutively express the nonclassic HLA class I molecule HLA-G. The HLA-G gene was originally isolated from a human lymphoblastoid cell line, but it is not expressed on any human cell type except the trophoblast, where it is expressed on the surface of the extravillous cytotrophoblast and secreted in its soluble form. HLA-G is associated with β_2-microglobulin, can interact with CD8, and has only a limited number of polymorphisms, in contrast to classic HLA molecules. It is found in highest levels in the first trimester and is markedly decreased in the third-trimester trophoblast. Recent studies have shown that B-cell activation in the context of HLA-G results in marked inhibition of natural killer (NK) cell activity. Thus, HLA-G may play a key role as a survival factor during early pregnancy.

IMMUNITY IN PREGNANCY

BACKGROUND: ALTERED
SUSCEPTIBILITY TO INFECTION
IN PREGNANCY

With the advent of antimicrobial therapy, many of the dangers posed by infection to maternal health have

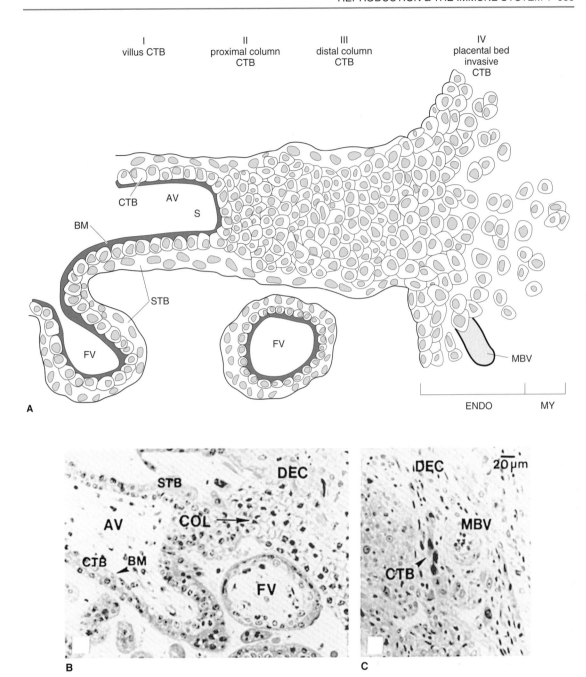

Figure 41–2. Trophoblast invasion at the maternal–fetal interface in the 10-week-old human placenta. **A:** Diagram showing floating villi and an anchoring villus with an associated cell column invading endometrium and myometrium of the uterine wall. The spatial organization of this tissue recapitulates the differentiation of cytotrophoblast along the invasive pathway. Zone I contains floating villi where mononuclear cytotrophoblast stem cells fuse to form the overlying syncytiotrophoblast layer past which maternal blood will percolate throughout gestation as part of the uteroplacental circulation. In an anchoring villus, cytotrophoblasts form cell columns that connect the fetal and maternal compartments of the placenta (zones II and III). After shallow penetration of the uterine wall, columns spread laterally and break up into clusters of cells that penetrate endometrium (also called decidua) and myometrium layers of the pregnant uterus in zone IV. These invasive cytotrophoblasts go on to invade and line maternal blood vessels, replacing endothelium and vascular smooth muscle in vessels of the inner one third of the uterine wall. **B** and **C:** Sections of a 10-week-old human placental bed biopsy showing all stages of cytotrophoblast differentiation along the invasive pathway. *Abbreviations:* FV = floating villi; AV = anchoring villus; ENDO = endometrium; MY = myometrium; CTB = cytotrophoblast; STB = syncytiotrophoblast; MBV = maternal blood vessel; DEC = decidua; S = stroma; BM = basement membrane; COL = column. (Reproduced, with permission, from Damsky CH, Fitzgerald ML, Fisher SJ: *J Clin Invest* 1992;89:210.)

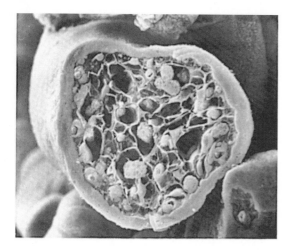

Figure 41–3. Scanning electron micrograph of a cross-fractured 10-week-old floating villus showing the villus core with its fetal vessels and numerous deep compartments formed by cytoplasmic processes of fixed stromal cells. Numerous Hofbauer cells are seen migrating between compartments. (Reproduced, with permission, from Castellucci M, Kaufmann P: *Placenta* 1982;3:269.)

been obscured. It is difficult to imagine that the single most common indication for therapeutic abortion prior to the late 1950s was tuberculosis. Indeed, infections against which host defenses are primarily cell-mediated, such as diseases caused by viruses, intracellular bacteria, fungi, protozoa, and helminths, have all been reported to be more likely acquired or reactivated and to be of greater virulence during pregnancy.

It is instructive to examine a few of the diseases to which pregnant women are more susceptible than nonpregnant controls. Until the 1960s, clinical poliomyelitis was two to three times more common in pregnancy, and the incidence of residual paralysis was significantly higher in pregnant patients. Hepatitis A occurs more commonly with a more fulminant course in pregnancy. One report from Africa notes a 40% rate of coma with 33% mortality among pregnant women compared with an 8% rate of coma and no mortality in nonpregnant controls. The frequency and severity of hepatitis B is thought to increase greatly during the last trimester. In the 1957 epidemic of influenza A, 50% of women of childbearing age who died in New York City were pregnant, even though they accounted for only 7% of women in that age group.

Pregnant women are much more likely to suffer the serious sequelae of malaria, including cerebral malaria, blackwater fever, acute renal failure, disseminated intravascular coagulation, pulmonary edema, and splenic rupture. In addition, plasmodia have a special affinity for placental tissue: A 46% placental infestation rate has been reported in an affected population that had only 17% positive peripheral blood

smears. Interestingly, resistance to malaria is promptly restored following parturition.

In endemic areas, coccidioidomycosis is a leading cause of maternal death. The risk of miliary tuberculosis is threefold higher in pregnancy, and leprosy is reported to progress rapidly in pregnant women. Host defense against the intracellular bacteria *Listeria monocytogenes* is almost entirely cell-mediated. Even though clinically significant infection with this organism usually occurs only in the immunocompromised, up to one third of cases are found in pregnant women, their fetuses, and neonates. Peripartum listeriosis generally starts with a flu-like prodrome and progresses to acute chorioamnionitis, resulting in abortion or premature labor and delivery. Placental histology reveals chorioamnionitis, and fetal autopsy shows gram-positive rods in the fetal liver, lungs, amniotic fluid, and blood. After delivery and evacuation of infected uterine contents, the maternal condition rapidly improves. Important findings in a murine model of placental listeriosis are discussed in the following section.

Proposed Mechanisms of Altered Immunity in Pregnancy

In the face of such impressive historic data on compromised host defenses during gestation, the exact role played by the gravid state in modulation of the immune response has remained elusive. In pregnancy, B-cell immunity is maintained at normal levels, and serum immunoglobulin levels are unchanged. In addition, some manifestations of cell-mediated immunity, such as delayed hypersensitivity, skin reactions, skin allograft rejection, and in vitro responses to mitogen, are unaltered in pregnancy.

Contemporary discussions of immune responses during pregnancy generally embrace a theory of depression of selective aspects of cell-mediated immunity thought to be necessary for maternal accommodation of the so-called fetal allograft. Unfortunately, many such discussions in the literature are highly speculative.

Local Immunosuppression at the Placenta & Adjacent Tissues

Experiments by Lu and Redline designed to study immunoregulatory mechanisms at the maternal–fetal interface during *L monocytogenes* infection in the pregnant mouse have yielded important information on cell-mediated immunity in pregnancy. Like the human, the adult mouse is able to mount an effective cell-mediated immune response to this intracellular parasite. During pregnancy, the maternal immune response in the liver and spleen was not impaired, even in the presence of overwhelming placental infection. In the placenta itself, large inflammatory infiltrates were identified in the maternal decidua; however, there was no inflammatory response in the fetal spongiotrophoblast and labyrinth layers of the murine placenta, despite the presence of large numbers of bacteria. This led to the conclusion that local events at the fetomaternal interface prevented an effective immune response and that the infected placenta might exert further detrimental effects by providing the *Listeria* a protected environment from which it could seed other maternal and fetal organs. Further work by this group has identified profound local deficits in macrophage function in the placenta, which cannot be accounted for by regional deficits in macrophage-activating cytokines nor by immunosuppressive trophoblast products. These investigators' speculation that mechanisms preventing optimal macrophage function in the murine placenta may have evolved, not to make the fetoplacental unit susceptible to intracellular infections but to protect it from rejection by the maternal immune system, is thought-provoking but as yet unproved.

Secretion of Placental Steroid Hormones

The placenta secretes high levels of estrogens and progesterone, which it synthesizes from maternal and fetal precursors, resulting in extremely high levels in the maternal–placental circulation and causing a marked increase in maternal systemic hormone plasma levels. Free and albumin-bound hydrocortisone, of fetoplacental-placental origin, also increase.

Steroid hormones have been shown in vitro to depress different aspects of cell-mediated immunity in a variety of experimental models, including inhibition of graft rejection and suppression of lymphocyte activation of macrophages. For example, Daynes and coworkers have found that hydrocortisone inhibits IL-2 production, yet enhances IL-4 production, by murine T cells activated at physiologic concentrations of the steroid. Additionally, T cells activated in the presence of physiologic concentrations of dehydroepiandrosterone (DHEA) will produce greater concentrations of IL-2. Other steroid hormones have varying effects on T-cell cytokine production. In general, glucocorticoids inhibit cytokine production and may account for their antiinflammatory effects. Notably, circulating glucocorticoid concentrations are increased during pregnancy. These alterations in circulating hormonal concentrations may be one mechanism by which systemic immunity is regulated during pregnancy.

Secretion of Placental Proteins

HCG is produced by the trophoblast, increases during the first trimester, and decreases through the remainder of pregnancy. Inconsistent experimental data and recent work with purified HCG suggest it has a minimal role in suppression of cell-mediated immunity in pregnancy. Alpha-fetoprotein (AFP) is secreted by the fetal liver into fetal serum and amniotic fluid in high levels during the second trimester and then plateaus. Physiologic levels of AFP can depress proliferative T-cell responses.

Intrinsically Decreased Lymphocyte Reactivity in Pregnancy

Although the clinical evidence for depressed cellular immunity during pregnancy is indisputable, opinion differs regarding changes in T-cell number, distribution, and reactivity during gestation. Some reports suggest a decrease in CD4 cells and others an increase in CD8 cells; cytotoxic activity of natural killer cells is said by others to be defective. Lymphocyte responsiveness to mitogens in vitro is moderately but significantly depressed in some studies but unchanged in others. Thymic involution, observed in other stressful conditions such as malnutrition and infection has been observed in rodents during the latter half of gestation coincident with rising plasma corticosteroid levels. No consistent or significant changes in B-cell immunity have been demonstrated during pregnancy.

SURVIVAL OF NORMAL PREGNANCY

Some authorities currently believe that for normal pregnancy to be established a T_H2-type response (see Chapter 9) must be induced by the maternal immune system at the maternal–fetal interface (Figure 41–4). In this manner, any adaptive maternal immune response would be apt to result in maternal antibody production and not in destructive cellular immunity that could damage trophoblast. Antibodies produced would not be harmless, but may actually aid in promotion of trophoblast implantation and remodeling of maternal endometrium. Animal and human studies, however, have found that pregnancy can occur and develop normally in the absence of maternal B cells or T cells, suggesting that adaptive immune responses during normal pregnancy are permissive rather than critical. On the other hand, innate immune responses by macrophages and NK cells in the pregnant endometrium (or decidua) appear to be critical to maintenance of normal pregnancy in inbred mouse strains. Moreover, recent data indicate that the innate immune system of women has increased activity during pregnancy. Although past dogma suggests that pregnancy is an "immunosuppressed" condition, newer data propose that pregnancy is characterized by marked changes in immunoregulation with enhanced innate immune activity and suppressed adaptive immunity. Determining those immunologic factors responsible for maintenance of normal pregnancy, as well as the pathophysiology of abnormal pregnancy, is the subject of ongoing research.

INFERTILITY & SPONTANEOUS ABORTION

With increased numbers of women of childbearing age; the routine availability of pregnancy diagnosis

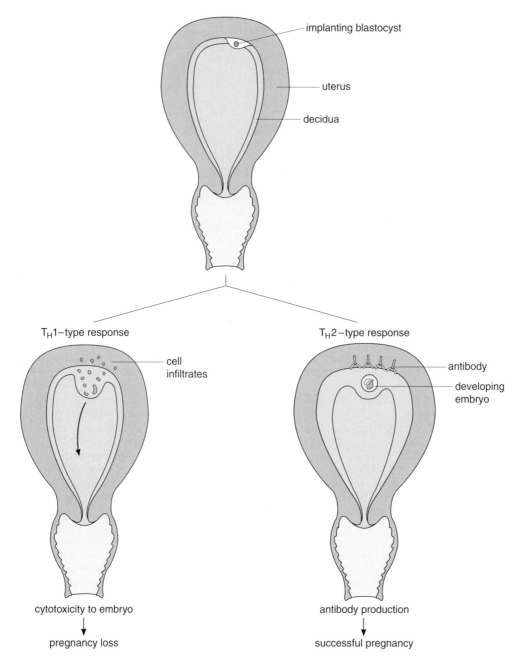

Figure 41–4. Immune responses evoked by early pregnancy. In this model, implantation of the conceptus results in a maternal immune response. One theory holds, that for the pregnancy to be successful, a T_H2-type response is necessary. Such a response results in inconsequential antibody production against trophoblast antigens. Should a T_H1-type response occur, however, embryotoxic factors such as IFNγ and TNFα mediates a cytotoxic, and lethal, response against the conceptus, leading to pregnancy loss.

before the first missed menstrual period; and significant numbers of couples electing to delay childbearing until they are older, statistically less fertile, and somewhat more likely to experience spontaneous pregnancy loss, the public perception that infertility and spontaneous abortion are worsening problems in the United States is not unfounded. Nevertheless, the rates of infertility and spontaneous abortion in this country are not increasing. Despite this fact, the number of couples seeking medical advice and treatment for infertility is increasing rapidly, to more than a million.

INFERTILITY

Infertility is the inability to establish pregnancy within a certain period of time, usually one year. Primary infertility refers to couples who have never achieved a pregnancy, whereas secondary infertility refers to those who have previously achieved a pregnancy but who are having difficulty doing so now. Documented causes of infertility include pelvic or tubal factors interfering with ovum transport, anovulation, abnormalities of the male reproductive system, and abnormal penetration of the cervical mucus by the sperm. For 10% of couples undergoing evaluation, no cause can be identified.

Immune Causes for Infertility

Antisperm antibodies have been studied since the early 1900s, when it was demonstrated that intraperitoneal injection of sperm into the female guinea pig induced antibody formation. Antisperm antibodies can be found in men and women in blood and lymphatic fluid (primarily IgG) and in local seminal or cervicovaginal secretions (primarily IgA). Development of these antibodies can occur in the male following traumatic or inflammatory disruption of the blood–testis barrier. Vaginal inoculation is far less likely to result in development of antisperm antibodies than is oral–genital intercourse. Interest in this field springs from two different clinical areas: first, the potential to identify a treatable cause of idiopathic infertility, and, second, development of a highly specific contraceptive method by vaccinating individuals "against" pregnancy by inoculation with sperm antigen.

Three types of assays have been used to detect antisperm antibodies: sperm agglutination assays, sperm immobilization assays, and assays that directly detect antibody. The source of sperm antigen determines whether antibodies of possible significance (eg, those directed against a sperm cell surface antigen) or of doubtful significance (those directed against internal antigen) will be detected. Many assays do not measure IgA, the predominant class of antigen in mucosal secretions. Agglutination assays can be falsely positive due the presence of amorphous material in semen or by serum proteins. Immobilization assays may be affected by complement sources (guinea pig sera) that are toxic to sperm. Immunoglobulin-specific techniques, such as enzyme-linked immunoabsorbent and immunofluorescence assays, can be highly quantitative but cannot yield information about the location of an antibody on the sperm surface, but other tests, such as immunobead and the mixed antiglobulin reaction with erythrocytes (MAR), can indicate the location of an antibody and can be used to evaluate immunoglobulin isotype, but do not provide quantitative information.

Depending on the assay used, antisperm antibodies are found in 1–12% of fertile women and in 10–20% of women with unexplained infertility. In the male, autoantibodies to sperm can be detected in both the seminal plasma and serum, and one half of men undergoing vasectomy form antisperm antibodies following the procedure. Importantly, data are not available that document significant differences in the presence or titers of antisperm antibodies in fertile and infertile populations.

Autoimmune disease of the testis and ovary is a known cause of infertility in domestic animals and is a likely cause of some forms of human infertility. Granulomatous disease and immune complexes can be found in the testis of infertile men and resemble changes seen in experimental autoimmune orchitis in mice. Ovarian autoantibodies and idiopathic oophoritis have been documented in women with premature ovarian failure. In addition, autoimmune orchitis and oophoritis have been identified as components of human polyendocrine and autoimmunity syndromes. Studies based on experimental autoimmune gonadal disease models have yielded new information on genetic control of organ-specific autoimmune disease and on antigen mimicry at the T-cell receptor.

Experimental autoimmune oophoritis is induced 2 weeks following immunization of rats with bovine ovarian homogenate or immunization with synthetic peptide fragments of ZP3, the sperm receptor protein on the zona pellucida (see the section on sperm–egg fusion). Disease can also be induced 2 days after adoptive transfer of T-cell lines and T-cell clones derived from lymph node cells from immunized, diseased mice to normal untreated recipients. These lines and clones are uniformly CD4 and produce IL-2, TNF, and IFNγ on stimulation. Interestingly, four randomly positioned amino acids in the peptide nanomer ZP3 330–338 are critical for induction of disease and T-cell response, but polyalanine peptide inserted with the critical ZP3 residues is fully capable of eliciting disease.

Experimental autoimmune orchitis is under polygenic control, involving *H*-2- and non-*H*-2-linked genes. Severe disease can be induced only by inoculation with homologous crude testis antigen and by adoptive transfer of T-cell lines and clones derived from lymph nodes of immunized mice. Manipulations of the normal immune system can also cause autoimmune gonadal disease. For example, neonatal murine thymectomy performed between day 1 and day 4 after birth can result in a variety of autoimmune sequelae, including autoimmune disease of the testis, ovary, thyroid, prostate, and stomach, suggesting that the neonatal T-cell repertoire is enriched with self-reactive T cells and that such novel disease models may be powerful tools for examining and manipulating mechanisms of self tolerance of a wide variety of potential autoantigens.

Immune Therapies for Infertility

Different therapies have been used to treat the infertile couple who show antisperm antibodies identified in either the male or the female. **Condom therapy** has been advocated to reduce exposure to antigen in women with antisperm antibodies. Pregnancy rates following specified periods of condom use vary from 11% to 56%; however, most studies do not include proper control groups. In fact, one study has documented a 44% rate of spontaneous pregnancy in couples who rejected condom contraception as a means of achieving pregnancy. Attempts to **process semen or wash sperm** to reduce the amount of antibody present in the ejaculate has not improved pregnancy rates, and techniques to chemically dissociate antibodies from sperm result in irreversible loss of sperm motility. One study evaluating the role of antisperm antibodies among infertile couples found that such determinations were not useful in the management of infertility. In couples who had antisperm antibodies, 23% achieved pregnancy without specific therapy for antisperm antibodies, whereas 24% of antisperm antibody-negative couples achieved pregnancy. These authors further concluded that antibody status in either partner was not a significant predictor of time to develop a pregnancy.

Intrauterine insemination (in order to bypass antibody present in the cervical mucus), **corticosteroid therapy, in vitro fertilization,** and **gamete intrafallopian transfer** have all been reported as successful therapies. Rare, but serious and unpredictable, complications, such as aseptic necrosis of the femur due to corticosteroids or anaphylactic shock after intrauterine insemination, can occur with these therapies, and none has been demonstrated effective in well-controlled, randomized trials. It would seem that the high spontaneous "cure" rate of this syndrome (ie, pregnancy without intervention), the difficulties involved in meaningful and standardized diagnostic evaluation of affected couples, and the large numbers of couples with unexplained infertility who might be subjected to these therapies would mandate such clinical trials in the near future. Until then, the detection of antisperm antibodies in couples with unexplained infertility can only be considered to be of unknown significance, and couples must be advised that prescribed treatments are of questionable benefit and carry the risk of serious complications.

RECURRENT SPONTANEOUS ABORTION

Background & Definitions

The occurrence of three or more spontaneous consecutive pregnancy losses defines this clinical syndrome. Given that a single clinically documented pregnancy carries a 15–20% chance of loss, some investigators believe that recurrent abortion is a chance phenomenon that occurs in about 0.5–1.0% of the population, and most clinicians find that no cause can be found for the majority of repetitive losses. Other researchers contend that a cause can be found for losses in over 60% of affected couples. The evaluation of women with two or more spontaneous pregnancy losses should include (1) a hysterosalpingogram for the evaluation of uterine anatomy, (2) parental karyotyping to evaluate for abnormal paternal chromosomal arrangements (eg, balanced translocations), (3) luteal phase evaluation (either with serum progesterone levels or endometrial biopsies), and (4) testing for antiphospholipid syndrome. It is important to note that, for couples with unexplained recurrent pregnancy loss, 60% or more will eventually carry a pregnancy successfully without specific therapeutic interventions. However, a small proportion of women who repetitively suffer first-trimester pregnancy losses and second-trimester fetal death appear to have an immunologic cause.

Antiphospholipid Syndrome

The **antiphospholipid syndrome** was first described in the early 1950s in women who were noted to have prolonged bleeding times that were not correctable by addition of normal plasma, history of hypercoagulability, false-positive Venereal Disease Research Laboratory (VDRL) syphilis test, and a history of recurrent pregnancy loss. In the following years, the lupus anticoagulant and the anticardiolipin antibody were characterized as acquired antibodies (IgG, IgA, or IgM), with specific activities against negatively charged phospholipids. They are thought to interact with thrombogenic adhesion molecules on endothelium, which would theoretically predispose to maternal thrombosis and placental infarction, resulting in placental insufficiency and pregnancy loss. For the lupus anticoagulant, diagnosis consists of prolongation of a phospholipid-dependent in vitro coagulation test, such as the activated partial thromboplastin time (aPTT) or the Russell viper venom time.

Women who suffer embryonic (< 10-weeks gestational age) or fetal death, in conjunction with a history of arterial or venous thrombosis, thrombocytopenia, and abnormal laboratory studies have antiphospholipid syndrome. Only 5% of women with recurrent pregnancy loss have evidence of antiphospholipid syndrome. Treatment for antiphospholipid syndrome during pregnancy includes anticoagulation with low doses of aspirin (≤ 81 mg/day) and subcutaneous heparin (either unfractionated or fractionated), along with intensive fetal surveillance. Even with these measures, pregnancies complicated by antiphospholipid syndrome are notable for an increased risk of severe early-onset preeclampsia, intrauterine growth restriction, and fetal distress, all necessitating early delivery before term for fetal behalf.

In normal obstetric populations, one or other of these antibodies are seen in 2% of women tested; in referral populations of women with recurrent pregnancy loss, this figure may approach 15%. The antiphospholipid syndrome, however, must be viewed as quite rare. More importantly, the presence of anticardiolipin antibody is of no significance in women without a history of recurrent (ie, at least three) pregnancy losses, and the presence of the even rarer lupus anticoagulant is of unknown significance in women without clinical histories of recurrent thromboses and pregnancy losses. Even in the presence of such histories, patients must be advised that studies showing benefit of therapies have used largely historic controls (often the patients themselves), so therapy is of necessity empirical and carries substantial risks. Other autoantibodies may be associated with recurrent pregnancy loss, but there is no consensus as to the potential role(s) of these antibodies nor the value of routine clinical determination for these antibodies.

IMMUNOTHERAPY

Approximately half of women who have recurrent pregnancy loss have a completely normal evaluation as detailed earlier. Given this finding, a purported immunologic cause has been advanced to account for repetitive pregnancy loss. Unfortunately, no specific testing or treatment has been found universally useful or accepted for this specific population. Older literature has invoked the concept of HLA homozygosity, or "sharing," between partners as a possible cause of recurrent pregnancy loss. In theory, HLA sharing has been said to lead to a decreased production of maternal "blocking" antibodies, which may appear in all successful pregnancies. One speculation is that these blocking antibodies were critical to normal pregnancy success by acting as an immunosuppressive agent. However, no studies have been performed to indicate that these antibodies were critical for pregnancy success or were merely epiphenomenal with normal pregnancy. Indeed, women with no B cells can reproduce successfully.

Based on these studies, immunotherapy, consisting of paternal white blood cell transfusion to the woman prior to conception, has been advanced as potentially enhancing the maternal immune response in a manner that will be beneficial for pregnancy outcome. This hypothesis is also based on older literature regarding renal transplantation, in which renal transplants appear to last longer and be less prone to rejection if the patient receives a white blood cell transfusion from the prospective donor prior to transplantation. Immunotherapy gained early favor in the mid-1980s on the basis of one randomized trial and was rapidly introduced into care by enthusiastic practitioners eager to provide an option for couples with this frustrating malady. Metaanalysis of four appropriately controlled randomized trials, however, found that the success rate for immunotherapy was 48%, but the untreated control population achieved pregnancy in 60% of cases. In another recent metaanalysis by the Recurrent Miscarriage Trialists Group of data from 15 centers found an increase in the number of live births from 60% in the control group to 70% in the treated group. They concluded that immunotherapy would have to be administered to 18 women in order to achieve one additional livebirth. This study suggested that immunotherapy may be of benefit for some women with recurrent pregnancy loss, however no current laboratory tests can reliably and reproducibly identify those women who may benefit from the procedure.

In the most recent and largest randomized controlled trial by the REMIS group, 193 women were randomized to placebo or immunotherapy. Among women who received immunotherapy, 36% achieved a live birth, whereas 48% of women who received placebo were successful. Because serious complications, such as graft-versus-host reactions and maternal blood group isoimmunization, have been reported from this therapy, this therapy for recurrent pregnancy loss has recently largely fallen into disfavor.

PROGESTERONE SUPPLEMENTATION

One treatment that may improve pregnancy outcome in women with recurrent pregnancy loss is empirical treatment with progesterone supplementation. Although older studies have not conclusively shown benefit, there is a reasonable scientific rationale for the use of supplemented progesterone. Recent studies have shown that progesterone has marked activities in regulating cytokine production. It has been shown that progesterone will inhibit T_H1-type responses and promote T_H2-type cytokine production in immune effector cells obtained from nonpregnant animals. Hence, if T_H2-type responses characterized pregnancy, the dramatic increases in maternal progesterone concentrations may be one factor that mediates this response. Maternal supplementation with progesterone may therefore be of use in some women with idiopathic recurrent pregnancy loss by correcting aberrant immune responses in decidua. However, there are no reliable methods of identifying women who may be at risk for such abnormal responses or who might benefit from progesterone supplementation.

Recurrent pregnancy loss and infertility are distressing problems that cause significant grief and suffering. Many couples presenting with these problems are panicked and desperate for a "cure." It is the duty of clinicians and scientists to thoroughly evaluate, educate, and protect these vulnerable individuals from empiric and potentially dangerous therapies whose benefits are largely unproved or have actually been disproved. In the case of therapies that may still be of value, the need for properly performed prospective trials has become imperative.

HIV INFECTION & THE REPRODUCTIVE SYSTEM

HETEROSEXUAL TRANSMISSION OF HUMAN IMMUNODEFICIENCY VIRUS

As a disease among women, acquired immunodeficiency syndrome (AIDS) was largely invisible until the late 1980s. Even up to the present day, most research on the disease has focused on adult males whose source of infection was most likely to be homosexual contact or intravenous drug use. Until it became apparent that growing numbers of women were being infected sexually, that the overwhelming majority of them were of reproductive age, and that they, when pregnant, were choosing to maintain their pregnancies, the reproductive health aspects of human immunodeficiency virus (HIV) infection and AIDS were not raised as a research priority.

In the United States today, heterosexual transmission of HIV-1 is the most rapidly rising cause of new infection, and women are being infected at a higher frequency than men. Worldwide, heterosexual contact is responsible for 70–80% of HIV infection, despite the inefficiency of this mode of transmission. Whereas one in four individuals exposed to *Neisseria gonorrhoeae* or hepatitis B develop disease, it is estimated that for a single contact, the infectivity of HIV-1 is 0.3%. Still, some individuals become infected after a single or few sexual contacts. Several cofactors have been found to increase the risk of acquiring disease through heterosexual contact. In the United States, male-to-female transmission is more efficient than female to male. It is generally agreed that compromise and alteration of vaginal mucosal immunity appear to have a significant influence on disease transmission. For example, postcoital bleeding, cervical ectopy (ie, migration of glandular endocervical epithelium from the endocervix to the ectocervix), lack of circumcision, genital ulcer disease, and infection with other sexually transmitted diseases have all been shown to be cofactors associated with transmission. In addition, receptive anal intercourse increases the risk of male-to-female dissemination of disease.

Infectivity appears to vary between specific HIV strains, and clinical stage of disease directly influences the amount of viral shedding in secretions. Susceptibility may be influenced by such unique factors as nutritional status, stage of menstrual cycle, or pregnancy. Both cell-associated and cell-free HIV are present in the cervicovaginal secretions and semen of asymptomatic HIV-infected individuals and AIDS patients. The fate of HIV-infected cells in ejaculate in the vagina is unknown. It is unlikely that infected cells can cross intact vaginal mucosa, and due to low vaginal pH, normal vaginal flora, lysozyme, and proteinases, latently infected cells in the ejaculate are unlikely to survive long enough to produce infectious virions, so that only cells producing infectious HIV particles at the time of inoculation are thought likely to contribute to sexual transmission.

The cellular targets of HIV during genital transmission are unknown. Because only a few CD4 T cells are present in the vaginal submucosa, the most likely targets are macrophages and Langerhans' cells. Cervical biopsy specimens from HIV-infected women show no evidence of epithelial cell infection by HIV. CD4-positive, class-II-bearing Langerhans' cells, dendritic cells, and macrophages present in the vaginal mucosa and submucosa may have a role in the sexual transmission of the virion (Figure 41–5). As antigen-presenting cells, they are well suited to disseminate virus from the mucosa to draining lymph nodes. In vitro, they have been shown to produce virus without exhibiting the cytopathic effects typical of T-cell infection. Thus, it is likely that infection and initial viral replication occurs in these local target cells, followed by further replication in draining lymph nodes before spread to more distant lymphoid tissues. There has been considerable speculation regarding the association of tissue trauma with spread of disease. It is unlikely that virus can gain direct entry into the bloodstream via breaks in the vaginal mucosa. Rather, it is more probable that blood cells (including CD4 T cells) escaping from the vasculature do not reenter the bloodstream but instead travel the same route as Langerhans' cells and macrophages, through the lymphatics to draining lymph nodes. Trauma and infection are likely to be associated with increased numbers of CD4 target cells in genital tissues and thus increase the efficiency of HIV transmission; these conditions, however, are unlikely to alter the route of infection.

Studies by A. I. Spira and colleagues of acute simian immunodeficiency virus (SIV) infection have yielded important insights into the sexual transmission of HIV-1. Four female rhesus macaques were inoculated intravaginally with the SIV mac251 strain. In situ polymerase chain reaction (PCR) amplification performed on tissue sections collected during the first 9 days after inoculation showed no evidence of infection of the epithelium itself. By day 2, evidence of infection appeared in cells of the lamina propria close to the basement membrane of stratified squamous epithelium of the vagina and ectocervix and the simple columnar epithelium of the endocervix. These submucosal cells had processes characteristic of antigen-presenting cells, contained class II antigens, but did not contain CD68, suggesting that they were dendritic cells or dendritic/T-cell syncytia. Provirus was detected in draining internal iliac lymph nodes by day 2, and in peripheral lymph nodes by day 5. Thus, it appears that productively infected submucosal dendritic cells are capable of quick dissemination of the

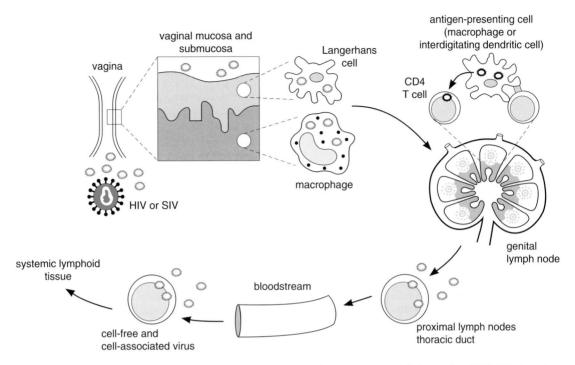

Figure 41–5. Viral dissemination during the genital transmission of human immunodeficiency virus (HIV). This hypothetical model depicts viral contact with the genital mucosa and infection of target cells, presumably macrophages or Langerhans' cells in the vaginal submucosa. Infected target cells move through lymphatic vessels to draining lymph nodes, enter the CD4 T-cell-rich lymph node paracortex, and present processed antigen, thus initiating an immune response. Viral replication occurs in the lymph node. Cell-free and cell-associated virus then travel via efferent lymphatics to proximal lymph nodes and the thoracic duct into the bloodstream, ultimately resulting in systemic infection. (Reproduced, with permission, from Miller CH et al: *Lab Invest* 1992;68:129.). *Abbreviation:* SIV = simian immuno- deficiency virus.

virus to draining lymph nodes followed by systemic dissemination shortly thereafter.

The question remains: If cells of the epithelium are not infected, how does HIV reach the lamina propria? Indeed, this group's observations reflect the inefficiency of HIV-1 transmission, prompting the researchers to suggest that transepithelial transport of HIV-1 is an important rate-limiting factor of HIV-1 transmission efficiency. In addition, they observed that viruses that can demonstrably infect epithelial cells, such as poliovirus, herpesvirus, and rhinovirus, are much more efficiently transmitted than HIV.

Current studies are aimed at demonstrating permeation of epithelium by free virus, Langerhans' cell binding and transport of virus, epithelial disruption by inoculation, and mechanisms not yet observed in the vagina that might be similar to intestinal M-cell transport of virus across epithelial cell barriers.

PERINATAL TRANSMISSION OF HIV

The rate of transmission of HIV from mother to infant varies widely. Diagnosis of HIV infection in the neonate is difficult because serologic studies are biased by the presence of maternally derived antibodies in neonatal serum. Prevalence studies of neonatal infection are based primarily on PCR and virus culture studies and have yielded rates of 11–60% transmission in different parts of the world. For diagnosis in the individual patient, it should be remembered that PCR is quite sensitive but can lack specificity, and virus culture is time-consuming and difficult to perform routinely. Transfer of HIV from mother to infant can occur in utero or after delivery. Even though HIV has been isolated from umbilical cord blood, amniotic fluid, placenta, and other fetal tissues, there is considerable disagreement in the literature about the frequency of HIV infection of fetal tissues. Some investigators find no virus in fetal tissues; others report detection of HIV genomic sequences in 30% of second-trimester abortuses, virtually identical to newborn transmission rates, and conclude that most vertical transmission occurs early in gestation. On the other hand, an observed delay in the ability to isolate HIV from neonatal serum until after 1 month of life suggests to some that transmission is most likely to occur at parturition, secondary to maternal-fetal transfusion, or fetal exposure to maternal secretions and blood during the delivery process.

HIV infection via breast milk is responsible for up to 40% of pediatric infections in the developing world. The mechanism of in utero and breast milk transmission of HIV is not understood. While transmission may correlate with absence of maternal antibody to the viral envelope, low maternal CD4 counts, p24 antigenemia and maternal viral load are highly predictive of the risk of vertical transmission. Although HIV has been detected in fetal and placental tissues by in situ hybridization, PCR, and immunohistochemistry, identification of viral particles in highly purified primary trophoblast culture has not yet been reported. In vitro, however, trophoblast cultures and human choriocarcinoma cell lines have been successfully infected by virus or virus-infected cells. The CD4 receptor is identified in some cell populations studied; however, significant literature exists suggesting that infection of the trophoblast can occur independently of the CD4-mediated pathway. Whatever the case, only low-level viral replication can be detected in these in vitro infected cells.

Given transplacental transmission of HIV, the exact route and mechanism of disease induction in the fetus is unclear. After 16–20 weeks gestation, mature T cells can be identified in fetal tissues and CD4, CD8 double-positive T-cell precursors are found even earlier. If early fetal infection occurs, it is unclear why entire $\alpha\beta$ T-cell populations are not eliminated. Different investigators speculate that infected T-cell precursors could go on to differentiate while latently infected; alternatively, transmission may occur much later in pregnancy.

PEDIATRIC HIV-1 INFECTIONS

Whatever the mode of transmission, the incubation period for perinatally acquired infection is comparatively short, with early-onset and late-onset patterns of disease presentation being reported. The early-onset group of infected infants develops disease early in life, between 3 and 8 months of age, and have a high mortality rate. For example, for infants in whom HIV is first diagnosed with *Pneumocystis carinii* pneumonia infection, median survival is 1 month; survival is somewhat longer with other initial presentations such as recurrent bacterial infections (50 months) and lobar interstitial pneumonia (72 months). Late-onset disease presents in older children and has a comparatively indolent course, closely resembling a lymphoproliferative disorder. Both late- and early-onset disease are commonly complicated by recurrent bacterial infections, ranging from recurrent otitis media to fulminant bacterial meningitis or pneumonia.

Most perinatal transmission appears to occur close to the time of delivery. It is now clear that antiretroviral therapy can lower the rate of vertical infection of fetuses and neonates by their HIV-1-infected mothers. The AIDS Clinical Trial Group protocol 076 showed that perinatal transmission was reduced from 25% in placebo-treated controls to 8% when zidovudine was administered to mothers prenatally, intrapartum, and to babies in the neonatal period. Further data show that the viral burden is highly correlated with vertical transmission rates.

In studies subsequent to the 076 trial, it has been found that cesarean delivery prior to labor is associated with an even lower rate of perinatal HIV transmission. Although these studies are retrospective in nature, perinatal transmission rate can be reduced to as low as 1–2% if abdominal delivery prior to labor and rupture of membranes is employed. However, these studies were performed in women receiving either no therapy or single-agent prophylaxis alone, usually AZT.

Since 1998, the goals of antiretroviral therapy in pregnancy have also focused on the control of maternal disease and the prevention of the emergence of antiretroviral resistance. Both of these goals require the use of potent combinations of three or more agents. To date, most antiretrovirals appear to be safe and well tolerated in pregnancy. In addition, their use has been associated with extremely low risk of perinatal transmission (<1% in preliminary reports), regardless of the route of delivery.

In the developing world, single- and double-drug strategies have been employed to interrupt perinatal and breast milk transmission of HIV-1. These strategies appear to be effective in controlled research settings, but their effect on transmission in clinical use has yet to be reported. There are reports of drug resistance among women who were perinatally exposed to one or more doses of single- and double-agent prophylaxis. Formula feeding has been shown to decrease mother-to-child transmission in one Kenyan study; however, even this intervention, costing about US $1000/baby, appears to remain far out of reach in the vast majority of the HIV-exposed children in the world.

PRETERM LABOR & DELIVERY

Perhaps the most pressing problem facing contemporary Western obstetrics is the issue of preterm birth. Despite recent advances in the pharmacologic control of uterine activity and the management of complications of prematurity, preterm birth continues to complicate approximately 10% of all deliveries in the United States and has not declined over the past 20 years. In fact, the rate of preterm births appears to be slowly climbing, even in the face of improved maternal and neonatal care.

One reason for the continuing problem of preterm birth is our poor understanding of the pathophysiology of the condition. Notably, the initiation of normal parturition (labor and delivery) at term in women is essentially unknown, although cortisol appears to have a central role in this process. Understandably then, the events leading to preterm parturition are not well delineated. One recent advance is the recognition that preterm labor constitutes a syndrome, in which there may be many causes. Among the possible causes of preterm labor is uterine overdistention (eg, twins), preterm premature rupture of the membranes (which must be distinguished from preterm labor with intact membranes), maternal trauma, uterine ischemia, uterine anomalies (space constraints on the developing fetus), and ascending intrauterine infection. A common theme to these possible causes is the concept that injury to the uterus in some form results in the final common pathway of uterine activity and then preterm labor.

Among the possible causes of preterm labor, some authorities estimate that up to 25% of instances of preterm labor may be due to intrauterine infection. In this model (Figure 41-6), ascending vaginal microbial flora infects the maternal and fetal gestational tissues (including decidua, fetal membranes, and placenta), and infection is then transmitted to the fetus. This infectious stimulus in some women then results in the uncontrolled elaboration of proinflammatory cytokines. These cytokines stimulate production of uterotonic arachidonic acid metabolites (eg, prostaglandin E2) in gestational tissues, leading to uterine contractions and preterm labor.

Supporting evidence for this hypothesis includes the following. First, many studies have shown that bacterial vaginosis, as characterized by overgrowth of anaerobic bacteria in the vagina, is associated with increased risk for preterm birth. Other bacterial infections in the vagina, for example Group B streptococcal infection, has also been associated with preterm birth in some studies. Second, several investigators have found that IL-1β, TNFα, IL-6, and IL-8 are produced by gestational tissues in response to bacterial products, indicating that human gestational tissues are rich sources of proinflammatory cytokines. Third, significantly increased concentrations of proinflammatory cytokines can be detected in the amniotic fluid of women with intrauterine infection. Fourth, histologic evidence of chorioamnionitis is significantly correlated with clinical evidence of intrauterine infection and increased proinflammatory cytokine concentrations in amniotic fluid. Fifth, antibiotic therapy in some studies has been shown to prolong pregnancy and improve neonatal outcome, particularly in those women who have preterm premature rupture of the membranes. Hence, intrauterine infection, although not proven beyond doubt, appears to play an important role in the pathophysiology of preterm birth.

Perhaps more important than the infectious agent itself is the maternal immune response to a bacterial stimulus. Gestational tissues appear to be particularly prone to exuberant inflammatory responsiveness to seemingly trivial infectious insults. This has led some authorities to postulate that some cases of preterm labor reflect an "intrauterine inflammatory response syndrome" or a "fetal inflammatory response syndrome," somewhat akin to the systemic inflammatory response syndrome noted in nonpregnant adults and children in which septic shock occurs but no definitive organism can be identified. As the maternal and fetal immune responses are better delineated, more specific and successful therapies may be forthcoming for the management of preterm labor.

PREECLAMPSIA

Preeclampsia, or toxemia in older literature, is a pregnancy-specific condition characterized by hypertension, proteinuria, and generalized edema. The condition usually occurs in the third trimester and worldwide is one of the most common causes of maternal mortality and morbidity. Delivery is currently the only cure for the condition. In early-onset cases prior to term that require delivery for cure, preeclampsia is also associated with significant neonatal mortality and morbidity rates. A hallmark feature of the pathophysiology of preeclampsia is endothelial cell activation, dysfunction, and then damage. Endothelial cell integrity is lost, resulting in transudation of fluid from intravascular spaces into tissues, leading to generalized edema. As a result, vasospasm occurs, leading to hypertension as well as proteinuria from the leakage of albumin due to glomerular damage. Preeclampsia is thus a systemic disease in which no organ system is left unaffected. One fascinating aspect of preeclampsia is the multiple possible presentations of the disease. Another is that no clear cause of the syndrome has yet been discovered. It has been said that preeclampsia is a "disease of theories" in which multiple possible causes have been postulated, yet none unequivocally proven. These possible causes include genetic, infectious, autoimmune, and, not surprisingly, immunologic.

Another characteristic hallmark of preeclampsia is poor trophoblast invasion, which usually occurs early in the second trimester. In normal pregnancies, trophoblasts will grow into maternal vessels at this time, resulting in wider diameter vessels with resultant increased maternal blood flow allowing for higher rates of exchange of nutrients, oxygen, and waste products. In women with preeclampsia, this outgrowth does not occur normally, resulting in blood vessels with a smaller diameter and a lessened potential for nutrient exchange. Histologically, features are evident suggestive of inflammatory cell infiltrates with foamy macrophages, much like seen in atherosclerosis. These findings have led to the theory that abnormal T-cell activity may contribute to the pathophysiology of the condition.

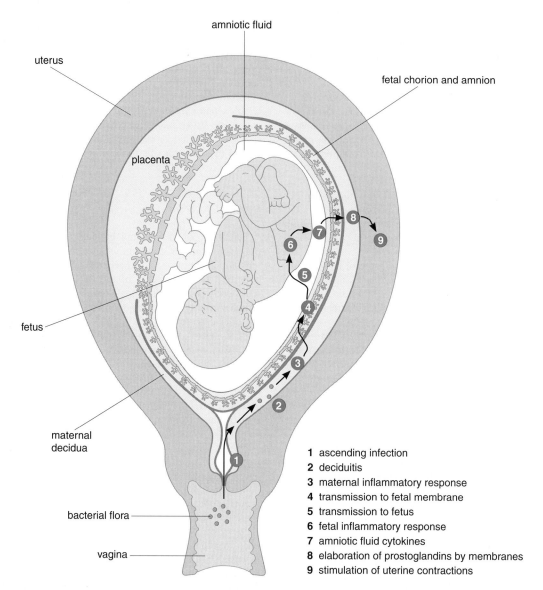

Figure 41–6. The intrauterine inflammatory response syndrome: Proposed pathophysiology of infection-mediated preterm birth. In this model, ascending infection from the vagina (1) traverses the cervix and results in maternal deciduitis (2). The resultant maternal inflammatory response (3) supports transmission of the infection to the fetal membranes and the fetus (4, 5). This fetal inflammatory response results in elaboration of amniotic fluid cytokines (6, 7). Both maternal and fetal inflammatory responses elicit the production of uterotonic arachidonic metabolites (8), leading to uterine contractions (9) and preterm birth.

Several other lines of investigation have led to a potential immunologic cause to preeclampsia. Preeclampsia tends to occur in first pregnancies, and the risk changes with changing paternity. Also, women with more exposure to seminal antigens (based on presumed sexual activity in monogamous relationships) have less risk of preeclampsia, suggesting that maternal response to antigens is blunted with more exposures such that women might become tolerant to paternal antigens with repeated sexual antigens.

Other findings suggest an immunologic component. Several studies have detected increased concentrations of maternal serum cytokines, including TNFα and IL-6. Additionally, IL-12 is elevated in the serum of women with severe preeclampsia. This finding is notable because IL-12 is critical in generating T_H1-type responses and because IL-12 is rarely found in the serum of normal women. The pathophysiology of preeclampsia may therefore reflect both increased innate and adaptive immunologic activity. One speculation is that one manifestation of the disease is a switch from a T_H2-type environment to a more T_H1-type environment.

Two major problems compromise studies on immunologic alterations and preeclampsia. First, there are no universally accepted definitions of preeclampsia, thus making comparisons of studies difficult. For example, it had been reported that NK cell activity is increased, decreased, or unchanged in different studies. Similarly, T-cell activation has been reported to be increased, decreased, or unchanged. The discrepancies in these studies result from the different definitions of preeclampsia being used and from the women in the studies being ascertained at different stages of a constantly changing condition. Second, it is difficult to determine cause or effect based on the studies. Given that every organ system is altered by preeclampsia, it would not be surprising to find that the immune system is changed as well, and in a fashion that contributes to the pathophysiology of the dis-

ease. However, assigning these changes as the cause of preeclampsia cannot be supported by any study.

CONCLUSION

As Medawar noted in 1952, and still is true today, every well-authenticated, clinically significant example of an immunization of the mother by its fetus has implicated antigen derived from either the red blood cell or platelet. Antigens responsible for the rapid and violent reactions provoked by grafting tissues from one individual to another are not part of maternal-fetal interactions. Precise characterization of the immunobiology of the maternal-fetal relationship properly begins with the detailed examination of the trophoblast and the tissues that it touches; further insight will be gained by attempts to understand the interactions of these tissues in light of contemporary cellular and molecular immunologic models.

REFERENCES

GENERAL

Gill TJ et al (editors): *Immunoregulation and Fetal Survival.* Oxford University Press, 1987.

Grimes DA: Technology follies: The uncritical acceptance of medical innovation. *JAMA* 1993;269:3030.

Medawar PB: Some immunological and endocrinological problems raised by the evolution of viviparity in vertebrates. *Symp Soc Exp Biol* 1953;7:320.

Strauss JF, Lyttle CR (editors): *Uterine and Embryonic Factors in Early Pregnancy.* Plenum Press, 1991.

REPRODUCTIVE TRACT ANATOMY & IMMUNITY

Bulmer D: The histochemistry of ovarian macrophages in the rat. *J Anat Lond* 1964;98:313.

Edwards JNT, Morris HB: Langerhans' cells and lymphocyte subsets in the female genital tract. *Br J Obstet Gynaecol* 1985;92:974.

Kutteh WH, Mestecky J: Secretory immunity in the female reproductive tract. *Am J Reprod Immunol* 1994;31:40.

Miller CH et al: Mucosal immunity, HIV transmission, and AIDS. *Lab Invest* 1992;68:129.

Ogra PL, Swtantarta SO: Local antibody response to polio-vaccine in the human female genital tract. *J Immunol* 1973;110:1307.

OVULATION & SPERMATOGENESIS

Adashi EY: Cytokine-mediated regulation of ovarian function: Encounters of a third kind. *Endocrinology* 1989; 124:2043.

Adashi EY: Editorial: With a little help from my friends—The evolving story of intraovarian regulation. *Endocrinology* 1995;136:4161.

Hurwitz A et al: Interleukin-1 is both morphogenic and cytotoxic to cultured rat ovarian cells: Obligatory role for heterologous, contact-independent cell–cell interaction. *Endocrinology* 1992;131:1643.

Kol S, Adashi EY: Intraovarian factors regulating ovarian function. *Curr Opin Obstet Gynecol* 1995;7:209.

Yule TD et al: Role of testicular autoantigens and influence of lymphokines in testicular autoimmune disease. *J Reprod Immunol* 1990;18:89.

FERTILIZATION, IMPLANTATION, & THE IMMUNE RESPONSE TO FETAL TISSUES

Castellucci M, Kaufmann P: A three-dimensional study of the normal human placental villous core: II. Stromal architecture. *Placenta* 1982;3:269.

Haimovici F et al: The effects of soluble products of activated lymphocytes and macrophages on blastocyst implantation events in vitro. *Biol Reprod* 1991;44:69.

Paria BC, Dey SK: Preimplantation embryo development in vitro: Cooperative interactions among embryos and role of growth factors. *Proc Natl Acad Sci U S A* 1990; 87: 4756.

Pijnenborg R et al: Trophoblast invasion and the establishment of haemochorial placentation in man and laboratory animals. *Placenta* 1981;2:71.

Rouas-Freiss N et al: Direct evidence to support the role of HLA-G in protecting the fetus from maternal uterine natural killer cytolysis. *Proc Natl Acad Sci U S A* 1997; 94:11520.

Saling PM: Mammalian sperm interaction with extracellular matrices of the egg. *Oxf Rev Reprod Biol* 1989;11: 339.

Stewart CL et al: Blastocyst implantation depends on maternal expression of leukemia inhibitory factor. *Nature* 1992;359:76.

Wassarman PM: Mouse gamete adhesion molecules. *Biol Reprod* 1992;46:186.

IMMUNITY IN PREGNANCY

Castellucci M et al: Mitosis of the Hofbauer cell: Possible implications for a fetal macrophage. *Placenta* 1987; 8:65.

Daynes RA et al: Regulation of murine lymphokine production in vivo. II. Dehydroepiandrosterone is a natural enhancer of interleukin 2 synthesis by helper T cells. *Eur J Immunol* 1990;20:793.

Daynes RA et al: Contrasting effects of glucocorticoids on the capacity of T cells to produce the growth factors interleukin 2 and interleukin 4. *Eur J Immunol* 1989; 19:3219.

Heyborne KD et al: Characterization of gamma delta T lymphocytes at the maternal–fetal interface. *J Immunol* 1992;149:2872.

Hunt JS et al: Evaluation of human chorionic trophoblast cells and placental macrophages as stimulators of maternal lymphocyte proliferation in vitro. *J Reprod Immunology* 1984;6:377.

Khayr WF et al: Listeriosis: Review of a protean disease. *Infect Dis Clin Pract* 1992;1:291.

Lu CY et al: Pregnancy as a natural model of allograft tolerance. *Transplantation* 1989;48:848.

McLean JM et al: Changes in the thymus, spleen and lymph nodes during pregnancy and lactation in the rat. *J Anat* 1974;118:223.

Redline RW, Lu CY: Role of local immunosuppression in murine fetoplacental listeriosis. *J Clin Invest* 1987;79: 1234.

Redline RW, Lu CY: Specific defects in the anti-listerial immune response in discrete regions of the murine uterus and placenta account for susceptibility to infection. *J Immunol* 1988;140:3947.

Rocklin RE et al: Immunobiology of the maternal–fetal relationship. *Ann Rev Med* 1979;30:375.

Sridama V et al: Decreased levels of helper T cells: A possible cause of immunodeficiency in pregnancy. *N Engl J Med* 1982;307:352.

Weinberg ED: Pregnancy-associated depression of cell mediated immunity. *Rev Infect Dis* 1984;6:814.

INFERTILITY & SPONTANEOUS ABORTION

Collins JA: Frequency and predictive value of antisperm antibodies among infertile couples. *Hum Reprod* 1993; 8:592.

Dudley DJ: Recurrent pregnancy loss and cytokines: Not as simple as it seems. *JAMA* 1995;273:1958.

Fraser EJ et al: Immunization as therapy for recurrent spontaneous abortion: A review and meta-analysis. *Obstet Gynecol* 1993;82:854.

Haas GG: Immunologic infertility. *Obstet Gynecol Clin North Am* 1987;14:1069.

Hill JA et al: T-helper 1-type immunity to trophoblast in women with recurrent spontaneous abortion. *JAMA* 1995; 273:1933.

Katz I et al: Cutaneous graft-versus-host-like reaction after paternal lymphocyte immunization for prevention of recurrent abortion. *Fertil Steril* 1992;57:927.

Kutteh WH et al: Antisperm antibodies: Current knowledge and new horizons. *Mol Androl* 1993;4:183.

Kutteh WH, Carr BR: Recurrent pregnancy loss. In: *Textbook of Reproductive Medicine,* Carr BR, Blackwell Richard E (editors). Appleton & Lange, 1993.

Luo AM et al: Antigen mimicry in autoimmune disease sharing of amino acid residues critical for pathogenic T cell activation. *J Clin Invest* 1993;92:2117.

Ober C et al: Mononuclear-cell immunisation in prevention of recurrent miscarriages: a randomized trial. *Lancet* 1999;354:365.

Mishell DR: Infertility. In: *Comprehensive Gynecology.* Herbst AL et al (editors). Mosby Year Book, 1992.

Recurrent Miscarriage Immunotherapy Trialists Group: Worldwide collaborative observational study and meta-analysis on allogeneic leukocyte immunotherapy for recurrent spontaneous abortion. *Am J Reprod Immunol* 1994;32:55.

Tung KSK, Lu CY: Immunologic basis of reproductive failure. In: *Pathology of Reproductive Failure.* Kraus FT et al (editors). Williams and Wilkins, 1992, pp 308–333.

Vazquez-Levin M et al: The effect of female antisperm antibodies on in vitro fertilization, early embryonic development, and pregnancy outcome. *Fertil Steril* 1991;56: 84.

HIV INFECTION, THE REPRODUCTIVE SYSTEM, & VERTICAL TRANSMISSION

Connor EM et al: Reduction of maternal–infant transmission of human immunodeficiency virus type 1 with zidovudine treatment. *New Engl J Med* 1994;331:1173.

Dickover RE et al: Identification of levels of maternal HIV-1 RNA associated with risk of perinatal transmission. Effect of maternal zidovudine treatment on viral load. *JAMA* 1996;275:599.

Garcia PM et al: Maternal levels of plasma HIV-1 RNA and the risk of pernatal transmission. Women and Infants Transmission Study Group *NEJM* 1999;341:394

Levy JA: Pathogenesis of human immunodeficiency virus infection. *Microbiol Rev* 1993;57:183.

Mestecky J et al: Mucosal immunity in the female genital tract: Relevance to vaccination efforts against the human immunodeficiency virus. *AIDS Res Hum Retroviruses* 1994;10,(supp 2):S11.

Miller CH et al: Mucosal immunity, HIV transmission, and AIDS. *Lab Invest* 1992;68:129.

Oxtoby MJ: Vertically acquired HIV infection in the United States. In: *Pediatric AIDS: The Challenge of HIV Infection in Infants, Children, and Adolescents,* 2nd ed. Pizzo PA, Wilfert CM (editors), Williams and Wilkins, 1994.

Spira AI et al: Cellular targets of infection and route of viral dissemination after an intravaginal inoculation of simian immunodeficiency virus into Rhesus macaques. *J Exp Med* 1996;183:215.

PRETERM LABOR & DELIVERY

Creasy RK: Preterm birth prevention: Where are we? *Am J Obstet Gynecol* 1993;168:1223.

Dudley DJ: Preterm labor: an intrauterine inflammatory response syndrome?. *J Reprod Immunol* 1997;36:93.

Hauth JC et al: Reduced incidence of preterm delivery with metronidazole and erythromycin in women with bacterial vaginosis. *New Engl J Med* 1995;333:1732.

Leveno KJ et al: The national impact of ritodrine hydrochloride for inhibition of preterm labor. *Obstet Gynecol* 1990;76:12.

Romero R et al: A fetal systemic inflammatory response is followed by the spontaneous onset of parturition. *Am J Obstet Gynecol* 1998;179:186.

PREECLAMPSIA

Dekker GA et al: Immune maladaptation in the etiology of pre-eclampsia: A review of corroborative epidemiologic studies. *Obstet Gynecol Survey* 1998;53:377.

Dudley DJ et al: Interleukin-12 concentrations are elevated in the serum of women with severe pre-eclampsia. *J Reprod Immunol* 1996;31:97.

Ness R et al: Heterogeneous causes constituting the single syndrome of pre-eclampsia: a hypothesis and its implications. *Am J Obstet Gynecol* 1996;175:1365.

Redman CWG et al: Pre-eclampsia: An excessive maternal inflammatory response to pregnancy. *Am J Obstet Gynecol* 1999;180:499.

Robillard P et al: Association of pregnancy-induced hypertension with duration of sexual cohabitation before conception. *Lancet* 1994;344:973.

Vinatier D et al: Pre-eclampsia: Physiology and immunological aspects. *Eur J Obstet Gynecol and Reprod Biol* 1995;61:85.

42 Mechanisms of Tumor Immunology

Philip D. Greenberg, MD

Tumor immunology is the study of (1) the antigenic properties of transformed cells, (2) the host immune responses to these tumor cells, (3) the immunologic consequences to the host of the growth of malignant cells, and (4) the means by which the immune system can be modulated to recognize tumor cells and promote tumor eradication. Although a potentially important function of the immune system would be to provide protection from the outgrowth of malignant cells, this represents a formidable and likely unsuccessful task with most cancers. Tumor cells have many immunologic similarities to normal cells, despite exhibiting abnormal propensities to proliferate, to spread throughout the host, and to interfere with normal organ functions. Thus, tumor cells present special problems to the host's immune system beyond those presented by other replicating antigens such as bacteria, which can more easily be distinguished as foreign.

Normal cells have a variable capacity to proliferate and to express differentiated functions. These cell activities are tightly coordinated within an organ or tissue, so that the rate of cell loss due to the natural death of mature differentiated cells is equal to the rate of appearance of new cells from the less mature proliferating cell pool. In some pathologic conditions, the stimulus for cell proliferation exceeds the requirement for cell replacement, resulting in organ hypertrophy from polyclonal expansion of cells proliferating in response to growth signals. Once the condition responsible for excess stimulation of cell growth terminates, however, the rate of cell proliferation decreases and the organ hypertrophy resolves. In contrast to this nonmalignant, regulated polyclonal cell growth, an individual cell may undergo a transforming event and acquire the potential to produce daughter cells that proliferate independent of external growth and regulatory signals. The autonomous growth of such transformed cells of monoclonal origin represents the basis of malignant disease. Many of the properties of tumor cells are summarized in Table 42–1. The protean effects of cancer reflect in large part the unrestrained growth of tumor cells that locally invade and disrupt normal tissue as well as metastasize and grow in distant organs.

Table 42–1. Common properties of tumor cells.

1. Failure to respond to the regulatory signals responsible for maintaining normal growth and controlling tissue repair
2. Autonomous growth without an absolute requirement for exogenous growth signals
3. Invasive growth through normal tissue boundaries
4. Metastatic growth in distant organs following entry into blood and lymph channels
5. Monoclonal origin, although genotypic and phenotypic heterogeneity may develop as tumor mass increases
6. Differences in appearance and membrane antigenic display from nontransformed differentiated cells of the same tissue origin

DEVELOPMENT OF TUMORS

The transformation of a normal cell to a malignancy can result from a variety of different causes, the particular nature of which helps determine if the immune system will effectively control the outgrowth of the tumor cells. These transforming events may occur spontaneously during cell division as random mutations or gene rearrangements; alternatively, they may be induced by a chemical, physical, or viral carcinogen.

Tumors induced by chemical carcinogens were initially described in the 18th century, when chimney sweeps were observed to have an unusually high incidence of carcinoma of the scrotum. Polycyclic aromatic hydrocarbons in soot and tar have since been found to be a major class of carcinogens, and retention of tar in the wrinkles of the scrotum was apparently responsible for these tumors. In fact, painting tar on epithelial cells became a useful experimental technique for inducing tumors in the laboratory. A second major class of carcinogens, the aromatic amines, was identified following the observation of a high frequency of bladder cancer among factory workers using aniline dyes. The mechanisms by which chemical carcinogens induce neoplastic transformation predominantly reflect the mutagenic activity of these compounds.

Evidence of tumor induction by physical carcinogens accrued rapidly following the discovery of x-rays and radioactivity in the late 19th century when many of the early radiologists developed skin cancer. The most dramatic evidence of radiation-induced carcinogenesis has been in survivors of the atomic bomb explosions at the end of World War II in Japan, who demonstrated an increased incidence of a wide range of tumors for more than 20 years after the nuclear holocaust. Such ionizing radiation directly injures cellular DNA, resulting in mutations, chromosomal breaks, and abnormal rearrangements. Another physical carcinogen, ultraviolet radiation, induces skin cancer on sun-exposed parts of the body, particularly in people with xeroderma pigmentosum, a disease in which the repair mechanism for ultraviolet-induced damage to DNA is defective.

Viral oncogenesis is of particular interest in tumor immunology because of the great likelihood that cells transformed by the introduction of viral genes will express new virus-associated antigens that can be recognized by the immune system. Oncogenic viruses can be subdivided into either DNA or RNA types, depending on the genetic information carried by the intact virus. Most cells infected by the potentially oncogenic DNA viruses, which include papovaviruses, herpesviruses, and adenoviruses, express all of the viral genes and support viral replication, which commonly results in cell lysis. Infection of cells nonpermissive for viral replication can result in integration of viral DNA into the host genome and expression of only some viral genes, however, so that lytic virus particles are not formed. Transformation results either from direct effects on expression or function of host genes by the integrated viral DNA or from aberrant splicing of transcribed viral RNA to produce new proteins that promote transformation. Several human DNA viruses have been found to contain potential oncogenes and have been associated with the development of malignancies. These include links between Epstein-Barr virus (EBV) and Burkitt's lymphoma, Hodgkin's disease and nasopharyngeal carcinoma, and between human papillomavirus and cervical, anogenital, and skin carcinomas.

Oncogenic RNA viruses contain genes for a polymerase called **reverse transcriptase,** which permits the use of the viral RNA as a template for transcription of a DNA copy that can be integrated into the host genome. Because this is a reversal of the normal DNA-to-RNA transcription of genetic information, these viruses are often referred to as **retroviruses.** RNA tumor viruses, which were first discovered in chicken tumors, appear to be responsible for a large number of naturally occurring cancers in many species. Some of these viruses contain directly transforming oncogenes, whereas others must activate host genetic material. A class of human retroviruses, the human T-cell leukemia viruses (HTLV), are responsible for a subset of T-cell leukemias, particularly cases occurring in a region of southern Japan where the infection is endemic. Many retroviruses, such as feline leukemia virus and HTLV, can spread horizontally from infected to normal hosts, and resistance to tumorigenesis in exposed hosts results in part from the generation of an immune response to virus-associated antigens.

Advances in molecular biology have provided the tools to better understand the events involved in transformation. Analogues to many of the viral oncogenes have been identified in the normal cellular genome, and in vitro studies of the analogues have demonstrated that activation of these cellular oncogenes can transform normal cells under appropriate conditions. The essential role of many cellular oncogenes in normal growth and development has been demonstrated, but abnormal expression or maintenance of these genes in an active state can result in transformation. This may occur by mutations, such as ones that interfere with regulation of the transcription or of the activity of the protein; by a translocation that places the oncogene next to an active cellular gene, such as is observed in B-cell tumors with the translocation of the c-*myc* oncogene next to an immunoglobulin V region gene; or by insertion of an active promoter that enhances expression, such as may occur following integration of a slowly transforming retrovirus. Oncogenes code for a wide variety of products including membrane receptors, signalling messengers, autocrine growth factors, inhibitors of apoptosis, and regulators of cell cycle progression and gene expression. The expression of some of these oncogene products, particularly those resulting from mutations of the normal protein, can render malignant cells sufficiently disparate from normal cells for detection by immunologic methods and potentially for elimination by immunologically directed attack.

ANTIGENS ON TUMOR CELLS

The field of tumor immunology is based in large part on the supposition that tumors express antigens that permit immunologic separation of malignant from normal cells. Although historically much skepticism surrounded this presumption, modern approaches facilitated by technologic advances in cellular and molecular immunology have convincingly demonstrated that many human tumors express antigens that can induce and be targets of cellular and humoral responses. The relevant tumor antigens fall into two major categories. **Unique tumor-specific antigens** are found only in tumor cells and therefore represent ideal targets for an immunologic attack. In contrast, **tumor-associated determinants** are found in tumor cells and also in some normal cells, but qualitative and quantitative differences in antigen expression permit the use of these antigens to distinguish tumor cells from normal cells.

A wide variety of cellular proteins have now been

identified to function as tumor antigens. Many distinct molecular mechanisms may result in the production of a tumor antigen. The most straightforward is a transforming event resulting in the production of a new protein, such as would occur following infection with a potentially oncogenic virus such as EBV, HTLV, or human papillomavirus (HPV). Similarly, point mutations or gene rearrangements affecting cellular oncogenes that promote the transformed phenotype, such as reported with *ras* and p53 in breast and colon cancer, *bcr–abl* in chronic myelogenous leukemia, or p16INK4 and CDK4 in melanoma, can result in the expression of new epitopes potentially recognizable by the immune system. Unique tumor antigens can also result from random mutations in cellular proteins as a consequence of genomic instability in transformed cells or uncovering normally nonexposed determinants, as observed with some complex branching glycolipid antigens in which deletion of a branch exposes a new antigenic determinant. Nonunique proteins that may nevertheless serve as tumor antigens can result from the aberrant expression of fetal or increased expression of differentiation antigens, such as that observed with the expression on human gastric carcinoma cells of ABO blood group antigens disparate from the host ABO blood type or of the melanoma-associated gene (MAGE) antigens in human melanoma cells, or from overexpression of oncogenic proteins, such as Her-2/Neu in breast and ovarian cancer.

New strategies to screen for novel or aberrantly expressed proteins have revolutionized the effort to identify tumor antigens. Molecular techniques, including cDNA and oligonucleotide arrays, have made it possible to efficiently screen tumor cells for the expression of potentially interesting tumor antigens and have identified antigens commonly expressed in particular tumor types as well as novel antigens resulting from mutations. Immunologic techniques, including the isolation of tumor-reactive T cells and antibodies from patients with cancer and the development of novel vaccination strategies, have made it possible to identify tumor antigens that clearly induce immune responses and to generate responses to antigens of interest.

Unique Tumor Antigens

These antigens can be detected only in tumor cells and not in other host cells. Identifying the presence of unique antigens in tumors from inbred mice was much simpler than for antigens in human tumors because of the ability to perform tumor transplantation studies. Advances in molecular biology, however, have improved the immunologic analysis of human tumors. Many tumors linked epidemiologically with viruses, viral genomes present in tumor cells have been isolated, viral proteins expressed in human tumors identified, and the resulting unique viral antigens demonstrated to be potentially immunogenic.

"Spontaneous" tumors, many of which may have actually been induced by exposure to environmental carcinogens, were perceived to have no predictable antigenic markers and therefore have posed a more difficult problem. Molecular and immunologic techniques are being used to characterize an ever-increasing number of potential target antigens, however. Improved methods to detect and recover low-frequency tumor-reactive T cells and antibodies from the blood, draining lymph nodes, and tumor masses of patients have provided the requisite immunologic reagents to screen expression libraries derived from tumor cells for immunogenic target antigens. The yield has included mutated oncogenes and proteins associated with the malignant phenotype as well as spontaneous mutations probably resulting from genomic instability characteristic of malignant cells.

Elucidation of the processing pathways for presentation of protein antigens in association with major histocompatibility complex (MHC) molecules to T cells has altered the foucs of the search for tumor-specific antigens. T cells recognize small peptides derived from intracellular degradation of cytosolic proteins that are inserted into a peptide-binding cleft in the MHC molecule and are then transported with the MHC molecule to the cell surface (see Chapter 6). Any abnormal cellular protein, not just a protein detected on the membrane, is therefore a potential immunogen. Thus, the presence in a tumor cell of a nonfunctional protein product of a mutated allele, such as often occurs with p53, could result in the immunogenicity of that product. Moreover, the difficulties previously encountered in detecting unique antigens on human tumors with monoclonal antibodies now appear to be predictable; the results do not imply that these tumors do not express unique antigens but, rather, that the use of molecular approaches to probe gene expression rather than surface phenotype are more likely to be productive, especially for antigens that can be targeted by T cells.

Tumor-Associated Antigens

Although it may not be possible to detect unique tumor antigens in all tumors, many tumors display antigens that distinguish them from normal cells. These tumor-associated antigens may be expressed by some normal cells at particular stages of differentiation, but the quantitative expression or the composite expression in association with other lineage or differentiation markers can be useful for identifying transformed cells. The identification of tumor-associated antigens has made quantum leaps in the last decade, beginning with the development of technologies to produce and screen monoclonal antibodies generated in mice in response to human tumors, progressing more recently with the development of SEREX (serologic analysis of antibody responses by expression cloning) technology to screen the human antibodies elicited by the tumor in cancer patients, and further advancing with the ability to analyze the differential display of genes in tumor cells as compared to normal cells. Many of the identified antigens are already invaluable diagnostically for distinguishing transformed from nontransformed cells and for defining the cell lineage of transformed cells, and many will likely prove to be attractive for targeting a therapeutic attack.

The best characterized human tumor-associated antigens are the oncofetal antigens. These antigens are expressed during embryogenesis but are absent or very difficult to detect in normal adult tissue. The prototype antigen is **carcinoembryonic antigen (CEA),** a glycoprotein found on fetal gut and human colon cancer cells but not on normal adult colon cells. Because CEA is shed from colon carcinoma cells and found in the serum, it was originally thought that the presence of this antigen in the serum could be used to screen patients for colon cancer. It soon became apparent, however, that patients with inflammatory lesions involving cells of endodermal origin, such as colitis or pancreatitis, as well as patients with other tumors, such as pancreatic and breast cancer, also had elevated serum levels of CEA. Despite these limitations, monitoring the fall and rise of CEA levels in colon cancer patients undergoing therapy has proven useful for predicting tumor progression and responses to treatment. Moreover, recent studies have suggested that T-cell responses can be elicited to CEA, and a clinical trial in patients with colon cancer is currently evaluating whether recombinant vaccines expressing CEA can induce T-cell responses to CEA that will eliminate residual cancer cells. Several other oncofetal antigens have been useful for diagnosing and monitoring human tumors. In particular, α-**fetoprotein,** an alpha globulin normally secreted by fetal liver and yolk sac cells, is found in the serum of patients with liver and germinal cell tumors and can be used as a marker of disease status.

One particularly interesting set of tumor-associated proteins have been termed cancer–testes antigens because they are detected only in malignant cells and germinal tissue. The best characterized include the MAGE family of proteins expressed in melanoma and many other tumors, and NY-ESO which is expressed by many carcinomas. Although the normal function of these proteins is largely unknown, the limited normal tissue expression renders them nearly unique tumor antigens. Indeed, T-cell and antibody responses to these proteins have been detected in many cancer patients, and they are being explored as targets of therapeutic responses.

Many other tumor-associated antigens, which have unknown function but very limited tissue distribution on normal cells, have been identified with monoclonal antibodies. Membrane glycoprotein and glycolipid antigens isolated from malignant melanoma cells appear to be relatively specific for these tumors, although some expression on normal cells such as

neuronal tissue has been detected. A glycoprotein found on human leukemia cells, called common acute lymphocytic leukemia antigen (CALLA, or CD10), has been detected at low levels on other cells such as granulocytes and kidney cells. Many other similar examples exist, and the use of such antigenic markers for diagnostic and therapeutic purposes has great promise.

The recent successes in isolation and cloning of tumor-reactive T cells from cancer patients, coupled with expression cloning of tumor genes and screening of the transfected targets for recognition by the T cells, has made it possible to identify tumor-associated antigens that a priori induce cellular immune responses. In melanoma, T-cell responses to several normal melanosomal proteins such as gp100 and tyrosinase, as well as MAGE proteins and mutated oncogenic proteins, have been characterized. Similar strategies have identified immunogenic proteins in breast cancer, ovarian cancer, lung cancer, and pancreatic cancer. Intentional immunization with candidate tumor antigens identified by molecular screening is yielding an ever-increasing number of immunogenic tumor proteins, such as telomerase, which is expressed in tumors to prevent senescence but is absent from most normal adult tissues. A major focus of tumor immunologists is designing strategies to provide or elicit therapeutic responses to these antigens in patients with a tumor that expresses the protein.

IMMUNOLOGIC EFFECTOR MECHANISMS POTENTIALLY OPERATIVE AGAINST TUMOR CELLS

Virtually all of the effector components of the immune system have the potential to contribute to the eradication of tumor cells. It is likely that each of these effector mechanisms can play a role in the control of tumor growth, but a particular mechanism may be more or less important, depending on the tumor and setting. The potential for mediating antitumor responses should become more evident by employing approaches to augment individual effector responses, such as by the adoptive transfer of large numbers of cells or the administration of cytokines or antibodies.

T Cells

The T-cell response is unquestionably the most important host response for the control of growth of antigenic tumor cells. It is responsible for both the direct killing of tumor cells and the activation of other components of the immune system. T-cell immunity to tumors reflects the function of the two T-cell subsets: class II-restricted T cells, which largely represent CD4 helper T (T_H) cells that mediate their effect by direct interaction with antigen-presenting cells (APC) and by the secretion of lymphokines to activate other effector cells and induce inflammatory responses, and class I-restricted T cells, which largely represent CD8 cytotoxic T (T_C) cells that can also secrete lymphokines but mediate their effect mostly by direct lysis of tumor cells.

The precise contribution of each T-cell subset and T-cell function to the antitumor response appears quite variable, but tumor-specific T cells from each subset are capable of mediating tumor eradication and have been detected in the peripheral blood of individual patients and in the cells infiltrating human tumors. Most tumor cells, however, express class I but not class II MHC molecules, and the T_H-cell subset cannot directly recognize these tumor cells. Therefore, such T_H-cell responses usually depend on APCs such as dendritic cells or macrophages to present the relevant tumor antigens in the context of class II molecules for activation. After antigen-specific triggering, these T cells futher activate dendritic cells and secrete lymphokines that activate T_C cells, macrophages, natural killer (NK) cells, and B cells and can produce other lymphokines, such as tumor necrosis factor (TNF), which may be directly lytic to tumor cells (see Chapter 9 and 10). In contrast to T_H-cells, the T_C-cell subset is capable of directly recognizing and killing tumor targets by disrupting the target membrane and disintegrating the nucleus. Only a minor fraction of class I-restricted CD8 T cells are capable of providing helper functions, however, and thus effective T_C-cell responses generally depend on class II-restricted CD4 T_H-cell responses to provide the necessary helper factors to activate and promote the proliferation of T_C-cells.

B Cells & Antibody-Dependent Killing

A potential role for host antibody responses in human tumor immunity was previously suggested by the occasional detection of tumor-reactive antibodies in the serum of patients. More recent sensitive approaches using SEREX screening strategies have suggested that antibody responses to tumor antigens may be much more common. Some of these antibodies are to surface antigens, such as the Her2-neu oncogene protein, and could have direct antitumor activity, whereas others are to intracellular proteins and could facilitate T-cell responses by enhancing processing and presentation by APC of tumor antigens released from dead tumor cells.

There are two major mechanisms by which antibodies may mediate tumor cell lysis. Complement-fixing antibodies bind to the tumor cell membrane and promote attachment of complement components that create pores in the membrane, resulting in cell disruption due to loss of osmotic and biochemical integrity. An alternative mechanism is antibody-dependent cell-mediated cytotoxicity (ADCC), in which antibodies, usually of the IgG class, form an intercellular bridge by binding via the variable region to a specific determinant on the target cell and via the Fc region to effector cells expressing Fc receptors. Many potential effector cells, including NK cells, macrophages, and granulocytes, can mediate the lytic event. ADCC is a more efficient in vitro lytic mechanism than complement-mediated cytotoxicity, requiring fewer antibody molecules per cell to kill. Preclinical immunotherapy studies with monoclonal antibodies of different isotypes (and thus different capacities to fix complement or mediate ADCC) have also suggested that ADCC may be the more important in vivo effector mechanism.

Natural Killer Cells

NK cells can kill a wide range of tumor targets in vitro (see also Chapter 9). The mechanism by which NK cells preferentially recognize and lyse transformed rather than normal targets is now becoming clearer with the increasing characterization of a broad array of inhibitory and activating receptors expressed by NK cells. The cytolytic potential of NK cells is largely contained by off signals delivered via families of inhibitory receptors that bind to class I molecules on potential target cells. Although this likely evolved to permit NK cells to distinguish, as a first line of defense, cells infected with viruses, which commonly down-regulate class I MHC molecules, many tumor cells also express low levels of class I and thereby release the inhibitory signal. The precise nature of the activating signal from tumor cells is less certain, but a variety of molecules such as CD48 and surface glycoproteins are candidates. Cytolysis by NK cells is mediated by the release of cytotoxic factor and the use of perforins to puncture holes in the target cell membrane. The cytotoxic activity of NK cells can be augmented both in vitro and in vivo with the lymphokines interleukin-2 (IL-2) and interferon, and via cross-linking the activating Fc receptor, and thus NK activity can be amplified by both immune T-cell and B-cell responses. Recent studies have demonstrated that augmentation of NK activity in visceral organs enhances resistance to the growth of metastases. Therefore, NK cells may provide a first line of host defense against the growth of transformed cells at both the primary and metastatic sites, as well as represent an effector mechanism recruited by T cells and B cells(or the pharmacologic administration of cytokines and antibodies) to supplement specific antitumor responses.

Additional cytotoxic effector cells that bear many similarities to but can be distinguished from classic NK cells have also been identified. Lymphokine-activated killer (LAK) cells can be induced by very high pharmacologic doses of IL-2, are phenotypically heterogeneous (including both NK and CD8 T cells), and kill a much broader spectrum of tumor targets than do NK cells, but their role during physiologic antitumor responses remains to be elucidated. NK T cells, another class of effector cells, express both NK- and T-cell markers and appear to be activated by recognition of nonclassical class I molecules via a relatively invariant T-cell receptor. These cells have been shown to be important in tumor resistance in murine models, and their role in human tumor biology is being actively investigated.

Macrophages

Macrophages are important in tumor immunity as antigen-presenting cells to stimulate the immune response and as potential effector cells to mediate tumor lysis. Resting macrophages are not cytolytic to tumor cells in vitro but can become cytolytic if activated with macrophage-activating factors (MAF). MAF are commonly secreted by T cells following antigen-specific stimulation, and therefore the participation of macrophages as effector cells in the absence of administration of cytokines may depend on T-cell immunity. This contention is supported by studies showing that macrophages isolated from immunogenic tumors undergoing regression exhibit tumoricidal activity, whereas macrophages isolated from progressing or nonimmunogenic tumors generally show no cytotoxic activity. T-cell lymphokines with MAF activity include interferon gamma, TNF, IL-4, and granulocyte-macrophage colony-stimulating factor (GM-CSF) (see Chapter 10).

The mechanisms by which macrophages recognize tumor cells and mediate lysis are not well defined, but activated macrophages may produce cytotoxic factors that mediate killing as well as bind to and lyse transformed cells in preference to normal cells. Binding by activated macrophages is an energy-dependent process dependent on trypsin-sensitive membrane structures. Several distinct lytic mechanisms appear to be operative, depending on the MAF responsible for activating the macrophages. These include intercellular transfer of lysosomal products, superoxide production, release of neutral proteinases, and secretion of the TNF. Studies in knockout mice have suggested that production of nitric oxide, which is a mediator of tumor apoptosis, may be the most critical effector mechanism employed by macrophages.

POTENTIAL MECHANISMS BY WHICH TUMOR CELLS MAY ESCAPE FROM AN IMMUNE RESPONSE

The concept of host immune surveillance, with the immune system providing the function of surveying the body to recognize and destroy frequently developing immunogenic tumor cells, was formally proposed by F. M. Burnet. The failure to demonstrate an increased appearance of immunogenic tumors in immunodeficient hosts incapable of tumor rejection has modified current views of immune surveillance, however. Although antigen-specific responses may provide a surveillance function for the development of certain tumors, such as those induced by oncogenic DNA and RNA tumor viruses, the immune system is much more efficient at recognizing infectious organisms than tumor cells as foreign. Thus, nonspecific effector populations, such as NK and NK T cells, rather than tumor antigen-specific immune responses, are now believed to be more important in the rejection of newly appearing tumor cells. The failure of the immune system to prevent the emergence of most tumors does not preclude the development of tumor-specific immune responses during the growth of established tumors. Indirect support for the presence of immunity to human tumors includes spontaneous regressions of tumors and regressions of metastatic lesions after removal of large primary tumors. Direct evidence of tumor immunity has been unequivocally provided by studies using sensitive in vitro methods to detect antibodies or T cells reactive with tumors in cancer patients. Thus, it seems likely that even though the emergence of many tumors may reflect a failure of immune surveillance and the absence of an immune response during early tumor growth, a potentially detectable but unfortunately ineffective immune response may still be generated during progressive growth of the tumor. Important goals in tumor immunology are to determine why such responses are ineffective and to devise methods to induce effective responses.

Many potential mechanisms permitting escape from immune destruction have been identified. Immunoselection of variant cells was initially suggested by analysis of the tumor cells present in a lesion, which often reveals heterogeneity with respect to morphology and surface phenotype. This has now been more definitively demonstrated in melanoma in which the generation of a T-cell response to one melanosomal protein has been associated with the outgrowth of tumors lacking this protein. The presence of such escape-variant cells is probably due to the inherent genomic instability of transformed cells, and preferential survival of these variant cells requires that the antigen being recognized is not associated with the malignant phenotype, such as a mutated oncogene. The failure to demonstrate immune selection in some cases could reflect the fact that, when the escape variant becomes the dominant population, the presence of an antitumor response is obscured by the loss of the tumor antigen in the analyzable target cells.

Antigenic modulation results in similar events to those described earlier, in that an immune response to a tumor antigen selects for the growth of antigen-negative cells. In this setting, however, antigen loss reflects only a phenotypic change in the tumor cell, and if the immune response is ablated, the antigen is reexpressed. Antigenic modulation resulting from antibody responses has been extensively reported, but modulation from T-cell responses has not yet been clearly identified.

As described in Chapter 6, the presentation of antigens by tumor cells for recognition by T cells requires the intracellular processing of proteins, with degradation to small, 8–9-amino-acid long, peptides that are transported to the endoplasmic reticulum and then inserted into a cleft in the class I MHC molecule for subsequent transport to the cell surface. Recent studies have shown that some tumor cells have defective antigen-processing machinery, with the results that class I molecules do not get loaded with peptides and transported to the surface, class I expression is low, and even potentially highly immunogenic tumor antigens cannot be presented to the immune system.

Tumor cells can nonspecifically interfere with the expression of immunity in the host using many mechanisms. Some tumor cells can release soluble factors that directly suppress immunologic reactivity. One well-studied phenomenon is the inhibition of immune responses by macrophages that have been modified as a result of residing in hosts bearing progressive tumors. This appears to be mediated largely via the spontaneous secretion of prostaglandins, and in vitro treatment of macrophages with the cyclooxygenase inhibitor indomethacin can overcome the inhibitory effects.

Patients with advanced cancer demonstrate increased susceptibility to opportunistic infections and can exhibit global depression of T-cell responses. Analysis of the T-cell receptor-signaling complex from T cells in such patients has demonstrated that this in part reflects a decrease in the amount of zeta chain present in T-cell receptor complexes. This defect, as well as the associated abnormal T-cell function, is reversible, further suggesting the notion that tumor growth can result in release of an immunosuppressive factor. The presence of abnormalities in the T-cell receptor complex with advanced disease has prompted analyses of T cells isolated from tumor sites at earlier stages of disease. Indeed, several studies have shown that T cells from draining lymph nodes or infiltrating tumors often have abnormally phosphorylated or absent zeta chains, which can render the T cell functionally nonreactive and would thus make the tumor appear nonimmunogenic. Recent studies in murine models with immunogenic tumors and large populations of reactive T cells that can be readily monitored have demonstrated that progressive tumors can selectively render the tumor-reactive T cells nonresponsive by mechanisms other than down-regulation of the zeta chain. Defining such mechanisms should facilitate strategies to detect and enhance antitumor responses.

The presence of tumor-specific suppressor T (T_S) cells may represent another reason for the difficulties in detecting tumor-specific immunity in cancer patients The major obstacle to understanding the role of T_S cells in tumor immunity has been the difficulty in isolating and characterizing such cells. Despite this difficulty, the biologic phenomenon of transferable antigen-specific T-cell-mediated suppression has been unequivocally demonstrated in vivo in animal models, and future studies will have to elucidate the bases for these observations.

One additional reason now emerging to explain the lack of an immune response to tumor cells derives from increased understanding of the functions of APCs. Tumor cells lack many of the essential qualities of professional APCs, such as expression of the costimulatory molecules CD80 and CD86 or production of the activating cytokine IL-12, and this may anergize rather than activate T cells. Molecular strategies in which tumor cells are modified to express these functions represent a promising means to elicit antitumor responses.

IMMUNOTHERAPY

Although the host immune system may often be inadequate for controlling tumor growth, the presence of identifiable tumor antigens in most tumor cells, the identification of a detectable but ineffective host response to many tumors, and an improved understanding of the mechanisms by which tumor cells evade immunity suggest that it may be possible to manipulate and amplify the immune system to promote tumor eradication. The recent technologic advances that permit isolation of lymphocyte subpopulations, identification and purification of tumor antigens, growth of selected antigen-specific T cells, amplification of immune responses with cytokines, and production of antibodies that can target surface tumor antigens have created a new potential and enthusiasm for the immunotherapy of tumors. Several distinct approaches to immunotherapy are being studied, and it seems likely that at least some of these approaches will soon become important modalities for the treatment of selected tumors.

Immunization to Tumor Antigens

Immunization of hosts bearing established progressing tumors with tumor cells or tumor antigen has generally been ineffective. in the past. Improved understanding of the requirements for T-cell activation and the special roles of dendritic cells (DC) in antigen presentation and the evolution of new vaccine technologies, however, has begun yielding more encouraging outcomes.

DC precursors can be readily isolated from the peripheral blood and expanded in vitro to large numbers with the appropriate cytokines. Such DC have been loaded with tumor antigens by a variety of means, including transfection, infection with recombinant viruses, incubation with the tumor protein or peptide, or phagocytosis of apoptotic tumor cells, and then inoculated into the patient to induce responses.

The optimal way to deliver DC remains to be clarified, but immune responses and clinical antitumor responses have already been observed.

An alternative approach has been to isolate tumor cells from a biopsy specimen, introduce cytokine genes and genes encoding costimulatory molecules expressed by professional APC, and then use these gene-modified tumor cells to immunize the host. Studies in mice with tumors expressing GM-CSF and costimulatory accessory molecules such as B7 have provided provocative results—protective T-cell responses to tumor cells previously perceived to be nonimmunogenic have been repeatedly detected. Approaches involving these methods are currently in human trials. Preliminary results of immunization with melanoma and renal cell tumors expressing GM-CSF, which presumably recruits and activates DC to present tumor antigens, have suggested that antitumor responses to established tumors can be achieved.

Another option being explored is to deliver tumor antigens in vivo in forms that will direct them to DC for presentation. These vary from the simplest approach in which the minimal peptide epitope encoding a tumor antigen is injected in an adjuvant or with GM-CSF, which has been shown to induce therapeutic T-cell responses in melanoma, to more complex approaches such as fusing the gene encoding the tumor antigen to the gene encoding GM-CSF and directly injecting the plasmid DNA or purified fusion protein.

Further development in vaccine technology, such as optimizing the immunostimulatory sequences in DNA vaccines, should increase the frequency with which antitumor responses are achieved. One promising new approach is the concurrent administration of a blocking antibody to CTLA-4 (cytotoxic T lymphocyte antigen 4) with a tumor vaccine—this prevents the normal dampening of T-cell responses that is mediated via signaling through CTLA-4. Complete rejection of established poorly immunogenic tumors has been reported following such vaccination in murine models, and clinical trials are currently being initiated with a prostate cancer vaccine in humans.

Adoptive T-Cell Therapy

Animal models have been developed in which hosts bearing advanced tumors can be treated by the transfer of tumor-specific syngeneic T cells. These models, in which syngeneic donor T cells immune to the tumor are used, have served as prototypes of what might be achievable if the host immune response to an autochthonous tumor could be selectively amplified. Complete tumor elimination following adoptive therapy requires an extended period, and the cells transferred must therefore be capable of persisting in the host to be effective. Noncytolytic lymphokine-producing class II-restricted CD4 T_H cells, as well as

directly lytic class I-restricted CD8 T_C cells, can mediate antitumor effects in these models, and optimal efficacy often requires both subsets. In settings in which only CD8 T_C are available, the administration of low-dose IL-2 has been shown to replace the helper function provided by CD4 T cells, to promote the in vivo survival and proliferation of the infused CD8 T cells, and to augment therapeutic efficacy.

There is now substantial experience with adoptive T-cell transfer in humans. The most completely analyzed studies have been for the treatment of virus-related diseases—in particular, cytomegalovirus (CMV) infection in immunocompromised bone marrow transplant recipients, human immunodeficiency virus (HIV) infection, and EBV-associated lymphoproliferative diseases. In these settings T cells specific for viral proteins have been isolated and expanded in vitro and then administered intravenously. The results have been encouraging and consistent with predictions from murine models. In particular, the T cells have been shown to effectively transfer immunity to the virus, to mediate antiviral effects, to traffic to lymph nodes, and to localize to sites of infection. The transfer of CD8 T_C in the absence of CD4 T_H has been shown to require the concurrent administration of low-dose IL-2 to persist and mediate prolonged antiviral activity.

This approach is also being explored in therapy of solid tumors. Although the initial efforts used lymphocytes isolated from tumor infiltrates that had been nonspecifically expanded in vitro with very high doses of IL-2, the use of tumor-reactive T cells propagated in vitro with sequential signals through the T-cell receptor (TCR) and the IL-2R is now becoming more routine. Studies in melanoma have demonstrated that these T cells localize to tumor sites and mediate antitumor effects, and suggests that this will become a valuable therapeutic modality. Additionally, the magnitude of in vivo T-cell responses that can be achieved by adoptive transfer far exceeds that induced by current vaccine technology. Thus, this approach can be used to enhance vaccine-induced responses, as well as to define the therapeutic limits that can be accomplished by vaccination to a particular tumor antigen.

T-cell therapy is also being evaluated in patients undergoing allogeneic bone marrow transplantation for malignant disease. In this setting, it has long been evident that patients who develop graft-versus-host disease as a consequence of donor T cells recognizing normal host tissues as foreign also benefit from a concurrent graft-versus-tumor effect. Strategies are being pursued to enhance the antitumor activity and diminish the toxicity to normal host tissues. One approach already in clinical trials involves the introduction of an inducible "suicide gene" in donor T cells, so that the cells can be ablated if toxicity becomes problematic. A more sophisticated approach, in which donor T cells are selected for recognition of proteins preferentially expressed by the tumor is currently being developed.

Administration of Monoclonal Antibodies

The development of the technology for generating monoclonal antibodies in the mid-1970s was expected to rapidly lead to the development of cancer therapeutics, but the initial results proved very disappointing. It became clear that many obstacles needed to be overcome, including the immunogenicity of murine proteins, modulation of target antigens, inadequate effector mechanisms to eliminate targeted cells, and biodistribution. These problems have been systematically addressed, and it appears that a new era for antibody therapy surrounded by much optimism is upon us. Two monoclonal antibodies, to CD20 and to Her2-neu, have already demonstrated efficacy and been approved as standard therapy for B-cell follicular lymphoma and metastatic breast cancer, respectively, and many other antibodies are under development.

The problem of host immune responses to administered antibodies of murine origin has been addressed by engineering chimeric antibodies with the murine antigen-binding CDR regions onto a human framework. More recently, strains of mice have been developed in which the mouse immunoglobulin locus has been replaced with the human gene, and such mice produce entirely human antibodies—such antibodies will shortly be entering clinical trials.

There are multiple mechanisms by which monoclonal antibodies (mAbs) can mediate antitumor activity, and enhancing these activities can increase the efficacy of mAb therapy. Initial efforts focused on improving ADCC activity because this appears to be a much more significant in vivo effector mechanism than complement-mediated lysis or opsonization. More recent studies have revealed advantages to targeting signaling molecules on tumors because cross-linking may lead directly to cell cycle arrest and apoptosis. This may indeed explain the observed clinical activity of antiidiotypic antibodies to the Ig receptor on B-cell lymphomas, anti-CD20 in B-cell lymphomas, and anti-Her2-neu receptor antibodies in breast cancer.

Several other approaches should also yield better therapeutic reagents. In vitro mutagenesis of the antibody-binding domain can yield mAbs with extraordinary affinity for the target antigen. Biodistribution can be improved by reducing the size of antibodies by removing much of the Fab and Fc portion and engineering multimers of the remaining antigen-binding Fv regions. Finally, cytotoxic molecules such as radionucleotides or toxins can be attached to these molecules to overcome problems of antigenic modulation and limiting host effector mechanisms by rapidly delivering a lytic signal.

Although each antibody will need to be carefully evaluated for toxicity and efficacy, mAb therapy is certain to become an increasingly important part of treatment regimens for cancer. In fact, preclinical studies suggest mAb therapy may be most effective when combined with standard treatments, and such regimens are currently being tested.

REFERENCES

Bluestone JA: Is CTLA-4 a master switch for peripheral T cell tolerance? *J Immunol* 1997;158:1989.

Boon T, Old LJ: Cancer tumor antigens. *Curr Opin Immunol* 1997;9:681.

Chambers CA, Allison JP: Costimulatory regulation of T cell function. *Curr Opin Cell Biol* 1999;11:203.

Cragg MS et al: Signaling antibodies in cancer therapy. *Curr Opin Immunol* 1999;11:541.

DeNardo SJ et al: A new era for radiolabeled antibodies in cancer? *Curr Opin Immunol* 1999;11:563.

Disis ML, Cheever MA: HER-2/neu oncogenic protein: Issues in vaccine development. *Crit Rev Immunol* 1998;18:37.

Gilboa E: The makings of a tumor rejection antigen. *Immunity* 1999;11:263.

Henderson RA, Finn OJ: Human tumor antigens are ready to fly. *Adv Immunol* 1996;62:217.

Hudson PJ: Recombinant antibody constructs in cancer therapy. *Curr Opin Immunol* 1999;11:548.

Kaplan DH et al: Demonstration of an interferon gamma-dependent tumor surveillance system in immunocompetent mice. *Proc Natl Acad Sci U S A* 1998;95:7556.

Kiessling R et al: Tumor-induced immune dysfunction [see comments]. *Cancer Immunol Immunother* 1999;48:353.

Kreitman RJ: Immunotoxins in cancer therapy. *Curr Opin Immunol* 1999;11:570.

Lanier LL: NK cell receptors. *Annu Rev Immunol* 1998;16:359.

Moretta A et al: Stimulatory receptors in NK and T cells. *Curr Top Microbiol Immunol* 1998;230:15.

Pardoll DM: Cancer vaccines. *Nat Med* 1998;4:525.

Pardoll DM, Topalian SL: The role of CD4+ T cell responses in antitumor immunity. *Curr Opin Immunol* 1998;10:588.

Riddell SR, Greenberg PD: Principles for adoptive T cell therapy of human viral diseases. *Annu Rev Immunol* 1995;13:545.

Rosenberg SA: A new era for cancer immunotherapy based on the genes that encode cancer antigens. *Immunity* 1999;10:281.

Sahin U et al: Serological identification of human tumor antigens. *Curr Opin Immunol* 1997;9:709.

Sherman LA et al: Strategies for tumor elimination by cytotoxic T lymphocytes. *Crit Rev Immunol* 1998;18:47.

Sotomayor EM et al: Tolerance and cancer: A critical issue in tumor immunology. *Crit Rev Oncog* 1996;7:433.

Timmerman JM, Levy R: Dendritic cell vaccines for cancer immunotherapy. *Annu Rev Med* 1999;50:507.

Toes REM et al: CD40-CD40 Ligand interactions and their role in cytotoxic T lymphocyte priming and anti-tumor immunity. *Semin Immunol* 1998;10:443.

Van den Eynde BJ, van der Bruggen P: T cell defined tumor antigens. *Curr Opin Immunol* 1997;9:684.

Velders MP et al: Active immunization against cancer cells: Impediments and advances. *Semin Oncol* 1998;25:697.

Whiteside TL: Signaling defects in T lymphocytes of patients with malignancy [see comments]. *Cancer Immunol Immunother* 1999;48:346.

Yee C et al: Prospects for adoptive T cell therapy. *Curr Opin Immunol* 1997;9:702.

43

Neoplasms of the Immune System

Susan K. Atwater, MD

GENERAL CONSIDERATIONS

Neoplasms of the immune system involve lymphocytes of B, T, and natural killer (NK) lineage; histiocytes; and antigen-presenting cells and are similar to other neoplasms in many respects, with some important differences. First, neoplastic lymphocytes may circulate in the peripheral blood and lymphatics, like their nonneoplastic counterparts; hence, many lymphoid neoplasms are disseminated at diagnosis. A traditional feature of benign tumors is that they remain localized and neither invade adjacent tissues nor metastasize. In other tissue types, tumors that disseminate throughout the body are characterized by an aggressive growth pattern and poor outcome. Neoplasms of the immune system, chiefly the chronic lymphoid leukemias and low-grade lymphomas, however, may not fit this pattern. These diseases frequently present with widespread systemic dissemination but remain slow-growing, indolent processes for many years.

A second feature of neoplasms of the immune system is that they may retain some functional characteristics of their normal counterparts (see Chapter 1). Neoplastic T cells may secrete cytokines; neoplastic plasma cells usually secrete immunoglobulins. Their functional behavior does not occur in response to a physiologic stimulus, however, as is true for normal cells. Hence, these cellular functions become autonomous and serve no useful purpose, often contributing to the ill health of the patient.

Hematologic neoplasms encompass not only the cell types already mentioned but disorders of myeloid cells and their precursors as well. Myeloid neoplasms are beyond the scope of this chapter, but the interested reader can find information about these disorders in some of the general references.

The purpose of this chapter is to focus on immunologic features of these neoplasms. Some general information is also provided, but for a more detailed clinical or pathologic description the reader should consult pathology or hematology/oncology texts.

CHARACTERISTICS OF MALIGNANT LYMPHOID CELLS

Clonality

Our current understanding of neoplasia is that it is a clonal process, in which a single cell undergoes malignant transformation via some genetic change and passes this change on to its progeny (see Chapter 42). The progeny are thus monoclonal, having a common cell of origin. Although neoplasia may involve a single transformative event in some instances, it is most commonly thought to be a multistep process, in which the first "hit" leads to a preneoplastic proliferation, and one or more additional genetic changes are required for definitive neoplasia. Even in an overt neoplasm, additional genetic changes may occur and lead to the development of drug resistance or a more aggressive type of tumor.

Although neoplasms are clonal processes as a general rule, exceptions occur in which polyclonal proliferations may behave aggressively in a manner similar to high-grade neoplasms, such as in lymphoproliferations following solid organ transplantation. Such exceptions are uncommon, however. Conversely, clonal populations of lymphoid cells may be noted when traditional clinical and histologic data show no evidence of a malignant process. Although many such proliferations may be preneoplastic, their clinical significance is often uncertain. Given these limitations, however, the establishment of clonality is an important component of the diagnostic evaluation of many lymphoid neoplasms.

Lineage Association

In general, hematologic neoplasms tend to show features of a particular cell lineage and can be recognized as T cell, B cell, or myeloid in nature. Also, to some degree, neoplasms tend to resemble discrete stages in normal cell development: For example, myeloma cells resemble normal plasma cells, leukemic lymphoblasts resemble normal T and B precursors, and so forth (Figure 43–1 and Tables 43–1 and 43–2).

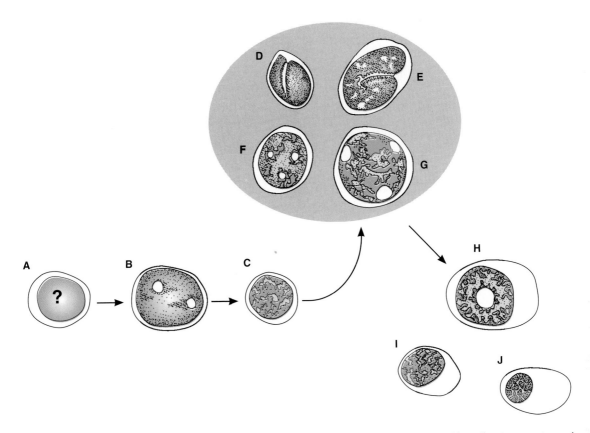

Figure 43–1. B-cell development. Lymphomas and leukemias of B lineage generally resemble cells, at some stage of normal B-cell development, both morphologically and immunophenotypically, to some extent. A simplified scheme of B-cell development is shown here. **A:** Pluripotent hematopoietic stem cells give rise to **B:** B precursors or B lymphoblasts in the bone marrow. Several immunophenotypic stages of B-precursor development are described in Table 43–1. **C:** Mature B cells may respond to an antigen stimulus by proliferating in germinal centers, giving rise to **D:** small cleaved, **E:** large cleaved, **F:** small noncleaved, and **G:** large noncleaved cell types. **H:** Immunoblasts, **I:** plasmacytoid lymphocytes, and **J:** plasma cells are found in terminal B-cell differentiation.

The greater the number of features one compares between normal and neoplastic cell populations, however, the more differences can be found. For example, neoplastic cells often express antigens from more than one cell lineage. In some cases, particularly with acute leukemias, multiple markers from each of two lineages may be present on the cells, producing a hybrid myeloid-lymphoid phenotype. Such mixed phenotypes are called **bilineal** if two or more populations are present within the neoplasm, each of a different

Table 43–1. Immunophenotypic stages of early B-cell differentiation.

Stage	Antigen(s)/Immunophenotype
0	CD34, HLA-DR
I	CD34, HLA-DR, TdT, CD19, CD10
II	HLA-DR (brighter), CD19, CD10 (dimmer)
III	HLA-DR, CD19, CD20, sIgM
IV	HLA-DR, CD19, CD20, CD21, CD22, ± sIgD

Abbreviations: HLA = human leukocyte antigen; TdT = terminal deoxynucleotidyl transferase; CD = clusters of differentiation.

Table 43–2. Immunophenotypic stages of early T-cell differentiation.

Multipotential thymic progenitors	CD7, CD13, CD33, CD34, CD45RA
Bipotential T/NK progenitors	CD7, cyCD3, CD13, cD33, CD34, CD38, CD45RA, ± CD2, ± CD5
Committed T-cell progenitors	CD1, CD2, cyCD3, CD5, CD7, CD13, CD28, CD34, CD38, CD45RA
Immature single-positive	CD1, CD2, cyCD3, CD4, CD5, CD7
Immature double-positive	CD1, CD2, cyCD3, CD4, CD5, CD7, CD8
Mature T cell	CD2, sCD3, CD5, CD7 *and either* (CD4+/CD8−) *or* (CD4−/CD8+)

Abbreviations: NK = natural killer; CD = clusters of differentiation.

lineage, and **biphenotypic** if a single population is present, showing coexpression of myeloid and lymphoid markers on the same cells. In other cases (eg, anaplastic large-cell lymphoma), cells may have lost the surface markers that indicate their lineage of origin, so that lineage determination then requires molecular diagnostic techniques.

When a cell population that has undergone malignant proliferation shows a combination of antigens that is not known to occur in normal cells, two possibilities are present: Either a normal cell counterpart exists but too few of these are present to have been detected during normal development, or no such normal cell counterpart exists. Often, the discovery of the normal cell counterpart is triggered by the recognition of the aberrant phenotype on neoplastic cells, as was the case for CD5 B cells and chronic lymphatic leukemia (CLL).

Aberrant Features

Just as neoplastic cells can express markers from more than one lineage, they may also express combinations of lineage-associated antigens that are not detectable, or present only on extremely rare cells, during normal cell development. For example, many leukemias of B lymphoblasts coexpress CD34, an antigen present on primitive hematopoietic progenitor cells and the very earliest normal B cells, along with CD22, a B-lineage-associated antigen present on the surface of only mature B cells. This combination is detectable only on a small percentage of normal B-cell precursors in bone marrow. Such differences can be useful in determining whether a proliferation of immature B cells in bone marrow is due to an increase in normal B precursors or acute leukemia.

Leukemia Versus Lymphoma

The term *leukemia* describes a hematologic neoplasm in which malignant cells are present in the bone marrow and the blood, whereas *lymphoma* describes a localized proliferation of lymphoid cells forming a solid tissue mass. Many hematologic neoplasms show both patterns of involvement, to varying degrees. Clinically, the neoplasm is usually described according to which growth pattern is predominant. For example, acute lymphoblastic leukemia, a disease that usually fills the bone marrow and gives rise to many circulating blasts, commonly also infiltrates lymph nodes. If a biopsy were performed on a sample from such a lymph node, a diagnosis of **lymphoblastic lymphoma** might be rendered if the pathologist had no knowledge of the blood or bone marrow findings. In this case, however, the best diagnosis for the patient is still acute lymphoblastic leukemia. In contrast, a lymphoma growing in a lymph node but only focally involving the marrow, with no peripheral blood involvement, is still called a lymphoma. In clinical practice, distinctions between

leukemia and lymphoma may thus be somewhat arbitrary. More important is the characterization of the type of neoplastic cell and the establishment of the correct diagnosis, so that appropriate therapy can be selected.

APPROACH TO DIAGNOSIS

A pathologic diagnosis is often regarded as *the* answer, despite the fact that wide variation exists in how neoplasms are diagnosed. Ancillary diagnostic modalities, such as immunophenotyping and cytogenetic and molecular analysis, may be essential to accurately characterizing some neoplasms, although morphologic examination may suffice for others. Equally important is the judicious weighing of all available data in a final assessment, especially when some data "fit the picture" better than others.

Morphologic Examination

Morphologic diagnosis has been the mainstay of diagnostic pathology for many decades. Although pathologists are often most familiar with hematoxylin–eosin-stained sections from paraffin-embedded tissue blocks, other preparations are often equally valuable, such as air-dried smears of blood or bone marrow cells stained with Wright's stain. In fact, hematopathologists consider these two techniques to be complementary, because each highlights different morphologic features of cells. For example, air-dried preparations are essential for the accurate diagnosis and classification of most leukemias. In contrast, examination of histologic sections is more important for the diagnosis and classification of non-Hodgkin's lymphomas, because sections provide information about the architecture of the tissues involved and the patterns of infiltration by abnormal cells. For example, the nodular growth pattern of a follicular center lymphoma would be seen histologically but cannot be appreciated if only a smear of cells is stained and examined.

Immunophenotypic Analysis

Cells can be characterized by detecting antigens in the cell membrane, cytoplasm, or nucleus using monoclonal antibodies directed against them. These antibodies are tagged with some compound to render them visible, usually either fluorochromes requiring analysis with either a flow cytometer or fluorescence microscope, or enzymes such as horseradish peroxidase or alkaline phosphatase that give rise to colored reaction products detectable in visible light under the microscope (see Chapters 15 and 16). Various methods of immunophenotypic analysis are available (Table 43–3), each with its advantages and drawbacks. In practice, it is best to have more than one method available and to select whichever method(s) give the most useful information for a given patient.

Table 43–3. Comparison of immunophenotyping methods.

Technique	Advantages	Disadvantages
Immunoperoxidase staining of frozen tissue sections	Tissue architecture visible Wide range of antibodies available	Cytomorphology not as good as with paraffin sections Technically difficult; not widely available
Immunoperoxidase staining of paraffin-embedded tissue sections	Tissue architecture visible Good cytomorphologic detail Widely available	Fewer antibodies available than with frozen sections or flow cytometry Surface immunoglobulin often fails to stain Two-color staining not widely available
Immunoperoxidase or immunoalkaline phosphatase staining of cytocentrifuge preparations	Excellent cytomorphology Cytoplasmic staining visible Good results with very few cells in sample	Tissue architecture not examined Two-color staining not widely available
Immunofluorescence by flow cytometry	Wide range of antibodies available Large numbers of cells examined Excellent immunoglobulin staining Ability to selectively analyze cell subpopulations Results available quickly Two- or three-color studies easy to perform	Tissue architecture not examined. Cytomorphologic detail visible only indirectly on cytocentrifuge preps from sample.

Monoclonal antibodies have been developed for a wide and ever-increasing variety of cell surface molecules; many of these are useful in clinical diagnosis. Six international workshops on human leukocyte differentiation antigens have been held, in which a standardized **cluster of differentiation,** or **CD,** nomenclature has been developed (see Appendix for CD table). Various antibodies recognizing the same antigen are grouped together within a cluster and referred to by the same CD number. Table 43–4 summarizes several commonly used antigens.

Immunophenotypic analysis using a variety of monoclonal antibodies can give information about how many cell populations are present within a sample, what the cell lineage and differentiation stage is of each population, and whether any of these populations show abnormal features (Tables 43–5 and 43–6). Answering these questions usually requires multiparametric analysis of some sort, in which several different parameters are measured for any given cell. Analysis using two simultaneous fluorochrome-tagged antibodies, each with a different color, is now commonplace in flow cytometry (see Chapter 16), and three- and four-color analysis are becoming more widely available. These allow precise dissection of cell types within a sample, maximizing the information obtained from the cell sample.

Clonality can be assessed in B-cell proliferations if the B cells express surface or cytoplasmic immunoglobulin. A reactive B-cell population contains a mixture of kappa-positive and lambda-positive B cells, and the ratio of kappa+ to lambda+ cells can be calculated. Nonneoplastic B-cell populations typically show κ:λ ratios from 1:1 to 2.5:1, whereas a monoclonal population contains light chains of only one type (Figure 43–2). Mixtures of monoclonal and polyclonal B cells can occur and increase or decrease the light-chain ratio in proportion to the number of monoclonal cells present. Light scatter properties of cells allow flow cytometric data to be examined selectively, looking at light-chain ratios of larger or smaller cells. Figure 43–3 shows a flow cytometric analysis of lymph node cells in which the smaller cells show a mixture of both light-chain types, but the larger cells are virtually all kappa-positive, indicating the presence of a monoclonal population within a mixed background of polyclonal lymphocytes.

Cytogenetic Analysis

Malignant cells are grown in short-term culture, and the chromosomes of cells in metaphase are spread out on a glass slide and stained so that the chromosomes show alternating regions of lightly and darkly staining DNA. Chromosomes can then be identified, and any rearrangements of chromosomes can be detected.

Using these methods, karyotypic abnormalities can be detected in almost all malignant neoplasms. These are somatic genetic changes, which are not present in nonneoplastic cells of that individual. In the case of hematolymphoid neoplasms, all of the cells within a tumor show the same or related chromosome abnormalities. This evidence strongly supports the notion that most neoplasms arise from a single altered cell, in which the somatic genetic changes somehow lead to a selective growth or survival advantage for the progeny of the original "mutant" cell. However, although neoplasms represent clonal growth from a single cell or origin, they are frequently not homogeneous because subpopulations evolve from the original clone due to the genetic instability of the neoplastic cells. **Primary** genetic changes are thought to occur early in the neoplastic process and may indeed

Table 43–4. Antigens useful in immunophenotypic analysis of lymphomas and lymphocytic leukemias.

Designation	Description
	B-Cell-Associated Antigens
sIg	Surface immunoglobulin, present on mature B cells and their neoplastic counterparts as well as on L3 ALL. Absent on plasma cells
cIg	Cytoplasmic immunoglobulin, present in plasma cells, some plasmacytoid lymphocytes and some immunoblasts
CD10	Also known as CALLA, the common *ALL* antigen, this antigen is present on many normal B-cell precursors and most cases of B-precursor ALL, but is also present on germinal center B cells and many cases of follicular center lymphomas, as well as on some T-ALL and T-LBL. However, it is not significantly present on mature circulating B cells
CD19	Expressed on B cells and their precursors from very early in development, but absent on plasma cells
CD20	Similar to CD19, though expression begins later in early B-cell development
CD22	Present in the cytoplasm in very early B-cell precursors, but not expressed on the surface until late in B-cell precursor development. Also present on mature B cells and their neoplastic counterparts, but absent on plasma cells
CD23	IgE Fc receptor; increased on EBV-infected B cells. Useful in distinguishing CLL (usually CD23+) from mantle cell lymphoma (usually CD23–)
CD79a	*mb*-1 protein, expressed in association with surface IgM. Highly specific marker for B lineage
	T- and NK Cell-Associated Antigens
CD1	Present on some normal thymocytes as well as Langerhans' cells; also on many T-lymphoblastic leukemias–lymphomas and Langerhans' cell histiocytosis
CD2	Sheep RBC "receptor"; present on thymocytes, mature T cells and mature NK cells. Present on most T- and NK-lineage neoplasms and occasional myeloid leukemias
CD3	Present in the cytoplasm of early thymocytes; expressed on the surface on mature T cells. Present in most T-lineage neoplasms. Cytoplasmic CD3 is detectable in nearly all T-lymphoblastic neoplasms
CD4	Helper–inducer T-cell subset, monocytes–macrophages and some dendritic cells; present on many T-lineage neoplasms
CD5	Immature and mature T cells and neoplasms
CD7	Immature and mature T and NK cells and neoplasms; also on 15–20% of acute myelogenous leukemia
CD8	Cytotoxic–suppressor T-cell subset; also many NK cells
CD16	IgG Fc receptor III; present on NK cells and granulocytes
CD56	NK cells, small T-cell subset, most T/NK angiocentric lymphomas; also some nonhematopoietic tumors
CD57	Some NK cells; also some nonhematopoietic tumors, especially of neuroendocrine origin
	Myeloid Lineage-Associated Antigens
CD11c	Monocytes–macrophages and NK cells. Although absent on mature resting B cells, CD11c is strongly expressed on hairy cell leukemia cells, and less strongly on some other low-grade B-cell neoplasms
CD13	Granulocytes, monocytes–macrophages, and their precursors; also on most acute myeloid leukemias
CD14	Monocytes–macrophages and their precursors; also on many myelomonocytic or monoblastic leukemias
CD15	Granulocytes, monocytes—macrophages, Reed-Sternberg cells of Hodgkin's disease
CD33	Granulocytes, monocytes–macrophages, and their precursors; also on most acute myeloid leukemias
	Miscellaneous
TdT	Terminal deoxyribonucleotidyl transferase is a nuclear enzyme that is active during rearrangement of immunoglobulin and T-cell receptor genes. It is found in nearly all lymphoblastic leukemias and lymphomas, but is not seen in mature B- or T-lineage neoplasms. It is also present in approximately 25% of acute nonlymphocytic leukemias
HLA-DR (Ia)	Class II HLA antigen; found on B lymphocytes and their precursors, monocyte–macrophage lineage cells, and activated mature T cells, as well as their neoplastic counterparts
Fc receptors	Receptors for Fc portion of immunoglobulin molecule. Plasma immunoglobulin binding nonspecifically to Fc receptors may interfere with measurement of light-chain expression patterns on B cells
CD25	IL-2 receptor; present on activated T cells. Generally expressed on adult T-cell leukemia–lymphoma cells but often absent or weak on Sézary cells
CD30	Ki-1 antigen, present on some activated B or T cells, and on the majority of anaplastic large-cell lymphomas and Hodgkin's disease
CD34	Present on multipotent hematopoietic stem cells and committed progenitors, but absent on more mature precursors. Expressed on many cases of ALL, lymphoblastic lymphomas, or AML, but absent in non-Hodgkin's lymphomas of mature B or T cells
Ki-67	Nuclear antigen expressed during the cell cycle but absent in G_0 cells. Fraction of Ki-67+ cells correlates with histologic grade in non-Hodgkin's lymphoma

Abbreviations: ALL = acute lymphoblastic leukemia; CD = clusters of differentiation; TdT = terminal deoxynucleotidyl transferase; HLA = human leukocyte antigen; EBV = Epstein–Barr virus; CLL = chronic lymphocytic leukemia; NK = natural killer.

be the event that causes the original neoplastic transformation. **Secondary** changes may or may not occur later in the disease and in some instances may be associated with disease progression.

Translocations are a common finding in hematologic malignancies and historically have provided clues to the location of oncogenes or tumor suppressor genes within the genome. Translocations involve

Table 43–5. Immunophenotypic characteristics of normal cell populations.

Cell Type and Source	Characteristics
Mature B cells (blood or lymph node)	Express CD19, CD20, CD22, HLA-DR, sIg Polytypic pattern of light-chain expression TdT-negative CD5 present on minority of cells CD10 absent in blood, present in germinal center B cells from lymph node CD11c is present only on small minority
Mature T cells	Express CD3, CD2, CD5 80–90% also express CD7 Mixture of CD4+ and CD8+ cells (CD4:CD8 ratio varies with clinical status of patient) TdT-negative
Bone marrow B cells	Many coexpress CD19 and CD10; some also express TdT Fewer are CD20+ or surface CD22+ These cells may be increased in number in some reactive settings
NK cells	Express CD2, CD7 Lack CD3 Express CD16, CD56, or CD57 Express CD11c
Thymocytes	Spectrum of differentiation stages; many coexpress CD4 and CD8, and express CD1 CD3+ and CD3– cells present; however, nearly all express CD2, CD5, and CD7

Abbreviations: CD = clusters of differentiation; HLA = human leukocyte antigen; TdT = terminal deoxynucleotidyl transferase; NK = natural killer.

breaks in two separate chromosomes (eg, chromosomes 14 and 18) and the rejoining of part of one chromosome to part of the other. These translocations are often reciprocal, with rejoining of the other halves as well. These events bring two different genes in close proximity to each other, often resulting in activation of one normally dormant gene by its close proximity to one that is actively being transcribed. The translocations may create fusion genes, coding for hybrid proteins whose amino and carboxy-termini originate from the two different genes. It is believed that most of these translocations are primary, in the sense that the fusion genes produced as a result of the translocation are integral to the pathogenesis of that particular leukemia or lymphoma. Table 43–7 shows several common cytogenetic abnormalities in lymphoid neoplasms along with their molecular correlates.

Burkitt's lymphoma and its leukemic counterpart, L3 acute lymphoblastic leukemia (ALL), provide examples of such recurring translocation. In nearly all cases of Burkitt's lymphoma or L3 ALL, translocations involving the long arm of chromosome 8 are seen, with the breakpoint occurring at 8q24. In most cases, the other chromosome involved is 14, with the breakpoint occurring at the locus of the immunoglobulin heavy-chain gene, 14q32. Breakpoints involving the kappa and lambda gene loci on chromosomes 2 and 22 are sometimes seen, however. This finding led to the identification of the c-*myc* protooncogene at 8q24. It is thought that when the c-*myc* oncogene is translocated adjacent to an immunoglobulin gene, the active enhancer of the latter gene deregulates the expression of c-*myc*, resulting in its constitutive activa-

Table 43–6. Commonly encountered immunophenotypic patterns and their significance.

Pattern	Significance
Light-chain restriction	A population of sIg+ or cIg+ B cells expressing only one light-chain type. This finding indicates the presence of a monoclonal population. However, this finding in and of itself is not tantamount to a diagnosis of malignancy (see text)
Polytypic light-chain expression	Both kappa+ and lambda+ B cells are present. Depending on other findings, results might either be most likely reactive, or suspicious for the presence of a small monoclonal population
T-cell antigen loss	When a majority population of T cells fails to express one or more pan T antigens, this finding is strong evidence for an abnormal and probably neoplastic process. Smaller populations with this finding are harder to interpret
CD5+ B cells	Normally present in blood in small numbers. However, if a majority of B cells are strongly CD5+, this suggests either CLL, small lymphocytic lymphoma, mantle cell lymphoma or (less likely) another process
CD11c+ B cells	Strong expression of CD11c on a majority population of B cells suggests the diagnosis of hairy cell leukemia, especially if CD22 is also strongly expressed. Weak CD11c expression on B cells is less specific
bcl-2+ germinal center B cells	*bcl*-2 protein (detectable in paraffin sections) is strongly expressed in the neoplastic follicular structures of follicular lymphomas, but is generally absent in reactive germinal centers
Mixture of normal-appearing T and B cells in a lymph node	Although this picture shows no evidence of an abnormal population, and indeed is a common result when reactive lymph node aspirates are analyzed, it may also be seen when neoplastic cells are a small minority of the total (as in Hodgkin's disease), or when a neoplasm is associated with fibrosis and not well represented in the sample sent for analysis

Abbreviations: CD = clusters of differentiation; CLL = chronic lymphocytic leukemia.

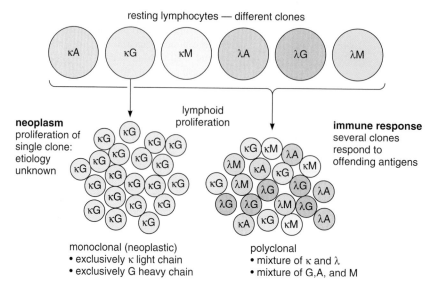

Figure 43–2. Monoclonal versus polyclonal proliferation of B lymphocytes. The monoclonal population contains one type of light and heavy chain in the example given κ and G chains), whereas the polyclonal population consists of lymphocytes containing both κ and λ light chains and several different heavy chains. (Reproduced, with permission, from Chandrasoma P, Taylor CR: *Concise Pathology.* Appleton & Lange, 1991.)

tion. Overexpression of c-*myc*, which encodes a protein active in mitogenesis, is thought to be the primary event in neoplastic transformation of Burkitt's lymphoma.

Cytogenetic information can help confirm the diagnosis of leukemia or lymphoma if a clonal karyotypic abnormality is found, although the absence of abnormalities does not exclude a diagnosis of neoplasia. A normal karyotype may be seen either when the neoplastic cells themselves have no visible karyotypic changes or when normal cells have preferentially grown out in short-term culture and the neoplastic cells have not been sampled for study.

Certain nonrandom chromosomal abnormalities are characteristic for a given diagnosis (eg, the t(8;14) translocation of Burkitt's lymphoma or the t(14;18) translocation seen in follicular center lymphomas). In addition, many abnormalities provide prognostic information, as seen in B-precursor ALL, in which both the t(9;22) and t(4;11) translocations have been shown to connote a particularly poor prognosis. In fact, in many cases, an ALL patient whose leukemic cells carry either of these translocations is often treated with bone marrow transplantation in first remission, in contrast to patients with good-prognosis ALL, who are generally not transplanted at that point.

Figure 43–3. Immunophenotypic analysis of a B-cell lymphoma. A 48-year-old man complained of an enlarged, nontender cervical lymph node that has been increasing in size over the past month and was 6 cm in diameter at the time of examination. A fine-needle aspiration biopsy of this mass showed scattered lymphocytes, mostly small and round with a few larger lymphocytes, within a bloody background. Because morphologic review was nondiagnostic, a sample was submitted for an immunophenotypic study. Cells were incubated with various fluorochrome-tagged monoclonal antibodies directed against B- or T-lymphoid cell membrane proteins and then analyzed on a flow cytometer. As each cell passed through the laser beam, scattered light was measured, as was light emitted by fluorochromes. Forward light scatter (FSC) is proportional to cell size, and side scatter (SSC) is proportional to the internal complexity of cells. Light scatter properties thus allow the user to correlate flow phenotypic findings with morphologic data. **A:** shows a plot of forward versus side scatter. Neutrophils, which appear in the upper half of the diagram, have high side scatter due to their granule content. A single broad population is present in the lower half of the diagram, where lymphocytes normally appear. Two analysis regions, or "gates," have been somewhat arbitrarily drawn, dividing this population into smaller, less complex cells (R1) and larger, more complex cells (R2). **B & C:** Smaller lymphoid cells within analysis region R1 are predominantly T cells expressing CD5; a lesser number express the B-cell-associated antigen CD19. These contain both kappa- and lambda-positive cells, with a κ:λ ratio of 2:1. **D & E:** The region containing larger cells contains mostly B cells, and virtually all of these express surface kappa light chains. The findings indicate the presence of a monoclonal population of large B lymphocytes within a background of smaller B and T lymphocytes. It is likely that nonneoplastic lymphocytes from the peripheral blood were admixed with lymphocytes from the neck mass.

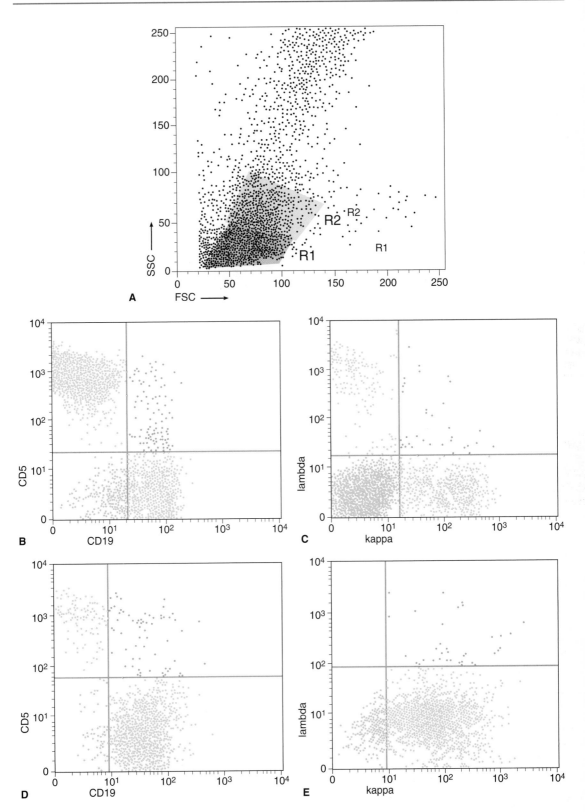

Although monoclonal B-cell populations may rarely be present in patients without overt malignancy, the clinical signs in this patient strongly favor a diagnosis of lymphoma. Further evaluation would be necessary to accurately characterize this process.

Table 43–7. Common cytogenetic abnormalities in lymphoid malignancies and their molecular correlates.

Cytogenetic Finding	Molecular Lesion	Diseases
t(14;18)(q32;q21)	Juxtaposition of *bcl*-2 adjacent to IgH gene with consequent *bcl*-2 overexpression	Follicular lymphomas, some diffuse B-cell lymphomas
t(8;14)(q24;q32) t(2;8)(p12;q24) t(8;22)(q24;q11)	Juxtaposition of c-*myc* with Ig heavy- or light-chain genes with consequent c-*myc* overexpression	Burkitt's lymphoma, L3 ALL
t(11;14)(q13;q32)	Fusion of *bcl*-2 (cyclin D1 gene) with Ig H gene	Mantle cell lymphoma
t(9;22)(q34;q11)	*bcr/abl* fusion	CML, some ALL
t(1;19)(q23;p13)	E2A/*PBX*1 fusion	Pre-B ALL (sIg–, cIg+)
12p13 abnl	Abnormalities involving *TEL*	Many B-precursor ALL
11q23 abnl	Fusion of *MLL/HRX* gene with various partners	Infant ALL, AML
14q11 abnl	α/δ T-cell antigen receptor gene	T-cell neoplasms
Trisomy 12	??	CLL
Hyperdiploidy	??	B-precusor ALL
3q27 abnl	*bcl*-6	Large-cell lymphomas
7q35 abnl	β T-cell antigen receptor gene	T-cell neoplasms
t(2;5)(p23;q35)	*NPM/ALK* fusion	Anaplastic large-cell lymphoma

Abbreviations: ALL = acute lymphoblastic leukemia; CML = chronic myelogenous leukemia; AML = acute myelogenous leukemia; CLL = chronic lymphocytic leukemia.

Molecular Genetic Analysis

Molecular analysis of DNA or RNA offers additional tools for detecting clonal populations and translocations (see Chapter 18). Its ability to detect clonal T-cell populations is especially critical because immunophenotypic methods for detecting T-cell clonality are not easily available. Detection techniques for B and T cells exploit the fact that during cell development, the immunoglobulin heavy chain undergoes somatic rearrangement within each B cell, giving rise to a slightly different rearranged gene for each cell. A similar process occurs in T cells in which T-cell receptor genes are rearranged.

In the Southern blot assay (see Chapter 18) to detect immunoglobulin gene rearrangements, DNA is first extracted and digested by restriction enzymes and then run on a gel to separate DNA fragments by size. These are incubated with a DNA probe that binds to the joining region of the immunoglobulin genes, whether these are germline or rearranged. In a population of reactive B cells, the B cells are polyclonal, and each has its own rearranged gene with a unique size. Hence, a smear of different fragment lengths binds the probe and is detected on the autoradiograph. In contrast, a monoclonal proliferation of B cells has identical rearranged immunoglobulin genes, and a single band is seen on the autoradiograph. A similar assay can detect monoclonal patterns of beta T-cell receptor gene rearrangement.

Translocations can be detected by Southern blot analysis as well, if a probe directed against the fusion gene is available. Translocations are also detectable by polymerase chain reaction (PCR) (see Chapter 18) if primers on either side of the breakpoint are available

and if the regions the primers recognize are not too widely separated. PCR detection of translocations is extremely sensitive, and its ability to detect minimal residual leukemia or lymphoma after therapy is the subject of many recent and ongoing research trials. PCR methods of detecting clonal populations via amplification of rearranged genes are also available now.

Integrating the Data

Patients whose clinical presentations are classic textbook examples of a disease are the exception rather than the rule. More commonly, most of the available data seem to fit one possible diagnosis, but some data do not fit the picture. Deciding how much weight to give each piece of information requires considerable experience.

THERAPY

Therapy and prognosis are interrelated. When response to a therapy varies, determining why becomes important so that those who respond poorly can be given alternative treatments. Prognostic indicators are developed that identify good and poor responders. In contrast, if a new treatment is found that cures everybody, the old prognostic indicators no longer predict outcome and lose their value. New therapies for neoplasms of the immune system are constantly being developed and compared, and although no neoplasm is 100% curable at present, significant advances have been made in the past few decades.

The therapy for treating neoplasms of the immune system is a combination of managing symptoms and signs (supportive therapy) and attempting to eradicate neoplastic cells through chemotherapy, radiation therapy, or surgical excision. Most patients are treated on prescribed protocols, which vary somewhat from center to center and have differing degrees of success depending on the type of neoplasm, the involved organ(s), and the extent of tumor spread.

Cytotoxic or other antitumor drugs in general affect DNA synthesis and are used in combination and in various delivery sequences to affect the maximum number of cells in S phase. The fact that proliferating cells are more vulnerable to cytotoxic therapy may explain why cure rates may be better with aggressive neoplasms than with low-grade ones. The latter may have an indolent, prolonged course in which remission may be readily induced but is often short-lived.

The selection of appropriate therapy is based on two major factors: cytologic-histologic type and extent of disease. The latter is determined by staging in Hodgkin's disease and the non-Hodgkin's lymphomas. The Ann Arbor Staging Classification for Hodgkin's disease defines four major stages (I–IV) extending from involvement of a single lymph node region (stage I) to disseminated involvement of distant extranodal organs (stage IV). Systemic symptoms such as fever, night sweats, and weight loss provide subcategories for the stages. Staging for non-Hodgkin's lymphomas is similar and uses history; physical examination; surgical and needle biopsies; and radiography, including tomography, radioisotope scans, computed tomography (CT) scans, and lymphangiograms. Because leukemias, by definition, involve bone marrow and peripheral blood, staging is not a factor, but cell type is.

Radiation Therapy

Radiation therapy is more central to the therapy of Hodgkin's disease than to the non-Hodgkin lymphomas. It plays an important role in localized disease, may be the only treatment used for low-grade lymphomas, and may be used in conjunction with chemotherapy in intermediate- and high-grade lymphomas.

Chemotherapy

The alkylating agent chlorambucil has been used alone since 1955 to treat indolent lymphomas and chronic lymphocytic leukemia (CLL). It is toxic, however, and may produce irreversible marrow suppression; it is also leukemogenic. Other drugs, such as cyclophosphamide, are also effective but are toxic. To increase effectiveness and reduce toxicity, combination chemotherapy was developed at the National Cancer Institute. The rationale for multiagent therapy is that drug-resistant cells arise spontaneously, and acquired resistance to a drug results from genetic mutation. Thus, exposure to several drugs may prevent the survival and proliferation of resistant cells. In addition, tumor cell death is related to dose intensity of drugs, so that a maximum dose of a maximum number of drugs over the shortest period should be most effective. This does not, however, avoid toxicity, and careful monitoring is required.

Bone Marrow Transplantation

Because of the ineffectiveness of radiation and chemotherapy in many patients with intermediate- and high-grade lymphomas or acute leukemias, a new therapeutic approach was needed. Both allogeneic and autologous bone marrow transplantation (see Chapter 52) have extended survival in some patients, particularly children.

Eradication of lymphomas or leukemic cells with high-dose chemotherapy and total-body irradiation (purging) is followed by the introduction of marrow-replenishing "stem cells." Techniques for purification of these multipotential cells from autologous marrow or peripheral blood have steadily improved, so that repopulation of the hematopoietic system is increasingly effective.

Other Agents

Purine nucleoside analogues are potent inhibitors of adenosine deaminase and have been found to be effective in several lymphoid malignancies. 2-Deoxycoformycin (pentostatin) and 2-chloro-2'-deoxyadenoside (2-CDA) are particularly effective in treating hairy cell leukemia, with clinical remissions seen in the majority of patients following treatment with either of these two agents. Fludarabine is especially effective in treating chronic lymphocytic leukemia, commonly inducing partial responses as well as some complete remissions even in patients whose disease is refractory to chlorambucil.

Therapy with monoclonal antibodies alone or coupled with radioisotopes or cellular toxins directed at lymphoma or leukemia antigens theoretically has great appeal and has been the subject of many clinical trials. These trials have had variable results, however, and currently this therapy is still investigational.

NEOPLASMS OF B & T LYMPHOCYTES

CLASSIFICATION OF LYMPHOMAS

"The urge to classify," wrote A. T. Hopwood in 1957, "is a fundamental human instinct; like a predisposition to sin, it accompanies us into the world and stays with us to the end." And although hematopathologists and their clinical colleagues alike share an interest in classifying lymphoid neoplasms, the two groups approach the task from slightly different perspectives. Pathologists, who see visual patterns in the different tumor types, are interested in a classification system that identifies these differing patterns as separate entities, which hopefully will lead to an increased understanding of what these patterns signify. Clinical hematologists and oncologists must decide how to treat the patient and want a simple, easy to use classification that reliably separates patients into prognostic categories.

Many classification systems for the non-Hodgkin's lymphomas have arisen over the past few decades, chief among them the Rappaport, Lukes-Collins, and Kiel classification systems. The International Working Formulation for Clinical Use was developed in 1982 as a way of communicating diagnoses across different systems (Table 43–8). It was not originally intended as a classification system itself but in practice has come to be used as such. It has proven useful in categorizing patients for multicenter clinical trials. More recently, in 1994, the International Lymphoma Study Group has developed the Revised European-American Lymphoma (REAL) classification, in which several provisional diagnostic entities are described (Table 43–9). This system is descriptive rather than proscriptive because it describes what hematopathologists are currently doing in their diagnostic practice. Although this system is sometimes viewed as more unwieldy than the Working Formulation, it describes several lymphoma types with distinct clinical and morphologic features, for which the question is whether they also will respond to treatment in a distinctive way. Both the Working Formulation and the REAL classification are referred to in this chapter. These two systems complement each other at the present time. Authors of the REAL classification have indicated the most important immunophenotypic, cytogenetic, and molecular features of each entity to be taken into consideration at diagnosis; these are summarized in Table 43–10. The World Health Organization Classification of Hematolymphoid Tumors is currently being revised to incorporate entities within the REAL Classification.

Table 43–8. International working formulation of Non-Hodgkin's lymphomas.

1. ML, small lymphocytic (SL)
   1a. Plasmacytoid (SL-P)
   1b. Consistent with CLL (SL/CLL)
2. ML, follicular, predominantly small cleaved cell (FSC)
3. ML, follicular, mixed small cleaved and large cell (FM)
4. ML, follicular, predominantly large cell (FL)
5. ML, diffuse, small cleaved cell (DSC)
6. ML, diffuse, mixed small cleaved and large cell (DM)
7. ML, diffuse, large cell (DL)
8. ML, large cell, immunoblastic (IBL)
9. ML, lymphoblastic (LBL)
10. ML, small noncleaved cell (SNC)
    10a. Burkitt's (SNC-B)
    10b. Non-Burkitt's (SNC-NB)

Abbreviations: CLL = chronic lymphatic leukemia.

Table 43–9. Revised European–American lymphoma (REAL) classification with corresponding working formulation subtypes.

Subtype	Working Formulation Equivalents
B-Cell Neoplasms	
Precursor B-lymphoblastic lymphoma–leukemia	LBL
B-cell CLL/PLL/SLL	SL, SL/CLL
Lymphoplasmacytoid lymphoma	SL-P
Mantle cell lymphoma	SL, DSC, FSC, DM, DL
Follicle center lymphomas, follicular	
Grade I	FSC
Grade II	FM
Grade III	FL
Follicle center lymphoma, diffuse	DSC, DM, DL
Marginal zone B-cell lymphomas	SL, DSC, DM
Hairy cell leukemia	—
Plasmacytoma–myeloma	—
Diffuse large B-cell lymphoma	DLC, IBL, DM
Burkitt's and Burkitt-like lymphomas	SNC-B, DLC, IBL
T-Cell Neoplasms	
Precursor T-lymphoblastic leukemia–lymphoma	LBL
T-cell CLL/T-cell PLL	SL, DSC, —
LGL leukemias (T and NK types)	SL, DSC, —
Mycosis fungoides/Sézary syndrome	—
Peripheral T-cell lymphomas, unspecified	DSC, DM, DL, IBL
Angioimmunoblastic T-cell lymphoma	DM, DL, IBL
Angiocentric lymphoma	DSC, DM, DL, IBL
Intestinal T-cell lymphoma	DSC, DM, DL, IBL
Adult T-cell leukemia–lymphoma	DSC, DM, DL, IBL
Anaplastic large-cell lymphoma	IBL

Abbreviations: LBL = lymphoblastic leukemia; SL = small lymphocyte; CLL = chronic lymphatic leukemia; SL-P = plasmatoid, small lymphocytic; DSC = diffuse, small cleaved; FSC = follicular, small cleaved cell; DM = diffuse, mixed cleaved cell; DL = diffuse, large cleaved cell; FM = follicular, mixed cleaved cell; FL = follicular, large cleaved cell; IBL = immunoblastic leukemia.

ACUTE LYMPHOBLASTIC LEUKEMIA & LYMPHOBLASTIC LYMPHOMA

Clinical Features

Acute lymphoblastic leukemia (ALL) and lymphoblastic lymphoma (LBL) affect both children and adults. In childhood, ALL accounts for the majority of acute leukemia cases. As discussed earlier, ALL

Table 43–10. Immunophenotypic and molecular features important in diagnosis of non-Hodgkin's lymphomas.

Subtype	Features Important in Definition of Entity[a]
B-Cell Neoplasms	
Precursor B-lymphoblastic lymphoma–leukemia	CD19+, TdT+, CD79a+, CD10±
B-cell CLL/PLL/SLL	B-cell assoc. antigen+, CD5+, CD23+, weak surface IgM
Lymphoplasmacytoid lymphoma	Cytoplastmic Ig+ (some cells), CD5–, CD10–
Mantle cell lymphoma	B-cell associated antigen+, CD5+, CD23–, presence of t(11;14) and/or cyclin D1 overexpression
Follicle center lymphomas	CD5–, CD43–, CD10±, usually surface Ig+, presence of t(14;18)
Marginal zone B-cell lymphomas	Cytoplasmic ig+ (in 40%), CD5–, CD10–
Hairy cell leukemia	CD5–, CD10–, CD23–, CD11c+ (strong), CD25+ (strong), CD103+
Plasmacytoma–myeloma	sIg–, cIg+, negative for most B-cell-associated antigens
Diffuse large B-cell lymphoma	B-cell associated antigen+, CD45±
Burkitt's and Burkitt-like lymphomas	sIgM+, B-cell-associated Ag+, CD10+, CD5–
T-Cell Neoplasms	
Precursor T-lymphoblastic leukemia–lymphoma	CD7+, cCD3+, TdT+, Ig–, B-cell-associated Ag–
T-cell CLL/T-cell PLL	T-cell-associated Ag+
LGL leukemias (T and NK types)	Both types: CD2+, CD16+, CD57±
	T-cell type: CD3+, CD56–
	NK type: CD3–, CD56±
Mycosis fungoides/Sézary syndrome	CD2/CD3/CD5+, CD4+, CD7– in most cases
Peripheral T-cell lymphomas (PTL), unspecified	Variable T-cell-associated antigen expression with frequent antigen loss
Angioimmunoblastic T-cell lymphoma	Same as for PTL
Angiocentric lymphoma	Same as for PTL
Intestinal T-cell lymphoma	CD3+, CD7+, CD103+
Adult T-cell leukemia–lymphoma	Usually CD4+, CD7–, CD25+ caused by HTLV-1
Anaplastic large-cell lymphoma	CD30+, EMA+ t(2;5) translocation

[a] Characteristic cell morphology is an essential component of defining these entities and is described in the text. Key to immunophenotypic designations: +: over 90% of cases positive; ±: over 50% of cases positive; ∓: less than 50% of cases positive; –: less than 10% of cases positive.

Abbreviations: CLL = chronic lymphatic leukemia; LGL = low-grade lymphoma; CD = clusters of differentiation; TdT = terminal deoxynucleotidyl transferase; NK = natural killer; HTLV = human T-lymphotropic virus; EMA = epithelial membrane antigen.

and LBL describe differing clinical presentations, both of which involve a proliferation of neoplastic lymphoblasts. Patients frequently present with cytopenias and circulating lymphoblasts in the blood. Lymph nodes are frequently enlarged, and in the case of T-ALL/LBL, an anterior mediastinal mass is commonly present. Within this group are several different types of ALL/LBL, each with distinctive immunophenotypic and cytogenetic features, which also differ in their clinical presentation. For example, the majority of infants with B-precursor ALL have a rearrangement of the maligannt lymphoblastic lymphoma (MLL) transcription factor at 11q23; these infants have a poor prognosis on conventional therapy and are often scheduled for bone marrow transplantation in first remission. In contrast, children with B-precursor ALL between 1 and 10 years of age usually have a favorable prognosis, especially in cases where

the blasts are hyperdiploid (with 51 or more chromosomes) and CD34+. These children are not generally offered bone marrow transplantation in first remission at this time because they often enjoy long-term clinical remissions, and the morbidity of the transplant procedure could lead to a worse outcome.

Morphologic Features

Lymphoblasts are of intermediate or large size, often with very high nuclear-cytoplasmic (N:C) ratios (eg, Figure 43–4A). Their chromatin is more finely distributed than the chromatin of mature lymphoid cells but may not be as smooth as that seen in myeloblasts. Nucleoli may or may not be present, and nuclear contours may be irregular in some cases. In a small minority of cases, ALL blasts may have abundant, deeply basophilic cytoplasm with frequent cytoplasmic vacuoles and multiple distinct nucleoli.

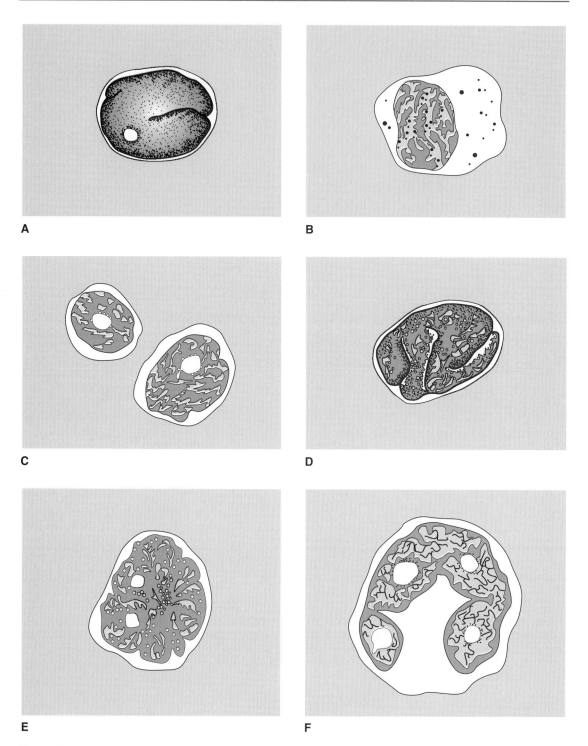

Figure 43–4. Morphology of selected T-cell neoplasms. **A:** T-lymphoblastic leukemia or lymphoma; **B:** large granular lymphocyte leukemia; **C:** T-prolymphocytic leukemia; **D:** Sézary's syndrome and mycosis fungoides; **E:** adult T-cell leukemia-lymphoma; and **F:** anaplastic large-cell lymphoma.

This morphologic pattern is associated with surface membrane immunoglobulin expression and c-*myc* rearrangements and is known either as ALL of FAB L3 type, or as Burkitt's lymphoma, depending on the clinical presentation. In both cases, the cells have an extremely high proliferative rate. Formerly, patients with this subtype responded poorly to conventional therapy, but more aggressive therapy protocols have led to markedly improved survival rates.

Immunophenotypic, Cytogenetic, & Molecular Features

Within the category of *acute lymphoblastic leukemia* are a variety of morphologically similar but biologically distinctive diseases, each with characteristic molecular, phenotypic, and clinical features. L3 ALL with surface immunoglobulin positivity and c-*myc* translocations were alluded to earlier. Some B-precursor ALL show a t(1;19) translocation involving the *E*2A and *PBX* genes; these typically express cytoplasmic μ heavy chains, but lack surface Ig, and have an intermediate prognosis. Philadelphia-positive ALL showing either the t(9;22) translocation or its molecular equivalent (a *bcr/abl* fusion gene) carry a particularly poor prognosis and are frequently treated more aggressively. Translocations involving the *MLL* (or *HRX*) gene at 11q23 may involve several partner genes, are frequently present in infant ALL, and connote a poor prognosis. One subtype of ALL with a relatively favorable outcome is characterized by **hyperdiploidy,** with a modal chromosome number of 51 or greater; this type of disease typically has a precursor-B (SIg-) phenotype often with weak or absent CD45 as well as CD34 positivity, is common in young children but not in infants, and responds well to conventional ALL therapy.

B-CELL CHRONIC LYMPHOCYTIC LEUKEMIA & SMALL LYMPHOCYTIC LYMPHOMA

Clinical Features

B-cell chronic lymphocytic leukemia (B-CLL) and small lymphocytic lymphoma (SLL) represent two different clinical presentations of this neoplasm of mature CD5 B cells. Patients are typically elderly or middle-aged adults who may or may not have associated peripheral cytopenias, organomegaly, or lymphadenopathy. Both diseases have an indolent clinical course, in which overall survivals of several years are commonplace. Despite its low rate of progression, however, the cells have low proliferative activity, and the disease is difficult if not impossible to eradicate with chemotherapy. Patients with anemia or thrombocytopenia at presentation have reduced survival rates compared with those with normal peripheral counts. Transformation to prolymphocytic leukemia or large-cell lymphoma supervenes in a number of patients and is associated with a poor prognosis.

Morphologic Features

Lymphocytes are usually small, with coarsely clumped chromatin, lacking nucleoli. Occasional patients may have larger cells that show the same characteristic nuclear features.

Immunophenotypic, Cytogenetic, & Molecular Features

The neoplastic cells have a mature B phenotype, in which surface immunoglobulin is present but typically very weak in staining intensity. CD5 is also characteristically positive, giving rise to speculation that B-CLL/SLL is the neoplastic counterpart of the few normal B cells that also express CD5. Pan B antigens CD20 and CD22 are weakly expressed as well. CD10 is absent, and CD11c weakly expressed. CD23 is present in the majority of cases, a feature that aids in distinguishing this disease from mantle cell lymphoma.

Comments

The diagnosis of B-CLL requires a peripheral lymphocytosis and the demonstration of a monoclonal CD5 B-cell population in the blood or bone marrow. In addition, some individuals may have monoclonal CD5 B cells present in their blood without an absolute lymphocytosis or other clinical sequelae. This has been termed *monoclonal lymphocytosis of uncertain significance,* and its true incidence is unknown; it is likely on a clinical spectrum with biologic similarity to B-CLL.

PROLYMPHOCYTIC LEUKEMIA

Clinical Features

Patients with prolymphocytic leukemia (PLL) are adults and typically present with splenomegaly and a high white blood cell count with many circulating prolymphocytes. Other peripheral counts are often decreased. Many patients present with de novo PLL; others have had a history of CLL that is undergoing a transformation to PLL.

Morphologic Features

Prolymphocytes are intermediate to large cells with clumped chromatin, moderate to low N:C ratios, and a prominent single central nucleolus. T-PLL cells tend to have irregular contours more often than B-PLL cells (eg, see Figure 43–4C). A small-cell variant of T-prolymphocytic leukemia has been described in which cells are small, and nucleoli may be less prominent than in classic T-PLL, appearing similar to CLL cells in some cases (see section on T-cell chronic lymphocytic leukemia.)

Immunophenotypic, Cytogenetic, & Molecular Features

Eighty percent of the cases of PLL is of B lineage, with bright surface immunoglobulin expression; many are also CD5+. Twenty percent are of T lineage, and most of these are CD4+. All are mature and lack terminal deoxynucleotidyl transferase (TdT).

Comments

Prolymphocytic leukemia is an aggressive disease that responds poorly to currently available therapies.

LYMPHOPLASMACYTOID LYMPHOMA & WALDENSTRÖM'S MACROGLOBULINEMIA

Clinical Features

Patients with lymphoplasmacytoid lymphoma (immunocytoma) may or may not have the typical clinical picture of Waldenström's macroglobulinemia, in which an excess of soluble monoclonal IgM circulates in the blood, increasing plasma viscosity and causing clinical symptoms. Most patients do have a monoclonal paraprotein of some kind, however. Patients are adults, who typically present with lymphadenopathy or organomegaly (or both), but who usually lack the lytic bone lesions or renal failure that are seen with plasma cell myeloma.

Morphologic Features

The lymphoid infiltrate consists of a mixture of small mature lymphocytes and plasmacytoid lymphocytes, with cytologic features intermediate between lymphocytes and plasma cells. A few typical plasma cells may also be present. Inclusions consisting of immunoglobulin may be present in the nucleus (Dutcher's bodies) or cytoplasm (Russell's bodies).

Immunophenotypic, Cytogenetic, & Molecular Features

Cells are of mature B lineage and typically lack CD5 or CD10 expression. Cells containing cytoplasmic immunoglobulin are typically present and correspond morphologically to cells showing plasmacytoid features.

Comments

Severe hyperviscosity is a medical emergency, often presenting with symptoms such as neurologic symptoms or visual loss due to retinal hemorrhages. Plasmapheresis is effective in reducing the amount of circulating IgM and reducing clinical symptoms.

MANTLE CELL LYMPHOMA

Clinical Features

Mantle cell lymphoma (MCL) affects older adults, with a marked male predominance. The lymphoma is frequently disseminated at diagnosis, with frequent involvement of blood and bone marrow. A subset of patients present with multifocal involvement of the GI tract known as lymphomatous polyposis. This appearance may mimic that of familial polyposis on colonoscopic examination.

Morphologic Features

The neoplastic cells in most cases are small to medium size with somewhat irregular nuclear contours and a mature chromatin pattern without nucleoli. The degree of nuclear irregularity is intermediate between the smooth contours of CLL/SL lymphocytes and the small cleaved cells of follicular lymphomas. Large cells are not seen within this infiltrate, in contrast to the case in follicular lymphomas. Also, proliferation centers are not seen, in contrast to the case in CLL/SL. A blastic variant is also described in which neoplastic cells appear similar to lymphoblasts but share the immunophenotype of other MCL. Histologically, many show a mantle zone pattern, in which neoplastic cells form widely expanded mantle zones around histologically benign germinal centers; however, a diffuse pattern is also recognized.

Immunophenotypic, Cytogenetic, & Molecular Features

Neoplastic cells have a mature B phenotype, expressing monotypic surface IgM and B-cell-associated antigens. They express the CD5 antigen; however, in contrast to CLL/SL, CD23 expression is characteristically absent. CD10 is usually, although not always, absent, and CD43 is usually positive. Many cases of MCL are associated with a t(11;14) translocation involving the immunoglobulin heavy-chain locus and the *bcl*-1 locus on chromosome 11. This latter locus involves the *PRAD*-1 gene, which encodes for cyclin D1, a cell cycle regulatory protein. MCLs lacking the t(11;14) on karyotypic analysis often show molecular evidence of *bcl*-1 gene rearrangement or cyclin D1 overexpression (or both). This translocation is thought to be a primary event in the pathogenesis of this lymphoma.

Comments

This type of lymphoma has been described under other names, including **mantle zone lymphoma, intermediate lymphocytic lymphoma,** and **centrocytic lymphoma.** The neoplastic cells are thought to be the neoplastic equivalent of the cells in the mantle zone of a normal lymphoid follicle. It was not included in the Working Formulation, and many cases have probably been misdiagnosed as CLL/SL or **diffuse small cleaved** lymphomas. Recognition of the frequency of t(11;14) translocations, and the relative specificity of this molecular lesion for MCL, have led to increased understanding of the biology of this lymphoma subtype. This lymphoma has a median survival of 3 years, considerably less than for low-grade lymphomas. Overall, 30–50% of patients show complete clinical responses to initial treatment, and promising results have been obtained with anti-CD20 monoclonal antibody therapy and bone marrow transplantation. Response to therapy is poorer than for large cell lymphoma, however, and optimal therapy has not yet been established. There is no evidence that any chemotherapy regimen produces durable long-term complete remissions.

FOLLICULAR CENTER LYMPHOMAS

Clinical Features

These lymphomas are most common in adults, presenting only rarely in children. Disseminated disease is frequently present at diagnosis, with multiple enlarged lymph nodes and frequent involvement of bone marrow and peripheral blood.

Morphologic Features

These lymphomas may show a nodular or diffuse pattern or show both patterns simultaneously. The nodules resemble normal germinal centers to an extent but are usually more closely packed and lack normal mantle zones or polarity. A characteristic feature is a decrease in the number of mitoses or tingible body macrophages compared with normal germinal centers, suggesting a lower proliferative activity than is seen in reactive settings. The infiltrates consist of a mixture of small cleaved cells (with irregular or cleaved nuclei) and larger cells that may have cleaved or noncleaved nuclei. The proportion of large cells is correlated with the aggressiveness of the lymphoma.

Immunophenotypic, Cytogenetic, & Molecular Features

The neoplastic cells are of mature B lineage and have a similar phenotype to reactive germinal center B cells, being frequently CD10-positive. Surface immunoglobulin is typically bright when present, although some may lack sIg. Most of these lymphomas have a rearrangement involving the *bcl*-2 oncogene and the immunoglobulin heavy-chain gene. Most but not all of these also result in a t(14;18) translocation visible on karyotype. The *bcl*-2 gene codes for a protein that protects cells against apoptosis. When this gene comes under the influence of the IgH promoter, the gene is constitutively activated and the high *bcl*-2 levels effectively immortalize the cells. Thus, even in neoplasms with very low proliferative activity, the cells accumulate progressively and may be hard to eradicate with conventional chemotherapy.

MARGINAL ZONE B-CELL LYMPHOMAS

Two distinct clinicopathologic entities are recognized within this group: (1) extranodal lymphomas of mucosa-associated lymphoid tissue (MALT) and (2) node-based monocytoid B-cell lymphomas. A third provisional category involves splenic marginal zone lymphomas, many of which may have circulating lymphocytes with cytoplasmic projections (the so-called **splenic lymphomas with villous lymphocytes**).

MALT LYMPHOMAS

Clinical Features

Adults are affected with MALT lymphomas, and there is a slight female predominance. Tumors are most often localized extranodal masses involving sites with glandular epithelium, most commonly the GI tract, salivary glands, thyroid, orbit, or lung. Most patients with salivary gland MALT lymphomas have a history of Sjögren's syndrome. Also, patients with gastric MALT lymphomas have a high incidence of infection with *Helicobacter pylori*.

Morphologic Features

The neoplastic cells, often called centrocyte-like cells, are small, with irregular nuclei somewhat similar to those of small cleaved follicular center cells but with more abundant pale-staining cytoplasm. They are similar to normal cells seen in the splenic marginal zone. MALT lymphomas show distinct histopathologic features similar to those seen in normal mucosa-associated lymphoid tissue (eg, small intestinal Peyer's patches). These include (1) the presence of neoplastic lymphocytes infiltrating epithelial structures, forming **lymphoepithelial lesions,** (2) concentration of plasma cells and plasmacytoid cells adjacent to epithelium, and (3) **follicular colonization,** or the presence of neoplastic centrocyte-like cells within otherwise reactive-appearing germinal centers. Mitoses are few, and most MALT lymphomas are low grade. Some, however, may show predominantly large cells.

Immunophenotypic, Cytogenetic, & Molecular Features

The neoplastic B cells typically express monotypic surface immunoglobulin and B-lineage-associated antigens. Because they lack CD5, CD10, or CD11c, they can be distinguished immunophenotypically from the neoplastic cells of most other lymphoproliferations of small B lymphocytes. Many cells also contain cytoplasmic immunoglobulin, in keeping with the frequent histologic finding of plasmacytoid differentiation. Trisomy 3 has been reported in many cases. Rearrangements of *bcl*-1 and *bcl*-2 are not seen.

Comments

Recently, an association of gastric MALT lymphomas with *Helicobacter pylori* infection has been reported, after which some patients with MALT lymphoma were treated with antibiotics. Surprisingly, many MALT lymphomas regress following eradication of the accompanying *H pylori* infection. The association between MALT lymphomas, *H pylori* gastritis, and Sjögren's syndrome has given rise to speculation that chronic antigenic stimulation plays an important role in pathogenesis of these neoplasms. Indeed, removal of the antigenic stimulus (as with eradication of *H pylori* infection) has led to regression of some of these lymphomas, suggesting that proliferation may often depend on ongoing antigenic stimulation.

MONOCYTOID B-CELL LYMPHOMAS NODE-BASED

Clinical Features

Most of the monocytoid B-cell lymphomas occur in patients with Sjögren's syndrome or extranodal MALT lymphomas; in fact, these may be the lymph nodal equivalent of MALT lymphomas. These also have an indolent clinical course.

Morphologic Features

Centrocyte-like cells, similar to those previously described for MALT lymphomas, are seen in parafollicular, perisinusoidal, or marginal zone pattern of distribution, altering but usually not effacing the nodal architecture.

Immunophenotypic, Cytogenetic, & Molecular Features

These features are similar to those of MALT lymphoma.

Comments

MALT lymphomas and monocytoid B-cell lymphomas are two clinical syndromes apparently involving the same type of neoplastic cell. Differing clinical presentations may be associated with different homing patterns of individual neoplastic clones.

HAIRY CELL LEUKEMIA

Clinical Features

Hairy cell leukemia affects adults, with a male predominance. Patients typically experience peripheral cytopenias and splenomegaly.

Morphologic Features

Neoplastic cells are medium-size to large, with low N:C ratios, abundant pale cytoplasm, and bland round to oval-shaped nuclei without nucleoli. On smear preparations, these cells may or may not show villous, or "hairy," cytoplasmic projections. Electron microscopy shows that these cells have interdigitating cytoplasmic processes, demonstrating that the projections seen on smear preparations are not merely due to technical artifact. In tissue sections, these cells often show a cytoplasmic "halo" of clear cytoplasm with distinct cell borders between adjacent cells.

Immunophenotypic, Cytogenetic, & Molecular Features

The cells have a mature B-lineage phenotype, with expression of B-lineage antigens and abundant surface immunoglobulin. They characteristically coexpress the monocyte/NK-associated antigen CD11c, usually with bright intensity, as well as the IL-2 receptor CD25.

Comments

For much of its history, hairy cell leukemia was referred to by the ungainly name of **leukemic reticuloendotheliosis,** and its cell of origin was unknown. Although we now know that this is a B-cell disease, a normal counterpart to the hairy cell has yet to be definitively identified. The disease has an indolent course, and whereas formerly it was considered impossible to eradicate from the marrow, newer treatment with purine analogues 2-chloro-2'-deoxyadenosine (2-CDA) and 2-deoxycoformycin result in clinical remission in 80–90% of patients. A few variant forms of hairy cell leukemia have been described; these also have been shown to respond well to these agents.

DIFFUSE LARGE B-CELL LYMPHOMA

Clinical Features

Large-cell lymphomas constitute 30–40% of non-Hodgkin's lymphomas in adults and may also be seen in children. Patients typically present with a single nodal or extranodal mass that may be rapidly enlarging. Although these tumors are aggressive neoplasms often with high proliferative activity, many are curable with chemotherapy.

Morphologic Features

All large-cell lymphomas have in common the presence of large lymphoid cells constituting the majority of cells present; most have some admixture of smaller lymphocytes. Traditionally, pathologists have recognized centroblastic and immunoblastic variants of large-cell lymphoma. Even when a group of expert pathologists attempts to distinguish between these entities, however, reproducibility of subclassification is poor. These entities are therefore grouped together in the REAL classification.

Immunophenotypic, Cytogenetic, & Molecular Features

Large-cell lymphomas may be of B- or T-cell type. Many T-cell lymphomas with distinct clinicopathologic features are described separately, however. All large-cell lymphomas are of mature type, lacking TdT expression. Many B-lineage large-cell lymphomas may show *bcl*-2 rearrangements, as has been described for follicular lymphomas; these patients have a less favorable outcome compared with patients whose cells lack *bcl*-2 rearrangements. In contrast, large-cell lymphomas containing rearrangements of the *bcl*-6 oncogene on chromosome 3q27 have a relatively favorable prognosis.

BURKITT'S & BURKITT-LIKE LYMPHOMAS

Clinical Features

Burkitt's lymphoma occurs in an endemic form in Africa, where it commonly affects the jaw or other facial bones, and a sporadic form in other parts of the world where patients typically present with intraabdominal tumors. In both cases, children are most commonly involved, and tumors tend to be rapidly expanding masses. Epstein–Barr virus (EBV) shows a strong association with the endemic form, and the EBV genome can be detected in over 90% of these tumors. A much lower proportion of sporadic cases are associated with EBV. Burkitt's and Burkitt-like lymphomas are also found in patients with acquired immunodeficiency syndrome (AIDS) or other patients with a history of immunosuppression.

Morphologic Features

Burkitt's lymphoma cells are medium-size with low N:C ratios, deeply basophilic cytoplasm with abundant vacuoles, and nuclei with multiple nucleoli. Diffuse monomorphic sheets of these tumor cells also contain abundant mitoses and tingible-body macrophages; these latter cells appear pale at low power and give rise to the typical "starry-sky" pattern often seen in this and other lymphomas. Burkitt-like lymphomas have similar features but may show larger cells or more pleomorphism, so that the distinction between Burkitt's and large-cell lymphoma is problematic.

Immunophenotypic, Cytogenetic, & Molecular Features

Burkitt's and most Burkitt-like lymphomas are of mature B-cell type, expressing surface immunoglobulin and lacking TdT. CD10 is expressed in most cases as well. Most contain a molecular rearrangement of the c-*myc* oncogene with an immunoglobulin gene, most often the heavy-chain gene. Many of these translocations are visible on cytogenetic examination as translocations involving 8q24 (see Table 43–7). These tumors show some of the highest proliferative activities seen in non-Hodgkin's lymphomas, as one would expect from the histologic appearance.

Comments

Burkitt's lymphoma and the L3 subtype of ALL are differing clinical presentations of the same cell type, with similar phenotypic and molecular features.

CLONAL PLASMA CELL DISORDERS

Plasma cell myeloma, or **multiple myeloma,** was recognized as a distinct clinicopathologic entity long before it was known that plasma cells were terminally differentiated B lymphocytes. Because plasma cells secrete immunoglobulin, clonal proliferations of plasma cells usually result in the excessive production of a single immunoglobulin type or often only a single light or heavy chain. These monoclonal paraproteins are detectable by serum electrophoresis or immunofixation as single sharp bands or peaks standing out from the background of reactive immunoglobulins. Often, the presence of monoclonal light chains is detectable in the urine whether or not a serum monoclonal paraprotein is present. These urine paraproteins have been referred to as Bence Jones proteins and may require urine immunofixation for detection (see Chapter 15).

The term **plasma cell dyscrasia** has been used as a generic term indicating any clinical syndrome in which an abnormal plasma cell population is found, whether or not the disease has obvious clinical signs of neoplasia. Clonal plasma cell proliferations form a clinical spectrum encompassing indolent and aggressive forms of disease. In many instances, the monoclonal paraprotein is responsible for the majority of clinical symptoms. Clinical evaluation of these syndromes should include routine laboratory tests, a measurement of serum viscosity, radiologic examination for the presence of lytic bone lesions, serum and urine electrophoresis, and renal function tests. Serum should be separated at 37°C because some paraproteins are cryoglobulins and precipitate at low temperatures (see Chapter 15).

PLASMA CELL MYELOMA

Clinical Features

Plasma cell myeloma usually affects only older adults; the disease is virtually unknown in children. Plasma cells form localized lytic bone lesions visible radiographically, and usually secrete a monoclonal immunoglobulin that can be detected on serum electrophoresis. Immunoglobulin light chains are frequently present in the urine (Bence Jones proteins). Anemia and renal failure are common clinical symptoms.

Morphologic Features

Infiltrates of plasma cells show a monomorphic appearance within any given patient, although wide morphologic variation is seen between patients. Plasma cells range from innocuous, normal-appearing plasma cells, to larger cells with prominent nucleoli, to cells with prominent cytoplasmic inclusions or other changes. In some instances, cells may be difficult to distinguish from plasmacytoid immunoblasts.

Immunophenotypic, Cytogenetic, & Molecular Features

Neoplastic plasma cells are similar to their normal counterparts in that most lack surface immunoglobulin; express abundant cytoplasmic Ig, CD38, and

PC-1; and lack most if not all surface B-cell antigens or CD45. In contrast, myeloma cells may express CD56, an adhesion molecule that is absent on normal plasma cells. Many myeloma populations show aneuploidy and a variety of cytogenetic abnormalities, including frequent abnormalities involving the immunoglobulin heavy-chain locus at 14q32.

Comments

Traditional therapy has been largely supportive, although aggressive cytotoxic therapy may prolong survival in selected patients. Autologous bone marrow transplantation is under investigation as a treatment modality. This procedure involves harvesting circulating CD34 stem cells from the peripheral blood. Most myeloma patients, however, have circulating small lymphocytes that can be shown to be monoclonal, expressing surface immunoglobulin of the same type as the myeloma cells. These cells are present in conventional stem cell harvests but may be absent from samples in which only CD34 cells have been selected for storage.

Recently, Kaposi's sarcoma-associated herpesvirus (KSHV) has been found within bone marrow dendritic cells in some patients with plasma cell myeloma, and in a lesser number of patients with MGUS.

SOLITARY PLASMACYTOMA

When a single plasmacytoma is found, the patient is assessed for other features of plasma cell myeloma. If no other sites of disease are identified, the patient is said to have a solitary plasmacytoma. These may occur in bone or soft tissue sites. The former has a high prevalence of paraproteinemia and is associated with a poorer prognosis as a result of progression to plasma cell myeloma. Extramedullary soft tissue plasmacytomas tend to have a more indolent course, usually show nonparaprotein, and only occasionally progress to plasma cell myeloma. Solitary plasmacytomas are usually treated with surgical excision or local radiotherapy.

MONOCLONAL GAMMOPATHY OF UNDETERMINED SIGNIFICANCE

A small percentage of otherwise healthy elderly people have small monoclonal paraproteins in either their serum or urine but lack other clinical features of myeloma. Although some of these people eventually develop myeloma, many do not, hence the name **monoclonal gammopathy of undetermined significance (MGUS)**. Patients with MGUS are commonly followed by hematologists at regular intervals to detect any evidence of progression to myeloma. Increasing levels of serum or urine paraprotein, or decreasing levels of normal immunoglobulins, often indicate progression to myeloma.

AMYLOIDOSIS

Deposits of amyloid may be associated with plasma cell neoplasms and dyscrasias. Amyloid is a complex substance containing fragments of an immunoglobulin light chain, especially the V region. Antibodies directed against this light chain may react with Bence Jones proteins. A nonimmunoglobulin component has a molecular weight of approximately 8000, with 76 amino acids, and is of unknown origin. Another component is a glycoprotein related antigenically to an α_1 globulin present in small amounts in normal human plasma.

Amyloid may arise from (1) the catabolism by macrophages of antigen-antibody complexes; (2) synthesis in situ of whole immunoglobulins or of light chains with reduced solubility; (3) genetic deletions of the light-chain gene, producing an anomalous protein with reduced solubility; of (4) separate synthesis of discrete regions of the light chain. Amyloid deposits may be detected in tissues by light microscopy as eosinophilic material on hematoxylin–eosin-stained sections. These deposits are birefringent with polarized light, and electron microscopy shows nonbranching fibrils, 8.5 nm wide and of various lengths. Special stains selectively stain the material.

A suggested classification of amyloidosis is presented in Table 43–11.

HEAVY-CHAIN DISEASES

Patients with this rare disease complex have paraproteins of one of the three major types of heavy chain (γ, μ, or α) in blood and urine; α-chain disease is the most common. Immunoelectrophoresis demonstrates that heavy chains, but not light chains, are present. There may be partial deletion of the Fc portion of the heavy chain, deletion in the hinge region, or a combination of the two.

α-Chain Disease

Patients commonly present with a severe malabsorption syndrome accompanied by chronic diarrhea, steatorrhea, weight loss, and hypocalcemia. They may have lymphadenopathy. The small intestine is infiltrated with plasma cells, lymphocytes, and histiocytes; these may appear to be benign initially, but as the disease progresses the plasmacytoid cells appear cytologically less mature and extend beyond the lamina propria. α-Chain disease is associated with abdominal lymphomas in patients living in the Mediterranean area, but the disease may occur in other geographic areas as well. Rare cases of involvement of the respiratory tract instead of the gastrointestinal tract have been reported.

Table 43–11. Classification of amyloidosis.

	Clinical Type	Sites of Deposition
Familial	Amyloid polyneuropathy (Portuguese, dominant inheritance)	Peripheral nerves, viscera
	Familial Mediterranean fever (recessive)	Liver, spleen, kidneys, adrenals
Generalized	Primary	Tongue, heart, gut, skeletal and smooth muscles, nerves, skin, ligaments
	Associated with plasma cell dyscrasia	Liver, spleen, kidneys, adrenals
	Secondary (infection, inflammation)	Any site
Localized	Lichen amyloidosis	Skin
	Endocrine-related (eg, thyroid carcinoma)	Endocrine organ (thyroid)
Senile		Heart, brain

γ-Chain Disease

Some patients with this disease may die within weeks of onset, and others may survive for more than 20 years. Commonly, the patients have a lymphoproliferative disorder with hepatosplenomegaly, lymphadenopathy, and uvular and palatal edema. Infection is common and is the usual cause of death. The patients have recurrent fevers, anemia, leukopenia, and atypical circulating lymphocytes.

μ-Chain Disease

IgM heavy-chain disease is seen in patients with long-standing B-CLL with progressive hepatosplenomegaly.

CRYOGLOBULINEMIA

A variety of serum and plasma proteins precipitate at low temperature. Some of these are nonimmunoglobulin cryoproteins such as cryofibrinogen, C-reactive-protein-albumin complex, and heparin-precipitable protein. The cryoimmunoglobulins may precipitate at temperatures as high as 35°C, so that during collection of blood, the specimen must be maintained at 37°C to avoid loss of a cryoprecipitated globulin (see Chapter 15). The rate at which the cryoglobulins precipitate may vary from minutes to days. Therefore, detection of cryoglobulins requires observation of the serum at 4°C for at least 72 hours.

Small amounts of polyclonal serum cryoglobulin is normally present in healthy individuals. Three types of pathologic cryoglobulins have been identified: type I (25%) includes monoclonal immunoglobulins (IgM and occasionally IgG and rarely IgA or Bence Jones protein); type II (25%) includes mixed cryoglobulins with a monoclonal IgM or occasionally IgG or IgA complexed with autologous normal IgG; and type III (50%) includes mixtures of polyclonal IgM and IgG. Patients with monoclonal type I cryoglobulins usually suffer from the symptoms of

their underlying disease (eg, multiple myeloma or Waldenström's macroglobulinemia). Patients with type II or III cryoglobulins may have immune complex disease with purpura, arthritis, and nephritis. These immune complexes often fix complement in vivo and in vitro.

BENIGN HYPERGAMMAGLOBULINEMIC PURPURA

This is a rare disease usually seen in young and middle-aged women. It is characterized by a dependent purpuric rash brought on by exercise or alcohol. Some of these patients have autoimmune disorders, particularly systemic lupus erythematosus or Sjögren's syndrome. The patients characteristically have a monoclonal IgG- κ paraprotein that acts as a rheumatoid factor, forming complexes with circulating IgG. Serum levels of IgA and IgM are normal or increased, and there are no findings of multiple myeloma. Treatment is directed at prevention and correction of the underlying autoimmune disorder. Severe symptoms may warrant plasmapheresis.

LARGE GRANULAR LYMPHOCYTE LEUKEMIAS

Clinical Features

Large granular lymphocytic leukemias (LGLL) are mostly indolent chronic leukemias that involve adults and produce an absolute increase in circulating large granular lymphocytes, usually with an absolute overall lymphocytosis as well. Peripheral cytopenias are common, especially neutropenia in T-cell cases. Many patients with T-cell LGLL have a history of rheumatoid arthritis or splenomegaly, and there is probably some overlap with Felty's syndrome in many cases. NK cell proliferations may be indolent or aggressive, and an association with EBV or systemic immunosuppression is often seen in the latter cases.

Morphologic Features

Most frequently, cells are similar to normal large granular lymphocytes, with low N:C ratios, clumped chromatin, and scattered distinct azurophilic granules (eg, see Figure 43–4B). In some cases, irregular nuclei, atypical nuclear features, or abnormal granules may be seen. If cell numbers are low, the peripheral smear may appear similar to the picture seen in acute viral reactions.

Immunophenotypic, Cytogenetic, & Molecular Features

Most cases of LGLL are of T-cell type, expressing CD3 as well as other pan T antigens, CD8, CD16, and usually CD56 or CD57 (or both). These are nearly always clonal and exhibit rearrangements of beta or less commonly gamma T-cell receptor genes. NK-LGLL are less common and lack CD3 expression; most are CD8+, but some are CD4–/CD8–. Clonality of NK-LGLL is difficult to study because T-cell receptor genes are uninformative. Some show clonal karyotypic abnormalities; these cases usually follow an aggressive clinical course.

T-CELL PROLYMPHOCYTIC LEUKEMIA

Clinical Features

Patients with this uncommon leukemia are usually older adults; typically present with a high WBC and splenomegaly; and may also have cutaneous, pleural or peritoneal involvement. The disease is rapidly progressive and associated with a poor prognosis.

Morphologic Features

Cells from the classical form of T-cell prolymphocytic leukemia (T-PLL) are medium-sized to large, often have irregular nuclear contours, and feature prominent nucleoli. A small cell variant of T-PLL is described in which cells are smaller and nucleoli are inconspicuous or even absent; these cases morphologically resemble B-cell CLL.

Immunophenotypic, Cytogenetic & Molecular Features

Cells have a mature T-cell phenotype, lacking TdT expression. In contrast to LGL leukemias, NK-related markers are absent. Most express CD4 but not CD8, although coexpression of CD4 and CD8 may be seen in a minority of cases. Cytogenetic abnormalities involving the beta T-cell receptor locus at 14q11 are frequently found.

Comments

The small cell variant of T-PLL includes cases formerly classified as "true T-cell CLL." The term *T-cell CLL* has fallen into disfavor because the name has been used inconsistently over the past two decades and could lead to confusion. Most cases described as T-cell CLL in the 1970s and 1980s would now be classified as LGL leukemias, a largely indolent disorder. It is essential to distinguish these from the more aggressive T-cell leukemias, which may look like CLL under the microscope but otherwise resemble T-PLL.

MYCOSIS FUNGOIDES & SÉZARY SYNDROME

Clinical Features

These indolent cutaneous lymphoproliferations occur in adults and may present as localized plaques or tumors (mycosis fungoides) or generalized erythroderma (Sézary syndrome). Scaling and fissuring of the skin on the palms and soles are common. Circulating neoplastic T cells are an expected component of Sézary syndrome and may either be absent or present in low numbers in mycosis fungoides. Mycosis fungoides may become more generalized and Sézary-like over time. Some patients go on to develop a more aggressive large-cell lymphoma.

Morphologic Features

The skin is densely infiltrated with lymphocytes, most with irregular nuclear contours, which occur adjacent to the epidermis and encroach on it (epidermotropism), and may form intraepithelial collections of lymphocytes known as Pautrier's microabscesses. On peripheral smears and touch preparations, lymphocytes have multiple nuclear infoldings producing a characteristic "cerebriform" appearance (eg, see Figure 43–4D). These infoldings are easier to appreciate in thin sections or in transmission electron micrographs. Mitoses are uncommon.

Immunophenotypic, Cytogenetic, & Molecular Features

Cells are of mature T-cell type, expressing pan-T antigens but lacking TdT. Most are CD4+, and most also lack expression of the pan-T antigen CD7. CD25, the IL-2 receptor, is usually absent, although occasional cases may show weak CD25 expression. CD25 expression, however (especially if bright), should suggest the diagnosis of adult T-cell leukemia-lymphoma. A variety of cytogenetic abnormalities have been described, none of which are characteristic for this disease.

ADULT T-CELL LEUKEMIA-LYMPHOMA

Clinical Features

This disease occurs in adults and is most common in Japan, the Caribbean, and to a lesser extent the southeastern United States. The disease is defined as a T-cell neoplasm caused by infection with human T-lymphotropic virus-1 (HTLV-1), a retrovirus; patients typically have circulating antibodies to HTLV-1, and their neoplastic lymphocytes can be shown to contain viral genomes. The acute form of this leukemia-lymphoma syndrome is by far the most common, in which patients usually present with hypercalcemia, a high WBC, organomegaly, lymphadenopathy, and frequent central nervous system involvement. Median survival is less than 1 year. A subacute form is described but is much less frequent.

Morphologic Features

Neoplastic lymphocytes show a variety of cell sizes, mostly medium-sized to large, and are characterized by frequently multilobed nuclei, sometimes showing a radial pattern (eg, see Figure 43–4E). Cells may also appear similar to cerebriform cells seen in cutaneous lymphomas. Chromatin is typically heavier than is seen in lymphoblastic malignancies, but both cell types may show prominent nucleoli.

Immunophenotypic, Cytogenetic, & Molecular Features

Cells have a mature T-cell phenotype, and although nearly all are CD4+, some have been shown to have a suppressor function in vitro. Many lack CD7 or other pan-T antigens. Expression of CD25 is characteristic. T-cell receptor genes are rearranged, and clonal integration of the HTLV-1 genome can be found.

PERIPHERAL T-CELL LYMPHOMAS

Peripheral T-cell lymphomas (PTL) includes a few distinct entities described in the following sections, as well as nondescript peripheral T-cell lymphomas not fitting these descriptions. All are neoplasms of mature T cells and commonly show pleomorphic histologic features in which atypical cells with irregular contours are present in a range of sizes.

ANGIOIMMUNOBLASTIC T-CELL LYMPHOMA

Clinical Features

Patients are adults who usually present with systemic symptoms, including fever, weight loss, a skin rash, generalized lymphadenopathy, and polyclonal hypergammaglobulinemia. Although these lymphomas may pursue an aggressive clinical course, spontaneous remissions have been described.

Morphologic Features

Histopathologic features are similar to angioimmunoblastic lymphadenopathy and include effacement of the nodal architecture; a hypocellular, or "pink," appearance at low power; absent or regressively transformed ("burnt-out") germinal centers; and a proliferation of small, branching blood vessels. Pleomorphic lymphocytes in a mixture of cell sizes are present in a background of histiocytes, eosinophils, and plasma cells and form sheets or aggregates in at least part of the infiltrate.

Immunophenotypic, Cytogenetic, & Molecular Features

Abnormal lymphocytes are of mature T lineage, showing variable loss of T-cell-associated antigens, and are usually CD4+. T-cell antigen receptor genes show a clonal rearrangement pattern, and EBV genomes can be detected in many of these tumors. Although no specific cytogenetic findings are described, trisomies 3 and 5 are often found.

Comments

The clinicopathologic spectrum between these lymphomas and angioimmunoblastic lymphadenopathy with dysproteinemia (AILD) suggest that cases of AILD without obvious lymphoma are nonetheless preneoplastic in nature. AILD and AILD-lymphomas may represent two aspects of a single biologic disorder of clonal T cells, in which only some cases fulfill traditional histopathologic criteria for a diagnosis of lymphoma.

ANGIOCENTRIC NK/T LYMPHOMA

Clinical Features

Rare in the United States, this disorder is common in Asia among adults, and frequently involves extranodal sites, especially the nose and paranasal sinuses. There is a clinical spectrum from indolent to aggressive behavior, and the proportion of large cells in the infiltrate may have some bearing on clinical behavior. Patients often develop hemophagocytic syndromes, for which the outcome is poor.

Morphologic Features

These tumors characteristically show an angiocentric and angioinvasive histologic pattern, with atypical lymphocytes invading vessel walls and forming cuffs around them. Not surprisingly, vessel lumina frequently become occluded, and ischemic necrosis is frequently noted in these tumors.

Immunophenotypic, Cytogenetic, & Molecular Features

These neoplasms have a mature T/NK phenotype, expressing the NK-related antigen CD56. Cells lack intact surface CD3 molecules and appear CD3– by flow immunophenotyping, but express CD3ε chains, which are detected by the polyclonal CD3 antibody reagent used commonly in paraffin-section immunohistochemistry. EBV genomes are frequently detectable in these cells.

Comments

These lymphomas bear some similarity to aggressive NK leukemias and may in fact represent their tissue counterpart.

INTESTINAL T-CELL LYMPHOMA

Clinical Features

Frequently patients with this lymphoma have had a history of gluten-sensitive enteropathy, and in fact the worldwide incidence pattern follows that of the enteropathy. Patients commonly present with abdominal pain or perforation and are found to have multiple intestinal ulcers. The clinical course is aggressive.

Morphologic Features

The intestinal ulcers consist of a pleomorphic admixture of small, medium, or large atypical cells that may infiltrate the overlying epithelium. Reactive histiocytic infiltrates or villous atrophy in adjacent mucosa may or may not be present.

Immunophenotypic, Cytogenetic, & Molecular Features

Cells have a mature T phenotype; many also express CD103. This latter feature is helpful in establishing the diagnosis.

Comments

Cases formerly described as "malignant histiocytosis of the intestine" are most likely examples of this type of T-cell lymphoma.

ANAPLASTIC LARGE-CELL LYMPHOMAS

Clinical Features

Anaplastic large-cell lymphomas (ALCL) affect both children and adults. Two clinical presentations are described: a primary cutaneous form localized to the skin without extracutaneous spread at diagnosis, and a systemic form involving lymph nodes and other organ sites as well as the skin in some cases. Some examples of the primary cutaneous form may regress, and this form may be difficult to distinguish from lymphomatoid papulosis in some cases.

Morphologic Features

Neoplastic cells are larger than most large lymphoma cells and show marked nuclear pleomorphism, with frequent wreath-like, horseshoe- or ring-shaped nuclei as well as multinucleated cells (eg, see Figure 43–4F). These cells may show a predominantly sinusoidal distribution pattern in lymph nodes. Neutrophils or macrophages may be present among neoplastic cells in some cases.

Immunophenotypic, Cytogenetic, & Molecular Features

Most cases of ALCL are of mature T lineage, showing clonal rearrangements of T-cell antigen receptor genes, although many lack T-lineage-associated antigens and can be difficult to characterize immunophenotypically. Strong expression of CD30 is a characteristic feature. A t(2;5) translocation has been identified in many cases and is relatively specific for this tumor type. The translocation involves a fusion of the *NPM* and *ALK* genes on chromosomes 5 and 2, respectively.

Comments

Prior to recognition of this lymphoma type, cases were often diagnosed as malignant histiocytosis or lymphocyte depletion Hodgkin's disease. Because lymphoma cells can show a somewhat cohesive appearance and are present in lymph node sinuses, confusion with metastatic carcinoma or melanoma is possible.

HODGKIN'S DISEASE

Hodgkin's disease comprises a group of lymphomas with unique clinical and histopathologic features, accounting for about one third of all lymphomas. Histologically, all forms of Hodgkin's disease are characterized by the presence of Reed-Sternberg cells and their variant forms. Reed-Sternberg cells (Figure 43–5) are very large cells with two or more nuclei or nuclear lobes, each of

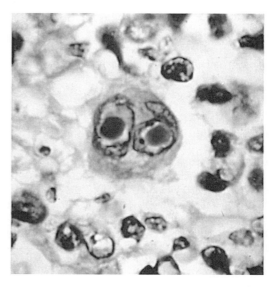

Figure 43–5. Hodgkin's lymphoma. High magnification of a classic Reed-Sternberg cell with two nuclei containing the typical nucleoli. (Reproduced, with permission, from Chandrasoma P, Taylor CR: *Concise Pathology.* Appleton & Lange, 1991.)

which contains a single large eosinophilic nucleolus. Their exact lineage is unknown. Variant forms have a single nucleus containing a similar nucleolus. Reed-Sternberg cells and variants are the neoplastic cells of Hodgkin's disease, and are characteristically present in a background of reactive cells (lymphocytes, histiocytes, eosinophils, and plasma cells). In most cases, the reactive cells far outnumber the neoplastic cells. It is believed that the reactive cells represent the host response to the neoplastic cells.

For many years, the disease was considered to be infectious rather than neoplastic because of its clinical course and pathology. The disease is now considered to be neoplastic because nonrandom chromosome abnormalities have been found in Hodgkin's disease tissue. An association with EBV has been found for some forms of Hodgkin's disease.

Clinical Features

The most common clinical presentation is one or more enlarged, nontender lymph nodes, most commonly in the cervical or supraclavicular node groups. Systemic symptoms, such as fever, chills, night sweats, or weight loss, also known as "B symptoms," are often present and imply a worse prognosis. Patients may also experience pruritus or pain in lymph nodes following ingestion of ethanol for reasons that are unclear. Splenomegaly is present in less than 20% of patients. Progression of disease is predictable, spreading first to adjacent nodal groups before involving more distant sites. This is in contrast to the progression of non-Hodgkin's lymphomas, in which noncontiguous sites may be involved with sparing of intervening node groups. Dissemination into parenchymal organs may occur later in the course of the disease. Clinical stage, or extent of tumor spread, is determined by physical examination, chest radiography, lymphangiogram, abdominal computed tomography (CT), and liver–spleen scan. Clinical stage is a lightly significant predictor of outcome and is used to determine the therapeutic approach. Histologic pattern is another important prognostic factor.

Morphologic Features

Four broad histologic subtypes are delineated by the Rye classification (Table 43–12): lymphocyte predominance, mixed cellularity, lymphocyte depletion, and nodular sclerosis. A nodular subtype of lymphocyte predominance Hodgkin's disease is recognized and is also known as the nodular L&H (lymphocytic and histiocytic) subtype. This subtype has an unusually indolent course and may represent a fundamentally different type of Hodgkin's disease (see later discussion). The mixed cellularity subtype shows typical Reed-Sternberg (RS) cells and their mononuclear variants within a background of lymphocytes, histiocytes, eosinophils, and plasma cells. The nodular sclerosis subtype shows broad bands of collagen fibrosis dividing the infiltrate into nodules at low power. Typical RS cells are admixed with lacunar RS variants, multilobed large cells with smaller nucleoli that may show retraction artifact in formalin-fixed sections. The lymphocyte-depletion variant shows abundant RS cells and variants with few background cells. Many cases formerly diagnosed as this subtype would now be considered to be anaplastic large-cell lymphoma.

Many cases of lymphocyte predominance Hodgkin's disease have a nodular pattern and are characterized by frequent L&H cells or "popcorn cells," an RS-like cell with less conspicuous nucleoli and a multilobated popcorn-like nuclear contour. Typical RS cells are extremely rare. Other cases within this subtype have a diffuse histologic pattern and may or may not have L&H cells.

Immunophenotypic, Cytogenetic, & Molecular Features

Except for the L&H cells of nodular lymphocyte predominance Hodgkin's disease, Reed-Sternberg cells and variants have a characteristic phenotype, ex-

Table 43–12. Rye classification of Hodgkin's disease.

Histologic Subtype	Percentage of US Cases	Predominant Features	Prognosis
Lymphocyte predominance	10	Young adult males, stage 1 or 2 at diagnosis; few Reed–Sternberg cells, good lymphocyte host response, connective tissue bands minimal	Excellent
Nodular sclerosis	60	Young females, stage 1 or 2 at diagnosis; predominant nodules due to wide bands or birefringent collagen, mediastinal mass, "lacunar" variants of Reed-Sternberg cells	Excellent
Mixed cellularity	20	Majority with stage 3 or 4 at diagnosis; abdominal involvement common, lymphocytes, plasma cells, eosinophils mixed with Reed-Sternberg cells, diffuse involvement of nodes	Good
Lymphocyte depletion	10	Older males, stage 3 or 4 at diagnosis; systemic symptoms, prolonged fever of unknown origin, abdominal and bone marrow involvement, numerous Reed-Sternberg cells, diffuse fibrosis, and few lymphocytes, indicating poor host response	Relatively poor

pressing CD30 and usually also expressing CD15, but typically lacking CD45. B- and T-associated antigens are also absent, and this feature is especially important in differentiating between lymphocyte depletion Hodgkin's disease and large-cell anaplastic lymphoma. In contrast, L&H cells of nodular lymphocyte predominance Hodgkin's disease are CD45+ and express B-lineage-associated antigens, and although they may or may not express CD30, they lack CD15 expression. These findings have given rise to the idea that nodular lymphocyte predominance Hodgkin's disease is a B-cell neoplasm, distinct from other forms of Hodgkin's disease. The cell of origin for classic Reed-Sternberg cells has been the subject of debate for some time, although recent evidence supports an origin from germinal center B cells.

NEOPLASMS OF MONONUCLEAR PHAGOCYTES & ANTIGEN-PRESENTING CELLS

Cells broadly characterized as histiocytes are of two types: mononuclear phagocytes and antigen-presenting cells. The former are derived from blood monocytes and differentiate into phagocytic cells. The latter comprise the dendritic and interdigitating reticulum cells found in lymphoid tissues, and Langerhans' cells present in the skin. Neoplasms of mononuclear phagocyte type with immature morphologic features are the monoblastic leukemias and the extramedullary myeloid tumors of monoblastic origin. These are discussed more fully in references covering acute nonlymphoid leukemias.

LANGERHANS' CELL HISTIOCYTOSIS

Langerhans' cell histiocytosis (LCH), also known as histiocytosis X, is by far the most common neoplasm of antigen-presenting cells. Until recently, it was unclear whether the etiology was neoplastic or reactive; however, clonality of the neoplastic cells has been demonstrated using an X chromosome inactivation assay. All share a similar histologic appearance characterized by the presence of plump Langerhans' cells with longitudinal nuclear grooves and abundant cytoplasm, admixed with eosinophils, lymphocytes, and rare plasma cells. Three clinical presentations are classically described and are briefly explained here, but the disease can present along a continuous clinical spectrum, frequently in a systemic manner in infants and in a more localized form in older children and adults. **Eosinophilic granuloma** typically presents as a solitary, slow-growing bone lesion in older children and adults, and has a benign clinical course. **Hand-Schüller-Christian** syndrome is a multifocal presentation occurring in children and showing involvement of the pituitary, with resulting diabetes insipidus. **Letterer-Siwe** syndrome describes the systemic multiorgan pattern of involvement seen in infants and carries the worst prognosis. Immunophenotypically, LCH cells are similar to normal Langerhans' cells in that they express the S100 antigen, CD1a, and CD4. Birbeck granules are visible by transmission electron microscopy.

Sarcomas of dendritic and interdigitating reticulum cells have been described and are extremely rare, presenting usually as localized masses in lymph nodes. Many have a spindle cell appearance similar to other soft tissue sarcomas. Immunohistochemical stains are required to demonstrate phenotypic features of reticulum cell origin.

MALIGNANT HISTIOCYTOSIS

Malignant histiocytosis (MH), a rare disease, is now considered to be even rarer than previously thought because many cases formerly diagnosed as MH would now be diagnosed as anaplastic large-cell lymphomas. In addition, a nonneoplastic proliferation of benign-appearing phagocytic histiocytes (described later in the chapter) has sometimes been confused with MH. The disease occurs in both children and adults and is characterized by widespread disease affecting the reticuloendothelial system, with frequent skin, bone, and GI tract involvement as well. Lymph nodes show a sinusoidal infiltrate of large cells with malignant nuclear features exhibiting phagocytosis. Diagnosis requires not only the characteristic morphologic findings and demonstration of histiocytic antigens (CD68, CD11c, CD14) via immunologic methods but also absence of B- and T-lineage-associated antigens.

HEMATOLOGIC PROLIFERATIONS IN IMMUNOSUPPRESSED PATIENTS

Patients with decreased systemic immune function, whether due to congenital immunodeficiency, HIV infection, or immunosuppressive therapy, have an increased risk of developing malignant lymphomas or lymphoma-like lymphoid proliferations (see Chapter 46). Each of these clinical settings is associated with distinct histopathologic and biologic findings. Patients on systemic immunosuppression following solid organ transplantation frequently develop B-cell proliferations. The risk for developing such a lesion is highest in patients with combined heart–lung transplants and is roughly correlated with the intensity of immunosuppression. Patients receiving cyclosporine or OKT3 therapy are at higher risk than other posttransplant patients. Although many of these lesions are monoclonal, many regress when immunosuppressive drugs are stopped, without the aid of cytotoxic chemotherapy. These are hence called **lymphoproliferative disorders** instead of malignant lymphomas. Epstein-Barr virus is present in the B lymphocytes and is thought to drive the proliferation of B cells unchecked by the usual immune surveillance, which limits B-cell proliferation in healthy people.

These posttransplant lymphoproliferative disorders show a spectrum of histopathologic changes. Most recently, three categories are recognized. **Plasmacytic hyperplasia** is a polyclonal proliferation without cytologic atypia, commonly involves the oropharynx, and generally regresses when immunosuppressive therapy is stopped. **Polymorphic hyperplasia** and **polymorphic lymphoma** show a mixed infiltrate of atypical lymphoid cells, small lymphocytes, and plasma cells; are generally monoclonal; and may or may not regress following cessation of immunosuppression. **Immunoblastic lymphomas** and **myeloma** are not only monoclonal but frequently contain additional genetic changes as well, such as c-*myc* translocations or *ras* oncogene mutations. These generally do not regress when immunosuppression is halted.

It is hypothesized that immunosuppression leads to reactivation of latent EBV infection, or perhaps an unchecked primary EBV infection, with expansion of multiple EBV-infected clones, producing at first a polyclonal proliferation. Clones with a selective growth advantage eventually overgrow the others, producing a monoclonal infiltrate. In some such proliferations, additional genetic changes to tumor suppressor genes or oncogenes may result in a fully malignant clonal neoplasm. This sequence of events is in keeping with the multistep pathogenesis that has been proposed for many other cancers.

HIV-infected individuals have an increased risk of developing lymphomas, and although all subtypes may be seen, three patterns are most common. The largest histologic subgroup is diffuse large-cell lymphomas of B lineage, with or without immunoblastic features. Although all are histologically malignant, both monoclonal and polyclonal varieties have been described. A second group consists of Burkitt's or Burkitt-like lymphomas. This group is associated with the t(8;14) translocation involving the c-*myc* oncogene, or its two variant translocations, as is also true for Burkitt's lymphomas in non-HIV-infected individuals (see Table 43–7). Central nervous system lymphomas constitute the third group and tend to occur later in the course of HIV/AIDS in patients with lower absolute CD4 counts than is true for the other lymphoma subtypes. Virtually all CNS lymphomas are associated with EBV infection, whereas other lymphoma subtypes contain both EBV+ and EBV-cases.

HIV infection in lymph nodes is associated with disruption of germinal center architecture, with follicular lysis, and eventual loss of germinal centers. HIV infection of antigen-presenting cells within germinal centers, with ensuing B-cell dysregulation, has been proposed to play a role in the pathogenesis of node-based HIV-related lymphomas. B cells in polyclonal lymphomas may possibly be proliferating in response to cytokines secreted by another cell population, possibly antigen-presenting cells.

BENIGN CONDITIONS MIMICKING OR ASSOCIATED WITH NEOPLASMS OF THE IMMUNE SYSTEM

A variety of lymphadenopathies may mimic lymphoma either clinically or morphologically. Some are considered truly benign, with little or no increased risk of subsequent lymphoma. This group includes typical follicular hyperplasia, most cases of angiofollicular lymph node hyperplasia (Castleman's disease), the lymphadenopathy seen in systemic lupus erythematosus, phenytoin (Dilantin) -associated lymphadenopathy, and most viral syndromes. Others may contain small clonal populations of T or B cells and are associated with an increased risk of subsequent lymphoma. These include the lymphoproliferations associated with Sjögren's syndrome and Hashimoto's thyroiditis and angioimmunoblastic lymphadenopathy. All of these may also show concomitant lymphoma at the time of diagnosis.

The hemophagocytic syndromes are a group of histologically benign but clinically aggressive disorders in which histiocytes show phagocytosis of erythrocytes, leukocytes, or platelets. Unlike malignant histiocytosis, the phagocytic cells have benign cytologic features. Patients typically present with fever, peripheral cytopenias related to increased cell destruction, lymphadenopathy or organomegaly, and frequently a component of chronic disseminated intravascular coagulation. The syndrome is associated with infection from a wide variety of agents, most commonly Epstein-Barr virus, and is often present in the setting of an underlying immune deficiency. Familial forms of hemophagocytic syndrome have been described and probably reflect a subtle familial immunodeficiency. T- or NK cell lymphomas and leukemias, most commonly angiocentric lymphomas, are frequently associated with a hemophagocytic syndrome. In these cases, EBV-infected neoplastic T cells are thought to release one or more cytokines, which stimulate reactive histiocytes and cause them to exhibit increased phagocytosis. The pathogenesis of infection-associated hemophagocytic syndromes probably involves release of similar cytokine(s) by reactive T lymphocytes.

REFERENCES

GENERAL
Brunning RD, McKenna RW: *Tumors of the Bone Marrow* (Atlas of Tumor Pathology series). Armed Forces Institute of Pathology Press, 1993.

Foucar K: *Bone Marrow Pathology.* ASCP Press, 1994.

Jaffe ES: *Surgical Pathology of the Lymph Nodes and Related Organs.* W. B. Saunders, 1995.

Warnke RA et al: *Tumors of the Lymph Nodes and Spleen* (Atlas of Tumor Pathology series). Armed Forces Institute of Pathology Press, 1995.

APPROACH TO DIAGNOSIS
Bain BJ: Routine and specialised techniques in the diagnosis of haematological neoplasms. *J Clin Pathol* 1995; 48:501.

Borowitz MJ et al: Predictability of the t(1;19)(q23;p13) from surface antigen phenotype: Implications for screening cases of childhood acute lymphoblastic leukemia for molecular analysis: A Pediatric Oncology Group study. *Blood* 1993;82:10.

European Group for the Immunological Characterization of Leukemias (EGIL): Proposals for the immunologic classification of acute leukemias. *Leukemia* 1995;9:1783.

Gelb AB et al: Detection of immunophenotypic abnormalities in paraffin-embedded B-lineage non-Hodgkin's lymphomas. *Am J Clin Pathol* 1994;102:825.

Hurwitz CA et al: Asynchronous antigen expression in B lineage acute lymphoblastic leukemia. *Blood* 1988;72:299.

Knapp W et al: Flow cytometric analysis of cell-surface and intracellular antigens in leukemia diagnosis. *Cytometry* 1994;18:187.

National Committee for Clinical Laboratory Standards. *Clinical Applications of Flow Cytometry: Immunophenotyping of Leukemic Cells; Proposed Guideline.* NCCLS Document H43-P, December 1993.

Pui C-H et al: Clinical and biologic relevance of immunologic marker studies in childhood acute lymphoblastic leukemia. *Blood* 1993;82:889.

Raimondi SC: Current status of cytogenetic research in childhood acute lymphoblastic leukemia. *Blood* 1993;81:2237.

Rassidakis GZ et al: Diagnosis and subclassification of follicle center and mantle cell lymphomas on fine needle aspirates: A cytologic and immunocytochemical approach based on the Revised European-American Lymphoma (REAL) Classification. *Cancer Cytopathol* 1999;87:216.

Romana SP: High frequency of t(12;21) in childhood B-lineage acute lymphoblastic leukemia. *Blood* 1995;86:4263.

Segal GH et al: CD5-expressing B-cell non-Hodgkin's lymphomas with *bcl*-1 gene rearrangement have a relatively homogeneous immunophenotype and are associated with an overall poor progosis. *Blood* 1995;85:1570.

Sullivan MP et al: Clinical and biological heterogeneity of childhood B cell acute lymphoblastic leukemia: Implications for clinical trials. *Leukemia* 1990;4:6.

MALIGNANT DISORDERS OF B & T LYMPHOCYTES
Bennett JM et al: Proposals for the classification of chronic (mature) B and T lymphoid leukemias. *J Clin Pathol* 1989;42:567.

Foucar K: Chronic lymphoid leukemias and lymphoproliferative disorders. *Mod Pathol* 1999;12:141.

Harris NL et al: A revised European-American classification of lymphoid neoplasms: A proposal from the International Lymphoma Study Group. *Blood* 1994;84:1361.

Jaffe ES: Hematopathology: Integration of morphologic features and biologic markers for diagnosis. *Mod Pathol* 1999;12:109.

National Cancer Institute Sponsored Study of Classifications of Non-Hodgkin's Lymphomas. *Cancer* 1982;49:2112.

Swerdlow SH: Small B cell lymphomas of the lymph nodes and spleen: Practical insights to diagnosis and pathogenesis. *Mod Pathol* 1999;12:125.

Zukerberg LR et al: Diffuse low-grade B-cell lymphomas: Four clinically distinct subtypes defined by a combination of morphologic and immunophenotypic features. *Am J Clin Pathol* 1993;100:373.

Acute Lymphoblastic Leukemia & Lymphoblastic Lymphoma (B- & T-Cell Types)
Cimino Get al: prognostic relevance of ALL-1 gene rearrangement in infant acute leukemias. *Leukemia* 1995; 9:391.

Copelan EA, McGuire EA: The biology and treatment of acute lymphoblastic leukemia in adults. *Blood* 1995; 85:1151.

Pui C-H et al: Biology and treatment of infant leukemias. *Leukemia* 1995;9:762.

Pui C-H et al: Childhood leukemias. *New Engl J Med* 1995;332:1618.

B-Cell Chronic Lymphocytic Leukemia & Small Lymphocytic Lymphoma
Caligaris-Cappio F: B-chronic lymphocytic leukemia: A malignancy of anti-self B cells. *Blood* 1996;87:2615.

O'Brien S et al: Advances in the biology and treatment of B-cell chronic lymphocytic leukemia. *Blood* 1995;85:307.

Pangalis GA et al: B-cell chronic lymphocytic leukemia, small lymphocytic lymphoma and lymphoplasmacytic lymphoma, including Waldenstrom's macroglobulinemia: A clinical, morphologic and biologic spectrum of similar disorders. *Semin Hematol* 1999;36:104.

Rozman C, Montserrat E: Chronic lymphocytic leukemia. *New Engl J Med* 1995;333:1052.

Mantle Cell Lymphoma
Banks PM et al: Mantle cell lymphoma. A proposal for unification of morphologic, immunologic, and molecular data. *Am J Surg Pathol* 1992;16:637.

Campo E et al: Mantle cell lymphoma. *Semin Hematol* 1999;36:115.

De Boer CJ et al: Cyclin D1 protein analysis in the diagnosis of mantle cell lymphoma. *Blood* 1995;86:2715.

Norton AJ et al: Mantle cell lymphoma: Natural history defined in a serially biopsied population over a 20-year period. *Ann Oncol* 1995;6:249.

Marginal Zone Lymphomas
Catovsky D, Matutes E: Splenic lymphoma with circulating villous lymphocytes/splenic marginal zone lymphoma. *Semin Hematol* 1999;36:148.

Dierlamm J et al: Marginal zone B-cell lymphomas of different sites share similar cytogenetic and morphologic features. *Blood* 1996;87:299.

Isaacson PG: Mucosa-associated lymphoid tissue lymphoma. *Semin Hematol* 1999;36:139.

Fisher RI et al: A clinical analysis of two indolent lymphoma entities: Mantle cell lymphoma and marginal zone lymphoma (including the mucosa-associated lymphoid tissue and monocytoid B cell subcategories): A Southwest Oncology Group study. *Blood* 1995;85:1075.

Bayerdorffer E et al: Regression of primary gastric lymphoma of mucosa-associated lymphoid tissue type after cure of *Helicobacter pylori* infection. MALT Lymphoma Study Group. *Lancet* 1995;345:1591.

Follicular Center Lymphomas

Symmans WF et al: Transformation of follicular lymphoma. Expression of p53 and bcl-2 oncoprotein, apoptosis and cell proliferation. *Acta Cytol* 1995;39:673.

Nathwani BN et al: Clinical significance of follicular lymphoma with monocytoid B cells. *Hum Pathol* 1999;30:263.

Hairy Cell Leukemia

Bouroncle BA: Thirty-five years in the progress of hairy cell leukemia. *Leukemia Lymphoma* 1994;14:1.

Chang KL et al: Hairy cell leukemia: Current status. *Am J Clin Pathol* 1992;97:719.

Plasma Cell Dyscrasias

Berenson JR et al: Multiple myeloma: the cells of origin—a two-way street. *Leukemia* 1998;12:121.

Ruiz AG, San MJ: Cell surface markers in multiple myeloma. *Mayo Clin Proc* 1994;69:684.

Chen BJ, Epstein J: Circulating clonal lymphocytes in myeloma constitute a minor subpopulation of B cells. *Blood* 1996;87:1972.

Lymphoplasmscytoid Lymphoma & Waldenström's Macroglobulinemia

Dimopoulos MA, Alexanian R: Waldenström's macroglobulinemia. *Blood* 1994;83:1452.

Diffuse Large-Cell Lymphoma

Hermine O et al: Prognostic significance of bcl-2 protein expression in aggressive non-Hodgkin's lymphoma. *Blood* 1996;87:265.

Offit K et al: Rearrangement of the *bcl-6* oncogene as a prognostic marker in diffuse large-cell lymphoma. *New Engl J Med* 1994;331:74.

Burkitt's & Burkitt-like Lymphomas

van Hasselt EJ, Broadhead R: Burkitt's lymphoma: A case file study of 160 patients treated in Queen Elizabeth Central Hospital from 1988 to 1992. *Paediatr Haematol Oncol* 1995;12:283.

LGL Leukemias

Loughran TP Jr: Clonal diseases of large granular lymphocytes. *Blood* 1993;82:1.

T-Prolymphocytic Leukemia & T-Cell CLL

Foon KA, Gale RP: Is there a T cell form of chronic lymphocytic leukemia? *Leukemia* 1992;6:867.

Matutes E et al: Clinical and laboratory features of 78 cases of T-prolymphocytic leukemia. *Blood* 1991;78:3269.

Matutes E, Catovsky D: Mature T-cell leukemias and leukemia/lymphoma syndromes: Review of our experience in 175 cases. *Leukemia Lymphoma* 1991;4:81.

Cutaneous T-Cell Lymphoma

Kim YH, Hoppe RT: Mycosis fungoides and the Sezary syndrome. *Semin Oncol* 1999;26:276.

Weinberg JM et al: The clonal nature of circulating Sézary cells. *Blood* 1995;86:4257.

Adult T-Cell Leukemia-Lymphoma

Shimoyama M: Diagnostic criteria and classification of clinical subtypes of adult T-cell leukemia-lymphoma. A report from the Lymphoma Study Group (1984–87). *Br J Haematol* 1991;79:428.

Peripheral T-Cell Lymphomas

Horning SJ et al: Clinical and phenotypic diversity of T cell lymphomas. *Blood* 1986;67:1578.

Cheng A-L et al: Direct comparison of peripheral T cell lymphoma with diffuse B-cell lymphoma of comparable histologic grades: Should peripheral T cell lymphomas be considered separately? *J Clin Oncol* 1989;7:725.

Anaplastic Large-Cell Lymphoma

Filippa DA et al: CD30 (Ki-1)-positive malignant lymphomas: Clinical, immunophenotypic, histologic and genetic characteristics and differences with Hodgkin's disease. *Blood* 1996;87:2905.

Kadin ME: Ki-1/CD30+ (anaplastic) large cell lymphoma: Maturation of a clinicopathologic entity with prospects of effective therapy. *J Clin Oncol* 1994;12:884.

Lamant L et al: High incidence of the t(2;5)(p23;q35) translocation on anaplastic large cell lymphoma and its lack of detection in Hodgkin's disease. Comparison of cytogenetic analysis, reverse transcriptase-polymerase chain reaction, and P-80 immunostaining. *Blood* 1996; 87:284.

Other T-Cell Neoplasms

Chan JKC: Peripheral T-cell and NK-cell neoplasms: an integrated approach to diagnosis. *Mod Pathol* 1999;12: 177.

Jaffe ES: Classification of natural killer (NK) and NK-like T cell malignancies. *Blood* 1996;87:1207.

HODGKIN'S DISEASE

Pan LX et al: Nodular lymphocyte predominance Hodgkin's disease: A monoclonal or polyclonal B cell disorder? *Blood* 1996;87:2428.

Stein H, Hummel M: Cellular origin and clonality of classic Hodgkin's lymphoma: Immunophenotypic and molecular studies. *Semin Hematol* 1999;36:253.

Weber-Mattiesen K et al: Numerical chromosome aberrations are present within the CD30+ Hodgkin and Reed-Sternberg cells in 100% of analyzed cases of Hodgkin's disease. *Blood* 1995;86:1484.

HISTIOCYTIC MALIGNANCIES

Willman CL et al: Langerhans-cell histiocytosis (Histiocytosis X)-A clonal proliferative disease. *New Engl J Med* 1994;331:154.

Cline MJ: Histiocytes and histiocytosis. *Blood* 1994;84: 2840.

BENIGN CONDITIONS MIMICKING NEOPLASMS

Cogan E et al: Brief report: Clonal proliferation of type 2 helper T cells in a man with the hypereosinophilic syndrome. *New Engl J Med* 1994;330:535.

Janka G: Infection- and malignancy-associated hemophagocytic syndromes. *Hematol/Oncol Clin North Am* 1998;12:435.

HEMATOLOGIC PROLIFERATIONS IN IMMUNOSUPPRESSED PATIENTS

Herndier BG et al: Pathogenesis of AIDS lymphomas. *AIDS* 1994;8:1025.

Knowles DM: Immunodeficiency-associated lymphoproliferative disorders. *Mod Pathol* 1999;12:200.

Bacterial Diseases

44

John L. Ryan, MD, PhD, & Steven J. Projan, PhD

Immunity to bacterial infections is mediated by both cellular and humoral mechanisms. Bacteria express many different surface antigens and secrete a variety of virulence factors (eg, toxins) that may trigger immune responses. Because the topic of bacterial immunity is vast, attention in this chapter focuses on three principal types of immunity to bacteria, with examples for which pathogenesis and host responses are well characterized.

1. The first is immunity to **toxigenic bacterial infections.** Bacterial exotoxins and endotoxins are important in the pathogenesis of specific diseases. Exotoxins are the sole virulence factor in certain toxigenic bacterial infections, and immunity directed against these toxins can completely prevent disease.

2. The second is immunity to **encapsulated bacteria.** These organisms evade phagocytosis by coating themselves with polysaccharide. Encapsulated bacteria may be gram-positive or gram-negative, and vaccines containing purified capsular antigens may generate protective immunity.

3. The third is immunity to **intracellular bacteria.** These bacteria avoid the host immune response because they grow inside cells, particularly phagocytes. The same evasive mechanism is used by many fungal and parasitic pathogens. Cellular immunity mediated by macrophages that are activated by specific lymphocytes and their products is the critical mode of host defense against this group of bacteria.

SERODIAGNOSIS

Serodiagnosis of bacterial diseases is of value only in specific circumstances. IgG antibody is long-lived, and its presence, although indicative of previous infection or immunization, gives little or no information on current bacterial infection. IgM antibody is usually produced within days to a few weeks after exposure to antigen, and thus its presence suggests recent exposure in most cases. As with viral diseases, serial determinations of antibody levels with rising titers are of greater diagnostic value, but because of the time intervals required, they are usually of little clinical value.

In general, culture of specific pathogens is required to confirm the diagnosis of a bacterial disease. Serologic tests may aid in diagnosis when diseases are caused by bacteria that are difficult to grow. *Brucella* is one such species. These organisms are difficult to culture from patients' specimens, and no useful delayed hypersensitivity skin test is available. A serum agglutination test for antibodies using *B abortus* antigen is often used to help diagnose brucellosis. Most mycobacteria are also difficult to grow, but antibody titers are not helpful in diagnosis. Thus, in contrast to viral and fungal pathogens, the serologic tests in bacterial infections remain primarily a tool for epidemiologic studies rather than for clinical diagnosis. Nevertheless, most bacteria induce specific antibody responses, which, in most cases, can be easily measured in serum. As discussed, these antibody responses are often critical in determining the host response to an infecting agent.

EXOTOXINS & ENDOTOXINS

Exotoxins are noxious proteins secreted by many bacteria. These toxins are often heat-labile and thus can be heat-inactivated for use as vaccines to prevent toxigenic bacterial disease. Many bacteria produce more than one protein exotoxin, making vaccine development more difficult. Endotoxins are somatic lipopolysaccharide-protein complexes. These complex antigens are located in the outer membrane of all gram-negative bacteria. Toxicologic activity is associated with the lipid A component of the endotoxin, whereas the serologic determinants are polysaccharides. Antibody directed against specific polysaccharides can be protective both by enhancing phagocytosis directly and by fixing complement for lysis. Unfortunately, from an immune standpoint, antigenic differences in the polysaccharide components of endotoxins exist among strains of bacteria. Thus, in general, infection with one strain does not generate protective immunity to reinfection with a different strain of the same species. IgM and IgG antibodies directed against the lipid A component of lipopolysaccharide have different capacities to neutralize the infectivity of gram-negative bacteria. It appears that IgM is a more potent neutralizing antibody than IgG. This is particularly true for cross-reacting antibody directed against core polysaccharide or lipid A determinants of gram-negative bacteria. Passive administration of human or murine IgM directed against core determinants of endotoxin has been attempted for treatment of gram-negative sepsis. These attempts have not been efficacious except in selected subgroups of patients.

TOXIGENIC BACTERIAL DISEASES

In this section, two groups of toxigenic diseases are considered. In the first group, an exotoxin is the sole virulence determinant, and vaccines directed at the exotoxin can generate effective immunity. In the second group, toxins are major virulence factors, but other pathogenic factors exist, making specific immune responses less effective in disease prevention (Figure 44–1). Antibody to toxins can neutralize the toxin by several mechanisms, including enhancing clearance by macrophages or blocking binding sites on toxin for its cellular receptors.

Clostridium Species

Clostridia are obligate anaerobic, spore-forming gram-positive rods, which cause a variety of clinical diseases. *Clostridium tetani* is the cause of tetanus. Disease occurs when spores are introduced into deep wounds from contaminated soil or foreign bodies.

After these spores germinate, a potent neurotoxin called tetanospasmin is produced. Tetanospasmin binds to the presynaptic membrane at the neuromuscular junction, it is then internalized and transported via the axon to the spinal cord. The toxin blockades neurotransmitter release from spinal inhibitory neurons leading to generalized muscular spasms, or **tetany.** A vaccine prepared from the inactivated toxin, termed *toxoid,* prevents disease by generating antibodies that neutralize the toxin. It is recommended that all children be immunized with tetanus toxoid soon after birth (see Chapter 50). Subsequent boosts of immunity to toxoid are required every 10 years during adult life to maintain a protective level of antibody. Antigenic variation in tetanus toxins does not appear to be significant because the single vaccine is protective.

Clostridium botulinum is another exotoxin-producing species for which immunity requires neutralizing antibodies to the toxin (antitoxin). *C botulinum* causes botulism, which is primarily a food-borne disease, occurring when toxin or spores are ingested from contaminated food. The botulinum toxin, which is quite heat-labile, acts by inhibiting the release of acetylcholine neurotransmitter at the neuromuscular junctions. This produces diplopia, dysphagia, and, in severe cases, respiratory arrest. Botulism is treated with antitoxin, which is equine antiserum directed against the three most common toxin serotypes: A, B, and E. A pentavalent toxoid (A, B, C, D, E) is distributed by the Centers for Disease Control and Prevention (CDC). This toxoid is

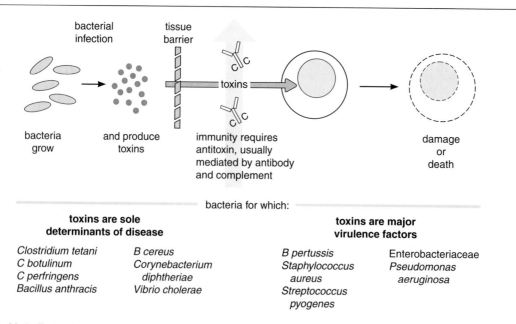

Figure 44–1. Toxigenic bacterial infections. In this group of bacterial infections, antibody to protein toxins and complement play a protective role in enhancing survival.

prepared from formalin-treated toxins, which are adsorbed to aluminum phosphate to enhance immunogenicity. Natural immunity does not occur, because immunogenic doses of these toxins are lethal. Recently, type A botulinum toxin (Botox) has been used both therapeutically and cosmetically for eyelid spasm and wrinkles because of its long-lived paralytic properties. At this point it is unclear whether repeated IM injection of active toxin elicts an immune response.

Several other *Clostridium* strains cause pyogenic infections that are mediated, in part, by cytopathic exotoxins. The most common are soft tissue infections caused by *Clostridium perfringens,* which releases a potent lecithinase called α toxin. This toxin has been associated with massive intravascular hemolysis in uncontrolled infection. It is associated with clostridial myonecrosis or, gas gangrene. *C perfringens* also secretes several other toxins, including a diarrheagenic enterotoxin (CPE) that is an important cause of food poisoning. Therapy with antitoxins has not been useful in treating diseases caused by *C perfringens* because the organism secretes such a wide variety of toxins.

Bacillus Species

Bacillus species are facultative anaerobic gram-positive rods that can form spores. They are similar to clostridia, except for their facultative anaerobic metabolism. One of the first pathogenic bacteria to be studied was *Bacillus anthracis,* the only nonmotile species in the genus. The disease anthrax is caused by human contact with animal products contaminated by *B anthracis.* Animals are infected by ingestion of the bacteria or spores in the environment. Pathogenicity depends on toxin production, and the disease can be prevented by vaccination against attenuated bacteria. Pasteur and Roux were the first to show that vaccination could prevent anthrax in animals. The anthrax exotoxin is complex, consisting of at least three components: protective antigen, edema factor, and lethal factor. The protective antigen, which is not toxic alone, induces immunity and is the major component of current vaccines. *B anthracis* has also been shown to have a polysaccharide capsule, which may contribute to the virulence of this organism.

Bacillus cereus represents another important toxigenic *Bacillus* species. It is a common cause of food poisoning. Several toxins, including a pyogenic toxin, enterotoxins, and a sphingomyelinase are produced. Little is known about protective immunity to these bacteria.

Corynebacterium diphtheriae

Corynebacteria are facultative anaerobic gram-positive rods that do not form spores. The most important species is *Corynebacterium diphtheriae,* the cause of diphtheria. This organism colonizes the mucous membranes of the posterior pharynx and elabo-

rates a potent exotoxin. The toxin kills cells by covalently linking adenosine diphosphoribose to elongation factor 2, which is required for cellular protein biosynthesis. Immunity to diphtheria depends on the presence of antibody to the toxin. Diphtheria toxoid, a formalin-inactivated toxin preparation, is currently used worldwide to vaccinate infants against diphtheria. Immunity to diphtheria is assessed by using the Schick test, in which small amounts of toxin and toxoid are injected intradermally at different sites. If no response is observed at either site after 48 hours, the patient is immune to the toxin (has circulating antitoxin) and is not hypersensitive to the toxoid. If necrosis occurs at the toxin site and response at the toxoid site, the patient does not have protective antibody. An immediate reaction at both sites indicates allergy to the proteins. A delayed reaction at one or both sites indicates cellular immunity to the proteins. The Schick test has been very useful in assessing immunity to *C diphtheriae,* but has been largely replaced by antibody titers. Nevertheless, it has provided insight into the importance of maintaining adequate circulating antibody to toxin to ameliorate or prevent clinical infection.

Vibrio cholerae

The vibrios are curved, gram-negative bacilli with polar flagellae. Infection with *Vibrio cholerae,* the agent of cholera, occurs after ingestion of contaminated water. Organisms multiply in the gut and release an enterotoxin (cholera toxin), which binds to epithelial cells and triggers massive secretion of fluid and electrolytes. Severe diarrhea may occur within hours after infection, and the fluid loss is often life-threatening, particularly among infants and young children. Cholera is unique among the toxigenic diseases in that antibody to the toxin does not fully prevent disease. Infection with *V cholerae* induces systemic and mucosal antibody. Mucosal IgA, which prevents attachment of the bacteria in the gut, may be the most important form of immunity. Cholera vaccines induce short-term protection and elicit only IgM and IgG responses unless administered orally. Neither IgM nor IgG functions well in the intestinal lumen. Despite extensive research an oral vaccine that confers long-lasting immunity has yet to be developed.

Bordetella pertussis

Pertussis (whooping cough) is caused by mucosal infection with *Bordetella pertussis,* a small, gram-negative coccobacillary organism that replicates in bronchial mucosa. Infection is characterized by paroxysmal coughing, which can result in significant morbidity in young children. *B pertussis* contains several antigens that may elicit immune responses, but the critical factors in immunity to this organism are not fully understood. Killed whole bacteria continue to be used as a vaccine, but acellular vaccines containing three to five components have proved efficacious and are in use. In fact a pertussis toxin toxoid by itself provides protective immunity. Pertussis vaccine is given in combination with diphtheria toxoid and tetanus toxoid (DPT) to infants at 2, 4, and 6 months of age, with boosters usually given 1 year later and again before the children begin to attend school. Immunity to pertussis is relatively short-lived, lasting only 3 years after completion of primary immunization or boosting. Antibody that prevents attachment of the bacteria to respiratory epithelium appears to be the first line of defense, with antitoxin providing further protection against a protein exotoxin produced by the bacteria.

The presence of *B pertussis* in the DPT combination vaccine may enhance the antibody response to both protein toxoids (DT) because the lipopolysaccharide in the outer membrane of *B pertussis* is a potent immune adjuvant. Thus, it is advantageous as well as convenient to use the combined vaccine, but the acellular form is better tolerated, producing fewer adverse reactions while maintaining efficacy.

Staphylococcus aureus

Staphylococci are facultative anaerobic, nonmotile gram-positive cocci that are most often seen as clusters in gram-stained specimens. *Staphylococcus aureus* is probably the single most prevalent pathogen in skin and soft tissue infections. Its virulence has been studied intensively, but the mechanism remains obscure. The primary line of defense against staphylococci is the polymorphonuclear leukocyte, which phagocytoses and kills the bacteria. *S aureus* produces a vast number of virulence factors, including secreted toxins, which have been shown to contribute to its pathogenicity. Production of coagulase, a factor that can bind and activate fibrinogen, defines the species *S aureus*. At least four separate hemolysins are also produced. A nonhemolytic leukocidin is cytotoxic for granulocytes. In addition, *S aureus* secretes several enterotoxins, a pair of related exfoliative toxin associated with epidermal necrolysis, and an exotoxin associated with the toxic shock syndrome.

The immune response to *S aureus* infections is inadequate in that previous infection does not protect the host from reinfection. Most clinical isolates of *S aureus* are capsule producers and among nosocomial isolates of methicillin-resistant *S aureus* (MRSA) two capsular types (5 and 8) predominate, but the capsular polysaccharides do not generate protective antibody. Conjugation of these polysaccharides to protein carriers, however, may elicit protective antibody. Similarly, antibodies to the toxic shock exotoxin and to the exfoliative exotoxins seem to prevent the specific clinical syndromes caused by these toxins. Pyogenic *S aureus* infections occur, however, despite the presence of multiple antibodies against cellular components in the host. Only the number and functional capacity of granulocytes are critically im-

portant in the defense against *S aureus*. Confounding the immune response to *S aureus* is protein A, which is produced by all strains. Protein A, which is anchored to the bacterial cell surface, binds to the Fc portion of IgG and may well provide immunologic camouflage for the bacteria, which blocks the immune response.

Another staphlococcal species associated with human disease is *S epidermidis*. This strain produces fewer toxins and is associated primarily with bacteremias in patients with plastic catheters or other indwelling devices. *S epidermidis,* as the name implies, is a major constituent bacterium of the skin flora. It adheres to catheters or other materials by means of extracellular polysaccharides, which inhibits the ability of granulocytes to function properly. Protective immunity to this organism also does not appear to develop because repeated infections may occur in susceptible hosts. Common to both *S aureus* and *S epidermidis* is a polysaccharide intercellular adhesin (PIA) that has been reported to be a protective antigen.

Streptococcus Species

Streptococci are a diverse group of catalase-negative, facultatively anaerobic gram-positive cocci that cause a variety of toxigenic and pyogenic infections in humans. *Streptococcus pyogenes* (a β-hemolytic, group A streptococcus)is the most important bacterial cause of pharyngitis. Late sequelae, such as rheumatic fever and glomerulonephritis, probably result from infection with certain hypervirulent strains of this species.

Most streptococcal infections do not confer immunity unless the syndrome is toxon-mediated, such as the streptococcal pyogenic exotoxins associated with scarlet fever and, more recently with toxic shock-like syndrome. The antigenic composition of streptococci is complex, with approximately 18 group-specific carbohydrate antigens lettered A–R. These antigens are useful for classifying streptococci, but they do not elicit protective immunity. Group A streptococci contain another set of type-specific M antigens, known as M proteins (more than 80 types exist). Genetic analysis of the "*emm* genes" which encode the various M proteins have replaced serology intyping with more than 90 "*emm* types" currently reported based on nucleotide sequences. These proteins are antiphagocytic factors and enhance the virulence of group A streptococci. The M proteins do generate protective IgG antibody, but because many serotypes of M protein exist, reinfection with another strain is common.

Streptococci of groups A, B, C, F, and G produce many extracellular products that may elicit protective immunity. Streptolysins O and S are cytopathic proteins that inhibit phagocytosis and killing by leukocytes. A variety of proteinases exist, including streptokinase and other degradative enzymes such as hyaluronidase and deoxyribonuclease, which enhance the pathogenicity of the organism. Antibodies may be produced to all of these factors during infection. The widely used Streptozyme test is a hemagglutination procedure that detects a variety of antibodies against streptococcal enzymes.

Group D streptococci have been reclassified as enterococci and are antigenically distinct from other streptococci in that they do not possess a group-specific carbohydrate antigen, but they do have a group-specific glycerol teichoic acid antigen. Because of their innate resistance to most antibiotics, enterococci have emerged as a leading cause of nosocomial infections in the United States.

Most of the streptococci that normally colonize the human oropharynx do not possess group-specific antigens and are classified in the viridans group. Many individual strains may be defined by biochemical tests, but none of these streptococci are prominent toxin producers. They are active in causing periodontal diseases and together with the staphylococci are the most common causes of infective endocarditis. Little is known about protective immunity to this diverse group of organisms. Recent research has focused on the use of recombinant strains of viridans streptococcus, *S gordonii,* as a live, attenuated adjuvant–antigen delivery system especially to produce a secretory IgA response.

Gram-Negative Rods

Gram-negative rods produce a variety of toxins and are responsible for many infectious diseases. The family Enterobacteriaceae comprises five major genera: *Escherichia, Klebsiella, Proteus, Yersinia,* and *Erwinia.* These are all glucose-fermenting, nonspore-forming bacilli. All members of the family Enterobacteriaceae, but particularly *Escherichia* and *Salmonella,* have undergone extensive immunologic analyses. They are serotyped on the basis of O antigens (polysaccharides associated with the lipopolysaccharide component of the outer membrane), K antigens (polysaccharide capsular components), and H antigens (proteins associated with flagella).

Some of these organisms are partially responsible for contributing to the immune pathogenesis of the spondyloarthropathies. The well-known association of the major histocompatibility complex (MHC) class I molecule human leukocyte antigen HLA-B27 and ankylosing spondylitis, as well the association of the disease with preceding enteric infection, has stimulated a search for molecular mimicry, that is, identity between epitopes on a bacterium and one in the human host. The immune response to *Klebsiella pneumoniae* elicits antibody that can bind to HLA-B27 on the surface of synovial lining cells. Similar molecular mimicry has been shown for *Shigella flexneri,* which produces an arthritogenic epitope that is shared by HLA-B27 antigen. Thus, the immune response to certain members of the Enterobacteriaceae may result in autoimmune disease in selected hosts.

Each member of the family Enterobacteriaceae contains an endotoxin. This endotoxin is a lipopolysaccharide–protein complex in the outer membrane and contains the O-specific serologic group. The biologically active components of the endotoxin are the lipid A and certain lipoproteins associated with the lipopolysaccharide.

Enterotoxins are also produced by many members of the Enterobacteriaceae, particularly *Escherichia coli. E coli* has at least two enterotoxins: an immunogenic heat-labile toxin structurally similar to cholera toxin, and a nonimmunogenic heat-stable toxin. More typical exotoxins are also related to certain strains of *E coli, Shigella,* and *Yersinia.*

Immunity to the Enterobacteriaceae is achieved early in life after colonization of the gut with *E coli.* Antibodies against K and O antigens are generated and are protective against autologous serotypes. Prior to the development of antibody, the neonate is susceptible to systemic and particularly to central nervous system infection by *E coli.* In adult life, these bacteria cause opportunistic as well as enteric diseases. Attempts to transfer passive immunity with antiserum to *E coli* have proved effective in both animal and some human studies. Antibodies directed against the endotoxin component may be able to help prevent the morbidity and mortality associated with sepsis in certain patient groups, but clinical trials to establish this have not yet been done.

Pseudomonas aeruginosa is the most clinically important nonfermenting gram-negative rod and has been the subject of extensive immunologic analysis. It characteristically produces exotoxin A, a cytolytic factor with a similar mechanism of action to diphtheria toxin. Antibodies directed against exotoxin A as well as the lipopolysaccharide appear to be important in immunity to infection with *P aeruginosa.* Different serotyping schemes have been used to define *P aeruginosa* for epidemiologic purposes. Multivalent vaccines containing several serotypes to protect immunocompromised patients from invasive *Pseudomonas* infection have been investigated but have not proven efficacious. *Pseudomonas* is a virulent opportunistic pathogen that commonly infects immunocompromised patients. The role of antibody to endotoxin in ameliorating human disease has been shown in animals by using homologous and heterologous antisera to protect them against lethal *P aeruginosa* infections.

Many of the gram-negative bacteria, including the enterics but also including *Pseudomonas aeruginosa,* use an ingenious method, referred to as type III secretion, to inject toxic exoproteins produced in the bacterial cytoplasm into host target cells. These target cells are often macrophages, and the toxins have been shown to severely affect host cells, often inducing apoptosis. Because they avoid the extracellular environment, these toxins and their toxoids have not given rise to protective immunity in animal models and are probably not viable vaccine candidates.

ENCAPSULATED BACTERIA

Bacteria that express capsular polysaccharide present a unique problem for the immune system. Capsular polysaccharide inhibits phagocytosis by both macrophages and polymorphonuclear leukocytes. Effective phagocytosis requires functional leukocyte receptors for the Fc region of immunoglobulin and C3b or C3bi (Figure 44–2). Opsonization of encapsulated bacteria with antibody and complement is necessary for phagocytes to efficiently ingest and kill these pathogens. The charge and hydrophilicity of unopsonized encapsulated bacteria inhibit phagocytosis by interfering with attachment of leukocytes and bacteria. Immaturity of humoral immunity in the very young and decline of humoral immunity in the elderly probably account for the susceptibility of individuals at these stages of life to invasive disease by encapsulated bacteria.

Bacterial vaccines hold great promise for enhancing immunity against encapsulated bacteria. Because polysaccharides are relatively poor immunogens, particularly in infants, complexes of protein with polysaccharides have proven to be more effective vaccines. Coupling of weak antigens with other types of adjuvants may also improves the efficacy of vaccines.

Streptococcus pneumoniae

Streptococcus pneumoniae strains, commonly called pneumococci, differ from other streptococci in that they contain complex polysaccharide capsules that consitute the major virulence determinant in the species. Pneumococci are respiratory pathogens that colonize upper airways and cause bronchitis or pneumonia after aspiration of respiratory secretions. The capsule inhibits alveolar macrophage phagocytosis and allows the pneumococcus to multiply in the lung. Patients with abnormal mucocillary reflexes or decreased alveolar macrophage function are more susceptible to pulmonary infection. Patients with decreased systemic clearance of bacteria are susceptible to disseminated disease.

Type-specific antibody is elicited and is protective, but there are more than 80 serotypes of pneumococci although relatively few of these serotypes represent a large majority of infectious strains. Thus, reinfection with a different serotype is common in susceptible persons. The polysaccharide capsule is sometimes cross-reactive with the capsular polysaccharides of different genera, including *Haemophilus* and *Klebsiella*. A vaccine containing capsular polysaccharide from the 23 most prevalent or virulent serotypes is available for adult patients at high risk for pneumococcal disease. Conjugated protein–polysaccharide vaccines containing the most common infecting serotypes have been developed and have been shown to prevent disease in young children.

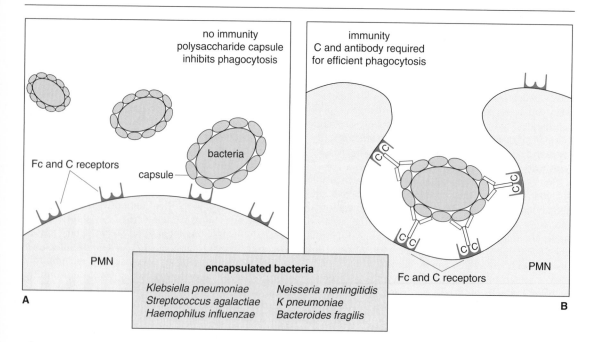

Figure 44–2. Encapsulated bacteria. **A:** Polysaccharide capsules allow bacterial multiplication by avoiding receptor-mediated phagocytosis. **B:** If specific antibody to the capsule is present, both antibody and complement serve as opsonins to enhance the uptake of bacteria by host phagocytes. *Abbreviation:* PMN = polymorphonuclear neutrophil.

Streptococcus agalactiae (Group B)

The group B streptococci are a leading cause of neonatal meningitis. Most disease is of late onset because of colonization, then subsequent infection of the infant occurs by members of the vaginal flora during parturition. Group B organisms contain four major capsular serotypes. Sialic acid, one of the carbohydrate components of group B streptococcal capsular polysaccharide, can block complement activation. This prevents a key nonspecific defense mechanism in infants who are without adequate antibody levels. Type-specific antibodies are protective for group B streptococcal disease. Both passive immunization with IgG antibody to capsular polysaccharides and active immunization with polysaccharides and protein–polysaccharide conjugates to prevent group B streptococcal disease in the neonatal period are under investigation, as is maternal immunization during pregnancy.

Haemophilus influenzae

Of the several species of *Haemophilus* that are known, *Haemophilus influenzae* is the most prevalent pathogen. Several distinct capsular serotypes have been defined, but type b *H influenzae* is responsible for most clinical disease. *H influenzae* is a respiratory pathogen that colonizes the oropharynx and causes bronchitis, pneumonia, or disseminated infection when local or systemic host defense factors are compromised. The type b capsule is a polyribitol phosphate. The susceptibility of a given host to infection is directly related to serum levels of bactericidal antibody. Maternal IgG is lost within a few months after birth, and natural antibody is acquired by 3–4 years of age. The development of natural antibody may be related to colonization and subsequent immunization with nonpathogenic members of the family Enterobacteriaceae that contain cross-reactive capsular polysaccharides. *H influenzae* type b capsular polysaccharide (polyriboseribitol phosphate, PRP) is a weak immunogen, and vaccines have not been effective in children younger than 2 years. However, conjugate vaccines with diphtheria toxoid, tetanus toxoid, and outer membrane proteins linked to PRP have proven effective in immunizing children between 6 months and 2 years of age. In few bacterial diseases has the protective role of antibody been so clearly demonstrated as in *H influenzae* type b disease. The widespread use of the new conjugate vaccines has nearly eradicated meningitis due to *H influenzae* in the United States.

Neisseria Species

These are gram-negative cocci containing high levels of cytochrome *c* oxidase. The two pathogenic species are *Neisseria gonorrhoeae* (gonococcus) and *Neisseria meningitidis* (meningococcus). Anticapsular antibody has no definite role in immunity to gonococci. Repeated infections with gonococci are quite common. Mucosal antibody directed against surface proteins appears to have some protective value, and the complement system is particularly important in the maintenance of bactericidal activity. The meningococcus normally inhabits the pharynx without producing disease. This provides a reservoir for outbreaks and produces some immunity in the host. The critical antigenic components of the meningococcus are capsular polysaccharides, and 13 distinct serotypes can elicit group-specific protective antibody. IgM antibody appears to be more protective than does IgG, perhaps because of its more potent complement-fixing activity. Patients deficient in the terminal complement components C6, C7, C8, or properdin are susceptible to recurrent neisserial infections. A polyvalent vaccine containing polysaccharide from groups A, C, Y, and W-135 is available. Group B capsular polysaccharides are cross-reactive with *E coli* capsular polysaccharides (K1 antigens), and no vaccine is available against this strain. The importance of antibody in protection against meningococcal disease is underscored by the peak incidence of disease, which occurs at about 1 year of age, when maternal antibody has waned and acquired antibody has not yet been produced.

Klebsiella pneumoniae

Klebsiella species are members of the family Enterobacteriaceae that are characterized by polysaccharide capsules with more than 70 serotypes. Although they are predominantly intestinal organisms that cause opportunistic infections, they are also associated with primary pneumonias. This is probably related to the ability of these bacteria to avoid phagocytosis in the absence of antibody. The capsular polysaccharides found in *Klebsiella* are related to those in *Streptococcus* and *Haemophilus*. The role of specific anticapsular antibodies in *Klebsiella* has not been elucidated. Immunity appears to be multifactorial, with disease most commonly occurring in debilitated patients with depressed host defenses.

Bacteroides fragilis

Bacteroides fragilis and closely related species are obligate anaerobic, nonspore-forming, gram-negative rods that colonize the intestinal tract and are often associated with intraabdominal abscess formation. Unless the mucous membrane barrier of the gastrointestinal or respiratory tract is damaged, *B fragilis* is an inocuous member of the normal flora. In the presence of tissue necrosis or trauma, *B fragilis* may be released into a relatively low-oxygen environment, allowing growth and elaboration of several enzymes that potentiate tissue damage. *B fragilis* also contains a capsular polysaccharide that is a key virulence factor in animal models of infection. The capsule mediates resistance to phagocytosis, and capsular antibody enhances the phagocytic killing of these bacteria.

INTRACELLULAR BACTERIAL PATHOGENS

Many bacteria have developed the ability to avoid host defense systems by invading cells so that serum antibody and complement cannot harm them and granulocytes cannot recognize them (Figure 44–3). Some of these bacteria can induce T-lymphocyte-mediated immunity in the same fashion as fungi, parasites, and viruses although this cytotoxic T-lymphocyte (CTL) response occurs less frequently after bacterial invasion than for viral infections. Serum antibody and complement are not markers of resistance for these bacteria. The presence of sensitized T lymphocytes and activated macrophages is the key factor in immunity. Microbial antigens are expressed on the surface of macrophages after the antigens are processed, in conjunction with products of the major histocompatibility complex. In this configuration, macrophages interact with T lymphocytes to produce macrophage-activating factors such as interferon gamma (IFNγ). This complex series of events is required for the expression of effective immunity to intracellular pathogens.

Salmonella Species

Salmonella species are members of the family Enterobacteriaceae and cause a significant proportion of enteric disease. Three major species (*Salmonella ty-* *phi, Salmonella choleraesuis,* and *Salmonella enteritidis*) exist. Based on serologic reactions, more than 1700 types of *S enteritidis* have been discovered. Most invasive disease, such as typhoid fever, is caused by *S typhi,* and it is of great interest that this is the only species of *Salmonella* with a surface capsular antigen. This capsule, therefore, is a key virulence factor for *S typhi.* Antibody against the capsule is not protective, and many typhoid carriers have circulating antibody. This reflects the ability of salmonellae to reside within cells of the reticuloendothelial system. Salmonellae usually enter the body by ingestion and cause enterocolitis if they are present in sufficient numbers to survive the acidic environment of the stomach. If they invade mucosal tissues, they can cause disseminated disease. Immunity to *Salmonella* involves activation of macrophages by sensitized T lymphocytes through lymphokine secretion. Circulating antibodies do not penetrate the cell to eradicate intracellular bacteria. Thus circulating antibody represents a marker of infection, but not of immunity.

Other Intracellular Bacterial Pathogens

Bacterial strains other than *Salmonella* that are intracellular pathogens include *Legionella, Listeria,* and *Brucella. Legionella pneumophila* and related strains are obligate intracellular parasites of macrophages. These bacteria exhibit optimal growth only within

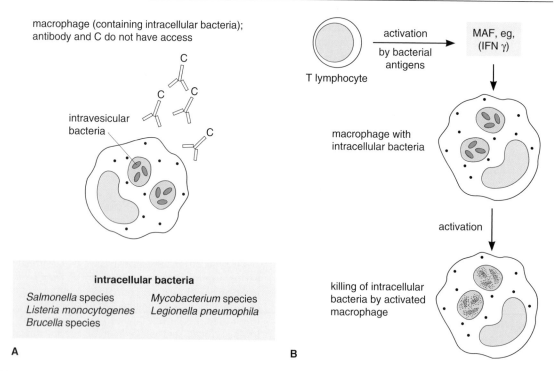

A

macrophage (containing intracellular bacteria); antibody and C do not have access

intravesicular bacteria

C C C C C

intracellular bacteria	
Salmonella species	*Mycobacterium* species
Listeria monocytogenes	*Legionella pneumophila*
Brucella species	

B

T lymphocyte

activation by bacterial antigens → MAF, eg, (IFN γ)

macrophage with intracellular bacteria

activation

killing of intracellular bacteria by activated macrophage

Figure 44–3. Intracellular bacterial pathogens. **A:** Antibody and complement have no access to intracellular pathogens. **B:** Lymphokines mediate macrophage activation, which allows the killing of these bacteria by both oxidative and nonoxidative mechanisms. *Abbreviations:* MAF = macrophage-activating factor; IFNγ = interferon gamma.

cells. Antibodies to serogroup-specific antigens are produced and are useful for diagnostic or epidemiologic studies, but they have not proved to be protective. Antigen-specific T-lymphocyte activation with release of IFNγ and other macrophage-activating factors enhances immunity to *Legionella.*

Listeria monocytogenes is a gram-positive rod similar to *Corynebacterium;* it causes meningeal infections or sepsis in adults and a variety of infections in neonates. Although antibody may play some role in preventing invasion, it is clear that the macrophage is the primary mode of defense against these bacteria. Investigations in animal models have demonstrated that T-lymphocyte function is important in macrophage activation for immunity to *Listeria.*

Brucella species are small coccobacillary gram-negative bacteria that resemble *Haemophilus* in appearance and are spread to humans through contact with animals (zoonosis). Three species are pathogenic for humans and cause systemic disease that may be chronic or subacute. The first is *Brucella abortus* from cattle, the second is *Brucella suis* from pigs, and the third is *Brucella melitensis,* usually from goats and sheep. Diagnosis is often made by serology, but antibody does not confer immunity. Immunity to *Brucella* species is conferred by activated macrophages produced by specifically sensitized T lymphocytes and lymphokines derived from them. The specific antigens that elicit cellular immunity to brucellosis have not been defined.

Mycobacterium Species

The genus *Mycobacterium* comprises a unique group of bacteria characterized by a lipid-rich cell wall that contains *N*-glycolylneuraminic acid. The major pathogenic strain is *Mycobacterium tuberculosis,* although *M avium* complex has emerged as a significant pathogen in patients with acquired immunodeficiency syndrome (AIDS). Prior to the use of HAART (highly active antiretroviral therapy) tuberculosis has been one of the great infectious scourges of humankind throughout history and remains a major world health problem today. One reason is that despite decades of excellent research into the immune mechanisms relating to tuberculosis, an effective vaccine has not been found. Bacillus Calmette-Guèrin (BCG), an attenuated *M bovis* strain, has been used for more than 60 years and is able to confer delayed cutaneous hypersensitivity but no clear-cut cellular immunity. Apparently, BCG lots used for vaccination vary widely, however, which has made evaluation of effectiveness problematic. Serum antibody plays no role in immunity to mycobacterial diseases. Sensitized T lymphocytes and activated macrophages are the critical factors in immunity. The components of the cell wall of *M tuberculosis* that may confer immunity have been analyzed in detail. Both proteins and polysaccharides have immunogenic potential, and some data support a substantive role for the polysaccharide components as the key epitopes for cellular immunity. A purified protein derivative is used as an intradermal antigen to measure delayed hypersensitivity to *M tuberculosis.* A positive delayed skin test demonstrates previous exposure to the bacteria and is often correlated with immunity. No one-to-one correlation exists between a positive skin test and immunity, however, and further definition of the protective antigens in the tubercle bacillus is needed before immunity to *M tuberculosis* can be understood.

The need to develop more effective vaccines against *M tuberculosis* has been accentuated by the recent striking increase in the incidence in AIDS patients of tuberculosis due to bacteria with multiple drug resistance.

Immunity to mycobacteria such as *M avium* complex and *M leprae* (the agent of Hansen's disease, ie, leprosy) is also mediated by cellular immunity, with serum components playing an insignificant role. The common occurrence of *M avium* complex infections in AIDS patients underscores the critical importance of cell-mediated immunity in resistance to mycobacterial infections.

CONCLUSIONS

Immunity to bacterial infections is extremely complex because of the diverse virulence factors used by bacteria to enhance their survival. In fact, a large number, if not a majority, of bacterial virulence factors are designed to either prevent or counteract host defenses. Primary nonspecific defense against bacterial infections is afforded by granulocytes, which ingest and kill most potential pathogens. Specific immunity is needed for protection against encapsulated or intracellular bacteria. This requires the development either of antibody, which can enhance killing by its opsonic or complement-fixing activity, or of T-cell immunity, which can activate the microbicidal activity of macrophages. In many infections, a complex interaction of immune mechanisms is required to achieve protective immunity. Thus, antibody, complement, granulocytes, lymphocytes, and macrophages are all needed to permit the development of protective immunity to many bacterial pathogens.

REFERENCES

GENERAL

Gorbach S et al (editors): *Infectious Diseases,* 2nd ed. WB Saunders, 1997.

Mandell GL et al (editors): *Principles and Practice of Infectious Diseases,* 5th ed. Chuchill Livingstone, 1999.

Sherris JC et al (editors): *Medical Microbiology: An Introduction to Infectious Diseases.* 2nd ed. Elsevier, 1990.

SPECIFIC

Bloom BR et al: Tuberculosis: Commentary on a reemergent killer. *Science* 1992;257:1005.

Daniel DM: Antibody and antigen detection for the immunodiagnosis of tuberculosis: Why not? What more is needed? Where do we stand today? *J Infect Dis* 1988; 158:678.

Densen P et al: Familial properdin deficiency and fatal meningococcemia. *N Engl J Med* 1987;316:922.

Dezfulian M et al: Kinetics study of immunologic response to *Clostridium botulinum* toxin. *J Clin Microbiol* 1987; 25:1336.

Facklam R et al: emm Typing and validation of provisional M types for group A streptococci. *Emerg Infect Dis* 1999; 5:247.

Fattom A et al: Laboratory and clinical evaluation of conjugate vaccines composed of *Staphyloccus aureus* type 5 and type 8 capsular polysaccharides bound to *Pseudomonas aeruginosa* recombinant exotoxin A. *Infect Immun* 1993;61:1023.

Fierer J: *Pseudomonas* and *Flavobacterium.* In: *Infectious Diseases and Medical Microbiology,* 2nd ed. Braude AI (editor). WB Saunders, 1986, p. 314.

Galan JE, Collmer A: Type III secretion machines: Bacterial devices for protein delivery into host cells. *Science* 1999;284:1322.

Gazapo E et al: Changes in IgM and IgG antibody concentrations in brucellosis over time: Importance for diagnosis and follow-up. *J Infect Dis* 1989;159:219.

Greenman RL et al: A controlled clinical trial of E5 murine monoclonal antibody to endotoxin in the treatment of gram-negative sepsis. *JAMA* 1991;266:1097.

Griffiss JM et al: Vaccines against encapsulated bacteria: A global agenda. *Rev Infect Dis* 1987;9:176.

Harriman GR et al: The role of C9 in complement-mediated killing of *Neisseria. J Immunol* 1981;127:2386.

Johnston RB: Recurrent bacterial infections in children. *N Engl J Med* 1984;310:1237.

Kasper DL: The polysaccharide capsule of *Bacteroides fragilis* subspecies *fragilis:* Immunochemical and morphologic definition. *J Infect Dis* 1976;133:79.

McCabe WR et al: Immunization with rough mutants of *Salmonella minnesota:* Protective activity of IgM and IgG antibody to the R595 (Re Chemotype) mutant. *J Infect Dis* 1988;158:291.

McKenney D et al: Broadly protective vaccine for *Staphylococcus aureus* based on an in vivo-expressed antigen. *Science* 1999;284:1523.

Orskov F, Orskov I: Enterobacteriaceae. In: *Infectious Diseases and Medical Microbiology,* 2nd ed. Braude AI (editor). WB Saunders, 1986.

Ryan KJ: Corynebacteria and other non-spore forming microoganisms. In: *An Introduction to Infectious Diseases.* Sherris JC (editor). Elsevier, 1984.

Santosham M et al: The efficacy in Navajo infants of a conjugate vaccine consisting of *Haemophilus influenzae* type b polysaccharide and *Neisseria meningitidis* outer-membrane protein complex. *N Engl J Med* 1991; 324:1767.

Schwimmbeck MD, Oldstone MBA: Molecular mimicry between human leucocyte antigens B27 and *Klebsiella. Am J Med* 1988;85(suppl 6A):51.

Ziegler EJ et al: Treatment of gram-negative bacteremia and septic shock with HA-1A human monoclonal antibody against endotoxin. *N Engl J Med* 1991;324:429.

Viral Infections

45

John Mills, MD

The interactions between viruses and the host immune system are not only complex and fascinating but also critical in determining the outcome of infection and strategies for its prevention.

With all other pathogens, viruses share the qualities of being complex, replicating immunogens that stimulate both cellular and humoral immune responses, which then influence the outcome of the infection. Virus infections may be broadly classified into those in which the host immune response eliminates the virus from the body (eg, influenza virus and poliovirus) and those in which the virus is able to persist despite the host immune response. Viruses may persist as a **latent infection,** with or without intermittent replication (eg, herpes simplex virus), or as a **chronic infection** (eg, HIV or hepatitis C virus). Viral genomes may be maintained either by integration into the host genome (eg, HIV) or independently within the cell (eg, herpes simplex virus).

Because viruses parasitize cellular metabolic processes during their own replication, they have a unique capacity to directly alter cell structure and function. Although it was once thought that the viral genome only specified those proteins required for intracellular replication as determined in vitro, it is now clear that many (if not most) viruses also carry genes that are dispensable for replication in cell culture but which play critical roles for in vivo pathogenesis. These "virulence factors" act by modulating either host immune responses or cell division and apoptosis. The generation of host immune responses can be inhibited (eg, the herpes simplex virus *ICP47* gene) or the effect of those responses on virus-infected cells can be blunted (eg, the HIV-1 Nef protein). Viruses also augment their replication by retarding apoptosis and regulating cell division (Table 45–1). The role of these viral proteins in pathogenesis is currently a topic of intense investigation.

The clinical features of infection by a specific virus are determined primarily by which cells are infected and by the cellular pathology induced by infection (eg, cytolysis). For many viruses, however, the host immune response to viral antigens induces additional injuries, called **immunopathic effects,** which are qualitatively different from directly **viropathic effects** and which may involve cells or organs that are uninfected by the virus. Much of the disease morbidity associated with some viruses is, in fact, secondary to the host immune response. Other viral infections may have late immunologic sequelae (Table 45–2).

INFLUENZA VIRUS

Major Immunologic Features

- Marked antigenic variation of viral surface proteins, resulting from mutation and recombination
- Cytolytic T lymphocytes (CTL) responsible for elimination of virus after infection in the naive host
- Serum antibodies to viral surface proteins mediate resistance to pneumonia; mucosal (IgA) antibodies protect against rhinotracheitis
- Several types of vaccines stimulate immune responses (primarily antibodies) and protect against disease

General Considerations

Influenza is a respiratory infection with systemic manifestations; it is caused by influenza viruses. The disease occurs chiefly in epidemics, predominantly during the winter months. Although all age groups are affected, the severity of the illness is greatest at the extremes of age, and the mortality rate is highest in the elderly and in individuals with underlying chronic cardiorespiratory disease. Recurrent epidemics of influenza contribute significantly to the premature death of patients in these risk groups.

Virology

Influenza virus has an envelope and an antisense RNA genome, which is segmented (seven to eight pieces) rather than continuous, as is found in most viruses. The virus has several important structural proteins (Table 45–3), and, in general, each genome segment specifies one protein.

Three types of influenza virus (A, B, and C) are known; the classification is based on the antigenic characteristics of the ribonucleoprotein and matrix pro-

Table 45–1. Some examples of strategies used by viruses to evade host immune responses and to regulate cell division and apoptosis.

Immune Response Blocked	Virus & Gene or Gene Product	Activity	Effect on Antiviral Immune Response
Antibody	CMV FcR protein	Expressed on CMV-infected cells; nonspecifically bind Fc portion of IgG	Blocks ADCC & possibly NK and CTL responses
	Measles NC	Binds to FcγRII on B lymphocytes, suppressing antibody production	Blocks synthesis of measles-specific antibodies
Complement	Vaccinia C21L	VCP binds C3b & C4b; blocks C' activation by both alternative and classical pathways	Reduces local inflammation; reduces activity of C'-dependent neutralizing antibody
Interferons	Vaccinia E3L Reovirus σ3 protein	Binds and sequesters dsRNA, blocking both activation of PKR and its inactivation of eIF2α by phosphorylation	Blocks activation of intracellular response to IFN (inhibition of protein synthesis and apoptosis)
	Influenza NS1	Blocks PKR binding to dsRNA by unknown mechanism, blocking PKR activation	Same as vaccina E3L
	Vaccinia K3L HCV NS5A/E2	Homologue of eIF2α, pseudosubstrate for PKR; blocks activation of PKR	Same as vaccina E3L
	HSVγ,34.5	Adaptor protein which dephosphorylates PKR-phosphorylated eIF2α, restoring its activity	Same as vaccina E3L
	HIV Tat	One-exon Tat (Tat72) binds PKR & inhibits its activity; two-exon Tat (Tat86) degrades IκB and augments NFκB transcription via a PKR-dependent mechanism	Same as vaccina E3L
	Vaccinia B8R	sIFN-Rγ which binds IFNγ & blocks interactions with cells	Blocks effects of IFNγ (eg, generation of cellular immune responses)
	Vaccinia B18R	sIFN-Rα which binds IFNα/β & blocks interactions with cells	Blocks antiviral effects of IFNα/β
	EBV BCRF1	IL-10 analog	Blocks IFN-γ production, reducing cellular immune responses
NK cells	HSV -? genes	HSV virus infects and inactivates NK cells	Directly reduces functional activity of NK cells
	CMV UL18 MCV MC080R	MHC class I homologue; expression on cells as decoy provides "self" signal to NK cells	Reduces NK lysis of CMV- or MCV-infected cells
	HIV Nef	Downregulates MHC class I types A & B (which blocks CTL) but not MHC class I types C & E	NK cells recognize MHC-C- & MHC-E-expressing cells as "self" and therefore do not lyse them
CTL	HSV UL41	Disrupts polysomes inhibiting cellular protein synthesis	Blocks synthesis of viral peptides and therefore MHC class I presentation of those peptides, reducing CTL susceptibility
	HSV US12/ICP47	Competes with viral peptides for TAP-binding site, blocking transport of peptides to MHC	Blocks MHC class I loading of viral peptides in ER, reducing cellular antigen presentation and CTL susceptibility

	CMV pp65	Phosphorylates a CMV protein (IE-1) which is a major CTL target, blocking its proteolysis and preventing MHC class I loading of peptides. No effect on IE-1 function otherwise	Same as HSV US12/ICP47
	CMV US6	Blocks viral peptide translocation to the ER by interfering with function of TAP complex	Same as HSV US12/CP47
	CMV US2/US11	Destabilizes MHC class I heavy chain, causing dislocation to cytosol where it is degraded	Reduces MHC class I antigen presentation and CTL susceptibility of infected cells
	CMV US3	Retains MHC class I complexes in ER	Same as US2/US11
	Adeno E3/19K	Binds to MHC class I via its ER lumenal domain, blocks transport of MHC-peptide complex to cell membrane (cytosolic retention signal)	Same as US2/US11
	HIV Nef protein	Selectively reduces expression of class I MHC-A & -B molecules (but not NK-signaling MHC-C & -E) by accelerating degradation in endolysosomes	Same as US2/US11
	HBV X	Augments FasL expression on HBV-infected cells which causes apoptosis of attacking CTL	Reduces CTL effectiveness
Interleukins	Vaccinia SPI-1 Cowpox crmA	Inhibits caspase 1 enzyme	Blocks conversion of pro-IL-1β to active IL-1β, inhibiting inflammatory responses and reducing febrile response
	Vaccinia B15R	Gene product is a sIL-1-R which binds IL-1β, blocking its binding to cells	Inhibits inflammatory responses and febrile response to infection and secretion
TNF	Vaccinia A53R	A sTNF-R which binds TNF, blocking its binding to cells	Blocks TNF-mediated cytolysis and immune enhancement
	CMV UL144	Integral membrane TNF receptor homologue	Function unknown -? Anti-apoptosis
	ASFV A238L	IκB homologue	Inhibits transcription off of TNF and IL-8 genes, blocking their synthesis & secretion
Chemotaxis	Vaccinia B29R	Soluble protein which binds CC, CXC, and C class chemokines, blocking their cell binding	Reduces leukocyte infiltration into sites of viral infection
	Swinepox K2R	Chemokine receptor expressed on cells; binds CC and ?CXC chemokines	Inactive signaling function, reducing leukocyte infiltration into sites of viral infection
	MCV MC148R	MIP-1β homologue which inhibits MIP-1β activity	Reduces leukocyte infiltration into sites of viral infection
	CMV US28	Integral membrane homologous to CCR5 & CXCR4	Function in CMV lifecycle unknown. Can mediate entry of HIV

(Continued)

Table 45-1. Some examples of strategies used by viruses to evade host immune responses and to regulate cell division and apoptosis. (*Continued*)

Immune Response Blocked	Virus & Gene or Gene Product	Activity	Effect on Antiviral Immune Response
Apoptosis inhibitors (also see TNF section)	Vaccinia SPI-1 & -2 Cowpox crmA	Serpin (serine protease inhibitor) which blocks ICE (caspase 1), other caspases & granzyme B	Decreased apoptosis (may also block apoptosis from CTL)
	MCV MC159	vFLIP which is a transdominant inhibitor of FADD and caspase 8	Same as vaccinia SPI-1
	Adeno E1B 19kDa	Blocks activation of FLICE caspase	Same as vaccinia SPI-1
	Adeno E1B-19K ASFV A 179L	Binds Bcl-2-interacting proteins which bind Bcl-2 family members (Bax, Bak & Bik), inactivating them	Decreased apoptosis
	Adeno E1B 55 kdA + E4 34kDa HPV E6	Binds p53 & accelerates its degradation, inhibiting p53-induced transcription	Decreased apoptosis, increased cell division and cell transformation
	HIV Nef	Binds p53 & many cellular kinases	Decreased apoptosis
Cell cycling	HIV Vpr	Mechanism unclear	Prolongs cell time in G2/M
	HIV Nef	Binds to and activates or inhibits *src* kinases	Drives cells into S phase and activates macrophages & T cell
	Adeno E1A HPV E7	Binds to retinoblastoma protein (pRB) and p300	Drives stationary cells into S phase and mitosis; would ultimately to apoptosis but for effects of Adeno E1B-19K
	CMV UL69	Unknown mechanism	Induces cells to accumulate in G1

Abbreviations: CMV = cytomegalovirus; FcR = receptor for Fc portion of IgG; VCP = vaccinia complement control protein; ADCC = antibody-dependent cellular cytotoxicity; NK = natural killer cells; CTL = cytotoxic T lymphocytes; C' = complement; HSV = herpes simplex virus; Adeno = adenovirus; PKR = interferon-induced protein kinase; IFN = interferon; sIFN-R = soluble interferon receptor; ICE = IL-1 converting enzyme; TNF = tumor necrosis factor; ASFV = African swine fever virus; MCV = molluscum contagiosum virus; TAP = transporters associated with antigen presentation; ER = endoplasmic reticulum; HBV = hepatitis B virus; HPV = human papilloma virus; vFLIP = virion FLICE (caspase 8) inhibitory protein.

Table 45–2. Viral infections with immunologic sequelae.

Acute Viral Infection	Immunologic Sequelae
Measles virus	Encephalitis (early), suba-cute sclerosing panen-cephalitis (SSPE) (late)
Rubella virus	Encephalopathy, arthritis
Hepatitis B virus	Polyarteritis nodosa, glomerulonephritis
Respiratory syncytial virus	Asthma (unproved asso-ciation)
Epstein–Barr virus	Guillain-Barré syndrome

teins, as well as other features. Influenza A virus is unique in part because it infects both humans and many other animals (pigs, horses, birds, and seals) and because it is the principal cause of pandemic influenza. When a cell is infected by two different influenza A viruses, the segmented RNA genomes of the two parental virus types mix during replication, so that virions of the progeny may contain RNA and protein from both parents (so-called "recombinants," even though they are really reassortants). Influenza A virus thereby varies its surface hemagglutinin and neuraminidase molecules by recombining with other strains (including animal strains) as well as by mutation. Like other viruses with an RNA genome, influenza virus has a high rate of mutation, which underlies its rapid **antigenic variation.** New epidemic strains are generated as the combined result of recombination (chiefly between animal and human strains) and mutation, which generate the required novel hemagglutinin and neuraminidase virion envelope proteins (Figure 45–1). Influenza B virus does not have an animal reservoir from which it can select novel hemagglutinin types, and thus the range of antigenic variation observed is narrower than that for influenza A virus. Influenza C virus appears to have only one serotype and differs from types A and B in some other features as well.

The principal targets for influenza virus infection are the ciliated epithelial cells of the upper and lower respiratory tract. Influenza virus infection kills these cells, which regenerate slowly during convalescence. Virus shedding terminates with recovery from infection, and neither chronic nor latent infection occurs.

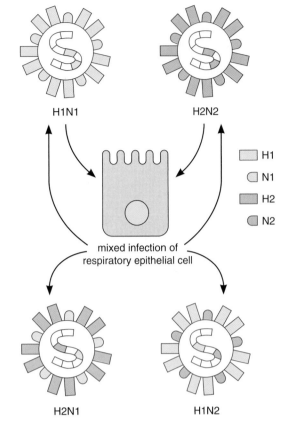

Figure 45–1. Schematic reproduction of genetic reassortment in influenza viruses. Shown are the major surface proteins and their corresponding gene segments.

Clinical Features

Influenza in humans is caused primarily by influenza A and B, with influenza C causing only infrequent infections with mild disease. Human Type A infections are caused virtually exclusively by the neuraminidase types N1 and N2 and hemagglutinin types H1, H2, and H3, although infections, some-

Table 45–3. Major proteins of influenza virus.

Protein	Location	Function
Hemagglutinin	Envelope (virion surface)	Ligand for cell receptor (sialic acid), facilitating binding of virus to cell surface
Neuraminidase	Envelope (virion surface)	Cleave cell receptor, releasing progeny virus from cell
Matrix protein	Internal	Stabilizes virus structure
M2	Envelope	Proton pore
RNA polymerase	Internal	Replicates RNA genome
Nucleoprotein	Internal	Stabilizes RNA within virion
NS1	Nonstructural	Inhibits host cell protein synthesis at mRNA level; blocks interferon effect (see Table 45–1)

times severe, have occurred with animal hemagglutinin types H5 and H9.

Influenza is spread through both aerosols and fomites. The clinical features of influenza are fever, cough, myalgia, headache, and malaise. Mild pharyngeal or conjunctival irritation is common, and gastrointestinal symptoms may occur as well, especially in children. There are no characteristic abnormalities on routine laboratory testing. Influenza may be diagnosed by culture of the virus from nasopharyngeal or pulmonary secretions, by direct detection of viral antigens on desquamated respiratory epithelial cells with labeled monoclonal antibodies, or by demonstration of an antibody response to the virus in convalescent-phase sera.

Immunologic Pathogenesis

Although influenza virus stimulates a vigorous host immune response, including specific antibodies and cytotoxic T cells, most of the clinical findings are probably due to the cytopathic effects of this virus and to vigorous stimulation of interferon alfa (IFNα) production. Recent studies in mice with experimentally induced influenza pneumonia suggest that the lung damage is secondary to interferon-gamma (IFNγ)-induced nitric oxide generation. In animal models of influenza, immunosuppression has a variable effect on the course of the infection, but virus replication is invariably prolonged. Patients with a wide variety of immunodeficiency disorders do not clearly show increased symptoms following influenza virus infection, although virus shedding may be prolonged, particularly in the context of cellular immune deficiency.

Cellular immunity, measured by either skin test reactivity or in vitro lymphocyte activation to antigens, is slightly depressed during acute influenza. This transient immunosuppression appears to have no clinical effects and does not alter antiviral immune responses. The mechanism is unknown, although it may be related to production of inhibitors of interleukin-1 (IL-1). In contrast, influenza virus infection suppresses normal pulmonary antibacterial defenses, so that patients recovering from influenza have a greatly increased risk of developing bacterial pneumonia. The mechanism of this effect is also unknown, but it may be the disruption of the mucociliary escalator combined with impaired function of pulmonary alveolar macrophages or neutrophils.

Infection with influenza virus stimulates interferon synthesis and also a vigorous CTL response, and both contribute to eradicating the virus. Antibody is also produced, but this appears to have only a marginal role in recovery from infection. Nude mice (which lack cellular immunity) cannot control influenza infection, and administration of antibody results in only transient cessation of virus shedding. In contrast, reconstitution of infected nude mice with cloned influenza-specific CTL eradicates the infec-

tion. Natural killer (NK) cells do not appear to play an important role in resistance to influenza.

Immunity to influenza is subtype-specific, long-lasting, and largely antibody-mediated. Antibodies directed against hemagglutinin and neuraminidase surface proteins are critical determinants of host resistance to influenza virus. Antibodies to the hemagglutinin prevent the virus from attaching to cells and neutralize infectivity. Alone, they can prevent infection. Antibodies to neuraminidase inhibit the release of virus from cells and its subsequent spread to other cells within the host or to other people. Although antineuraminidase antibodies do not prevent infection, they ameliorate disease.

The influenza virus M2 protein is found on the surface of the virion and infected cells, like the hemagglutinin and neuraminidase. In contrast to them, however, the M2 protein is highly conserved between strains. Antibodies to the M2 protein are protective in animals, suggesting that the M2 protein might be used as an influenza vaccine that would protect against all serotypes.

In mice, serum antibodies to influenza prevent pulmonary infection but not rhinotracheitis; in contrast, mucosal IgA antibody (to the hemagglutinin and neuraminidase) is primarily responsible for resistance to upper respiratory infection. The limited data available from humans suggest that this is true in humans as well.

Influenza is associated with a number of postinfectious disorders, including encephalitis, myopericarditis, Goodpasture's syndrome, and Reye's syndrome. The pathogenesis of these complications is unknown.

Treatment

A new class of drugs, neuraminidase inhibitors, has recently become available to treat influenza. The prototype is zanamavir, but others are in development. These drugs inhibit influenza neuraminidase and prevent release of virions from infected cells (in a manner similar to neuraminidase antibody); they are effective against both influenza A and B for both treatment and prophylaxis. The older antiinfluenza drugs, amantadine and rimantadine, inhibit the function of the influenza proton channel protein (M2) and thereby block intracellular virion uncoating, but as they are active only against influenza A, they have achieved little clinical use and are now chiefly of historical interest.

Prevention

Resistance to influenza infection and disease is largely mediated by antibodies (chiefly to the hemagglutinin), whereas recovery from infection is facilitated largely by influenza-specific CTL. The antibody response is largely highly serotype-specific (with the exception of M2 antibodies discussed earlier), whereas the CTL response tends to be broader as it is directed toward viral proteins, such as the nucleoprotein, which are highly conserved amongst strains.

Two types of influenza vaccines are now available: purified subunit hemagglutinin vaccines and live attenuated vaccines. Prototypes of both were first developed in the 1940s, shortly after the discovery of influenza virus in 1933.

Current subunit vaccines are prepared from semi-purified hemagglutinin derived from virus grown in embryonated eggs and inactivated with formalin or β-propiolactone. These vaccines must be given parenterally (usually intramuscularly) and chiefly stimulate a serum-neutralizing IgG antibody response. These vaccines do not significantly protect against influenza infection, but do prevent disease, especially severe disease. They are highly type-specific, however, and their composition therefore changes each year. A typical recent vaccine included type A H3 and H1 hemagglutinins as well as a type B hemagglutinin. Influenza C is not included because of its minor public health importance.

Current subunit vaccines cause minor local reactions but are relatively free of serious side effects. The swine influenza subunit vaccine (administered widely in the United States 1976 because of a suspect imminent epidemic) was associated with a relatively high risk of Guillain-Barré syndrome, a complication almost certainly due to an immunologic response to virion components. Current subunit influenza vaccines appear to cause only about a 1.7-fold increase in the incidence of this syndrome (one additional case per million vaccinees). Transient slight bronchospasm has also been reported from influenza vaccine; the mechanism is unknown but may also be immunologic.

Recently a live attenuated, intranasally administered influenza vaccine has also been shown to be safe and to be highly effective for the prevention of influenza. It will almost certainly be licensed shortly. This vaccine has been attenuated by adapting the virus to grow at subnormal temperatures (so-called "cold-adapted" strains). In clinical trials a trivalent (A H1, A H3, and B) vaccine was highly effective at preventing both severe and mild influenza in children, but was somewhat less effective in adults. The only side effect observed so far is an increased incidence of upper respiratory symptoms in the week following immunization. One clinical trial in which adults were immunized with combined subunit and live attenuated influenza vaccines suggested that this regimen was superior to inactivated vaccine alone.

RESPIRATORY SYNCYTIAL VIRUS

Major Immunologic Features

- Moderate antigenic variation of viral surface proteins
- Imperfect immunity, resulting in repeated infections throughout life

- Bronchospasm in infected infants, perhaps as a result of IgE antibodies to respiratory syncytial virus
- Passive immunoprophylaxis with a neutralizing humanized mouse monoclonal antibody protects infants against severe disease

General Considerations

Respiratory syncytial virus (RSV) causes respiratory infections in children and adults. Infections occur in annual epidemics, commonly during the winter or rainy months. The disease causes severe pneumonia and bronchiolitis in infants, whereas upper respiratory infection predominates in adults.

Virology

RSV is an enveloped virus with a continuous, negative-stranded RNA genome. On the basis of antigenic and sequence analysis of the virion surface glycoproteins, F and G, two major groups (A and B) have been identified, both of which have subgroups, although the exact number is still uncertain. Most of the observed antigenic variation is in the G protein. The virus infects respiratory epithelium and causes extensive cytopathology, including characteristic syncytia. Recovery from infection is complete, and neither latent nor chronic infection occurs.

Clinical Features

The virus is spread through airborne droplets and by interpersonal contact through fomites. In infants 2–24 months of age, RSV infection is frequent and is often associated with lower respiratory tract disease. It is the most common cause of bronchiolitis-pneumonia associated with bronchospasm and air trapping (Figure 45–2). The severity of disease is greatest in premature infants and those with underlying chronic cardiorespiratory conditions. Infection is diagnosed by recovery of the virus in tissue culture, by identification of viral antigens on desquamated respiratory epithelial cells with monoclonal antibodies, or by documentation of a serum antibody response. Elderly adults, particularly if institutionalized, and immunocompromised patients of all ages are also at risk of severe RSV lower respiratory tract disease.

Immunologic Pathogenesis

Infection with RSV stimulates both humoral and cellular immunity. Eradication of established infection is primarily but not exclusively a function of intact CTL because patients with defective cellular immunity may become persistently infected with the virus. Antibody (against the F and G proteins) appears to partially protect against reinfection and disease, and maternal IgG antibody transferred transplacentally to the fetus confers some protection against disease early in life. Passive transfer of antibody to either the F or G proteins, but particularly the former, is protective in experimental RSV infection and in in-

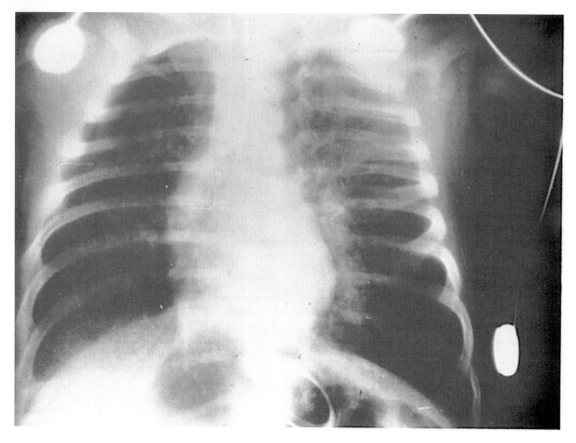

Figure 45–2. Chest radiograph of a 1-year-old child with bronchiolitis due to respiratory syncytial virus, showing diffuse hyperinflation and air trapping with a left upper lobe infiltrate.

fants. The lung collectin SP-A neutralizes RSV in vitro by binding the F glycoprotein of the virus and may ameliorate infection.

The wheezing and air trapping associated with RSV bronchiolitis is probably due to a combination of direct RSV cytopathology and immunopathology. RSV stimulates an IgE response (effectively, an allergy to the virus,) which causes mast cell degranulation. Clinical studies have shown that the severity of bronchiolitis was directly proportional to the quantity of mast cell products in bronchial secretions. RSV infection of epithelial cells stimulates secretion of the eosinophil chemoattractants RANTES and MIP-1α; the recruited eosinophils also bind to and are degranulated by RSV-infected cells. In experimental animals, administration of CD8-expressing, RSV-reactive T cells worsens pulmonary lesions in infected animals while simultaneously accelerating resolution of the infection. In vitro studies have also shown that RSV infection of lymphocytes and macrophages can directly depress the function of these cells, perhaps restricting the protective antiviral immune response.

The best evidence that RSV bronchiolitis has an immunopathic component comes from a clinical trial conducted in the 1960s showing that infants who had received a parenterally administered, formalin-inactivated, highly immunogenic RSV vaccine paradoxically had worse disease following RSV infection than infants who had received a placebo. This vaccine predominantly induced a T_H2-type immune response (vs the T_H1-type response usually associated with RSV infection), and also stimulated high titers of antibody to the F protein which was ineffective as it lacked neutralizing activity.

Treatment

A nucleotide analogue, ribavirin, has been shown to accelerate the recovery of children with RSV infection and is licensed for this indication in the United States. The drug is aerosolized and administered by inhalation. Because of its high cost and marginal efficacy, this drug is generally used only for children who are at risk for severe morbidity or mortality from RSV infection.

Prevention

Many efforts to produce a vaccine have been made because of the morbidity and mortality rates associated with RSV infection in infants. Unfortunately, the adverse outcome of the clinical trials of the formalin-inactivated RSV vaccine in the 1960s significantly retarded vaccine development.

In experimental animals, RSV infection can be prevented by immunization with purified F or G proteins (or subunits thereof), or by administration of live attenuated RSV. Although a purified F protein vaccine was immunogenic in children and adults and showed some evidence of producing protection from disease, this vaccine was not immunogenic in seronegative young infants. However, clinical development of a purified F protein vaccine is continuing in older, high-risk children (eg, those with cystic fibrosis) and in the elderly. Immunization with F and G proteins, alone or with other virion proteins, may also be possible using DNA vaccines.

In young children and infants, live attenuated RSV vaccines have received the most attention. A number of attenuated strains have been studied in phase I clinical trials; however, it has proven difficult to find strains that are sufficiently attenuated for very young infants and still able to infect (and induce a protective immune response) in older infants. A two-vaccine strategy has been proposed, with young infants being given a highly attenuated variant, followed by a less-attenuated strain when they are older.

A breakthrough in prevention of RSV infection has been achieved recently by studies showing that RSV disease can be prevented by prophylactic administration of either high-titer human RSV immunoglobulin or by neutralizing monoclonal antibodies. Both of these strategies affect severe RSV disease and the requirement for hospitalization more than they do on RSV morbidity overall. Human RSV immunoglobulin is quite inconvenient to administer because it needs to be given intravenously every month. The humanized murine neutralizing F antibody (palivizumab), however, can be given conveniently as a monthly intramuscular injection. It is currently recommended that one or the other passive immunoprophylactic strategy be implemented in high-risk children (eg, those with prematurity or chronic cardiorespiratory disease) during the RSV season.

MEASLES VIRUS

Major Immunologic Features
- A single viral serotype; either infection or immunization results in lifelong immunity
- Acute infection depresses cellular immunity
- Rash caused by cellular immune response to virus in the skin
- "Unbalanced" immune response to inactivated measles vaccine may produce atypical and severe disease after natural infection

General Considerations
Measles virus causes an important acute exanthem of childhood and, rarely, a chronic, slowly progressive neurologic disease, **subacute sclerosing panencephalitis** (SSPE), which may follow decades after an acute infection. The highly infectious virus is spread via respiratory secretions. Acute infection is associated with significant morbidity and mortality, especially in individuals in developing countries. An effective live, attenuated vaccine is available; if used widely, it could prevent nearly all cases.

Virology
Measles virus is a paramyxovirus with an envelope and a negative-stranded RNA genome. It has a genome and protein composition typical of paramyxoviruses; the major envelope glycoproteins are a fusion (F) and attachment-hemagglutinin (H) protein. The H protein attaches to the cell receptor for measles virus, CD46. Only one serotype exists, although minor sequence changes may occur in the surface glycoproteins of the virus. Acute infection of cells results in their death, commonly accompanied by syncytial giant-cell formation.

Clinical Features
After an incubation period of 9–11 days, during which the virus undergoes subclinical replication at unknown sites, perhaps in the lymphoreticular system, viremia occurs (virus is carried primarily in monocytes) and patients develop fever, cough, coryza, and conjunctivitis. Within 1 or 2 days, an erythematous, maculopapular rash develops, which quickly spreads over the entire body. In malnourished children, the disease is severe, and enteritis is prominent. The main complications are bacterial superinfections, such as otitis media and pneumonia, and a postinfectious encephalomyelitis. Deaths from measles, rare in developed countries, are usually due to intercurrent bacterial infections.

Decades after the primary infection, a very small proportion of individuals develop SSPE, a chronic, progressive neurologic disorder due to persistent infection of the central nervous system. SSPE is caused by clonal variants of measles virus with defects that interfere with virion assembly and budding. As a consequence, extracellular virus is not produced, and infected cells do not produce viral antigens on their surface and thus are not removed by immune surveillance. A low-grade, persistent infection results in gradual neurologic injury by unknown mechanisms. SSPE is particularly common in those who acquired measles before the age of 2 years and is very rare after measles vaccination.

The diagnosis of measles can be made clinically in most cases. Lymphopenia is a characteristic laboratory abnormality in acute cases. The diagnosis may be confirmed by recovering the virus from blood or oropharyngeal secretions in tissue culture, by demonstrating viral antigen on leukocytes or respiratory epithelium, or by documenting the development of IgG antibodies to the virus during convalescence. The presence of IgM antibody to measles virus during the illness also confirms the diagnosis.

Immunologic Pathogenesis

Resistance to measles virus infection is primarily attributable to serum IgG-neutralizing antibodies, specifically to the F and H envelope glycoproteins. Protective antibodies resulting from infection persist for life, as do those from immunization unless the vaccine was given prior to 1–2 years of age. In contrast, control of measles virus replication following infection is predominantly a function of cellular immunity (specifically, CTL) although antibodies can contribute to recovery from infection. Patients with defects in cellular immunity often develop rapidly progressive fatal infections, but those with isolated agammaglobulinemia recover normally.

Measles was the first virus infection to be associated with suppression of immune responses (von Pirquet observed transient loss of tuberculin reactivity in patients with measles in 1908), and measles is now recognized as a major cause of transient but clinically significant impairment of cellular immunity. The mechanisms by which measles virus induces cellular immunodeficiency are complex and include downregulation of IL-12 synthesis, a major cytokine involved in stimulating cellular (T_H1-type) immune responses, functional impairment and apoptosis of CD40-activated dendritic cells and associated T lymphocytes, and blocking proliferation of lymphocytes through G0/G1 cell cycle arrest.

Measles also has complex effects on humoral immunity. Binding of the measles virus nucleocapsid to FcγRII on B lymphocytes blocks antibody synthesis; however, patients with measles virus infection tend to exhibit polyclonal B-cell activation and elevated immunoglobulin concentrations.

The mechanism of the postviral encephalitis that can complicate measles has been clarified by the development in Michael Oldstone's laboratory of a CD46-transgenic mouse model for measles infection. (Mouse cells are resistant to measles infection because they fail to express CD46; CD46-transgenic cells become susceptible.) CD46-transgenic mice infected with measles virus develop encephalitis associated with expression of measles virus antigens; infiltration of CD4, CD8, and B lymphocytes and macrophages; and increased synthesis of the chemokines regulated on activation, normal T expressed and secreted (RANTES), and interferon-inducible protein-10 (IP-10); and the cytokines IL-6, TNFα and IL-1β. These findings suggest that the encephalitis represents a mixture of measles virus cytopathology and immunopathology.

One of the most striking immunopathologic syndromes related to measles virus was the "atypical" measles seen following immunization with formalin-inactivated measles vaccine. These vaccines stimulated protective neutralizing antibodies and were widely administered in the 1960s. Later it was apparent, however, that the protective antibodies waned within a few months, and if these individuals were subsequently infected with measles virus, a disease syndrome distinct from classical measles, called "atypical" measles, developed in up to half of the infected subjects. The inactivated measles vaccines were withdrawn within a few years as a result. Atypical measles was characterized principally by a prolonged high fever, an atypical and severe rash, and pneumonitis. Recent studies in nonhuman primates have shown that this disease results from a nonprotective measles antibody response in the absence of a CTL response. The rash is due to immune complex deposition, complement activation, and eosinophil infiltration.

Prevention

Passive administration of pooled human IgG (immune serum globulin or intravenous immunoglobulins) is not a long-term control measure but is useful for postexposure prophylaxis of nonimmune subjects. It prevents measles even if given up to 1 week after exposure.

Current measles vaccines are live, attenuated viruses given parenterally. They are extremely effective and prevent disease in more than 95% of those immunized. Because measles virus is extremely infectious and highly communicable, however, herd immunity requires that more than 98% of the population have protective antibodies. Thus, control of the disease requires high compliance with immunization guidelines. All children should be immunized unless they have a congenital or acquired defect in cellular immunity contraindicating live virus vaccination.

HUMAN HERPESVIRUS 8 (HHV-8)

Major Immunologic Features

- HHV-8 infects B lymphocytes
- Cancers due to HHV-8 (eg, Kaposi's sarcoma) appear virtually exclusively in the context of immunosuppression

Virology

Human herpesvirus type 8 (HHV-8), also called the Kaposi's sarcoma herpesvirus, is a gamma herpesvirus (like Epstein-Barr virus) and the most recently discovered member of the human herpesvirus family. It is the causal agent of Kaposi's sarcoma and some other unusual malignancies. The virus was discovered in 1994 by Moore and colleagues using a novel system that permits selective amplification of foreign genetic sequences from host tissue (representational difference analysis). Subsequently HHV-8 has been grown in cell culture like other viruses, where it has been shown to infect B (CD19-expressing) lymphocytes, endothelial cells, and the spindle cells characteristic of Kaposi's sarcoma. Like some other members of the herpesvirus family, the HHV-8 genome encodes homologues of human cytokines and chemokines, and proteins that regulate signal transduction, cell cycling, and apoptosis.

Clinical Features & Diagnosis

HHV-8 appears to be spread predominantly by sexual intercourse, and in the developed world appears to be found primarily amongst homosexual men. In developing countries the virus is found in both men and women. Because the virus replicates in B lymphocytes, it can be transmitted via transfusion of leukocyte-containing blood products; however, this appears to be unusual because of the donor deferral and testing programs in most developed countries. HHV-8 does not appear to be transmitted by plasma or plasma products. Transmission via sharing of needles (during injecting drug use) is also possible, but has not yet been documented by good epidemiologic studies. Rarely the infection has been transmitted by organ donation.

No clinical syndrome has yet been identified in association with acute HHV-8 infection. Chronic infection appears to be asymptomatic. Surprisingly, although HHV-8 infects B lymphocytes, no immune dysfunction has yet been reported in infected patients.

HHV-8 infection can be diagnosed by detecting either HHV-8 antibodies in blood or HHV-8 sequences in peripheral blood cells (chiefly B lymphocytes) or tissue (eg biopsies of Kaposi's sarcoma tissue). Current serologic tests detect antibodies to antigens produced during either lytic (replicative) and latent infections by immunofluorescence of enzyme-linked immunoassay; testing by immunoblotting (Western blotting) has also been described. Serologic tests are more sensitive than detection of HHV-8 sequences in peripheral blood mononuclear cells for diagnosing HHV-8 infection. Unfortunately, the available serologic tests, although suitable for seroepidemiologic studies, are still insufficiently sensitive and specific for definitive diagnosis of individual patients. For example, up to 20% of patients with Kaposi's sarcoma who have HHV-8 genetic sequences demonstrated in the sarcoma tissue will be seronegative using some current HHV-8 antibody assays.

A proportion of patients infected with HHV-8 will develop malignancies, chiefly Kaposi's sarcoma. Virtually all patients with Kaposi's sarcoma have HHV-8 infection, and the virus is found in high concentration in sarcoma tissue. Other malignancies associated with HHV-8 infection include primary effusion B-cell lymphomas and multicentric Castleman's disease. Primary effusion lymphomas are interesting because Epstein–Barr coinfection appears to be virtually universal, and the burden of HHV-8 genomes in the tumors is very high (up to 80 viral genome copies per cell). A reported association between HHV-8 and multiple myeloma remains very controversial. HHV-8-related malignancies tend to appear either in the context of severe cellular immunodeficiency (eg, the late stages of HIV infection, or drug-induced immunosuppression related to organ transplantation) or in the very elderly. Whether occurrence in the latter group represents disease due to immunosuppression or a prolonged incubation period is unknown. Likewise, the mechanism by which these tumors are induced is unknown, although HHV-8, like other herpesviruses, has recognized oncogenic gene sequences.

There is no validated treatment for HHV-8 infection or its cancer sequelae. HHV-8 is susceptible to foscarnet in vitro, and anecdotal data suggest that long-term foscarnet therapy may either prevent Kaposi's sarcoma or reduce the likelihood of its development. No preventive measures are available other than preventing infection through safe sexual practices and screening blood and organ donors.

HEPATITIS A VIRUS

Hepatitis A virus (HAV) is closely related to other picornaviruses (small, nonenveloped RNA viruses) such as poliovirus. There is only a single serotype. HAV is transmitted primarily by the fecal-oral route. Following ingestion, the virus travels via the bloodstream to the liver, probably the exclusive site of virus replication. Replication in the liver results in a brief period of viremia (5–10 days) and shedding of virus in the stools for 1–2 weeks. The infection resolves completely in all cases, except for rare instances of fatal infection. In contrast to HBV, chronic or latent infection does not occur. Resolution of infection is dependent on intact cellular immunity because patients with cellular immunodeficiency may experience prolonged virus shedding and disease, similar to the situation with other enteroviruses (see the section on Poliovirus).

The incubation period of HAV infection averages 30 days and ranges from 10 to 50 days. Most infections, especially those in children, are asymptomatic, although evidence of "chemical" hepatitis is usually found on laboratory testing. Liver cell injury is thought to be due primarily to the host cellular immune response, as in HBV infection. The mortality rate during acute infection is about 0.1% overall, but it is lower in children and increases with increasing age.

HAV infection generates a vigorous antibody response, which protects against reinfection and serves as the basis for diagnosis. Detection of the transient anti-HAV IgM response is the single most useful test for acute infection, whereas detection of the long-lasting anti-HAV IgG response is the best marker for past infection and resistance to subsequent infection.

Unlike HBV, no serologic test is available for HAV antigen.

Resistance to HAV infection is mediated solely by serum antibody to the virus. This has been demonstrated by studies showing passive transfer of protection by immune globulin that contains antibody to HAV. Protection from HAV infection can be achieved with pooled human IgG given every 3–6 months. The intramuscular preparation is usually used, although intravenous immune globulin is also effective. Protection from illness may also be achieved by administration of IgG within 1 week following exposure to HAV. An inactivated HAV vaccine grown in cell culture is now licensed in many countries; it is entirely safe and provides long-lasting protective antibodies. At present it is recommended primarily for residents of developed countries who are traveling to developing countries and who otherwise would have received immune globulin for protection. In the future, it may become part of the recommended panel of vaccines for universal immunization.

HEPATITIS B VIRUS

Major Immunologic Features
- Single viral serotype, with eight major subtypes
- Liver damage secondary to antiviral cellular immune response
- Acute and chronic immune complex disease possible
- Infection and immunization usually result in long-lasting, complete resistance
- Prevention of perinatal transmission by passive antibody administration followed by active immunization

General Considerations

Hepatitis B virus (HBV) is a major cause of acute and chronic hepatitis as well as hepatocellular carcinoma. The virus causes either acute, self-limited infection or a chronic infection that may be lifelong. Chronic carriers may remain infectious for life and are the major reservoir for the virus.

Virology

HBV is a nonenveloped DNA virus with a unique structure and mode of replication. It is related to several other animal hepatitis viruses, which collectively are known as hepadnaviruses. They contain double-stranded DNA with a nicked or single-stranded region, and they replicate via an RNA intermediate. Virion genomic DNA is synthesized from the RNA intermediate by a virion-encoded RNA-dependent DNA polymerase, structurally closely related to the reverse transcriptases of retroviruses, which are enveloped viruses with an RNA genome. The major proteins of HBV are the surface antigen (HBsAg) and core antigen (HBcAg). Although over eight sub-types of the virus are recognized, this distinction is rarely of clinical importance. Following infection, the virus replicates primarily in hepatocytes, with production of large amounts of excess surface antigen, HBsAg, which then circulates in the blood. Acute infection may resolve, with complete elimination of the virus or may be followed by chronic persistent infection in which viral cDNA persists and replicates either as an episome or integrated into the host genome. Persistent infection is associated with a high risk of hepatic carcinoma.

Epidemiology

Chronic HBV infection is a worldwide public health problem, particularly in Asia. More than 350 million individuals worldwide have chronic HBV infection; in the United States nearly 1.5 million people are carriers of HBV; more than 1 million persons die each year from HBV-related liver disease.

HBV is transmitted almost exclusively by sexual contact, use of injectable drugs, transfusion of blood or blood products, tattooing, acupuncture, and perinatal transmission (from infected mothers to their infants at birth). The incubation period varies from 3–4 weeks to 6 months; generally it is 1–2 months.

Pathology

Acute HBV infection is characterized histologically by ballooning and degeneration of hepatocytes, with focal necrosis of hepatocytes and lymphocytic infiltration of parenchyma and portal tracts. More extensive central necrosis results in necrotic zones that bridge portal tracts or join portal areas to central veins, so-called **bridging necrosis.** In chronic infection with minimal chronic hepatitis, the limiting plate (between the portal tract and the parenchyma) and lobular architecture are preserved. **Piecemeal necrosis** may be observed as a result of disruption of the limiting plate. In more severe cases erosion of the limiting plate exceeds 25%, and more extensive lobular changes (similar to those observed in acute hepatitis including bridging necrosis) are found. Ongoing hepatocellular injury increases the risk of progression to macronodular cirrhosis.

Immunopathogenesis

HBV is not cytopathic, and hepatocyte injury occurs largely as a result of this immune response to the virus. (Other noncytopathic mechanisms also contribute to viral clearance). The differences in the clinical outcome of HBV infection are determined by the initial immune response.

A vigorous polyclonal cytotoxic T-lymphocyte response against HBV capsid and envelope proteins occurs during acute self-limited HBV infection, resulting in virtual clearance of viral DNA from the blood. Recent data suggest that traces of HBV persist after recovery, however, resulting in maintenance of CTL responses for decades. During acute infection T_H2

lymphocytes amplify B cells that produce neutralizing antibodies against HBsAg. This anti-HBs facilitates removal of HBsAg from the blood. More important in the effective immune response against HBV is the development of T_H1 lymphocytes that recognize HBV antigens presented in the context of major histocompatibility complex (MHC) class II molecules on antigen-presenting cells and interact with CTLs. These CTLs in turn recognize HBV epitopes presented by MHC class I molecules on HBV-infected hepatocytes. Apoptosis has also been implicated in destruction of infected hepatocytes by activated CTLs. Cytokines released by these activated CTLs, especially TNFα and IFNγ, directly or indirectly inhibit HBV replication within the infected cell.

In contrast, the virus-specific CTL response is less vigorous in chronic HBV infection. Incomplete clearance of HBV and ongoing hepatic injury of variable severity ultimately result in the activation of the process of hepatic fibrosis and subsequent development of cirrhosis and hepatocellular carcinoma. The CTL response is probably also the cause of the hepatic injury that occurs in patients with chronic HBV infection.

Ongoing chronic hepatitis may underlie the development of hepatocellular carcinoma, a terminal complication of inflammation and fibrosis, resulting from progressive genomic errors in hepatocytes and unregulated growth and repair mechanisms leading to hepatocyte dysplasia. HBV encodes a multifunctional protein (pX) required for viral transcription that has been implicated in the development of hepatocellular carcinoma through activation of mitogenic signaling pathways.

Clinical Features

HBV infection of adults usually results in a self-limited disease that is often asymptomatic. Some 10–20% of individuals with acute HBV infection have symptomatic hepatitis, but only 1% of those develop fulminant hepatitis. In some patients with acute HBV infection simultaneous synthesis of HBsAg and anti-HBs results in immune complex disease, manifested as rash, arthralgias and arthritis, and, rarely, glomerulonephritis.

Chronic infection accounts for less than 5% of adult HBV infections. Infection during infancy or childhood is associated with a high risk of persistent infection, however. Asians are at higher risk than whites for developing chronic infection, and cirrhosis and hepatocellular carcinoma account for more than 50% of deaths in Asian men with chronic HBV infection. Chronic infection with persistent viral replication is a risk factor for progressive liver disease. HIV coinfection may prolong infectivity. Hepatoma is a risk associated with chronic HBV infection, particularly in patients with HBV-related cirrhosis. A small proportion of patients with chronic HBV infection develop complications of antigen–antibody complex disease such as polyarteritis nodosa and glomerulonephritis.

Diagnosis

HBV infection is diagnosed by the detection of HBsAg in serum during acute and chronic infection. HBsAg usually disappears within 1–6 months of infection; its persistence signifies chronic carrier state. The antibody response to HBsAg may be delayed for several months after infection (usually appearing 1–3 months after disappearance of HBsAg, the so-called window period) and is seldom useful for diagnosis of acute HBV infection (see Table 45–4 and Figure 45–3). The detection of anti-HBc-IgM can be used to confirm acute infection; it is present in serum during the window period.

The diagnosis of chronic infection is made by the presence in the serum of HBsAg and anti-HBc in the absence of anti-HBs. Active viral replication and high infectivity is indicated by the presence of HBeAg and DNA polymerase activity. HIV coinfection prolongs HBeAg positivity. HBeAg may spontaneously clear over time during chronic infection, with the appearance of anti-HBe.

Treatment

Patients with chronic HBV infection with evidence of active viral replication (HBeAg and HBV DNA-positive), chronic liver disease on biopsy, and elevated alanine aminotransferases are treated with IFNα. Recent studies show better response rates when IFNα is used in combination with lamivudine,

Table 45–4. Use of HBV markers for the diagnosis of hepatitis.

Markers Present in Serum			
HBsAg	IgM Anti-HBcAg	Anti-HBsAg	Diagnosis
+	+	−	Acute HBV infection
−	+	−	Acute HBV infection (after HBsAg has disappeared)
+	−	±	Chronic HBV infection
−	−	+[a]	Past HBV infection or HBV vaccination Indicates immunity

[a] IgG-class anti-HBcAg also present if infection has occurred (not present following immunization).

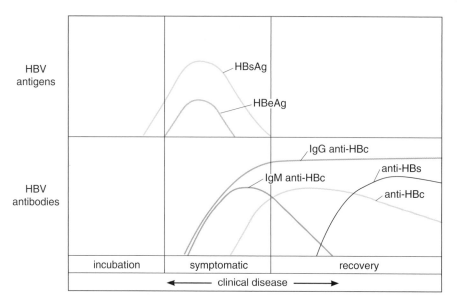

Figure 45–3. Schematic showing temporal pattern of viral markers, illness, and antibody response in acute HBV infection.

an oral nucleoside analogue also used to treat HIV infection. These compounds significantly improve liver histology, reduce HBV DNA and serum alanine aminotransferase levels, and increase the HBeAg seroconversion rates, compared with placebo. Other compounds undergoing clinical evaluation include famciclovir and adefovir dipivoxil. As has become clear during treatment for HIV, combination therapy for HBV is necessary to prevent emergence of resistance.

Liver transplantation is an option for patients with end-stage liver disease due to HBV. Patients who are HBV DNA-negative have a good prognosis following liver transplantation.

Prevention

Cytotoxic T lymphocytes are critical to recovery from HBV infection and elimination of the virus. In contrast, resistance to HBV infection is mediated effectively by antibody to HBsAg alone. Either passive administration of antibody to HBsAg or eliciting anti-HBsAg by immunization with inactivated or recombinant HBsAg confers resistance to infection.

Preventive measures for HBV infection employ either pooled human immune serum globulin with high titers of antibody to HBsAg (hepatitis B immune globulin) or HBV vaccine. The latter consists of HBsAg, either purified from the plasma of chronic carriers or prepared by recombinant DNA techniques. Both types of vaccines are extremely safe and induce protective antibodies in more than 95% of individuals immunized.

Control measures may be implemented either in anticipation of infection or after infection has already

occurred; the latter is known as **postexposure prophylaxis.** Postexposure prophylaxis is highly effective and is indicated when a susceptible individual has been exposed to someone with active infection (ie, a patient with HBsAg in the blood), for example through sexual contact or a needlestick injury. It is also indicated postpartum to infants born to mothers with HBV infection. Passive immunity is achieved immediately by administration of hepatitis B immune globulin. Then active immunity is stimulated by administration of HBV vaccine. The only circumstance in which antigenic variation in HBV has been clinically significant is in postexposure prophylaxis of infants born to HBV-infected mothers, in which vaccine-induced escape mutants have occasionally been observed.

Preexposure immunization against HBV infection was formerly recommended only for individuals at high risk of HBV infection, but the consensus now is that universal hepatitis B immunization has a favorable cost–benefit ratio and should be instituted in all countries. Integration of HBV vaccination into routine infant immunization programs is recommended for all countries with intermediate to high levels of HBV endemicity; in countries with low endemicity, universal immunization of adolescents may be considered an alternative to infant immunization.

HEPATITIS C

Major Immunologic Features

- HCV-specific immune responses critical for viral clearance and pathogenesis

- HCV genetic variability contributes to viral persistence through immunologic escape
- HIV coinfection may worsen the prognosis of chronic HCV infection

General Considerations

Hepatitis C (HCV) is an important cause of acute and chronic hepatitis, linked to the development of cirrhosis and hepatocellular carcinoma. With the development of serologic tests for hepatitis A and B it became evident that a number of cases of hepatitis, particularly posttransfusion hepatitis, were due to another agent. These cases were designated non-A, non-B hepatitis. HCV is the major cause of posttransfusion non-A, non-B hepatitis. As a result of the discovery in 1989 of HCV and its molecular characterization, a number of immunologic assays were developed to assist in diagnosis.

Virology

HCV is a single-stranded, positive-sense RNA virus, discovered in 1989 and originally considered to be a member of the Flaviviridae. HCV was discovered by extracting all of the nucleic acid from the plasma of a chimpanzee with non-A, non-B hepatitis, then reverse transcribing the RNA into DNA and cloning of the product. The RNA encodes a single, large polyprotein encoded by an open reading frame that is proteolytically cleaved. The open reading frame encodes three N-terminal HCV structural proteins (C, E1, and E2) and six nonstructural (NS) C-terminal proteins (including NS2, NS3, NS4, and NS5) that are required for viral replication. Regions encoding the E1 and E2 envelope proteins are highly variable. Six major genotypes have been identified, with at least 50 subtypes. Type 1 is the most prevalent in the United States. The clinical outcome and response to therapy is associated with genotype. Within an infected individual a number of genetically distinct variants or quasi-species also occur. More complex quasi-species correspond to longer duration of infection, higher plasma levels of virus, and poorer response to therapy.

Epidemiology

The distribution of HCV worldwide is fairly uniform, with the frequency of infection in blood donors ranging from 0.2–1.5%. About 4 million individuals are infected in the United States, 20–25% of whom are likely to develop cirrhosis. HCV infection is now the major cause for liver transplantation in the United States. No nonhuman reservoir has been identified.

Transmission is predominantly via percutaneous exposure, in particular, the injection of illicit drugs, but also by transfusion of HCV-contaminated blood products, needlestick injuries in health care workers, and HCV-infected organ transplantation. Community-acquired infections also occur in which the route of transmission is less clear. Maternal–fetal transmission is not a major risk factor for transmission, possibly because patients with chronic HCV infection often have fairly low levels of viremia. HIV coinfection may increase the risk of vertical transmission. Sexual transmission remains a subject of contention.

Immunopathogenesis

Although hepatocytes and B lymphocytes are thought to be infected with HCV, no cellular receptor has been conclusively identified. Recent data show that HCV binds to CD81 via its envelope protein E2, but it is unclear whether this binding is followed by viral entry and infection.

Similar to HBV, the immune response to HCV antigens is considered to be responsible for viral clearance and disease pathogenesis. Viral clearance in acute infection is due to a strong CD4 and CD8 T-cell response, particularly CD8 CTL activity within the liver. Viral persistence is associated with a weak antiviral immune response to viral antigens with lack of eradication of infected cells. In addition, a high rate of HCV genetic variability occurring during viral replication is thought to contribute to viral persistence. This high genetic variability of HCV is of major importance in facilitating viral escape from immune surveillance. HCV also encodes proteins that facilitate evasion of immune surveillance. A poor cytokine response has also been considered to contribute to lack of clearance of HCV from the liver. HCV-specific CD4- and CD8- mediated responses are vigorous during chronic infection, suggesting that persistence may occur even in the presence of an active T-cell response. HCV-specific CD8 CTL not only play a role in eradicating viral infection, they also cause the liver injury once chronic infection is established. The viral core protein has been demonstrated in the transgenic mouse model to induce hepatocellular carcinoma.

Clinical Features

Similar to hepatitis B, acute HCV infection is often asymptomatic (about 60%), or it may present as typical acute hepatitis; fulminant hepatitis is rare. Chronic infection occurs in about 85% of patients with HCV infection. Patients who are chronic carriers may never develop fibrosis, whereas others progress to chronic active hepatitis with cirrhosis. Factors that influence the progression of HCV include age of infection, gender, and immune status. Chronic HCV infection is characterized by fluctuating serum transaminases. Liver biopsy is recommended to evaluate disease severity before antiviral treatment is started. HIV coinfection may worsen the prognosis of HCV infection by enhancing HCV replication. Progression to cirrhosis occurs in about 10% of patients, and regular screening for hepatocellular carcinoma is indicated in these patients. The average time from infection to development of hepatocellular carcinoma is 30 years. Liver transplantation is considered in patients with end-stage liver disease. Recurrence of HCV infection after transplantation is almost universal, but this does not appear to affect survival.

HCV infection is also associated with mixed cryoglobulinemia, porphyria cutanea tarda, membranoproliferative glomerulonephritis, Sjögren's syndrome and diabetes mellitus.

Diagnosis

Diagnosis of infection is made by HCV antibody testing or direct detection of HCV RNA in serum. Second- and third-generation enzyme immunoassays and recombinant immunoblot assays, which include the 5-1-1 and c100-3 antigens, the c22-3 core antigen, and the c33c nonstructural antigen derived from NS3, and, for the third-generation assays, a recombinant NS5 antigen, are highly sensitive for the detection of HCV antibodies. Positive results with the immunoassays are rare earlier than 12 weeks from infection, however.

Quantitative reverse transcription of HCV RNA followed by PCR of the cDNA (RT-PCR) is used in many clinics in the management of HCV to monitor the progress of therapy.

Treatment

Patients with chronic HCV infection who have elevated serum aminotransferase levels and compensated liver disease may be treated with IFNα alone or in combination with ribavirin. Significant benefit is gained from treatment with IFNα, which directly inhibits the replication of HCV intracellularly, resulting in sustained virologic and biochemical responses in 20–40% of patients who receive a 12-month regimen. Response rates are lower in patients infected with genotype 1 HCV who have high serum HCV RNA levels and evidence of cirrhosis. Combination therapy with ribavirin further improves the beneficial response as indicated by a decrease in serum alanine aminotransferase levels and HCV RNA. As proteolytic processing of the HCV polyprotein is catalyzed by the viral serine protease located within the N-terminal region of nonstructural protein 3 (NS3), new therapies using serine protease inhibitors are being investigated.

No vaccine is available to prevent HCV infection.

OTHER HEPATITIS VIRUSES

Delta Hepatitis (HDV)

A defective RNA virus, hepatitis delta virus (HDV), can replicate only in HBV-infected cells, and thus causes infection only in patients with HBV infection. The delta virus genome codes for only one protein, delta antigen, and following replication, genomes of the progeny are packaged in HBsAg. HDV may be cotransmitted with HBV or may superinfect patients with chronic HBV infection.

HDV is transmitted primarily by injection of illicit drugs, although it may also spread by sexual contact. HDV coinfection usually results in more severe HBV disease than HBV alone. HDV superinfection of patients chronically infected with HBV often results in marked worsening of the chronic hepatitis. Diagnosis is made by the detection of antibody to HDV in serum. No specific treatment is available. HDV infection is prevented by hepatitis B immunization

Hepatitis E

HEV, a positive-sense RNA virus encoding three open reading frames that resembles caliciviruses, is the main cause of enterically transmitted non-A, non-B hepatitis. Zoonotic as well as human-to-human transmission of HEV is suspected. Molecular cloning of the viral genome led to the development of diagnostic tests, including an enzyme-linked immunosorbent assay (ELISA) for antibody and reverse transcriptase polymerase chain reaction (RT-PCR) for HEV RNA. Newer assays using a truncated variant of HEV surface proteins are more sensitive and specific in detecting HEV antibodies than the current ELISA. Women who contract HEV infection during the third trimester of pregnancy have a high risk of fulminant hepatitis.

Hepatitis G

Hepatitis G virus (HGV) is a newly identified RNA virus within the Flaviviridae. Up to 10% of blood donors have evidence of infection by PCR. HGV can cause persistent viremia but is not hepatotropic and does not seem to have an important role in liver disease. Most HGV infections are not associated with hepatitis. Sexual transmission, blood transfusion and maternal–fetal transmission of HGV have been documented. Patients receiving chronic renal dialysis and recipients of renal transplants appear to be at high risk for HGV infection. HGV does not appear to worsen the course of concurrent hepatitis A, B, or C.

Transfusion-Transmitted Virus

In 1997, transfusion-transmitted virus (TTV), a novel single-stranded DNA virus, was reported in patients with posttransfusion hepatitis of unknown cause in Japan. This nonenveloped, single-stranded virus has wide sequence diversity and has been classified into 16 genotypes. The prevalence of antibodies to TTV in healthy subjects is high, and changes in TTV DNA titer are not linked to alanine aminotransferase levels, suggesting that TTV is not hepatopathogenic.

RABIES VIRUS

Rabies virus infection is enzootic in many wild animal species, including foxes, skunks, and bats. It can infect many domestic animals (dogs are the most commonly infected), although infection of domestic animals is unusual in developed countries because of the widespread application of control measures. When rabies virus infects humans, generally as the result of an animal bite, the resulting disease is virtually 100% fatal. Hence, preventive measures are of the utmost importance.

Rabies is the type species of the genus Lyssavirus (lyssavirus 1); at least six other lyssaviruses occur, and some can cause a rabies-like illness in humans (eg, the Australian bat lyssavirus). Although only one serotype is detectable by the usual clinical criteria, studies with monoclonal antibodies have identified strains with differing geographic and host ranges. Following a bite wound, the virus replicates in muscles and nerves, extends centripetally along peripheral nerves over a period of days to months or even years, finally reaching the spinal cord and central nervous system. At this stage the hyperexcitability and hydrophobia characteristic of rabies occur. No effective antiviral drugs are available, and even with maximum supportive care, virtually every affected individual dies.

Because of the tremendous epidemiologic and public health implications of a case of rabies, the clinical diagnosis of rabies must be supported by laboratory data. Viral antigens can be detected by immunofluorescence with specific antisera or monoclonal antibodies in the brains of animals and humans and in corneal epithelial cells of humans. This technique is more sensitive than the histopathologic demonstration of Negri bodies. Detection of rabies virus genomic RNA in tissue following amplification by RT-PCR can be used for diagnosis or, if coupled with sequencing or type-specific primers, for subtyping rabies strains. A diagnosis can also be made by demonstrating a rise in antibody titer following infection, although this is less useful clinically.

Animal data support a role for the host immune response in the pathogenesis of rabies. Although immunosuppression of animals prior to infection shortens the latency period and increases the mortality rate, immunosuppression after infection may delay mortality, even though brain virus titers are increased. In immunosuppressed animals with high brain virus titers, administration of rabies hyperimmune serum markedly worsens disease, further supporting the role of the immune system in production of illness.

Antibody to the virus surface glycoprotein (G protein) is protective. Individuals with serum antibody elicited by immunization are resistant to infection, and protection from disease can be achieved even after infection by administration of hyperimmune animal or human antibodies. These antibodies are effective only if given shortly after infection, and their efficacy is increased by local administration around the site of the bite wound, suggesting that they act by local neutralization of the virus.

The first rabies vaccines were prepared by Pasteur in 1880, who used virus that had been adapted to growth in rabbit neural tissue and then inactivated by heating and drying. A wide variety of rabies vaccines are available worldwide. They fall into two general types: those grown in animal brains (eg, rabbit, monkey, mouse) and those grown in cell culture (eg, human diploid fibroblasts, chick embryo cell culture). All are inactivated. Brain-derived vaccines are widely used in developing countries, and although they are effective, they cause a relatively high incidence of postvaccination allergic encephalitis. Cell culture vaccines are used exclusively in developed countries; the first of these, the diploid fibroblast-derived vaccine, causes a low (6%) incidence of allergic reactions, whereas the chick embryo cell culture-derived vaccine appears to be free of such reactions. DNA vaccines against rabies are safe and effective in nonhuman primates and may represent the future of human rabies vaccines. Poxvirus recombinants expressing the rabies virus G protein infect animals and induce rabies immunity if given by mouth and can be distributed in food bait. These latter vaccines have been useful in controlling rabies in feral animal populations.

POLIOVIRUS

Poliovirus is the cause of poliomyelitis, an acute encephalomyelitis that results in asymmetric paralysis with muscle atrophy. Although cases of paralysis almost certainly due to poliovirus have been recognized for thousands of years, the 20th century has seen a marked increase in the incidence of the disease and a change from endemic to epidemic spread. Development of poliovirus vaccine in the middle of the 20th century and its widespread application in developed countries have resulted in the virtual elimination of the disease in vaccinated populations.

Poliovirus is a member of the picornavirus family, which consists of small, nonenveloped positive-stranded RNA viruses and includes other enteroviruses (echovirus, coxsackievirus, etc), rhinoviruses, and HAV. Although closely related by structure, mode of replication, and RNA sequence homology, these viruses exhibit tremendous antigenic diversity, and little or no serologic relatedness or cross-resistance occur among them. Poliovirus has three noncross-reactive serotypes: serotypes 1, 2, and 3. Infection generates a vigorous cellular and humoral immune response to the coat proteins of the virus.

Patients infected with poliovirus and the other enteroviruses shed large amounts of virus in the feces, often for periods of weeks or months. Infection is transmitted when a susceptible individual ingests food or water contaminated by infected feces. The virus replicates in the intestinal tract, and viremia occurs; this is followed by seeding of the spinal cord and central nervous system. Although most patients (>99%) recover without sequelae, the remainder suffer some degree of motor nerve dysfunction, which varies from minimal weakness of an extremity to severe paralysis of all major muscle groups. Partial or complete recovery may occur after the acute illness.

Resolution of infection and elimination of the virus appear to require intact cellular immune mechanisms because patients with defective cellular immunity continue to shed poliovirus as well as other enteroviruses for months or years after infection. Antibodies, however, play some role in recovery from infection because patients with isolated hypogammaglobulinemia also experience persistent enterovirus infections. Resistance to disease is mediated by neutralizing serum antibody to virion surface antigens. Administration of pooled human immune serum globulin containing antibodies to poliovirus prevents the disease, even if given a few days after exposure. In addition, inactivated vaccines that stimulate humoral but not cellular immunity are also highly protective. Intestinal infection can still occur in the presence of serum antibodies; however, viremia with seeding of the central nervous system does not occur. Intestinal mucosal IgA (coproantibody) antibody to poliovirus is stimulated by natural infection and immunization with live attenuated (Sabin-type) vaccine and prevents infection.

The first poliovirus vaccine consisted of tissue culture-grown suspensions of poliovirus types 1–3 inactivated with formalin. Although inactivated (Salk) vaccine is highly effective for preventing paralytic poliomyelitis, it has several disadvantages. It requires parenteral injection (hence, an increased cost for needles and syringes); booster doses are required to maintain immunity; and it does not displace wild-type poliovirus circulating in the community. Live, attenuated (Sabin) vaccine can be given orally; it does not routinely require booster doses; and when immunization is widespread in a community, the vaccine virus displaces the wild-type virus in the environment, thus reducing the risk of paralytic disease among the unimmunized. Live poliovirus may rarely revert to virulence, however, producing paralytic disease in vaccinees or their contacts.

Both inactivated and live attenuated poliovirus vaccines are manufactured and used today, although either one or the other is usually selected by national vaccination programs. The choice between live and inactivated virus vaccine is often the subject of heated debate, but either type of vaccine will virtually eliminates paralytic poliomyelitis if used extensively. Widespread polio immunization has already eradicated poliomyelitis in the Americas and Australasia; the World Health Organization has set in place a program to eradicate poliovirus infection worldwide by early in the 21st century. Active investigation is also under way to improve both the live attenuated and inactivated vaccines.

REFERENCES

GENERAL

Farrell HE, Davis-Poynter NJ: From sabotage to camouflage: Viral evasion of cytotoxic T lymphocyte and natural-killer cell-mediated immunity. *Semin Cell Dev Biol* 1998;9:369.

Granville DJ et al: Interaction of viral proteins with host cell death machinery. *Cell Death Differ* 1998;5:653.

Gale M, Katze MG: Molecular mechanisms of interferon resistance mediated by viral-directed inhibition of PKR, the interferon-induced protein kinase. *Pharmacol Ther* 1998;78:29.

Ploegh HL: Viral strategies of immune evasion. *Science* 1998;280:248.

Smith GL et al: Vaccinia virus immune evasion. *Immunol Rev* 1997;159:137.

Spriggs MK: One step ahead of the game: Viral immunomodulatory molecules. *Ann Rev Immunol* 1996;14: 101.

Taylor DR et al: Inhibition of the interferon-inducible protein kinase PKR by HCV E2 protein. *Science* 1999;285:107.

Tyler KL, Fields BN: Pathogenesis of viral infections. In: *Virology,* 3rd ed. Fields BN et al (editors). Lippincott-Raven Publishers, 1996.

Whitton JL, Oldstone MBA: Immune response to viruses. In: *Virology,* 3rd ed. Fields BN et al (editors). Lippincott-Raven Publishers, 1996.

INFLUENZA VIRUS

Belshe RB et al: The efficacy of live attenuated, cold-adapted, trivalent, intranasal influenza virus vaccine in children. *N Engl J Med* 1998;338:1405.

Bender BS, Small PA: Influenza: Pathogenesis and host defense. *Semin Respir Infect* 1992;7:38.

Klenk HD, Rott, R: The molecular biology of influenza virus pathogenicity. *Adv Virus Res* 1988;34:247.

Lasky T et al: The Guillain-Barré syndrome and the 1992–3 and 1993–4 influenza vaccines. *N Engl J Med* 1998;339: 1797.

Murphy BR, Webster RG: Orthomyxoviruses. In: *Virology,* 3rd ed. Fields BN et al (editors). Lippincott-Raven Publishers, 1996.

Neirynck S et al: A universal influenza A vaccine based on the extracellular domain of the M2 protein. *Nat Med* 1999;5:1157.

Nichol KL et al: Effectiveness of live, attenuated intranasal influenza virus vaccine in healthy working adults. *JAMA* 1999;282:137.

RESPIRATORY SYNCYTIAL VIRUS

Collins PL et al: Respiratory syncytial virus. In: *Virology,* 3rd ed. Fields BN et al (editors). Lippincott-Raven Publishers, 1996.

Crowe JE, Jr: Immune responses of infants to infection with respiratory viruses and live attenuated respiratory virus candidate vaccines. *Vaccine* 1998;16:1423.

Domachowske JB, Rosenberg HF: Respiratory syncytial virus infection: Immune response, immunopathogenesis and treatment. *Clin Microbiol Rev* 1999;12:298.

Mills J: Immunotherapy and immunoprophylaxis of respiratory syncytial virus infections. *Curr Opin Infect Dis* 1995;8:473.

MEASLES VIRUS

Griffin DE, Bellini WJ: Measles virus. In: *Virology,* 3rd ed. Fields BN et al (editors). Lippincott-Raven Publishers, 1996.

Karp CL et al: Mechanism of suppression of cell-mediated immunity by measles virus. *Science* 1999;273:228.

Manchester M et al: Characterization of the inflammatory response during acute measles encephalitis in NSE-CD46 transgenic mice. *J Neuroimmunol* 1999;96:107.

Naniche D et al: Cell cycle arrest during measles virus infection: A G0-like block leads to suppression of retinoblastoma protein expression. *J Virol* 1999;73:1894.

Polack FP et al: Production of atypical measles in rhesus macaques: Evidence for disease mediated by immune complex formation and eosinophils in the presence of fusion-inhibiting antibody. *Nat Med* 1999;5:629.

HEPATITIS A VIRUS

Hollinger FB, Ticehurst JR: Hepatitis A virus. In: *Virology,* 3rd ed. Fields BN et al (editors). Lippincott-Raven Publishers, 1996.

Lemon SM: Hepatitis A virus: Current concepts of the molecular biology, immunobiology and approaches to vaccine development. *Rev Med Virol* 1992;2:73.

HEPATITIS B VIRUS

Chisari FV: Hepatitis B virus biology and pathogenesis. *Mol Genet Med* 1992;2:67.

Ferrari C et al: Immune pathogenesis of hepatitis B. *Arch Virol Suppl* 1992;4:11.

Hollinger FB: Hepatitis B virus. In: *Virology,* 3rd ed. Fields BN et al (editors). Lippincott-Raven Publishers, 1996.

Main J et al: Treatment of chronic viral hepatitis. *Antivir Chem Chemother* 1998;9:449.

Menne S, Tennant BC: Unraveling hepatitis B virus infection of mice and men (and woodchucks and ducks). *Nat Med* 1999;5:1125.

Rehermann B et al: The hepatitis B virus persists for decades after patients' recovery from acute viral hepatitis despite active maintenance of a cytotoxic T-lymphocyte response. *Nat Med* 1996;2:1104.

HEPATITIS C VIRUS

Cooper S et al: Analysis of a successful immune response against hepatitis C virus. *Immunity* 1999;10:439.

Pileri P et al: Binding of hepatitis C virus to CD81. *Science* 1998;282:938.

RABIES VIRUS

Dietzschold B et al: Rhabdoviruses. In: *Virology,* 3rd ed. Fields BN et al (editors). Lippincott-Raven Publishers, 1996.

Dreesen, DW. A global review of rabies vaccines for human use. *Vaccine* 1997;15:S2.

King AA, Turner GS: Rabies: A review. *J Comp Pathol* 1993;108:1.

Lodmell DL et al: DNA immunization protects nonhuman primates against rabies virus. *Nat Med* 1998;4:49.

POLIOVIRUS

Melnick JL: Enteroviruses: Polioviruses, coxsackieviruses, echoviruses, and newer enteroviruses. In: *Virology,* 3rd ed. Fields BN et al (editors). Lippincott-Raven Publishers, 1996.

HUMAN HERPESVIRUS TYPE 8 (HHV-8).

Chang Y et al: Identification of herpesvirus-like DNA sequences in AIDS-associated Kaposi's sarcoma. *Science* 1994;266:1865.

Moore PS et al: Molecular mimicry of human cytokine and cytokine response pathway genes by KSHV. *Science* 1996;274:1739.

Martin JN et al: Sexual transmission and the natural history of human herpesvirus 8 infection. *N Engl J Med* 1998; 338:948.

Regamey N et al: Transmission of HHV-8 infection from renal-transplant donors to recipients. *N Engl J Med* 1998; 339:1358.

Sitas F et al: Antibodies against HHV-8 in black South African patients with cancer. *N Engl J Med* 1999;340: 1863.

Cesarman E, Knowles DM: The role of HHV-8 in lymphoproliferative diseases. *Semin Cancer Biol* 1999;9:165.

46

AIDS & Other Virus Infections of the Immune System

Suzanne Crowe, MD, MBBS, FRACP, & John Mills, MD

Although measles virus infection has been recognized for decades as a cause of immunosuppression, Epstein-Barr virus (EBV) was the first pathogen shown to cause immune dysfunction as a result of directly infecting cells of the immune system. Since then, other viruses, especially herpesviruses and retroviruses, have been identified that can infect cells of the immune system and produce immune suppression, immune stimulation, or both. The discovery of the human immunodeficiency virus (HIV), which primarily infects immune cells, has provided additional impetus for understanding the mechanisms by which virus infection results in immune dysfunction.

HUMAN IMMUNODEFICIENCY VIRUS

Major Immunologic Features
- CD4 cells of the immune system, including T lymphocytes, monocyte–macrophages, follicular dendritic cells, and Langerhans' cells, infected
- Progressive global defects of humoral and cell-mediated immunity
- CD4 (helper–inducer) T lymphocytes depleted
- Polyclonal activation of B lymphocytes with increased immunoglobulin production
- Disease progression despite vigorous humoral and cell-mediated responses to the virus

General Considerations
The acquired immune deficiency syndrome (AIDS) was first recognized in 1981. The identification of HIV as the causative agent of AIDS in 1983–1984 was rapidly followed by characterization of this virus and the target cells it infects and by elucidation of the multiple consequences of infection. Epidemiologic studies have identified the major populations at risk of acquiring infection and the routes by which the virus can be transmitted. The clinical illnesses associated with HIV infection have been classified, and therapeutic strategies to treat or suppress them have been designed. By 1985, diagnostic kits had been developed for the detection of antibody to HIV, potentially therapeutic compounds were being screened for in vitro activity against this virus,

and clinical trials for safety and efficacy of these potential drugs had begun. In 1987, only 6 years after the initial recognition of the AIDS epidemic and 3 years after identification of HIV, zidovudine (2′-azido-3′-deoxythymidine [AZT]), the first antiretroviral agent, was licensed by the US Food and Drug Administration for treatment of HIV infection.

Infection with HIV results in an acquired defect in immune function, especially involving cell-mediated immunity. Infected individuals may be asymptomatic or have progressive disease associated with recurrent opportunistic infections, certain cancers, severe weight loss, and central nervous system degeneration. Over the past few years the use of potent combinations of antiretroviral drugs (highly active antiretroviral therapy, HAART) together with the ability to monitor treatment responses by quantifying HIV RNA in plasma has remarkably altered the prognosis of HIV infection. HAART has dramatically reduced the incidence of opportunistic infections and improved survival.

The recognition of the viral etiology of AIDS has stimulated immunologists to investigate the pathogenesis of the disease. Rational development of effective antiretroviral compounds can be aided by knowledge of the mechanisms by which HIV can damage the immune system. Although research on HIV has provided us with more pathogenetic information than we have on any other virus, the genesis of the characteristic and profound immune dysfunction caused by HIV still remains incompletely understood.

Etiology
A. Virology: HIV is a member of the retrovirus family, a group of enveloped viruses possessing the enzyme reverse transcriptase. This enzyme allows the virus to synthesize a DNA copy of its RNA genome. HIV was previously termed *human T-lymphotrophic virus type III* (HTLV-III), *lymphadenopathy-associated virus* (LAV), and *AIDS-related virus* (ARV). Molecular characterization of these retroviruses demonstrated their relatedness, however, and they are regarded as variants of the same virus. HIV has been subclassified within the lentivirus family, a group of nontransforming retroviruses with a long latency pe-

riod from infection to the onset of clinical features, similar morphologic features, and nucleotide sequence homology. Other members of the lentivirus family include visna and caprine arthritis-encephalitis viruses, which cause chronic, progressive neurodegenerative disease in sheep and goats, respectively. The clinical picture of lentivirus infection in sheep and goats is fairly similar to that resulting from HIV infection in humans and is characterized by a slow and progressive disorder of the immune system and the brain. HIV is also closely related to simian immunodeficiency virus (SIV), which causes an AIDS-like illness in macaque monkeys. There are two types of HIV: HIV-1 is most prevalent in central Africa, the United States, Europe, and Australia; HIV-2 is found in west Africa, parts of Europe, and less commonly elsewhere. As a result of mutation and recombination events, a number of defined variants of HIV-1 and HIV-2 have now been defined. There are two groups of HIV-1: the M (major) group, which predominates worldwide and is subdivided into at least nine subtypes or clades (A to I) based primarily on *env* (and *gag*) sequence differences, and the O (outlier) group, which consists of a smaller number of divergent strains. HIV-2 has been similarly subdivided into subtypes. At the molecular level, HIV-2 more closely resembles SIV, supporting data that suggest that HIV originated from primate lentiviruses. When compared with HIV-1, HIV-2 has a longer clinical latency period from the time of infection to the development of symptoms and has a lower rate of vertical transmission (Table 46–1; Figure 46–1).

B. Genomic Organization: HIV consists of an inner core, containing an RNA genome, surrounded by a lipid envelope. The HIV genome (Figure 46–2)

Table 46–1. Classification of retroviruses.

Oncoviruses	Lentiviruses	Spumiviruses
Avian retroviruses	Visna/maedi virus	Human foamy virus
Bovine leukemia virus	Caprine arthritis encephalitis virus	Simian foamy virus
Murine retroviruses	Equine infectious anemia virus	
Feline leukemia virus	HIV-1 and HIV-2	
HTLV-I and HTLV-II	Simian immunodeficiency virus	

Abbreviations: HTLV = human T-cell leukemia virus; HIV = human immunodeficiency virus.

contains the standard retroviral structural genes, *env, gag,* and *pol,* encoding the viral envelope proteins, viral core protein, and viral enzymes (reverse transcriptase, integrase, and proteinase), respectively. HIV and SIV possess at least six other genes, a feature that makes them unique among retroviruses. Many of these gene products are made as precursor proteins, which must be cleaved by viral proteinases or cellular enzymes later in the replicative cycle. Within the DNA provirus, the viral genes are flanked by long terminal repeats (LTR) at both the 5′ and the 3′ ends. The LTR contains enhancer and promoter elements, which are necessary for transcription. Cellular factors that modulate transcription bind to sequences within the U3 domain of the LTR. HIV is initially transcribed into a full-length messenger ribonucleic acid (mRNA), which is translated into the structural Gag and Pol proteins. Production of singly and multiply spliced mRNA is necessary for the syn-

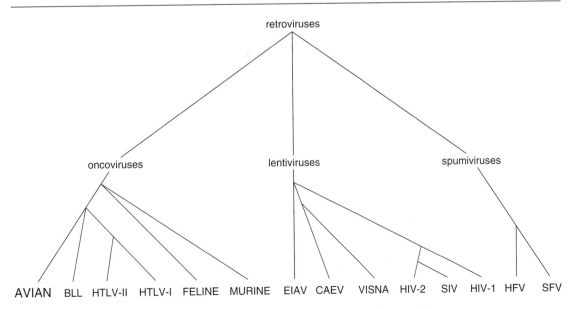

Figure 46–1. Schematic evolutionary relationships among retroviruses.

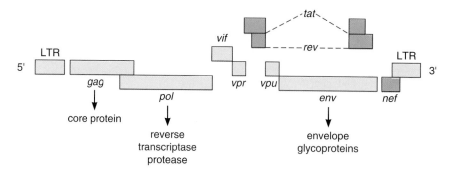

Figure 46–2. Genomic organization of HIV. The 9.6-kb genome of HIV consists of both structural and regulatory sequences (see text for details). HIV has a far more complex genome than that of many other retroviruses.

thesis of the envelope proteins and accessory proteins, respectively.

The *gag* and *env* genes encode a number of proteins that are fundamentally responsible for virion structural integrity and entry into cells. The *env*-encoded gp160 is cleaved to form gp120 and gp41, and these extensively glycosylated proteins are responsible for binding to CD4 and a chemokine receptor on the cell surface and subsequent fusion of virus with cell membranes, respectively. A translational frameshift between *gag* and *pol* results in production of the Gag-Pol polyprotein Pr160$^{gag/pol}$, which is cleaved by protease to yield reverse transcriptase and RNase H, integrase, and protease. This frameshifting event occurs at a frequency of 5–10% of Gag synthesis due to a slippage sequence, causing the ribosome to slip back 1 nucleotide (-1 frameshifting) and translate the *pol* coding sequence, thus bypassing the *gag* termination codon. Gag polyprotein Pr55^{gag} encodes mature capsid proteins MA (p17), CA (p24), p2, NC (p7), p1, and p6 through proteolytic cleavage by the virus-encoded protease.

The first of the additional gene products to be recognized was the transactivating protein Tat, a positive-feedback regulator of HIV replication, which can accelerate viral protein production several 1000-fold. Tat binds to TAR (transactivating response) structures within the R domain of the LTR at both the DNA and RNA levels. The *rev* gene encodes proteins that regulate viral mRNA expression. The Rev protein permits unspliced mRNA to leave the nucleus and thus inhibits transcription of the regulatory genes while enhancing expression of the viral structural genes. Rev protein binds to the Rev-responsive element (RRE), within the *env* gene. Additional Rev monomers are required to assemble on the RRE because multimerization is necessary for Rev function. The product of the virion infectivity gene, *vif*, increases viral infectivity and may be responsible for the efficient cell-to-cell transmission observed with HIV. The *nef* gene is critical for HIV pathogenicity. A number of functions of Nef have been elucidated, including down-modulation of CD4 and major histocompatibility complex (MHC) class I expression on the surface of T lymphocytes, interaction with cellular serine-threonine kinases MAPK/ERK and tyrosine kinases including the Src family members lck and hck through SH3 domains, and enhancement of viral infectivity. The role of Nef in HIV pathogenesis is clear from experiments both in macaques, in which *nef*-deleted strains of SIV were less pathogenic than wild-type virus, and from data regarding a cohort of HIV-infected long-term slow-progressors who were all infected with a strain of HIV-1 that has deletions in the *nef* region. Two further genes have been described: the *vpr* (viral protein R) gene, and the *vpu* (viral protein U) gene. The *vpr* gene is considered to play a role in the regulation of viral and cellular gene expression and may be important in viral assembly and infection of macrophages. It also induces apoptosis through cell-cycle arrest. The gene *vpu* influences release of HIV from the cell surface and contributes to CD4 degradation within the endoplasmic reticulum (see Figure 46–2).

C. Pathogenesis of Infection: HIV infection affects predominantly the immune system and the brain. The dominant immunologic feature of HIV infection is progressive depletion of the CD4 (helper–inducer) subset of T lymphocytes, thereby reversing the normal CD4:CD8 ratio and inexorably causing immunodeficiency. The depletion of CD4 lymphocytes is predominantly due to the tropism of HIV for these and other CD4-bearing cells because the CD4 cell surface molecule functions as a receptor for the virus. The CD4 lymphocyte is necessary for the proper functioning of the immune system. It interacts with antigen-presenting cells, B cells, cytotoxic T cells, and natural killer (NK) cells (see Chapter 9). Thus, it is easy to see that infection and depletion of this cell population could induce profound immunodeficiency. Early in situ hybridization studies suggested that only very few (about 1 in 10,000) CD4 lymphocytes contain replicating HIV. More recently, studies of peripheral blood lymphocytes have demonstrated that up to

1 in 10 of these cells are infected with HIV, particularly in persons with advanced disease. Although the data are limited, the number of infected cells in tissues appears to be larger than that in peripheral blood.

The finding that the CD4 molecule is present on cells other than helper-inducer T lymphocytes was accompanied by evidence that HIV could infect other cell populations that expressed this molecule on their surface. Other cells susceptible to HIV infection include monocyte–macrophages, microglial cells, Langerhans' cells, and other bone-marrow-derived cells, and immortalized B cells. Whether HIV is able to infect macrophages or lymphocytes (cell tropism) is determined largely by the amino acid sequence of the HIV envelope.

The chemokine receptors CCR5 and CXCR4 have been identified as major coreceptors for HIV-1. Following binding of gp120 to specific epitopes (V1 region) of the CD4 molecule on the cell surface, a conformational change occurs in gp120 that permits binding to either CCR5 or CXCR4 receptors. This exposes the fusion domain on gp41, allowing HIV to fuse with host cell plasma membranes and enter the cell. Macrophage-tropic (M-tropic), nonsyncytium-inducing strains of HIV-1 use the CCR5 coreceptor for HIV entry, whereas T-cell line (T-tropic) syncytium-inducing strains of HIV-1 enter via CXCR4 coreceptor. As a result of this finding, these strains are now called "R5" and "X4" strains, respectively. Other molecules, including Fc receptors, complement receptors, and galactosyl ceramide receptor, may act as accessory receptors for HIV on some cell types, such as macrophages, fibroblasts, brain astrocytes, and oligodendrocytes. The first cellular targets of HIV infection are thought to be Langerhans' cells and other tissue dendritic cells within the lamina propria. Where studied, the strains of HIV found in newly infected patients are almost always macrophage-tropic (R5), which infect dendritic cells more efficiently than X4 strains. Infected dendritic cells carry the virus to deeper tissues and to regional lymph nodes where infection spreads to CD4-expressing T lymphocytes. Shortly after this systemic dissemination occurs. Cells of macrophage lineage are thought to provide an important reservoir for HIV in vivo and may contribute to the pathogenesis of the immune deficiency by functioning abnormally. For example, HIV-infected macrophages poorly phagocytose organisms such as *Candida albicans, Toxoplasma gondii,* and *Mycobacterium avium complex.* Although the pathogenesis of immune dysfunction associated with HIV infection is incompletely understood, it is likely that the process occurs through collective dysfunction of both antigen-presenting cells, such as macrophages, and T lymphocytes, especially the CD4 subset.

The loss of CD4 lymphocytes, which is characteristic of HIV infection, occurs largely as a result of apoptosis, or programmed cell death. Other mechanisms also contribute to the death of uninfected CD4 T cells, including cell fusion with HIV-infected cells, the development of pores in the cell membrane of the infected lymphocyte as HIV buds from the cell surface, the accumulation of unintegrated viral DNA within the cell cytoplasm, and the killing of both uninfected CD4 T cells (innocent bystanders) that have found free HIV envelope glycoprotein gp120 and HIV-infected cells expressing gp120 by gp120-specific clones of cytotoxic lymphocytes.

Recent data show that from the time of infection huge numbers of virions are produced every day, with rapid turnover of both HIV virions (half-life approximately 6 hours) as well as infected T cells (half-life less than 1.5 days). Although the level of HIV RNA in plasma may be low during the time of clinical latency, limited data suggest that considerable amounts of virus are produced in tissues, particularly in the lymph nodes.

Activated CD4-expressing T lymphocytes that are productively infected with the HIV are responsible for about 99% of plasma HIV RNA (viral load). These cells are also exquisitely susceptible to antiretroviral therapies. Cells of macrophage lineage contribute only about 1% of viral load, but are more resistant to therapy, due to longer half-life and to their location in tissues such as the brain into which antiretroviral drugs penetrate poorly. Thus these cells are considered to be an important reservoir of HIV in infected individuals.

During acute infection the viral load is often extremely high. Once cytotoxic T lymphocyte (CTL) and other immune responses develop, the viral load declines. About 9 months after infection a balance is achieved between the host immune response and the virus; this is reflected by a relatively stable concentration of HIV RNA in plasma and is termed the **virologic set-point.** A high set-point is associated with a poor prognosis and vice versa.

HIV replication within monocyte-macrophages occurs at a leisurely pace compared with that within lymphocytes, with little cytopathology, supporting their role as a viral reservoir in vivo. Resting T lymphocytes can also be infected with HIV, but the virus replication cycle is blocked at the reverse transcription step. If the cell is activated within a few days, infectious virus is produced; otherwise, the infection is aborted. These nonactivated lymphocytes provide an additional reservoir of HIV in infected persons. Through studies of patients receiving HAART, long-lived resting memory CD34-expressing CD4 lymphocytes have also been shown to be a reservoir of HIV. Infectious virus can be recovered from these cells in the blood of persons who have had extremely low levels of plasma HIV RNA (less than 50 copies/mL) for months or years. The factors that trigger latently infected cells to produce virus are not completely known. A number of intracellular and viral factors can influence the production of HIV.

These include cellular transcription factors such as the DNA-binding protein NFκB, as well as cytokines, including tumor necrosis factor alpha (TNFα) and the colony-stimulating factors GM-CSF and M-CSF, which have been found to augment HIV replication. A number of viruses (herpes simplex virus, cytomegalovirus, adenovirus, human T-lymphotropic virus type I, Epstein-Barr virus, and hepatitis B virus) stimulate HIV replication in vitro, but these findings have not been substantiated clinically. In addition, HIV regulatory genes themselves can influence viral production.

Early in infection, when the individual is asymptomatic, macrophage-tropic strains of HIV are isolated predominantly from peripheral blood. At this stage, the virus generally does not produce the characteristic cytopathology of multinucleated giant cells or syncytia in cell culture and is described as nonsyncytium-inducing (NSI). A change in viral phenotype from NSI to syncytium-inducing may occur at approximately the same time as decline in CD4 numbers and the onset of HIV-related clinical disease. In a number of individuals, however, progression of disease occurs without a change in viral phenotype. The tropism of the viral strains also broadens to include T lymphocytes and other cell populations as disease progresses. Another major feature of HIV infection is involvement of the central nervous system. The clinical findings range from minor memory defects to personality changes to progressive, fatal dementia. The mechanism of brain damage is obscure. Because there is no evidence to support direct neuronal infection with HIV, it is more likely that soluble factors such as quinolinic acid or TNFα secreted by infected cells that transport the virus to the brain may alter the function of neurons and contribute to the dementia. In infected brain tissue, HIV has been detected in multinucleated giant cells composed predominantly of monocyte–macrophages and in microglia, suggesting a major pathogenetic role for these cells. An alternative hypothesis is that HIV may competitively inhibit neuroleukin from binding to neurons. This neurotrophic factor shares homology with a conserved region of the HIV envelope glycoprotein, gp 120.

Epidemiology

Transmission of HIV has been documented to occur via both homosexual and heterosexual contact, administration of infected blood or blood products, artificial insemination with infected semen, exposure to blood-containing needles or syringes, and transmission from an infected mother to her fetus or to the infant during or after birth (Table 46–2). Male-to-female transmission is more commonly reported than female-to-male transmission. Transmission from mother to offspring occurs by transplacental passage of the virus at the time of delivery, in utero or, through breast feeding, with estimates for the preva-

Table 46–2. Individuals at risk of HIV infection.

High risk
Homosexual and bisexual men
Injecting drug users who share needles or syringes
Sexual partners of people in high-risk groups
Children born to infected mothers, especially those not receiving antiretroviral drugs
Blood transfusion recipients in countries where blood bank testing is unavailable
Low risk
Health care workers, including nurses, doctors, dentists, and laboratory staff

lence of transmission of HIV from an infected mother to her child varying from 15 to 30%. Antiretroviral therapy of mother and infant can reduce the risk of vertical transmission to 5% or less. The diagnosis of HIV in a neonate can be difficult (see the section on neonatal diagnosis). Health care workers are at risk of HIV infection, but this risk is considered to be very low (approximately 1:250 HIV-positive needlestick exposures results in infection). Epidemiologic data do not support transmission of HIV by casual contact, insects, or sharing of utensils (tableware, toothbrushes, etc). No data suggest aerosolized transmission of the virus. HIV can be detected in saliva samples from HIV-infected persons, at extremely low titer (less than one infectious particle per milliliter). Similarly, urine, feces, sweat, tears, and amniotic fluid are considered unlikely to transmit HIV because of their extremely low viral titers.

In central and western Africa and Asia, cases of AIDS are equally distributed among men and women, and heterosexual transmission (especially from infected female prostitutes to their clients) is thought to account for the majority of cases. Risk factors associated with HIV infection in heterosexuals include large numbers of sexual partners, prostitution, sex with prostitutes, a history of sexually transmitted disease such as a gonorrhea or syphilis, and genital ulceration of any cause. Although both bowel mucosa and cervical epithelium can be infected with HIV, the chance of infection is markedly increased if abrasions or ulceration are present. Other risk factors include multiple use of needles or syringes in health clinics and ritualistic practices in which unsterilized instruments are used; these include scarification, tattooing, and ear-piercing.

Exposure to HIV does not always result in infection. One exposure may be sufficient to cause infection, however, depending on inoculum size, route of entry, and perhaps, host factors. The dose to infect 50% of exposed individuals (ID_{50}) is unknown for humans, but it is presumed to be low (<10–100 virions). Both cell-free and cell-associated viruses are infectious. About 50% of HIV-infected individuals not receiving antiretroviral therapy will contract AIDS over a 10- to 12-year period from the time of infection. The latency period (from time of infection to onset of disease) may vary according to viral inoculum, virulence of the infecting strain, route of entry, and age of the patient.

Individuals who are homozygous for a 32-nucleotide deletion in the CCR5 gene are extremely resistant to HIV-1 infection. Only a handful of cases of HIV infection in CCR5 delta-32 homozygotes have been reported worldwide; these individuals were infected with CXCR4-using (X4) strains of HIV-1. (Heterozygotes for this mutation have low levels of CCR5 expression on cells and have no resistance to infection but a slower rate of HIV disease progression compared with normals.) Other genetic determinants of susceptibility to HIV infection or disease progression include HLA types, other mutations in chemokine or chemokine receptor genes, and mutations resulting in low levels of the serum collectin mannose-binding protein.

Clinical Features

A. Acute HIV Mononucleosis: Following infection with HIV, an individual may remain asymptomatic or develop an acute illness that resembles infectious mononucleosis. This syndrome usually occurs within 2–6 weeks after infection, with reported periods ranging from 5 days to 3 months. The predominant symptoms are fever, headache, sore throat, malaise, and rash. Clinical findings include pharyngitis (which may be exudative and may be accompanied by mucosal ulceration); generalized lymphadenopathy; a macular or urticarial rash on the face, trunk, and limbs; and hepatosplenomegaly (Table 46–3). During the acute illness, antibodies to HIV are generally undetectable. Although the illness is often severely incapacitating, requiring bedrest or even hospitalization, some individuals experience only mild symptoms and do not seek medical attention.

Acute infection with HIV has also been associated with neurologic disease, including meningitis, encephalitis, cranial nerve palsies, myopathy, and peripheral neuropathy. These findings are usually accompanied by features of the acute HIV mononucleosis syndrome.

B. Symptomatic HIV Infection: The development of HIV-related symptoms is regarded as evidence of progressive immune dysfunction. Constitutional symptoms and signs include persistent fever, night sweats, weight loss (but insufficient weight loss to fulfill the Centers for Disease Control and Preven-

tion [CDC] criteria for AIDS) unexplained chronic diarrhea, eczema, psoriasis, seborrheic dermatitis, herpes zoster, oral candidiasis, and oral hairy leukoplakia. The last two conditions are regarded as poor prognostic indicators and herald progression to AIDS. HIV-related thrombocytopenia (defined as a platelet count of <50,000/μL without other known causes) is found in less than 10% of individuals, usually does not result in a bleeding diathesis, and does not herald disease progression.

C. AIDS: The criteria for diagnosis of AIDS have been defined by the CDC and comprise certain opportunistic infections and cancers, HIV-related encephalopathy, HIV-induced wasting syndrome, and a broader range of AIDS-indicative diseases in individuals who have laboratory evidence of HIV infection. The CDC has now altered the definition to include adults and adolescents with diagnosed HIV infection who have a CD4 lymphocyte count of less than 200 cells/μL of blood or a CD4 T-lymphocyte level of less than 14% regardless of clinical symptoms. In addition, pulmonary tuberculosis, recurrent bacterial pneumonia, and invasive cervical cancer have been added to the list of AIDS-defining conditions.

The most common opportunistic infections encountered are *Pneumocystis carinii* pneumonitis; disseminated cryptococcosis; toxoplasmosis; mycobacterial disease (both *Mycobacterium avium* complex infection and tuberculosis); chronic, ulcerative, recurrent herpes simplex virus infection; disseminated cytomegalovirus infection; and histoplasmosis (Table 46–4). Patients with AIDS also have a higher incidence of *Salmonella* bacteremia, staphylococcal infections, and pneumococcal pneumonia. Children with AIDS may develop opportunistic infections such as *P carinii* pneumonia, but they have a higher incidence of lymphocytic interstitial pneumonitis and recurrent bacterial infections than adults do.

The most common cancer diagnosed in AIDS patients is Kaposi's sarcoma, a neoplasm or neoplasm-like disease involving endothelia and mesenchymal stroma. Once common in AIDS patients, this tumor is now less frequently seen as a presenting illness. The reason for this is obscure. A herpesvirus (HHV-8) is the causal agent of Kaposi's sarcoma. Late in the course of immune dysfunction, high-grade B-cell lymphomas are encountered; these are generally resistant to therapy.

Table 46–3. Clinical features of acute HIV infection.

Fever and sweats
Myalgia and arthralgia
Malaise and lethargy
Lymphadenopathy and splenomegaly
Pharyngitis
Anorexia, nausea, and vomiting
Headaches and photophobia
Macular rash

Table 46–4. Common opportunistic infections encountered in AIDS patients.

Pneumocystis carinii pneumonia
Toxoplasmosis
Mycobacterium avium complex disease
Disseminated *Mycobacterium tuberculosis* infection
Persistent, ulcerative herpes simplex virus infection
Disseminated cytomegalovirus infection
Cryptococcal meningitis

Laboratory Diagnosis

A. Serology:

1. Seroconversion. During the early phase of the primary illness, antibodies to HIV are not detected in the serum; they generally appear 3–4 weeks after infection. IgM antibodies, detected by immunofluorescence, generally precede IgG antibody detection by Western immunoblot. During seroconversion, antibodies directed against the various viral proteins do not develop simultaneously. Those directed against HIV p24 (core) and gp41 (transmembrane) proteins can be detected before those directed at the *pol* gene products on Western blot.

HIV antigenemia (predominantly HIV p24, measured by enzyme immunoassay) usually precedes seroconversion. The serum or plasma p24 antigen assay is licensed for diagnosis of HIV infection. Methods to detect p24 antigen by enzyme-linked immunosorbent assay (ELISA) involve an acid dissociation technique to remove the antigen from complexed antibody.

Quantitative reverse transcriptase polymerase chain reaction (RT-PCR) and branched-chain DNA assays are used to quantify HIV RNA in plasma. In patients with acute HIV infection with undetectable antibody by ELISA, the plasma viral load usually is very high (>100,000 copies/mL). These tests are currently not licensed to diagnose HIV infection due to lack of specificity. False-positive results in viral load assays, usually less than 3000 copies/mL, have been reported.

2. Screening for HIV. ELISA is the basic screening test currently used to detect antibodies to HIV. Recombinant virion proteins or synthetic peptides are immobilized on plastic beads or multiwell trays. Test serum containing antibodies to HIV bind to these viral proteins. An enzyme-linked antihuman antibody added to the reaction binds to the complex and is detected colorimetrically. The ELISA is both highly sensitive (> 99%) and highly specific (> 99% in high-risk populations). The genomic diversity between HIV-1 and HIV-2 is greatest within the envelope region. Because significant homology exists between the *gag* and *pol* gene products of the subtypes of HIV, HIV-2 can usually be detected by HIV-1 ELISAs. Early HIV-1 ELISA tests performed poorly in detecting antibodies to HIV-2 and to group O HIV-1. Current ELISA tests have included antigens that efficiently detect HIV-2 and most group O infections.

3. Confirmatory Tests. A repeatedly reactive ELISA should be confirmed by either a Western blot or, less commonly, immunofluorescence assay. Because of its high sensitivity, a negative ELISA does not usually warrant confirmatory testing. The Western blot detects specific antibodies directed against the various HIV proteins. Purified viral proteins are run on a polyacrylamide gel, transferred to a nitrocellulose membrane, and then reacted with the test serum. Antibodies to HIV present in the serum bind

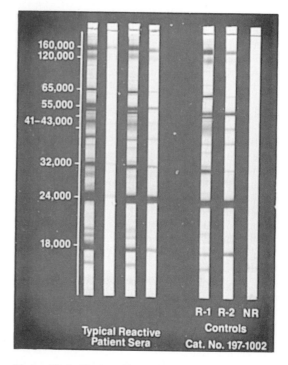

Figure 46–3. Western blot analysis. Reactive sera typically contain demonstrable antibodies to envelope proteins gp160, gp120, and gp41, as well as to core proteins p55 and p24 and to reverse transcriptase p32. Detection of antibody to p24 alone is insufficient to meet the diagnostic criteria for a positive Western blot and may be due to a nonspecific reaction. Alternatively, a reactive band at 24,000 may represent an early serologic response during seroconversion. (Photograph courtesy of Bio-Rad Laboratories, Richmond, CA.)

to the specific viral protein (Figure 46–3). Interpretation of HIV western blot reactions is partly subjective, and criteria are established to designate positive, indeterminate, and negative reactions. In general, antibodies to at last two or three critical virion proteins (p24, gp41, and gp120/160) constitute a positive result, and the absence of antibodies to any HIV protein is reported as negative.

B. Neonatal Diagnosis: Neonates with HIV infection pose a difficult serodiagnostic problem because maternal IgG antibody crosses the placenta. Thus, the infant passively acquires anti-HIV antibody, which may persist for up to 15 months. Although the level of antibody in uninfected infants gradually declines, this occurs too slowly to be of clinical value in the context of making treatment decisions. Detection of serum p24 antigen in the infant confirms the diagnosis of HIV infection. In addition, culture of virus from peripheral blood or tissue, detection of HIV cDNA in peripheral blood mononuclear cells, or plasma HIV RNA in plasma may be helpful, although these are not tests licensed for HIV diagnosis. The predictive value of specific IgM antibodies in the diagnosis of neonatal and perinatal infection awaits clarification. Culture of the virus from peripheral blood or tissue or demonstration of HIV antigen is therefore necessary to be confident of the diagnosis of HIV infection in asymptomatic infants born to HIV-infected mothers. The PCR, which amplifies HIV genome present in cells or serum, provides a useful adjunct to diagnosis.

Immunologic Findings

A. CD4 Lymphocyte Depletion: The immunologic hallmark of AIDS is a defect in cell-mediated immunity, characteristically associated with a decrease in the number and function of the CD4 T lymphocytes. CD4 T lymphocytes are functionally separated into the T_H1 subset, which produces interferon gamma (IFNγ) and IL-2, and the T_H2 subset, which produces IL-4, IL-6, and IL-10. In advanced HIV infection, the T_H1 subset is markedly decreased in number.

CD4 cell numbers range in a spectrum in all clinical stages of HIV infection: occasional asymptomatic individuals have very low counts, whereas rarely the values are normal in individuals with AIDS. Individuals who present with Kaposi's sarcoma may have higher CD4 cell counts than those who initially present with AIDS-defining opportunistic infections. CD4 cell levels are of prognostic value: The risk of progression to AIDS in a given time interval increases as the CD4 count declines. The CD4 number can also provide a guide to the risk of development of individual opportunistic infections and malignancies (Figure 46–4). Not unexpectedly, certain infections with organisms of high virulence (eg, *Mycobacterium tuberculosis*) are manifest when the CD4 count is well preserved, whereas others with organisms of lower virulence (eg, *M avium* complex) tend to occur only when the CD4 number is much lower. In general the CD4 lymphocyte number is less than 200 cells/μL of blood at the time of AIDS diagnosis, and with the routine use of prophylaxis for common opportunistic infections and antiretroviral drugs, the CD4 number is in fact commonly lower than 100/μL at the onset of the first AIDS-defining illness. With the use of HAART, many patients are experiencing a rise in CD4 counts from less than 100 cells/μL to well above 200 cells/μL. In these patients, clinicians are cautiously discontinuing prophylactic treatments such as trimethoprim–sulfamethoxazole (used to prevent *Pneumocystis carinii* pneumonia and *Toxo-*

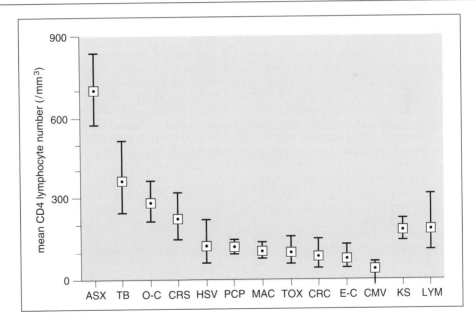

Figure 46–4. The mean CD4 lymphocyte numbers and approximately 95% confidence intervals for individuals with asymptomatic HIV infection, oral candidiasis, or AIDS-defining opportunistic infections or malignancies. Assessments were performed between 2 months preceding or 1 month following diagnosis of the illness, with 55% being determined at the time of diagnosis. A total of 307 events in 222 patients were examined. *Abbreviations:* ASX = asymptomatic infection; TB = disseminated tuberculosis; O-C = oral candidiasis; CRS = *Cryptosporidium;* HSV = recurrent mucocutaneous herpes simplex virus; PCP = *P carinii* pneumonia; MAC = disseminated *M avium* complex; TOX = *T gondii* encephalitis; CRC = cryptococcal meningitis; E-C = esophageal candidiasis; CMV = cytomegalovirus retinitis; KS = Kaposi's sarcoma; LYM = lymphoma. (Reproduced, with permission, from Crowe SM et al: Predictive value of CD4 lymphocyte numbers for the development of opportunistic infections and malignancies in HIV-infected persons. *J Acquir Immune Defic Syndr* 1991;4:770.)

plasma encephalitis as well as bacterial infections), even though the full CD4 T lymphocyte repertoire is not restored after therapy.

The CD4:CD8 ratio invariably becomes inverted primarily as a consequence of CD4 lymphocyte depletion. A variety of other conditions, however, including infection with EBV, hepatitis B virus, and cytomegalovirus (CMV), can cause inversion of the CD4:CD8 ratio, primarily owing to an increase in the CD8 subset. Thus, this ratio is of no diagnostic value.

B. Abnormal Delayed-Type Hypersensitivity Responses: Delayed-type hypersensitivity responses are usually normal in the early phase of HIV infection and decreased or absent in patients with advanced disease.

C. T-Cell Proliferative Responses: The normal in vitro proliferative responses of CD4 T lymphocytes to soluble antigens (eg, tetanus toxoid) and mitogens (eg, concanavalin A, phytohemagglutinin, or pokeweed mitogen) are impaired in HIV-infected individuals, especially AIDS patients. This abnormality may be due to a selective loss of a subset of CD4 lymphocytes, to defective antigen presentation by monocyte–macrophages, or to direct viral suppression of CD4 lymphocyte function. In contrast to individuals experiencing progression of HIV infection, those with long-term nonprogressive disease frequently have strong HIV-specific CD4 proliferative activity. Responses to mitogens tend to vary in HIV-infected individuals and are less severely impaired than responses to antigen. Antigen responses but not mitogen responses strictly require the interaction of the CD4 molecule on the surface of the lymphocyte with the class II MHC molecule. The HIV envelope glycoprotein (gp120) binds to the CD4 molecule, and its presence could interfere with the interaction with the class II MHC molecule, thus explaining why mitogen responses are less impaired than antigen responses.

D. Cytotoxic Lymphocyte Responses: Cells infected with HIV provide a target for lysis by the various types of cytotoxic cells, including MHC-restricted cytotoxic lymphocytes, MHC-nonrestricted NK cells, and lymphokine-activated cells. Cytotoxic T lymphocyte (CD8 or CD4) responses and NK cell activity are present but quantitatively defective in cells from HIV-infected individuals with late stages of infection. Long-term nonprogressors of HIV infection have high precursor frequencies of HIV-specific CTL with broad specificity, including recognition of HIV core proteins, compared with CTL responses in progressors. HIV disease progression may be due to mutations within CTL recognition epitopes resulting in "escape mutants" that evade CTL control. Although the number of NK cells is relatively normal compared with that in uninfected controls, and binding of these cells to their target is unimpaired, their cytotoxic capacity is moderately diminished. Recent in vitro studies suggest that reduced NK activity may

be restored by IL-12. Cytotoxic CD8 cells kill infected cells of the same class I MHC type that express HIV proteins (envelope, core, and some regulatory proteins). In addition to this cytotoxic role, CD8 lymphocytes can suppress HIV replication in CD4 lymphocytes through production of soluble factors.

E. B-Cell Responses:
1. Polyclonal B-cell activation resulting in hypergammaglobulinemia is commonly found in HIV-infected individuals, resulting predominantly in increases in serum IgG1, IgG3, and IgM levels. This spontaneous secretion of immunoglobulin by B cells is not always present, and in HIV-infected infants panhypogammaglobulinemia may occur.

2. Autoantibodies directed against erythrocytes, platelets, lymphocytes, neutrophils, nuclear proteins, myelin, and spermatozoa have been found in patients infected with HIV. In some instances these have been associated with disease (eg, HIV-associated thrombocytopenia and peripheral neuropathy).

3. Sera of HIV-infected individuals contain high levels of antibodies that react with monomeric HIV envelope glycoproteins, especially gp120. These antibodies, however, react poorly with the native, oligomeric envelope glycoprotein that is present on the surface of the virion. It has been particularly difficult to neutralize the infectivity of primary HIV-1 isolates.

4. The enhancement of in vitro HIV infection by antibodies has been reported, although the in vivo significance of this phenomenon is uncertain. Antibody-enhanced viral uptake is mediated by Fc and complement receptors.

5. B-cell proliferative responses to T-cell-independent specific B-cell mitogens (eg, formalinized *Staphylococcus aureus* Cowan 1 strain) are impaired.

6. Despite depression of helper T-cell function and abnormalities of humoral immunity, HIV-infected individuals at early stages of infection can often mount appropriate antibody responses to commonly used vaccines. A decrease in response to hepatitis B vaccine, pneumococcal vaccine, and influenza vaccine, however, is generally found as HIV disease progresses.

Vaccination (pneumococcal, influenza, etc) increases the viral load in HIV-infected individuals whose immune function allows them to develop a specific response to the vaccine. Some recent studies (but not all) have found that vaccination of HIV-infected individuals, especially those with preserved CD4 counts, can increase HIV RNA in plasma for weeks to months following vaccination.

The HIV-infected monocyte–macrophage is an important reservoir for HIV in vivo. Phagocytosis and killing of organisms, antigen presentation, and chemotaxis are moderately impaired. Macrophages also play a role in the pathogenesis of AIDS-related dementia, possibly mediated by secretion of quinolinic acid (Table 46–5).

Table 46–5. Potential role of macrophages in the pathogenesis of AIDS.

Act as target for HIV
Provide reservoir for HIV
Contribute to immune deficiency through abnormal function
    Defective phagocytosis
    Defective chemotaxis
    Defective antigen presentation
    Abnormal cytokine production
Contribute to T-cell depletion through a cell fusion process[a]

[a] Shown in vitro only.

G. Other Immunologic Responses: Other abnormal immunologic parameters include decreased lymphokine production (in particular, IL-2 and IFNγ), decreased expression of IL-2 receptors, and an increase in the level of circulating immune complexes. Elevated serum levels of β_2-microglobulin and neopterin are of some prognostic importance in predicting progression to AIDS.

H. Hematologic Findings: Subjects with acute HIV infection generally have leukopenia with an atypical lymphocytosis. Transient thrombocytopenia occurs in some patients. With disease progression, the total leukocyte count falls, with an associated lymphopenia, reflecting depletion of CD4 lymphocytes. The hemoglobin and hematocrit decrease as a result of anemia due to chronic disease, the presence of an opportunistic infection, or related to therapy. Mild thrombocytopenia is common.

Differential Diagnosis

Acute HIV mononucleosis must be distinguished from infectious mononucleosis caused by EBV, CMV infection, and less commonly, rubella, secondary syphilis, hepatitis B, human herpesvirus type 6 infection, and toxoplasmosis (Table 46–6). Once there is evidence of immunodeficiency, it should be ascertained that this is an acquired rather than a congenital defect and that no other underlying explanation is possible for the clinical and immunologic manifestations, such as hematologic cancer or tissue transplantation. Any individual with laboratory-confirmed HIV infection and a definitively diagnosed disease that meets the CDC criteria for AIDS is considered to have AIDS, however, regardless of the presence of other potential causes of immune deficiency.

Table 46–6. Differential diagnosis of acute HIV infection.

EBV infectious mononucleosis
CMV infection
Rubella
Secondary syphilis
Hepatitis B
Toxoplasmosis
Human herpesvirus type 6

Abbreviations: HIV = human immunodeficiency virus; EBV = Epstein–Barr virus; CMV = cytomegalovirus.

Treatment

A. Life Cycle of HIV: The initial phase of the replicative cycle of HIV involves binding of specific epitopes of cell surface CD4 molecules to defined regions of virion gp120. Following this, HIV enters the cell and is uncoated. Viral RNA is then used as a template by reverse transcriptase to make a minus-strand DNA copy, thus forming an RNA-DNA hybrid. Soon thereafter, the RNA strand is degraded by the ribonuclease H activity of reverse transcriptase. A positive DNA strand is synthesized, and the linear double-stranded DNA molecule changes conformation to become circular. Some of this DNA migrates to the nucleus and subsequently becomes integrated into the cellular DNA to form the HIV provirus, through the action of the viral integrase. Cellular transcription factors that bind to HIV LTR depend on the activation of the lymphocyte; differentiation of monocytes into macrophages is associated with increased replication of HIV; cytokines can influence HIV replication through the previously mentioned mechanisms as well as by their independent activities. The replication cycle continues with the translation of viral genomic RNA and viral proteins from unspliced, singly spliced, and multiply spliced mRNA species. These proteins undergo posttranslational protein cleavage and glycosylation. The final stage of assembly of viral proteins occurs during or shortly after budding of the virion through the cell membrane, with acquisition of envelope during the budding process (Figure 46–5).

B. Antiretroviral Therapy: The complicated machinery used by HIV in its replicative cycle has provided many specific target sites for potential intervention (Table 46–7). Because reverse transcriptase is not normally present in human cells, selective inhibitors of this enzyme have been a major focus of drug development. Zidovudine (AZT) is the prototype nucleoside analog reverse transcriptase inhibitor (NRTI). It is a thymidine analog that requires phosphorylation by host nucleoside kinases to the triphosphate derivative within the infected cell for it to be active. Once phosphorylated, the drug inhibits the virus-encoded reverse transcriptase enzyme because it has about 100 times the affinity for this enzyme as it does for the host DNA polymerase. Zidovudine further prevents HIV replication by becoming incorporated into the transcribed DNA strand and thus preventing further HIV DNA synthesis. Other NRTIs include didanosine (ddI), zalcitabine (ddC), stavudine (d4T), lamivudine (3TC), and abacavir. In countries where there is ready access to antiretroviral therapies, two NRTIs are generally used in combination with either a nonnucleoside reverse transcriptase inhibitor (NNRTIs), such as nevirapine, delavirdine, or efavirenz, or a protease inhibitor, such as indinavir, ritonavir (now commonly used in combination with another protease inhibitor), saquinavir, nelfinavir, or amprenavir. In such a combination these drugs are re-

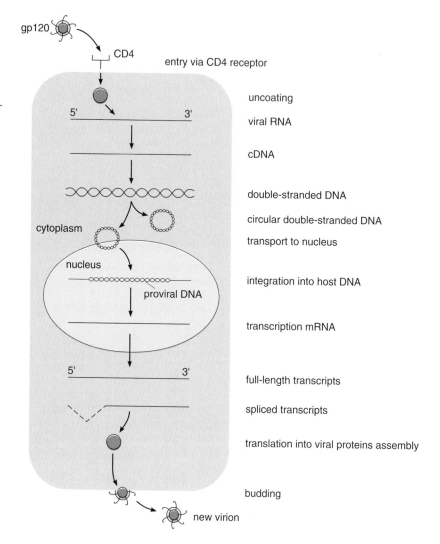

gp120

CD4

entry via CD4 receptor

uncoating

5'   3'   viral RNA

cDNA

double-stranded DNA

circular double-stranded DNA

cytoplasm

transport to nucleus

nucleus

integration into host DNA

proviral DNA

transcription mRNA

5'   3'   full-length transcripts

spliced transcripts

translation into viral proteins assembly

budding

new virion

Figure 46–5. Replicative cycle of HIV. Lifelong infection is a consequence of the viral replicative cycle.

ferred to as highly active antiretroviral therapy (HAART).

Timing of commencement of antiretroviral therapy depends on a combination of factors, including CD4 lymphocyte numbers, viral load, and clinical symptoms. Patient readiness for therapy is also a major factor because the timing of medications and their administration in relationship to food and other drugs make adherence difficult. In general, if the viral load exceeds 5000–10,000 copies/mL and the CD4 count is falling or is below 500 cells/μL, virtually every clinician would advise commencing therapy. A number of ongoing clinical trials seek to determine whether commencement of HAART during the acute HIV infection can reset the virologic set-point to a lower level and thus alter long-term prognosis.

Agents acting at other sites in the replicative cycle (including integrase inhibitors) are in development.

C. Monitoring of Patients With HIV Infection: The CD4 count gives an indication of the level of damage that has already occurred to the immune system as a result of HIV infection. As such, it is predictive of disease progression independent of plasma viral load measurements, which indicate how rapidly the damage is occurring. When monitoring patients, the CD4 count should almost always be measured in conjunction with viral load. Generally, changes to the CD4 count develop relatively slowly after commencement of therapy, and the CD4 numbers may continue to rise over a period of many months or years while the viral load remains suppressed.

Viral load levels should be measured in conjunc-

Table 46–7. Classes of antiretroviral drugs licensed for the treatment of HIV infection.

Drug	Class	Requires Intracellular Phosphorylation for Activity	Resistance Mutations (codons)
Zidovudine	NRTI	Yes	441, 67, 70, 210, 215, 219 of RT
Didanosine	NRTI	Yes	65, 74, 75, 184 of RT
Zalcitabine	NRTI	Yes	65, 69, 74, 75, 184 of RT
Stavudine	NRTI	Yes	75 of RT
Lamivudine	NRTI	Yes	184 of RT
Abacivir	NRTI	Yes	65, 74, 115, 184 of RT
Nevirapine	NNRTI	No	98, 100, 103, 106, 108, 181, 188, 190 of RT
Delavirdine	NNRTI	No	103, 181 of RT
Efavirenz	NNRTI	No	100, 101, 103, 108, 179, 181, 188 of RT
Saquinavir	PI	No	10, 48, 54, 63, 71, 73, 82, 84, 90 of Pr
Ritonavir	PI	No	20, 32, 33, 36, 46, 54, 63, 71, 82, 84, 90 of Pr
Indinavir	PI	No	10, 20, 24, 32, 46, 54, 63, 71, 73, 82, 84, 90 of Pr
Nelfinavir	PI	No	30, 36, 46, 63, 71, 77, 84, 88, 90 of Pr
Amprenavir	PI	No	10, 46, 47, 50, 84 of Pr

Abbreviations: NRTI = nucleoside analog reverse transcriptase inhibitor; NNRTI = nonnucleoside reverse transcriptase inhibitor; PI = protease inhibitor; RT = reverse transcriptase; Pr = protease.

tion with CD4 counts about 1 month after commencement of therapy to ensure a decline of at least 1 $\log_{10}$ copies/mL. Ideally, the viral load should be suppressed to less than 50 copies/mL. In patients who have been previously exposed to multiple antiretroviral regimens, neither a decline of 1 $\log_{10}$ copies/mL nor suppression to undetectable levels may be possible. Regimens must then be tailored to achieve the best results in any individual patient. An increase in viral load after a period of suppression may be due to a number of causes including nonadherence with the regimen, lack of absorption of medication or interaction with other concomitant medications, lack of potency of drug combination, or the development of HIV strains resistant to the antiretroviral drugs being used. In patients not requiring treatment or in those stable on antiretroviral therapy, viral load and CD4 counts are generally monitored every 2–3 months. Common methods used to measure viral load are RT-PCR and branched DNA assay.

In patients for whom therapy has failed or those who are newly infected with HIV, it may be useful to obtain an HIV genotype or phenotype assessment of drug susceptibility to guide therapy. The HIV genotype tests detect mutations within the reverse transcriptase and protease genes. Expert advice is usually required to analyze the data. HIV phenotype testing will provide an IC_{50} or IC_{90} value for each drug against which the patient's strain of HIV is tested, when compared with wild-type HIV. These tests are in use in only some clinics.

D. Immunorestorative Therapy: Attempts to restore the defective immune system have, to date, generally been ineffective. The alleged immune stimula-

tor inosine pranobex (Isoprinosine) has been associated with only transitory immunologic benefit; bone marrow and peripheral blood lymphocyte transplantation is not regarded as useful because the transplanted cells also become infected with HIV. The augmentation of immune responses by IL-2 and IL-12 is currently being investigated. Recombinant interleukin-2 has been found in clinical trials to cause a large increase in CD4 lymphocyte numbers, when administered with an antiretroviral agent. Inhibitors of cytokines (eg, pentoxifylline, a TNFα inhibitor) may provide additional immune and antiviral benefit. It is possible that combination therapy with an immunomodulatory agent together with one or more antiretroviral agents will be more effective than either alone. In certain patients with Kaposi's sarcoma, administration of high-dose IFNγ has been beneficial. Interferon inducers, such as the mismatched doubledstranded RNA compound Ampligen, are effective in inhibiting HIV replication in vitro. Early clinical trials with this drug suggested temporary clinical improvement with restoration of immune responses, but these studies have not been confirmed. G-CSF is commonly used in patients who develop neutropenia due to drugs or opportunistic infection. GM-CSF is less frequently used in patients due to concern that it may increase HIV replication within macrophages. It has, however, been used successfully to augment macrophage function in conjunction with HAART as adjunctive therapy in some patients with drugresistant opportunistic infections.

Passive immunotherapy to enhance HIV-specific humoral immunity is being evaluated in a number of clinical trials. Approaches have included the use of humanized monoclonal antibodies directed against either the CD4-gp120-binding site of the viral envelope or the immunodominant V3 loop of HIV gp120.

Another approach to boost or augment the immune response to HIV has been the use of a therapeutic vaccine administered to persons already infected with HIV. Jonas Salk, the polio vaccine pioneer, developed a vaccine made from inactivated HIV (without the envelope); studies suggested that it is safe and that it can boost delayed hypersensitivity responses to vaccine antigens. A number of other candidate vaccines have been tested in clinical trial with only modest results. The immunogens included envelope proteins made in insect and mammalian cell systems, as well as novel approaches such as HIV core protein produced so that the HIV p24 is presented to the immune system as a virus-like particle. A vaccine comprising an avipox vector expressing Gag and Pol in addition to IFNγ enter phase 1 clinical trials in the year 2000 in HIV-infected persons with preserved CD4 counts and low viral load who are receiving antiretroviral therapy (HAART).

Prevention

A. Vaccines: The development of an effective vaccine has been hampered by the genomic diversity of HIV (Table 46–8). Strains of HIV vary in their nucleic acid sequence by up to 20% as a result of high-frequency point mutations that occur during the replication of the virus. An estimate of the error rate of HIV reverse transcriptase is 1 in 10,000 nucleotides, which translates into about one mutation in the viral genome in every newly produced virion. This variation is most evident in the envelope region of HIV. Of interest, certain regions are conserved between different isolates (eg, the region of gp120 that interacts with CD4), and other regions of the envelope are highly variable. Unfortunately, the major antigenic epitopes (and therefore, predictably, the major protective epitopes) are in the regions associated with the highest degree of strain-to-strain variation. This includes the immunodominant third variable loop (V3) within gp120. The V3 loop contains the GP-GRA amino acid sequence, which is regarded as the principal neutralizing domain. This genomic diversity is one of the many major obstacles hampering vaccine development because an effective vaccine should provide protection against all strains of HIV.

Table 46–8. Obstacles to development of HIV vaccine.

Genomic diversity of HIV strains
Progression of infection despite vigorous immune response
    Transmission of HIV in vivo by cell fusion as well as by
      cell-free virus
Lack of a good animal model
Potential enhancement of HIV replication by neutralizing
    antibody

Another impediment to vaccine development is the fact that HIV is spread from cell to cell via a fusion process as well as by cell-free virus.

Prophylactic HIV vaccines under development use strategies similar to those employed for development of other vaccines. The earliest vaccines tested were purified recombinant envelope proteins (eg, gp160, gp41, or gp120) given to eliciting neutralizing antibodies. Despite the results of early clinical trials with these vaccines suggesting that the neutralizing antibody responses were disappointingly low, not broadly reactive, and poorly active toward primary isolates, phase III efficacy trials of a gp120-based vaccine are underway in the United States and Thailand and are scheduled for completion in 2001.

The most promising current approaches for an HIV vaccine appear to be recombinant vectors that, on injection, result in the in situ synthesis of HIV antigens. This strategy mimics in vivo replication of HIV and therefore stimulates both humoral and cellular immune responses. The most popular vectors are poxviruses (eg, modified vaccinia Ankara, fowlpox, or avipox) or "naked" DNA vaccines; the principal HIV antigens have been *gag, pol,* and *env* gene products and Nef. The immune response to these live vectors can be directed and stimulated by the coexpression of cytokine genes, most notably IFNγ and interleukin-12, used because of their ability to stimulate T_H1-type immune responses thought to be important for control of HIV infection. These vector-based vaccines have been successful at preventing SIV infection of macaques, and several variants are slated for clinical trials in 2000. A number of other HIV vaccines strategies are being pursued, including inactivated whole-virus vaccines.

Live attenuated vaccines have been remarkably successful at controlling or eradicating other viral infections, including smallpox and polio. These vaccines also have the advantage of being inexpensive to manufacture and generally producing long-term immunity with a relatively small number of immunizations. Development of a live attenuated HIV vaccine, however, remains a daunting task, due to the high mortality and long incubation period of HIV infection and the lack of a suitable animal model to test attenuation. Studies of deletion mutants of SIV in macaques and of a *nef*-LTR-deleted Australian strain of HIV in a cohort of blood transfusion recipients, however, have clearly shown that it is possible to make attenuated (albeit not yet fully attenuated) strains of SIV and HIV. A handful of investigators are continuing to pursue this option for HIV vaccine development.

B. Education: The major thrust of strategies to prevent HIV infection lies in education of individuals about practicing safer sex, in which the transmission of bodily fluids (specifically semen, vaginal secretions, and blood) is prevented, and not sharing needles or syringes.

CYTOMEGALOVIRUS

Major Immunologic Features

- Increased CD8 lymphocyte numbers and transient suppression of CD4 lymphocyte numbers and cell-mediated immunity
- Decreased MHC class I antigen expression and induction of Fc receptors in CMV infection
- Numerous virus gene products blunt host immune responses

General Considerations

Cytomegalovirus (CMV) is a member of the herpesvirus family, a group that includes the human pathogens EBV, herpes simplex virus types 1 and 2, varicella-zoster virus, and human herpesviruses types 6–8, as well as many animal pathogens. Similar to other herpesviruses, CMV is associated with persistent, latent, and recurrent infection, the last being due to reactivation of latent virus. CMV remains latent in monocytes, granulocyte-monocyte progenitor cells, and perhaps in other cell types.

The prevalence of infection within a community varies with socioeconomic status, being as low as 40% in upper strata and approaching 100% in lower groups.

Clinical Features

Infection with CMV can result in a variety of clinical syndromes, depending partially on the immune state of the infected individual (Table 46–9). In healthy subjects, infection is usually subclinical, occasionally causing an infectious mononucleosis-like syndrome resembling that due to EBV or primary HIV infections (however, pharyngitis is unusual). Often allergic skin rashes develop to antibiotics, similar to that observed during acute EBV infection. If infection is acquired in utero, following primary maternal infection, the infant may be born with cytomegalic inclusion disease (CID), which has features of hepatosplenomegaly, microcephaly, chorioretinitis, thrombocytopenia, and jaundice. Although only about 5–10% of infants with prenatal infection are born with CID, another 2–5% develop abnormalities, such as deafness, spasticity, intellectual retardation, and dental defects within the first 2 years of life. Asymptomatic perinatal infection may be acquired as a result of exposure to CMV in the birth canal or through breastfeeding.

Patients with defective cellular immunity, such as those with AIDS or those being treated with im-

Table 49–9. Clinical manifestations of CMV infection.

Prenatal infection
  Cytomegalic inclusion disease
Immunocompetent host
  Subclinical infection
  CMV mononucleosis
Immunocompromised host
  Disseminated CMV: retinitis, esophagitis, colitis, pneumonitis, other sites

munosuppressive drugs, are prone to disseminated CMV infection. In this instance, the infection involves predominantly the retinas, gastrointestinal tract (especially the colon, esophagus, and liver), and lungs. Such individuals often have progressive disease, despite high levels of serum-neutralizing antibody. Reactivation of CMV infection also appears to trigger graft-versus-host disease in many cases. Organ transplant recipients develop generalized and occasionally fatal CMV disease more commonly following primary than reactivated infection. In vitro studies have shown clearly that coinfection by CMV and HIV augments HIV replication. Thus, it was speculated that CMV might be a cofactor augmenting the pathogenicity of HIV and shortening the incubation period (between infection and development of AIDS). Although to date there is no clinical evidence that such is the case, this biologically plausible hypothesis remains under study.

Immunologic Findings

IgM antibodies are produced following initial infection and generally persist for 3–4 months. IgG antibodies appear at the same time, peak about 2 or 3 months after infection, and persist for many years and often for life. Although the antibody response is directed against many virion proteins, neutralizing antibodies are primarily directed against the envelope glycoproteins, especially gB and gH. Although neutralizing antibodies play no role in control of established CMV infection, there is good evidence that they can prevent infection.

Primary CMV infection is followed by activation of both CTL, whose function is to specifically destroy CMV-infected cells, and NK cells. The CTL response to CMV is targeted against a variety of virion antigens. Both the NK and CTL responses appear to play a role in controlling established CMV infection; the role of CTL has recently been reinforced by studies showing protection from CMV infection by passive infusion of CMV-specific CTL in bone marrow transplant recipients. Not surprisingly, there is good evidence that susceptibility to CMV infection is at least partly genetically determined.

CMV infection, however, also results in a general impairment of cellular immunity, characterized by impaired blastogenic responses to nonspecific mitogens and specific CMV antigens, diminished cytotoxic ability, and elevation of the CD8 lymphocyte subset with a moderate but transient decrease in the number of CD4 lymphocytes. Cytomegalovirus, and probably other herpesviruses, encode numerous proteins that enable the virus to evade the host immune responses (see also Table 45–1). These include proteins that block effective antibody responses (eg, expression of membrane Fc receptors on infected cells) and reduce the effectiveness of NK and CTL attack on virus-infected cells. Most impressively, CMV has an extraordinary array of proteins that foil CTL responses by numerous mechanisms (see Table 45–1). CMV also expresses analogs of TNF and chemokine receptors whose function is currently unknown. Interestingly, the CMV chemokine receptor analog is also a functional receptor for HIV-1, perhaps explaining why cells normally not susceptible to HIV infection might become so when CMV-infected.

In the immunocompetent individual, specific defects in the cell-mediated immune response are restored within a few months following infection. Seropositive individuals, however, may intermittently excrete CMV for many years or perhaps for life, owing to low-grade chronic infection or reactivation of latent infection.

Primary CMV infection in immunocompromised individuals results in a severely blunted immune response to the virus. Contrariwise, reactivation of latent CMV infection usually results from immunosuppression, especially that due to major organ transplantation (eg, heart, lung, bone marrow) and HIV infection. Reactivation of infection in the context of immunosuppression does not result in any predictable changes in CMV serology.

The immaturity of the immune response in infants with congenital or perinatal infection results in chronic excretion of CMV in nasopharyngeal secretions and urine. The immune response in these children is eventually restored coincident with cessation of viral excretion.

Treatment & Prevention

Three antiviral agents are now available for treating CMV infection: ganciclovir, foscarnet, and cidofovir; they are used only for treating severe CMV infections in immunocompromised patients. These drugs are effective for treatment of established CMV infection, as well as for "chemosuppression"-prevention of reactivation of latent infection by long-term therapy. CMV pneumonitis in bone marrow transplant recipients responds poorly to antivirals alone and is usually treated with an antiviral plus intravenous immunoglobulin. CMV pneumonitis probably results from a combination of direct viral cytopathology and a host autoimmune response, and the intravenous immunoglobulin is thought to act as an immunomodulator, not as an antiviral. Use of adjunctive immunoglobulin as treatment for other types of CMV infections has not been beneficial. Reactivation of latent CMV infection and the resulting disease can be largely prevented by a chemosuppression strategy in which patients at risk of reactivation are given antivirals (eg, ganciclovir) before and during the period of severe immunosuppression.

Passive immunoprophylaxis with either CMV hyperimmune globulin or CMV-specific CTL has been shown to prevent CMV infection or disease. A live attenuated CMV vaccine (the Towne strain) is apathogenic, but has not clearly shown protective efficacy, and attempts are currently underway to construct subunit CMV vaccines, using the gB and gH envelope glycoproteins.

EPSTEIN-BARR VIRUS

Major Immunologic Features

- B lymphocytes target cells
- Atypical T-cell lymphocytosis
- Heterophil antibodies produced
- In vitro transformation of B lymphocytes

General Considerations

EBV is a member of the herpesvirus family and, as such, can establish persistent and latent infection. EBV also can transform B lymphocytes and has clinically relevant oncogenic potential. Primary infection, which may be subclinical, results in a lifelong carrier state.

Pathogenesis

The virus initially replicates within the pharyngeal epithelium, with subsequent infection of B lymphocytes in subjacent lymphoid tissue. Circulating lymphocytes are responsible for generalized infection. Following the acute infection, EBV remains latent within the B-lymphocyte population; these cells most probably provide a lifelong reservoir of the virus. Intermittent seeding of the pharyngeal epithelia, with low-level replication within these cells, allows potential transmission of infection to susceptible members of the community.

The incubation period varies from 3 to 7 weeks; most commonly adolescents and young adults develop symptomatic infection.

Shedding of EBV from salivary tissue declines following acute infection but probably persists for life. Recently, EBV has been found in both semen and cervical epithelium, suggesting the possibility of sexual transmission. Transmission of EBV by blood transfusion and bone marrow transplantation has been rarely described.

Clinical Features

In 1964, Epstein, Achong, and Barr described the presence of viral particles in fibroblasts cultured from tissue from a patient with Burkitt's lymphoma. Since then, this virus has been causally associated with acute infectious mononucleosis, nasopharyngeal carcinoma, lymphomas in immunocompromised individuals, X-linked lymphoproliferative syndrome (Duncan's syndrome), and two HIV-related conditions (oral hairy leukoplakia and lymphocytic interstitial pneumonitis) (Table 46–10). EBV has been proposed as the cause of the chronic fatigue syndrome, but no evidence supports this association.

Infectious mononucleosis is the most common illness caused by EBV. This disease occurs most frequently in young adults. Typical features include

Table 46–10. Diseases associated with EBV.

Infectious mononucleosis
Burkitt's lymphoma
Nasopharyngeal carcinoma
Lymphomas in immunocompromised host
X-linked lymphoproliferative syndrome
Oral hairy leukoplakia[a]
Lymphocytic interstitial pneumonitis[a]

[a] In HIV-infected individuals.

fever; sore throat, often with exudate; rash; generalized lymphadenopathy; and splenomegaly. Chemical hepatitis is present in most patients, and a few develop frank jaundice. Patients with infectious mononucleosis have a much higher incidence of drug-induced skin rashes than normals. Although ampicillin is the drug traditionally associated with rash in this context, a wide variety of other antibiotics and drugs present a risk nearly as high. This propensity is not unique to acute EBV infection because it is also seen in CMV mononucleosis and during HIV infection.

Rare complications of infectious mononucleosis include hemolytic anemia, aplastic anemia, encephalitis, Guillain–Barré syndrome, myocarditis, nephritis, and hepatic failure.

In immunodeficient patients, primary EBV infection can cause a variety of conditions, including uncomplicated mononucleosis, a benign polyclonal B-cell hyperplasia, and both polyclonal and monoclonal B-cell lymphomas.

EBV is definitely the causative agent of a number of cancers: Burkitt's lymphoma, nasopharyngeal cancer, immunosuppression-induced lymphomas, and Duncan's syndrome. EBV coinfection is also universal in the HHV-8-associated primary effusion B-cell lymphomas (see HHV-8 section). The mechanisms by which EBV causes these tumors are multiple and complex, and beyond the scope of this chapter; however, oncogenesis is uniformly associated with long-standing infection.

Laboratory Diagnosis of Infectious Mononucleosis

Usually a mild leukopenia precedes the development of a leukocytosis (and absolute lymphocytosis) during the second to third week of illness. From 50 to 70% of the lymphocytes are atypical. IgM heterophil antibodies, which agglutinate sheep erythrocytes, are found in the sera of more than 90% of individuals with infectious mononucleosis. They persist for 3–6 months.

The pattern of antibody response to EBV initially reflects the synthesis of viral antigens involved in cell lysis, notably the early antigens (EA), viral capsid antigens (VCA), and EBV-induced membrane antigens (MA). VCA and MA are classified as late antigens because their expression is suppressed in the presence of inhibitors of DNA synthesis. The appear-

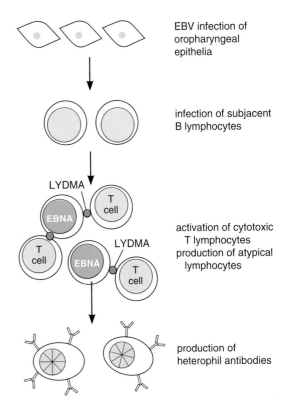

Figure 46–6. Pathogenesis of infectious mononucleosis. Following infection of oropharyngeal epithelia, EBV infection spreads to the subjacent B lymphocytes. Activation of cytotoxic T lymphocytes by EBV antigens results in the appearance of atypical lymphocytes in the peripheral blood. *Abbreviations:* LYDMA = lymphocyte-detected membrane antigen; EBNA = Epstein-Barr nuclear antigen; EBV = Epstein-Barr virus.

ance of antibody directed against the EBV nuclear antigen (EBNA) usually occurs weeks to months after infection. EBNA is present in all cells containing the viral genome, whether latently or productively infected (Figure 46–6).

Immunologic Features of EBV Infection

Following EBV infection, most patients mount a vigorous humoral and cellular immune response. The humoral immune response is directed against a variety of viral proteins (Figure 46–7); antibodies to viral MA and gp350 proteins are neutralizing but probably do not play a role in controlling established infection. In addition, perhaps because EBV encodes an IL-10 homologue that stimulates B-cell replication, EBV infection is associated with polyclonal hyperglobulinemia. The cellular immune response to EBV is extremely vigorous; in fact, the atypical lymphocytes so characteristic of this disease are primarily activated CD8, EBV-specific CTL, and NK cells. Control of acute EBV infection is probably due primarily to the

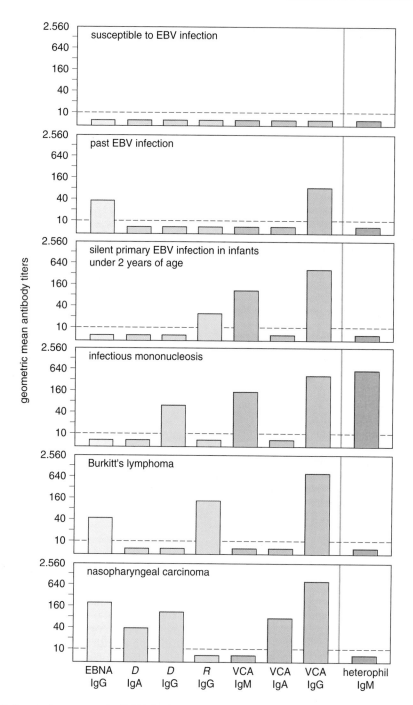

Figure 46–7. Serologic response to EBV infection. Typical antibody patterns are observed in different clinical conditions caused by EBV. *Abbreviations:* EBV = Epstein-Barr virus; D = diffuse; R = restricted; EBNA = Epstein-Barr nuclear antigen; VCA = viral capsid antigen; Ig = immunoglobulin.

CTL response. Individuals with severe cellular immunodeficiency, such as renal transplant recipients, may develop fulminant EBV infection or B-cell malignancies following primary infection. In addition, a rare, X-linked inherited immune defect occurs that predisposes to severe, often fatal EBV infection (Duncan's syndrome; X-linked lymphoproliferative disease).

EBV infects B lymphocytes through binding to the CD21 molecule on the cell surface. CD21 is expressed on a variety of cells besides mature B lymphocytes, including follicular dendritic cells, and pharyngeal and cervical epithelia. CD21 is a receptor for the C3d component of complement as well as for EBV. Following infection, large numbers of atypical lymphocytes appear within the circulation that are not, in fact, virus-infected B cells but result from polyclonal activation of CD8 cells (see Figure 46–6). These activated T cells, which are not MHC-restricted or EBV-specific, are responsible for preventing the unchecked expansion of EBV-transformed B lymphocytes. In addition, EBV-specific, MHC-restricted cytotoxic T cells are produced. Of interest, these cells appear to specifically recognize virus-infected B lymphocytes expressing **lymphocyte-determined membrane antigen (LYDMA),** without requiring MHC restriction. The true specificity of cytotoxic T-cell responses in infectious mononucleosis remains to be completely elucidated. The mechanism for viral persistence may involve inhibition of the normal replicative cycle of EBV within B cells prior to the expression of LYDMA, the target antigen for cytotoxic T cells. Some of the recognized complications of acute EBV infection, such as drug-induced skin rashes, hemolytic anemia, and Guillain–Barré syndrome, are almost certainly due to immunopathic mechanisms.

Treatment & Prevention

Therapy for infectious mononucleosis is symptomatic. Although EBV is susceptible to acyclovir in vitro, the drug is of little or no clinical benefit. Oral hairy leukoplakia (an HIV-associated EBV infection), however, responds clinically and virologically to acyclovir. Because EBV-associated tumors carry EBV antigens, scientists are attempting to use EBV-specific CTL to treat these tumors. A subunit vaccine to stimulate EBV CTL in patients with EBV-related lymphomas is undergoing clinical study at present.

Because EBV infection is associated with tumors of public health significance in many parts of the world (eg, Burkitt's lymphoma in Africa; nasopharyngeal cancer in China), efforts are underway to develop vaccines to prevent EBV infection altogether, or to limit EBV replication following infection (and hopefully thereby to decrease the risk of oncogenesis). A subunit vaccine containing EBV gp350 (the major virion membrane protein that stimulates neutralizing antibody) and peptide-based vaccines to stimulate EBV-specific CTL are both under development.

HUMAN T-CELL LEUKEMIA VIRUS TYPES I & II

The field of human retrovirology is relatively young. In 1980, the first human retrovirus was isolated in the United States from the T lymphocytes of two black men with aggressive T-cell cancers. This virus, now called human T-cell leukemia virus I (HTLV-I), has since been causatively linked with adult T-cell leukemia (ATL) and an incurable progressive neuromyelopathy called tropical spastic paraparesis or HTLV-1-associated myelopathy (HAM). HTLV-II has been associated with unusual T-cell malignancies in humans.

HTLV-I is a type C retrovirus of the oncornavirus family (see Table 46–1). Like other oncornaviruses, HTLV-I may transform (immortalize) cells following infection, although unlike acutely transforming oncornaviruses, it lacks a specific oncogene. HTLV-I preferentially infects T cells although other cell types can be infected in vitro. Infected T cells are transformed by an unknown mechanism, and it is the proliferation of these transformed cells (which contain the HTLV-I provirus, an integrated DNA copy of the retroviral RNA genome) that results in ATL and perhaps other tumors. The transformed T lymphocytes are usually CD4 (rarely, CD8), express many activation markers, and produce numerous cytokines.

ATL is caused by oligoclonal proliferation of transformed T lymphocytes and is clearly associated with clinically significant immunosuppression. In contrast, HAM is most likely an autoimmune disease, and HTLV-I infection has also been associated with autoimmune arthritis and uveitis. Nothing is known about the immunologic mechanisms involved, however.

Endemic HTLV-I infection exists in parts of the Caribbean region, Japan, and Africa. Worldwide, up to 20 million persons are estimated to be infected with HTLV-I. The modes of transmission of HTLV-I are virtually identical to those for HIV: via infected blood, through sexual contact, and from mother to child. There is no direct evidence for transplacental transmission of HTLV-I; however, transmission to the infant commonly occurs via the mother's milk, analogous to transmission of bovine leukemia virus.

There is a high rate of infection with HTLV-II in certain populations, including injecting drug users. Screening of blood bank donations in the United States for HTLV-I/II began in 1988. Seroprevalence ranged from 0 to 0.1%. Because HTLV-I is difficult to distinguish serologically from HTLV-II, assays that detect both together have been developed. HTLV-I/II infection is usually detected by enzyme immunoassay, with positives being confirmed by immunoblotting. Differentiation between HTLV-I and HTLV-II infection can be made by immunoblot but is more reliably determined by PCR amplification of provirus.

HUMAN HERPESVIRUS 6

Human herpesvirus (HHV) 6 is a herpesvirus with a genome closely related to that of human cytomegalovirus, which infects predominantly T lymphocytes. Two variants are recognized, HHV-6A and HHV-6B, which are genetically closely related but clinically and epidemiologically distinct. HHV-6A is not known to cause disease, whereas HHV-6B is the major cause of exanthem subitum and other illnesses, primarily in children. HHV-6 infects predominantly the CD4 subset of T lymphocytes, although it does not use CD4 itself as the receptor (unlike HIV). HHV-6 infection of T cells causes cytomegaly and syncytium formation, induces CD4 expression, and may down-regulate CD3/T-cell receptor (TCR) expression. HHV-6 also suppresses IL-2 synthesis, blocking proliferation of lymphocytes in response to antigenic stimulation. Infection of macrophages suppresses a variety of functions of these cells.

Primary infection with HHV-6 usually occurs in childhood. HHV-6A infection appears to be asymptomatic, whereas HHV-6B causes exanthem subitum (roseola infantum; sixth disease) and undifferentiated febrile illnesses. Primary infection with HHV-6B accounts for 15–40% of children presenting to hospital emergency departments with febrile illnesses. Primary infection of adults with HHV-6 is rare, but infectious mononucleosis-like syndromes have been reported. A variety of other syndromes due to primary HHV-6B infection have been reported involving the respiratory tract, central nervous system, liver, and reticuloendothelial system. Reactivation of latent HHV-6 infection in immunosuppressed patients (especially those receiving bone marrow transplants) has been associated with febrile episodes, pneumonitis, and graft rejection, although the etiologic relationship remains unproven. Interestingly, despite infection of CD4-bearing lymphocytes like HIV, there is no evidence that HHV-6 causes clinically important immunosuppression.

REFERENCES

HUMAN IMMUNODEFICIENCY VIRUS

Berger EA et al: Chemokine receptors as HIV-1 coreceptors; Roles in viral entry, tropism and disease. *Annu Rev Immunol* 1999,17:657.

Crowe SM et al: Predictive value of CD4 lymphocyte numbers for the development of opportunistic infections and malignancies in HIV-infected persons. *Acquir Immune Defic Syndr* 1991;4:770.

Desrosiers RD: Strategies used by human immunodeficiency virus that allow persistent viral replication. *Nat Med* 1999,5:723.

Heilman CA, Baltimore D: HIV vaccines—Where are we going? *Nat Med* 1999,4(Suppl 5):532.

Ho DD et al: Rapid turnover of plasma virions and CD4 lymphocytes in HIV-1 infection. *Nature* 1995;373:123.

Levy JA: *HIV and the Pathogenesis of AIDS.* ASM Press, 1994.

CYTOMEGALOVIRUS

Benedict CA et al: Cutting edge: A novel viral TNF receptor superfamily member in virulent strains of human cytomegalovirus. *J Immunol* 1999;162:6967.

Britt WJ, Alford CA: Cytomegalovirus. In: *Virology,* 3rd ed. Fields BN et al (editors). Lippincott-Raven, 1996.

Hengel H et al: Cytomegaloviral control of MHC class 1 function in the mouse. *Immunol Rev* 1999;168:167.

Pleskoff O et al: Identification of a chemokine receptor encoded by human cytomegalovirus as a cofactor for HIV1 entry [see comments] *Science.* 1997;276:1874.

Ploegh HL: Viral strategies of immune evasion. *Science.* 1998;280:248.

Tay CH et al: The role of LY49 NK cell subsets in the regulation of murine cytomegalovirus infections. *J Immunol* 1999;162:718.

EPSTEIN-BARR VIRUS

Hanto DW: Classification of Epstein-Barr virus-associated post-transplant lymphoproliferative diseases: Implications for understanding their pathogenesis and developing rational treatment strategies. *Annu Rev Med* 1995; 46:381.

Moss DJ et al: Potential antigenic targets on Epstein-Barr virus-associated tumors and the host response. *CIBA Found Symp* 1994;187:4.

Rickinson AB, Kieff E: Epstein-Barr virus. In: *Virology,* 3rd ed. Fields BN et al (editors). Lippincott-Raven, 1996.

Tosato G et al: Epstein-Barr virus as an agent of hematological disease. *Baillieres Clin Haematol* 1995;8:165.

HUMAN T LYMPHOTROPIC VIRUS TYPE I

Cann AJ, Chen ISY: Human T-cell leukemia viruses type I and II. In: *Virology,* 3rd ed. Fields BN et al (editors). Lippincott-Raven, 1996.

Hollsberg P, Hafler DA: Pathogenesis of diseases induced by human lymphotropic virus type I infection. *N Engl J Med* 1993;328:1173.

HUMAN HERPESVIRUS TYPE 6

Caserta MT, Hall CB: Human herpesvirus-6. *Annu Rev Med* 1993;44:377.

Pellett PE, Black JB: Human herpesvirus 6. In: *Virology,* 3rd ed. Fields BN et al (editors). Lippincott-Raven, 1996.

Fungal Diseases

47

Thomas F. Patterson, MD, & David J. Drutz, MD

Fungal infections are called **mycoses.** Fungi are eukaryotes: they possess a true nucleus containing several chromosomes, bounded by a nuclear membrane. Bacteria are prokaryotes, with a single linear chromosome and no true nucleus. The principal sterol of the fungal cell membrane is ergosterol, the target of amphotericin B and the antifungal azoles and triazoles. Fungal cell walls differ from those of bacteria by lacking peptidoglycans, teichoic acids, and lipopolysaccharides (endotoxin). In their place are the external and antigenic **peptidomannans** embedded in matrices of α- and β-**glucans;** structural rigidity is provided by sheets, disks, or fibrils of **chitin** (poly β-1,4-*N*-acetylglucosamine). RNA-typing studies have established a relationship between true fungi and *Pneumocystis carinii,* an organism initially classified as a protozoan based on growth characteristics. *P carinii* has chitin and β-glucans in its wall and contains a fungal-specific protein elongation factor 3, but it lacks ergosterol, responds poorly to most traditional antifungal agents, and appears morphologically distinct from fungi. Although data establish the molecular similarity of *P carinii* to fungi, differences clearly exist so that additional classification is still needed. Other organisms that lack an in vitro culture system such as *Loboa loboi* and *Rhinosporidium seeberi* are presumed to be fungi, but molecular analysis is needed to identify their correct phylogeny.

There are thousands of fungi in nature, but relatively few are pathogenic for normal humans. Table 47–1 lists common mycoses according to the usual sites of infection. **Superficial** mycoses usually occur on the body external to common immunologic influences. Cutaneous mycoses produce delayed hypersensitivity responses to the local presence of keratinolytic fungi. **Subcutaneous** and **systemic** mycoses represent successful challenges to major immunologic host defense mechanisms. Some systemic mycoses (eg, blastomycosis, coccidioidomycosis, histoplasmosis, and paracoccidioidomycosis) are caused by primary pathogens, theoretically capable of infecting anyone in an endemic area. Others (eg, candidiasis, cryptococcosis, aspergillosis, and mucormycosis [zygomycosis]) are caused by opportunistic pathogens, which seldom cause life-threatening tissue invasion in the absence of impaired host defense. Most fungal infection is acquired from environmental sources. Other fungi, such as *Pityrosporum (Malassezia)* and *Candida* spp., may result from endogenous colonizing sources. Yeasts such as *Candida albicans, C glabrata, C tropicalis,* and other *Candida* spp. cause infection from environmental sources and may be associated with nosocomial transmission, frequently through hand transmission. Most primary invasive mycoses are acquired by the inhalation of specialized forms (conidia and spores) that are progeny of filamentous soil forms of the fungi. Once inhaled, some fungi reproduce in the body in the original filamentous (mycelial, hyphal) form. Others adopt specialized forms (yeasts, spherules, and endospores) more suitable for host survival and tissue invasion. Opportunistic fungi, however, can cause overwhelming infection in patients with impaired host defenses, including those with acquired immunodeficiency syndrome (AIDS), organ and bone marrow transplants, and hematologic malignancy. Mycoses that exist in nature as an infectious mold and invade tissues as a yeast (or yeast-like form such as spherules or endospores) are called **dimorphic fungi** (see Table 47–1). A major attribute of all opportunistic filamentous fungi is the tendency to invade blood vessels **(angioinvasion),** with resultant tissue infarction (Table 47–2).

Immunity to the mycoses is principally cellular, involving neutrophils, macrophages, lymphocytes, and probably natural killer (NK) cells. With the possible exception of the dermatophytes and *Rhizopus arrhizus,* the principal etiologic agent of mucormycosis (zygomycosis), fungi are not susceptible to direct killing by antibody and complement. Patients with neutropenia or defective neutrophil function appear predisposed to hematogenously disseminated infection with yeast-like fungi (eg, *Candida* spp, *Trichosporon beigelii*), or with filamentous fungi (eg, *Aspergillus,* agents causing mucormycosis, and *Fusarium* spp). Patients with defective cell-mediated immunity (CMI) (eg, patients with AIDS) are predisposed to mucosal candidiasis or hematogenously disseminated cryptococcosis, histoplasmosis, and coccidioidomycosis (Table 47–3). Allergy to fungi is discussed in Chapters 26–29.

Table 47–1. Common mycoses according to usual sites of disease production.

Site and Disease	Etiologic Agents	Origin	Invasive Form	Pathophysiologic Basis	Principal Clinical Features
Superficial mycoses Pityriasis (tinea) versicolor	Malassezia furfur	Hair follicle (yeasts)	Yeasts or mycelia	Decreased epithelial turnover allows normal flora to produce disease	Hypopigmented or hyperpigmented macular skin lesions
Malassezia	Malassezia furfur	Hair follicle (yeasts)	Yeasts	Obstructed hair follicles are damaged by follicular flora	Acneiform folliculitis
Tinea nigra	Exophiala werneckii	Soil (mycelia)	Mycelia	Hyperhidrosis permits infection from environment	Brown-black nonscaly macules (especially on palms)
White piedra	Trichosporon beigelii	Soil, skin (mycelia)	Mycelia and yeasts	Poor personal hygiene permits infection from environment or by normal flora	Soft whitish nodules on hair shaft
Black piedra	Piedraia hortae	Soil (mycelia)	Mycelia	Poor personal hygiene permits infection from environment	Hard gritty black nodules on hair shaft
Cutaneous mycoses Dermatophytosis	Epidermophyton, Trichophyton, and Microsporum spp	Soil and animal fur (mycelia)	Mycelia	Etiologic agents are keratinolytis; infection is potentiated by warmth, moisture, and occlusion; cutaneous inflammation is due to delayed-hypersensitivity reaction	Tinea pedis (scaly, vesicular, ulcerative), tinea cruris (dry, red, scaloped, expanding), tinea corporis (ring worm); tinea barbae (suppuration, beard), tinea capitis (scalp; resembles seborrhea), tinea unguium (nails)
Subcutaneous mycoses Chromoblastomycosis	Cladosporium, Fonsecaea, Philaophora, and Rhinocladiella spp	Soil (mycelia)	Mycelia and sclerotic bodies	Traumatic implantation	Papules, warty tumors, plaques, cauliflower-like growths
Mycetoma	Acremonium, Exophiala, Leptosphaeria, Madurella, Microsporum, and Pseudallescheria spp	Soil (mycelia)	Mycelia and grains	Traumatic implantation	Swelling, draining fistulae, pus, and grains
Sporotrichosis	Sporothrix schenckii	Vegetation (mycelia)	Yeasts	Traumatic implantation	Subcutaneous nodules along lymphatics

(Continued)

Table 47–1. *(continued)*.

Site and Disease	Etiologic Agents	Origin	Invasive Form	Pathophysiologic Basis	Principal Clinical Features
Systemic invasive mycoses Primary pathogens Blastomycosis	*Blastomyces dermatitidis*	Soil (mycelia)	Yeasts	Inhalation of conidia	Pulmonary, spreading to skin, bones, male reproductive tract
Coccidioidomycosis	*Coccidioides immitis*	Soil (mycelia)	Spherules and endospores	Inhalation of arthroconidia	Pulmonary, spreading to skin, bones, joints, meninges
Histoplasmosis	*Histoplasma capsulatum*	Soil (mycelia)	Yeasts	Inhalation of microconidia	Pulmonary, spreading to reticuloendothelial system, mucous membranes, adrenals
Paracoccidioidomycosis	*Paracoccidioides brasiliensis*	Soil (mycelia)	Yeasts	Inhalation of conidia	Pulmonary, spreading to reticuloendothelial system, skin, mucous membranes, adrenals
Opportunistic pathogens Candidiasis	Principally *Candida albicans, C tropicalis, C glabrata,* and *C parapsilosis*	Mucosal surfaces (yeasts, pseudomycelia)	Yeasts, pseudomycelia, mycelia	Local extension; bloodstream invasion from colonization sites (mucosal disruption)	Mucosal site, spreading to eyes, skin, kidneys, myocardium, other sites
Cryptococcosis	*Cryptococcus neoformans*	Soil (yeast, basidiospores [sexual form])	Yeasts	Inhalation of desiccated yeasts or basidiospores	Pulmonary, spreading to meninges, brain, bone skin
Aspergillosis	*Aspergillus fumigatus, A flavus, A terreus,* and *A niger,* principally	Soil (mycelia)	Mycelia	Inhalation of conidia	Invasive pulmonary or sinus disease, leading to hematogenous dissemination
Mucormycosis (zygomycosis)	*Rhizopus, Rhizomucor, Absidia, Cunninghamelia, Mortierella, Saksenaea* and *Mucor* spp	Soil (mycelia)	Mycelia	Inhalation of spores	Invasive sinus or pulmonary disease, leading to hematogeneous dissemination

(continued)

Table 47–1. Common mycoses according to usual sites of disease production *(continued)*.

Site and Disease	Etiologic Agents	Origin	Invasive Form	Pathophysiologic Basis	Principal Clinical Features
Pneumocystosis	*Pneumocystis carinii*	Unknown	Cysts and trophozoites	Inhalation of infective particles or arousal from latency	Progressive interstitial lung disease with or without cysts, pneumothorax
Phaeohyphomycosis	Approximately 40 genera of pigmented fungi (eg, *Alternaria, Bipolaris, Cladosporium, Exserohilum, Phialophora, Wangiella*)	Soil (mycelia)	Mycelia	Inhalation or implantation of common environmental fungi (pigmented; dematiaceous)	Invasive sinus or pulmonary disease, leading to hematogenous dissemination
Hyalohyphomycosis	Diverse nonpigmented fungi (eg, *Fusarium, Paecilomyces, Pseudallescheria, Scopulariopsis*)	Soil (mycelia)	Mycelia	Inhalation or implantation of common environmental fungi (nonpigmented)	Invasive sinus or pulmonary disease, leading to hematogenous dissemination

Salient features of the superficial, cutaneous, and subcutaneous mycoses may be found in Tables 47–1 to 47–4. The major systemic invasive mycoses found in the Western hemisphere are described in the following section.

SYSTEMIC INVASIVE MYCOSES: PRIMARY PATHOGENS

BLASTOMYCOSIS

Major Immunologic Features

- Yeasts large, single, and broad-based; commonly exceed the size of phagocytes
- Islands of suppuration (microabscesses) amid granulomas
- Neutrophils and CMI may play important and concomitant roles in host defense
- Severe, widely disseminated infection possible in patients with defective CMI, including those with AIDS

General Considerations

Blastomycosis is an inhalation-acquired mycosis that can produce primary pulmonary infection or hematogenously disseminated disease involving predominantly skin, bones, and the male genitourinary tract. *Blastomyces dermatitidis* is a spherical multinucleated yeast with thick walls and single broad-based buds. The mycelial form is a soil organism found on river banks predominantly in the south central United States and around the Great Lakes. A closely related fungus occurs in Africa. Infection occurs by inhalation of fungal microconidia in endemic areas (eg, by hunters, trappers, campers, or boaters). Sporadic and occasional common-source outbreaks occur, for example, from soil from damp areas such as a beaver dam or a river bank. Endemic areas are defined by the occurrence of cases and by seroconversions. There is no reliable skin test to gauge population exposures and establish the epidemiology of infection. There is no known genetic predisposition or convincing sex or age prevalence. Men are more susceptible than women to progressive pulmonary or hematogenous disease. Blastomycosis is an infrequent complication of AIDS although overwhelming disseminated infection may occur as a late complication.

Pathology

See Table 47–2.

Clinical Features

A. Signs and Symptoms: Primary exposure may be asymptomatic, or it may produce an influenza-like syndrome. Pneumonia, pleuritis, pulmonary cavitation, and mediastinal adenopathy may occur. Hematogenous dissemination may occur in the presence or absence of apparent pulmonary disease. Favored sites of metastatic infection include skin (papules, pustules, or verrucous granulomas that heal

Table 47–2. Pathologic features of subcutaneous and systemic mycoses.

Mycosis	Predominant Location of Fungi	Suppuration	Granulomas	Caseation	Fibrosis	Calcification	Other
Subcutaneous Chromomycosis	Extracellular (sclerotic bodies)	Dominant	Dominant	Rare	Dominant	Rare	PH; transdermal elimination.
Mycetoma	Extracellular (grains)	Dominant	Dominant	Rare	Dominant	Rare	Grains surrounded by immune complex deposition (Splendore–Hoeppli phenomenon)
Sporotrichosis	Intracellular and extracellular (yeasts)	Dominant	Dominant	Occasional	Occasional	Rare	Asteroid bodies with Splendore–Hoeppli phenomenon)
Systemic Primary pathogens Blastomycosis[a]	Extracellular (yeasts)	Dominant	Dominant	Rare	Occasional	Occasional	PH
Coccidioidomycosis	Extracellular (spherules)	Dominant (endospores)	Dominant (spherules)	Rare	Occasional	Occasional	PH
Histoplasmosis	Intracellular (yeasts)	Rare	Dominant	Occasional	Dominant	Dominant	Proliferative end-arteritis (lungs)
Paracoccidioidomycosis[a]	Extracellular (yeasts)	Dominant	Dominant	Rare	Dominant	Occasional	PH
Opportunistic pathogens Cryptococcosis[a]	Extracellular (yeasts)	Rare	Dominant	Rare	Rare	Rare	Extensive accumulation of extracellular capsular material may distort local anatomy

(continued)

Table 47–2. Pathologic features of subcutaneous and systemic mycoses *(continued).*

Mycosis	Predominant Location of Fungi	Suppuration	Granulomas	Caseation	Fibrosis	Calcification	Other
Candidiasis[b]	Intracellular (yeasts), extracellular (pseudomycelia mycelia)	Dominant	Rare	Rare	Rare	Rare	Granuloma formation common only in CMC[c]
Aspergillosis[b]	Extracellular (mycelia)	Dominant	Rare	Rare	Rare	Rare	Angioinvasion and infarction
Mucormycosis (zygomycosis)[b]	Extracellular (mycelia)	Dominant	Rare	Rare	Rare	Rare	Angioinvasion and infarction
Pneumocystosis	Extracellular (trophozoites, cysts)	Rare	Rare	None	Occasional	Rare	Foamy intraalveolar infiltrate and alveolar epithelial damage

Abbreviations: PH = pseudoepitheliomatous hyperplasia of skin and mucosal lesions; CMI = cell-mediated immunity.
[a] Severely depressed CMI is often associated with poor granuloma formation and increased suppuration with increased numbers of microorganisms (blastomycosis, coccidioidomycosis, paracoccidioidomycosis) or with gelatinous masses of encapsulated fungi (cryptococcosis).
[b] Severe neutropenia is often associated with loss of suppurative tissue response.
[c] Chronic mucocutaneous candidiasis.

centrally and extend peripherally); bone (lytic lesions, especially vertebrae and long bones, with or without draining sinuses); and prostate, testis, and epididymis. Central nervous system infection occurs in about 5% of cases, (40% in patients with AIDS, where disseminated, progressive infection with extensive pulmonary involvement occurs). Gastrointestinal tract involvement almost never occurs.

B. Laboratory Findings: These include leukocytosis, abnormal chest radiograph, and evidence of specific organ dysfunction at metastatic loci. Diagnosis is established by finding large budding yeasts on smears or histologic sections and by recovering the fungus in culture.

C. Immunologic Diagnosis: See Table 47–4. With the possible exception of antibody directed against the A antigen, immunologic tests lack either sensitivity or specificity.

D. Differential Diagnosis: This includes diverse granulomatous infectious diseases (eg, other mycoses and tuberculosis), sarcoidosis, and pulmonary cancer.

E. Treatment: Itraconazole is highly effective and has fewer side effect than ketoconazole when used to treat chronic, indolent forms of blastomycosis. For patients with meningitis or acute life-threatening infections, intravenous amphotericin B is preferable.

F. Prevention: No vaccine is available.

G. Complications and Prognosis: Untreated extrapulmonary blastomycosis carries a 20–90% mortality rate; with therapy it is less than 10%. Mortality rates in AIDS patients with disseminated infection are high, however. Most relapses occur within 1 year of treatment, but they have been documented after as long as 9 years.

COCCIDIOIDOMYCOSIS

Major Immunologic Features
- Inhaled arthroconidia have antiphagocytic surface and are highly infectious
- Spherules exceed the size of phagocytes and have an antiphagocytic surface
- Endospores released in packets that exceed the size of phagocytes
- Mixed granulomas and suppuration
- Primary infections signaled by erythema nodosum or erythema multiforme
- Negative skin test (coccidioidin, spherulin) and high complement fixation antibody titer suggest hematogenous dissemination
- Disease much more severe in patients with defective CMI (including in AIDS)
- Infection confers solid immunity

Table 47–3. Effect of common immunologic abnormalities on disease course of common mycoses.

Mycosis	Reduction in PMN[a]	Reduction in CMI[b]	Other
Superficial Pityriasis (tinea) versicolor	None	None	Lipid hyperalimentation therapy is associated with *Malassezia furfur*[c] and pulmonary vasculitis, especially in infants
Pityrosporum folliculitis	None	None	Treatment
Tinea nigra	None	None	
White piedra	Hematogenous dissemination of *Trichosporon beigelii*[d]	None	
Black piedra	None	None	
Cutaneous Dermatophytosis	None	Increased severity and chronicity of *T rubrum* infection	
Subcutaneous Chromomycosis	None	None	
Mycetoma	None	None	
Sporotrichosis	None	Increased in severity and likelihood of dissemination	
Systemic, invasive Primary pathogens Blastomycosis	None	Increase in severity and likelihood of dissemination	Frequency of meningitis is increased in patients with AIDS
Coccidioidomycosis	None	Definite increase in severity and dissemination	Possible increase in severity and dissemination in second and third trimesters of pregnancy
Histoplasmosis	None	Definite increase in severity and dissemination	
Paracoccidioidomycosis	None	Probable increase in severity or likelihood of dissemination	
Opportunistic pathogens Candidiasis	Hematogenous dissemination	Increased severity of mucosal disease	
Cryptococcosis	None	Definite increase in severity and dissemination	
Aspergillosis	Invasive paranasal sinus and respiratory infection, and hematogenous dissemination	Possible increase in severity	
Mucormycosis (zygomycosis)	Invasive paranasal sinus and respiratory infection, and hematogenous dissemination	Possible increase in severity	Diabetic ketoacidosis predisposes to invasive paranasal sinus infection
Pneumocystosis	None	Drastic increase in incidence and severity in AIDS	
Phaeohyphomycosis	Invasive paranasal sinus infection and hematogenous dissemination	None	
Hyalohyphomycoses	Invasive paranasal sinus infection and hematogenous dissemination	None	

Abbreviations: AIDS = acquired immunodeficiency syndrome; CMI = cell-mediated immunity.

[a] <500 PMN/dL.

[b] Principally AIDS. Histoplasmosis, coccidioidomycosis, and cryptococcosis also occur with increased severity and/or extent of dissemination in patients with other causes of depressed CMI (eg, immunosuppression for organ transplantation).

[c] *Malassezia* is a lipophilic fungus. Lipid hyperalimentation therapy allows them access to the bloodstream. Patients with *Malassezia* fungemia do not have tinea versicolor or folliculitis.

[d] Patients with *Trichosporon beigelii* sepsis do not necessarily have white piedra.

Table 47–4. Immunologic diagnosis of subcutaneous and systemic mycoses.

| Mycosis | Serologic Tests | | Delayed-Hypersensitivity Skin Test[1] | Comments[2] |
	Antibody	Antigen		
Subcutaneous Chromoblasto-mycosis	None	None	None	Diagnosed by characteristic clinical appearance and histopathology. Specific etiologic diagnoses requires culture.
Mycetoma	None	None	None	Diagnosed by characteristic clinical picture. Specific etiologic diagno-sis microscopic exami-nation of grains and cultures of grains and biopsy material.
Sporotrichosis	EIA, TA, LPA (sen-sitive/specific) CF, ID (less sensitive)	None	Investigational only	Serologic tests generally valuable only in extracutaneous and disseminated infection. A slide latex agglutination titer of ≥1:8 is presumptive evidence of dissemi-nated or systemic infection.
Systemic Primary patho-gens Blastomycosis	ID, CF (blastomycin as antigen); ID, CF EIA (A ant-igen)	None	Blastomycin (mycelial phase), BASWS (investi-gational only)	The blastomycin skin test and serologic tests lack sensitivity and specificity. Tests for antibody to A antigen are more specific (especially ID and EIA).
Coccidioido-mycosis	IgM (TP, IDTP, LPA); IgG (CF, IDCF) (coccidio-idin as antigen)	Experimental only	Coccidioidin (my-celial phase), sph-erulin (spherule phase)	IgM tests positive early and tran-siently; IgG tests positive later and more persistently. A CF antibody titer in blood >1:16 suggests hematogenous dissemi-nation, especially if skin tests are negative. A positive CF titer in the cere-brospinal fluid is virtually diagnos-tic of meningitis.
Histoplasmosis	CF (whole yeast cells as antigen); CF (histoplasmin as antigen); ID (histoplasmin as antigen); LPA (histoplasmin as antigen)	Useful for antigen detection in urine serum CSF (see text); avail-able in Indian-apolis commer-cially	Histoplasmin (my-celial phase), his-tolyn CYL (yeast phase)	A positive histoplasmin skin test can artificially elevate CF antibody titers and produce a positive ID test ("m" band). Histolyn YCL is less likely to do this. An ID antibody "h" band suggests active infection. An LPA antibody titer ≥1:32 suggests active infection. A CF antibody titer ≥1:32 or a fourfold titer rise suggests active infection. *Histoplasma* polysaccharide antigen highly sensitive and specific for disseminated infection.

(Continued)

General Considerations

Coccidioidomycosis is an inhalation-acquired my-cosis that can produce primary pulmonary infection, progressive pulmonary disease, or hematogenously disseminated disease involving predominantly skin, subcutaneous tissues, bones, joints, and meninges.

Coccidioides immitis is characterized uniquely by large spherules that rupture to release hundreds of en-dospores, which, in turn, mature to more spherules. The mycelial form of *C immitis* is found in the soil of semidesert areas of the United States (eg, California, Arizona, and Texas), contiguous areas of Mexico,

Table 47–4. Immunologic diagnosis of subcutaneous and systemic mycoses *(continued)*.

| Mycosis | Serologic Tests | | Delayed-Hypersensitivity Skin Test[a] | Comments[b] |
	Antibody	Antigen		
Paracoccidioi-domycosis	ID, CIE (simple, more specific); CF, EIA (sensitive; less specific)	None	Various "paracocci-dioidins" (mycelial phase), investigational only	Elevated precipitin titers (transient) precede elevated CF titers (more persistent). The number and duration of precipitin bands directly proportional to disease activity. The CF titer directly proportional to the severity of illness. The skin test commonly negative with active disease.
Opportunistic pathogens Cryptococco-sis	IFA, EIA, TA	Capsular polysac-charide (LPA, EIA)	"Cryptococcin" (investigational only)	Cryptococcal skin tests and tests for antibody lack sensitivity and specificity. The LPA for cryptococcal antigen is highly sensitive and specific. Rare (low-titer) cross-reactivity with *Trichosporon beigelii*. A positive cerebrospinal fluid test is diagnostic of cryptococcal meningitis.
Candidiasis	Multiple, diverse serologic tests (precipitins, agglutinins most common); CIE, IHA, IFA, RIA, ID, LPA	Mannan (LPA, EIA, RIA, coagglutin-ation), enolase 48-kd cytoplasmic protein (LIA, EIA, DIA), undefined heat-labile gly-coprotein antigen (LPA), D-arabini-tol, D-mannose (GLC)	Oidiomycin	Skin tests lack diagnostic value (healthy persons are positive). Antibody tests lack sensitivity and specificity, especially in immuno-suppressed patients. Mannan antigen tests positive in low titer, generally too late in the course of illness to be useful diagnostically. Heat-labile antigen lacks sensitivity and specificity in immunocompro-mised patients.
Aspergillosis	Multiple, diverse serologic tests (precipitins most common)	Galactomannan and related anti-gens (RIA, EIA)	"Aspergillin"	More than 90% of patients with ABPA have positive *Aspergillus* skin tests and precipitin. More than 90% of patients with as-pergilloma have precipitin. Serologic tests for antibody lack sensitivity and are without value in patients with invasive aspergillosis. Galactomannan antigen is not of proven efficacy in diagnosis.
Mucormycosis (zygomyco-sis)	EIA, ID	None	None	Serologic tests for zygomycosis have been unsuccessful.

Abbreviations: BASWS = an alkali-soluble, water-soluble blastomycosis skin test preparation; BF = bentonite flocculation; CIE = counterimmunoelectrophoresis; CF = complement fixation; DIA = dot immunoassay; EIA = enzyme immunoassay; ID = immuno-diffusion; IDCF = immunodiffusion with the CF antigen; = IDTP = immunodiffusion with the TP antigen; IFA = indirect immunofluor-escence assay; IHA = indirect hemagglutination; GLC = gas–liquid chromatography; LIA = liposomal immunoassay; LPA = latex particle agglutination; PHA = passive hemagglutination; RIA = radioimmunoassay; TA = tube agglutination; TP = tube precipitin; YCA = whole yeast cell agglutination.

[a] Skin tests are predominantly of epidemiologic importance, defining loci of endemicity. A positive skin test indicates only that infection has occurred in the past. Some skin tests (especially histoplasmin) can influence serologic test results.

[b] In vitro correlates of CMI (eg, lymphocyte blastogenesis and migration inhibition) have been studied extensively, but are insufficiently standardized for routine diagnostic use.

and scattered areas of Central and South America. Infection occurs by inhalation of arthroconidia in endemic areas (eg, by tourists, travelers, farmers, archeologists, or construction engineers).

Sporadic and, occasionally, common-source outbreaks occur (eg, dust storm in central California). Endemic areas are defined by skin test (coccidioidin, spherulin) reactivity. Susceptibility to hematogenous dissemination is greatest at the extremes of age. It is also positively correlated with male sex, race (especially blacks and Filipinos), deficient CMI, and hormonal status (it occurs more often in the second and third trimesters of pregnancy than in the first). The growth of *C immitis* is stimulated by estrogen. There is a suspected HLA-related susceptibility to infection (HLA-A9).

Pathology

See Table 47–2.

Clinical Features

A. Signs and Symptoms: Primary exposure may be asymptomatic (60%) or associated with an influenza-like syndrome. In some patients (especially white women) transient arthralgias, erythema nodosum, or erythema multiforme (also known as valley fever, and desert rheumatism) may occur. Similar immunologic phenomena have been observed with histoplasmosis and blastomycosis. Pneumonia, pleuritis, and pulmonary cavitation may occur; cavitary lung disease may be chronic or progressive. Hematogenous dissemination usually occurs in the absence of apparent pulmonary disease. Among the usual manifestations of metastatic infection are skin lesions, including nodules, ulcers, sinus tracts from deeper loci, and verrucous granulomas. Also involved are bones, joints, tendon sheaths, and meninges. Meningitis may be the sole apparent locus of metastasis. The gastrointestinal tract is rarely involved.

In patients with AIDS, disease is more acute and more severe. Manifestations of fungemia, including hematogenous (miliary) pneumonia, adult respiratory distress syndrome (ARDS), cellulitis, and papulopustular skin lesions in a hematogenous pattern, may dominate. Meningitis is commonly present.

B. Laboratory Findings: These include leukocytosis, eosinophilia (including cerebrospinal fluid), abnormal chest film, and evidence of specific organ dysfunction at metastatic loci. **Diagnosis** is established by demonstrating endosporulating spherules on smears and histologic sections and by recovering the fungus in cultures.

C. Immunologic Diagnoses: See Table 47–4. Immunologic tests are useful in diagnosis and prognosis. Negative delayed-hypersensitivity skin tests and an elevated (or rising) complement fixation (CF) titer suggest hematogenous dissemination. An elevated CF titer in the cerebrospinal fluid is virtually diagnostic of coccidioidal meningitis, which is often culture-negative. An immunodiffusion test for complement fixing (IDCF) IgG antibody to *C immitis* correlates well with traditional CF tests. Antibodies are detected 2–6 weeks after onset of infection and parallel the extent of infection. Coccidioidin (and presumably spherulin) skin testing in a patient with active erythema nodosum may produce a violent, necrotic skin test reaction.

D. Differential Diagnosis: This includes diverse granulomatous infectious diseases (eg, mycoses, tuberculosis), sarcoidosis, and cancers.

E. Treatment: Amphotericin B is the drug of choice in immunocompromised patients acutely ill with hematogenous dissemination; it must be given intrathecally for meningitis. Ketoconazole, itraconazole, and fluconazole are useful for long-term maintenance therapy of nonmeningeal disease. Fluconazole and itraconazole have both been used successfully in disseminated infection, including that of the central nervous system (CNS), but slow response and eventual relapse after discontinuation of therapy is common. Even in nonmeningeal disease, azole therapy must be continued for 6–12 months after resolution of infection. The poor efficacy of amphotericin B in meningeal disease has led to the use of fluconazole, which offers the potential advantage of high cerebrospinal fluid levels, or itraconazole in CNS infection. Lifelong azole therapy for meningeal disease is usually required because relapses are very common.

F. Prevention: A spherule vaccine has failed to demonstrate effective protection.

G. Complications and Prognosis: Most patients recover spontaneously from primary infection. Erythema nodosum and erythema multiforme are considered particularly good prognostic signs. Some 2–4% of primary infections go on to progressive cavitary lung disease poorly responsive to antifungal drugs, or to hematogenously disseminated disease. Meningitis is fatal without therapy. AIDS-associated infections require lifelong suppressive therapy to prevent relapse.

HISTOPLASMOSIS

Major Immunologic Features

- Reticuloendothelial system disease with tiny yeasts residing in macrophages
- Granulomas with or without caseation
- Possible partial immunologic basis (subintimal arterial proliferation; pulmonary infarction) for cavitary lung disease
- More severe in patients with defective CMI (including those with AIDS)
- Reactivation of latent infection possible in patients with AIDS
- Prominent calcification and fibrosis during healing
- Occasional waning of immunity to reinfection

General Considerations

Histoplasmosis is an inhalation-acquired mycosis that can produce primary pulmonary infection, progressive pulmonary disease, or hematogenously disseminated disease involving predominantly the reticuloendothelial system, mucosal surfaces, and adrenal glands. *Histoplasma capsulatum,* a tiny intracellular yeast, is a soil saprobe (mycelial form) that is found worldwide. It is particularly common in river valleys of the southeastern and central United States. It grows particularly well in soil fertilized by bird droppings and bat guano, especially in caves. Infection occurs by inhalation of microconidia in endemic areas, for example, by farmers, cave explorers, tourists, or construction workers. Sporadic and, occasionally, common-source outbreaks occur (eg, during construction in Indianapolis). Reactivation of latent infection is common in patients with advanced AIDS; patients living in nonendemic regions may develop active histoplasmosis from exposure to *H capsulatum* many years earlier in an endemic area. A positive delayed-hypersensitivity skin test is extremely common in endemic areas. Hematogenous dissemination is especially common at the extremes of age. Progressive pulmonary disease, strongly resembling tuberculosis, is especially likely in white men with chronic obstructive pulmonary disease. There is no known genetic predisposition.

Pathology

See Table 47–2.

Clinical Features

A. Signs and Symptoms: Primary exposure may be asymptomatic or associated with a flu-like syndrome. Pneumonia, pleuritis, pulmonary cavitation, and mediastinal adenopathy may occur. Except in infants, hematogenous dissemination usually occurs in the absence of apparent pulmonary disease. Favored sites of metastatic infection include the reticuloendothelial system (hepatosplenomegaly; lymphadenopathy; bone marrow involvement with anemia, leukopenia, and thrombocytopenia); mucous membranes (oronasopharyngeal ulcerations); gastrointestinal tract (malabsorption); and adrenals (adrenal insufficiency). An intense fibrotic response during healing may lead to fibrous mediastinitis. Calcification is common at healed loci ("buckshot" granulomas of the lungs; splenic calcifications). A presumed ocular histoplasmosis syndrome is described in persons in endemic regions, which may represent a hyperactive immunologic response to histoplasmin antigen. In patients with AIDS, disease is more acute and may be fulminating, resembling bacterial septicemic shock. Manifestations include hematogenous (miliary) pneumonia, ARDS, disseminated intravascular coagulation (DIC), hematogenously distributed papulopustules, and meningitis.

B. Laboratory Findings: These include leukocytosis or leukopenia, thrombocytopenia, and anemia.

There is evidence of specific organ dysfunction at metastatic loci. **Diagnosis** is established by the presence of intracellular yeasts on smears (eg, buffy coat smears in AIDS patients); histologic specimens (eg, mucosal biopsies); or cultures of sputum, blood, bone marrow, and liver biopsy material.

C. Immunologic Diagnoses: See Table 47–4. Serologic tests may be useful in assessing disease activity and, less frequently, in establishing the diagnosis. A positive histoplasmin skin test may spuriously induce elevated antibody titers detected serologically. The detection of polysaccharide antigen in urine, blood, or CSF may be especially helpful in diagnosis and in assessing the response to therapy.

D. Differential Diagnosis: This includes diverse granulomatous infectious diseases (eg, mycoses, tuberculosis, leishmaniasis, and toxoplasmosis), sarcoidosis, Whipple's disease and other causes of malabsorption, and lymphohematogenous cancer. *Penicillium marneffei,* a dimorphic fungus with a yeast-like intracellular form, is an emerging pathogen in AIDS patients in Southeast Asia. The disease, penicilliosis, and the fungus, bear a superficial resemblance to histoplasmosis and its causative fungus.

E. Treatment: Amphotericin B is the drug of choice in treating immunocompromised patients acutely ill with hematogenous dissemination. Itraconazole is highly effective for nonmeningeal, non-life-threatening forms of the disease and has fewer side effects than does ketoconazole. Fluconazole is less active than itraconazole, but at higher doses it may be used in patients intolerant of itraconazole. AIDS-associated infections require lifelong suppressive therapy to prevent relapse.

F. Prevention: No vaccine is available.

G. Complications and Prognosis: Most primary infections resolve spontaneously. Progressive cavitary pulmonary disease is difficult to treat and may contribute to death from underlying pulmonary insufficiency. Hematogenous dissemination is generally fatal in the absence of therapy. Relapses are common in those with severe underlying immunodeficiency. Adrenal insufficiency may occur years after the original disease is quiescent.

PARACOCCIDIOIDOMYCOSIS

Major Immunologic Features

- Large, multiply budding yeasts may exceed size of phagocytes
- Mixed granulomas and suppuration
- Possibly more severe with defective CMI.

General Considerations

Paracoccidioidomycosis is an inhalation-acquired mycosis that can produce primary pulmonary infection or hematogenously disseminated disease involving predominantly the skin, mucous membranes, reticuloendothelial system, and adrenals. *Paracoccidioides brasiliensis* is a large, spherical, uninucleate yeast with highly characteristic multiple buds attached by narrow necks (wagon wheel appearance). The mycelial form is a soil saprobe only rarely recovered from the area where it is endemic in tropical and subtropical forests of Latin America, particularly Brazil, Venezuela, and Colombia. Paracoccidioidomycosis is the most common systemic mycosis in South America. Infection occurs by inhalation of conidia and is most common among agricultural workers. The disease is sporadic. Skin test surveys suggest that men and women are equally susceptible, but men are 12–48 times as likely to experience hematogenous dissemination, perhaps because physiologic concentrations of estrogen can prevent the conversion of conidia to invasive yeasts. In Brazilians, HLA-B40 antigen is more common in patients than in controls; in Colombians, HLA-A9 and -B13 are more common. Paracoccidioidomycosis is uncommon in AIDS patients.

Pathology

See Table 47–2.

Clinical Features

A. Signs and Symptoms: Primary exposure may be asymptomatic, or pneumonia, pleuritis, pulmonary cavitation, and mediastinal adenopathy may occur. Hematogenously disseminated disease occurs in two main forms. In the **juvenile** pattern (3–5% of cases), the primary pulmonary infection disseminates rapidly, with predominant reticuloendothelial system involvement. In the **adult** form (90% of cases), fungi, presumably aroused from latency, give rise to progressive localized lung disease, skin and mucocutaneous lesions, reticuloendothelial system infection, and adrenal involvement. Oropharyngeal mucosal invasion is characteristic, with ulcerating lesions that involve most of the oral adventitia. Lesions are so painful that eating is difficult; tooth loss is common. Involvement of the gastrointestinal tract may lead to malabsorption; adrenal involvement can produce adrenal insufficiency.

B. Laboratory Findings: These include leukocytosis and evidence of specific organ dysfunction at metastatic loci. Diagnosis is established by demonstrating multiple-budding yeasts on smears or histologic sections and by recovering the fungi in culture.

C. Immunologic Diagnosis: See Table 47–4. Serologic tests are of use in monitoring the course of established disease.

D. Differential Diagnosis: This includes diverse granulomatous infectious diseases (eg, mycoses, tuberculosis, leishmaniasis, yaws, and syphilis), sarcoidosis, and cancer.

E. Treatment: Both ketoconazole and itraconazole are useful. Itraconazole has become the drug of choice because of its improved side effect profile and shorter required duration of therapy. Sulfonamides have traditionally been used and offer a less expensive alternative.

F. Prevention: No vaccine is available.

G. Complications and Prognosis: Disseminated paracoccidioidomycosis is generally fatal in the absence of therapy. Disease that was originally acquired asymptomatically may present as disseminated infection years after the infected individual has emigrated from the area where the infection is endemic. Length of therapy is critical because relapses are common. Most patients require 1–2 years of therapy, which may be guided by serial serology.

SYSTEMIC INVASIVE MYCOSES: OPPORTUNISTIC PATHOGENS CANDIDIASIS

Major Immunologic Features

- Source of infection usually the normal host flora
- Intact mucosal barriers major nonspecific host defense mechanism
- Phagocytes ingest yeasts but attack pseudomycelia and mycelia by extracellular apposition
- Neutropenia predisposes to hematogenous dissemination
- Defective CMI predisposes to invasive mucosal disease
- Thrush, esophagitis, and vaginitis major presenting features of AIDS
- Chronic mucocutaneous candidiasis specific syndrome in patients with defective immunoregulation

General Considerations

Candidiasis is a general term for diseases produced by *Candida* species and encompasses colonization, superficial infection (eg, thrush, vaginitis, cystitis, and intertrigo), deep local invasion (eg, esophagitis), and hematogenous dissemination (eg, to the eyes, skin, kidneys, and brain). The species that most commonly cause candidiasis are *C albicans* (yeasts, pseudomycelia, and mycelia), *C tropicalis* (yeasts and pseudomycelia), and *C (Torulopsis) glabrata* (yeasts only). *Candida* species are found in nature, but human infection usually arises from normal flora. *C albicans, C tropicalis,* and *C glabrata* are commonly found on mucous membranes (eg, vagina, and gastrointestinal tract) but rarely on the skin. Vaginal colonization is increased by diabetes mellitus, pregnancy, and the use of oral contraceptive agents. Carriage at all sites is increased by antibiotics. Hematogenous dissemination occurs most commonly in a setting of neutropenia or gastrointestinal mucosal disruption after repeated abdominal surgery. Neonates may be colonized or infected by passage through a colonized birth canal; premature infants in intensive care units are at particularly high risk for life-threatening *Candida* sepsis. Nosocomial transmission of candidal infection may occur with hand transmission, a common exogenous source of the organism. Vaginal colonization occurs after menarche. Disseminated infection occurs in both sexes and at all ages as a function of immunologic impairment. **Chronic mucocutaneous candidiasis,** described in the following section, shows a familial tendency in about 20% of cases. In about 50% of cases there is associated endocrinopathy (eg, hypoparathyroidism, hypoadrenalism, hypothyroidism, or diabetes mellitus). The cause of this association is unknown (see Chapter 24).

Pathology
See Table 47–2.

Clinical Features
A. Signs and Symptoms: Mucosal candidiasis is characterized by thrush, laryngitis, esophagitis, gastritis (especially in patients with drug-induced hypochlorhydria), vaginitis, cystitis, and intestinal candidiasis (the assumed source of hematogenous dissemination in most neutropenic patients). Vulvovaginitis is probably the most common overall manifestation of *Candida* infection. Chronic mucocutaneous candidiasis is manifested by persistent infection of skin, scalp, nails, and mucous membranes and is often accompanied by chronic dermatophyte infections. Associated findings include alopecia, depigmentation, cheilosis, blepharitis, keratoconjunctivitis, corneal ulcers, and cutaneous horn formation. Hematogenously disseminated candidiasis can be either acute or chronic. The acute syndrome is characterized by involvement of the eyes (chorioretinitis), muscles (myalgias), skin (macronodular skin lesions), and kidneys (parenchymal destruction, papillary necrosis, and bezoar formation). Hematogenous (miliary) pulmonary infection is common, but *Candida* aspiration pneumonia is rare. Other manifestations include myocardial abscesses, meningitis, cerebral abscesses, and arthritis. Chronic disseminated candidiasis occurs most commonly in patients recovering from neutropenia who remain febrile despite broad-spectrum antibacterial therapy. Imaging studies reveal abscesses in the liver, spleen, lungs, and kidneys. The former designation of this syndrome as "hepatosplenic" candidiasis is not adequately descriptive and should be dropped.

B. Laboratory Findings: These include leukopenia or leukocytosis and evidence of specific organ dysfunction at metastatic loci. Diagnosis is established by direct histologic demonstration of fungal tissue invasion or recovery of fungi in culture from normally sterile areas (or both). Candidemia should be regarded as indicative of invasive infection in all but the most exceptional circumstances. Candiduria indicates cystitis more frequently than it indicates progressive renal infection.

C. Immunologic Diagnosis: See Table 47–4. Serologic tests are not helpful in neutropenic patients.

D. Differential Diagnosis: This includes diverse septicemic syndromes (eg, *Staphylococcus aureus* and *Pseudomonas aeruginosa* infections) and diverse opportunistic infectious diseases of neutropenic patients, including mycoses.

E. Treatment: Topical imidazoles are used for treating thrush and vaginitis, ketoconazole or fluconazole for vaginitis or progressive mucocutaneous infection, amphotericin B or fluconazole for deep local invasive infection or hematogenous dissemination, and amphotericin B plus flucytosine (depending on renal function) for managing disseminated infections that involve the eyes or central nervous system. Fluconazole may be useful as prolonged follow-up therapy of acute or chronic disseminated candidiasis. It has similar efficacy in the treatment of candidemia in nonneutropenic patients. Amphotericin B, however, remains the standard therapy for neutropenic patients and those with complicated infections and infection due to some species of *Candida* other than *C albicans*. Candiduria can usually be cured by removal of a urinary catheter plus a short course of fluconazole or intravesicular amphotericin B.

F. Prevention: Prophylactic administration of nystatin or ketoconazole to immunocompromised patients has not been clearly shown to prevent *Candida* infections. Prophylactic ketoconazole may actually predispose to infection by *C tropicalis, C glabrata,* or *Aspergillus* spp, which are not susceptible to ketoconazole. Similarly, prophylactic fluconazole may predispose to infections with *C krusei* or *C glabrata;* however, fluconazole prophylaxis has decreased the incidence of candidemia in patients undergoing bone marrow transplantation or induction chemotherapy for hematologic malignancy.

G. Complications and Prognosis: Chronic mucocutaneous candidiasis can be ameliorated but not cured by chronic ketoconazole therapy. *Candida* endocarditis is essentially incurable without valve replacement. Empirical amphotericin B therapy in febrile neutropenic patients has led to an improved prognosis for recovery in these patients, whose illness is otherwise extremely difficult to diagnose and who often die untreated. Reversal of neutropenia is the most important single predictor of recovery from infection.

CRYPTOCOCCOSIS

Major Immunologic Features
- Unencapsulated environmental yeasts acquire a capsule in lungs
- Encapsulated yeasts evade phagocytosis
- Free capsular polysaccharide triggers suppressor cells, down-regulating host defenses

- Disease much more common and severe in patients with defective CMI, particularly those with AIDS
- Detection of free capsular polysaccharide extremely helpful in diagnosis

General Considerations

Cryptococcosis is an inhalation-acquired mycosis that is initiated by symptomatic or asymptomatic pulmonary infection. In patients with altered CMI, dissemination to the meninges is common. Less common sites of hematogenous dissemination include skin, bones, eyes, and prostate. *Cryptococcus neoformans* is an encapsulated yeast with four serotypes (A, B, C, and D) based on antigenic differences in the capsular polysaccharide. Virulence is linked to encapsulation and the capacity to synthesize melanin. Cryptococci are ubiquitous, and the disease occurs worldwide. Serotypes A and D are most commonly found in avian habitats (eg, in pigeon dung); serotypes B and C may be associated with eucalyptus trees. Serotype A causes most disease worldwide; serotype D is common only in Europe. Disease caused by serotypes B and C is found predominantly in subtropical areas (most commonly Australia but also including southern California). Serotypes A and D are the most common causes of cryptococcal infection in immunocompromised patients and are overwhelmingly the most common serotypes recovered from patients with AIDS. Studies with poorly standardized "cryptococcin" skin tests suggest that asymptomatic infection may be common. Immunosuppression (including AIDS) causes the disease to emerge from apparent latency. Some 6–13% of AIDS patients develop a *C neoformans* infection. Cryptococcosis is more common in males, even excluding the current AIDS population. Infection is rare in children. The disease is sporadic. There is no known genetic predisposition. Most patients with infection have underlying immunosuppression.

Pathology

See Table 47–2.

Clinical Features

A. Signs and Symptoms: Cryptococcal infection commonly presents as isolated meningitis. Disease of the lungs is generally not apparent, even though this is the site of fungal entry. In patients who present with pulmonary infection, however, meningeal involvement may be inapparent or absent. The most common manifestations of pulmonary cryptococcosis are solitary or multiple infiltrates or nodules. Cryptococcal meningitis is commonly a subtle or subacute process characterized by headache, impaired mentation, optic neuritis or papilledema, cranial nerve palsies, and seizures. Hydrocephalus may lead to progressive mental deterioration. In patients with AIDS, meningeal involvement may also be subtle, despite disproportionately huge numbers of fungi in the cerebrospinal fluid. In addition, manifestations of widespread hematogenous dissemination may also be present (eg, diffuse skin lesions, miliary pulmonary infiltrates, ARDS) and may lead rapidly to death. Other sites of hematogenous dissemination include the skin (particularly prominent in AIDS patients), bones, prostate, kidneys, and liver.

B. Laboratory Findings: Meningitis is usually low grade, with lymphocytosis and low sugar levels in cerebrospinal fluid. The diagnosis is usually established by cryptococcal antigen detection, India ink stains, and positive cultures of the cerebrospinal fluid. Organisms may also be cultured from blood, skin lesions, urine, and prostatic secretions.

C. Immunologic Diagnosis: See Table 47–4. Demonstration of cryptococcal antigen in cerebrospinal fluid or blood is extremely helpful in establishing the diagnosis. In AIDS patients, antigen titers are extremely high.

D. Differential Diagnosis: The differential diagnosis of pulmonary cryptococcosis includes diverse infections and cancers. Cryptococcal meningitis may be confused with diverse chronic hypoglycorrhachic syndromes, including tuberculosis or coccidioidomycosis. Symptoms may be erroneously attributed to a primary psychiatric disorder. In AIDS patients the differential diagnosis includes the gamut of opportunistic infections commonly encountered in this disorder.

E. Treatment: Because of its rapidity of action, amphotericin B, with or without flucytosine, should be used to initiate therapy. Fluconazole may be substituted once the infection has stabilized. AIDS-associated infection requires lifelong suppressive therapy to prevent relapse.

F. Prevention: The widespread use of fluconazole in patients with AIDS appears to have resulted in an overall decreased incidence of cryptococcal infections. Fluconazole prophylaxis significantly reduced the number of cryptococcal infections in a prospective clinical trial, but long-term prophylaxis is expensive and may lead to the emergence of fluconazole-resistant yeasts.

G. Complications and Prognosis: Patients with any alteration in mental status at the time of presentation are more likely to die than those with normal mentation. Elevated intracerebral pressures have been associated with increased morbidity and mortality associated with cryptococcal meningitis. Large-volume spinal taps and drugs (eg, steroids or acetazolamide) may be needed to reduce intracranial pressures. The likelihood of cure is inversely proportional to the severity of underlying immunosuppression. Although the cryptococcal antigen test is very helpful in establishing a diagnosis, the decrease in antigen titer may not be proportionate to the extent of clinical therapeutic response. Thus, disappearance of antigen from cerebrospinal fluid may not be a realistic therapeutic goal.

ASPERGILLOSIS

Major Immunologic Features

- Infection caused by inhalation of conidia (common environmental contaminants)
- Conidia ingested and killed by alveolar macrophages
- Phagocytes attack mycelia by extracellular apposition
- Neutropenia or neutrophil dysfunction predisposes to respiratory tract invasion, angioinvasion, and hematogenous dissemination
- Balls of fungi may colonize previously damaged respiratory tissues (aspergilloma)
- Allergy may develop to inhaled conidia or to fungi colonizing the bronchial tree (atopic asthma, extrinsic allergic alveolitis, allergic bronchopulmonary aspergillosis)

General Considerations

Aspergillosis is a term that encompasses colonization, allergy, or tissue invasion. In addition, *Aspergillus* spp produce mycotoxins. Aflatoxin (*A flavus*) is linked epidemiologically to hepatocellular carcinoma; gliotoxin (*A fumigatus*) is toxic to macrophages and cytotoxic T cells. The focus of this section is on **invasive aspergillosis.** Allergic bronchopulmonary aspergillosis (ABPA) is discussed in Chapter 28. *Aspergillus* spp are among the most common environmental saprophytic fungi. Only a few thermotolerant species are pathogenic for humans, most notably *A fumigatus, A flavus, A terreus,* and *A niger. Aspergillus* infections occur worldwide. Outbreaks of invasive aspergillosis have followed exposure to conidia released by hospital construction, contaminated air-conditioning ducts and filters, and fireproofing materials above false ceilings. Invasive infection occurs in both sexes at all ages as a function of immunologic impairment. There is no known genetic predisposition.

Pathology

See Table 47–2.

Clinical Features

A. Signs and Symptoms: Invasive pulmonary aspergillosis occurs characteristically in immunosuppressed, neutropenic patients. Widespread bronchial ulceration, parenchymal invasion, and angioinvasion lead to patchy necrotizing pneumonia, thrombosis, and infarction. Suggestive clinical features include pleuritic chest pain with hemoptysis in a febrile, neutropenic patient on broad-spectrum antibiotics. Widespread metastatic infection may occur. Infarcted lung tissue may contain necrotic sequestrae that resemble aspergillomas. A similar process may take place in the paranasal sinuses, resulting in a clinical picture identical to that of rhinocerebral mucormycosis (see the following section). An **indolent,**

semiinvasive pulmonary infection occasionally occurs in immunocompetent patients with underlying chronic obstructive pulmonary disease. Ulcerative tracheobronchitis occurs in patients with AIDS and as a complication of lung transplantation and is characterized by ulcerative endobronchial lesions that may require bronchoscopy for diagnosis.

B. Laboratory Findings: These include neutropenia, abnormal chest or sinus radiographs, and evidence of specific organ dysfunction at metastatic loci. **Diagnosis** depends on histologic demonstration of tissue invasion by an exclusively mycelial fungus. Cultivation of *Aspergillus* spp from respiratory secretions may reflect only transient colonization, but in a high-risk patient (eg, febrile, neutropenic patient with pulmonary infiltrates) it may be an important clue to the diagnosis of infection; blood cultures are rarely positive.

C. Immunologic Diagnosis: See Table 47–4. Serologic tests for antibody are not useful in diagnosis of invasive aspergillosis; antigen and polymerase chain reaction (PCR) tests are promising but still experimental. Skin tests and precipitin titers are required for the diagnosis of ABPA (see Chapter 28).

D. Differential Diagnosis: This includes diverse opportunistic pulmonary infections (bacterial and fungal), pulmonary infarction, diverse septicemic syndromes, and rhinocerebral mucormycosis.

E. Treatment: Amphotericin B is the only drug of proven therapeutic value for treating severely immunosuppressed patients. It must be used early and aggressively if the patient is to survive. Itraconazole may be useful for long-term follow-up therapy or in treating patients whose disease is not acutely life-threatening. Liposomal forms of amphotericin B reduce the toxicity of amphotericin therapy and allow higher doses of drug to be given, which may improve the outcome of some patients with this disease.

F. Prevention: Hospital rooms with enclosed filtered ventilation systems provide some degree of protection from environmental fungi.

G. Complications and Prognosis: Invasive aspergillosis is commonly fatal. An aggressive approach to diagnosis and treatment is essential. Surgical debulking of infected, infarcted tissues may be of particular value. Empirical amphotericin B therapy in febrile neutropenic patients who are not responding to broad-spectrum antibacterial agents is commonly used in an attempt to prevent this and other opportunistic mycoses. Reversal of neutropenia is the single most important predictor of recovery from this infection.

MUCORMYCOSIS (ZYGOMYCOSIS)

Major Immunologic Features

- Infection caused by inhalation of spores
- Spores ingested and prevented from germinating by alveolar macrophages

- Phagocytes attack mycelia by extracellular apposition
- Acidotic states predispose to invasive paranasal sinus infection
- Neutropenia predisposes to paranasal sinus, pulmonary, and disseminated infection

General Considerations

Mucormycosis is a suppurative opportunistic mycosis that produces predominantly paranasal sinus (rhinocerebral) disease in patients with acidosis and rhinocerebral, pulmonary, or disseminated disease in patients with neutropenia. The most common etiologic agent is *Rhizopus arrhizus;* others include *Rhizomucor, Absidia, Cunninghamella, Mortierella, Saksenaea* spp, and, rarely, *Mucor.* These are all common environmental contaminants. Colonization and infection are uncommon in healthy persons; mucormycosis is less common than invasive aspergillosis in immunocompromised patients. Infection occurs sporadically; clusters of infection are sporadic but rare. Wound infections may occur, and CNS infection may complicate intravenous drug abuse. Invasive infection occurs in both sexes and all ages as a function of acidosis or immunosuppression. There is no known genetic predisposition.

Pathology

See Table 47–2.

Clinical Features

A. Signs and Symptoms: These are virtually identical to those of invasive aspergillosis. Rhinocerebral mucormycosis accounts for about 50% of all cases; more than 75% of cases occur in patients with acidosis, especially diabetic ketoacidosis. Increasing numbers of cases are being seen, however, in association with neutropenia and immunosuppression. Early clinical features include nasal stuffiness, bloody nasal discharge, facial swelling, and facial and orbital pain. Later manifestations include orbital cellulitis, proptosis, endophthalmitis, orbital apex syndrome, cranial nerve palsies, and cerebral extension.

B. Laboratory Findings: These include acidosis (principally diabetic ketoacidosis), neutropenia, abnormal paranasal sinus or chest radiographs, and evidence of specific organ dysfunction at sites of local extension (central nervous system) or metastatic loci. **Diagnosis** requires histologic demonstration of tissue invasion by an exclusively mycelial fungus. Cultures are positive in fewer than 20% of patients, and positive cultures may represent fungal contaminants.

C. Immunologic Diagnosis: See Table 47–4. There are no useful tests available.

D. Differential Diagnosis: This includes diverse opportunistic paranasal sinus (aspergillosis, phaeohyphomycosis, hyalohyphomycosis) and pulmonary bacterial and fungal infections.

E. Treatment: Amphotericin B is the only drug

of proven value. Aggressive surgical debridement is required for paranasal sinusitis or rhinocerebral mucormycosis. The efficacy of hyperbaric oxygen for treating devitalized tissues is controversial.

F. Prevention: No effective preventive measures are known.

G. Complications and Prognosis: Rhinocerebral mucormycosis advances at an extremely rapid rate; an aggressive approach to diagnosis and treatment is essential. Survival is more likely in the setting of diabetic ketoacidosis than that of neutropenia.

PNEUMOCYSTOSIS

Pneumocystis carnii, the etiologic agent of pneumocystosis, has been considered a protozoan organism based on morphologic appearance. Molecular evidence shows that it is not a protozoan, however, but shares homology with fungi. Distinct differences between true fungi and *P carnii* exist, however (eg, lack of ergosterol in the cyst wall, distinct morphologic characteristics, lack of response to antifungal agents), suggesting that additional classification is needed.

Major Immunologic Features

- Infection apparent only in patients with impaired CMI or in infants with severe protein-calorie malnutrition (marasmus)
- Most common index diagnosis for AIDS
- Predominantly alveolar and interstitial; extrapulmonary spread distinctly rare

General Considerations

Pneumocystis carinii pneumonia (PCP) is an apparently inhalation-acquired disease, but the environmental form of the pathogen has never been identified. PCP occurs predominantly in patients with impaired CMI and is classically the defining opportunistic infection for AIDS. *P carinii* is a unicellular eukaryote with a proposed life cycle consisting of trophozoites and cysts. It can be maintained transiently in cell culture but has never been cultivated independently in cell-free media. Seroepidemiologic studies indicate that more than two thirds of normal children have acquired antibody to *P carinii* by 3–4 years of age. Clinical attributes of the presumed infecting event are unknown, and autopsy studies have failed to provide evidence of residual pulmonary microorganisms in persons who have died of unrelated causes. The occurrence of PCP in immunocompromised adults could represent either new infection or arousal of inapparent disease from latency. When PCP occurs in infants with AIDS or marasmus, it is assumed to represent primary infection. Common-source outbreaks of PCP have occurred, suggesting that infection may be spread by aerosol. Most cases, however, appear to be sporadic. Diverse animal species harbor *P carinii,* as evidenced by spontaneous occurrence of PCP in response to immunosuppression. There is no evidence of spread from animals to humans; there are antigenic differences among human and animal strains. Prevalence is directly related to the occurrence of marasmus or impaired CMI. Neutropenia is not a risk factor. There is no independent age or sex-related susceptibility. Approximately 75% of AIDS patients experience at least one episode of *P carinii* pneumonia if no prophylaxis is given. There is no known genetic predisposition.

Pathology

See Table 47–2.

Clinical Features

A. Signs and Symptoms: These include fever, cough, and shortness of breath, especially in patients with prolonged fatigue and weight loss.

B. Laboratory Findings: These include CD4 T-cell counts generally below 200/mL; elevated serum lactic dehydrogenase level; and diffuse alveolointerstitial infiltrates on chest radiograph, sometimes with cystic changes or pneumatoceles. Hypoxemia and alveolar-to-arterial O_2 tension differences are common, especially in response to exercise. Gallium lung scanning is sensitive but not specific. **Diagnosis** is established by visualizing characteristic organisms in expectorated or induced sputum, bronchoalveolar lavage fluid, or lung biopsy specimens obtained transbronchially or by open thoracotomy.

C. Immunologic Diagnosis: See Table 47–4. There are several experimental techniques for detecting an antibody response to *P carinii* or free *P carinii* antigen. A monoclonal antibody immunofluorescence method specific for *P carinii* has enhanced recognition of the organism (over that by Giemsa and fast silver stains) in clinical specimens.

D. Differential Diagnosis: This includes the numerous opportunistic pulmonary infections in patients with AIDS or profoundly depressed CMI, including tuberculosis, histoplasmosis, cryptococcosis, toxoplasmosis, cytomegalovirus infection, bacterial pneumonia, lymphomas, and Kaposi's sarcoma.

E. Treatment: Trimethoprim-sulfamethoxazole (TMP-SMZ) and intravenous pentamidine isethionate are both effective for the treatment of *P carinii;* however, TMP-SMZ is associated with fewer and milder side effects, particularly in patients without AIDS. Other drugs shown to be effective include dapsone, TMP–dapsone, trimetrexate, clindamycin–primaquine, and atovaquone. Corticosteroids are useful in the prevention and treatment of *P carinii*-induced ARDS.

F. Prevention: *P carinii* prophylaxis is central to the clinical management of AIDS. A regimen of TMP-SMZ given daily or three days per week is highly effective. Aerosolized pentamidine administered once monthly is also effective. No vaccine is available.

G. Complications and Prognosis: Aggressive use of prophylaxis in AIDS patients and immune reconstitution associated with highly active antiretroviral therapy (HAART) is decreasing the frequency of PCP as an index diagnosis. Aerosolized pentamidine may delay or change its presentation to less easily recognized forms (eg, apical cystic disease and hematogenously disseminated disease, both of which are now extremely rare. Pneumothorax is a late but important complication.

REFERENCES

GENERAL

Dixon DM et al: Development of vaccines and their use in the prevention of fungal infections. *Med Mycol* 1998;36:57.

Minamoto GY, Rosenberg AS: Fungal infections in patients with acquired immunodeficiency syndrome. *Med Clin North Am* 1997;81:381.

Morrison VA et al: Non-candidal fungal infections after bone marrow transplantation. Risk factors and outcome. *Am J Med* 1994;96:497.

Patel R, Paya CV: Infections in solid organ transplant recipients. *Clin Microbiol Rev* 1997;10:86.

Patterson TF: Editorial response: Approaches to the therapy of invasive mycoses-the role of amphotericin B. *Clin Infect Dis* 1998;26:339.

Vanden Bossche H et al: Antifungal drug resistance in pathogenic fungi. *Med Mycol* 1998;36(suppl 1):119.

White TC et al: Clinical, cellular, and molecular factors that contribute to antifungal drug resistance. *Clin Microbiol Rev* 1998;11:382.

PITYROSPORUM & MALASSEZIA INFECTION

Gueho E et al: The role of *Malassezia* species in the ecology of human skin and as pathogens. *Med Mycol* 1998;36(Suppl 1):220.

WHITE PIEDRA

Assaf RR, Weil ML: The superficial mycoses. *Dermatol Clin* 1996;14:57.

Hajjeh RA, Blumberg HM: Bloodstream infection due to *Trichosporon beigelii* in a burn patient: Case report and review of therapy. *Clin Infect Dis* 1995;20:913.

DERMATOPHYTOSIS

Elewski BE: Onychomycosis: pathogenesis, diagnosis, and management. *Clin Microbiol Rev* 1998;11:415.

Weitzman I, Summerbell RC: The dermatophytes. *Clin Microbiol Rev* 1995;8:240.

CHROMOMYCOSIS

Elgart GW: Chromoblastomycosis. *Dermatol Clin* 1996; 14:77.

MYCETOMA

Rivitti EA, Aoki V: Deep fungal infections in tropical countries. *Clin Dermatol* 1999;17:171.

SPOROTRICHOSIS

Kauffman CA: Sporotrichosis. *Clin Infect Dis* 1999;29:231.

BLASTOMYCOSIS

Davies SF, Sarosi GA: Epidemiological and clinical features of pulmonary blastomycosis. *Semin Respir Infect* 1997;12:206.

Bradsher RW: Therapy of blastomycosis. *Semin Respir Infect* 1997;12:263.

COCCIDIOIDOMYCOSIS

Cox RA, Magee DM: Protective immunity in coccidioidomycosis. *Res Immunol* 1999;149:417.

Stevens DA: Coccidioidomycosis. *N Engl J Med* 1995;332:1077.

HISTOPLASMOSIS

Wheat J: Histoplasmosis. *Medicine* (Baltimore) 1997; 76:339.

PENICILLIUM MARNEFFEI INFECTION

Cooper CR Jr, McGinnis MR: Pathology of *Penicillium marneffei.* An emerging acquired immunodeficiency syndrome-related pathogen. *Arch Pathol Lab Med* 1997; 121:798.

CANDIDIASIS

Edwards JE Jr et al: International conference for the development of a consensus on the management and prevention of severe candidal infections. *Clin Infect Dis* 1997;25:43.

Rangel-Frausto MS et al: National epidemiology of mycoses survey (NEMIS): Variations in rates of bloodstream infections due to *Candida* species in seven surgical intensive care units and six neonatal intensive care units. *Clin Infect Dis* 1999;29:253.

CRYPTOCOCCOSIS

Casadevall A et al: Antibody and/or cell-mediated immunity, protective mechanisms in fungal disease: An ongoing dilemma or an unnecessary dispute? *Med Mycol* 1998;36(Suppl 1):95.

Powderly WG: Recent advances in the management of cryptococcal meningitis in patients with AIDS. *Clin Infect Dis* 1996;22(Suppl 2):S119.

Saag MS et al: A comparison of itraconazole versus fluconazole as maintenance therapy for AIDS-associated cryptococcal meningitis. National Institute of Allergy and Infectious Diseases Mycoses Study Group. *Clin Infect Dis* 1999;28:291.

van der Horst CM et al: Treatment of cryptococcal meningitis associated with the acquired immunodeficiency syndrome. National Institute of Allergy and Infectious Diseases Mycoses Study Group and AIDS Clinical Trials Group. *N Engl J Med* 1997;337:15.

ASPERGILLOSIS

Denning DW: Invasive aspergillosis. *Clin Infect Dis* 1998;26:781.

Patterson JE et al: Hospital epidemiologic surveillance for invasive aspergillosis: Patient demographics and the utility of antigen detection. *Infect Control Hosp Epidemiol* 1997;18:104.

Verweij PE et al: Current trends in the detection of antigenemia, metabolites and cell wall markers for the diagnosis and therapeutic monitoring of fungal infections. *Med Mycol* 1998;36(Suppl 1):146.

MUCORMYCOSIS (ZYGOMYCOSIS)

Gonzalez CE et al: Disseminated zygomycosis in a neutropenic patient: Successful treatment with amphotericin B lipid complex and granulocyte colony-stimulating factor. *Clin Infect Dis* 1997;24:192.

Holland J: Emerging zygomycoses of humans: *Saksenaea vasiformis* and *Apophysomyces elegans. Curr Top Med Mycol* 1997;8:27.

Lee FY et al: Pulmonary mucormycosis: The last 30 years. *Arch Intern Med* 1999;159:1301.

PNEUMOCYSTOSIS

Hughes WT: Current issues in the epidemiology, transmission, and reactivation of *Pneumocystis carinii. Semin Respir Infect* 1998;13:28.

PHAEOHYPHOMYCOSIS

de Hoog GS: Significance of fungal evolution for the understanding of their pathogenicity, illustrated with agents of phaeohyphomycosis. *Mycoses* 1997;40(Suppl 2):5.

Sutton DA et al: U.S. case report of cerebral phaeohyphomycosis caused by *Ramichloridium obovoideum (R mackenziei):* Criteria for identification, therapy, and review of other known dematiaceous neurotropic taxa. *J Clin Microbiol* 1998;36:708.

Parasitic Diseases

48

James H. McKerrow, MD, PhD, & Stephen J. Davies, BVSc, PhD

Parasitic diseases such as malaria, schistosomiasis, and leishmaniasis are among the most important health problems in developing countries. Not only is an understanding of the immunology of parasitic disease essential to controlling these diseases by immunization—the study of the host response to parasites continues to lead to important discoveries about the immune response itself. For example, the response to schistosome (blood fluke) eggs by infected mice represents one of the best experimental models for studying the formation and regulation of granulomatous inflammation. Immature schistosomes (schistosomula) and eggs have also provided an in vitro experimental model for elucidating the function of the eosinophil. New models of regulation of cytokine production and the role of cytokines in the immune response have come from studies of leishmaniasis—a protozoan parasite infection.

Immune responses to the complex antigenic structures of parasites have diverse manifestations and do not always lead to complete protective immunity. Parasites have complex life cycles involving multiple states and often multiple hosts or vectors. Not only can each stage of the parasite present multiple antigenic targets but more than one stage may be present in the host at a given time. Furthermore parasite infections are chronic—often persisting for years or even decades. Unfortunately, as is often the case with infectious diseases, the immune response to parasites can even produce more serious disease than the parasite itself. Examples are the hepatic granulomas of schistosomiasis, antigen-antibody complex glomerulonephritis in quartan malaria, and antibody-mediated anaphylactic shock from a ruptured hydatid cyst or from too-rapid killing of filarial microfilariae.

Some of the most fascinating and perplexing aspects of parasitic disease are the variety of mechanisms by which the parasite evades the immune response (Figure 48–1). A parasite can "hide" within a host's own cells, as in leishmaniasis, produce successive waves of progeny with different surface antigens, as in African trypanosomiasis, or disguise itself as "self" with host antigens, as occurs in schistosomiasis. Nonspecific immunosuppression, due to a variety of stimuli, is characteristic of a number of parasitic infections. The ability of parasites to adapt to the host environment is the essence of successful parasitism, and it increases immeasurably the difficulty of developing immunization procedures against parasitic infection.

THE IMMUNE RESPONSE TO PROTOZOA

Protozoa are important agents of worldwide disease. Falciparum malaria, for example, is still considered one of the most lethal diseases in humans despite massive efforts at eradication and control. These parasites also offer unlimited immunologic challenges, the immune responses induced being as diverse as the protozoa themselves. In developing countries, especially in Africa, malaria and trypanosomiasis take enormous tolls of life and are significant barriers to economic development. Amebiasis, giardiasis, and toxoplasmosis are widespread even in highly developed countries. The use of immunosuppressive drugs to treat cancer and to prevent rejection of transplanted organs has resulted in activation of otherwise subclinical infections with protozoa such as *Toxoplasma*. Finally, the global epidemic of acquired immune deficiency syndrome (AIDS) has led to exacerbation of preexisting parasitic infections as well as complicated multiple infections by protozoa like *Cryptosporidium, Toxoplasma,* and *Microsporidia.*

MALARIA

Major Immunologic Features
- Complex partial humoral and cellular immunity occurs with multiple exposure
- Significantly higher mortality rates from cerebral malaria for nonimmune individuals in endemic areas
- Species-specific protective IgG antibody produced against merozoites after multiple infections

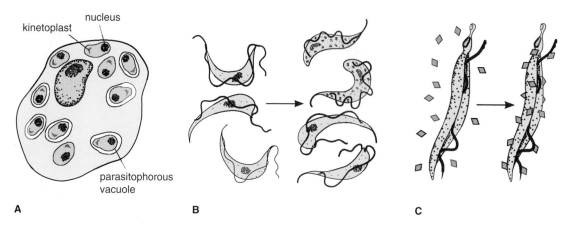

Figure 48–1. Some of the devious ways in which parasites evade the host immune response. **A:** Living within a host cell (*Leishmania* living in macrophage within a parasitophorous vacuole). **B:** Rapidly changing surface antigens (trypanosomes). **C:** "Camouflaging" surface with host antigens.

- Vaccine development hindered by genetic variability in immune response to specific antigens.

General Considerations

Human malaria is caused by species of *Plasmodium.* It is transmitted by female anopheline mosquitoes that ingest the sexual forms of the parasite in blood meals. The infective **sporozoites** develop in the mosquito and are injected into the definitive (human) host when bitten by the insect. In the human, the parasites first develop in an exoerythrocytic form, multiplying within hepatic cells without inducing an inflammatory reaction. The progeny, or **merozoites,** invade host erythrocytes to begin the erythrocytic cycle and initiate the earliest phase of clinical malaria. The **gametocyte** is the sexual stage taken up by the mosquito.

Destruction of erythrocytes occurs on a 48-hour cycle with *Plasmodium vivax* and *Plasmodium ovale* and every 72 hours with *Plasmodium malariae.* The characteristic chills-fever-sweat malarial syndrome follows this cyclic pattern, being induced by synchronous rupture of infected erythrocytes by the mature asexual forms (schizonts), releasing merozoites that quickly invade new erythrocytes. *Plasmodium falciparum,* although classically thought to occur on a 48-hour cycle, is, in fact, frequently not synchronous. In contrast to the exoerythrocytic stage, the erythrocytic merozoites induce an array of humoral responses in the host, as demonstrated by complement fixation, precipitation, agglutination, and fluorescent antibody reactions.

In *P vivax* and *P ovale* infections, relapse after a period of dormancy may result from periodic release of merozoites from the liver (**hypnozoites**), owing to the lack of an immune response to the intracellular parasites. When the erythrocytic cellular and humoral protection is deficient (from concurrent infection, age, trauma, or other debilitating factors), the reappearing blood-stage forms induce a new round of clinical malaria until the erythrocytic cycle is again controlled by a humoral and T-cell host response. This is a true relapse, as opposed to a recrudescence of erythrocytic infection. Relapses can occur for up to 5 years with some strains of *P vivax* and possibly 2–3 years for *P ovale. P malariae* appears to recur only as a recrudescent erythrocytic infection, sometimes appearing 30 or more years after the primary infection. *P falciparum* may have a short-term recrudescence but does not develop a true relapse from liver-developed merozoites.

Blackwater fever, formerly a common and rapidly fatal form of falciparum malaria among colonists in Africa, has declined in frequency with reduction in quinine therapy. It is associated with repeated falciparum infection, inadequate quinine therapy, and possibly genetic factors more frequently found in whites. The resulting rapid, massive hemolysis of both infected and uninfected erythrocytes is thought to result from autoantibodies from previous infections that react with autoantigens (perhaps an erythrocyte-parasite-quinine combination) derived from a new infection with the same falciparum strain. With increased use of quinine to prevent or treat chloroquine-resistant falciparum malaria, blackwater fever may again increase in frequency in coming years.

Quartan malaria, caused by *P malariae,* has been associated with a serious complement-dependent, antigen-antibody immune complex reaction producing glomerulonephritis and nephrosis in African children, which results in edema and severe kidney damage unless the disease is arrested early. After loss of the edema, persistent symptomless proteinuria or slowly deteriorating renal function is common. Stable remissions with corticosteroid therapy occur when proteinuria is restricted to only a few classes of protein, and histologic changes are minimal. Patients with poorly controlled generalized proteinuria, however, probably do not benefit from antimalarial or immunosuppressive therapy. Chronic *P malariae* infection probably triggers an autoimmunity perpetuating the immune complex glomerulonephritis, but the antigen involved is not yet identified.

Innate, nonacquired immunity to malaria is well demonstrated. Africans or African Americans lacking Duffy blood group antigen Fy(a–b–) are immune to *P vivax* because this genetic factor appears to be necessary for successful merozoite penetration of the human erythrocyte by this plasmodial species. Intracellular growth of the malaria parasites is also affected by the hemoglobin molecular structure. Sickle cell (SS) hemoglobin inhibits growth of *P falciparum*. This genetic factor is widespread in areas of Africa hyperendemic for falciparum malaria. Although prevalence of infection appears unaffected by the sickling trait, *severe* infections in individuals with hemoglobin A/S (sickle cell trait) are very much reduced compared with those in individuals who are nonsickling homozygous. Similarly, *P falciparum* growth is retarded in erythrocytes with the fetal hemoglobin (F)—hence the selective advantage of β-thalassemia heterozygotes, in whom postnatal hemoglobin F declines at a lower than normal rate. Other red cell abnormalities such as glucose-6-phosphate dehydrogenase deficiency appear to be protective of the erythrocyte and thereby reduce the severity of plasmodial infection.

Immunity to *P falciparum* malaria is species- and strain-specific. If immune individuals migrate to other, geographically distinct endemic areas, they may acquire new disease. Both acquired and innate specific or nonspecific resistance to malaria is influenced by a number of genetic traits that reflect strong selective pressure in areas with specific mosquito-human-*Plasmodium* combinations. A very gradual long-term resistance to hyperendemic falciparum malaria is acquired in African populations. The resistance develops years after the onset of disease among nearly all children older than 3 months of age. Initial passive protection is present owing to transplacental maternal IgG. Nonetheless, malaria deaths in Africa are estimated at a million a year, chiefly among children younger than 5 years. Even after surviving a childhood infection, a large proportion of adults remain susceptible to infection and show periodic parasitemia, even though their serum contains antiplasmodial antibodies, some with demonstrated protective action. Susceptibility to a low-level chronic infection provides the population with a protective **premunition** or prevention of subsequent infection. It is believed that in hyperendemic areas of Africa, nearly all residents harbor a continuous series of falciparum infections of low to moderate pathogenicity throughout their lives. Antibodies are produced that inhibit the entry of merozoites into erythrocytes. All immunoglobulin classes are elevated in the serum of malaria patients, but IgG levels appear to correlate best with the degree of malaria protection (or control of acute manifestations).

In addition to the variables of parasite genetics and vector biology, it is clear that human populations vary significantly in their ability to mount an immune response to the malaria parasite. This realization has somewhat dampened the optimism for early development of a subunit vaccine against malaria because preliminary clinical trials of the first vaccine candidate were disappointing, raising fears that subunit vaccines would be poorly immunogenic in many individuals in a target population. Genetic variability in induction of immune response by a vaccine is by no means a new observation. Even to a very effective recombinant vaccine like that against hepatitis B, responses follow a bell-shaped curve, with some individuals failing to produce sufficient levels of antibodies in the standard vaccination protocol. The situation in malaria is even more heterogeneous in inbred strains of mice as well as in outbred human populations. In mice, the variability in immune response is linked to variability in the major histocompatibility complex (MHC). Immune response to malaria in humans, however, is probably also regulated by genes outside the MHC region that have yet to be fully defined. Currently three vaccination strategies are still being pursued: antisporozoite to prevent liver cell infections, antimerozoite to prevent red blood cell infections, and antigametocyte to block transmission.

The failure to induce protective antibodies in vaccinated individuals led research investigators to focus on the role of cell-mediated immunity, and especially T cell-derived cytokines, already known to be important in control of other parasitic diseases. One striking observation indicates that our understanding of the immune response to malaria is still incomplete. Despite the fact that specific individuals with low T-cell counts and malaria infections were studied, HIV infection had no significant effect on the course of malaria, nor has malaria a significant effect on the course of HIV infection. This suggests that humoral immunity may indeed be important in control of malaria or that other types of T cells, for example γδ T cells, generate cytokines that can control malaria but are not affected in HIV infection. CD8 T-cell responses to hepatocyte stages may also be important for control because antibody-inducing vaccines targeting sporozoites have not been successful to date.

TOXOPLASMOSIS

Major Immunologic Features

- Specific antibody present
- Nonspecific increase in serum immunoglobulins
- Widespread natural acquired immunity; major mechanism probably cell-mediated immunity

- Disseminated *Toxoplasma* a frequent complication in HIV-infected individuals with low T-cell counts

General Considerations

Toxoplasma infection in humans is generally **asymptomatic.** It has been estimated that as much as 40% of the adult population in the world is infected, as are all species of mammals that have been tested for the presence of this ubiquitous parasite. Clinical disease, which develops in only a small fraction of those infected, ranges from benign lymphadenopathy to an acute and often fatal infection of the central nervous system. The developing fetus and the aged or otherwise immunologically compromised host are most vulnerable to the pathologic expression of massive infection and resulting encystation in the eye or brain. Damage to the fetus is greatest during the first trimester when the central nervous system is being organized, and nearly all such instances end in fetal death. Infection of the mother during the second trimester may produce hydrocephaly, blindness, or varying lesser degrees of neurologic damage in the fetus. Most cases of fetal infection occur during the third trimester, resulting in chorioretinitis or other ophthalmic damage, reduced learning capacity or other expressions of central nervous system deficit, or asymptomatic latent infection that may become clinically apparent years later. Women exposed *before* pregnancy—as indicated by a positive indirect immunofluorescent or Sabin-Feldman dye test—are thought to be unable to transmit the infection in utero.

The **diagnosis** of toxoplasmosis is made in most cases by serology. A positive test for IgM antibodies appears approximately 5 days after infection, and IgG antibody at approximately 1–2 weeks. Because the IgG antibodies may persist for months to years, the presence of IgM antibodies is diagnostically more useful. A single high titer is indicative of acute infection. For confirmation, two specimens are generally drawn at a 3-week interval and tested simultaneously. A serial rise in titer is a reliable indication of recent infection.

In **ocular** toxoplasmosis, no rise in titer is observed, but a negative serology can be used to rule out chorioretinitis. The IgM serology can also be used during pregnancy and on cord blood, but serologic positivity may be suppressed by immunosuppressive therapy or in patients with AIDS.

Toxoplasmosis is an example of a **zoonosis.** Many potential sources of infection have been suggested, including tissue cysts in raw or partially cooked pork or mutton and oocysts passed in feces of infected cats (the true final hosts). Yet these sources seem insufficient to account for such large numbers of infections. The major reservoirs of infection are therefore unknown. *Toxoplasma* infection usually occurs through the gastrointestinal tract, and the protozoa can apparently penetrate and proliferate (as rapidly multiplying tachyzoites) in virtually every cell in the body. They ultimately produce cysts filled with minute slow-growing infective bodies (bradyzoites) that remain viable for long periods. Following a successful cellular and humoral immune response, only encysted parasites can survive.

The **tachyzoites** of *Toxoplasma* and the **promastigotes** of *Leishmania* (discussed in the following section) are two examples of parasite protozoa that replicate inside human macrophages. These protozoa are, of course, not the only infectious agents that can replicate inside a cell of the human immune system (Figure 48–2). The retrovirus that produces AIDS is the best known example, but in many ways the adaptation of protozoan parasites, which are themselves eukaryotes, is even more remarkable. *Toxoplasma* invades a cell in a process that is independent of normal phagocytosis. The tachyzoite attaches to the cell membrane and induces changes in membrane topology as well as secretion from the specialized parasite structures called **rhoptries.** The parasite enters the cell through a moving membrane junction and forms a parasitophorous vacuole in the cytoplasm. This vacuole is a specialized structure that is probably the result of rhoptry secretions and that contains no recognizable host membrane proteins.

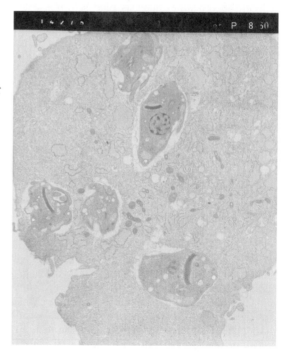

Figure 48–2. Electron micrograph (×10,125) of amastigotes of *Trypanosoma cruzi* infecting a host cell. Five dark amastigotes, the black bar-like kinetoplast is seen. This is a complex of circular DNA that includes genes coating for the parasite's mitochondrial enzymes. Hiding a replicating life cycle stage within the host cell cytoplasm is one way in which parasites evade the immune response.

The "parasite nature" of the vacuole prevents it from becoming acidified or fusing with host cell lysosomes. Before invasion, parasites become coated with extracellular matrix proteins like laminin which, by interacting with host cell integrins (cell surface receptors), inhibit phagocytosis and the oxidative burst of macrophages that could result in parasite killing.

The ability of macrophages to kill intracellular parasites is greatly increased if the parasites are first exposed to antibody. In that case, the antibody-coated *Toxoplasma* is recognized by the Fc receptors of the macrophage. This triggers normal phagocytosis and the formation of reactive oxygen and nitrogen intermediates that ultimately kill the parasite.

An intact immune system is necessary for protection against *Toxoplasma;* thus, immunosuppression to control transplant rejection or malignancies, or infection with HIV, may result in active toxoplasmosis. This phenomenon may result either from the elimination of sensitized lymphocytes previously limiting an inapparent infection or from inability of the immunosuppressed host to mount an adequate protective response to new infection.

LEISHMANIASIS

Leishmania is a genus of obligate intracellular parasites that infect macrophages of the skin and viscera to produce disease in both animals and humans. Sandflies, the principal vectors, introduce the parasites into the host while taking blood meals. In leishmaniasis, a range of host responses interact with a number of parasite leishmanial species and strains to produce a panoply of pathologic and immunologic responses. Leishmaniasis teaches two important lessons: (1) Different species or strains of the same parasite can produce dramatically different diseases in a given host and (2) Genetic differences in the host can also lead to vastly different immune responses to infection by the same parasite.

1. CUTANEOUS LEISHMANIASIS

Major Immunologic Features
- Cell-mediated immunity critical
- Little or no specific serum antibody

General Considerations
Old World cutaneous leishmaniasis, or **tropical sore,** is caused by several forms of *Leishmania: L tropica, L major,* and *L aethiopica.* These agents induce an immune response characterized by nonprotective antibody but strong cell-mediated immunity. In cutaneous leishmaniasis, the patient's immune response chiefly determines the form taken by the clinical disease; however, the strain of parasite may also determine part of the host response. If the patient mounts an adequate but not excessive cell-mediated immune response to the parasite, healing of the ulcerative lesions and specific protection result. If cell-mediated immunity to the parasite is inadequate or suppressed, however, the result may be diffuse cutaneous disease, in which there is little chance of spontaneous cure. In the Old World, this condition is due chiefly to *L aethiopica* in East Africa. A similar form, caused by *L mexicana* subsp *pifanoi,* occurs in Venezuela, again in specifically anergic patients. On the other hand, an excessive cell-mediated immune response produces **lupoid** or **recidiva** leishmaniasis, caused by *L tropica,* in which nonnucleated lymphoid nodules form at the edge of the primary lesion; these lesions persist indefinitely, although parasites are not easily demonstrated. Recidiva leishmaniasis may occur from 2 to 10 years after the initial lesion. Thus, a spectrum of host responses to cutaneous leishmaniasis exists, ranging from multiple disseminated parasite-filled ulcers or nodules (anergic response) to single, spontaneously cured immunizing sores, to recidiva hyperactive host responses with few or no parasites (allergic response).

Cutaneous leishmaniasis of the New World is caused by a number of leishmanial pathogens now divided into two species complexes: *Leishmania mexicana* (subdivided into four or more subspecies) and *Leishmania braziliensis* (subdivided into four or more subspecies). The parasite subspecies (considered distinct species by many specialists) are distinguished on the basis of growth characteristics in the vector and in culture, isoenzyme electrophoresis patterns, kinetoplast DNA analysis, lectin-binding specificities, excreted factor serotyping, and monoclonal antibody probes. Geographic factors, hosts, and the character of the disease produced in humans are also important.

The most significant clinical distinction in the *L mexicana* complex is the high frequency of ear cartilage lesions (**chiclero ulcer**) and rare diffuse cutaneous leishmaniasis. In the *L braziliensis* complex, metastatic lesions develop, usually within 5 years of healing of the initial ulcer, which itself may be large, persistent, and disfiguring. Nasal cartilage and other nasopharyngeal tissues are attacked and destroyed by this subsequent massive ulceration (**espundia),** which may erode away much of the face and cause death by septic bronchopneumonia, asphyxiation, or starvation. This manifestation of American leishmaniasis is frequently nonresponsive to treatment. Parasites are abundant in the early stages of espundia but subsequently are rare, whereas persistent infiltration of giant cells, plasma cells, and lymphocytes is characteristic. Delayed and perhaps immediate hypersensitivity and circulating antibody levels are higher in espundia than in cases of the primary lesion alone. The mucocutaneous form is thought to be an allergic or abnormal immunologic manifestation of infection with the type subspecies *L braziliensis.*

The Montenegro hypersensitivity skin test (also called Leishmanin test), which uses promastigotes of *Leishmania* as antigen, is rapidly positive with cutaneous leishmaniasis, particularly the New World forms. Assays for lymphocyte proliferation or production of cytokines such as interferon gamma are also positive. Dermal response to kala-azar is slower, becoming positive only after cure of the visceral infection. Serodiagnosis of cutaneous leishmaniasis is still unsatisfactory because of low serum antibody levels and, in Latin America, because of cross-reactions with Chagas' disease antibodies. An exciting advance in field analysis of species (*L mexicana* versus *L braziliensis* complexes) is the application of nonradioactive species-specific DNA probes. Using the polymerase chain reaction (PCR), the *Leishmania* species infecting a patient can be determined from a small amount of parasite material in a cutaneous lesion.

The varying clinical courses that infection with *Leishmania* spp. can produce constitute a paradigm for the immune response to intracellular parasites. *Leishmania* enter cells by a different pathway than do the *Toxoplasma* organisms discussed in the previous section. *Leishmania* promastigotes enter passively through phagocytosis into macrophages. One of the unusual features of this infection is the predilection of the organisms for infection of the macrophage, a cell which is itself key to the host immune response. *Leishmania* have adapted to replication in an unusual environment, the phagolysosomal vacuoles. Never-

theless, in those cases of spontaneous cure of cutaneous leishmaniasis, parasite killing does occur. Recent studies in a mouse model of infection have begun to shed light on this interplay between host and intracellular parasite. First, a single dominant genetic locus, called Bcg, appears to govern whether or not mice are resistant to infection both by *Leishmania* and *Mycobacterium*. This locus includes a gene that codes for a membrane channel protein that may be key in the transport of precursors of nitric oxide or oxygen radicals used by the macrophage for parasite killing. It is noteworthy that lessons from studying the immune response to intracellular parasites can cross-fertilize research on host response to *Mycobacterium* and other fungal or bacterial infections in which macrophages play a key role.

T-cell products are also key to a successful host response to *Leishmania*. Interferon gamma is critical to parasite killing. In *L major* infections of mice, two CD4-positive T-cell subtypes have been identified. In genetically resistant mice, the T_H1 subtype predominates (Figure 48–3). This T-cell population produces interferon gamma in its cytokine repertoire. In contrast, genetically susceptible mice have a predominant T_H2 T-cell subtype response with no production of interferon gamma, but rather cytokines like IL-5, IL-4, and IL-10. Although the existence of distinct T-cell subtypes in human infections is more controversial, the mouse studies point out how a particular cytokine profile is key to activating infected macrophages to successfully kill the intracellular parasites. This work

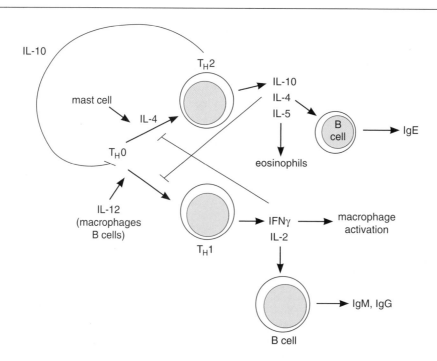

Figure 48–3. Cytokine production by T_H1 and T_H2 subtypes of CD4 T cells.

has had pragmatic application, in that administration of recombinant interferon gamma enhances patient response to chemotherapy in cases of visceral leishmaniasis.

2. VISCERAL LEISHMANIASIS

Major Immunologic Features
- Delayed hypersensitivity only after spontaneous recovery or chemotherapy
- Polyclonal B-cell proliferation with increased non-specific immunoglobulin levels
- Parasites in cells throughout the body produce systemic disease, characterized by leukopenia and splenomegaly and release of cachectin (TNFα)

General Considerations

The immune response to visceral leishmaniasis (**kala-azar**)—caused by various subspecies of *Leishmania donovani* (considered separate species by some authorities)—is significantly different from that of cutaneous leishmaniasis, although the parasites are distinguishable only by enzyme analysis using zymodemes or other forms of molecular characterization. Massive **polyclonal hypergammaglobulinemia** with little or no evidence of cell-mediated immunity is the rule in visceral leishmaniasis. No quantitative relationship exists between the elevated serum immunoglobulin and antiparasite antibodies, which are, moreover, not species-specific. The elevated immunoglobulin diminishes rapidly when treatment begins. Delayed cutaneous hypersensitivity to parasite antigens becomes demonstrable only after spontaneous recovery or treatment, which suggests that cell-mediated mechanisms play a role in the resolution of the infectious process. Under certain circumstances, dermal "leishmanoid" occurs after kala-azar symptoms resolve. Nodules containing many parasites form papules as a result of incomplete or defective cell-mediated immunity, or a persistent allergic reaction to parasite antigens. Many cases of severe disseminated infection in individuals with HIV have now been reported in Mediterranean countries. This underscores the importance of cell-mediated immunity in controlling disease.

AFRICAN TRYPANOSOMIASIS

Major Immunologic Feature
- Succession of parasite populations in bloodstream, each with a different antigenic coating

General Considerations

Trypanosoma brucei subsp *gambiense,* also called *T gambiense,* is the agent of chronic Gambian or West African **sleeping sickness.** *Trypanosoma brucei* subsp *rhodesiense,* also called *T rhodesiense,* is the agent of acute Rhodesian or East African sleeping sickness. Both cause human disease, and the Rhodesian form is most responsible for denying vast areas of Africa to human occupation, chiefly in the flybelt regions where the tsetse fly vectors are found. Tsetse-borne trypanosomes (*Trypanosoma brucei* subsp *brucei* as well as several other species) infect domestic animals with similar or even greater virulence. This dual threat—one to humans and the other to domestic animals, especially cattle—has had an enormous effect on human history in Africa. The great herds of wild herbivores, once abundant everywhere, have survived in this region because of their natural tolerance to heavy infections. The trypanosomes multiply extracellularly in successive waves in the human and animal bloodstream but produce very little disease in spite of their numbers. Only when the parasites enter the central nervous system does the ravaging disease, sleeping sickness, develop. It is this pathologic phase of an otherwise harmless chronic or recurrent infection to which humans and domestic animals succumb and which most native antelope and other herbivores resist.

Greatly increased levels of **immunoglobulins,** especially of the IgM class, are regularly present in infected humans and animals. The increased immunoglobulin levels, which do not correlate positively with protection, may result from B-cell stimulants produced by the trypanosomes themselves or by the increased IgG production by helper T cells, which act nonspecifically to increase immunoglobulin levels. A large proportion of the immunoglobulin in infected hosts is nonspecific in nature.

Although trypanosomes are continually exposed to the host immune system in the bloodstream, they evade the host's defenses. The first hint of how this is accomplished was noted in 1910, when the periodicity of fever in patients with trypanosomiasis was correlated with a sharp rise and fall in the number of trypanosomes found in the blood. More recently, it was discovered that when individual organisms are cloned in culture, each clone displays a unique antigenic surface protein. When organisms first enter the host (Figure 48–4), the host immune system generates antibodies against the predominant surface antigen (variable surface glycoprotein [**VSG**]). Antibodies can kill over 90% of the original infecting trypanosome population. Not all of the trypanosomes are killed because some have switched on a different VSG antigen not recognized by the initial immune response. This switch occurs spontaneously and can be detected in immune-deficient mice. It is therefore not dependent on the host immune response. The switch occurs very rapidly, so that by 5 days into an infection, parasites with more than one antigen type can be detected. By 6 days, as few as 15% of the trypanosomes may still have the initial surface VSG. This switching from one VSG to another explains the waves of parasitemia and periodicity of the fever

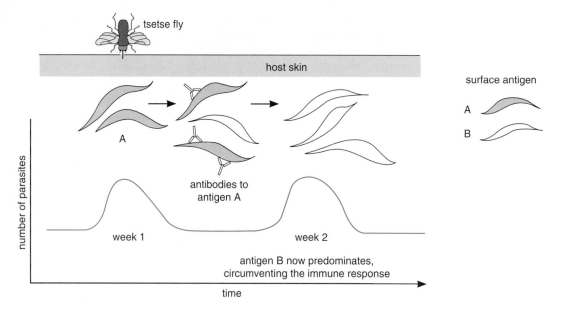

Figure 48–4. Antigenic variation and parasitemia in trypanosomiasis.

characteristic of trypanosomiasis. The potential VSG repertoire is unknown, although parasites derived from a single parent trypanosome have been found with more than 100 distinct VSGs.

Recombinant DNA techniques have revealed in part the mechanism by which the trypanosome can so quickly switch its surface coat.

One copy of the VSG gene is located on a specific trypanosome chromosome (Figure 48–5). If that VSG is to be expressed, a copy is made of the gene, and it is translocated to another chromosome close to the telomere. In this new location—and only in the new location—it is transcribed into messenger RNA to which a 35-nucleotide sequence is added. This small

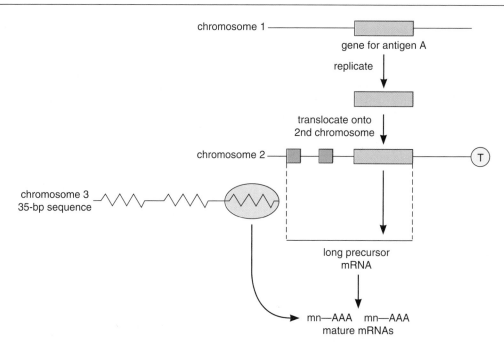

Figure 48–5. Molecular mechanism of antigenic diversity in trypanosomiasis.

35-nucleotide sequence has been transcribed from yet another site where many of these small sequences are found closely linked to one another. Most trypanosome proteins have this small sequence at the beginning of their message. It is therefore assumed necessary for expression of the messenger RNA. Some of the VSGs come from genes that are already near the telomere, however, and therefore do not translocate before expression. Although the mechanism of "gene jumping" and subsequent expression has been elucidated, the exact mechanism by which one VSG is switched to another is still unclear. Understanding this switching mechanism might provide a means of interrupting the ability of trypanosomes to change their antigenic disguises.

Serodiagnosis of trypanosomiasis is possible by using indirect immunofluorescence, enzyme-linked immunosorbent assay (ELISA), indirect hemagglutination, direct agglutination, gel precipitation for IgM titration, and gel precipitation using trypanosomal antigen. Nevertheless, none of these methods are yet suitable for field studies or surveys in Africa.

Specific antibodies to trypanosomes can either lyse the parasites or clump them. Clumping allows for more efficient removal of the parasites by the reticuloendothelial system. It is controversial whether humans or domestic animals living in endemic areas develop resistance to infection, although epidemiologic observations suggest that resistance does arise. The fact that there are healthy human carriers of *T rhodesiense*—which usually produces a fatal infection—implies that some protective mechanism must exist. One possible clue to this mechanism is the dense packing of VSG on the surface membrane of trypanosomes which "hides" other surface molecules from the immune response. Furthermore, "immune-privileged" sites such as the flagellar pocket—a partially enclosed space at the base of the flagellum of kinetoplast parasites—are the major site for protein secretion or endocytosis by the parasite.

Suppression of immune responses to other unrelated antigens may be observed during trypanosomal infections. Whether suppression results from exhaustion of B cells, the presence of suppresser T cells, a lack of helper T cells, or the availability of fewer T cells to interact with new antigens is unknown.

The multiplicity of antigenic variants observed during field studies in bovines makes vaccination an unlikely solution to trypanosomiasis unless common antigens can be found.

THE IMMUNE RESPONSE TO HELMINTHS

Multicellular parasites, by reason of their size, more complex tissue and organ structure, and varied and active metabolism, include very complex host responses. Further complicating the picture is the fact that several forms of the parasite may be present in the host, each eliciting a unique immune response. Helminth infections also exhibit a phenomenon called "aggregated distribution" in which some individuals in a given population harbor the majority of parasites (often with multiple species).

The primary antigens of helminths may often be metabolic byproducts, enzymes, or other secretory products. For example, the eggs of *Schistosoma mansoni* have been shown to secrete unique antigens that induce granuloma formation; the various stages of developing nematodes have stage-specific antigens, often molting fluids, to which the host responds in various ways; and the granules in the stichocytes, special cells located in the "neck" of *Trichuris trichiura*, elicit specific antibody.

Trematodes, cestodes, and nematodes probably all share common antigens. The two most frequent responses to helminths—eosinophilia and IgE (reaginic) antibody—are both T-cell-dependent. Moreover, certain helminths have been shown to potentiate the immune response to other antigens, perhaps by common metabolic byproducts acting as nonspecific adjuvants.

TREMATODES

Trematodes are important pathogens of humans and domestic animals. Fascioliasis debilitates and kills domestic animals in large numbers and renders the livers unfit for human consumption. Schistosomiasis is a major disease of humans. The lung flukes of the genus *Paragonimus* cause central nervous system complications in humans if they encyst in the brain. In the lung, considerable mechanical damage results. *Opisthorchis* (*Clonorchis sinensis*), the fish-borne Chinese liver fluke, causes much morbidity both in Asia and among recent emigrants from endemic areas, producing infection that may last the lifetime of the host.

SCHISTOSOMIASIS

Major Immunologic Features

- Humoral (IgE, IgM, IgG) and cellular (eosinophils, lymphocytes, macrophages) responses to invading worms
- Serum sickness-like acute disease may develop (Katayama fever)
- Chronic disease from granulomatous reaction to eggs with subsequent fibrosis
- Developing larvae and adult worms evade immune response by camouflaging their surface with host antigens

Schistosomiasis in humans is caused by *S mansoni, S japonicum, S haematobium,* and *S mekongi.* The advent of new high dams in many areas of the world, especially Africa, has increased the prevalence of schistosomiasis, because the additional irrigation made possible by the dams has vastly enlarged the habitat of the **freshwater snails** that serve as intermediate hosts to the worms. The life cycle of this parasite depends on skin penetration of the definitive host by infective larvae produced in large numbers in the snail. Because attempts to reduce snail populations have largely failed, infection has become rampant in these areas. *S mansoni,* now widespread in Africa and the Middle East, has also spread extensively in South America where it was introduced by the slave trade. *S haematobium* is found in all watered areas of Africa and the Arabian peninsula. *S japonicum* is found in the Yangtze River watershed in China, where it has been subjected to a vast control effort but is still common in Szechwan province and may be returning to the main river valley. It is also common in the central Philippines. A purely animal-infecting (zoophilic) form is found in Taiwan. *S mekongi,* a newly described species similar to *S japonicum,* causes human disease in Thailand, Laos, and Cambodia, with a scattering of cases in Malaysia, recently described as *S malaysiensis.* A focus of *S japonicum* in Sulawesi (Celebes) may prove to be a distinct species.

The schistosomes that infect humans have the following **life cycle:** Infected humans and animals excrete eggs that hatch in water, releasing **miracidia;** these actively penetrate snails in which several generations of multiplying larvae (**sporocysts**) develop. These in turn produce great numbers of fork-tailed cercariae, the stage infective for humans, which leave the host snail at the rate of 300–3000 per day. The **cercariae** penetrate the skin of the definitive host, leaving the tail outside, and enter the bloodstream as minute motile immature **schistosomula,** which migrate in 3–8 days to the lungs and eventually to the liver. Further development and adult worm pairing take place about 5 weeks after skin penetration. The paired mature schistosomes then migrate against the venous flow into the mesenteric or vesical venules, where eggs are deposited. The embryo (**miracidium**) within the egg secretes proteases that may facilitate passage through the blood vessel and adjacent tissue into the lumen of the intestine (or bladder in the case of *S haematobium*). Alternatively, some investigators have suggested that the granuloma produced by the host around the egg "chaperones" it through the wall of the intestine. Egg movement is also probably aided by peristalsis of the intestine or contractions of the bladder.

Unfortunately, not all the eggs reach the lumen of the intestine or bladder. Some become trapped in the submucosa, and others do not leave the bloodstream but instead are carried with the venous flow to the liver portals, or by collateral circulation to other organs of the body. Because of their size, eggs reaching the liver become trapped in the portal venules and do not enter into the sinusoids. When eggs are trapped in the liver, the wall of the intestine, or the bladder, they elicit a **granulomatous inflammation** that is the hallmark of the chronic stage of schistosomiasis. An early infiltrate of neutrophils and lymphocytes may be seen around eggs, but distinctive granulomas containing a core of macrophages and eosinophils, surrounded by a cuff of lymphocytes, appear shortly. The early stages of inflammation may be seen by 6 weeks, but granulomas reach their maximal cellularity within 9–12 weeks. Later, an increasing number of fibroblasts or lipocytes (**Ito cells**) can be seen in association with the granulomas, and the cellular lesion is slowly replaced by collagen. In the liver, older lesions become periportal scars. Because numerous eggs are deposited, a circumferential periportal fibrosis called Symmer's clay pipestem fibrosis develops, particularly well demarcated in *S mansoni* infection. This fibrosis blocks normal blood flow from the portal venous system to the sinusoids, resulting in portal hypertension and its complications.

Granuloma formation is initiated by soluble proteins secreted through pores in the eggshell by the embryonic miracidium. These soluble egg products, some of which have been purified, are used in one serodiagnostic test for schistosomiasis. As might be expected from the diverse cells that make up the granuloma, the mechanisms of granuloma formation, modulation, and subsequent fibrosis are complex. Pleiotropic cytokines are involved, as well as factors from the egg itself that may be both chemotactic and mitogenic for fibroblasts. The importance of cellular immunity in granuloma formation has been underscored by the observation that both the granulomatous reaction to schistosome eggs and subsequent periportal fibrosis are absent or significantly diminished in thymic-deficient ("nude") mice and in mice with severe combined immunodeficiency (SCID). SCID mice have no functional T and B cells, and in the absence of a granulomatous response, schistosome eggs produce a frequently fatal acute hepatotoxic effect. One conclusion made from these observations was that the granulomatous reaction to the eggs protects the host from diffusible egg products that can directly damage liver cells. On the other hand, an unexpected observation was that an intact cellular immune response was necessary for egg production by schistosome females and passage of eggs through the intestinal wall. Injection of supernatant from cultures of T-cell clones led to reconstitution of the host granulomatous response as well as egg production and transmission. This suggested that specific T-cell-derived cytokines were required as key elements in the host–parasite interplay. These observations confirm that the host–parasite relationship is an extremely intricate, complicated, and evolved phenomenon in which elements of the host immune response are sometimes subverted by the parasite for its own replication and transmission.

Although the immune response to schistosome eggs is the central immunopathologic mechanism in chronic schistosomiasis, it is not the only immune response of importance in schistosome infection. In some previously infected individuals, invading cercariae may elicit a dermatitis with features of both immediate and delayed hypersensitivity. This response is similar to the **"swimmers' itch"** produced by schistosomes that also infect nonhuman hosts including other mammals and birds. These enter the skin of previously sensitized individuals. Some schistosome species may produce an acute form of schistosomiasis **(Katayama fever)** characterized by fever, eosinophilia, lymphadenopathy, diarrhea, splenomegaly, and urticaria. This appears to be an anaphylactic (IgE) or serum sickness (IgG) reaction. In fact, cases of glomerulonephritis secondary to schistosome antigen–antibody complexes have been reported.

An important unresolved question is whether protective immunity to schistosomiasis develops in humans after infection. Studies in Kenya and Gambia have shown that schistosome-infected individuals in an endemic area who had been treated with antischistosomal drugs showed an age-dependent resistance to reinfection. Children were much more easily reinfected than were adults, suggesting that true human immunity can be acquired with age. Identification of "resistant" groups of children may help to identify important parasite antigens. Augmentation of the response to these antigens would be one rational approach to vaccine development. Schistosomiasis is primarily a disease of children and teenagers. The most severely affected individuals, although rare, do not survive to adulthood.

The question of immunity to reinfection has been studied intensively in animal models. Two models in particular have been used. In the first of these, called the **concomitant immunity model,** mice are infected with 20–30 normal *S mansoni* cercariae 6 weeks prior to challenge. In the second, called the **attenuated vaccine model,** mice are immunized by 400–500 cercariae attenuated by 20–50 krad of gamma radiation 2 weeks before challenge. The mechanisms by which the host eliminates the challenge infection may be different in each of these two models. Studies with the concomitant immunity model in mice or in rats, a naturally nonpermissive host, emphasized the importance of specific antiparasite IgG and eosinophils. In fact, these models help to elucidate many of the cellular functions of eosinophils. **Eosinophilia** is a common denominator in helminth parasite infections, and histologic examination of parasites and host tissue invariably confirms the presence of numerous eosinophils around dead or dying organisms. On the other hand, studies with the attenuated vaccine model pointed to macrophages as the principal effector cells, as well as T_H1 responses in elimination of the chal-

lenge infection. Whether one or both of these mechanisms is key in the human immune response to schistosome infection remains an active area of research and debate.

By comparing normal with various immune-deficient mouse strains, the cellular and antibody requirements of vaccine immunity have been investigated. Vaccinated mice with T-lymphocyte deficiencies, as well as mice immunosuppressed from birth, have a sharply diminished resistance to a challenge infection. On the other hand, mice deficient in complement, mast cells, natural killer (NK) lymphocytes, and IgE show no difference in resistance compared with normal controls. In a theme common to many parasitic infections, CD4 T cells secreting interferon gamma and macrophages appear key to killing larvae in vaccinated mice.

The exact site of killing schistosomula in vaccinated mice remains controversial. Most studies indicate that killing occurs in the lungs; however, some evidence also exists for immune killing in the skin.

Immunologic diagnosis of schistosome infection in the absence of egg excretion by the host can be accomplished in various ways, both humoral and cellular. Stage-specific humoral responses can be used to produce circumoval precipitation; schistosomal growth inhibition or death; and complement fixation, hemagglutination, and various precipitation reactions. None of these reactions can be positively correlated with protection. Immediate and delayed cutaneous hypersensitivity develop in most individuals during the course of the disease, although the specificity of these reactions is often suspect because of antigens that cross-react with those of other worms. The purification of novel antigenic fractions and sensitive ELISA or radioimmunoassays, however, may improve the specificity of tests based on these responses.

CESTODES

Two types of immune response to cestodes occur. One is directed against the intestinal lumen-dwelling adult tapeworms such as *Diphyllobothrium latum* and *Taenia saginata,* which have restricted, nonhumoral immunogenic contact. The response is chiefly cell-mediated, is induced primarily by the scolex, affects growth and strobilation of challenge worms, and varies considerably with the host species. The other is directed against migratory tissue-encysting larval tapeworms such as *Hymenolepis nana* (in its intravillous larval phase), *Echinococcus granulosus* (hydatid cysts), and *Taenia solium* (cysticercosis), which have intimate and continuous tissue contact and induce a strong parenteral host response detectable as serum antibody, which is strongly protective against reinfection. Serodiagnostic tests are available only for the larval tissue cestode parasites, and humoral responses that protect the challenged host have only recently been described for this form of cestode parasitism. ELISA for serodiagnosis of cysticercosis—with some cross-reactivity—has been developed.

ECHINOCOCCOSIS

Major Immunologic Features
- IgE elevated
- Anaphylaxis may occur after rupture of hydatid and release of cyst fluids
- Casoni skin test of questionable use
- Diagnostic antibody present

General Considerations

The most serious human cestode infection is caused by *Echinococcus*. These tiny tapeworms do not produce pathologic lesions in the definitive host, the dog, but severe complications occur when their eggs are ingested by humans and other animals. Humans may become infected by accident, and the disease incidence can be particularly high in rural communities dominated by sheep farming, even in developed countries. The larval form of the tapeworm hatches from the egg in the intestine of the intermediate host, for example, humans, and then claws its way through the intestinal mucosa and is transported through the lymphatic and blood vessels to sites in which it grows to enormous proportions, although it is enclosed by a heavy cyst wall laid down by both the host and the parasite. In humans, *Echinococcus* normally forms fluid-filled cysts in the liver, but these can also occur in the lungs, brain, kidneys, and other parts of the body. **Hydatid cysts** are highly immunogenic and result in production of higher titers of IgE and other immunoglobulins. If a cyst is ruptured, anaphylactic response to the cyst fluid can cause death. Little or no immune protection is elicited by this highly immunogenic cestode, because the hydatid cysts remain alive for years, and in animals they increase in number as the host ages. Humans are usually a dead-end host, for the cysts must be eaten by a canid to become sexually mature. There is some evidence that complement-mediated lysis of protoscoleces (the numerous future scoleces in hydatid fluid or "hydatid sand") might be protective in the infected human or other intermediate host.

The Casoni skin test indicates past or present echinococcosis. It consists of intradermal injection of hydatid cyst fluid, resulting in both immediate and delayed hypersensitivity. The specificity of this test is in doubt because of cross-reactions with other helminths. Heating the cyst fluid slightly increases the specificity of the test. Serodiagnosis can be made by hemagglutination, complement fixation, and flocculation tests, ELISA, and radioimmunoassay, using serum from the patient and specially fractionated antigenic components made from cyst fluid. These tests are not species-specific.

NEMATODES

Nematodes are the commonest, most varied, and most widely distributed helminths infecting humans. As with other parasites, immunogenicity is a reflection of the degree and duration of parasite contact with the host's tissues. Even with the intestinal lumen dwellers such as *Ascaris,* there is a migratory larval phase in which such contact is made—in most cases, in the pulmonary capillaries and alveolar spaces. The hookworms of humans (*Ancylostoma duodenale* and *Necator americanus*) also undergo a migration, except that the infective larvae enter via the skin or buccal mucosa rather than as hatchlings in the small bowel. *Strongyloides stercoralis,* the small intestinal roundworm of humans, undergoes a similar hookworm-like migration (as well as a stage of internal autoinfection or reinvasion via the mucosa of the large intestine).

The immature stages are particularly immunogenic, probably because of their high production of antigens from secretory glands and of enzymes or other products from these metabolically active stages. Commercially prepared vaccines are available only for nematodes, and all are living larval worms, irradiated to arrest their development but not their immunogenicity. One especially effective vaccine is against the cattle lungworm, *Dictyocaulus viviparus.* Another important group of human parasites are the filariae (chiefly *Wuchereria bancrofti, Brugia malayi, Loa loa, Onchocerca volvulus,* and the related guinea worm, *Dracunculus medinensis*). Diagnosis of these infections is often difficult, in part because of the presence of common antigens that preclude highly specific immunologic tests. **Hypersensitivity** reactions may occur after drug treatment (eg, with diethylcarbamazine for *Onchocerca*) in which large numbers of dead or dying microfilariae produce severe skin reactions and edema or dangerous reactions in the eye, and (in the case of *Loa*) when dead adult worms may induce severe central nervous system reactions.

1. TRICHINOSIS

Major Immunologic Features
- Positive skin tests for immediate and delayed hypersensitivity
- Diagnostic antibody

General Considerations

Trichinosis is acquired by ingestion of the infective larvae of *Trichinella spiralis* in uncooked or partially cooked meat. Pork is the primary source of infection in humans. The larvae are released from their cysts in the meat during digestion and rapidly develop into adults in the mucosa of the host's small intestine. After copulation in the lumen, the males die and the females return to the intestinal mucosa, where for about 5–6 weeks they produce 1000–1500 larvae per female, which migrate through the lymphatic system to the bloodstream. These larvae travel in the blood to all parts of the body and develop in voluntary muscles, especially in the diaphragm, tongue, masticatory and intercostal muscles, larynx, and the eye. Within the sarcolemma of striated muscle fibers, the larvae coil up into cysts whose outer walls are rapidly laid down by host histiocytes. Larvae may remain viable and infective for as long as 24 years, even though the cysts calcify. The encysted larvae apparently do not elicit immune protection. The migrating larvae and adult forms of the parasite excrete antigens that appear to be responsible for induction of the strong protection from subsequent challenge infections. An important expression of host resistance is active expulsion of developing or adult worms from the gut of a parasitized host—the so-called **self-cure phenomenon.** This occurs when a new infection initiates a host response, resulting in elimination of the old infection—the opposite of concomitant immunity.

The expulsion of *T spiralis* in humans appears to follow the mechanism proposed by Ogilvie and coworkers for the rodent hookworm, *Nippostrongylus brasiliensis.* A two-step mechanism is proposed: antibody-induced metabolic damage that blocks feeding by the worms followed by worm expulsion induced by activated lymphocytes. Both antibodies and cells are probably required for full expression of intestinal resistance, and the effect is synergistic rather than additive. As in the case of leishmaniasis, discussed earlier, CD4 lymphocytes of the T_H1 subtype may be the effector cells in cellular immunity via their production of interferon gamma.

Trichinella infection sometimes presents characteristic clinical symptoms, such as edema of the eyelids and face, but often presents less specific clinical signs such as eosinophilia, which can also be suggestive of several other parasitic infections. Specific immunodiagnostic tests may thus be of great importance. The **bentonite flocculation test** for human trichinosis is of value because of its high degree of specificity. A skin test **(Bachman intradermal test)** produces both immediate and delayed responses.

Infection of humans with *Trichinella* initially elicits IgM antibody followed by an IgG response. IgA antibody has been reported, which is not surprising, because the female worms are in the intestinal mucosa, although the locally produced protective gut antibodies probably are IgG rather than IgA or IgM. This antibody reaction against the feeding worms is complement-independent and, as noted, precedes the rapid expulsion of the antibody-damaged worms by T lymphocytes.

Although *Trichinella* is extremely immunogenic in its hosts, it can also exert an immunosuppressive action. Certain viral infections are more severe during infection with this parasite, and skin grafts show delayed rejection. On the other hand, cellular immunity to bacille Calmette–Guérin (BCG) seems to be potentiated when *T spiralis*-infected mice are less susceptible to *Listeria* infections.

2. ASCARIASIS

Major Immunologic Features
- Specific antibody detectable
- Elevated IgE

General Considerations

Ascaris, the giant roundworm of humans, is a lumen-dwelling parasite as an adult and causes little inconvenience to the host except in the heaviest infections although even single adult worms may produce mechanical damage by entering the bile or pancreatic ducts, or penetration through an amebiasis intestinal lesion may result in peritonitis. Ingestion of eggs is followed by their hatching and penetration of the mucosa by the larvae that eventually reach the lung via the bloodstream. In a previously infected host, hypersensitivity reactions in the lung resulting from high levels of IgE antibody can cause serious pneumonitis. Acute hypersensitivity to *Ascaris* antigens often develops in laboratory workers and makes it virtually impossible for them to continue working with the nematode.

Cases of sudden death in Nigeria have been ascribed to *Ascaris*-induced **anaphylactic shock** syndrome, heretofore rarely diagnosed or recognized. Death probably resulted from the worm's release of a substance causing mast cell activation and degranulation because degranulated mast cells were found throughout the body tissues in these children, or from interaction of a specific IgE antibody with *Ascaris* allergen at the mast cell surface. Allergy in ascariasis may underlie many of the symptoms of *Ascaris* infection, including abdominal pain.

3. FILARIID NEMATODES

Major Immunologic Features
- Induction of host immune response to adults or microfilariae leads to disease

General Considerations

Filariid nematodes are introduced into the human host by insect vectors. Those of the genus *Brugia* or *Wuchereria* are spread by a mosquito vector, whereas *Onchocerca volvulus* is transmitted by a blackfly. Although the stages of each life cycle are similar, the type of disease produced varies considerably. A common theme is that morbidity is due primarily to the **host immune response** to the parasite, rather than to any toxic product of the parasite itself.

O volvulus is the causative agent of **onchocerciasis,** or African river blindness. This is the major cause of blindness in endemic areas of West Africa and Central America. Infectious larvae that are deposited by a blackfly bite migrate in the subcutaneous tissue and develop into adults in approximately 1 year. The adults elicit an unusual fibrogenic host response resulting in a subcutaneous collagenous nodule in which the worm lives. The female produces large numbers of microfilariae, which migrate out of the nodule and are distributed widely in subcutaneous tissue. This dispersal of microfilariae increases the likelihood that they will be picked up again by the in-

sect vector to continue the life cycle. Humans react to migrating microfilariae by production of both circulating antibody and cellular immunity. An intense delayed hypersensitivity-like reaction to dead or dying microfilariae can lead to a disseminated skin reaction or a more serious eye disease. Microfilariae can enter all chambers of the eye and elicit a keratitis or retinitis, which over a period of years can lead to total blindness.

Parasites of the genera *Brugia* and *Wuchereria,* in contrast, produce **lymphatic filariasis.** In this case, damage is caused by adult worms residing in lymphatics, most commonly in the groin. Over time, the lymphatic lumen may be compromised by scarring leading to blockage of lymph drainage from the lower extremities and production of a disfiguring condition called **elephantiasis** that characterizes severe chronic disease.

REFERENCES

GENERAL

Ash C: Macrophages at the centre of infection. *Parasitol Today* 1991;7:2.

Cox FEG, Liew EY: T-cell subsets and cytokines in parasitic infections. *Parasitol Today* 1992;8:371.

Desowitz RS: *Ova and Parasites. Medical Parasitology for the Laboratory Technologist.* Harper & Row, 1980

Finkelman FD, Urban, JF Jr: Cytokines: Making the right choice. *Parasitol Today* 1992;8:311.

Kay AB et al: Leukocytes activation initiated by IgE-dependent mechanisms in relation to helminthic parasitic disease and clinical models of asthma. *Int Arch Allergy Appl Immunol* 1985;77:69.

Klei TR: Experimental immunologic studies on lymphatic filariasis. In: *Molecular & Immunological Aspects of Parasitism.* Wang CC (editor). American Association for the Advancement of Science, 1991.

Scott P: IL-12: Initiation cytokine for cell-mediated immunity. *Science* 1993;260:496.

Soulsby EJL (editor): *Immune Responses in Parasitic Infections: Immunology, Immunopathology, and Immunoprophylaxis.* Vol 1: *Nematodes.* Vol 2: *Trematodes and Cestodes.* Vol 3: *Protozoa.* Vol 4: *Protozoa, Arthropods, and Invertebrates.* CRC Press, 1987.

SERODIAGNOSTIC TESTS

Center for Infectious Diseases. *Reference and Disease Surveillance.* CDC, 1985.

Sun T: *Pathology and Clinical Features of Parasitic Diseases,* Masson Monograph in Diagnostic Pathology. Vol 5. Masson, 1982.

FILARIASIS

Orihel TC, Eberhard M:. Zoonotic filariasis. *Clin Microbiol Rev* 1998;11:366.

LEISHMANIASIS

Reiner SL et al: T_H1 and T_H2 cell antigen receptors in experimental leishmaniasis. *Science* 1993;259:1457.

Scott P, Sher A: A spectrum in the susceptibility of leishmanial strains to intracellular killing by murine macrophages. *J Immunol* 1986;136:1461.

MALARIA

Butcher GA: HIV and malaria: A lesson in immunology? *Parasitol Today* 1992;8:307.

Greenwood B et al: Why do some African children develop severe malaria? *Parasitol Today* 1991;7:277.

Hoffman SL et al: From genomics to vaccines: Malaria as a model system. *Nat Med* 1998;4:1351.

Riley EM et al: The immune recognition of malaria antigens. *Parasitol Today* 1991;7:5.

Wahlgren M et al: Waves of malarial variations. *Cell* 1999; 96:603.

SCHISTOSOMIASIS

Cheever AW: Schistosomiasis: Infection versus disease and hypersensitivity versus immunity. *Am J Pathol* 1993; 142:699.

Damian RT et al: *Schistosoma mansoni:* Parasitology and immunology of baboons vaccinated with irradiated cryopreserved schistosomula. *Int J Parasitol* 1985;15:333.

Hagan P, Wilkins HA: Concomitant immunity in schistosomiasis. *Parasitol Today* 1993;9:3.

Pearce EJ et al: The initiation and function of T_H2 responses during infection with Schistosoma mansoni. *Adv Exp Med Biol* 1998;452:67.

Stadecker MJ, Colley DG: The immunobiology of the schistosome egg granuloma. *Parasitol Today* 1992;8:218.

Yazdanbakhsh M: Common features of T cell reactivity in persistent helminth infections: Lymphatic filariasis and schistosomiasis. *Immunol Lett* 1999;65:109.

TRYPANOSOMIASIS

Bangs JD: Surface coats and secretory trafficking in African trypanosomes. *Curr Opin Microbiol* 1998;1:448.

Burleigh BA, Andrews NW: Signaling and host cell invasion by Trypanosoma cruzi. *Curr Opin Microbiol* 1998;1:461.

Donelson JE, Turner MJ: How the trypanosome changes its coat. *Sci Am* 1985;252:44.

Esser KL, Schornblecher MJ: Expression of two variant surface glycoproteins on individual African trypanosomes during antigen switching. *Science* 1985;229:290.

Kierszenbaum F: Chagas' disease and the autoimmunity hypothesis. *Clin Microbiol Rev* 1999;12:210.

Parsons M et al: Antigenic variation in Africana trypanosomes: DNA rearrangements program immune evasion. *Immunol Today* 1984;5:43.

49

Spirochetal Diseases: Syphilis & Lyme Disease

Linda K. Bockenstedt, MD

INTRODUCTION

The Spirochaetaceae family of microbes are long, helically curved, gram-negative bacilli that contain flagella-like axial fibrils enclosed within a loosely attached outer sheath. The axial fibrils facilitate the motility of the organism, which move in a wave-like, undulating fashion. Spirochetes can be separated morphologically into the genera *Treponema, Borrelia,* and *Leptospira,* each of which contains organisms pathogenic for humans. *Treponema* include the causal agents of syphilis, pinta, yaws, and bejel; *Borrelia* include the vector-borne agents of relapsing fever and Lyme disease; and *Leptospira* species cause leptospirosis. The entire genomes of the syphilis spirochete, *Treponema pallidum,* and the Lyme disease agent, *Borrelia burgdorferi,* have recently been sequenced. Remarkably, these organisms appear to be devoid of known virulence genes and toxins, and, in the case of *T pallidum,* require the import of host molecules to sustain basic biologic functions needed for life. A striking feature of these spirochetes is the proportion of genes dedicated to the production of proteins with the potential to be surface-exposed. Of unknown biologic function, these genes are believed to be crucial for infectivity and for spirochete evasion of host immune defenses. In this chapter, the clinical syndromes of syphilis and Lyme disease are described as illustrative examples of the immunopathogenesis of spirochetal infections.

SYPHILIS

General Considerations

Syphilis, a sexually acquired infection with the spirochete *T pallidum,* was described in epidemic proportion in Europe in the late 15th century and was demonstrated to be of spirochetal origin in 1905, when the organisms were first visualized microscopically in fluid smears from secondary syphilis lesions. The disease reached peak incidence rates in the late 1940s (66.4 cases/100,000 persons), just prior to the introduction of penicillin therapy. Incidence rates rapidly declined to 3.9 cases/100,000 persons by 1956, but have fluctuated since despite the availability of effective antibiotics and the institution of public health measures. Over 3.5 million cases of syphilis are estimated to occur annually worldwide. The heightened transmission of other sexually acquired infections, especially HIV, in patients with active syphilis underscores the important need to prevent the development of this disease.

Clinical Features

Primary Syphilis. Like most spirochetal infections, syphilis has episodes of clinically apparent disease punctuated by periods, often spanning years, of asymptomatic latent infection. The disease is acquired by direct contact of mucosal surfaces or abraded skin with infectious lesions. Spirochetes disseminate widely throughout the host within hours of infection, although disease generally presents weeks later at the spirochete entry site. The classic primary syphilitic lesion is a single **chancre** appearing in the anogenital region 2–6 weeks after infectious contact. The chancre appears first as a painless, indurated papule that expands and ulcerates, forming a sharply demarcated border surrounded by a clean base. This lesion is teeming with spirochetes and highly infectious. It persists for 2–6 weeks, then heals spontaneously. Extragenital lesions have an atypical appearance, with induration mild or absent and pain a prominent symptom. Primary syphilis is often accompanied by regional painless lymphadenopathy.

Secondary Syphilis. Secondary syphilis occurs on average 8 weeks after resolution of the primary chancre; as many as 60% of patients may not recall a primary lesion. Although it can present as a distinct stage, secondary syphilis often overlaps temporally with primary syphilis, a feature that likely reflects the disseminated nature of the infection at the time of clinical presentation. The regions most commonly affected symptomatically include the skin, head and neck areas, and gastrointestinal tract. The skin rash of secondary syphilis is often mild and mimics other dermatologic conditions, appearing as a maculopapular, follicular, or pustular rash. Syphilis is one of the few infectious dermatologic conditions that involve the palms and soles. Other features of secondary syphilis include pharyngitis and mucous patches. The mucous patch appears as a painless ulcerative lesion involving the buccal mucosa, tongue, or lips. Condylomata lata are papular lesions in the genital area. Ocular involvement can present as a multitude of inflammatory conditions, including episcleritis, keratitis, uveitis, optic neuritis, and pupillary changes. Spirochete invasion of the meninges can lead to aseptic meningitis, which may be asymptomatic; cranial neuropathies most often involve the facial and auditory nerves and can lead to sensorineural deafness. Gastrointestinal symptoms include anorexia, nausea, and vomiting; jaundice may be present in as many as 10% of patients, but overt hepatitis is rare. Painless lymphadenopathy accompanies signs and symptoms of secondary syphilis in 75% of patients and is especially prevalent in the head and neck region (suboccipital, cervical, and posterior auricular nodes). Systemic symptoms at this stage include varying degrees of malaise, headache, and low-grade fever. Despite intermittent arthralgias and vague bone pain, syphilis rarely causes frank arthritis.

Latent and Tertiary Syphilis. After a latent period of months to years, about 15% of untreated individuals develop tertiary signs of infection. Prior to the antibiotic era, **gumma** formation was the most common complication of late syphilis. Now rarely seen, these granulomatous lesions appear as indurated nodules in the skin and can ulcerate; gummatous visceral involvement can also occur, especially in the respiratory and gastrointestinal tracts, and in the bones. More serious manifestations involve the cardiovascular and nervous systems. **Syphilitic aortitis** begins within 5–10 years of primary infection and can lead to aortic insufficiency and aneurysm formation. Aortitis most commonly involves the ascending aorta and is due to spirochete invasion of the vessel wall and secondary chronic inflammation. Neurologic involvement can be asymptomatic or present as **meningovascular disease** (aseptic meningitis or diffuse encephalitis), **tabes dorsalis,** or **paresis.** Meningovascular disease usually presents with signs and symptoms of meningitis, followed within days to weeks by diffuse encephalitis. Tabes dorsalis involves the dorsal spinal cord early in its course, leading to fleeting lower extremity pains and paresthesia. Later, loss of position and vibratory sensation leads to a positive Romberg sign and wide-based gait. Paresis begins with memory impairment that progresses to dementia with psychotic features. The frequency of these complications has diminished due to the earlier diagnosis and more frequent use of antibiotics for other infections.

T pallidum can be passed transplacentally to the developing fetus and cause fetal demise, birth defects, or latent infection of the newborn. The gestational stage at which maternal–fetal transmission occurs determines whether significant congenital abnormalities arise; mothers with latent infection can still transmit infection to the fetus.

Pathogenesis

Because *T pallidum* cannot be grown in culture, much of our understanding of syphilis immunopathogenesis has derived from studies of the human condition, animal models of primary disease, and limited in vitro data with tissue-extracted spirochetes. On exposure to epithelial surfaces, spirochetes attach and penetrate through endothelial cell layers. Tissue invasion is believed necessary for treponemal virulence, although the mechanisms through which it occurs are unknown. All stages of syphilis are characterized by vascular involvement (periarteritis and obliterative endarteritis), and treponemes appear to have a predilection for the perivascular and vascular tissues. Histopathology of primary chancres reveals numerous spirochetes and cellular infiltrates initially composed of T lymphocytes, followed within days by macrophages and plasma cells. Testicular inoculation of rabbits with the Nichols strain of *T pallidum* results in acute orchitis due to T-lymphocyte infiltration beginning 6 days after infection, followed by macrophages at day 10. The appearance of macrophages correlates with clearance of spirochetes and healing of the lesions. In vitro studies have shown that macrophages ingest *T pallidum* rather slowly (over hours), and killing requires the presence of immune serum; these findings suggest that opsonizing antibody is important for efficient uptake and destruction of spirochetes. Activation of macrophages is likely facilitated by cytokines released from T lymphocytes. Few studies have examined cytokine production in syphilis; interleukin 2 (IL-2) has been detected in primary chancres, and lymphocyte culture supernatants contain macrophage-activating factors, including interferon gamma (IFNγ).

T pallidum-specific antibodies arise early in infection and can be detected in serum as well as in diseased tissues. Antibodies are first directed toward a limited array of treponemal antigens (especially the 37- and 47-kD antigens and the flagellin protein), but specificities expand broadly by secondary and early latent syphilis. *T pallidum* infection induces antibodies that inhibit attachment of spirochetes to cells, and IgG from syphilitic humans can immobilize and kill *T pallidum* in vitro in the presence of complement. Antibody also enhances phagocytosis of treponemes by neutrophils and macrophages. Demonstration that *T pallidum*-specific antibody alone can confer protective immunity has been difficult, but several recent studies have provided convincing evidence. A striking feature of *T pallidum* is its relatively low density of outer membrane proteins. Antibody directed against *T pallidum* rare outer membrane proteins (TROMPs) can lead to their surface aggregation and subsequent treponemal death. Naturally acquired immunity to *T pallidum* infection correlates with the level of antibodies to TROMPs. Recently, a multigene family, termed *T pallidum* repeat *(tpr),* has been identified that is related to the major surface protein *(msp)* genes of *T denticola.* This latter family encodes for proteins that are surface-exposed porins and mediate binding to host cells. Antibodies raised against the variable domain of recombinant Tpr K (a *tpr* dominantly transcribed in the Nichols strain of *T pallidum*) opsonize treponemes for phagocytosis and markedly alter the development of primary lesions in rabbits after challenge infection; all rabbits become infected, however. It has been hypothesized that recombination of different conserved domains of *tpr* genes with previously silent variable domains can lead to the expression of antigenic variants. This hypothesis explains the observation that *T pallidum* harvested from rabbit testes during the resolution phase of orchitis are resistant to phagocytosis. Antibodies that arise naturally to the dominant Tpr present on disease-inciting treponemes would be incapable of binding to Tpr variants expressed on treponemes that adapt to persist in the host. Thus, treponemes may evade host defenses by expressing levels of surface proteins below the threshold required for induction of an immune response or for killing after antibody binding and by antigenic variation of the proteins themselves.

Although humoral immunity is required for host defense against treponemal infection, antibody responses can cause disease. Circulating immune complexes present in secondary syphilis may contribute to the pathology of skin lesions and their deposition within the kidney is one cause of the rare syphilitic nephropathy. Although antibodies to cardiolipin, an anionic phospholipid, are a hallmark of early syphilis and provide the basis for nontreponemal tests for the disease, they are not associated with clot formation or the development of antiphospholipid antibody syndrome.

T pallidum elicits T-cell responses that can be detected by in vitro lymphoblast transformation assays and by histologic examination of diseased tissues. Although some in vitro studies suggest that T cells from syphilitic patients and infected animals are depleted in the circulation or functionally suppressed in vitro, careful kinetic studies in the rabbit model of syphilis suggest that these responses are intact for at least 6 weeks after inoculation. Moreover, histologic analysis shows that T cells are recruited to sites of disease. In the primary chancre, CD4 T cells predominate cellular infiltrates, whereas in secondary lesions, CD8 T cells are more prevalent. Gummas seen in tertiary syphilis represent typical delayed-type hypersensitivity reactions, with granuloma formation characterized by palisading lymphocytes and central necrosis. Thus, the ability to detect T-cell responses may depend on the location from which they are sampled (peripheral blood, draining lymph node, or diseased tissue) relative to the stage of disease. The exact role T cells play

in disease expression is unclear, as underscored by studies of HIV-infected patients who acquire syphilis. The majority of such patients exhibit identical syphilitic disease patterns as HIV-negative individuals, even when CD4 T-cell counts fall below 500/μL. One study, however, showed that HIV-infected males, but not females, were more likely to present with secondary syphilis, and there is debate about whether response to antibiotics is impaired in HIV-infected individuals treated for syphilis.

Acquired immunity to syphilis arises slowly and is believed to involve both humoral and T-cell-mediated immunity. Fifty percent of patients with previously treated latent syphilis do not develop primary chancres on reinfection, and in the rabbit model of syphilis, complete resistance to new infection develops only after 3–6 months of infection. Passive transfer of immune serum and immune splenic T cells can partially protect hamsters from challenge infection with *T pallidum.* The combined effects of specific humoral and T-cell-mediated immunity are believed to maintain the latent phase of syphilis. This notion is supported by the finding of high titer *T pallidum*-specific antibody in the sera of patients with latent syphilis. It has been postulated that the eventual loss or lowering of *T pallidum*-specific antibody responses permits reactivation of disease and tertiary manifestations.

Diagnosis

The intermittent and varied clinical manifestations of untreated syphilis has led to its nickname, the "great imitator." The diagnosis of syphilis should be suspected in patients who are at risk for sexually transmitted diseases; these include the urban poor, individuals engaged in recreational drug use, and those from developing countries, where rates of syphilis are high. Because *T pallidum* cannot be successfully grown in culture, other methods are routinely used for the diagnosis of syphilis. Dark-field microscopy of fluid smears from involved skin and tissues can reveal the presence of spirochetes, but even direct fluorescent analysis using *T pallidum*-specific antibody cannot distinguish this treponeme from other pathogenic *Treponema* species. Two groups of serologic tests are useful in establishing the diagnosis of syphilis. Nontreponemal tests detect antibodies to a complex of lecithin, cholesterol, and cardiolipin and are useful for screening for possible exposure to *T pallidum.* These tests, the Venereal Disease Research Laboratory (VDRL) test and rapid plasma reagin (rpr), become positive within 4–6 weeks of infection and are positive in 70% of patients with primary disease and all patients with later stages. They lack specificity, however, and many conditions—age, pregnancy, drug addiction, malignancy, autoimmune disease (especially systemic lupus erythematosus and antiphospholipid antibody syndrome), and viral infections—can yield positive tests in the absence of true *T pallidum* infection. Serologic tests specific for treponemal infection include the serum fluorescent-treponemal antibody absorbance test (FTA-ABS) and the microhemagglutination test, which use *T pallidum* organisms as a source of antigen. Positive nontreponemal tests should be confirmed using the treponemal tests, which have higher sensitivity and specificity. False-positive tests have been reported in pregnant patients and when autoimmune disease or viral infections (especially Epstein-Barr virus and parvovirus) are present. The diagnosis of neurosyphilis is based on VDRL, cell counts, and protein levels within cerebrospinal fluid. All pregnant patients should be screened for syphilis, and infants born to seropositive mothers should be evaluated with quantitative nontreponemal serologic tests. Because of the high association between HIV infection and syphilis, individuals should be screened for both. Both VDRL and rpr titers correlate with disease activity; titers are expected to fall by two to three dilutions within 3 months of successful therapy and become negative by 12 months. *T pallidum*-specific tests remain positive for life in 75% of patients treated for primary syphilis and all patients with later stages of the disease. The relationship between stage of disease and serologic test results is depicted in Figure 49–1.

Treatment & Prognosis

Penicillin remains the drug of choice for treatment of all stages of syphilis; alternative antibiotics, such as tetracycline derivatives, erythromycin, and ceftriaxone, can be used in patients allergic to penicillin, but require greater compliance and may not be as efficacious. There is no documented acquisition of penicillin resistance by *T pallidum,* although the organism may have the genetic potential to develop resistance. The dosages and duration of therapy are empiric and based on clinical experience; in general, later stages of the disease require larger doses of antibiotics for longer periods of time. About 50% of patients with syphilis experience a **Jarisch-Herxheimer (J-H) reaction** after antibiotics are initiated. The J-H reaction manifests as a sudden worsening of signs and symptoms, with fever occurring within 12 hours of antibiotics and resolving within 24 hours. This phenomenon responds symptomatically to antipyretics but cannot be prevented by pretreatment with antihistamines and does not appear to be a drug reaction per se. Although the cause of the reaction is unknown, it is widely held to be due to the release of treponemal lipoproteins and secondary induction of an inflammatory response (see Lyme disease pathogenesis section for more detailed discussion regarding the immuno-

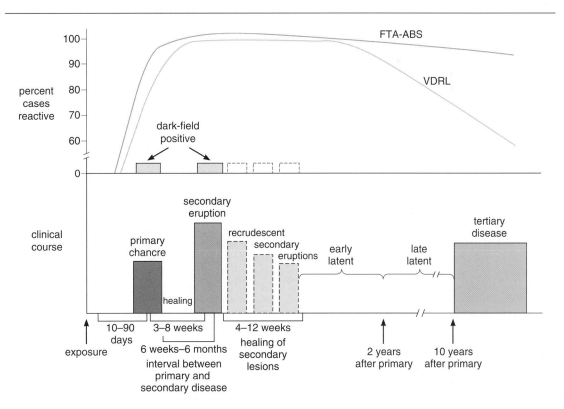

Figure 49–1. The course of untreated syphilis. (Reproduced, with permission, from Joklik WK et al (editors): *Zinsser Microbiology,* 20th ed. Appleton-Century-Crofts, 1992.) Abbreviations: FTA-ABS = fluorescent-treponemal antibody absorbance test; VDRL = Venereal Disease Research Laboratory.

logic properties of spirochetal lipoproteins). Studies of the natural history of untreated syphilis suggest that about a third of patients develop tertiary manifestations, with gummas and cardiovascular syphilis more common than neurosyphilis. Males are more likely to develop tertiary syphilis and have higher mortality rates than women. Irreversible tissue damage is characteristic of tertiary and congenital disease, even with antibiotic therapy.

Prevention

A five-point syphilis control plan, initiated in 1937, has been generally successful in controlling the disease. This plan employs a number of containment strategies, including public education, surveillance, and aggressive treatment of afflicted individuals and their partners. Public education campaigns are directed toward recognition of disease and implementation of preventive measures such as use of condoms and safe sex practices. Screening at-risk populations, especially drug users and patients with other sexually transmitted diseases, is more cost-effective than screening the general population as a whole. All pregnant women must be screened for syphilis; routine premarital screening, however, is no longer required. Prompt treatment of affected individuals, partner notification, and prophylactic treatment of sexual contacts are essential to limit spread of the disease. Although syphilis is readily responsive to antibiotic therapy, public health concerns regarding transmission of other sexually acquired diseases (especially HIV) have intensified research interest in the development of an effective syphilis vaccine. The recent sequencing of the *T pallidum* genome may facilitate this endeavor.

LYME DISEASE

General Considerations

Lyme disease is a multisystem disorder caused by infection with the tick-transmitted spirochete, *Borrelia burgdorferi*. Since its initial recognition as a clinical entity in 1977 in the region of Lyme, Connecticut (after which it is named), Lyme disease has increased in incidence and expanded geographically so that it is now the most common vector-borne disease in the United States. More than 95,000 cases have been reported since CDC surveillance began in 1982. Although early infection is usually responsive to antibiotics, delay in diagnosis and disseminated infection can lead to recurrent or chronic manifestations that are inexplicably more difficult to cure. The potential for chronic, disabling signs and symptoms has made Lyme disease a major public health concern.

Areas endemic for Lyme disease have environmental features that favor the passage of *Borrelia burgdorferi* between its two principal hosts: ticks and mammals. *Borrelia burgdorferi* is transmitted by hard-shelled ticks of the *Ixodes* family. These tiny ticks pass through three developmental stages—larvae, nymph, and adult—during their 2-year life span. Ticks feed only once per developmental stage and acquire infection with *Borrelia burgdorferi* during ingestion of a blood meal from an infected host. Because infection is not passed transovarially in ticks, a competent reservoir for spirochetes is necessary to maintain *B burgdorferi* in nature. The reservoir host varies regionally, with small rodents such as the white-footed mouse serving this role in the northeastern United States. Larvae feed preferentially on small rodents and are the first stage to acquire infection, whereas adult ticks feed almost exclusively on deer (hence the common name "deer tick"). The promiscuous feeding pattern of the nymph typically allows for transmission of infection to humans. The seasonal occurrence of Lyme disease (late spring through early fall) parallels the feeding pattern of the nymphal tick.

Clinical Manifestations

As a subacute pathogen, *B burgdorferi* is not a particularly aggressive organism and requires its hosts (mammal and tick) to survive in order to maintain its own persistence in nature. Disease is due largely to the host immune response to spirochete products, especially lipidated outer membrane proteins (Osps), rather than to tissue injury from the pathogen itself. Lyme disease occurs in stages that reflect the in vivo maneuvering of the spirochete as it adapts to and persists in the mammalian host. Spirochetes deposited within the skin during tick feeding can remain localized to the inoculation site, or they may disseminate through the connective tissue of the skin and via the bloodstream to distant organ sites. Once spirochetes penetrate the vasculature, all tissues can become infected at least transiently. Clinically apparent disease is most prevalent in the skin, heart, joints, and nervous system.

Early, Localized Lyme Disease. The hallmark of early, localized Lyme disease is the skin rash, **erythema migrans** (EM). EM manifests at the site of tick bite within 3–30 days and presents classically as an expanding, erythematous lesion (>4 cm in diameter) with central clearing. The rash is nonpruritic and relatively asymptomatic, although it can be associated with a tingling sensation. Less classic EM presents without the bull's eye appearance as a single flat, macular lesion or with necrotic, vesicular, or ulcerating centers. Localized EM can be associated with systemic flu-like symptoms such as fatigue, malaise, arthralgia and myalgia, headache, and stiff neck. Overt signs of inflammation outside of the skin are absent (eg, in the joints and cerebrospinal fluid), and spirochetes cannot be cultured from sites other than the leading margin of the EM lesion. Systemic symptoms are therefore believed to be due to cytokines released during the acute-phase response rather than to true disseminated infection.

Acute Disseminated Lyme Disease. Dissemination of spirochetes from the skin is clinically apparent within weeks to months of initial infection. In animal models, and presumably humans, spirochetes can infect all tissues; disease in humans presents primarily in the skin, joints, heart, and nervous system. Inflammatory changes can rarely occur in other sites, as, for example, the eye (panophthalmitis, keratitis) and muscle (focal myositis). Spirochetes in the skin can give rise to EM lesions distant from the tick inoculation site; secondary lesions are generally smaller than the primary lesion. Acute Lyme arthritis is monoarticular, affecting the knee in 80% of cases, followed by the shoulder, ankle, elbow, and temporomandibular joint. It is unusual for Lyme arthritis to involve more than three joints or to cause disease in the small joints of the hands and feet. Arthritis typically begins with the sudden onset of pain and swelling in the afflicted joint, with massive effusions (>50–100 mL) common. The degree of pain is disproportionately less than the amount of swelling, reminiscent of the asymmetric arthritis of the seronegative spondyloarthropathies. The inflammation subsides in days to weeks (median 8 days) even without antibiotic therapy. Untreated patients may have recurrent attacks in the same joint. Synovial fluid is inflammatory, with a marked predominance of neutrophils. In addition to arthritis, periarticular inflammation of tendons and bursae is often present. This gives rise to episodic tendinitis and bursitis, especially around joints afflicted with arthritis. Heel pain and sausage digits can be seen.

Neurologic abnormalities characteristic of acute disseminated Lyme disease involve both the peripheral and central nervous systems and include cranial neuropathies, peripheral radiculopathies, and meningitis. Unilateral Bell's palsy, due to involvement of cranial nerve VII, is the most common cranial neuropathy; Lyme disease is one of the rare causes of bilateral facial palsy. Other cranial nerves may be involved, especially those affecting ocular muscle function, but involvement of the lower cranial nerves (IX–XII) is uncommon. Peripheral nervous system disease presents most often as a mild, patchy, sensorimotor neuropathy. Painful peripheral radiculoneuropathies that follow dermatomal distributions have also been described and typically present with unilateral involvement of the extremity. Untreated patients with unilateral radiculopathy can develop involvement of the opposite extremity with time, giving the appearance of a symmetric disorder. Neurophysiology tests show abnormalities in sensory nerves, and limited biopsy data reveal epineural perivascular inflammation. Patients with meningitis present with headache and meningeal signs. Cerebrospinal fluid analysis reveals a lymphocytic pleocytosis with normal glucose and occasionally oligoclonal bands. *Borrelia burgdorferi*-specific intrathecal antibodies are often present and provide a useful diagnostic tool to distinguish neuroborreliosis from other forms of lymphocytic meningitis. Spirochete penetration into the subarachnoid space with secondary inflammation is believed to be the cause of meningitis. Rarely, mild encephalitis accompanies meningitis, indicating central nervous system involvement.

Carditis occurs in 8% of patients with disseminated Lyme disease and characteristically presents as varying degrees of atrioventricular heart block that can progress to complete heart block. Placement of a temporary pacemaker may be necessary, but permanent pacemakers are rarely required in the absence of underlying conduction system disease. Myopericarditis due to *B burgdorferi* penetration of the heart tissue and secondary lymphoplasmacytic infiltrates can lead to cardiac dysfunction, but chronic cardiomyopathy is rare. Valvular heart disease is absent.

Features of disseminated Lyme disease can occur sequentially or concomitantly. Fatigue and migratory musculoskeletal pain are dominant symptoms at this stage. As with localized EM, signs of disseminated Lyme disease resolve spontaneously without specific therapy, although spirochetes persist within tissues. Fatigue generally remains. The majority of patients with acute disseminated Lyme disease have objective signs of disease and positive serologic tests for *B burgdorferi*.

Chronic Lyme Disease. A small proportion (<10%) of patients with acute Lyme disease develop chronic signs and symptoms involving the skin, joints, or nervous system. The skin lesion acrodermatitis chronica atrophicans (ACA) has been reported in 10% of Lyme disease patients in Europe. This lesion appears first as erythema and pigmentation, followed by hypopigmentation and atrophy of the skin, giving it a cellophane-like quality. The *B burgdorferi* serotype *B afzelii* can be cultured from ACA lesions; this serotype is found primarily in Europe and accounts for the rarity of this skin manifestation in the United States. The inflammatory phase of ACA responds readily to antibiotics.

Ten percent of patients with intermittent oligoarthritis develop persistent joint inflammation with pannus formation and bony destruction. Histopathology of the synovium reveals features similar to rheumatoid arthritis, with fibrous deposition, villous hypertrophy, vascular proliferation, and mononuclear cell infiltration. Patients with chronic Lyme arthritis have high-titer *B burgdorferi*-specific IgG and are more likely to have specific antibody to the spirochete lipoprotein Osp A than patients with other manifestations of Lyme disease. Tests for rheumatoid factor and antinuclear antibodies are negative. Patients with chronic arthritis unresponsive to antibiotics have a higher frequency of HLA-DR4 and HLA-DR2 compared with those who respond to therapy. It is currently debated whether chronic arthritis is due to persistent infection, continued immune responses to poorly degraded *B burgdorferi* antigens, or infection-induced autoimmunity.

About 5% of patients with untreated Lyme disease develop chronic neurologic symptoms, primarily subtle cognitive dysfunction, meningoencephalitis, or sensorimotor neuropathies. Neuropsychiatric testing in some cases reveals chronic organic brain dysfunction. Reports of Alzheimer's disease and multiple sclerosis-like syndromes are anecdotal. Persistent infection or irreversible neurologic damage could potentially explain these signs and symptoms.

Pathogenesis

Lyme disease begins when spirochetes present in tick salivary glands are deposited within the skin during tick feeding. Spirochetes reside in the midgut of unfed ticks and travel during the first 24 hours of tick feeding through the hemolymph to the tick salivary glands. Plasminogen, present in mammalian extracellular fluids ingested by the tick, facilitates this process. Spirochetes change phenotypically during their migration from tick midgut to salivary gland and also after deposition within the host. The outer surface proteins (Osps) A and B are dominantly expressed by spirochetes in the midgut, whereas those populating the salivary gland express abundant amounts of Osp C. Other lipoproteins, including decorin-binding protein A (DbpA), may be up-regulated in this process. DbpA binds decorin, a mammalian protein decorating collagen fibers; it is believed that DbpA facilitates attachment of spirochetes to the connective tissue matrix in the skin. Tick saliva contains immunosuppressive and anticoagulant properties that could increase spirochete infectivity. After replicating locally, spirochetes penetrate through the dermal layers of the skin and enter blood vessels where they disseminate widely. Disease severity is determined by a combination of factors, including spirochete virulence and number, and host genotype. A striking feature of *B burgdorferi* infection in humans and in animal models is the paucity of organisms present in diseased sites relative to the inflammatory response. Recent studies have shown that the lipidated Osps of *B burgdorferi* (and *T pallidum* lipoproteins) are potent stimulants of innate immune cells and can incite local inflammation when injected intradermally. Lipoproteins bind via their lipid moiety to the pattern recognition receptor Toll-like receptor 4 (TLR4) and, through a cascade of signaling events, activate NFκB to cause cell activation; the lipopolysaccharide coreceptor CD14 augments this response. *B burgdorferi* can up-regulate adhesion molecules, including E-selection, vascular cell adhesion molecule (VCAM)-1, and intercellular adhesion molecule (ICAM)-1 on vascular endothelial cells, facilitating the influx of innate immune cells to sites of infection. Spirochetes also up-regulate cytokines from endothelial cells, glial cells, and synovial cells. Indeed, much of the acute inflammation seen in Lyme disease may be stimulated by Osps, and regulation of Osp expression during the course of infec-

tion likely plays a significant role in disease activity. Nearly 10% of the genome is composed of genes that could potentially encode lipoproteins. Although the majority of Osps serve unknown biologic functions, their abundant representation within the genome suggests that they are critically important for spirochete biology.

Phagocytic cells readily ingest and kill *B burgdorferi* in vitro, releasing inflammatory mediators, including reactive oxygen intermediates (ROI), nitric oxide (NO), and cytokines in the process. Neither ROI nor NO appears essential for killing, because spirochetes are still killed by cells from patients with chronic granulomatous disease that do not produce ROI, and animals treated with inhibitors of nitric oxide synthase to abrogate NO production remain resistant to disease.

Specific B- and T-cell immunity is elicited by *B burgdorferi* infection, although the magnitude of these responses may vary according to spirochete virulence, pathogen burden, and host genetic factors. The mouse model of Lyme borreliosis has proven useful in determining the role of specific immunity in Lyme disease pathogenesis. Experimentally infected mice reproducibly develop acute arthritis and carditis within 2 weeks of spirochete inoculation; as in humans, disease undergoes regression even though spirochetes persist in tissues. Inflammatory infiltrates are composed largely of innate immune cells: Neutrophilic infiltrates predominate in joints, and macrophage infiltration of the base of the heart is characteristic of murine Lyme carditis. *B burgdorferi* causes similar disease manifestations in severe combined immunodeficient (SCID) mice, which lack B and T cells, confirming the important role of innate immune responses in the pathology associated with Lyme disease. In contrast to immunocompetent mice, disease does not regress in SCID mice. The components of specific immunity that mediate disease regression differ according to the site examined. Passive transfer of *B burgdorferi*-specific IgG is sufficient to induce arthritis regression in SCID and B-cell-deficient mice, but has no effect on carditis. In contrast, adoptive transfer of CD4 T cells into mice selectively deficient in αβ TCR+T cells facilitates carditis regression.

Although not required for arthritis regression, *B burgdorferi*-specific T cells can modulate arthritis severity. Studies using mice genetically deficient in CD4 or CD8 T cell subsets have suggested that both subsets can exacerbate arthritis in mice, and *B burgdorferi*-specific CD4 T cells can cause severe destructive arthritis in hamsters. The role of CD4 T helper (T_H) cells and their associated cytokines in disease is complex. *B burgdorferi*-specific T_H1 cells that produce proinflammatory cytokines, including IFNγ, can be found in patients with chronic Lyme disease and in mouse strains susceptible to severe disease, suggesting that T_H1 responses are detrimental to the host. This notion is supported by the dominance of T_H2 cell responses in one disease-resistant mouse strain (BALB/c). *B burgdorferi* elicits primarily T_H1 cells in the disease-resistant C57BL/6 mouse, however. Kinetic analysis of T_H cytokine responses in disease-resistant strains suggests that early proinflammatory cytokines may be beneficial to the host by promoting activation of innate immune cells, thereby facilitating the clearance of spirochetes. The antiinflammatory action of T_H2 cells, notably IL-4 production, correlates with accelerated regression of established disease, suggesting that their role is to reduce the inflammatory responses after spirochetes have been cleared. In this regard, it is noteworthy that a CD4 T_H1 cell line can protect mice against challenge infection, and neutralization of IL-12, a cytokine promoting T_H1 responses, results in a modest attenuation of disease at the expense of enhancing spirochete burden.

The Role of Autoimmunity in Lyme Disease.
Controversy surrounds whether chronic Lyme disease reflects persistent infection versus infection-induced autoimmunity. The frequent inability to detect spirochetes in chronically diseased tissues either by culture in vitro or by polymerase chain reaction (PCR) amplification of spirochete DNA suggests that in some cases, immune responses persist after the spirochete has been eliminated. Host responses are appropriate, if, for example, they are directed toward poorly degraded spirochetal antigens, or inappropriate (autoimmune), if they are perpetuated by host antigens resembling spirochete components (molecular mimicry). Specific immune responses to Osp A have been implicated in the development of treatment-resistant Lyme arthritis. High-titer Osp A antibodies and Osp A-specific T cells are more prevalent in patients with treatment-resistant Lyme arthritis, particularly those expressing HLA-DR4 or HLA-DR2 alleles. A peptide of Osp A from *B burgdorferi* has significant homology to human leukocyte function-associated antigen (LFA)-1, and T cells specific for the Osp A peptide can respond to human LFA-1 in vitro. Synovial T cells reactive with this epitope of Osp A can be detected in patients who have progressed to chronic, treatment-resistant Lyme arthritis, especially among individuals bearing HLA-DR4. LFA-1 is an adhesion molecule expressed throughout the body, and levels of expression are increased on inflamed synovium. It has been postulated that local major histocompatibility complex (MHC) class II presentation of the cross-reactive LFA-1 peptide perpetuates the Osp A T-cell response in the absence of spirochetes (and Osp A), thereby leading to chronic synovitis. Although supporting a role for molecular mimicry in the induction of chronic Lyme arthritis, these findings do not explain the apparent localization of autoimmunity to a single site when LFA-1 is expressed in other tissues and the ability of synovectomy to cure arthritis.

Cross-reactive antibodies to neuronal components may contribute to neuropathy and CNS dysfunction characteristic of chronic neuroborreliosis. Naturally arising antibodies to *B burgdorferi* flagellin can bind human heat shock protein 60 and immunization with *Borrelia* glycolipids can induce antibodies that bind host gangliosides in vitro. Despite these in vitro observations, there is no evidence that cross-reactive antibodies bind host tissue in vivo, and these antibodies do not cause disease in animal models.

Spirochete Persistence.
In both animal models and humans, spirochetes can persist in tissues in the absence of clinically apparent disease. These "host-adapted" spirochetes have been observed in extracellular locations within connective tissue in the absence of acute inflammation. At this stage, the host serum contains antibodies that can prevent new infection, but that immunity is unable to clear established infection. The spirochete could persist in the face of a protective immune response through antigenic variation and by gaining access to immunoprivileged sites. Although spirochetes can penetrate cells in vitro, there is no direct evidence that they persist intracellularly in vivo. In contrast, spirochetes are known to rapidly change Osp expression when passing from tick to mammal; modulation of surface expression of antigens by host-adapted spirochetes may therefore be an evasion strategy employed to avoid recruitment of innate immune cells and to prevent the binding of borreliacidal antibodies. A number of *B burgdorferi* proteins appear to be expressed exclusively in vivo, and antibodies to some of these can provide protection against tick-borne spirochete challenge. *B burgdorferi* also possesses a gene cassette, the *vls* locus, that is capable of producing hundreds of protein variants through the recombination of a single gene with a group of nonexpressed genes. This system is analogous to the genes (*vmp*) encoding variable membrane protein of *B hermsii,* the agent of relapsing fever, although the recombination occurs in a random nature as opposed to the programmed rearrangements of the vmps. Antibodies to vls protein variants can be found in mice infected with *B burgdorferi,* indicating that the genes are expressed in vivo and their products are immunogenic. It has been estimated that a single *B burgdorferi* spirochete can give rise to hundreds of variants through genetic recombination of vls genes.

Diagnosis

The diagnosis of Lyme disease should be considered in an individual who has had environmental or occupational exposure to ticks and who presents with clinical features described earlier. Culture of *B burgdorferi* is the gold-standard for documentation of infection, but, except when performed on biopsy specimens of EM lesions, this method is relatively insensitive. Other methods such as PCR of body fluids or tissues for spirochete DNA are available only in specialized centers; urine antigen tests are of unproven accuracy. Serologic tests (enzyme-linked immunosorbent assay [ELISA] and immunoblot) are available commercially; although sensitive and specific, they are not standardized among laboratories and can only be used to confirm exposure to *B burgdorferi,* not prove active infection. *B burgdorferi* shares many proteins in common with other bacteria for which antibodies may cross-react and yield false-positive tests. One of the earliest antigens targeted by antibodies is the 41-kd flagellar protein; antiflagellin antibodies are seen in other conditions involving flagellated organisms, including those due to oral spirochetes. *B burgdorferi* is a sticky organism, and hypergammaglobulinemia or high-titer IgM antibodies (eg, rheumatoid factor) can give rise to false-positive tests. Patients with early Lyme disease can have negative serologic tests if they are treated early or their sera is examined prior to the development of detectable levels of anti-*B burgdorferi* antibodies. Patients with disseminated disease are generally seropositive. Immunoblots should be performed in patients who test positive by ELISA to confirm the presence of antibodies characteristic of *B burgdorferi* infection. It is anticipated that recombinant forms of *B burgdorferi* antigens expressed in vivo will be incorporated into serologic tests and enhance their sensitivity and specificity. The Centers for Disease Control has published guidelines for the use of serologic testing to support the diagnosis of Lyme disease.

Differential Diagnosis

The protean manifestations of Lyme disease have resulted in its nickname, the "new great imitator." EM remains the single most characteristic feature of Lyme disease, but may be overlooked or absent; other skin conditions, including erythema multiforme and common insect bites, can be mistaken for EM. The Lyme disease vaccine, which retains the lipid moiety of Osp A, can give rise to an EM-like lesion within hours to days of vaccination. Joint inflammation resembles the arthritis of the seronegative spondyloarthropathies and juvenile rheumatoid arthritis. Even in areas endemic for *B burgdorferi,* viral causes of Bell's palsy and aseptic meningitis are more common than Lyme disease. Musculoskeletal pain and fatigue must be distinguished from fibromyalgia and chronic fatigue syndrome. Because the diagnosis is largely based on clinical presentation, with serologic tests providing supporting evidence, it is critical that appropriate risk factors for acquiring the disease are present and that other causes of signs and symptoms have been excluded.

Treatment & Prognosis

Oral therapy with amoxicillin or doxycycline for 2–4 weeks is effective in early disease and for treating isolated Bell's palsy. Disseminated infection is generally treated with intravenous antibiotics to ensure adequate CNS penetration, but oral therapy has been used in acute arthritis with equivalent outcomes. As a rule, the duration of disease prior to institution of antibiotic therapy predicts time to response; chronic neurologic or arthritis manifestations may take months to resolve in some patients, and some may fail to respond. The most common cause of failure to respond to antibiotics is an inaccurate diagnosis of Lyme disease. Lyme disease can result in fibromyalgia and chronic fatigue that is unresponsive to antibiotic therapy.

Prevention

Strategies for prevention of Lyme disease include (1) environmental measures; (2) methods for decreasing human exposure to ticks; and (3) vaccination. Elimination of wooded and brushy areas can deter deer from populating the region, and spraying properties with insecticides can reduce the local tick population. For individuals in endemic areas, wearing clothing that limits skin exposure to ticks, use of insect repellent sprays containing DEET, and daily personal surveillance for ticks can reduce the risk of acquiring Lyme disease. A Lyme disease vaccine that uses the *B burgdorferi* Osp A lipoprotein as a vaccine antigen has recently received FDA approval for adults. Immunization requires three injections to achieve nearly 80% efficacy in preventing Lyme disease, but protective antibody titers wane rapidly. It is anticipated that yearly boosters will be required to maintain protective immunity. Osp A expression is diminished on spirochetes prior to their deposition within the mammal, and the vaccine has no effect on spirochetes that have entered the host. Instead, spirochetes are killed by borreliacidal Osp A antibodies that enter the tick midgut during the first 24 hours of feeding; thus, the vaccine prevents transmission of the spirochete. Phase I–III studies have demonstrated that the vaccine is relatively safe; however, because Osp A immune responses have been linked to chronic arthritis, concern exists over long-term effects, especially with frequent vaccination. Other *B burgdorferi* antigens, notably the in vivo expressed proteins Osp C and DbpA, are under investigation as candidate vaccine antigens.

REFERENCES

SPIROCHETES

Norris SJ, Larsen SA: *Treponema* and other host-associated spirochetes. In: *Manual of Clinical Microbiology,* 6th ed. Murray PR et al (editors). ASM Press, 1995.

Joklik WK et al: The spirochetes. In: *Zinsser Microbiology.* Joklik WK et al (editors): Appleton & Lange, 1992.

SYPHILIS

Singh AE, Romanowski B: Syphilis: Review with emphasis on clinical, epidemiologic, and some biologic features. *Clin Microbiol Rev* 1999;12:187.

Fraser CM et al: Complete genome sequence of *Treponema pallidum,* the syphilis spirochete. *Science* 1998;281:375.

Radolf JD et al: *Treponema pallidum*: Doing a remarkable job with what it's got. *Trends Microbiol* 1999;7:7.

Blanco DR et al: Cellular and molecular pathogenesis of syphilis. In: *Microbial Determinants of Virulence and Host Response,* Ayoub EM et al (editors). American Society of Microbiology, 1990.

Lukehart SA: Immunology and pathogenesis of syphilis. In: *Advances in Host Defense Mechanisms,* Gallin JI, Fauci AS (editors). Raven Press, 1992.

Centurion-Lara A et al: *Treponema pallidum* major sheath protein homologue Tpr K is a target of opsonic antibody and the protective immune response. *J Exp Med* 1999;189:647.

Blanco DR et al: Immunization with *Treponema pallidum* outer membrane vesicles induces high-titer complement-dependent treponemicidal activity and aggregation of *T pallidum* rare outer membrane proteins (TROMPs). *J Immunol* 1999;163:2741.

Centers for Disease Control and Prevention: 1998 guidelines for treatment of sexually transmitted diseases. *MMWR Morb Mortal Wkly Rep* 1998;47:28.

St. Louis ME: Strategies for syphilis prevention in the 1990s. *Sex Transm Dis* 1996;23:58.

LYME DISEASE

Radolf JD: Role of outer membrane architecture in immune evasion by *Treponema pallidum* and *Borrelia burgdorferi. Trends Microbiol* 1994;2:307.

Fraser CM et al: Genomic sequence of a Lyme disease spirochete, *Borrelia burgdorferi. Nature* 1997;390:580.

Barbour AG, Zuckert WR: New tricks of tick-borne pathogen. *Nature* 1997;390:553.

Bockenstedt LK, Malawista SE: Lyme disease. In: *Clinical Immunology: Principles and Practice,* Rich RR (editor). Mosby-Year Book Inc., 1996.

Evans J: Lyme disease. *Curr Opin Rheumatol* 1998;10:339.

Seiler KP, Weis JJ: Immunity to Lyme disease: Protection, pathology and persistence. *Curr Opin Immunol* 1996; 8:503.

Zhang J-R et al: Antigenic variation in Lyme disease borreliae by promiscuous recombination of VMP-like sequence cassettes. *Cell* 1997;89:275.

Brightbill HD et al: Host defense mechanisms triggered by microbial lipoproteins through toll-like receptors. *Science* 1999;285:732.

Hirschfeld M et al: Inflammatory signaling by *Borrelia burgdorferi* lipoproteins is mediated by toll-like receptor 2. *J Immunol* 1999;163:2382.

Kalish RA et al: Association of treatment-resistant chronic Lyme arthritis with HLA-DR4 and antibody reactivity to Osp A and Osp B of *Borrelia burgdorferi. Infect Immunol* 1993;61:2774.

Kamradt T et al: Dominant recognition of a *Borrelia burgdorferi* outer surface protein A peptide by T helper cells in patients with treatment-resistant Lyme arthritis. *Infect Immunol* 1996;64:1284.

Gross D et al: Identification of LFA-1 as a candidate autoantigen in treatment-resistant Lyme arthritis. *Science* 1998;281:703.

Centers for Disease Control and Prevention: Recommendations for test performance from the second national conference on serologic diagnosis of Lyme disease. *MMWR Morb Mortal Wkly Rep* 1995;44:590.

Steere AC et al: Vaccination against Lyme disease with recombinant *Borrelia burgdorferi* outer-surface lipoprotein A with adjuvant. Lyme Disease Vaccine Study Group. *New Engl J Med* 1998;339:209.

Sigal LH et al: A vaccine consisting of recombinant *Borrelia burgdorferi* outer-surface protein A to prevent Lyme disease. *New Engl J Med* 1998;339:216.

Centers for Disease Control and Prevention: Recommendations for the use of Lyme disease vaccine. *MMWR Morb Mortal Wkly Rep* 1999;48:1.

Section IV.
Immunologic Therapy

Immunization

50

Moses Grossman, MD & Abba I. Terr, MD

The goal of immunization in any one individual is the **prevention** of disease. The goal of immunization of populations is the **eradication** of disease. Immunization has accounted for spectacular advances in health around the world. Childhood immunizations are part of routine health care; the government has financed the purchase of vaccines for the public, and all states have laws requiring proof of immunization as a condition for school entry. As a result, poliomyelitis, diphtheria, and tetanus have all but disappeared in developed nations; measles, rubella, and pertussis are now rare. Smallpox has been eradicated, and the World Health Organization has made poliomyelitis the next target for eradication.

HISTORICAL OVERVIEW

For centuries we have known that individuals who recover from certain diseases are protected from reinfection. The moderately successful but hazardous introduction of small quantities of fluid from the pustules of smallpox into the skin of uninfected persons (variolation) was an effort to imitate this natural phenomenon. Edward Jenner's introduction of vaccination with cowpox virus (1796) to protect against smallpox was the first documented use of a live, attenuated viral vaccine and the beginning of modern immunization. Robert Koch demonstrated the specific bacterial cause of anthrax in 1876, and the causes of several common illnesses were rapidly identified thereafter. Successful immunizations followed (Table 50–1).

TYPES OF IMMUNIZATION

Immunization may be **active:** administration of an antigen (usually as a modified infectious agent or toxin) for active production of immunity or **passive:** administration of antibody-containing serum or sensitized cells for passive protection of the recipient.

ACTIVE IMMUNIZATION

Active immunization results in the production of antibodies directed against the infecting agent or its toxic products; it may also initiate cellular responses mediated by lymphocytes and macrophages. The most important protective antibodies include those that inactivate soluble toxic protein products of bacteria (antitoxins), facilitate phagocytosis and intracellular digestion of bacteria (opsonins), interact with the components of serum complement to damage the bacterial membrane and hence cause bacteriolysis (lysins), or prevent the proliferation of infectious virus (neutralizing antibodies). Newly appreciated are the antibodies that interact with components of the bacterial surface to prevent adhesion to mucosal surfaces (antiadhesins). Some antibodies may not be protective and, by "blocking" the reaction of protective antibodies with the pathogen, may actually depress the body's defenses.

Antigens react with antibodies in the bloodstream and extracellular fluid and at mucosal surfaces. Antibodies cannot readily reach intracellular sites of infection where viral replication occurs. They are effective against many viral diseases in two ways, however: (1) by interacting with the virus before initial intracellular penetration occurs and (2) by preventing locally replicating virus from disseminating from the site of entry to an important target organ, as in the spread of poliovirus from the gastrointestinal tract to the central nervous system or of rabies virus from a puncture wound to peripheral neural tissue. Lymphocytes acting alone and antibody interacting with lymphoid or monocytic effector K cells may

Table 50–1. Historical milestones in immunization.

Variolation	1721
Vaccination	1796
Rabies vaccine	1885
Diphtheria toxoid	1925
Tetanus toxoid	1925
Pertussis vaccine	1925
Viral culture in chick embryo	1931
Yellow fever vaccine	1937
Influenza vaccine	1943
Viral tissue culture	1949
Poliovaccine, inactivated (Salk)	1954
Poliovaccine, live, attenuated (Sabin)	1956
Measles vaccine	1960
Tetanus immune globulin (human)	1962
Rubella vaccine	1966
Mumps vaccine	1967
Hepatitis B vaccine	1975
Smallpox eradicated	1980
First recombinant vaccine (hepatitis B)	1986
Conjugate polysaccharide vaccine for *H influenzae* B	1988
Poliomyelitis eliminated from Western Hemisphere	1994
Varicella-zoster vaccine	1995
Hepatitis A vaccine	1995
Rotavirus vaccine	1998
Lyme disease vaccine	1999

also recognize surface changes in virus-infected cells and destroy these infected "foreign" cells.

Types of Vaccines

The agent used for active immunization is termed *antigen, immunogen,* or *vaccine.* It may consist of **live, attenuated** viruses (measles virus) or bacteria (bacillus Calmette–Guérin [BCG]) or **killed** microorganisms (*Vibrio cholerae*). It may also be an **inactivated** bacterial product (tetanus toxoid) or a specific single **component** of bacteria (polysaccharide of *Neisseria meningitidis*). Such a polysaccharide component may be conjugated to a protein in order to produce immunogenicity at an earlier age (conjugated *Haemophilus influenzae*). It may be a **recombinant DNA** segment (hepatitis B virus), in which case it would be expressed in another living cell (yeasts, *Escherichia coli*). In each case, it usually contains—in addition to the desired antigen—other ingredients including other antigens, suspending fluids that may be complex and may contain protein ingredients of their own (tissue culture, egg yolk), preservatives, and adjuvants for enhanced immunogenicity (aluminum, protein conjugate). Undesirable reactions may occur not only to the antigen itself but also to these added components.

Active immunization with living organisms is generally superior to immunization with killed vaccines in inducing a long-lived immune response. A single dose of a live, attenuated virus vaccine often suffices for reliable immunization. Multiple immunizations are recommended for poliovirus in case intercurrent enteroviral infection or interference among three simultaneously administered virus types in the trivalent vaccine prevents completely successful primary immunization. The persistence of immunity to many viral infections may be explained by repeated natural reexposure to new cases in the community, the unusually large antigenic stimulus provided by infection with a living agent, or other mechanisms such as the persistence of latent virus.

All immunizing materials—live organisms in particular—must be properly stored to retain effectiveness. Serious failures of smallpox and measles immunization have resulted from inadequate refrigeration prior to use. Agents presently licensed for active immunization are listed in Table 50–2.

Factors in Immunization

Primary active immunization produces a protective antibody level more slowly than the incubation period of most infections and must therefore be performed prior to exposure to the causative agent. By contrast, "booster" reimmunization in a previously immune individual provides a rapid secondary (anamnestic) increase in immunity.

Previous infection can also substantially alter the response to an inactivated vaccine. For example, volunteers who have recovered from cholera or who live in a cholera-endemic area respond to parenteral immunization with an increase in anticholera secretory IgA, which is not seen in immunized control subjects.

The **route** of immunization may be an important determinant of successful vaccination, particularly if nonreplicating immunogens are used. Thus, immunization intranasally or by aerosol, which stimulates mucosal immunity, often appears to be more successful than parenteral injection against viral or bacterial respiratory challenges.

The route of administration recommended by the manufacturer and approved by the FDA should be used. Vaccines containing **adjuvants** such as aluminum hydroxide should always be given deep into the muscle, ideally in the anterolateral portion of the upper thigh, and not subcutaneously.

The **timing** of primary immunization, the interval between doses, and the timing of booster injections are based on both theoretic considerations and empiric vaccine trials. The resulting recommendations should be followed closely. Many factors are involved. For instance, the age at which measles immunization is administered in the United States was changed from 12 to 15 months because the persistent maternal antibody, although present in small amounts only, was shown to interfere with active antibody formation by the child. Ironically, now that most mothers have induced immunity rather than naturally acquired measles antibody, their lower antibody titer may require that childhood immunization be changed back to 12 months of age.

Because of the clonal nature of immunity, it is possible—and, in fact, routine practice—to give many different antigens simultaneously. Some antigens are premixed (measles, mumps, rubella [MMR] and

Table 50–2. Vaccines for active immunization.

Disease	Product	Type of Agents (Route of Administration)
Cholera	Cholera vaccine	Killed bacteria (Sc, IM, ID)
Diphtheria	DTP, DTaP, DT (adsorbed for child under age 7) also available in combination with conjugated *H influenzae* vaccine; Td (adsorbed) for all others.	Toxoid (IM)
Haemophilus influenzae infections	Polysaccharide capsule conjugated with protein	Polysaccharide protein conjugate (IM)
Hepatitis A	Hepatitis A vaccine	Inactivated hepatitis A virus (IM)
Hepatitis B	Hepatitis B vaccine (human carriers). (Recombinant DNA, produced in yeast cells	Recombinant antigen or formalin-treated purified antigen (IM)
Influenza	Influenza virus vaccine. Monovalent or bivalent (chick embryo). Composition of the vaccine is varied depending on epidemiologic circumstances	Killed whole or split virus types A and B (IM)
Japanese encephalitis	Japanese encephalitis vaccine	Inactivated virus derived from mouse brain (SC)
Measles[a]	Measles virus vaccine, live (chick embryo)	Live attenuated virus (SC)
Meningococcus	Meningococcal polysaccharide vaccine (combination vaccine against groups A, C, Y, and W135)	Polysaccharide (SC)
Mumps[b]	Mumps virus vaccine, live (chick embryo)	Live virus (SC)
Pertussis	DTP, DTaP	Killed bacteria. Also an "acellular" vaccine containing two or more antigens but not the whole cell (IM)
Plague	Plague vaccine	Killed bacteria (IM)
Pneumococcus	Pneumococcal polysaccharide vaccine, polyvalent	Polysaccharide (SC, IM)
Poliomyelitis	Poliovirus vaccine, live, oral, trivalent (monkey kidney, human diploid)	Live virus types I, II, III (oral)
	Poliomyelitis vaccine, inactivated	Killed virus types I, II, III (IM)
Rabies	Rabies vaccine (human diploid)	Killed virus (IM or ID [preexposure only])
Rubella[b]	Rubella virus vaccine, live (human diploid)	Live attenuated virus (SC)
Smallpox	Smallpox vaccine (calf lymph, chick embryo). (Available from CDC)	Live vaccinia virus ID)
Tetanus	DTP, DT (adsorbed) for children under age 7; Td, T (adsorbed) for all others	Toxoid (IM)
Tuberculosis	BCG vaccine	Live attenuated-*Mycobacterium bovis* (ID, SC)
Typhoid	Typhoid vaccine	Killed bacteria (SC)
		Live attenuated bacteria (oral)
Varicella	Varicella vaccine	Live attenuated virus (SC)
Yellow fever	Yellow fever vaccine (chick embryo)	Live virus (SC)
Lyme disease	Lyme disease vaccine	*Borrelia burgdorferi* lipidated protein A (IM)
Rotavirus infantile gastroenteritis	Rotavirus vaccine rhesus-based tetravalent	Live virus modified by gene reassortment (oral)

Abbreviations: DTP = diphtheria, tetanus, pertussis; DT = diphtheria, tetanus; SC = subcutaneous; IM = intramuscular; ID = intradermal.
[a] Consult manufacturer's package insert for further information.
[b] Combination vaccines are available.

diphtheria, pertussis, tetanus [DPT]), whereas others may be given on the same day at different sites (MMR and varicella-zoster [VZV]). Live virus vaccines that are not given on the same day, however, should be given at least 1 month apart.

Splenectomy may markedly impair the primary antibody response to thymus-independent antigens such as bacterial polysaccharides, although many splenectomized patients respond normally to polysaccharide antigens because of priming by natural exposure prior to splenectomy.

Technique of Immunization

When administering subcutaneous or intramuscular vaccines, it is essential to pull back on the syringe before depressing the plunger to make certain that they will not be injected intravenously, resulting in lessened immunizing effect and increased untoward reactions. It is particularly important to use a sufficiently long needle (usually >1 in.) for intramuscular delivery of adjuvant-containing (eg, alum [aluminum phosphate]-adsorbed) vaccines to prevent subcutaneous necrosis.

Recent studies of injection techniques suggest that the anterolateral thigh or deltoid site is preferable to the buttocks to avoid sciatic nerve damage or delivery into fat.

The intradermal route of immunization is under intensive study as a means of obtaining an earlier or greater immune response with the same amount of antigen or of inducing a satisfactory immune response with a smaller quantity of expensive immunogens, such as the hepatitis B and rabies vaccines.

Adverse Reactions & the Risk-Benefit Ratio

All vaccines approved and licensed in the United States have been shown to be safe and effective. Each, however, has also been shown to cause adverse reactions. Sometimes these are minimal in occurrence rate and severity, as in tetanus toxoid. Historically, some immunizing agents produced adverse reactions that were so severe they would be unacceptable today; variolation and the original rabies vaccine made from spinal cord material are two examples. Smallpox vaccination with vaccinia virus carried a very acceptable risk at a time when smallpox posed an imminent and serious threat. Now that smallpox is eradicated, the risk-benefit ratio of the vaccine is infinite. At present, the most controversial vaccine in routine use is the whole-cell pertussis vaccine. It is only about 70% effective for protection, causes very frequent minor reaction, and occasionally produces serious neurologic reactions. It is still used, however, because the risk–benefit ratio is acceptably low. Japan, the United Kingdom, and Sweden have experienced a significant rise in the fatality rate from pertussis since the use of the vaccine was discontinued. This whole-cell vaccine is currently being supplanted by an acellular pertussis vaccine, which is at least as effective but with fewer side effects.

Unique Hazards of Live Vaccines

Because of their potential for infection of the fetus, live vaccines should *not* be given to a pregnant woman unless she is in immediate high risk of infection (eg, a poliomyelitis epidemic). A pregnant woman traveling in an area where yellow fever is endemic *should* be immunized because the risk of infection exceeds the small theoretic hazard to fetus and mother. If yellow fever vaccination is being performed solely to comply with a legal requirement for international travel, however, the woman should seek a waiver with a letter from her physician.

Live vaccines, can cause serious or even fatal illness in an immunologically incompetent host. They generally should not be given to patients receiving corticosteroids, alkylating drugs, radiation, or other immunosuppressive drugs or to individuals with known or suspected congenital or acquired defects in cell-mediated immunity (eg, severe combined immunodeficiency disease, leukemias, lymphomas, Hodgkin's disease, and HIV infection). Patients with pure hypogammaglobulinemia and normal cell-mediated immunity usually tolerate viral infections and vaccines well but have a 10,000-fold excess of paralytic complications over the usual one case per million recipients, in part because of the frequent reversion of attenuated poliovirus strains to virulence in the intestinal tract. Because live poliovirus is shed by recipients, it should not be given to household contacts of these patients either.

Even in immunocompetent hosts, live vaccines may result in mild or, rarely, severe disease.

The early measles vaccines caused high fever and rash in a significant proportion of recipients. The mild, recurrent arthralgia or arthritis that can follow rubella immunization may represent the consequences of a secondary rather than a primary infection in an individual who has low levels of antibodies not detected by all assays and who has in vitro evidence of cell-mediated immunity.

Because passage through the human intestinal tract occasionally results in reversion of oral attenuated poliovirus vaccine (particularly type III) to neurovirulence, paralytic illness has occurred in recipients or, rarely, their nonimmune contacts, especially adults. The success of live polio vaccines in preventing widespread natural infection has resulted in the paradox that the vaccine itself now accounts for a large portion of the few cases of paralytic poliomyelitis seen each year in theUnited States. Killed (Salk) vaccine also appears to be effective in abolishing polio. The major advantages of live (Sabin) vaccine, which sustain its use despite the small risk of paralysis (5 cases per million doses in nonimmune recipients), are its ease of administration and more durable immune response. It is likely that a schedule combining the sequential administration of both vaccines will be introduced within the next few years.

Live vaccines may contain undetected and undesirable **contaminants.** Epidemic hepatitis resulted in the past from vaccinia and yellow fever vaccines containing human serum. More recently, millions of people received SV40, a simian papovavirus contained in live or inactivated poliovirus vaccine prepared in monkey kidney tissue culture. Although a virus closely related to SV40 has been isolated from the brains of patients with progressive multifocal leukoencephalopathy, a lethal degenerative disease, there is no known history of polio immunization in these cases. A suspected risk of cancer in children of mothers who received inactivated polio vaccine during pregnancy was not confirmed in a 20-year follow-up of a large number of childhood recipients. SV40 can now be detected and excluded from human viral vaccines, but other undetected viruses might be transmitted by vaccines grown in nonhuman cell lines. Yellow fever vaccine has been reported to be probably contaminated with avian leukosis virus. Bacteriophages and probably bacterial endotoxins have also been shown to contaminate live virus vaccines, although without known hazard thus far.

Live viral vaccines probably do not interfere with tuberculin skin testing, although they depress some measurements of lymphocyte function.

Unlike live vaccines, inactivated vaccines may safely be given to immunocompromised hosts, although they may not dependably elicit an adequately protective immune response.

The risk–benefit ratio of live measles vaccine is sufficiently low to recommend its use in patients with human immunodeficiency virus (HIV) infection— even immunocompromised patients.

Other Adverse Effects

Allergic reactions may occur on exposure to egg protein (in measles, mumps, influenza, and yellow fever vaccines) or antibiotics or preservatives (eg, neomycin or mercurials) in viral vaccines. Patients with known IgE-mediated sensitivity to a vaccine component (eg, egg albumin in yellow fever vaccine grown in eggs) should not receive the vaccine unless successfully desensitized (in cases when immunization is essential). Occasionally, the product of a different manufacturer does not contain the offending allergen. Improvements in antigenicity and better purification procedures in vaccine production decrease the amount and number of foreign substances injected and result in fewer side effects.

Reporting Adverse Effects & Legal Liability

Litigation arising from adverse reaction to vaccines has greatly increased the cost of vaccines in recent years. This threat to development and production of new vaccines prompted the passage of the National Childhood Vaccine Injury Act of 1986, which provides for compensation of those injured by adverse reactions and also mandates that certain adverse effects be reported and that physicians use vaccine information pamphlets prepared by the Centers for Disease Control and Prevention (CDC) for information on benefits and risks of vaccines. These pamphlets are mandatory when government-purchased vaccine is used and can be obtained by calling 1-800-PIK-VIPS (1-800-745-8477). They are also available on the internet at *http://www.cdc.gov/.* Physicians and clinics purchasing their own vaccines may prepare their own information pamphlets.

The reportable events are listed in Table 50–3. Reports are to be made to the Vaccine Adverse Event Reporting System, 1-800-822-7267. Preventable adverse effects can be minimized by reading vaccine labels, storing vaccines carefully, using the correct method of administration at the proper site, and being aware of contraindications, particularly by identifying immunocompromised hosts.

PASSIVE IMMUNIZATION

Immunization may be accomplished passively by administering either preformed immunoreactive serum or cells.

Antibody, either as whole serum or as fractionated, concentrated immune (gamma) globulin that is predominantly IgG, may be obtained from human or animal donors who have recovered from an infectious disease or have been immunized. These antibodies may provide immediate protection to an antibody-deficient individual. Passive immunization is thus useful for individuals who cannot form antibodies or for the nonimmunocompromised host who might develop disease before active immunization could stimulate antibody production, which usually requires at least 7–10 days.

Additionally, passive immunization is useful when no active immunization is available, when passive immunization is used in conjunction with vaccine administration (eg, in rabies vaccination), in the management of specific effects of certain toxins and venoms, and, finally, as an immunosuppressant.

Antibody may be obtained from **humans** or **animals,** but animal sera produce an immune response in humans that leads to rapid clearance of the protective antibodies from the circulation of the recipient and the risk of allergic reactions, particularly serum sickness or anaphylaxis (see later section). Thus, to obtain a similar protective effect, much more animal antiserum must be injected compared with human antiserum (eg, 3000 units of equine tetanus antitoxin versus 300 units of human tetanus immune globulin).

Human Immune Globulin

This preparation is derived from alcohol fractionation of pooled plasma. The antibody content of im-

Table 50–3. Vaccine injury table.

Illness, Diability, Injury, or Condition Covered	Latent Period[a]
I. DTP; P; DT; Td; or tetanus toxoid; or in any combination with polio; or any other vaccine containing whole-cell pertussis bacteria, extracted or partial-cell pertussis bacteria, or specific pertussis antigen(s):	
A. Anaphylaxis or anaphylactic shock	4 hours
B. Encephalopathy (or encephalitis)	72 hours
C. Any sequela (including death) of an illness, disability, injury, or condition referred to above which illness, disability, injury, or condition arose within the time period prescribed.	Not applicable
II. (a). Measles, mumps, rubella, or any vaccine containing any of the foregoing as a component:	
A. Anaphylaxis or anaphylactic shock	4 hours
B. Encephalopathy (or encephalitis)	5–15 days (not less than 5 days and not more than 15 days) for measles, mumps, rubella, or any vaccine containing any of the foregoing as a component.
C. Residual seizure disorder in accordance with subsection (b)(3)	5–15 days (not less than 5 days and not more than 15 days) for measles, mumps, rubella, or any vaccine containing any of the foregoing as a component.
D. Any sequela (including death) of an illness, disability, injury, or condition referred to above which illness, disability, injury, or condition arose within the time period prescribed.	Not applicable
II. (b). In the case of measles, mumps, rubella (MMR), measles, rubella (MR) or rubella vaccines only:	
A. Chronic arthritis	42 days
B. Any sequela (including death) of an illness, disability, injury, or condition referred to above which illness, disability, injury, or condition arose within the time period prescribed.	Not applicable
III. Polio vaccine (other than inactivated polio vaccine):	
A. Paralytic polio	
In a nonimmunodeficient recipient	30 days
In an immunodeficient recipient	6 months
In a vaccine associated community case	Not applicable
B. Any acute complication or sequela (including death) of an illness, disability, injury, or condition referred to above which illness, disability, injury, or condition arose within the time period prescribed.	Not applicable
IV. Inactivated polio vaccine:	
A. Anaphylaxis or anaphylactic shock	4 hours
B. Any acute complication or sequela (including death) of an illness, disability, injury, or condition referred to above which illness, disability, injury, or condition arose within the time period prescribed.	Not applicable

Abbreviations: DTP = diphtheria, tetanus, pertussis; P = pertussis; DT = diphtheria, tetanus; Td = combined tetanus and diphtheria toxoid (adult type).
[a]Time of first symptom or manifestation of onset or of significant aggravation after vaccine administration.

mune globulin is almost all of the IgG isotype and reflects the infection and immunization experience of the donor pool. Three types of preparations are available: standard immune gamma globulin for intramuscular use (IMIG), standard immune globulin adapted for intravenous use (IVIG), and specific immune globulins with a known high content of antibody against a particular antigen; the last may be available for intravenous or intramuscular use.

Immune globulin should be given only for those indications where efficacy has been established. Although its side effects are minimal, the administration is painful, and rare anaphylactoid reactions have been described. It is not useful for the immunologically normal child or adult with frequent viral infections. There is no evidence that HIV infections can be transmitted by the administration of immune globulin. ***Caution:*** The intramuscular form should *never* be given intravenously; very serious systemic reactions may result from the presence of high-molecular-weight aggregated immunoglobulins.

IVIG is derived from the same pool of adult donors and also consists almost solely of IgG antibodies. The immune globulin has been adapted to intravenous use by eliminating high-molecular-weight complexes that may activate complement in the recipient. The advantages of the intravenous route are the ability to administer large doses of immune globulin, the more rapid onset of action, and the avoidance of intramuscular injections, which are painful and may be contraindicated because of a tendency to bleed. IVIG is particularly valuable as replacement therapy for antibody deficiency disorders and for the management of idiopathic thrombocytopenic purpura and Kawasaki disease. The cost, however, is approximately five times that of IMIG. Approximately 2.5% of patients receiving IVIG experience side effects of fever or vasoactive phenomena (usually vasodilatation), but these reactions can usually be prevented by slow administration of the material. IVIG has been used in formal clinical trials and informally for a number of other diseases with autoimmune features or of uncertain cause because of its ability to block cellular Fc receptors, but proof of efficacy in these cases remains unknown. Currently it is in short supply.

Special Preparations of Human Immune Globulin

Many preparations with a high titer of a specific antibody are available. These are prepared either by hyperimmunizing adult donors or by selecting lots of plasma tested for a high specific antibody content. Most of these are available in the intramuscular form; a few for intravenous use (Table 50–4).

Animal Sera & Antitoxins

These preparations are used only when human globulin is not available, because they carry a much higher risk of anaphylactic reactions. They are usually prepared from hyperimmunized horses or rabbits.

No antiserum of animal origin should be given without carefully inquiring about prior exposure or allergic response to any product of the specific animal source. Whenever a foreign antiserum is administered, a syringe containing aqueous epinephrine, 1:1000, should be available. If allergy (to foreign antiserum) is suspected by history or shown by skin testing and no alternative to serum therapy is possible, desensitization may be attempted as outlined in Chapter 30.

The various materials available for passive immunization, of both human and animal origin, are detailed in Table 50–4.

Passive Immunization in Noninfectious Diseases

A. Prevention of Rh Isoimmunization: Rh-negative women are at hazard of developing anti-Rh antibodies when Rh-positive erythrocytes enter their circulation. This occurs regularly during pregnancy with an Rh-positive fetus, whether the pregnancy ends in a term or preterm delivery or in abortion. It may also occur with other events listed here. The development of anti-Rh antibodies threatens all subsequent Rh-positive fetuses with **erythroblastosis.** This can be prevented by administration of Rh immune globulin to the mother.

Rh-negative females who have not already developed anti-Rh antibodies should receive 300 μg of Rh immune globulin within 72 hours after obstetric de-

Table 50–4. Materials available for passive immunization. (All are of human origin unless otherwise stated.)

Disease	Product[a]
Black widow spider bite	Antivenin widow spider, equine (IM,IV)
Botulism	ABE polyvalent antitoxin, equine (IM, IV)
Cytomegalovirus	CMV immune globulin (IV)
Diphtheria	Diphtheria antitoxin, equine (IM)
Hepatitis A	Immune globulin (IM)
Hepatitis B	Hepatitis B immune globulin (HBIG) (IM)
Hypogamma-globulinemia	Immune globulin (IM, IV)
Measles	Immune globulin (IM)
Rabies	Rabies immune globulin[b] (IM)
Rh isoimmunization (erythroblastosis fetalis)	Rh_o (D) immune globulin (IM)
Snakebite	Antivenin coral snake, equine. Antivenin rattlesnake, copperhead, and moccasin, equine (IV)
Tetanus	Tetanus immune globulin[c] (IM)
Vaccinia	Vaccinia immune globulin (IM)
Varicella	Varicella-zoster immune globulin (VZIG) (IM)[d]

Abbreviations: ABE = antibotulinum toxin, equine; CMV = cytomegalovirus; HBV = hepatitis B virus; IM = intramuscular; VIG = vaccinia immunoglobulin.
[a] Route of administration.
[b] Antirabies serum, equine, may be available but is much less desirable.
[c] Bovine and equine antitoxins may be available but are not recommended. They are used at 10 times the dose of tetanus immune globulin.
[d] Contact the regional blood center of the American Red Cross.
Note: Passive immunotherapy or immunoprophylaxis should always be administered as soon as possible after exposure to the offending agent. Immune antisera and globulin are always given intramuscularly unless otherwise noted. Always question carefully and test for hypersensitivity before administering animal sera.

livery, abortion, accidental transfusion with Rh-positive blood, chorionic villus biopsy, and, probably, amniocentesis, especially if the needle passes through the placenta. This passive immunization suppresses the mother's normal immune response to any Rh-positive fetal cells that may enter her circulation, thus avoiding erythroblastosis fetalis in future Rh-positive fetuses; it may protect in a nonspecific manner as well, analogous to the "blocking" effect of high-dose IgG in ameliorating autoimmune diseases such as idiopathic thrombocytopenic purpura. Even if more than 72 hours has elapsed after exposure, Rh immune globulin should still be administered because it is effective in at least some cases. Some investigators have also suggested the administration of anti-Rh globulin to Rh-negative newborn female offspring of Rh-positive mothers to prevent possible sensitization from maternal-fetal transfusion.

A significant number of Rh isoimmunizations occur during pregnancy rather than at the time of delivery. This can be almost completely prevented with anti-Rh globulin at 28 weeks of gestation. The American College of Obstetricians and Gynecologists recommends routine administration of 300 μg of Rh immune globulin at 28 weeks of gestation and again at delivery as soon as it is determined that the infant is Rh-positive. Prior to 28 weeks of gestation, any condition associated with fetomaternal hemorrhage (abortion, amniocentesis, ruptured ectopic pregnancy) should be treated with Rh immune globulin (a 50-μg "minidose" is used before 12 weeks and a standard 300-μg dose is used thereafter). A larger dose is necessary when a significant fetomaternal hemorrhage (more than 25 μg/mL of incompatible cells) has taken place.

B. Serum Therapy of Poisonous Bites: The toxicity of the bite of the black widow spider, the coral snake, and crotalid snakes (rattlesnakes and other pit vipers) may be lessened by the administration of commercially available antivenins. These are of equine origin, so the risk of serum sickness is high and the possibility of anaphylaxis must always be considered.

Antisera for scorpion stings and rarer poisonous bites, especially of species foreign to North America, may also be available.

Information on the use and availability of antivenins is often available from Poison Control Centers, particularly those in cities having large zoos, such as New York and San Diego. A Snakebite Trauma Center has been established at Jacobi Hospital in New York ([212] 430-8183). In addition, an antivenin index listing the availability of all such products is maintained by the Poison Control Center in Tucson, Arizona ([602] 626-6016 or 626-6000).

C. Kawasaki Syndrome: This severe disease, a form of generalized vasculitis, produces coronary artery aneurysms that may result in myocardial infarction in a significant number of cases. IVIG 400 mg/kg daily for 5 days given as early as possible during the acute phase of the disease substantially improves the outcome. A single 2-g/kg dose of IVIG administered over 10 hours is equally efficacious.

D. Thrombocytopenic Purpura: In this disease, IVIG is given because it presumably prolongs platelet survival by blocking Fc receptors for IgG on macrophages that ingest antibody-coated platelets.

Hazards of Passive Immunization

Illness may arise from a single injection of foreign serum but more commonly occurs in patients previously injected with proteins from the same or a related species. Reactions range in severity from **serum sickness** (see Chapter 28) arising days to weeks following treatment to acute **anaphylaxis** (see Chapter 27). **Demyelinating encephalopathy** has been reported.

Rarely, the administration of human immune globulin is attended by similar allergic reactions, particularly in patients with **selective IgA deficiency** (see Chapter 21). Viral hepatitis may be transmitted by whole human plasma or serum but not by the purified gamma globulin fraction.

The administration of intact lymphocytes to promote cell-mediated immunity is hazardous if the recipient is immunologically depressed. The engrafted donor cells may reject the recipient by the graft-versus-host reaction (see Chapter 52).

COMBINED PASSIVE-ACTIVE IMMUNIZATION

Passive and active immunization are often undertaken simultaneously to provide both immediate, transient protection and slowly developing, durable protection against rabies or tetanus. The immune response to the active agent may or may not be impaired by the passively administered antibodies if the injections are given at separate sites. Tetanus toxoid plus tetanus immune globulin may give a response superior to that generated by the toxoid alone, but after antiserum has been given for rabies, the course of active immunization is usually extended to ensure an adequate response.

Parenterally administered live virus vaccines, such as measles or rubella virus, should not be given until at least 6 (and preferably 12) weeks after the administration of immune globulin.

CLINICAL INDICATIONS FOR IMMUNIZATION

Immunizing procedures are among the most effective and economical measures available for preservation and protection of health. The decision to immunize a specific person against a specific pathogen is a complex judgment based on an assessment of the risk of infection, the consequences of natural unmodified illness, the availability of a safe and effective immunogen, and the duration of its effect.

HERD IMMUNITY

The organism that causes tetanus is ubiquitous, and the vaccine directed against it has few side effects and is highly effective, but only the immunized individual is protected. Thus, immunization must be universal. By contrast, a nonimmune individual who resides in a community that has been well immunized against poliovirus and who does not travel has little opportunity to encounter wild (virulent) virus. Here the immunity of the "herd" protects the unimmunized person because the intestinal tracts of recipients of oral polio vaccine fail to become colonized by or transmit wild virus. If, however, a substantial portion of the community is not immune, introduced wild virus can circulate and cause disease among the nonimmune group. Thus, focal outbreaks of poliomyelitis have occurred in religious communities that refuse immunization.

ANTIGENIC SHIFT & ANTIGENIC VARIATION

Each immunologically distinct viral subtype requires a specific antigenic stimulus for effective protection. Immunization against adenovirus infection has not benefited civilian populations subject to many differing types of adenovirus, in contrast to the demonstrated value of vaccine directed against a few epidemic adenovirus types in military recruits. Similarly, immunity to type A influenza virus is transient because of major mutations in surface chemistry of the virus every few years (antigenic shifts). These changes render previously developed vaccines obsolete and may not permit sufficient production, distribution, and use of new antigen in time to prevent epidemic spread of the altered strain. Antigenic variation may also be an important impediment to immunization against HIV infection.

SOME SPECIFIC DISEASES

Pertussis

Several acellular vaccines used in Japan for the past 12 years are saline suspensions of two or more antigens: formalin-treated lymphocyte proliferative factor (pertussis toxin) and filamentous hemagglutinin. The degree of protection afforded by acellular vaccine appears to be about the same as or better than that for the whole-cell product, and minor reactions (fever, pain) are less frequent. Acellular pertussis vaccine (in combination with diphtheria and tetanus toxoids [DT]) has been licensed for children older than 15 months. Licensing for younger children awaits the evaluation of already completed studies.

Poliomyelitis

Two forms of polio vaccine are available. The live, attenuated oral (Sabin) vaccine, used in the United States and many parts of the world, is cheap, effective, and easily administered. Infection causing paralysis occurs in only 1 per 7 million immunodeficient recipients or members of their households. The killed virus vaccine (Salk) is also effective, particularly in

the new "enhanced" form. It requires injection and gives a shorter duration of immunity but is free of the danger of producing paralysis in the recipient or household members. Immunodeficient individuals should receive the killed vaccine. Adults who have never been immunized are protected by herd immunity in developed countries and should therefore be immunized with the killed (Salk) vaccine prior to travel to areas endemic for polio.

Hepatitis A

Although hepatitis A virus (HAV) vaccine was licensed in the United States in 1995, the disease remains the most important viral infection preventable by widespread vaccination. Routine HAV vaccine is recommended for all high-risk groups, including travelers to countries with endemic disease, sexually active homosexual males, users of injected street drugs, children in communities with high rate of infection, and persons with chronic liver disease (because of the risk of acute liver failure by the virus) or clotting factor disorders. HAV vaccination may be considered for control of the spread of disease to noninfected persons during disease outbreaks in communities or institutions.

Postexposure prophylaxis with HAV immune globulin (IG) 0.02 mL/kg is recommended for persons exposed to HAV within 2 weeks who have not previously been immunized with the HAV vaccine at least 1 month prior. The index patients, but not the contacts, should be screened for anti-HAV IgM to verify the diagnosis. IG may also be recommended in other situations in which the disease is confirmed, such as household or sexual contacts, day care employees, or fellow food handlers.

Hepatitis B

Vaccine for hepatitis B has been available for a number of years and is used for special populations—health care workers, infants of surface antigen-positive mothers. A 1992, recommendation for universal immunization against hepatitis B in infancy has been widely adopted.

Influenza

Annual administration of the inactivated vaccine for the current strains of influenza virus continues to be the principal means of prevention and reduction in severity of this disease in selected populations at risk of serious morbidity, complications and mortality. This includes all persons ≥ 65; those < 65 with chronic cardiovascular or pulmonary disorders, with recent hospitalization for certain other chronic diseases, or who reside in chronic-care facilities; those ≤ 18 on long-term aspirin therapy (because of the risk of Reye syndrome); and women who will likely be in the second or third trimester of pregnancy during the expected influenza season. To avoid transmission to these persons, vaccination is also recommended for all health care personnel with patient contact; personnel of chronic-care, home care, or assisted living facilities; and household contacts of those at high risk.

The vaccine should not be administered at the time of an acute febrile illness or to a person with a documented anaphylactic sensitivity to any component of the vaccine. The majority of egg-sensitive persons will not have an allergic reaction to the small quantity of egg protein in the vaccine, but all such persons should be evaluated with proper skin testing, preferably by a trained allergist familiar with the technique and interpretation of testing and possible desensitization if warranted.

Influenza and pneumococcal vaccines can be administered concurrently but at different sites.

Rabies

Three inactivated rabies virus vaccines are licensed for use in the United States for both preexposure and postexposure prophylaxis by the intramuscular route: human diploid cell vaccine (HDCV), rabies vaccine adsorbed (RVA) and purified chick embryo vaccine (PCEC). All three are of similar efficacy and safety. HDCV can also be given intradermally, but for preexposure use only. Two antirabies IgG preparations from hyperimmunized human donors (rabies immune globulin, RIG) are also available at a recommended dose of 20 IU/kg.

Postexposure prophylaxis consists of a single administration of RIG surrounding the wound site if possible and the remainder IM, followed by the vaccine 1 mL IM on days 0, 3, 7, 14, and 28. If previously vaccinated, the vaccine only is given 1 mL IM on days 0 and 3. **Preexposure** vaccination for persons at high risk of exposure to potentially rabid animals consists of primary immunization by IM or intradermal route followed by booster vaccination at 6- to 24-month intervals depending on antibody status and degree of occupational exposure.

Cholera

Cholera immunization offers only temporary and incomplete protection. It is of little use to travelers and should be given only when the risk of exposure is high or in fulfillment of local regulations.

Varicella

An attenuated strain of varicella-zoster virus (VZV) vaccine was licensed in the United States in 1995 and recommended for routine immunization of all children between the ages of 12 and 15 months. It can be administered simultaneously with MMR vaccine but not in the same syringe. It should be required prior to the child's entrance into a day care facility or school in the absence of a documented infection with immunity. It is effective in preventing infection or modifying disease severity in susceptible persons within 3 days of exposure without increased

risk of adverse effects from the vaccine. It is recommended for all susceptible health care workers and those in other high-risk environments.

This live virus vaccine is contraindicated in cellular immunodeficiency. Selected children with asymptomatic HIV infection whose age-specific CD4 T-cell counts are ≥ 25% of predicted may be immunized with two doses 3 months apart. It should not be given to persons with bone marrow or lymphatic malignancies.

Adverse reactions are rare and most frequently a skin rash. More serious illnesses reported following vaccination are generally similar to those following the natural disease but of lower frequency. Transmission of the vaccine virus is very rare and induces a mild disease in an immunocompetent recipient.

Lyme Disease

A newly developed recombinant *Borrelia burgdorferi* lipidated outer-surface protein A vaccine for Lyme disease has recently been licensed for use. It is administered in three doses over 1 year and is recommended only for those who live in endemic areas during the disease transmission season.

Rotavirus Disease

Rotavirus infects nearly all children < 5 years of age worldwide and is the most common cause of severe gastroenteritis in this age group. A multivalent oral, live rotavirus vaccine was licensed for use in the United States in 1998 for routine administration at ages 2 months, 4 months, and 6 months. It significantly decreases disease incidence, severity, and mortality. Like all live viral vaccines, it should not be given to immunocompromised infants.

AGE AT IMMUNIZATION

The **natural history of a disease** determines the age at which immunization is best undertaken. Pertussis, polio, and diphtheria often infect infants; immunization against these diseases is therefore begun shortly after birth. Serious consequences of pertussis are uncommon beyond early childhood, and pertussis vaccination is not usually recommended after 6 years of age. Because the major hazard of rubella is the congenital rubella syndrome, and because nearly half of congenital rubella cases occur with the first pregnancy, it is very important to immunize as many females as possible prior to puberty. In this way the theoretic hazard of vaccinating a pregnant female and endangering the fetus is avoided, although inadvertently immunized fetuses have thus far not been reported to be damaged by their exposure to the attenuated virus.

The **efficacy of immunization** may also be age-related. Failure may occur because of the presence of interfering antibodies or an undeveloped responsiveness of the immune system. Infants cannot be reliably protected with live measles, mumps, or rubella vaccines until maternally derived antibody has disappeared. Because a proportion of children immunized as late as 1 year of age fail to develop antibody after measles vaccination, the age recommended for measles vaccine administration had been changed to 15 months. Because measles is becoming a rare disease in the United States, however, most mothers have shorter lasting vaccine-derived antibodies rather than disease-induced antibodies. Thus it makes sense to go back to the 12-months immunization schedule, particularly if the infant is likely to be exposed, usually through travel. Furthermore, delay in immunization is attended by a decrease in the number of children actually immunized, which approximates the improved rate of seroconversion. Infants frequently develop severe infections with *Haemophilus influenzae* type b, pneumococci, or meningococci, but injecting them with purified capsular polysaccharide has failed to reliably yield a good antibody response, despite the excellent activity of the same antigen in older children and adults. This issue has now been addressed by the development of several conjugated *H influenzae* vaccines (polysaccharide conjugated to protein). A similar effort is under way for *Neisseria meningitidis* and *Streptococcus pneumoniae* polysaccharide vaccines.

Recommendations for Childhood Immunization

Despite the extraordinary effect of immunization in the developed world, the World Health Organization (WHO) estimates that of every 1000 children born today, 5 are crippled by poliomyelitis, 10 die of neonatal tetanus, 20 die of pertussis, and 30 die of measles and its complications. A rational program of immunization against infectious diseases begins in childhood, when many of the most damaging and preventable infections normally appear. Table 50–5 summarizes the current guidelines for immunization in childhood recommended by the Advisory Committee on Immunization Practices (ACIP) and the American Academy of Pediatrics. The need for childhood immunization has increased because unimmunized individuals in a partially immune population are less exposed to such childhood diseases as measles and mumps and therefore develop them later than they otherwise would. When these illnesses do occur in adolescence or adulthood, they are often diagnostically bewildering to the physician unprepared for such illnesses in this age group.

The patient should have an up-to-date **record** of all immunizations. Physicians should have a recall system or other means to identify children who are due for immunizations. It is *not* necessary to restart an interrupted series of vaccinations or to add extra doses. If the vaccine history is unknown and there are no obvious contraindications, the child or adult

should be fully immunized appropriately for his or her age. Reimmunization poses no significant risk.

WHO recommends an accelerated immunization program for developing countries: at birth, oral poliovirus and BCG; at ages 6, 10, and 14 weeks, oral poliovirus and DTP; at age 9 months, measles (to be repeated in the second year of life if given before age 9 months).

Immunization of Adults & the Elderly

Childhood immunization programs have significantly decreased the incidence of preventable infections in developed countries. Optimal immunization of adult populations has not yet been achieved, however. Much disease preventable by immunization continues to exist. Table 50–6 lists the most important immunizations for the adult and elderly population.

SIMULTANEOUS IMMUNIZATION WITH MULTIPLE ANTIGENS

The simultaneous inoculation of the nonliving antigens of diphtheria, tetanus, and pertussis (DPT) elicits a response equal to that seen with their separate injection. Similarly, the single injection of a mixture of live, attenuated measles, rubella, and mumps viruses elicits good responses to each component of the mixture. Between 2 and 14 days following the administration of one live virus vaccine, however, there is a period of suboptimal response to a subsequently injected live virus vaccine. Live vaccines that are not given simultaneously should be given at least 4 weeks apart if time permits. The administration of cholera and yellow fever vaccines within 1–3 weeks of each other decreases the antibody response to both agents. These immunizations also should be given at the same time or at least 4 weeks apart.

The recent addition of conjugated *H influenzae* vaccine and recombinant hepatitis B vaccine to childhood immunizations has created a serious problem with multiple needle sticks necessary at each well-baby visit. This has stimulated the production of combined vaccines, such as DPT and conjugated *Haemophilus* vaccine. Several combinations are commercially available, and more are under way.

IMMUNIZATION FOR FOREIGN TRAVEL

Foreign travel immunization planning includes the current status of the traveler and the requirements of the area to be visited. Infectious diseases such as measles that are rare in the United States are rampant in developing countries. Thus, travelers (children, in particular) should be up to date on their routine immunizations and boosters.

Table 50–5. Recommended childhood immunization schedule[a]—United States, January–December 2000.

Vaccine	Birth	1 mo	2 mos	4 mos	6 mos	12 mos	15 mos	18 mos	24 mos	4–6 yrs	11–12 yrs	14–16 yrs
							Age					
Hepatitis B[b] (Hep B)	Hep B											
		Hep B				Hep B					Hep B	
Diphtheria and tetanus toxoids and pertussis[c]		DTaP	DTaP	DTaP			DTaP			DTaP	Td	
Haemophilus influenzae type b[d] (Hib)		Hib	Hib	Hib		Hib						
Polio[e]		IPV	IPV		IPV					IPV		
Measles–mumps–rubella[f]						MMR				MMR	MMR	
Varicella[g]						Var					Var	
Hepatitis[h]									Hep A in selected areas			

☐ Range of recommended ages for vaccination.

⬭ Vaccines to be given if previously recommended doses were missed or were given earlier than the recommended minimum age.

▨ Recommended in selected states and/or regions.

Note: On October 22, 1999, the Advisory Committee on Immunization Practices (ACIP) recommended that Rotashield (rhesus rotavirus vaccine-tetravalent [RRV-TV]), the only U.S.-licensed rotavirus vaccine, no longer be used in the United States (*MMWR,* Vol. 48, No. 43, November 5, 1999). Parents should be reassured that children who received rotavirus vaccine before July 1999 are not now at increased risk for intussusception.

[a]This schedule indicates the recommended ages for routine administration of licensed childhood vaccines as of November 1, 1999. Any dose not given at the recommended age should be given as a "catch-up" vaccination at any subsequent visit when indicated and feasible. Additional vaccines may be licensed and recommended during the year. Licensed combination vaccines may be used whenever any components of the combination are indicated and the vaccine's other components are not contraindicated. Providers should consult the manufacturers' package inserts for detailed recommendations.

[b]**Infants born to hepatitis B surface antigen (HBsAg)-negative mothers** should receive the first dose of hepatitis B vaccine (Hep B) by age 2 months. The second dose should be administered at least 1 month after the first dose. The third dose should be administered at least 4 months after the first dose and at least 2 months after the second dose, but not before age 6 months. **Infants born to HBsAg-positive mothers** should receive Hep B and 0.5 mL hepatitis B immune globulin (HBIG) within 12 hours of birth at separate sites. The second dose is recommended at age 1–2 months and the third dose at age 6 months. **Infants born to mothers whose HBsAg status is unknown** should receive Hep B within 12 hours of birth. Maternal blood should be drawn at delivery to determine the mother's HBsAg status; if the HbsAg test is positive, the infant should receive HBIG as soon as possible (no later than age 1 week). **Al children and adolescents (through age 18 years)** who have not been vaccinated against hepatitis B may begin the series during any visit. Providers should make special efforts to vaccinate children who were born in or whose parents were born in areas of the world where hepatitis B virus infection is moderately or highly endemic.

[c]The fourth dose of diphtheria and tetanus toxoids and acellular pertussis vaccine (DTaP) can be administered as early as age 12 months, provided 6 months have elapsed since the third dose and the child is unlikely to return at age 15–18 months. Tetanus and diphtheria toxoids (Td) is recommended at age 11–12 years if at least 5 years have elapsed since the last dose of diphtheria and tetanus toxoids and pertussis vaccine (DTP), DTaP, or diphtheria and tetanus toxoids (DT). Subsequent routine Td boosters are recommended every 10 years.

[d]Three *Haemophilus influenzae* type b (Hib) conjugate vaccines are licensed for infant use. If Hib conjugate vaccine (PRP-OMP) (PedvaxHIB or ComVax [Merck]) is administered at ages 2 months and 4 months, a dose at age 6 months is not required. Because clinical studies in infants have demonstrated that using some combination products may induce a lower immune response to the Hib vaccine component, DTaP/Hib combination products should not be used for primary vaccination in infants at ages 2, 4, or 6 months unless approved by the Food and Drug Administration for these ages.

[e]To eliminate the risk for vaccine-associated paralytic poliomyelitis (VAPP), an all-inactivated poliovirus vaccine (IPV) schedule is now recommended for routine childhood polio vaccination in the United States. All children should receive four doses of IPV: at age 2 months, age 4 months, between ages 6 and 18 months, and between ages 4 and 6 years. Oral poliovirus vaccine (OPV) (if available) may be used only for the following special circumstances: 1) mass vaccination campaigns to control outbreaks of paralytic polio; 2) unvaccinated children who will be traveling in <4 weeks to areas where polio is endemic or epidemic; and 3) children of parents who do not accept the recommended number of vaccine injections. Children of parents who do not accept the recommended number of vaccine injections may receive OPV only for the third or fourth dose or both; in this situation, health-

Table 50–6. Vaccines and toxoids[a] recommended for adults, by age groups, in the United States.

Age group (years)	Vaccine/toxoid					
	Td[b]	Measles	Mumps	Rubella	Influenza	Pneumococcal Polysaccharide
18–24	X	X	X	X		
25–64	X	X[c]	X[c]	X		
≥65	X				X	X

[a]Refer also to sections in text on specific vaccines or toxoids for indications, contraindications, precautions, dosages, side effects, adverse reactions, and special considerations.
[b]Td, tetanus and diphtheria toxoids, adsorbed (for adult use), which is a combined preparation containing <2 flocculation units of diphtheria toxoid.
[c]Indicated for persons born after 1956.

National health authorities may require an international certificate of vaccination against cholera or yellow fever from travelers, usually depending on the presence of these diseases in countries on their itinerary. Cholera vaccination may be given by any licensed physician, but it is not very effective, and not generally recommended unless required. The completed certificate must be validated with an official stamp. Yellow fever vaccination may be administered and the certificate validated only at an officially designated center, which may be located by contacting the state or local health department. In addition to these legal requirements, all adults should be adequately immunized against measles, tetanus, and diphtheria and to undergo additional immunizations (against poliomyelitis, typhoid, hepatitis A, and meningococcal meningitis) if they are visiting areas where the frequency of illness in the population or the level of sanitation increases the risk of infection. Travelers should be immunized against plague if contact with wild rodents or rabbits in an endemic rural area is anticipated and to hepatitis B if sexual contacts are anticipated in Southeast Asia or sub-Saharan Africa. Japanese B encephalitis is prevalent in a number of Asian countries (China, India, Thailand, Japan, Nepal, and others). It is mosquito-borne, so travelers to these destinations who anticipate exposure to mosquitoes should consider immunization. An inactivated vaccine has recently been licensed in the United States.

Travelers to malaria-endemic areas should be specifically advised to use mosquito repellents, malaria chemoprophylaxis, and acute therapy of presumptive infections.

No special immunizations are generally recommended for persons traveling from the United States to Western Europe, Canada, Australia, or Japan. Detailed suggestions of the US Public Health Service (CDC) are given for each country in its *Health Information for International Travel Supplement* (see References and in its Web site at *http://www.cdc.gov/*).

VACCINES FOR SPECIAL POPULATIONS

The greatest application of vaccines is in routine immunization of children and adults in large population groups. Some vaccines, however, are used only for populations at greater hazard of exposure to disease by virtue of geography, occupation, or special circumstance. The armed forces use an oral adenovirus vaccine containing types 4 and 7, as well as a polyvalent meningococcal vaccine, for all recruits.

Veterinarians and animal handlers usually receive preexposure rabies vaccination, whereas postexposure rabies immunization is appropriate for the general public. Hepatitis B vaccine is recommended for those with increased occupational, household, or lifestyle risks.

---

care providers should administer OPV only after discussing the risk for VAPP with parents or caregivers. During the transition to an all-IPV schedule, recommendations for the use of remaining OPV supplies in physicians' offices and clinics have been issued by the American Academy of Pediatrics (*Pediatrics,* Vol. 104, No. 6, December 1999).
[f] The second dose of measles, mumps, and rubella vaccine (MMR) is recommended routinely at age 4–6 years but may be administered during any visit, provided at least 4 weeks have elapsed since receipt of the first dose and that both doses are administered beginning at or after age 12 months. Those who previously have not received the second dose should complete the schedule no later than the routine visit to a health care provider at age 11–12 years.
[g] Varicella (Var) vaccine is recommended at any visit on or after the first birthday for susceptible children, ie, those who lack a reliable history of chickenpox (as judged by a health care provider) and who have not been vaccinated. Susceptible persons aged ≥13 years should receive two doses given at least 4 weeks apart.
[h] Hepatitis A vaccine (Hep A) is recommended for use in selected states and regions. Information is available from local public health authorities and *MMWR,* Vol. 48, No. RR-12, October 1, 1999.
Use of trade names and commercial sources is for identification only and does not constitute or imply endorsement by CDC or the US Department of Health and Human Services.
Source: Advisory Committee on Immunization Practices (ACIP), American Academy of Family Physicians (AAFP), and American Academy of Pediatrics (AAP).

VACCINES CURRENTLY IN DEVELOPMENT

Many vaccines are currently in various stages of development. New ones produced by recombinant DNA technology can be anticipated; the first to be licensed and marketed is hepatitis B recombinant vaccine. Synthetic analogues of antigen and possibly antiidiotype antibodies may be developed in the future.

Effective vaccines against hepatitis A, Lyme disease, and rotavirus are the most recent ones to be licensed and available, although their full application remains to be determined. Vaccines against cytomegalovirus, herpes simplex virus, gonococci, *Plasmodium, Pseudomonas aeruginosa,* respiratory syncytial virus, *Shigella,* and many other pathogens are undergoing active development in the laboratory and in clinical trials. An effort is under way to conjugate the polysaccharide capsule of pneumococci to protein in a manner analogous to what has been accomplished with *H influenzae.*

Special immunoglobulin pools high in specific antibodies are being developed. The use of monoclonal antibodies in clinical practice is discussed in Chapter 53.

HIV INFECTION

Active efforts are under way to develop a recombinant DNA vaccine using HIV viral components.

Among the many current strategies being investigated are the use of the gp120 subunit, fusion of HIV envelope proteins with the T-cell HIV receptor complex (CD4 and coreceptor), and insertion of HIV genes into live canarypox vaccine followed by boosting with gp100 subunit. Candidate vaccines have been targeted both for prevention of HIV infection in uninfected individuals and for boosting the immune response of those already infected. Many obstacles stand in the way of the effort, among them the frequent antigenic shift of this virus (see Chapter 46). The current recommendation for HIV-infected individuals is that they receive all the normal childhood immunizations (see Table 50–4), with the exception that polio immunization be restricted to the inactivated form (Salk). This is principally to protect other members of the household who may be seriously immunocompromised. Live measles vaccine is recommended, despite the theoretic hazard, because of the severe form of measles infection that occurs in HIV-infected children. Vaccines against influenza and *S pneumoniae* should also be administered to the appropriate individuals in this group.

REFERENCES

Ad Hoc Working Group Standards for Pediatric Immunization Practices: *JAMA* 1993;269:1817.

American Academy of Pediatrics: *Report of Committee on Infectious Diseases.* 1994 AAP Elk Grove Village, IL 60009-0927.

Barnett ED, Chen R: Children and international travel: Immunizations. *Pediatr Infect Dis J* 1995;14:982.

Cherry JB: Acellular pertussis vaccines: A solution to the pertussis problem. *J Infect Dis* 1993;168:21.

CDC: Recommendations for use of *Haemophilus* b conjugate vaccines and a combined diphtheria, tetanus, pertussis, and *Haemophilus* b vaccine. *MMWR* 1994; 42:(RR013).

CDC: Prevention and Control of influenza. *MMWR* 1999:48(No. RR-4)

CDC: Prevention of hepatitis A through active or passive immunization. *MMWR* 1999:48(No. RR-12)

CDC: Prevention of varicella. *MMWR* 1999:48(No. RR-6)

CDC: Human rabies prevention—United States, 1999. *MMWR* 1999:48(No. RR-1)

CDC: Recommendations for the use of Lyme disease vaccine. *MMWR* 1999:48(No. RR-7)

CDC: Rotavirus Vaccine for the prevention and control of Rotavirus gastroenteritis among children. *MMWR* 1999:48(No. RR-2)

CDC: Recommendations of the international task force for disease eradication. *MMWR* 1993;42:RR16.

CDC: *Health Information for International Travel 1998.* HHS Publication. (Revised annually.)

Edwards KM, Decker MD: Combination vaccines: Hopes and challenges. *Pediatr Infect Dis J* 1994;13:345.

Gilsdorf JR: Vaccines: Moving into the molecular era. *J Pediatr* 1994;125:339.

Katz SL: Prospects for childhood immunizations in the next decade. *Pediatr Ann* 1993;22:733.

Lieu TA et al: Cost effectiveness of a routine varicella vaccination program for U.S. children. *JAMA* 1994; 271:375.

Loewenson PR et al: Physician attitudes and practices regarding universal infant vaccination against hepatitis B infection in Minnesota: Implications for public health policy. *Pediatr Infect Dis J* 1994;13:373.

Nichol KN et al: The effectiveness of vaccination against influenza in healthy working adults. *N Engl J Med* 1995;333:889.

Rabinovich R, Robbins A: Pertussis vaccines: A progress report. *JAMA* 1994;271:68.

Schmitt HJ et al: Efficacy of acellular pertussis vaccine in early childhood after household exposure. *JAMA* 1996;275:37.

Stiehm ER: New developments: Recent progress in the use of intravenous immunoglobulin. *Curr Prob Pediatr* 1992;22:335.

Shann F, Steinhoff MC: Vaccines for children in rich and poor countries. *Lancet* 1999;354,suppl7.

Szilagyi PG et al: Missed opportunities for childhood vaccinations in office practices and the effect on vaccine status. *Pediatrics* 1993;91:1.

51

Allergy Desensitization

Dale T. Umetsu, MD, PhD

Allergen desensitization (allergen immunotherapy, hyposensitization) is primarily used to treat IgE-mediated diseases by injections of allergen extracts. It is an adjunct to symptomatic drug therapy and is effective when allergen avoidance is not possible. Because allergen immunotherapy functions as an antigen-specific immune modifier, many consider immunotherapy for allergy as "vaccine" therapy.

Since 1911 it has been extensively used in allergy practice to treat hay fever and allergic asthma. Numerous controlled clinical trials establish the effectiveness of allergen immunotherapy in allergic rhinitis and Hymenoptera venom anaphylaxis. Short-term desensitization has been accomplished in some cases of penicillin, insulin, and other drug allergy. It is not effective in T-cell-mediated allergy, such as contact dermatitis (poison ivy or poison oak), or for immune complex disease (Arthus reaction or serum sickness).

METHODS

Gradually increasing quantities of allergen protein are injected subcutaneously once or twice a week or alternatively daily or every 30 minutes (rush immunotherapy, especially for Hymenoptera, insulin, or penicillin allergy) until a maximally tolerated dose (generally 100,000 times the initial dose, equivalent to 2–100 µg of the major allergen) is achieved. The injections are then continued once every 3–4 weeks (every 4–8 h in penicillin allergy). Several studies have demonstrated that clinical benefit begins after several months of injections for inhalant allergy and progresses thereafter. Prolonged clinical benefit appears to be sustained following discontinuation of immunotherapy after 3–4 years of injections. Current guidelines generally recommend that the course of immunotherapy be continued in patients with inhalant allergy for at least 2 or 3 successive years after a significant reduction in symptoms has occurred. Allergen immunotherapy for Hymenoptera venom anaphylaxis is highly effective in reducing or eliminating serious reactions from stings throughout the period of active treatment at maintenance dosage. The effect persists following discontinuation after 3–5 years of maintenance injections.

Allergen immunotherapy is individualized based on the clinical history and allergen-specific testing. Immunotherapy allergens are extracted from active constituents from animals, plants, or insects (Hymenoptera venoms). They are usually water-soluble proteins and many are standardized by in vivo and in vitro assays against defined allergens. The current crude or partially purified extracts will probably be replaced in the future by recombinant proteins. In most instances, the allergens are diluted in glycerin to reduce proteolysis and degradation. Because most atopic patients are allergic to multiple allergens, treatment of patients generally consists of mixtures of allergens. Such mixtures may reduce allergen extract potency because of excessive dilution and degradation of allergenic activity by proteases in fungal and insect extracts.

EFFICACY

The efficacy of allergen immunotherapy in seasonal and perennial allergic rhinitis and allergic asthma, with specific IgE antibody against pollens, fungi, dust mites, or animal dander has been demonstrated in multiple double-blind placebo-controlled studies. The treatment reduced allergic rhinitis symptom scores, use of rescue medications for rhinitis, particularly at the peak of the pollen season (Figure 51–1), and to a somewhat lesser extent it reduced symptoms of asthma and the need for asthma medications. These effects are allergen-specific and require high doses of maintenance therapy.

Hymenoptera insect venom anaphylaxis responds exceedingly well to immunotherapy: 95% of treated patients are protected from reactions to deliberate or unintentional stings, whereas about 50% of untreated or placebo-treated control patients continue to experience systemic reactions to stings. Immunotherapy for documented IgE-mediated penicillin allergy, generally with rush protocols occurring over several hours, is also very effective. Although experimental desensitization protocols are proceeding for food allergy, the risk of serious anaphylaxis has dampened enthusiasm for treatment of this problem.

uation of pharmacologic therapy in allergic individuals results in recurrence of symptoms on reexposure to allergen. Because immunotherapy alters the underlying specific immune response (see later discussion), its effect persists long after the injections have been discontinued and may result in cure for some individuals, particularly those with venom sensitivity.

SAFETY

Allergen immunotherapy for IgE-mediated diseases can result in immediate localized and systemic reactions, including life-threatening anaphylaxis. Reactions are most common during the dose escalation phase at or near the maintenance level, and as many as 2–20% of patients may develop systemic reactions over the course of immunotherapy. Both immediate (local or generalized urticaria, wheezing, or anaphylaxis within 30 minutes) and late reactions (localized swelling, or wheezing within 6–18 h) reactions can occur. These may occur more frequently during the seasons of high pollen and mold spore counts, in patients with asthma [especially if the 1-second forced expiratory volume (FEV_1) is less than 80% of predicted], and during rush immunotherapy. Potentially fatal reactions usually begin within 30 minutes after the injection, so patients should be treated in facilities equipped to treat anaphylaxis and closely observed for 20–30 minutes after each injection. Between one and five deaths occur per year in the United States from allergy injection treatment or skin testing. Risk factors for fatal reactions to allergen immunotherapy include labile or symptomatic asthma, errors in dosage, first injections from a new vial of extract, concomitant use of β-adrenergic-blocking agents for unrelated diseases, and home administration of immunotherapy. Other immediate adverse effects include vasovagal reactions, infections, or injury from malplacement of the needle. There are no proven instances in which allergen desensitization produced systemic immune complex disease or other late sequelae.

IMMUNOLOGIC MECHANISMS

Several immunologic effects are induced in allergic patients by successful immunotherapy, including allergen-specific antibody and T-cell responses.

IgE, IgG, & Skin Test Reactivity

During the dose escalation phase of allergen immunotherapy, serum allergen-specific IgE levels rise, sometimes accompanied by a temporary worsening of symptoms. During the maintenance phase, serum allergen-specific IgE declines along with a reduction in the size of immediate phase and gradual elimination of the late-phase skin test reactions to the aller-

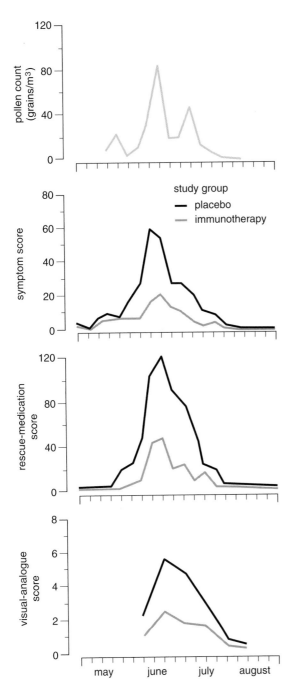

Figure 51–1. Median weekly pollen counts and symptoms, rescue-medication, and visual-analogue scores for placebo and immunotherapy patients. From Durham et al: Long-term efficacy of grass-pollen immunotherapy. *New Engl J Med* 1999;341:468.

Allergen immunotherapy, unlike pharmacologic and allergen avoidance therapy, may improve the natural course of allergic disease and asthma. Discontin-

gen. Improvement of symptoms with pollen immunotherapy is associated with a blunting of the usual seasonal rise in allergen-specific IgE.

During conventional allergen immunotherapy, allergen-specific IgG antibody is usually, but not always, induced. The antibody is often called "blocking antibody" because it inhibits the effect of IgE antibody in the passive transfer (Prausnitz–Küstner) skin test and in in vitro histamine release assays, presumably by competing with IgE for allergen binding. Although allergen-specific IgG levels in serum have been used in the past to monitor the success of venom immunotherapy, its presence does not always correlate with clinical efficacy suggesting that other immunologic mechanisms are responsible for ameliorating the disease. Blocking antibodies of the IgA isotype may also be detected in the serum of treated patients, but their significance is unclear. Some studies suggest that the quantity of blocking antibody of the IgG4 subclass may correlate better with clinical improvement than that of other IgG subclasses, but this remains controversial. Blocking antibody persists in serum during maintenance treatment, then gradually diminishes after treatment is stopped.

Immune Modulation, CD4 T-Cell Subsets, & Other Regulatory Cells

The goal of allergen immunotherapy is increasingly seen as the conversion of pathologic allergen-specific immune responses into protective ones (**immune modulation or immune deviation**). There is increasing evidence that nonallergic individuals do not necessarily lack immune responses against allergens, but rather that they actively suppress the development of harmful allergic inflammation on exposure to allergens. CD4 T_H2 cells (ie, those secreting IL-4, IL-5, and IL-13) play a critical role in the pathogenesis of chronic inflammation in allergic disease and asthma. Successful immunotherapy is associated with reduced function of allergen-specific T_H2 cells, and often with the development of allergen-specific T_H1 cells (ie, those producing IFNγ). It is unclear if immunotherapy converts allergen-specific T_H2 cells directly into T_H1 cells, or if it simply induces allergen-specific T_H1 cells de novo from naive uncommitted T cells, whereas the number of T_H2 effector cells regress by attrition. The assumption, nevertheless, is that T_H1 cells protect against allergic disease by dampening the activity of T_H2 effector cells and inhibiting IgE antibody production.

The evidence for a salutary effect of T_H1 cells in allergic disease and asthma is strong but indirect. T_H1 cells inhibit the proliferation and therefore the development of T_H2 cells, and IFNγ inhibits IgE synthesis in some instances. Reduced IFNγ secretion in neonates is associated with the subsequent development of atopy. Individuals predisposed toward the production of T_H1 cytokines (eg, patients with multiple sclerosis) appear less likely to develop allergic

disease. Infection with *Mycobacterium tuberculosis,* which induces a T_H1-dominated protective immune response also reduces the likelihood of developing atopy. T_H1 cells from experimental animals reduce mucus production and airway eosinophilia, but they fail to directly inhibit T_H2 cell-induced airway hyper-reactivity and may in fact exacerbate airway inflammation.

Other immunologic mechanisms may be important. For example, immune modulation by allergen immunotherapy may induce allergen-specific CD8 T cells, or regulatory T_H cells secreting TGFβ or IL-10 (termed **T_H3 or T_R1** cells), which may be more important than T_H1 cells in down-regulating allergic inflammation and preventing atopy in normal individuals. This would be consistent with the fact that T-cell proliferative responses to allergen decrease after completion of allergen immunotherapy, suggesting that anergy (unresponsiveness) or deletion (possibly due to apoptosis) of allergen-specific T cells may occur. It is also possible that the efficacy of desensitization may require a combination of several immunologic changes, including the indication of T_H1 and T_H3 cells and the inhibition of mast cells, thereby reducing the production of histamine and PGD_2. Whatever the precise mechanism, of desensitization, it is specific for the allergens injected, dose-related, and requires repeated and prolonged parenteral antigen administration.

FUTURE STRATEGIES

Although allergen immunotherapy is effective in reducing allergic symptoms and unique in its capacity to improve the natural course of the disease, treatment failures do occur, and a complete course of immunotherapy requires years of injections. A continuing effort has therefore been made to improve its efficacy and to reduce the risk of reactions and the number of injections, through the use of adjuvants; different routes of administration; and by chemical alteration, modification, or polymerization of the allergen.

MODIFIED ALLERGENS

In theory, increasing the immunogenicity of the injected allergens while decreasing their allergenicity (the binding of the treatment allergen to IgE) should permit injections of high doses without the need for a dose escalation phase. This has been accomplished by polymerizing allergens using urea, formaldehyde or glutaraldehyde. Studies both in humans and mice have demonstrated that polymerized allergens can rapidly induce immune deviation or modulation by converting allergen-specific IL-4 producing T_H2 lymphocytes into allergen-specific T_H1 cells, and reducing allergen-specific IgE. Commercial interest is dimmed, however, by the significant difficulty of producing uniform lots of these modified proteins. More recently, recombinant allergens have been generated with cysteine residues removed by site-directed mutagenesis. These modified allergens do not possess disulfide bonds, lack the normal secondary/tertiary structure, and have 100-fold reduced IgE binding, but they are capable of stimulating T cells. The effectiveness of these allergens in therapy for allergic rhinitis is not yet clear. Allergen covalently linked to polyethylene glycol (PEG) has also been used to effectively reduce side effects of grass pollen extracts. PEG conjugation of enzymes and other proteins, however, appears to reduce their immunogenicity.

PEPTIDE IMMUNOTHERAPY

A new strategy for desensitization was introduced several years ago using peptide fragments of allergens. T cells recognize only a few immunodominant fragments of antigens or allergens, generally 12–15 amino acid residues in length, presented in the binding groove of major histocompatibility complex (MHC) class II antigens expressed on antigen-presenting cells (see Chapter 6). Because such peptides lack the tertiary structure of the native allergens, they have significantly reduced binding to allergen-specific IgE and reduced capacity to trigger degranulation in mast cells compared with native allergen. This allows for administration of much larger allergen doses (particularly on a molar basis), much more rapidly than is possible with conventional (complete) allergen. Immunodominant peptides have been identified by stimulation of T-cell clones using overlapping peptide-mapping analysis of T-cell epitopes from allergic patients. Injections of these immunodominant peptides results in functional inactivation or anergy in allergen-specific CD4 T cells. The T-cell unresponsiveness appears to occur because T-cell stimulation with peptides in vivo occurs in the absence of the usual costimulation, by molecules on the antigen-presenting cell, such as B7.1, B7.2, and CD40. Several clinical trials have shown efficacy with the immunodominant peptides for cat and ragweed allergen, but transient late-occurring reactions (1–6 h after injection) have been observed, possibly from activation and then inactivation of allergen-specific T cells. The injected peptides occasionally induce IgE antibodies. The T-cell anergy induced by peptide therapy appears to be unique.

ADJUVANTS

The idea that converting allergen-specific T_H2 responses into T_H1 responses (immune deviation) results in protection against allergic disease has spawned many attempts to use adjuvants to enhance T_H1 responses. Many of these attempts have focused on two cytokines, IL-12 and IL-18, which potently induce IFNγ production in CD4 T cells in a synergistic fashion. They may also play a role in eliminating allergen-specific T_H2 cells.

Administration of the IL-12 and IL-18 also activates many allergen-nonspecific cells (eg, NK cells, $\gamma\delta$ T cells and $\alpha\beta$ T cells), however, raising concern that the elevated IFNγ production in responding cells may activate autoreactive cells and result in autoimmune disease. The effects of IL-12 or IL-18 could be allergen-specific, however, by covalently linking the allergen with IL-12 as **fusion proteins,** which would direct the IL-12 activity toward allergen-specific cells.

Naked DNA vaccines containing the cDNA for the major antigenic determinants might enhance specific T_H1 responses (immune enhancement). DNA constructs that include sequences with CpG motifs (immunostimulatory sequences, ISS) efficiently induce IL-12 and IL-18 production. For allergen immunotherapy fusion of the CpG motifs with the allergen cDNA could limit the cytokine effects to allergen-specific cells. Finally, if mechanisms such as tolerance or suppression are important in the down-regulation of allergic disease, administration of cytokines such as IL-10 and TGFβ, or methods to induce these cytokines in antigen-specific cells may also be effective in immunotherapies for allergic disease and asthma.

ALTERNATIVE ROUTES OF ADMINISTRATION

Protocols for oral, sublingual, bronchial inhalation, and intranasal immunotherapy for aeroallergen sensitivity have been developed, but the results of clinical trials to date have been largely negative. Recent studies of oral immunization indicate that high doses induce deletion or apoptosis of antigen-specific T cells, whereas low doses induce the development of regulatory cells, often with the production of IL-4, IL-10, and TGFβ. Thus, improved methods of oral therapy may provide a safe and effective means to treat allergic diseases and asthma.

SUMMARY

Allergen immunotherapy has been a method for treating allergic disease for more 90 years. It is the only available therapy that has a strong potential for altering the natural course of the disease and perhaps curing allergy. Our knowledge of the mechanism of action of allergen immunotherapy is rapidly improving, and new, more effective immunotherapies are likely in the near future.

REFERENCES

Bousquet J, et al: Allergen immunotherapy: Therapeutic vaccines for allergic diseases. *Ann Allergy Asthma Immunol* 1998;81:401.

Creticos PS: Immunotherapy with allergens. *JAMA* 1992; 268:2834.

Durham SR et al: Long-term clinical efficacy of grass-pollen immunotherapy. *N Engl J Med* 1999;341:468.

Faria AM, HL Weiner: Oral tolerance: Mechanisms and therapeutic applications. *Advan Immunol* 1999;73:153.

Hansen G et al: Allergen-specific T_H1 cells fail to counterbalance T_H2 cell-induced airway hyperreactivity but cause severe airway inflammation. *J Clin Invest* 1999; 103:175.

Jutel M et al: Bee venom immunotherapy results in decrease of IL-4 and IL-5 and increase of IFN-gamma secretion in specific allergen-stimulated T cell cultures. *J Immunol* 1995;154:4187.

Pene J et al: Immunotherapy with Fel d 1 peptides decreases IL-4 release by peripheral blood T cells of patients allergic to cats. *J Aller Clin Immunol* 1998;101:571.

Rocklin RE et al: Generation of antigen-specific suppressor cells during allergy desensitization. *N Engl J Med* 1980;302:1213.

Rolland J, R O'Hehir: Immunotherapy of allergy: anergy, deletion, and immune deviation. *Curr Opin Immunol* 1998;10:640.

Roman M et al: Immunostimulatory DNA sequences function as T helper-1-promoting adjuvants. *Nat Med* 1997;3:849.

Secrist H et al: Allergen immunotherapy decreases interleukin 4 production in CD4+ T cells from allergic individuals. *J Exp Med* 1993;178:2123.

Seder RA, S Gurunathan: DNA vaccines—Designer vaccines for the 21st century. *N Engl J Med* 1999;341:277.

Umetsu DT, RH DeKruyff: T_H1 and T_H2 CD4$^+$ cells in human allergic diseases. *J Aller Clin Immunol* 1997;100:1.

Yeung VP et al: Heat killed *Listeria monocytogenes* as an adjuvant converts established T_H2-dominated immune responses into T_H1-dominated responses. *J Immunol* 1998;161:4146.

Clinical Transplantation

52

Manikkam Suthanthiran, MD, Peter Stock, MD, Fraser Keith, MD,
Charles Linker, MD, & Marvin R. Garovoy, MD

Transplantation of organs is a life-enhancing and technologically advanced form of therapy in medical practice today.

The first successful renal transplant was performed in 1954. Advances in histocompatibility testing and immunosuppressive drug therapy made it a clinical reality in the 1960s. Improved use of immunosuppressive drugs (prednisone and azathioprine) reduced infectious complications and mortality. The 1970s witnessed the beneficial effects of blood transfusions and antilymphocyte globulin (ALG) as graft-enhancing treatments. The 1980s was the era of cyclosporine and the advent of monoclonal antibody therapy, which greatly improved the success rate of kidney, heart, liver, lung, and pancreas transplants. The 1990s added immunosuppressive drugs (tacrolimus and mycophenolate mofetil) and, more recently, "humanized" monoclonal antibodies to the α chain (CD25) of the IL-2 receptor, and rapamycin, an immunosuppressant that blocks growth factor signal transduction. Transplant outcome has become so promising that it is now being offered early in the care of many patients with chronic and debilitating diseases.

KIDNEY TRANSPLANTATION

Patients with end-stage renal disease can be considered for renal transplantation. Absolute contraindications are those that interfere with the safe administration of anesthesia or immunosuppressive therapy, such as debilitating cardiopulmonary disease, cancer, and untreated peptic ulcer or infection. Preoperative immunologic evaluation includes ABO blood grouping, histocompatibility testing of the patient's and potential donor's human leukocyte antigens (HLA) and the degree of haplotype matching (see Chapters 16 and 17), state of presensitization to HLA antigens, and viral serology (hepatitis B and C viruses, human immunodeficiency virus, cytomegalovirus, and Epstein-Barr virus). Evaluation to rule out contraindications includes voiding cystourethrography and dental, pulmonary, and cardiac status.

ABO Testing

ABO testing is performed on all recipients and potential donors. The ABO system is present on the vascular endothelium of the graft as well as on erythrocytes. Transplanting across the ABO barrier produces very rapid graft rejection owing to preformed isohemagglutinins that injure the vascular endothelium and elicit a coagulation reaction in situ. Blood transfusion compatibility rules also apply to renal transplantation: For a type O recipient the donor should be type O; for a type A recipient the donor may be type A or O; for a type B recipient the donor may be type B or O; and for a type AB recipient the donor may be type A, B, or O. It is possible to overcome the ABO barrier by plasmapheresis to lower the natural titer of anti-A or anti-B antibodies and by administration of cyclophosphamide to prevent new antibody formation, but long-term graft survival has been disappointing.

Living Related & Unrelated Donor Transplantation

All recipients and their potential donors should have complete testing for HLA-A, -B, -C, -DR, and -DQ antigens (see Chapter 17). Family typings usually determine the genotype or haplotype (chromosome) assignment for each identified antigen. The value of **haplotype matching** (zero, one, or two) was established clinically; a sibling matched for two haplotypes and a parent or sibling matched for one haplotype achieve 90% graft survival at 1 year. Because of improved immunosuppression, zero-haplotype-matched family members can now also achieve 90% graft survival at 1 year. The benefits of matching are best seen in long-term outcome. The half-life (time for 50% of grafts functioning at 1 year to fail) is 26.9 years for two-haplotype-matched grafts, but only 12.2 years for one-haplotype-matched living related donor grafts. Recently, living unrelated (spouse, friend) transplants have become an established and acceptable source of donors.

Typically, the donor is highly motivated and altruistic. Provided there is ABO compatibility, a good outcome can be expected, and further improvement of graft survival is also seen between those recipient-donor pairs who share one or more HLA antigens.

Presensitization

Prior exposure to transplantation antigens can lead to sensitization manifested by the development of **cytotoxic antibodies** against HLA antigens and a poorer graft outcome. Moreover, presensitized patients who receive second and subsequent transplants are more likely to reject these grafts than are those who receive a primary graft. This is especially likely in patients who rejected their first graft in < 3 months. Whether repeated rejection is caused by specific sensitization to transplantation antigens or reflects a high immune reactivity of the recipient is under investigation.

The most likely causes of formation of anti-HLA antibodies are pregnancy and previously rejected grafts. To monitor the extent of anti-HLA antibodies produced, serum from each recipient is collected monthly and tested in a manner known as **screening.** The patient's serum is crossmatched against a panel of lymphocytes obtained from many individuals. The number of individuals whose cells are killed is often expressed as a percentage of the panel (eg, 10% panel-reactive antibody). By this procedure, it is possible to determine the extent of presensitization, that is, the likelihood that the recipient will have a positive crossmatch, assuming that the transplant organ is taken from the same genetic pool of donors as the lymphocyte panel. In addition, knowing which HLA antigens on the lymphocyte panel cells have been lysed makes it possible to analyze the specificities of the antibodies in the serum that are responsible for the positive reactions.

Crossmatching

The crossmatch test is used to determine the presence of any preformed antibodies (presensitization) to donor HLA antigens by using the patient's most recent serum and donor lymphocytes (see Chapter 19). Positive crossmatches are a contraindication to transplantation because they are associated with very early and uncontrollable rejection episodes, leading to irreversible graft loss.

Cadaveric Transplantation

When the recipient has no family members as potential donors, the opportunity exists to receive a kidney from a recently deceased individual (cadaveric transplantation). Recipients referred for this type of treatment undergo comparable immunologic evaluation of ABO grouping, HLA typing, and antibody screening and are then placed on a waiting list.

When a potential cadaveric donor's organs are harvested, a section of spleen, some lymph nodes, and peripheral blood are collected for determining the donor ABO blood group and HLA antigens. Recipients on the waiting list can then be crossmatched against the donor tissues, using the patient's current serum and the recipient's highest reacting serum within the past 2 years to exclude the possibility of a positive crossmatch. Recipients who are ABO-compatible and crossmatch-negative become available for further consideration. Often, a second round of crossmatch testing occurs among this smaller pool of recipients, in which additional past sera are chosen to be certain of no hidden presensitization. From among the ABO-compatible, crossmatch-negative recipients, the best matched recipients may then be selected. Additional criteria, such as length of time on the waiting list, urgency of medical condition, whether this is a first or second transplant, and age of recipients are considered in organ allocation.

Donor Evaluation & Procedures

Candidacy for **living donation** is determined by evaluating the potential donors for heart disease, renal dysfunction, diabetes, infection, and malignancy. A preoperative angiogram guides selection of the right or left kidney for living donation. Factors that influence the choice of kidney are operating safety for the donor, vascular and internal anatomy, and occasionally differential creatinine clearance by renal scan. The living donor nephrectomy procedure includes a flank incision through which the kidney and vascular pedicle are removed. The ureter and all periureteral soft tissue are removed to preserve the ureteral blood supply and prevent distal ureteral avascular necrosis.

Donors who have undergone uninephrectomies experience no long-term change in survival or lifestyle. Because improved immunosuppression and preoperative conditioning have increased success rates of living donor transplantation, it is now possible to consider living donors who share two, one, or no haplotypes with the recipient. With the increasing demand for kidneys, many centers are now performing transplants from living unrelated donors. A 90% 1-year survival rate can be achieved. Evaluation of donor motivation and psychologic factors is necessary.

Cadaveric donors can be considered when they are determined to be neurologically dead and free from metastasizing tumors, kidney dysfunction, or active infection (particularly with hepatitis viruses or HIV). The criteria for who is positive for hepatitis C antibody are evolving. Hemodynamic stabilization with volume expansion and the conservative use of vasopressors and desmopressin acetate maintain optimal organ function. Both kidneys are removed with renal arteries and veins frequently left en bloc with the donor aorta and vena cava. Both ureters are removed, including all periureteral soft tissue to include the ureteral blood supply and prevent distal ureteral avascular necrosis. Samples of spleen and lymph nodes are also removed for donor tissue typing and crossmatching against potential recipients.

The removed kidney is flushed with preservation fluid to remove all donor blood, and it can be stored by either of two methods. Cold storage involves storing in ice to maintain subphysiologic temperatures. Alternatively, the aorta or renal arteries are cannulated, and a cold mixed-electrolyte solution is instilled by continuous cold pulsatile perfusion. Cadaver renal transplantation within the first 48 hours (cold ischemia time) after donor nephrectomy is preferred. Graft survival rates are progressively lower with increases in cold ischemia time.

Blood Transfusion

In the past, recipient **preconditioning** with blood transfusion led to improved graft survival, but with improved immunosuppressive protocols, the benefits have been more difficult to demonstrate. Furthermore, many now believe that the infectious risks associated with blood transfusions outweigh the potential benefits.

Transplant Surgery

The **operative procedure** for the recipient includes an incision over the iliac fossa through which the graft is placed in the retroperitoneal position against the psoas muscle (Figure 52–1). A renal artery anastomosis to either the internal or external iliac artery and renal vein anastomosis to the external iliac vein are standard. Ureteroneocystostomy involving anastomosis of the ureter to bladder mucosa

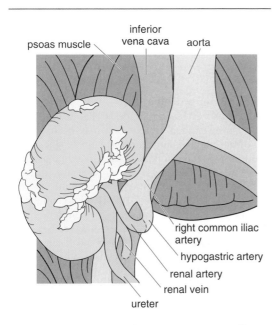

Figure 52–1. Technique of renal transplantation. (Reproduced, with permission, from Way LW (editor): *Current Surgical Diagnosis & Treatment,* 9th ed. Originally published by Appleton & Lange. Copyright © 1991 by The McGraw-Hill Companies, Inc.)

through an anterior cystotomy incision is a usual approach. The ureter is often passed through a short submucosal tunnel in the bladder wall to prevent vesicoureteral reflux.

Postoperatively, hemodynamic stability is achieved with central venous pressure monitoring and careful fluid and diuretic management. Careful monitoring of urine output, electrolytes, blood urea nitrogen, and serum creatinine to evaluate renal function is mandatory. All cadaveric kidneys have some degree of acute tubular necrosis, ranging from very mild to very severe. Dialysis is required in approximately 20% of cadaveric renal transplant recipients during the early period of severe acute tubular necrosis (usually 5–10 days). Recipients who require dialytic support in the first week of transplantation (delayed graft function group) have inferior short-term as well as long-term graft survival rates compared with those who do not require dialysis. Acute tubular necrosis is rare in patients receiving related-donor transplants because donor nephrectomy and recipient transplant are performed sequentially, minimizing cold-storage time.

Postoperative Immunosuppression

Postoperative immunosuppression is the most variable aspect of recipient care. Standard treatment to prevent rejection includes **corticosteroids** and additional immunosuppression depending on the type of allograft and tissue match (see Chapter 53). **Cyclosporine** (5–15 mg/kg/d) has clearly improved allograft success in recipients of cadaveric and some related-donor transplants, but it is nephrotoxic, and monitoring of drug dosages and serum drug levels (100–400 μg/mL) is required.

Azathioprine, an antimetabolite that interferes with new DNA formation in proliferating cells, is frequently used (1–2 mg/kg/d) in combination with prednisone and cyclosporine. It is potentially hepatotoxic, whereas **cyclophosphamide** is a nonhepatotoxic alternative. **Antilymphocyte globulin** (ALG; 10–20 mg/kg) and **antithymocyte globulin** (ATG; 10–20 mg/kg) from serum of animals immunized with human lymphocytes or thymocytes, respectively, are potent immunosuppressive reagents. These heterologous animal proteins can be made in horses, sheep, goats, or rabbits. Monoclonal antilymphocyte antibodies against specific T-cell subsets are also in clinical use. **Lymphoplasmapheresis** occasionally is used to remove recipient lymphocytes and immunoglobulin while immunosuppressive drugs are concurrently administered. Local graft irradiation has been used but has not provided reliable immunosuppression. Recently, a number of newer immunosuppressive agents with different mechanisms of action have been approved (**tacrolimus, mycophenolate mofetil**) on the basis of their ability to reduce acute rejection in the first 6 months after transplantation.

Rejection

Classic signs and symptoms of **acute** rejection include swelling and tenderness over the allograft and decrease in renal function. Systemic manifestations such as temperature elevation, malaise, poor appetite, and generalized myalgia can be seen. Decrease in renal function is diagnosed by a decrease in urine volume, increasing blood urea nitrogen and creatinine levels, poorly controlled hypertension, fluid retention, and radiographically by ultrasonography (blurring of corticomedullary junctions, increased resistive index, prominent pyramids) and by radionuclide renal scans showing decreased uptake and excretion of the tracer.

In the presence of a decline in renal function, however, the differential diagnosis includes prerenal azotemia and obstruction, acute tubular necrosis, pyelonephritis, and other drug-induced toxicity. In addition, recurrence of the primary renal disease and de novo glomerulonephritis can be late causes of decreased renal function. Renal biopsy is frequently performed to histologically and precisely diagnose the cause of graft dysfunction (Figures 52–2, 52–3).

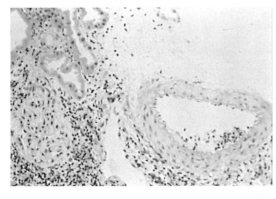

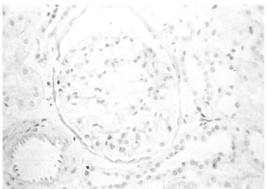

Figure 52–2. Top: Early acute rejection showing focal mononuclear cellular infiltrate in the interstitium and in the wall of a blood vessel. **Bottom:** Appearance of normal renal biopsy specimen with glomeruli, arterioles, and tubules.

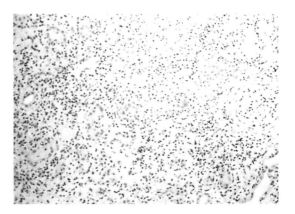

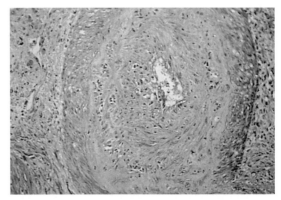

Figure 52–3. Top: Acute rejection-severe. Diffuse mononuclear cellular infiltrate throughout the interstitium. **Bottom:** Chronic rejection. Fibroobliterative changes in an arteriole and reduction of vascular lumen.

PATHOLOGY OF GRAFT REJECTION

Mechanisms of Rejection

A. Acute: Evidence suggests that at least two pathways of antigen presentation may be operative. The **direct path** of antigen presentation suggests that blood-borne and donor antigen-presenting cells ("passenger cells") in grafts provide the primary stimulus. These are dendritic cells and monocytes expressing allogeneic class I and II HLA molecules. The **indirect path** of antigen presentation suggests that host (recipient) antigen-presenting cells (APC) can present shed allogeneic class I and II HLA antigens from donor parenchymal cells. Both donor and host APCs provide second signals, interleukin-1 (IL-1), and IL-6, which aid in triggering lymphocyte activation (Figure 52–4). IL-1 not only is involved in the activation of helper-inducer CD4 T cells but probably also is important for the activation of unprimed cytotoxic CD8 T cells and B lymphocytes. The activation of helper-inducer T cells by alloantigen is necessary but not sufficient to the development of cell immune responses against the graft. Also required is a costim-

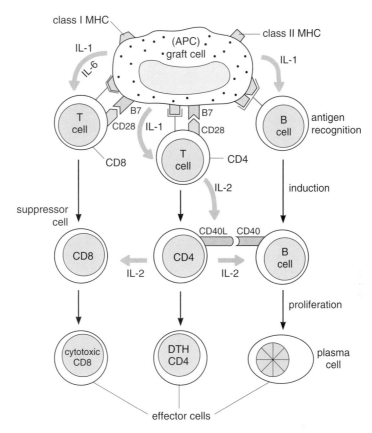

Figure 52–4. Generation of allograft rejection response (primary). *Abbreviations:* MHC = major histocompatibility class; APC = antigen-presenting cell; DTH = delayed-type hypersensitivity.

ulating signal by the interaction of other molecules on the APC and T lymphocyte. The best studied is the B7 family of molecules on the APC (B7.1/7.2, now called CD80/86), which must bind to the CD28 molecule on T lymphocytes. Together, interaction of the T-cell receptor/major histocompatibility class (MHC—signal 1) with the costimulus (signal 2) stabilized by cell adhesion molecules (intercellular adhesion molecule [ICAM]-1/leukocyte function-associated antigen [LFA]-1) supports full T-lymphocyte activation (Figure 52–5).

Once activated, these cells release IL-2, which is an essential cofactor in the activation of both CD8 T cells and B cells. As a consequence of exposure to antigen plus costimulating signals, clonal proliferation and maturation of alloantigen-reactive cells takes place. This leads to the development of effector T cells, which migrate from lymphoid tissue via the blood to all tissues, including the graft, where they mediate damage to antigen-containing sites, and antibody, which is released into the blood or produced locally within the graft, where it has access to these antigens (Figure 52–6).

The precise mechanism by which T cells destroy the graft is still under study. Effector T cells that can destroy graft tissue develop from both CD8 and CD4 subclasses (see Figure 52–6). The results are similar except that CD8 T cells recognize HLA-A and HLA-B antigen-bearing cells, whereas CD4 T cells recognize HLA-DR antigen-bearing cells. Both CD4 and CD8 subclasses of effector cells probably can directly destroy graft cells by classic cytotoxic T-cell mechanisms. Another important consequence of T cell-activation, however, is their release of other lymphokines, especially interferon gamma (IFNγ), which can produce two important effects. First, IFNγ induces increased expression of HLA-A, -B, and -DR on graft tissue, which potentially makes the graft more vulnerable to effector mechanisms. Second, it activates monocytes to mediate a destructive delayed hypersensitivity response against the graft.

Hence, T cells can directly cause target cell injury or activate macrophages, resulting in nonspecific destruction. Lymphokines in addition to IL-2 and IFNγ are released from activated T cells; they include IL-4 and IL-5, which play a role in directing B-cell pro-

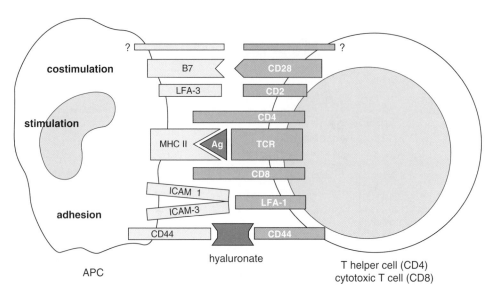

Figure 52–5. Schematic representation of costimulatory and adhesion molecules on the surface of antigen-presenting cells (APC) and T lymphocytes. *Abbreviations:* MHC = major histocompatibility class; ICAM = intercellular adhesion molecule; LFA = leukocyte function-associated antigen; TCR = T-cell receptor.

duction of antibody. Antibody-mediated damage may then take place directly through complement activation or by recruitment of antibody-dependent cell-mediated cytotoxic (ADCC) effector cells (see Figure 52–6). Most of the cells that arrive in the graft early after transplantation are lymphocytes, which migrate out of the capillary and venous beds, but after 4–7 days a remarkably heterogeneous collection of cell types appears. Those of the lymphocytic series predominate over the monocyte-macrophage and include also a few polymorphonuclear neutrophils. Although a variety of cell types are present, there is some evidence that early rejection of solid-tissue allografts is associated with T lymphocytes having direct cytotoxic activity against donor target cells. A significant number of B lymphocytes, null cells, and monocytes also appear in the early infiltrate, and although cytotoxic T-cell activity is easily demonstrated at first, later stages of rejection may involve a non-T killer cell. In all phases, the presence of antibodies and ADCC effector cells makes this mechanism an additional possibility. Macrophages appear to play an effector and suppressor role, whereas some B lymphocytes become activated and begin immunoglobulin synthesis in situ. When the host has been primed to donor antigens before transplantation, an accelerated process, often marked by antibody-mediated vasculitis, may result.

Recent applications of anti-T-cell monoclonal antibodies as diagnostic reagents in staining biopsy specimens and in vivo as therapy add considerable support to the key role of T lymphocytes in most cases of rejection. When immunofluorescence or immuno-peroxidase techniques are used with renal graft biopsy specimens, 50–90% of the infiltrating cells generally express CD3 and CD2, with variable proportions of CD4 and CD8 cells. Although the peripheral blood often shows an increased proportion of CD4 cells in association with acute rejection episodes, many investigators relate rejection in the kidney to a preponderance of CD8 cells. More precisely, the grafts of patients experiencing irreversible rejection show a preponderance of CD8 cells in the blood and perivascular areas (ratio of CD4 to CD8 cells <1.0). When peripheral blood CD4:CD8 ratios are higher, perivascular ratios are also higher, and rejection usually is reversible with therapy. High-dose corticosteroids, given either intravenously (methylprednisolone, 1 g/d for 3 days) or orally (prednisone, 5–10 mg/kg/d for 5 days) are often used to treat acute rejection. Corticosteroids function through several pathways. They reduce the capacity of APCs to express class II antigens and to release IL-1. They also inhibit the alloactivation of T cells and consequently the release of IL-2. Their effect on migration and function of effector cells, as well as their capacity to block the release of IFNγ, may explain their efficacy in reversing acute rejection. In this regard, they are known to produce lymphocytopenia, especially of CD4 T cells, by delaying transit of lymphocytes through marrow and lymphoid tissues.

If there is no response or only a partial response to corticosteroids, polyclonal antibodies (eg, ATG) may be given (10–20 mg/kg/d for 5–14 days). ATG lyses lymphocytes, especially T cells, making it an excellent agent for treatment of acute rejection. ATG, how-

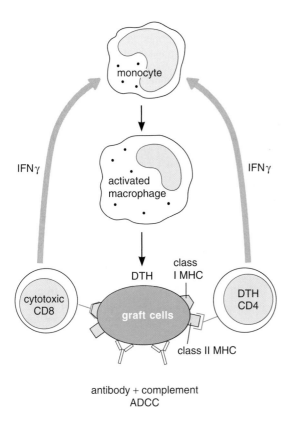

Figure 52–6. Effector mechanisms of allograft rejection. *Abbreviations:* MHC = major histocompatibility class; ADCC = antibody-dependent cell-mediated cytotoxicity; DTH = delayed-type hypersensitivity; IFN = interferon.

ever, may cause anaphylaxis, serum sickness, and fever. Biologic effects also vary because there is no effective measure for standardization.

More commonly, monoclonal antibodies (muromonab-CD3) are used to treat rejection refractory to steroids. This is a mouse IgG2 monoclonal antibody to the human T-cell surface molecule CD3. Not only is it effective for the treatment of initial bouts of rejection, but rejection episodes that are resistant to high-dose steroids usually respond to 5 mg/d intravenously for 10 days. This anti-CD3 initially causes an acute T-lymphocyte depletion as the antibody-coated T lymphocytes are opsonized and eliminated by the reticuloendothelial system. After 48 hours of therapy, T lymphocytes slowly return to the circulation; however, the T-cell receptor/CD3 complex is modulated (cleared) from the cell surface. Without a sufficient number of CD3 molecules present, T-cell activation is impaired. One side effect of therapy may be the production of antimouse antibodies in a small percentage of patients, which can limit the effectiveness of a subsequent course of therapy. Prolonged or high-dose muromonab-CD3 therapy has been associated with an increased incidence of lymphoproliferative disease. In the future, monoclonal antibodies against lymphokine receptors and adhesion molecules as well as soluble cytokine receptors may be found useful. Figure 52–7 shows the site of action of some of the currently approved immunosuppressive drugs.

B. Hyperacute: Preformed anti-ABO isohemagglutinins or anticlass I HLA antibodies, when present

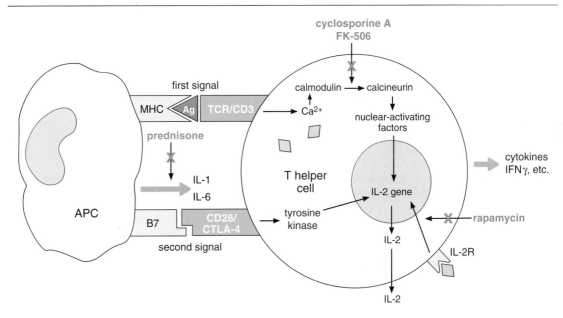

Figure 52–7. Schematic representation of the molecular sites of action of some currently available immunosuppressive agents. *Abbreviations:* APC = antigen-presenting cell; CTLA = cytotoxic T lymphocyte antigen; MHC = major histocompatibility class; IL = interleukin; IFN = interferon; TCR = T-cell receptor.

in sufficient quantity, bind to the vascular endothelium and trigger a cascade of immunologic events. Initially, fixation of complement components and complement activation ensues, followed by activation of the clotting pathway. This series of events, if severe enough, can result in microthrombi within glomerular capillary loops and arterioles, leading to severe ischemia and necrosis of the graft. At present, there are no effective means of treating this lesion once it begins. Emphasis is therefore placed on prevention by careful assessment of ABO blood type and donor-specific sensitization to HLA antigens by crossmatch testing prior to transplantation.

C. Chronic: Chronic rejection, which can occur months to years after transplantation, is characterized by a narrowing of the vascular arterial lumen owing to growth of endothelial cells that line the vascular bed (see Figure 52–4). The actual control mechanisms for this response are unknown but may include immunologic injury signals, monocyte release of IL-1, and platelet and endothelial cell release of platelet-derived growth factor. Initially, the proliferating endothelial cell lesion is reversible, but once it progresses to fibrotic changes within the blood vessel wall itself, it is unresponsive to current modes of immunosuppression, leading to graft ischemia, extensive interstitial fibrosis, and ultimate loss of renal function. Because no specific therapy is available for this form of rejection, emphasis is on prevention by seeking the greatest possible degree of histocompatibility between recipients and donors.

Outcome

Survival of patients after renal transplantation is superior to that of patients undergoing dialysis. In most series, patient survival at 2 years is 90–95%. Graft survival, defined as allograft function adequate to maintain life without dialysis, is 85% at 2 years in cadaveric renal allograft recipients treated with current immunosuppressive regimens. Related-donor transplants have a greater than 90% success rate at 2 years.

Surviving renal allografts have normal function, with mean creatinine levels of less than 2 mg/dL in most series. A functioning allograft therefore affords the recipient an optimal chance for normalization of health and is associated with minimal morbidity and mortality rates.

LIVER TRANSPLANTATION

Experimental liver transplantation in large animals beginning in the early 1950s established its feasibility and potential problems. The first human liver transplant was performed in 1963. Initially unsuccessful, liver transplantation later became a successful procedure because of improved surgical techniques, intraoperative management, and methods of immunosuppression. In 1999, more than 4000 liver transplants were performed in the United States, and over 100 liver transplant centers exist at this time. These numbers will likely further expand with increasing numbers of living related liver transplants.

From results of experimental liver transplantation in animals, liver grafts were initially thought to be immunologically privileged, however, rejection is commonly encountered in human liver transplantation. In certain strains of pigs and rats, liver grafts between the same donor and recipient combination have prolonged survival even though allogeneic kidney allografts are rejected within a short time. In addition, animals tolerate subsequent skin grafts from the same donor for prolonged periods but promptly reject third-party skin grafts. These effects are specific to only limited strains. There is evidence that long-term induction of tolerance to the transplanted liver occurs naturally. According to a hypothesis proposed by Thomas Starzl, lymphoid cells from the donor organ migrate to the periphery and set up a state of **chimerism,** the development of host tolerance to the transplanted tissue. Immunosuppression has been successfully withdrawn in some chimeric recipients, but others have rejected the organ following withdrawal. The functional significance of the chimeric state and its association with graft acceptance remains unclear. The mechanism of liver transplant rejection and the expression of MHC antigens on the surface of liver cells and bile duct cells are distinctly different from that of the kidney and other whole organs.

Indications

Liver transplantation is indicated when an individual's disease process is likely to progress to death within 2 years or when the compromise in life-style is so severe as to merit the risk of transplant. Although some diseases are known to be fatal in the long term, it is only recently that short-term survival can be predicted in primary biliary cirrhosis and sclerosing cholangitis.

Signs and symptoms of progressive liver deficiency include malaise, weight loss, encephalopathy, ascites, coagulopathy, hypoalbuminemia, hyperbilirubinemia, and renal insufficiency. Complications of cholestatic disease include intractable pruritus, metabolic bone disease, recurrent biliary sepsis, and xanthomatous neuropathy. Progressive complications of portal hypertension (gastroesophageal bleeding, ascites) in liver deficiency require intervention. With the development of transjugular intrahepatic portasystemic shunts (TIPS), variceal bleeding and refractory ascites can often be managed effectively until a donor organ becomes available. TIPS is effective in the pretransplant setting to control variceal bleeding and refractory ascites. It can, however, exacerbate the encephalopathy and is used most effectively as a bridge to transplantation. At present, many potential liver transplant recipients die before a suitable organ becomes available.

Current trials of a bioartificial liver to support patients with acute decompensation of the liver use porcine hepatocytes to filter the blood, similar in concept to hemodialysis for renal insufficiency. If successful, this could be used as a bridge to liver transplantation in fulminant hepatic failure or as a temporary support for a recoverable toxic insult (eg, acetaminophen toxicity).

The most common indication for liver transplant in the adult population to date has been chronic active hepatitis. Others include primary biliary cirrhosis, alcoholic cirrhosis, fulminant hepatic failure, hemochromatosis, Wilson's disease, Budd-Chiari syndrome, biliary atresia, and inborn errors of metabolism. Some patients with hepatocellular tumors or cholangiocarcinomas have received transplants, and a few have survived for 3–5 years.

Preliminary data suggest that selected patients with localized hepatocellular tumors can achieve successful transplants using chemoembolization followed by transplantation. Patients with antigen-positive chronic active hepatitis B frequently have recurrent hepatitis B antigenemia following transplantation. In the past, large numbers of these patients developed recurrent hepatitis and cirrhosis, although the rapidity of progression of chronic active hepatitis leading to cirrhosis and liver failure has been questioned. The use of hepatitis B hyperimmune globulin (HBIG) and lamivudine has dramatically improved the results of transplantation for hepatitis B. It remains unclear how long the recipients need to be treated. Patients transplanted for hepatitis C also are at risk for disease recurrence. To date no therapy has been effective in preventing the recurrence of hepatitis C although trials with interferon and ribavirin therapy on a prophylactic basis following liver transplantation are currently in progress. Although liver transplantation for alcohol-related liver failure was initially controversial, this has become more widely accepted because of the increasing evidence that results are comparable to those of other causes of liver failure. Most transplant centers require that these patients remain abstinent from alcohol for 6–12 months and that they can comply with posttransplant treatment regimens.

The most common diagnosis for which liver transplantation is performed in infants and children is **extrahepatic biliary atresia.** This disease occurs in 1:8000 to 1:12,000 live births in the United States. Children commonly undergo the Kasai procedure, which has long-term effectiveness in one third to one half of all patients. For patients with failed hepaticojejunostomy, liver transplantation is the only viable solution. Other indications for liver transplants in children are inborn errors of metabolism such as α_1-antitrypsin deficiency, tyrosinemia, and Wilson's disease. As outcomes have improved, liver replacement

has been used to treat liver-based inborn errors of metabolism that result in extrahepatic organ system failure. For example, one patient with homozygous familial hypercholesterolemia has received a heart-liver transplant, and several patients with oxalosis and renal involvement have received combination liver-kidney transplants. For infants and smaller children, living related donors have been used with increasing frequency with success approximating that of cadaveric transplantation. Although no immunologic advantage has been noted to date, increased availability of organs has led to more optimal timing of the transplant and decrease in pretransplantation mortality.

With expanding waiting lists for liver transplants and increasing numbers of patients dying on the waiting list, several transplant centers are splitting livers for transplantation into two recipients. Similarly, success with living donor liver transplants from adult to children is being expanded to include adult to adult transplants. This technique requires the transplant of an entire hepatic lobe in order to provide enough liver tissue to avoid hepatic insufficiency immediately following transplantation. Because of the significant donor risks associated with a right or left hepatic lobectomy, this strategy is currently being utilized on a limited basis. With more experience, living donation for adult liver transplants will likely expand and provide an important alternative to the limited pool of cadaveric donors.

Contraindications to liver transplantation vary from center to center. General guidelines are the exclusion of potential recipients whose disease conditions are associated with poor prognosis. These include extrahepatic malignancy, evidence of metastatic disease, and rapid recurrence of hepatitis B or C in potential retransplant candidates. HIV positivity has been a relative contraindication to liver transplantation. With improvements in antiretroviral therapy for the treatment of HIV, however, several centers are proceeding with trials of transplantation in the HIV-positive recipient with undetectable viral loads and adequate CD4 counts. Further contraindications include behavioral and social issues that may predict a poor outcome because of noncompliance. Examples are active substance abuse and the recipient's inability to meet the rigors of postoperative management (compliance and medication protocol) or postoperative follow-up. Finally, medical contraindications to liver transplantation include advanced cardiopulmonary disease, anatomic considerations that preclude surgical reconstruction, and active infection, especially with fungal pathogens.

Procedure

Orthotopic liver transplantation is the most commonly used method to date. The host liver is removed and replaced with the transplanted liver in the orthotopic position. Heterotopic transplantation, in which the native liver is left in place and the transplanted liver is placed at an ectopic site, is less frequently performed, because the clinical results have been less successful.

Several surgical strategies have evolved to increase the number of available organs required for the rapidly expanding waiting list. Split-liver transplantation can be performed between two adults, but it has more frequently been accomplished between an adult and a child. The child generally receives segments 2 and 3, with segments 4–8 given to adult recipients. For adult-to-children living donor transplants, the most frequent technique involves the donation of segments 2 and 3. For adult-to-adult living donor transplants, the entire right lobe is frequently required to provide enough hepatic mass to support the recipient following transplantation. As with the standard orthotopic liver transplantation, efforts should be made to minimize both the cold and warm ischemic times, in an effort to maximize initial allograft function and minimize the potential for ischemic damage to the biliary system.

The standard procurement procedure for cadaveric livers includes a flush with heparinized University of Wisconsin (UW) solution followed by cold preservation. UW solution enables the liver to be preserved for more than 20 hours in some cases. This has greatly expanded the ability to transport organs long distances and to use back-up recipients if the first one proves unacceptable for transplantation. To minimize the risk of intrahepatic biliary strictures associated with prolonged hepatic preservation time, however, an attempt is made to transplant within 12 hours after harvest. The recipient hepatectomy is technically the most difficult phase of the transplant operation because of frequent portal hypertension, previous surgery, and coagulopathy. Often excessive bleeding occurs due to numerous adhesions at the operative site. The liver is mobilized although not removed until the donor organ is brought into the operative field and examined. The anhepatic phase is the time of greatest physiologic stress, because at this point the liver is removed and clamping of the portal vein and vena cava results in decreased venous return to the heart. This may in part be overcome by the use of venovenous bypass, which serves to bypass the splanchnic circulation and the infrahepatic vena caval circulation. Many centers, however, do not use venovenous bypass during the anhepatic phase, which lasts from the time when the host liver is removed until the vascular clamps are released, reperfusing the new liver. The revascularization phase requires attention to hemostasis. Revascularization involves supply to the liver via either the portal vein or the hepatic artery, or both, depending on the individual's anatomy and stability on venovenous bypass. The specific type of arterial revascularization depends on the blood supply to the donor organ. Complex revascularization may be required if multiple arteries are

supplying the donor liver. The bile duct is reconstructed using a choledochocholedochostomy, preferably when the recipient's common duct is of good quality, or a choledochojejunostomy if the recipient's duct is of poor quality (eg, in biliary atresia) or of marked unequal size compared with the donor's common bile duct (Figure 52–8). Improvements in surgical technique, new technologic advances such as the venovenous bypass, the availability of UW solution, and the ability to control coagulation have decreased operative mortality rates and expanded the preservation time.

Outcome

Early graft failure, also known as **primary nonfunction,** may be a devastating complication if the patient does not receive a second transplant. The previously described liver assist device has potential utility in the setting of primary nonfunction. In preliminary clinical trials, the liver assist has provided a successful bridge to retransplantation following primary nonfunction. Primary nonfunction encompasses a spectrum ranging from no graft function (and certain death without retransplantation) to a liver whose function is mildly impaired at the outset but regains function within the first few days or weeks after transplantation. Factors related to primary nonfunction include the nature of the donor's injury, the donor's retrieval operation, the preservation solution, the length of preservation, host immunologic factors, the transplant operation, and host cardiovascular status. One established factor associated with primary nonfunction is the presence of moderate to extensive fat deposits in the donor's liver. When fatty infiltration of the liver is suspected, a biopsy specimen should be taken. The pathologic confirmation of moderate to extensive fat should preclude the use of such livers. Donor hypernatremia is a risk factor shown to be an independent variable for primary nonfunction. Perhaps the best predictor of poor graft function is the surgeon's initial impression of the donor liver at the time of procurement.

Infectious complications after transplantation are frequent. Survival after infection relates to the type of offending organisms. Bacterial infections from pulmonary, bladder, and vascular sites usually respond to antibiotics, but fungal or viral infections may be associated with higher mortality and morbidity rates. As mentioned previously, the use of HBIG and lamivudine has dramatically improved the results following transplantation for hepatitis B. The development of resistant strains of virus remains a problems, which will be dealt with by the development of newer efficacious antiviral agents (eg famciclovir).

Rejection is common after liver transplantation and may be seen in over 50% of patients when defined by histologic means alone (see later discussion). It can be readily diagnosed (see later discussion) by frequent percutaneous biopsies and is easily

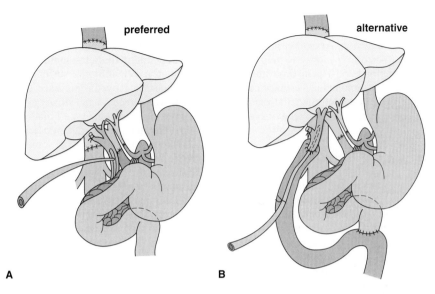

Figure 52–8. Liver transplantation. **A:** The preferred method and **B:** the alternative technique are shown. The donor suprahepatic vena cava, infrahepatic vena cava, portal vein, and hepatic artery are anastomosed end to end to the corresponding recipient vessels. **A:** When the recipient's common duct is intact and the size matches the donor's common duct, a choledochocholedochostomy is performed. **B:** When the recipient duct is not intact (eg, biliary atresia or sclerosing cholangitis), a choledochojejunostomy is used.

and successfully treated when diagnosed early. Although rejection is common during the early post-transplant period (see later discussion), the rejection is generally easily reversed with steroids. The requirement for monoclonal antibodies (eg, anti-CD) for steroid-resistant rejection is rare. Unlike rejection following renal transplantation, early rejection following liver transplants is not usually sufficiently detrimental to affect the long-term function of the liver. Late failure is due to chronic failure or recurrence of the original disease. A particularly virulent type of rejection that is associated with damage to or disappearance of bile ducts may be connected with early graft loss. The survival rate at 1 year following liver transplantation ranges between 80 and 90% and is about 70% at 5 years.

Crossmatching

Decisions regarding the suitability of the donor organ for liver transplantation are currently based on ABO blood matching and organ size. HLA antigen typing is not used to match donors and recipients, although an inverse relationship between matching and survival has been reported. Many liver transplants are performed in small adults, so the donor liver must be of an appropriate size to fit into the abdominal cavity. The use of livers that are made surgically smaller has drastically changed the approach to transplant in small recipients. The use of partial grafts from live donors is an extension of the work with pared-down organs from cadavers. Crossmatches are not routinely

performed preoperatively but occasionally have been performed retrospectively. Only a few instances of hyperacute rejection have been reported when the liver recipient has preformed antibodies against the donor. The reason for the apparent resistance of the liver to hyperacute rejection is unknown. It has been suggested that the liver is not sensitive to preformed antibodies or that the liver mass itself results in dilution of the antibody titer to a level that is not harmful. Occasionally, liver-kidney transplants in recipient-donor combinations with a positive crossmatch become negative on completion of the liver transplant. Increased antibody fixation to the graft has not been demonstrated. Loss of cytotoxic antibodies, however, could be due to the formation of soluble immune complexes. Alternatively, it may be that the blood loss associated with the liver transplant operation may dilute the antibody titers.

Rejection

Although rejection is readily diagnosed by percutaneous **biopsy,** other causes of hepatic malfunction must be considered. Biliary obstruction, vascular thrombosis, viral hepatitis, drug toxicity, and recurrence of the underlying disease must all be excluded. Signs and symptoms of rejection include fever, abdominal pain, ascites, hepatomegaly, and decreased appetite, all of which are nonspecific. Laboratory abnormalities do not predict for rejection but include elevation of serum bilirubin, alkaline phosphatase, and transaminases. During the first 2 weeks following liver transplant, there is poor correlation between elevation in liver functions, and biopsies are sometimes necessary to rule out rejection. After this initial period, the decision to perform a biopsy is predicated on abnormal liver function tests. The **histopathologic features** that suggest rejection include a mixed cellular portal infiltrate with bile duct epithelial damage and central vein or portal vein endothelial damage.

Immunosuppression

Treatment of rejection includes use of methylprednisolone, antilymphoblast globulin, monoclonal antibody, and immunosuppressant drugs, based on an assessment of the severity of the rejection.

Current protocols at most transplantation centers call for cyclosporine and prednisone with or without azathioprine as prophylaxis against rejection. Tacrolimus, another IL-2 inhibitor, has been used as an alternative to cyclosporine, and in some institutions has been the primary agent. As mentioned earlier, patients have been switched from cyclosporine to tacrolimus for recurrent rejection problems. The antimetabolite mycophenolate mofetil has been very effective in preventing rejection of cadaveric renal transplants and is currently being used as potential replacement for azathioprine in the initial immunosuppressive regimens following liver transplantation. The long-term necessity of mycophenolate mofetil remains unclear, and this agent is frequently tapered off in immunosuppressive regimens at 6 months in the setting of viral hepatitis or history of malignancy.

The use of cyclosporine and tacrolimus may be limited by their nephrotoxicity, which is compounded in patients with recent hepatorenal syndrome. It is in the setting of renal insufficiency that newer nonnephrotoxic agents may have an important role. The IL-2 receptor inhibitors as well as sirolimus may provide adequate immunologic protection until the renal function recovers following transplantation. In this way, the nephrotoxic agents can be avoided until renal recovery is complete. Advances in the field of immunosuppression are eagerly awaited to avoid the complications of the currently used immunosuppressive drugs.

PANCREAS TRANSPLANTATION

Unlike liver transplantation, which often is life-saving, pancreas transplantation can be considered only life-enhancing at present. An important goal of pancreas transplantation is the prevention of progression of the secondary sequelae of diabetes—nephropathy, neuropathy, and retinopathy—by providing biologically responsive insulin-producing tissue. Pancreas transplantation can be performed with the whole organ, a segmental graft, or dispersed islets of Langerhans. Most uremic diabetic patients improve considerably with a kidney transplant, but

other long-term complications of diabetes, such as retinopathy, angiopathy, and neuropathy, do not improve. The **autoimmune** pathogenesis of **type I insulin-dependent diabetes mellitus** is evidenced by mononuclear cell infiltrate surrounding the islets of Langerhans, and by the presence of circulating autoantibodies directed against islet cytoplasm and cell surface antigen in some type I diabetics (see Chapter 34). Autoantibodies to glutamic acid decarboxylase (GAD) identified in the sera of some diabetic patients may be important in the pathogenesis of diabetes. The disease is also strongly associated with other organ-specific autoimmune endocrinopathies and with HLA-DR3 and -DR4 and -DQμ3.2 alleles. Pancreatic tissue appears to be very immunogenic when transplanted into type I diabetic patients. The contribution of recurrent autoimmune disease following pancreatic transplantation remains to be determined.

Indications

Ideally, pancreas transplantation should be performed before the patient has developed any secondary complications of diabetes. Not all diabetic patients suffer from them, however. Only about 40% of individuals with type I diabetes develop uremia. It has been difficult to balance the risk of long-term immunosuppression against the risks of developing systemic complications of diabetes. Therefore, until recently, pancreas transplantation has been performed on patients who were uremic and required a **simultaneous renal transplant.** Several centers, however, now perform pancreas transplants in patients who have neither uremia nor kidney transplantation but have other progressive secondary complications that outweigh the risk of long-term immunosuppression. Solitary pancreas transplantation, either in the nonuremic diabetic patient or following successful renal transplantation, was previously limited by poor graft survival presumably because of the inability to detect rejection without a simultaneously transplanted kidney. With improved immunosuppressive regimens and better monitoring techniques for rejection, results of **solitary pancreas transplants** have approximated simultaneous pancreas-renal transplants in selected centers. It can be anticipated that this procedure will be performed with increasing frequency in patients with poorly controlled diabetes.

Procedure

For the whole-organ or segmental graft, the pancreas is removed from the donor and preserved in cold storage so that it can be transported from a distant retrieval site to the facility where transplantation is to take place. Preservation time in UW solution has exceeded 20 hours. Pancreas transplantation can either be done simultaneously with implantation of the kidney or sequentially in a postkidney-transplant patient with stable renal function. Simultaneous implantation of the kidney allows kidney function and kidney biopsy to be used as markers for rejection. Various surgical techniques are used for implantation of the pancreas graft, either as a whole organ with a small button of donor duodenum or as a distal segment of the pancreas (Figure 52–9).

Most frequently, the whole organ is transplanted **heterotopically** to the iliac fossa. With improvement in surgical technique and immunosuppressive regimens, exocrine drainage is increasingly achieved via the donor's duodenum to the recipient's jejunum or ileum. The technique of exocrine drainage via the recipient's bladder is still used, predominantly in solitary pancreas transplants, when a simultaneously transplanted kidney is not available as another marker of rejection. Drainage to the recipient's bladder permits monitoring of the urine amylase, which is useful for gauging rejection of the pancreas.

Another technical variation of the pancreas transplant is venous drainage of the transplanted pancreas into the recipient's portal circulation via the mesenteric vein. The benefits of portal drainage remain to be determined, including minimizing the hyperinsulinemia associated with systemic drainage via the iliac vein.

Outcome

The major **complications** following pancreas transplantation are infection, vascular thrombosis, preservation injury, rejection, and pancreatitis. Overall graft function and patient survival rates have improved steadily since the first human pancreas transplant was performed in 1966. The present overall pancreas graft survival at 1 year is over 80% in patients with a simultaneous kidney transplant. As mentioned earlier, with stricter matching criteria, better techniques for monitoring rejection, and improvements in immunosuppressive regimens, selected centers have reported graft survival approximating that for simultaneous pancreas-renal transplants.

Crossmatching & Immunosuppression

Pancreas transplant donors and recipients are typed and matched for ABO and HLA antigens, and a transplant is not performed if the crossmatch is positive. The exact role of tissue typing has not been clearly defined. In simultaneous pancreas-kidney transplant, both organs are not uniformly rejected, but rejection of their kidney graft can frequently be used to predict ongoing rejection of the pancreas. Nonetheless, in some instances the pancreas fails (presumably owing to rejection) while the kidney graft continues to function. HLA-DR matching is clearly beneficial in isolated cadaveric pancreas transplantation.

Rejection of the vascularized pancreatic allograft is recognized by a **loss of blood glucose control.**

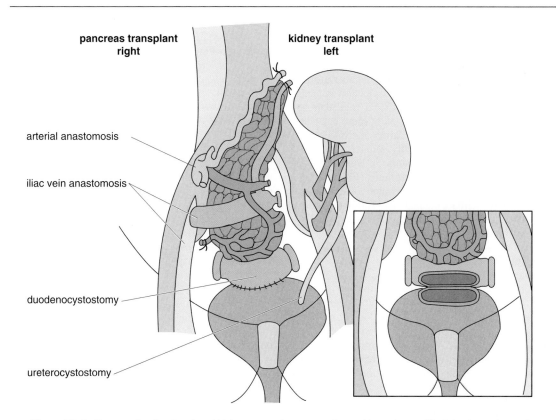

Figure 52–9. Pancreaticoduodenal and kidney transplant, as performed in patients with diabetic nephropathy.

This is unfortunately a relatively insensitive and late finding. Disappearance of insulin from the circulation usually parallels the plasma glucose levels and is not an early indicator of rejection. Corticosteroid immunosuppression also tends to cause diabetogenic effects. Serum amylase levels have not been useful in diagnosis of rejection. In transplants drained into the urinary system, however, **low urinary amylase** usually precedes changes in blood glucose levels, therefore allowing time for institution of antirejection therapy.

The current practice at some centers is to perform a **biopsy** of the graft when there is a question of rejection. **Vasculitis** is the only certain histologic evidence for rejection because parenchymal fibrosis and inflammatory cell infiltrate may indicate a foreign body reaction, particularly in grafts with polymer-injected ducts or grafts associated with recurrent disease. Successful immunosuppression for pancreas transplantation appears to be more difficult than for kidney or liver transplantation.

Currently used immunosuppressive regimens for pancreas transplantation have dramatically decreased the incidence of rejection previously noted at several centers. An early rejection episode of either the kidney or pancreas approximated 80% just 3 years ago. The addition of tacrolimus and mycophenolate mofetil to the maintenance immunosuppressive regimens has decreased this to less than 20%, prompting several centers to reinitiate the transplantation of a solitary pancreas in the nonuremic recipient. Rejection is usually treated with intravenous bolus corticosteroids, an increase in the oral prednisone dose, or a course of OKT 3. Currently, many centers are reporting the prevalence of a single rejection episode following simultaneous pancreas-renal transplant at approximately 80%. Although most of these episodes are reversible with the administration of OKT 3, it is clear that these patients initially require more immunosuppression than recipients of only kidney transplants. The addition of tacrolimus (FK 506) and mycophenolate mofetil to the immunosuppression protocols may facilitate management following either solitary pancreas transplantation or simultaneous pancreas-renal transplantation.

Islet Cell Transplantation

A successful placement of isolated islets between nonidentical donor-recipient pairs has been a goal for some time. Survival of isolated islet allografts is shorter than that of allografts of skin, kidney, or heart regardless of placement site. Syngeneic grafts produce insulin and reverse hyperglycemia, virally induced diabetes, diabetes induced by beta cell toxins, and spontaneous diabetes in BB rats and NOD mice, but autografts cannot be used in most clinical situations.

Islet cells are obtained from either adult or fetal pancreas. The fetal pancreas contains less connective tissue, yielding more viable islets but still not sufficient to render a recipient normoglycemic. Islets are retrieved by mechanical separation followed by enzymatic digestion, usually with collagenase, then density gradient centrifugation to remove as much nonislet tissue as possible. Even purified islets contain dendritic cells and other cells capable of supporting an immune response. Attempts to reduce the immunogenicity of islet tissue have included treatment with anticlass II monoclonal antibody or irradiation and culturing of pure islets in an oxygen-rich atmosphere. Encapsulation of individual islets within a semipermeable biologic membrane to exclude immunocompetent cells has been successful in rats and mice. Islet tissue derived from genetically manipulated mice deficient for MHC class I antigens has been transplanted across major histocompatibility barriers, markedly prolonging survival. Adenoviral transduction of islets to express immunoregulatory molecules such as CTLA4-Ig has been used to protect islets from the immune response. Although islet transplantation has been slow to develop as a therapy for type I diabetes, success of allotransplanted islets from a single cadaveric donor has been reported. The advent of nonislet-toxic immunosuppressive regimens will transform islet transplantation to a clinical reality. Recent demonstration of islet allotransplantation in primate models across major histocompatibility barriers has been accomplished using nonislet toxic antibodies blockade directed against the CD40-CD40 ligand costimulatory pathway. With further improvements in nonislet-toxic regimens, methods of tolerance, and gene therapy, islet transplantation will reach its full potential.

HEART TRANSPLANTATION

The first human heart transplant in 1964 using a chimpanzee donor was a technical success, but the recipient died from inadequate cardiac output a few hours later. The second and third attempts in 1967 were also unsuccessful. In 1968, more than 100 heart transplants were performed with a 1-year survival rate of 20%, reflecting the primitive state of knowledge about recipient-donor selection and immunosuppressive management. The few groups that remained clinically active throughout the 1970s slowly filled these gaps. The advent of cyclosporin in the 1980s markedly reduced the risk of death from acute rejection and infection during the first few months following transplantation, resulting in an almost exponential worldwide growth in both the number of patients undergoing transplantation and the number of transplant centers, until 1988 when further increases were limited by the available supply of donor hearts.

In 1983, the International Society for Heart and Lung Transplantation (ISHLT) began a registry of patients undergoing all forms of thoracic organ transplantation. The 1999 report listed 48,541 patients who had undergone cardiac transplantation since the registry was begun. Annually, about 3500 patients throughout the world undergo transplants in more than 300 centers, most of which are in the United States.

Recipient Selection

Cardiac transplantation is performed in selected patients who have an **imminently life-threatening** cardiac disease that is not amenable to conventional medical or surgical treatment. The main indications are coronary artery disease and idiopathic dilated cardiomyopathy in adults, and congenital heart disease and cardiomyopathy in children. All age groups have been transplanted successfully, and operative techniques have been developed for even the most complex congenital cardiac venous and arterial malformations. The current operative mortality is less than 10% for most patients. Elevated pulmonary vascular resistance, congenital heart disease, repeat heart transplantation, and ventilator or circulatory assist device dependence at transplant are the most important early risk factors for mortality.

The only **absolute contraindications** are irreversible pulmonary vascular disease, uncontrollable infection or cancer, and a separate life-threatening disease. **Relative contraindications** include age over 65 years; advanced generalized organ dysfunction (CNS, hepatic, or renal) from poor cardiac function; and a recent pulmonary infarct or a separate disease process that would significantly affect or be affected by immunosuppression (eg, cholelithiasis, peptic ulcer disease, diverticulosis, peripheral vascular disease). Patients with a history of medical noncompliance or who are at increased risk of noncompliance because of drug or alcohol addiction or psychiatric conditions are not good candidates for any organ transplantation.

Donor Selection

Cardiac donors are heart-beating brain-dead cadavers with good cardiac function and without significant history or risk factors for cardiac disease. Donors and recipients are matched for ABO blood group compatibility and body size. Prospective donor-recipient crossmatching is performed only if pretransplant recipient screening reveals an elevated panel-reactive antibody (> 15%) or a highly specific HLA antibody specificity. The extreme shortage of cardiac donors in recent years has led to considerable relaxation in the criteria for donor suitability. Currently, donor age > 50 years is acceptable if cardiac function is satisfactory and any coronary disease is either mild or amenable to conventional coronary artery bypass or angioplasty. Ventricular hypertrophy, requirement for moderate inotropic support, and short periods of severe hypotension or cardiac arrest are also no longer absolute exclusions, provided echocardiographic and visual assessment of cardiac function are satisfactory.

Organ Procurement

Hearts are usually procured during donor multiorgan retrieval at sites remote from the recipient. The coronary circulation is flushed with a cold electrolyte solution, and then the heart is stored in the same solution at 4°C until it is implanted in the recipient. With current techniques, the maximal safe duration of ex vivo preservation is about 6 hours, but preferably less than 4 hours. High-speed civilian jet travel allows for donor hearts procured within a radius of 2000 miles from the transplant center.

Operative Procedure

Two operative techniques are possible for cardiac transplantation. Both require temporary cardiopulmonary bypass support. In the **heterotopic,** or "piggy-back," technique, the recipient's heart remains in its usual location and the donor heart is connected in a parallel configuration in the right pleural space. In the **orthotopic** technique the recipient's ventricles are completely excised and the donor's heart is positioned in its normal mediastinal location. The former is technically more difficult, offers few advantages over the orthotopic technique, and is now performed infrequently. Cardiac function is often impaired in the first few days following transplantation. In most cases this responds to pharmacologic treatment, and resting hemodynamics in the late post-transplant period are remarkably normal in the absence of allograft rejection.

Immunosuppression & Allograft Monitoring

The usual maintenance immunosuppressive regimen following heart transplantation today consists of a combination of cyclosporine or tacrolimus, azathioprine, and corticosteroids. Some groups have also begun replacing azathioprine with mycophenolate mofetil. The dosages of the individual drugs are adjusted to produce the desired level of immunosuppression (targeted blood levels, WBC, acute rejection episodes) and minimal toxicity (infections, renal function, hepatic function, bone marrow suppression, malignancy) or side effects. Because chronic corticosteroid use has been implicated in many of the late metabolic, skeletal, and ocular complications, many groups have successfully weaned patients from corticosteroids without increasing alloreactivity or compromising graft function. Antilymphocyte sera and monoclonal anti-T-cell antibodies have been used for treatment of steroid-resistant rejection or as induction therapy.

The clinical signs of **allograft dysfunction** are fatigue, dyspnea, fever, hypotension, arrhythmias, added heart sounds, increased jugular venous pressure, and pulmonary rales. They usually appear late in the course of acute cardiac rejection. The EKG findings of acute rejection are nonspecific. There is no reliable test of peripheral blood leukocyte function or activation for detecting acute rejection in its early stages. Thus monitoring alloreactivity following cardiac transplantation depends almost exclusively on the histologic examination of small pieces of myocardium removed during transvenous endocardial biopsies performed throughout the rest of the recipient's life at intervals that parallel the expected risk of rejection: weekly during the first 1–2 months after transplant, and at 3–6 month intervals beyond the first year. The biopsy specimens are graded histologically, and treatment of acute rejection usually begins once there is evidence of myocyte damage or persistent inflammation.

Chronic rejection in cardiac transplantation is manifested as coronary vasculopathy. It usually presents as heart failure or arrhythmias rather than angina because of the persistent denervation of the allograft. It consists of diffuse concentric intimal hyperplasia of both epicardial and intramyocardial vessels. The consequences of acute myocardial infarction and ischemic myocardial dysfunction are the same as those of atherosclerotic coronary artery disease. Detection is usually by periodic coronary angiography or, more recently, intracoronary ultrasound.

Complications

Primary graft failure, rejection, infection, and neoplasia are the major obstacles to successful heart transplantation. During the first posttransplant year primary graft failure, acute rejection, and infection account for more than 90% of the deaths. **Hyperacute** rejection has been documented only rarely and then usually on the basis of postmortem examination. **Acute** cellular rejection, on the other hand, occurs frequently, and treatment is required in more than 70% of patients during the first year after transplant. Fortunately most episodes resolve with high-dose pulse steroid therapy without any permanent loss of allograft function. As the incidence of acute rejection diminishes to a low but stable level beyond the first year, **chronic** rejection emerges as the major cause of late mortality. The occurrence of angiographically detectable **coronary artery disease** in the allograft may be as high as 40% at 4 years posttransplant, and there is currently no specific treatment to either prevent or halt its progression. Interestingly, this disease is seen almost exclusively in recipients who develop HLA antibodies in the posttransplant period, suggesting that humoral rejection mechanisms may be important and providing some impetus for an appropriate immunosuppressive treatment.

Infection continues to be an important early and late cause of morbidity and mortality. The range and sites of opportunistic infections and the risk factors are quite similar to those seen with other solid-organ transplants. The allograft itself is fairly resistant to infection. Although CMV and toxoplasma will occasionally be identified in endocardial biopsies, serious bacterial and fungal infections seldom involve the heart except as a terminal event.

Malignancy is also an important cause of morbidity and mortality among cardiac transplant recipients. The range and sites of tumors parallel that observed in other solid-organ transplants. The incidence of malignancy seems to correlate more with the overall degree of immunosuppression than with specific drugs. Given the generally more intense immunosuppression in heart transplant recipients than in most other recipients, it is perhaps not surprising that more tumors are seen in this population.

Results

Currently, the average patient and graft survivals in the ISHLT registry are 79.4, 65.2, and 45.8% at 1, 5, and 10 years, respectively. At 2 years after transplantation 85% of recipients are in New York Heart Association Functional Class I and 13% are in Class II. Up to 60% have been able to return to work or school full time.

COMBINED HEART-LUNG & LUNG TRANSPLANTATION

Before 1980, more than 35 pulmonary transplantations including 3 combined heart-lung transplants were performed in humans, with a median survival of less than 2 weeks. One patient survived for 10 months but with poor graft function. The excellent results with cyclosporine-based immunosuppression protocols in both animal and human cardiac transplantation in the early 1980s encouraged investigators at Stanford University to revive combined heart-lung transplantation first in primates and shortly thereafter in humans. In these early experiments healing of the supracardial tracheal anastomosis was almost always successful, whereas in previous isolated lung transplantation bronchial anastomotic complications (eg, dehiscence or stenosis) were the major cause of death in those who survived beyond the first week. Thus combined heart-lung transplantation was initially thought to be the safest operative procedure for all patients with end-stage cardiopulmonary or pulmonary disease, and isolated lung transplantation was abandoned. Canine experiments at the University of Toronto, however, revealed the adverse effects of high-dose perioperative corticosteroid therapy, the neutral effect of cyclosporine therapy, and the beneficial effect of omental wrapping on bronchial anastomotic healing. This resulted in the first successful human single-lung transplant there in 1983 in a patient with pulmonary fibrosis, and in the past 15 years single-lung transplantation has emerged as the preferred procedure for most types of end-stage pulmonary disease. Patients with pulmonary sepsis (cystic fibrosis, bronchiectasis) require bilateral lung replacement and now undergo either combined heart-lung or simultaneous bilateral single-lung transplantation.

The ISHLT also maintains a registry for patients undergoing combined heart-lung and lung transplantation. By 1999, 2510 patients had undergone combined heart-lung transplantation at 124 centers, 5347 patients had undergone single-lung transplantation, and 3751 patients had undergone bilateral lung replacement at 153 centers. As in cardiac transplantation, the major limiting factor affecting further transplantation remains limited donor organ availability.

Recipient Selection

The **indication** for combined heart-lung or lung transplantation is still the presence of an **end-stage disease** for which no alternative treatments can restore satisfactory survival or function. Major clinical categories include (1) pulmonary vascular disease, either primary pulmonary hypertension or Eisenmenger's syndrome secondary to congenital heart disease; (2) restrictive lung disease including idiopathic pulmonary fibrosis; (3) obstructive lung disease such as emphysema secondary to α_1-antitrypsin deficiency; and (4) diseases such as bronchiectasis and cystic fibrosis that produce a mixed restrictive and obstructive picture. All age groups have undergone transplantation successfully, and the indications for single-lung transplantation have been extended to include patients with Eisenmenger's syndrome and correctable intracardiac shunts (atrial septal defect, ventricular septal defect, patent ductus arteriosus).

Absolute contraindications for single or bilateral lung transplantation include concomitant cardiac failure, particularly severe right ventricular dysfunction; uncontrollable infection or cancer; and the presence of a separate life-threatening disease. Preoperative low-dose steroids, prior intrathoracic surgery, and tracheostomy are **relative contraindications.** A few ventilator-dependent patients have undergone transplantation successfully, but the presence of severe cachexia or multiorgan failure has invariably proven fatal.

Donor Selection

Lung donors are heart-beating brain-dead cadavers with good pulmonary function, no evidence of pulmonary sepsis, and a negative history or risk factors for pulmonary disease. Obviously, combined heart-lung donors must also satisfy the requirements for cardiac donation. Donors and recipients are matched in terms of approximate size, including thoracic dimensions, and ABO compatibility. If pretransplant screening of the recipient for HLA antibodies is positive, a preoperative cross-match is also preformed. For single-lung transplantation, unilateral lung disease in the donor is not necessarily a contraindication, provided function of the contralateral lung is satisfactory.

Organ Procurement

Combined heart-lung or lung procurement almost always occurs as part of a donor multiple-organ retrieval from the same donor at a site remote from the recipient. The heart and both lungs can be retrieved as a single block of tissue or separated and used in as many as three recipients. Although several techniques have proved effective for lung preservation, the simplest and most commonly used is the cold flush technique. A potent pulmonary vasodilator, prostacyclin or prostaglandin E1, is administered prior to flushing the pulmonary circulation with a cold electrolyte or blood-electrolyte solution, and the lungs are inflated and stored in the same solution at 4°C until they are ready to be implanted in the recipient. Lungs procured in this way can be safely maintained for up to 10 hours, which markedly extends the safe procurement radius over that available for cardiac transplantation, providing additional time for sequential bilateral lung transplantation and HLA typing or crossmatching if they are required.

Operative Procedure

In the combined heart-lung transplant procedure the recipient's lungs, left atrium, and both ventricles are excised and replaced with donor tissue. The airway is then reattached at the lower end of the trachea. This requires a major surgical dissection with temporary cardiopulmonary bypass support and can be complicated by bleeding or injury to the phrenic or recurrent laryngeal nerves. Single or bilateral single-lung transplants are technically simpler and do not always require temporary cardiopulmonary bypass support. The pulmonary artery and a cuff of left atrial tissue surrounding the pulmonary veins are used for the vascular anastomoses, and the airway is reattached at the level of the main stem bronchus. In neither technique is the bronchial circulation directly reestablished. The success of single and bilateral lung transplantation in patients with primary pulmonary hypertension has also led to use of pulmonary transplantation combined with simultaneous cardiac repair in patients with congenital heart disease and Eisenmenger's physiology.

Immunosuppression & Allograft Monitoring

Following lung transplantation the usual **maintenance immunosuppression** consists of cyclosporine or tacrolimus, azathioprine or mycophenolate mofetil, and corticosteroids. The dosages of the individual drugs are adjusted to optimize immunosuppression and minimize toxicity and side effects. Some physicians withhold routine corticosteroid therapy for 2–3 weeks following transplantation to allow for trachealbronchial healing, while others believe that with modification of the bronchial anastomotic technique routine postoperative corticosteroid therapy is not detrimental. In addition, the direct access to the allograft epithelium afforded by the airway has presented an opportunity to try aerosolized delivery of corticosteroids and cyclosporine.

Clinical signs of **acute pulmonary rejection** are dyspnea, tachypnea, fever, rales, hypoxemia, reduced 1-second forced expiratory volume (FEV_1), and pulmonary infiltrates. They mimic those of pulmonary infection, and differentiation of the two is crucial, although both may coexist within the allograft. Periodic bronchoscopy as part of their routine posttransplant surveillance is extremely useful in this regard. A histologic grading system for both acute and chronic pulmonary rejection has been adopted to determine when to augment immunosuppression. **Chronic rejection** in lung allografts manifests as bronchiolitis obliterans that presents as either an asymptomatic decline in expiratory airflow rates or in more advanced cases as unremitting dyspnea. The small airways are obstructed and eventually obliterated of small airways by chronic inflammation and fibrosis.

Noninvasive pulmonary function tests, including exercise oximetry, are extremely sensitive and reliable to monitor allograft function. Because both pulmonary infection and rejection cause declines in airflow rates and gas transfer, many practitioners use a surveillance program of daily home spirometry with or without oximetry. These data can even be transmitted electronically to the transplant center to facilitate early detection, treatment, and recovery, or at least prevention of further loss of allograft function.

The role of radiologic techniques (chest x-ray films, various types of CT scans, ventilation-perfusion scans) in allograft surveillance is still being defined, in addition to their usefulness in the diagnosis of mediastinal lymphadenopathy, pleural-based processes, pulmonary nodules, or indeterminate pulmonary infiltrates.

Complications

Technical problems with bleeding and graft dysfunction are important early sources of morbidity and mortality for the lung or combined heart-lung recipient. These, together with acute rejection and infection, account for more than 90% of deaths in the first posttransplant year. Acute pulmonary rejection occurs frequently, and asynchronous rejection of the heart and lungs may occur in recipients of combined heart-lung transplantation. At least 30% of the operative survivors ultimately develop symptoms and signs of chronic pulmonary rejection (obliterative bronchiolitis), usually in a progressively downhill and ultimately fatal course. One of the most important risk factors for the development of obliterative bronchiolitis is the frequency and severity of acute pulmonary rejection within the first 6–12 months after transplant. Some heart-lung recipients have also developed **coronary artery disease** in their allograft.

Infection is an important early and late cause of morbidity and mortality for all solid-organ transplants, but the lung recipient is particularly predisposed to pulmonary infections. The allograft's normal defense mechanisms are chronically suppressed by immunosuppressive drugs, the airway denervation, and abnormal mucociliary clearance resulting from the surgery. Primary cytomegalovirus (CMV) pneumonitis is life-threatening in this population, leading some to recommend donor-recipient CMV matching. Some form of CMV prophylaxis for recipients at risk during the first few months after transplant is almost universally recommended. CMV infection may also be a risk factor for the later development of chronic rejection.

Cancer within the allograft and elsewhere is also a significant long-term risk for the lung recipient. The overall degree of immunosuppression is probably more important than is any specific drug. Like heart transplant recipients, these patients require more intensive immunosuppression than do other recipients of solid-organ transplants.

Results

Currently, the average patient and graft survival in the ISHLT registry are 61% and 40% for combined heart-lung transplantation at 1 and 5 years, respectively; 70.8% and 40.4% for single-lung transplantation at 1 and 5 years, respectively; and 71.7% and 49.4% for bilateral lung transplantation at 1 and 5 years, respectively. Major risk factors common to all groups are retransplantation and ventilator dependence at the time of transplant.

BONE MARROW TRANSPLANTATION

Bone marrow transplantation began in 1968 when a few patients with severe combined immunodeficiency disease (SCID), Wiskott-Aldrich syndrome, or advanced leukemia received infusions of marrow from HLA-identical siblings. Previous observations in animals had shown that matching the donor and recipient at the MHC loci reduced the incidence of graft-versus-host (GVH) disease and improved survival rates. Many patients have now survived for more than two decades after bone marrow transplantation for a variety of malignant and nonmalignant hematologic diseases. Laboratory and clinical advances in histocompatibility typing, prevention of GVH disease, supportive care, and reduction of the risk of relapse have made bone marrow transplantation a realistic and successful form of treatment for several previously uniformly fatal diseases (Tables 52–1 and 52–2).

Until recently, most **bone marrow donors** have been either identical twins (syngeneic) or genotypically HLA-identical individuals (allogeneic). Only 30% of patients, however, can be expected to have an HLA-identical donor, but the use of marrow from

Table 52–1. Diseases treatable
by bone marrow transplantation.

Allogeneic/Syngeneic	Autologous
Aplastic anemia	Leukemia
Leukemia	AML
AML	ALL
ALL	Multiple myeloma
CML	Non-Hodgkin's lymphoma
Myelodysplasia	Hodgkin's disease
Multiple myeloma	Solid tumors
Non-Hodgkin's lymphoma	Breast
Hodgkin's disease	Testicular
Immunodeficiencies	Neuroblastoma
Common variable	
SCID	
Wiskott–Aldrich syndrome	
Agranulocytosis	
Osteopetrosis/genetic	
diseases	

Abbreviations: AML = acute myelogenous leukemia; ALL = acute lymphoblastic leukemia; CML = chronic myelogenous leukemia; SCID = severe combined immunodeficiency disease.

partially matched family members or phenotypically matched unrelated donors is increasingly successful. The National Marrow Donor Program (NMDP) has HLA-typing information on more than 4 million volunteer donors, and 70% of chronic leukemia patients can now find a suitable donor through this registry. For diseases not involving the marrow, autologous transplantation allows the use of high-dose chemoradiotherapy and avoids the risk of GVH disease. Studies of monoclonal antibodies to leukemic and other malignant cells or of in vitro chemotherapy give promise that such marrow "purging" techniques could greatly extend the benefit of autologous transplantation to patients assumed to have indiscernible neoplastic cells remaining in the marrow.

Indications & Results

A. SCID: Bone marrow transplantation is the treatment of choice for children with congenital SCID and

Table 52–2. Genetic diseases treatable
by bone marrow transplantation.

SCID
Wiskott–Aldrich syndrome
Fanconi's anemia
Kostmann's syndrome
Chronic granulomatous disease
Osteopetrosis
Ataxia–telangiectasia
Diamond–Blackfan syndrome
Mucocutaneous candidiasis
Chédiak–Higashi syndrome
Cartilage–hair hypoplasia
Mucopolysaccharidosis
Gaucher's disease
Thalassemia major
Sickle cell anemia

Abbreviation: SCID = severe combined immunodeficiency disease.

its variants. No immunosuppressive conditioning is necessary for HLA-matched transplants. Partially matched recipients require conditioning, usually with cyclophosphamide and busulfan. The **removal of T cells** from donor marrow by lectin agglutination or monoclonal antibody and complement lysis enables parents to serve as donors for haploidentical children with these disorders.

B. Aplastic Anemia: Severe aplastic anemia has a mortality rate of 90% when treated with supportive care alone. Allogeneic bone marrow transplantation increases survival to 60% overall and to 80% in patients younger than 30 years. Furthermore, if patients are able to avoid pretransplantation transfusions—and hence presensitization—the overall actuarial survival at 10 years increases to 80–90%. Unlike leukemia, rejection of the donor marrow in aplastic anemia had been a major cause of failure in the past (15–30% versus 1% for leukemia); this is probably due to the underlying autoimmune nature of the aplasia in some patients, to presensitization by transfusions, and to the lack of radiotherapy in the standard and conditioning regimen. Adding ATG to cyclophosphamide reduces graft rejection without causing excessive toxicity.

For patients without marrow donors or for those over age 60 years, the treatment of choice is immunosuppressive therapy with ATG combined with cyclosporine. This produces responses and 5-year survival in 60% of patients. Long-term survivors may develop myelodysplasia, however, reflecting underlying bone marrow injury. High-dose cyclophosphamide (200 mg/kg) without stem cell support has recently been reported to produce comparable results and is an alternative treatment.

C. Acute Myelogenous Leukemia: Acute myelogenous leukemia (AML) is now a curable malignancy, both in children and adults. With improvements in supportive care, adults up to age 60 should be considered curable. After an initial complete remission with intensive chemotherapy, several potentially curative options are available. Nonablative intensive chemotherapy offers a 30–40% chance of long-term survival.

For patients with histocompatible siblings, allogeneic bone marrow transplantation in first remission offers a 60% long-term cure rate, but with a 20–25% treatment-related mortality rate in the first 6 months. The improved disease control (15–20% relapse rate compared with 55–65% for chemotherapy) is due both to the high-dose ablative chemoradiotherapy and to an alloimmune "graft-versus-leukemia" (GVL) effect of the marrow graft.

For patients without suitable donors or in older patients, autologous bone marrow transplantation offers the advantage of improved disease control from ablative therapy. In the absence of GVL, however, the relapse rate would be expected to be higher than in allogeneic bone marrow transplantation. Autologous bone marrow transplantation is a far less morbid procedure, with treatment-related mortality less than 5%, and preliminary results showing relapse rates of 20–40% and long-term survival in 40–70% of cases. The choice of allogeneic versus autologous transplant depends on risk factors associated with the patient's leukemia, primarily those associated with the cytogenetics of the leukemia.

D. Chronic Myelogenous Leukemia: During the last 50 years, patients with chronic myelogenous leukemia (CML) had no hope for cure or improved survival. Data now clearly show that allogeneic bone marrow transplantation provides a 60–80% relapse-free survival in the chronic phase of CML. Results are more favorable when the transplant is performed within 1 year of diagnosis in patients younger than 30 years, wherein the disease-free survival is 80%. Results in patients with more advanced CML are inferior. For patients without suitable sibling donors, a search for a matched correlated donor should be performed through the NMDP.

E. Acute Lymphoblastic Leukemia: Acute lymphoblastic leukemia (ALL) is now a curable malignancy in both children and adults. Conventional nonablative chemotherapy is curative in 60–90% of children and 30–60% of adults, depending on a number of factors. Allogeneic bone marrow transplantation is usually reserved for patients in second remission or in those with high-risk cytogenetics that predict a poor outcome with conventional therapy. Allogeneic bone marrow transplantation offers a 30–50% cure rate in second remission. Autologous bone marrow transplantation is not as successful as in AML but remains one option for patients without donors and should be recommended to patients destined to do poorly with conventional chemotherapy.

Procedure: Bone marrow aspirated from the iliac crests of a donor is entirely regenerated in 8 weeks. Because the amount harvested is less than 20% of the total, the donor is not harmed immunologically or hematologically. Multiple aspirations of 5 mL each, yielding a total of 10 mL/kg of the recipient's body weight (600–1200 mL), are obtained in a single procedure under general or epidural anesthesia. The marrow is drawn through heparinized needles and placed into heparinized, buffered culture medium. This mixture is then gently filtered through fine stainless steel mesh screens to produce a single-cell suspension. Nucleated-cell counts are checked to ensure the adequacy of the withdrawn marrow. If the donor and recipient are ABO-compatible, 2×10^8 to 6×10^8 nucleated marrow cells/kg of the recipient's weight are infused intravenously together with erythrocytes (erythrocyte volume of 20–30%). If the donor and recipient are not ABO-compatible, the erythrocytes must be removed from the donor's marrow in vitro.

In recent years, stem cells for **allogenic trans-plantation** have been increasingly collected from the peripheral blood rather than by bone marrow harvesting. The donors are treated with 4–5 days of subcutaneous granulocyte colony-stimulating factor (G-CSF) and undergo leukopheresis on the fourth or fifth day. In 80% of cases, a single day's collection yields an adequate stem cell dose (CD34 $> 3 \times 10^6$/kg of the recipient's weight). As in autologous transplantation, the use of blood stem cells speeds engraftment and reduces short-term toxicity. Despite the tenfold higher CD3 cell dose in the graft, the risk of acute GVH disease has not increased. Preliminary studies suggest a higher risk of chronic GVH disease.

For **autologous transplantation,** the use of peripheral blood stem cells has virtually replaced the harvest of pelvic bone marrow. Progenitor cells are mobilized and collected as described earlier, either alone or with chemotherapy. The collection of $> 5 \times 10^6$/kg CD34-positive cells ensures reliable prompt engraftment. The use of peripheral blood stem cells, as opposed to pelvic bone marrow, has sped engraftment and reduced morbidity and mortality significantly.

Except in patients with SCID, destruction of the recipient's immune system is necessary to prevent rejection and to allow transplantation of an entirely new hematopoietic system, including new immunocompetent cells. This is usually accomplished by giving cyclophosphamide, 50–60 mg/kg for 4 or 2 days (the higher dose for patients not receiving total-body irradiation). The dose of total-body irradiation is 1000–1400 cGy, which is usually administered in fractions over 3–5 days rather than in a single dose, to reduce toxicity to the lungs and eyes. This combination of chemotherapy and radiotherapy provides a potent immunoablative and antineoplastic function for most cancer patients.

A new development in the field of allogenic transplantation is the use of nonmycophenolate preparation regimens. The use of immunosuppressive drugs such as fludarabine and mycophenolate mofetil have allowed significant reductions in the dose of radiation and chemotherapy required to allow engraftment. These new less toxic preparation regimes promise to greatly extend the number of candidates for allogenic transplantation.

Following preparative chemoradiotherapy and infusion of the marrow, patients are extremely vulnerable to infections. The early and aggressive use of broad-spectrum antibiotics and amphotericin B is critical. The role of trimethoprim-sulfamethoxazole in preventing *Pneumocystis carinii* pneumonia is clearly established. Ganciclovir is effective in reducing the risk of CMV infections and pneumonitis. Platelet transfusions, on the other hand, are given to keep the platelet count above 15,000/μL to prevent serious spontaneous hemorrhage. All blood products must be irradiated to prevent GVH disease caused by viable lymphocytes in transfused cellular components or plasma.

Engraftment is heralded by a rising leukocyte count and the appearance of circulating mature neutrophils 2–4 weeks after transplantation. In general, all hematopoietic and immune cells of the recipient are replaced by donor cells, although rare examples occur of mixed "chimerism," most often in children who receive transplants for immunodeficiency diseases. As peripheral counts improve, antibiotics can be discontinued and transfusions become unnecessary. Patients can be discharged when they can be observed closely as outpatients for at least the first 100 days after transplantation.

Posttransplantation Complications

The major obstacles to successful bone marrow transplantation are GVH disease, infections, interstitial pneumonia, venoocclusive liver disease, and relapse of the underlying disease. GVH disease and infections are responsible for 10–30% of morbidity and mortality in the first 100 days following transplantation.

Graft-Versus-Host Disease

The presence of immunocompetent donor cells in an immunocompromised host is a prerequisite for graft-versus-host (GVH) disease. In patients who are HLA-identical with their donors, the occurrence of GVH disease is attributed to "minor," presently undetectable differences in histocompatibility.

Acute GVH disease in humans consists of skin rash, severe diarrhea, and jaundice. Immunocompetent CD8 T cells can be found in biopsy specimens of organs rich in surface DR antigens: the skin, intestine, and liver. are The skin rash of acute GVH disease usually begins at the time of engraftment, 10–28 days after transplantation as a fine, diffuse, erythematous, macular rash often beginning on the palms, soles, or head and spreading to involve the entire trunk and sometimes the extremities. In severe GVH disease, the rash can become desquamative—the clinical equivalent of an extensive second-degree burn. Watery diarrhea is associated with malabsorption, cramps, and gastrointestinal bleeding when severe. Hyperbilirubinemia results from inflammation of small bile ducts and is usually accompanied by an elevated serum alkaline phosphatase. Elevations of alanine aminotransferase and aspartate aminotransferase are mild to moderate. A staging and grading system for GVH disease developed at the University of Washington has become standard (Table 52–3).

Successful prevention of acute GVH disease began with the use of methotrexate after transplantation. Initially, approximately 50% of patients treated with methotrexate alone developed acute GVH disease within 10–70 days after grafting, and up to half of these died. Therapy with both methotrexate and cyclosporine has reduced the risk of acute GVH disease to 20–40%, with only 5–10% of cases being severe (grade III–IV). Cyclosporine is continued for the first

Table 52–3. Clinical staging of graft-versus-host disease by organ system.

Stage	Skin	Liver	Gastrointestinal Tract
+	Maculopapular rash <25% body surface	Serum bilirubin 2–3 mg/dL	>500 mL diarrhea/d
+ +	Maculopapular rash 25–50% body surface	Serum bilirubin 3–6 mg/dL	>1000 mL diarrhea/d
+ + +	Generalized erythroderma	Serum bilirubin 6–15 mg/dL	>1500 mL diarrhea/d
+ + + +	Generalized erythroderma with bullous formation and desquamation	Serum bilirubin >15 mg/dL	Severe abdominal pain with or without ileus

6 months after transplantation. Infusions of ATG, prednisone, and monoclonal antibodies have been used with limited success to treat established acute GVH disease. T-cell depletion of donor marrow is highly successful in reducing GVH disease, but with an increased risk of rejection, higher relapse rate of leukemia, and increased risk of fungal infections.

Chronic GVH disease affects 25–45% of patients surviving longer than 180 days. It is more frequent in older patients and in those with preceding acute GVH disease. It resembles the spectrum of rheumatic or autoimmune disorders, and its main clinical effect is to produce severe immunodeficiency, leading to recurrent and life-threatening infections, like those in the congenital and acquired immunodeficiency syndromes. Treatment with prednisone, alone or in combination with immunosuppressives, can effectively reverse many of the manifestations of chronic GVH disease in 50–75% of affected patients. If the patient survives for 3–5 years, the manifestations of chronic GVH disease usually resolve.

Chronic GVH disease has a beneficial effect of reducing relapse of malignant disease, presumably through an alloimmune GVL effect. Infusions of donor lymphocytes have relapses of chronic myeloid leukemia after allogenic transplantation.

Venoocclusive Disease of the Liver

High doses of chemoradiotherapy, such as that used to condition patients prior to marrow transplantation, can cause a fibrous obliteration of small hepatic venules, known as venoocclusive disease of the liver, in about 20% of patients. Manifestations are hepatomegaly, ascites, hepatocellular necrosis, and encephalopathy within 8–20 days after transplantation.

It resolves in 60% of patients but is fatal in 5–20%. There is no effective treatment.

The most important risk factor is the presence of hepatitis before transplantation, which, by serology and natural history, is usually non-A, non-B viral hepatitis associated with transfusions. Patients with transaminasemia before bone marrow transplantation are three to four times more likely to develop venoocclusive disease than are those with normal serum liver enzymes. Venoocclusive disease must be distinguished from GVH disease of the liver and from viral and fungal infections.

Infections

Infectious complications of bone marrow transplantation are from the lack of granulocytes and lymphocytes following ablation by the pretransplant conditioning regimen. Because full recovery of these two major elements of the immune system occurs separately following transplantation, the risk of infection can be separated into **three distinct phases** (Table 52–4).

The **first,** and most dangerous, phase is the 2–4-week period prior to engraftment, when no circulating leukocytes are present. During this time, patients are at risk for both bacterial and fungal infections, which can advance extremely rapidly and cause death. Clinical experience and trials over the past 15 years have led to the aggressive, empirical use of broad-spectrum antibiotics (both antibacterial and antifungal). The recent increase in infections by resistant species of staphylococci, especially *Staphylococcus epidermidis* responsive only to vancomycin, is probably from the use of tunneled, central intravenous catheters. As a result, vancomycin is added to the antibiotic regimen.

Two to 4 weeks after transplantation, the marrow begins to export granulocytes successfully to the blood; when the absolute neutrophil count reaches 500/μL and is rising, the greatest threat of bacterial infection is past. The **second** phase of potential infectious complications is from the paucity and immaturity of lymphocytes, and the greatest risk is fungal and viral infections during the second and third posttransplant months. An especially prominent and potent pathogen is *Aspergillus fumigatus,* which can cause vascular invasion in the lungs and brain. Even when treated with amphotericin B, the infection is difficult to eradicate and may be fatal. The most prominent viral pathogen is CMV. Ganciclovir prophylaxis has had a major effect, so that CMV pneumonitis, formerly uniformly fatal, can now be effectively treated with ganciclovir plus intravenous immunoglobulin.

The **third** phase of infectious complications occurs after the third month and lasts until lymphocyte maturation occurs. This parallels the neonatal period and takes 6–18 months. During this time, the ratio of CD4 to CD8 T cells is abnormal, T cells respond poorly to antigens, and immunoglobulin production is abnormal. This leads to a risk of infection by encapsulated bacteria such as pneumococci because of a lack of opsonic immunoglobulins. The higher risk of viral infection diminishes as T-cell function gradually improves. Patients must remain relatively isolated until the immune system has fully recovered. Those with chronic GVH disease may never recover full immune function. The majority of surviving patients, however, do recover full immunity and lead lives free from infection, requiring no antibiotics or other supplements. Unlike patients with solid-organ transplants, they do not need to take immunosuppressive medications to ensure engraftment because the immune and hematopoietic systems are replaced. Once tolerance is achieved (by about 6 months after transplantation), all medications can gradually be discontinued, and patients are able to live completely normal lives.

Table 52–4. Sequence of infections after bone marrow transplant.

Phase	Infection
I Up to engraftment	Gram-positive cocci/central lines Gram-negative bacteria *Candida* *Aspergillus*

II
After initial engraftment
	Fungal
	  Aspergillus
	  Candida esophagitis
	Viral
	  CMV
	  Adenovirus
	  EBV
	  Respiratory syncytial virus, enterovirus, parainfluenza, papovaviruses

III Late	Sinopulmonary (sicca syndrome, IgA deficiency) *Streptococcus pneumoniae/Haemophilus influenzae* Varicella-zoster virus

Abbreviations: CMV = cytomegalovirus; EBV = Epstein–Barr virus.

BONE TRANSPLANTATION

Bone is more commonly transplanted than any other tissue. In general, bone-grafting operations are performed to promote healing of nonunited fractures, to restore structural integrity of the skeleton, and to facilitate cosmetic repair. Human skull defects larger than 2–3 cm are closed by neurosurgeons to protect the brain and restore bone integrity. Plastic surgeons, oral surgeons, and periodontists use fresh autografts and freeze-dried allografts in oral and maxillofacial surgery. Various bone grafts are used to promote stability of the spine and to correct spinal deformity. Autografts and allografts are used to repair the appendicular skeleton (arms and legs). When autograft sources are insufficient, allogeneic bone may be used but only in combination with an autograft, which provides a greater degree of early repair. Bone is procured for implantation by aseptic removal or by removal and subsequent sterilization by ethylene oxide or gamma irradiation. Except for a fresh autograft, all other bone tissues are used after freezing, which reduces immunogenicity.

Posttransplantation Course

After grafting, one of three courses can be followed: (1) the bone graft may become viable, acquiring the mechanical, cosmetic, and biologic characteristics of adjacent bone; (2) it may partially or completely resorb without satisfactory new bone formation, leaving disfigurement or instability; or (3) it may become sequestrated, encapsulated, and treated by the host as a foreign body. The most likely graft to achieve optimal function in humans is the fresh autograft; however, allogeneic implants are becoming more widely used.

A bone graft transferred to a recipient undergoes several adaptive phases before ultimate incorporation into the skeletal system. Osteogenesis from surviving cells of the graft itself is characteristic only of fresh autografts. By contrast, cells from an allograft usually elicit antibody production and cell-mediated immunity and start to decay. These alloimplants slowly revascularize by invasion of capillary sprouts from the host bed during the process of resorption of the old matrix. Finally, in both autografts and allografts, osteoinduction occurs by the process of recruitment of mesenchyme-type cells into cartilage and bone under the influence of a diffusible bone morphogenetic protein derived from the bone matrix. Bone morphogenetic protein is a recently discovered glycoprotein of MW 17,500. The target cell for its activity is an undifferentiated, perivascular mesenchymal cell whose protein synthesis is reprogrammed in favor of new bone formation.

Temporally, healing of bone grafts follows a well-known pattern. For the initial 2 weeks, an inflammatory response occurs, associated with infiltration of the graft by vascular buds and the presence of fibrous granulation tissue, osteoclast activity, and osteocyte autolysis. There occurs a "creeping substitution" of graft bone, manifested as differentiation of mesenchymal cells into osteoblasts that deposit osteoid over devitalized trabeculae. Dead trabeculae are later remodeled internally. Thus, through appositional new bone formation, the graft is strengthened. In contrast to cancellous bone, cortical bone grafts undergo a somewhat longer period of resorption and slower appositional phases of new bone formation. This results in only half strength being acquired during the first 6 months and full strength 1–2 years after grafting.

Immunologic Rejection

Because bone is a composite of cells, collagen, ground substance, and inorganic minerals, all but the minerals are potentially immunogenic. Cell surface transplantation antigens associated with the MHC are the most potent immunogens within osteochondral allografts and are found on cells of osteogenic, chondrogenic, fibrous, neuronal, fatty, hematopoietic, and mesenchymal origin. Cell-rich marrow contributes significantly to immunogenicity.

Fresh allogeneic bone can sensitize the host and cause the production of circulating antibodies. Nevertheless, cellular immunity is thought to be more important than humoral antibodies in causing rejection of allogeneic bone transplants. Cartilage seems to resist destruction by antibody and cellular resorptive mechanisms, but if an immune response by the recipient develops, this protection is only relative, and a low-grade, slow, immunologically mediated inflammatory response ensues, characterized by an increase in synovial fluid, leukocyte counts, antibody response, and pannus reactions.

Rejection of allogeneic bone (cortical or cancellous) elicits a response that delays healing at the site of osteosynthesis and blocks revascularization, resorption, and appositional new bone formation. Clear-cut rejection or failure of the graft occurs in only about 10% of bone grafts.

Immunosuppression

Temporary systemic immunosuppression has been used because MHC antigens are present in bone for only 2–3 months after transplantation. Drugs that have successfully allowed bone union include azathioprine, corticosteroids, cyclosporine, and cyclophosphamide. Because of side effects and the low rate of graft failure, these drugs are no longer routinely used in human musculoskeletal transplantation. A promising new technique to diminish the antigenicity of grafts uses a temporary biodegradable cement that coats the donor bone and hides the bone cell antigens until these cells have died and their MHC antigens have deteriorated.

Clinical Recovery

Early ambulation and mild exercise stimulate blood flow and osteogenesis within the graft. External splinting helps to stabilize the graft. Education of the patients in proper posture, weight-bearing, turning, and exercise has been helpful in allowing sufficient time for healing.

FUTURE OF TRANSPLANTATION

The current shortage of hearts, livers, and lungs is a major impediment to offering transplantation to the growing number of eligible recipients. Stimulated by this urgent need, research into the use of xenogeneic organs (from species other than humans) is proceeding. In addition to the usual rejection problems, a more severe form of hyperacute rejection and problems associated with transmission of animal viruses must be overcome before this approach can become a clinical reality.

Closer to implementation, however, are transplants of specific types of cells that can be used to replace missing genes or enzymes. One can imagine transplanting hepatic parenchymal cells for their synthesis of clotting factors, proteins, and even hematopoietic stem cells.

REFERENCES

KIDNEY TRANSPLANTATION

Cho YW, Terasaki PI: In: *Long Term Survival in Clinical Transplants.* Terasaki P (editor). UCLA Tissue Typing Laboratory, 1988.

Halloran PF et al: The molecular immunology of acute rejection: An overview. *Transplant Immunol* 1993;1:3.

Mizel SB: The interleukins. *FASEB J* 1989;3:2379.

Roake J: Dendritic cells and the initiation of the immune response to organ transplants. *Transplant Rev* 1994;8:37.

Solez K et al: International standardization of criteria for the histologic diagnosis of renal allograft rejection: The Banff working classification of kidney transplant pathology. *Kidney Int* 1993;44:411.

Suthanthiran M, Strom TB: Renal transplantation. *N Engl J Med* 1994;331:365.

Terasaki PI et al: High survival rates of kidney transplants from spousal and living unrelated donors. *N Engl J Med* 1995;333:333.

Warvariv V, Garovoy MR: Transplantation immunology. In: *Textbook of Internal Medicine.* Kelley WN (editor). Lippincott, 1989, p. 752.

LIVER TRANSPLANTATION

Busuttil RW et al: Right lobe living donor liver transplantation. *Ann Surg* 1999;229:313.

Casino C et al: Recurrence of hepatitis C virus infection after orthotopic liver transplantation: role of genotypes. *New Microbiol* 1999;22:11.

Cattral MS et al: Outcome of long-term ribavirin therapy for recurrent hepatitis C after liver transplantation. *Transplantation* 1999;67:1277.

Herrero JO et al: Risk factors for recurrence of hepatitis C after liver transplantation. *Liver Transpl Surg* 1998; 4:265.

Lo CM et al: Minimum graft size for successful living donor liver transplantation. *Transplantation* 1999;68: 1112.

Marcos A et al: Right lobe living donor liver transplantation. *Transplantation* 1999;68:798.

Rela M et al: Split liver transplantation. *Br J Surg* 1998; 85:881.

Perillo R et al: Multicenter study of lamivudine therapy for hepatitis B after liver transplantation. Lamivudine Transplant Group. *Hepatology* 1999;29:1581.

Riordan SM et al: Extracorporeal support and hepatocyte transplantation in acute liver failure and cirrhosis. J *Gastroenterol Hepatol* 1999;14:757.

Sheiner PA et al: The efficacy of prophylactic interferon alfa-2b in preventing recurrent hepatitis C after liver transplantation. *Hepatology* 1998;28:831.

PANCREAS & ISLET CELL TRANSPLANTATION

Jordan ML et al: Long-term results of pancreas transplantation under tacrolimus immunosuppression. *Transplantation* 1999;67:266.

Kenyon NS et al: Long-term survival and function of intrahepatic islet allografts in rhesus monkeys treated with humanized anti-CD154. *PNAS* 1999;96:8132.

Kirk AD et al: Treatment with humanized monoclonal antibody against CD154 prevents acute renal allograft rejection in nonhuman primates. *Mature Med* 1999;5:686.

Reddy KS et al: Surgical complications after pancreas transplantation with protal-enteric drainage. *J Am Coll Surg* 1999;189:305.

Stratta RJ: Review of immunosuppressive usage in pancreas transplantation. *Clin Transplant* 1999;13:1.

Sutherland DE et al: Report from the International Pancreas Transplant Registry 1998. *Trans Proc* 1999;31:597.

HEART & LUNG TRANSPLANTATION

Bourge RC et al: Pretransplantation Risk Factors for Death after Heart Transplantation: A Multiinstitutional Study. *J Heart Lung Transplant* 1993;12:549.

Heng, D et al: Bronchiolitis Obliterans Syndrome: Incidence, Natural History, Prognosis, and Risk Factors. *J Heat Lung Transplant* 1998;17:1255.

Hosenpud, JD et al: The Registry of the International Society for Heart and Lung Transplantation: Sixteenth Official Report—1999. *J Heart Lung Transplant* 1999; 18:611.

ISHLT: A working formulation for the standardization in the diagnosis of heart and lung rejection. *J Heart Lung Transplant* 1992;9:587.

O'Connell JB et al: Cardiac Transplantation: Recipient Selection, Donor Procurement, and Medical Follow-up. *Circulation* 1992; 86:1061.

Maurer J et al: International Guidelines for the Selection of Lung Transplant Candidates. *J Heart Lung Transplant* 1998;17:703.

Trulock EP: Management of Lung Transplant Rejection. *Chest* 1993;103:1566.

BONE MARROW TRANSPLANTATION

Attal M et al: A prospective, randomized trial of autologous bone marrow transplantation and chemotherapy in multiple myeloma. *N Engl J Med* 1996;335:91.

Blay JY et al: The international prognostic index correlates to survival in patients with aggressive lymphoma in relapse: Analysis of the PARMA trial. *Blood* 1998; 92:3562.

Buckley RH et al: Hematopoietic stem-cell transplantation for the treatment of severe combined immunodeficiency. *N Engl J Med* 1999;340:508.

Deeg HJ et al: Long-term outcome after marrow transplantation for severe aplastic anemia. *Blood* 1998;91:3637.

Ferrant A et al: Karyotype in acute myeloblastic leukemia: Prognostic significance for bone marrow transplantation in first remission: A European group for blood and marrow transplantation study. *Blood* 1997;90:2931.

Gale RP et al: Survival with bone marrow transplantation versus hydroxyurea or interferon for chronic myelogenous leukemia. *Blood* 1998;91:1810.

Guillaume T et al: Immune reconstitution and immunotherapy after autologous hematopoietic stem cell transplantation. *Blood* 1998;92:1471.

Haioun C et al: Benefit of autologous bone marrow transplantation over sequential chemotherapy in poor-risk aggressive non-Hodgkin's lymphoma: Updated results of the prospective study LNH87-2. *J Clin Oncol* 1997; 15:1131.

Linker CA et al: Autologous bone marrow transplantation for acute myeloid leukemia using 4-hydroperoxycyclophosphamide-purged bone marrow and the busulfan/etoposide preparative regimen: A follow-up report. *Bone Marrow Tranplant* 1998;22:865.

Matthews DC et al: Phase I study of ^{131}I-Anti-CD45 antibody plus cyclophosphamide and total body irradiation for advanced acute leukemia and myelodysplastic syndrome. *Blood* 1999;94:1237.

Nademanee A et al: Results of high-dose therapy and autologous bone marrow/stem cell transplantation during remission in poor-risk intermediate and high-grade lymphoma: International index high and high-intermediate risk group. *Blood* 1997;90:3844.

Radich J et al: Detection of *bcr-abl* transcripts in Philadelphia chromosome-positive acute lymphoblastic leukemia after marrow transplantation. *Blood* 1997;89:2602.

Ratanatharathorn V et al: Phase III study comparing methotrexate and tacrolimus (Prograf, FK506) with methotrexate and cyclosporine for graft-versus-host disease prophylaxis after HLA-identical sibling bone marrow transplantation. *Blood* 1998;92:2303.

Ringden O et al: Peripheral blood stem cell transplantation from unrelated donors: a comparison with marrow transplantation. *Blood* 1999;94:455.

Sweetenham JW et al: High-dose therapy and autologous stem-cell transplantation for adult patients with Hodgkin's disease who do not enter remission after induction chemotherapy: Results in 175 patients reported to the European group for blood and marrow transplantation. *J Clin Oncol* 1999;17:3101.

BONE TRANSPLANTATION

Prolo DJ, Rodrigo JJ: Contemporary bone graft physiology and surgery. *Clin Orthop* 1985;200:322.

53

Immunosuppressive, Antiinflammatory, & Immunomodulatory Therapy

John Imboden, MD, James S. Goodwin, MD, John Davis, Jr. MD, MPH, & David Wofsy, MD

This chapter reviews current pharmacologic approaches to immune-mediated and inflammatory diseases. Broadly speaking, immunosuppressive drugs inhibit cell- or humoral-mediated immune responses, and antiinflammatory drugs suppress the functions of nonspecific inflammatory cells, such as macrophages, neutrophils, basophils, and mast cells. In practice, the distinction between immunosuppressive and antiinflammatory drugs is not always clear, because drugs may affect more than one cell type and because of the extensive interactions between the immune response and inflammation. In addition to these agents, advances in biotechnology have produced an array of novel protein drugs that have created opportunities to manipulate the immune system in ways that were not previously possible. The first generation of these so-called immunomodulators is now in clinical practice.

IMMUNOSUPPRESSIVE AGENTS

John Imboden, MD, & John Davis, Jr., MD, MPH

CYTOTOXIC AGENTS

As their name indicates, cytotoxic agents have the capacity to kill cells. These drugs were introduced into clinical practice for the treatment of neoplastic diseases. Appreciation of their immunosuppressive abilities followed, eventually leading to their use in the treatment of immune-mediated diseases and of transplant rejection. The decision to use these drugs should not be undertaken lightly because each medication carries with it the risk of serious toxicity, including susceptibility to infection and the development of neoplasia.

Folate Antagonists

Methotrexate is the only folate antagonist in current clinical use. Its parent compound, aminopterin, was used successfully in 1948 for the treatment of childhood leukemia. The first extensive experience with folate antagonists in nonneoplastic disease came with the use of methotrexate for the treatment of psoriasis. Controlled studies demonstrated the efficacy of low-dose, weekly methotrexate in treating rheumatoid arthritis in the 1980s. Now methotrexate is the disease-modifying drug most widely prescribed for the treatment of rheumatoid arthritis in the United States, and it is used in a variety of other immune-mediated diseases as well. Low-dose, weekly methotrexate appears to have both antiinflammatory and immunosuppressive effects.

Methotrexate, a folate analog, affects folate-dependent pathways. Most notably, it inhibits the enzyme dihydrofolate reductase, thereby preventing the reduction of oxidized folates to tetrahydrofolate. Several important synthetic pathways require fully reduced folates as cofactors, including the pathway for synthesis of thymidylate, which is necessary for DNA synthesis. Inhibition of dihydrofolate reductase, therefore, blocks proliferating cells in the S phase, leading to their death. Provision of leucovorin—a metabolically active, fully reduced folate—bypasses the block of dihydrofolate reductase and can "rescue" cells from methotrexate-induced death.

Inhibition of dihydrofolate reductase accounts for much of the antineoplastic activity of methotrexate and for many of its side effects. It is not clear, however, whether inhibition of dihydrofolate reductase accounts for the efficacy of methotrexate in rheumatoid arthritis and other inflammatory diseases. Currently, the weight of evidence suggests that other effects of methotrexate are more important. In the low doses used to treat immune-mediated disease, methotrexate does not appear to cause reduction of T or B lymphocytes, as might be expected if cytotoxic effects were critical. The relevant targets of low-dose methotrexate have not been defined with precision, but an attractive candidate is the enzyme 5-amino-imidazole-4-carboxamide ribonucleotide (AICAR) transformylase. Inhibition of AICAR transformylase leads to accumulation of AICAR, which in turn stimulates the extracellular release of adenosine. Adenosine has a number of antiinflammatory and immunomodulatory effects that may contribute to the therapeutic effects of methotrexate.

Methotrexate is used to treat a wide range of inflammatory conditions, including rheumatoid arthritis, psoriasis, the spondyloarthropathies, polymyositis, systemic lupus, multiple sclerosis, Crohn's disease, vasculitis, and graft-versus-host disease. The most extensive use is in rheumatoid arthritis. Approximately 70% of rheumatoid patients have a clinical response to methotrexate. Complete remissions, however, are rare, and even patients with substantial clinical responses often have some residual joint inflammation. Responses can be sustained for years, but the disease invariably returns when methotrexate is discontinued.

When used in the treatment of inflammatory disease, methotrexate is given as a weekly pulse that is usually administered orally. The doses are low relative to chemotherapy regimens for neoplastic disease. Following oral administration, the majority of methotrexate is eliminated through the kidney, and the drug should be used with caution in the setting of renal insufficiency. Methotrexate also is converted intracellularly to polyglutamate forms. Intracellular methotrexate polyglutamates are retained for prolonged time intervals and are potent inhibitors of dihydrofolate reductase and AICAR transformylase.

Toxicity is a major limitation to the use of low-dose, weekly methotrexate. In the initial studies of rheumatoid arthritis, up to 60% of patients reported side effects attributable to the drug. The most common toxicities result from inhibition of dihydrofolate reductase and the consequent death of proliferating cells: mucositis (manifested as oral ulceration, dyspepsia, and diarrhea) and bone marrow suppression (leading to cytopenias). Oral folate substantially reduces the incidence of mucositis and cytopenias and does not appear to diminish the efficacy of methotrexate in rheumatoid arthritis. Folate supplements, now in common use, do not protect against methotrexate-induced pulmonary toxicity, however, which is a hypersensitivity reaction, or hepatotoxicity. The latter correlates with cumulative dose and, after years of therapy, can cause hepatic fibrosis that leads to frank cirrhosis in a small minority of patients. Methotrexate is teratogenic and should never be used in pregnancy or in the absence of adequate contraception. Although unusual, opportunistic infections can occur with low-dose, weekly methotrexate. Several studies reported the development of low-grade B-cell lymphomas that regressed simply with discontinuation of methotrexate.

Purine Analogs

6-mercaptopurine (6-MP) was the first of this class to be used clinically. **Azathioprine,** an imidazole derivative of 6-MP, is the purine analog in current use for immunosuppression. The newer nucleoside analogs **fludarabine** and **cladribine** have been used in preliminary studies of refractory immune-mediated disease.

Azathioprine is a "pro-drug" that is converted to active 6-MP in vivo. 6-MP, an S-phase-specific agent, inhibits DNA synthesis, probably by interfering with the salvage pathway of purine synthesis and by blocking de novo purine synthesis. Derivatives of 6-MP also can be incorporated into DNA, but the significance of this is unclear. The administration of azathioprine can cause a lymphopenia of both T and B cells and can inhibit both cell-mediated and humoral immunity. Azathioprine blocks primary immune responses more effectively than secondary responses.

Azathioprine is approved by the US Food and Drug Administration (FDA) for the prevention of renal allograft rejection and for the treatment of rheumatoid arthritis. For several decades, it has been a mainstay for the prevention of graft rejection following renal and other organ transplantation. Although the availability of alternative forms of immunosuppression has diminished its use, azathioprine continues to be used widely to prevent transplant rejection, often in combination with prednisone and cyclosporine. Despite FDA approval, azathioprine rarely is the drug of first choice for treating rheumatoid arthritis, and it is not used nearly to the same extent for managing that disease as methotrexate, sulfasalazine, or hydroxychloroquine. Azathioprine, however, has an important role in the management of a wide range of other immune-mediated diseases, including systemic lupus erythematosus, polymyositis, inflammatory bowel disease, multiple sclerosis, and bullous pemphigoid. In these settings, azathioprine often facilitates lowering of the corticosteroid dose needed to control disease activity and thus is considered "steroid-sparing."

Azathioprine is administered orally. Because azathioprine and its metabolites are excreted by the kidney, the drug should be used carefully in the presence of renal insufficiency. An important pathway in the metabolism of 6-MP, the active form of azathioprine, is its conversion to inactive 6-thiouric acid by the enzyme xanthine oxidase. Because allopurinol inhibits xanthine oxidase, allopurinol potentiates the toxicity of azathioprine. Azathioprine should be used at reduced doses and with extreme caution in patients who are also taking allopurinol.

The major toxicity of azathioprine is myelosuppression, particularly leukopenia. Gastrointestinal disturbances, usually manifested as nausea and vomiting, occur in a sizable minority. Another important toxicity is hepatitis, which usually reverses with discontinuation of the drug. Azathioprine is immunosuppressive even in the absence of leukopenia and also is associated with an increased incidence of lymphoproliferative disorders, particularly in renal transplant patients.

The newer nucleoside analogs **fludarabine** and **cladribine** selectively target lymphocytes and are used primarily for the treatment of low-grade lymphoproliferative diseases: hairy cell leukemia, chronic lymphocytic leukemia, and follicular lymphomas. These drugs cross the plasma membrane by a facilitated transport mechanism and are phosphorylated by the enzyme deoxycytidine kinase to triphosphate derivatives, which cause DNA strand breaks and interfere with DNA repair processes. Because lymphocytes have an unusually high ratio of deoxycytidine kinase to 5′ nucleotidase, they accumulate higher levels of triphosphate metabolites and are more susceptible than other cell types to the cytotoxic effects of these drugs. Indeed, fludarabine and cladribine produce significant and prolonged lymphopenia of naive and memory lymphocytes in vivo. Initial studies suggest that fludarabine and cladribine may be effective in treating severe rheumatoid arthritis, lupus nephritis, and other refractory immune-mediated diseases but carry an increased risk of infection, particularly with herpes zoster.

Alkylating Agents

The alkylating agents, particularly **cyclophosphamide,** are important components of the armamentarium against the severest forms of immune-mediated disease. These drugs cross-link macromolecules, forming covalent linkages by alkylation of such moieties as phosphate groups and amino groups. Alkylating agents are toxic for resting (G_0) cells but show greatest toxicity for actively proliferating cells. These cytotoxic effects appear to derive largely from the cross-linking of DNA.

Cyclophosphamide is both antiinflammatory and immunosuppressive. Administration of cyclophosphamide reduces the numbers of lymphocytes, with B cells exhibiting greater sensitivity than T cells. Cyclophosphamide usually depresses humoral immunity, particularly primary antibody responses. It has variable effects on cell-mediated immunity. Primary immune responses are inhibited more readily by cyclophosphamide than are secondary immune responses.

Pioneering studies at the National Institutes of Health in the 1970s demonstrated a dramatic effect of cyclophosphamide on the survival rate of patients with Wegener's granulomatosis and formed the foundation for use of cyclophosphamide in other severe immune-mediated diseases. Currently, cyclophosphamide is the mainstay of therapeutic regimens for life-threatening vasculitides, including Wegener's granulomatosis, microscopic polyarteritis, polyarteritis nodosa, and isolated angiitis of the central nervous system. It also is used for managing severe end-organ involvement, particularly renal disease, in systemic lupus, and for pulmonary fibrosis, both idiopathic and secondary to rheumatic disease.

Cyclophosphamide itself does not have alkylating capability and must undergo activation through metabolism by the mixed-function oxidase system in the liver. Cyclophosphamide and its metabolites are excreted by the kidney and accumulate in the presence of renal insufficiency. When used for immune-mediated diseases, cyclophosphamide is administered either in low doses orally or in monthly intravenous pulses. Low-dose oral regimens appear to be more efficacious for the suppression of disease activity but carry the risk of greater toxicity. Monthly intravenous pulses are better tolerated but are less effective. Daily oral cyclophosphamide is used for managing active Wegener's granulomatosis and other systemic vasculitides. Lupus nephritis is commonly treated with monthly intravenous cyclophosphamide, as are other severe manifestations of lupus.

Toxicity is a major concern with cyclophosphamide therapy and necessitates a careful weighing of the potential risks and benefits. A common serious complication of cyclophosphamide is marrow suppression, particularly neutropenia. Acrolein, a renally excreted cyclophosphamide metabolite, is toxic to the bladder and can cause severe hemorrhagic cystitis, particularly in patients on oral cyclophosphamide regimens. Hydration and the use of intravenous mesna, which binds and inactivates acrolein, help to minimize the risk of cystitis following pulse intravenous cyclophosphamide. Cyclophosphamide therapy substantially increases the long-term risk of carcinoma of the bladder. Premature ovarian failure and oligospermia are common with cyclophosphamide therapy. Other toxicities include gastrointestinal disturbances, alopecia, pulmonary fibrosis, and the development of leukemias, lymphomas, and other neoplasms. Cyclophosphamide therapy, especially in combination with corticosteroids, carries an increased risk of infection.

A second alkylating agent, **chlorambucil,** is also used in the treatment of immune-mediated disease, but not nearly to the same extent as cyclophosphamide. Although only a few head-to-head comparisons have been made, chlorambucil appears to be less immunosuppressive and less effective than cyclophosphamide. It is administered orally and shares many of the toxicities of cyclophosphamide, with the notable exception of hemorrhagic cystitis.

MYCOPHENOLATE MOFETIL

Mycophenolate mofetil, a recently introduced immunosuppressive agent, is used for the prevention of rejection following allogeneic organ transplantation. Mycophenolate mofetil is converted in vivo to mycophenolic acid, an active metabolite that inhibits inosine monophosphate dehydrogenase, thereby blocking the de novo synthesis of purines. Because lymphocytes rely on the de novo pathway but other cells can use the salvage pathway of purine production, mycophenolic acid affects T and B cells to a greater extent than other cell types. In vitro, mycophenolic acid inhibits the proliferative responses of lymphocytes to mitogens and alloantigens.

Mycophenolate mofetil is administered either orally or through intravenous infusion. The parent drug is hydrolyzed rapidly to the active form, mycophenolic acid, which is then converted to inactive metabolites. Studies comparing mycophenolate mofetil and azathioprine found that, when used in combination with corticosteroids and cyclosporine, fewer episodes of renal allograft rejection occurred with mycophenolate mofetil than azathioprine. Graft survival and mortality, however, were not significantly different between the two regimens. Currently, mycophenolate mofetil is approved for use following renal or cardiac transplantation. The relative selectivity of mycophenolate mofetil for lymphocytes suggests that this drug may be useful in the treatment of autoimmune diseases, but experience with mycophenolate mofetil for this indication is limited.

LEFLUNOMIDE

The FDA recently approved **leflunomide** for the treatment of rheumatoid arthritis. After oral administration, leflunomide is converted to an active metabolite that inhibits dihydro-orotate dehydrogenase, a key enzyme in the de novo synthesis of pyrimidines. T cells rely on the de novo pathway as a major source of pyrimidine and so are particularly sensitive to the effects of leflunomide. Prospective, double-blind studies indicate that the efficacy of leflunomide is comparable to that of methotrexate in the treatment of rheumatoid arthritis. Experience with the use of leflunomide for other immune-mediated disorders is very limited. Leflunomide is usually well tolerated; toxicities include gastrointestinal side effects, rash, alopecia, and abnormal liver function tests.

CYCLOSPORINE, TACROLIMUS, & SIROLIMUS

These immunosuppressive agents interfere with signaling pathways during T-cell activation. Critical to their action is the formation of an intracellular complex with cytosolic proteins known as **immunophilins**—**cyclophilin** in the case of cyclosporine and **FK-binding protein-12** (FKBP12) for tacrolimus and sirolimus. The drug-immunophilin complex inhibits the signaling pathway.

Cyclosporine interferes with a key step in the activation of T cells and is a potent immunosuppressant. It has had a major effect on the field of organ transplantation and also has an important role in the treatment of a variety of immune-mediated disorders.

Cyclosporine is an unusual, cyclic polypeptide of 11 amino acids isolated from the fungus *Tolypocladium inflatum Gams.* Quite lipophilic, the drug enters cells and binds cyclophilin, a cytoplasmic protein. Cyclophilin is a peptidyl-prolyl cis-trans isomerase involved in the folding of proteins, but the immunosuppressant effects of cyclosporine are not due to the inhibition of the isomerase activity of cyclophilin. Rather, the cyclosporine-cyclophilin complex acquires the ability to inhibit calcineurin, a calcium-activated serine phosphatase that plays a critical role in the relay of signals from T-cell antigen receptor (TCR) to the nucleus (Figure 53–1).

Stimulation of the TCR triggers an increase in the concentration of intracellular free calcium, which activates calcineurin. Activated calcineurin dephosphorylates cytoplasmic NF-AT (nuclear factor of activated T cells), a DNA-binding protein involved in the transcription of genes encoding lymphokines (eg, interleukin-2 [IL-2]) and cell-surface molecules (eg, CD40 ligand) induced during T-cell activation. Dephosphorylation of cytoplasmic NF-AT reveals its nuclear localization sequences, leading to the translocation of NF-AT from the cytosol to the nucleus where it acts in concert with other factors to promote gene transcription.

By inhibiting calcineurin, the cyclosporine-cyclophilin complex prevents the dephosphorylation of NF-AT and blocks the translocation of NF-AT to the nucleus. Phosphorylated NF-AT remains in the cytosol, unable to promote gene transcription. Because many key TCR-induced responses, such as the production of IL-2, are NF-AT-dependent events, cyclosporine is a potent inhibitor of T-cell activation. It is also relatively selective for T cells. Cyclophilin, calcineurin, and (despite its name) NF-AT are not T-cell-specific, but T cells express relatively low levels of calcineurin (only 5000 molecules per cell compared with 200,000 molecules per cardiac muscle cell), rendering them more sensitive to inhibition by cyclosporine.

Cyclosporine usually is administered orally. Because absorption is variable, blood levels are often used to monitor therapy. The drug is extensively metabolized by the liver and is eliminated mainly in the bile.

The major use of cyclosporine is to prevent the rejection of organ transplants. Cyclosporine also has proven efficacy in a range of immune-mediated diseases, including graft-versus-host disease, psoriasis, refractory rheumatoid arthritis, Behçet's disease, polymyositis, and membranous glomerulonephritis.

Nephrotoxicity is a major limitation to the use of cyclosporine. Other toxicities include hypertension, abnormal liver function tests, neurologic side effects

normal signal transduction for IL-2 transcription

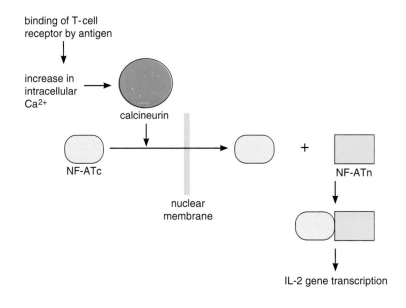

action of cyclosporin A

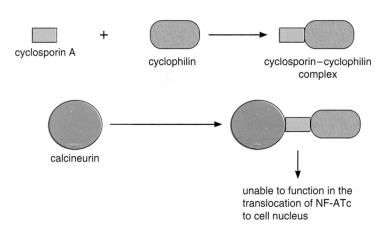

Figure 53–1. Mechanisms involved in normal signal transduction and the action of cyclosporine. Binding of the T-cell receptor by a ligand initiates an increase in intracellular calcium. This activates calcineurin, which in turn dephosphorylates the cytoplasmic component of nuclear factor of activated T cells (NF-ATc). Dephosphorylation translocates NF-AT to the nucleus, where it acts in conjunction with other transcription factors (designated here as NF-ATn) to initiate the transcription of the IL-2 gene. Cyclosporine acts as an immunosuppressant by binding to an immunophilin, cyclophilin. This complex inhibits calcineurin and prevents it from dephosphorylating NF-ATc, thereby blocking the nuclear translocation of NF-AT.

including tremor and convulsions, hirsutism, gingival hypertrophy, and gastrointestinal disturbances. Particularly when used in combination with other immunosuppressants, cyclosporine therapy is associated with an increased incidence of lymphomas and carcinoma of the skin.

Tacrolimus (formerly known as **FK506**) is a macrolide antibiotic and a potent inhibitor of T-cell activation. Although structurally unrelated, cyclosporine and tacrolimus share a similar mechanism of action and have a common target: calcineurin. Tacrolimus forms a complex with FKBP12, an immunophilin that, like cyclophilin, is a peptidyl-prolyl cis-trans isomerase. The tacrolimus-FKBP12 complex in turn inhibits calcineurin and prevents the dephosphorylation of cytoplasmic NF-AT. Like cyclosporine, tacrolimus therefore blocks the entry of NF-AT into the nucleus of activated T cells and inhibits NF-AT-dependent transcription.

Tacrolimus is approved by the FDA for the prevention of liver allograft rejection. It is also used as an alternative to cyclosporine for prophylaxis of rejection in recipients of renal and other organ transplants. Like cyclosporine, tacrolimus may be effective in immune-mediated disease such as psoriasis and severe rheumatoid arthritis, but the experience in these disorders is limited. The toxicity profile of tacrolimus is similar to that of cyclosporine.

Sirolimus (also known as **rapamycin**) is another macrolide antibiotic with immunosuppressive properties. Sirolimus is structurally related to tacrolimus and, like tacrolimus, binds FKBP12. Unlike tacrolimus and cyclosporine, however, sirolimus does not inhibit calcineurin but acts at a much later stage in T-cell activation, blocking IL-2-induced progression from G1 to S phase of the cell cycle. The sirolimus-FKBP12 complex inhibits mTOR (mammalian target of rapamycin; also designated RAFT1), a serine kinase involved in the relay of signals from the IL-2 receptor for the regulation of protein synthesis. Not surprisingly, in view of their

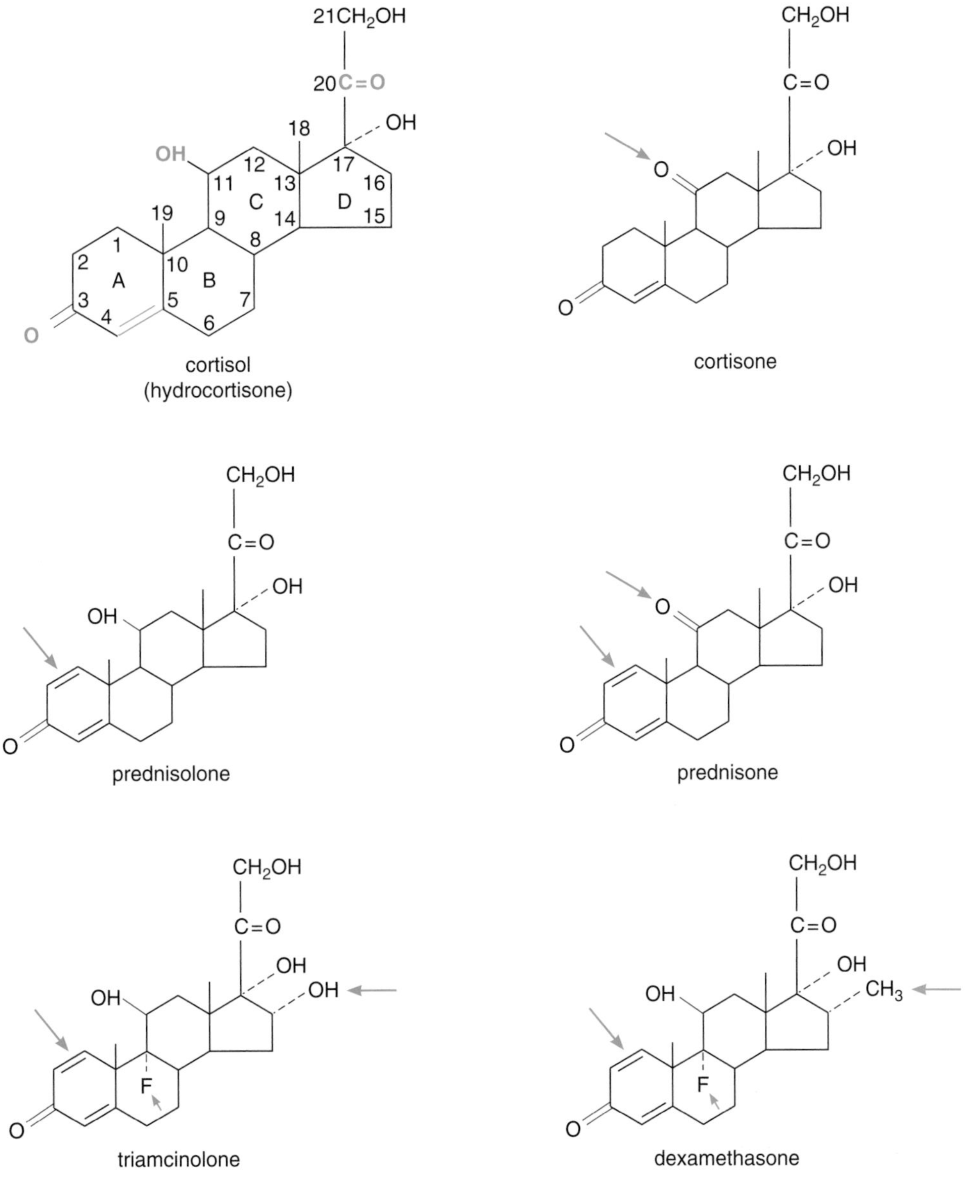

Figure 53–2. Structures of corticosteroid hormones and drugs. The arrows indicate the structural differences between cortisol and each of the other compounds.

different targets, cyclosporine and sirolimus appear to have synergistic effects in the inhibition of T-cell function. Recently the FDA approved sirolimus for use in combination with cyclosporine and corticosteroids for the prevention of acute renal allograft rejection.

ANTIINFLAMMATORY DRUGS

James S. Goodwin, MD

CORTICOSTEROIDS

Glucocorticoids are the most powerful drugs currently available for the treatment of inflammatory diseases, but their use is associated with significant toxicity. The discovery of corticosteroids was a major advance in the treatment of inflammatory diseases. Since the first successful use in 1948 of hydrocortisone (cortisol), the principal glucocorticoid of the adrenal cortex, for suppression of the clinical manifestations of rheumatoid arthritis, numerous compounds with glucocorticoid activity have been synthesized and are presently standard therapy for many immunologic and nonimmunologic inflammatory conditions.

Pharmacology & Physiology

Corticosteroids are 21-carbon steroid hormones derived from the metabolism of cholesterol. Figure 53–2 shows the structures of the commonly used synthetic corticosteroids. The activity of corticosteroids depends on the presence of a hydroxyl group on carbon-11. Two of the most commonly used corticosteroids, cortisone and prednisone, are inactive until converted in vivo to the corresponding 11-hydroxyl compounds—cortisol and prednisolone.

The clinical potency of the various synthetic steroids depends on their rate of absorption, concentration in target tissues, affinity for steroid receptors, and rate of metabolism and subsequent clearance. Table 53–1 shows the half-lives and relative poten-

cies of the commonly used glucocorticoid preparations. Most are well absorbed after oral administration. Corticosteroid uptake is not usually affected by intrinsic intestinal diseases, and food intake does not influence absorption. Approximately 90% of endogenous circulating cortisol is bound with high affinity to the plasma protein corticosteroid-binding globulin. Another 5–8% is bound to albumin, a high-capacity but low-affinity reservoir for steroids. Most synthetic steroids, with the exception of prednisolone, have a low affinity for corticosteroid-binding globulin and are bound predominantly to albumin. Only the small fraction of circulating corticosteroids that are not protein-bound are free to exert a biologic action, whereas those associated with proteins are protected from metabolic degradation.

Corticosteroids are metabolized in the liver. Hydroxylation of the 4,5 double bond and ketone groups and subsequent conjugation with glucuronide or sulfate render steroids inactive and water-soluble. The kidney excretes 95% of the conjugated metabolites, and the remainder are lost in the gut. Individual differences exist in the half-lives of synthetic steroids, and patients receiving those with prolonged clearance may be at increased risk for side effects from therapy. Clearance rates of corticosteroids are also affected by other drugs and disease states. Phenytoin, phenobarbital, and rifampin can increase steroid clearance by inducing hepatic enzyme activity. Estrogen therapy and estrogen-containing oral contraceptives impair the clearance of administered steroids and may decrease the steroid requirement. In patients with liver diseases, the metabolism of corticosteroids is not significantly altered, and dose adjustments are not necessary. Dose adjustments are also generally not necessary for patients with kidney disease. Corticosteroids can lower plasma salicylate levels by enhancing their renal clearance. Patients on fixed-dose salicylate therapy may develop rapid increases to toxic levels of serum salicylate when glucocorticoids are withdrawn or tapered.

Mechanism of Action

All steroid hormones, including vitamin D, corticosteroids, sex hormones, and mineralocorticoid, act by binding to high-affinity receptors in the cytoplasm

Table 53–1. Half-life relative potency of commonly used glucocorticoids.

Glucocorticoid	Plasma Half-Life (min)	Relative Glucocorticoid Potency	Relative Mineralocorticoid Potency
Cortisol	80–120	1.0	1.0
Cortisone	80–120	0.8	0.8
Prednisone	200–210	4.0	0.25
Prednisolone	120–300	5.0	0.25
Triamcinolone	180–240	5.0	0
Dexamethasone	150–270	30–150	0

(Figure 53–3). The steroid–receptor complex, in turn, has a high affinity for nuclear interphase chromosomes and thus binds to chromosomal DNA. This triggers DNA transcription, with the formation of messenger RNA, leading to new protein synthesis. The specific genes transcribed and proteins produced after exposure to steroid hormones vary with the different steroid hormones and also with the target cell. Specificity of cell response is manifested in at least two ways. (1) The steroid-receptor complex binds to specific regulatory sequences, which, in turn, leads to transcription of the particular genes containing those sequences. Presumably the steroid–receptor complex binding vitamin D attaches to regulatory sequences on different genes from those used by the complex binding cortisol. (2) Only a small portion of the genome is capable of induction by steroid hormone because it is contained in an "unraveled" portion of chromatin sensitive to digestion with DNAse. This unraveled portion differs depending on the cell type.

The mechanism of steroid action outlined in Figure 53–3 is consistent with the delay in appearance of the pharmacologic or physiologic effects after drug administration. Some effects of glucocorticoids and other steroids are rapid, however, implying that other mechanisms of action may also be operating.

Cells exposed to glucocorticoids synthesize and release a phospholipase A_2-inhibitory glycoprotein, now termed lipomodulin. The inhibition of phospholipase A_2 leads, in turn, to a reduction in the release of arachidonic acid, thereby slowing production of arachidonic acid metabolites. Lipomodulin appears to be a family of molecules, one of which was re-cently cloned and found to have potent antiinflammatory actions. Thus, the antiinflammatory actions of glucocorticoids may be related, at least in part, to lipomodulin-induced reduction of arachidonic acid metabolites—the prostaglandins and leukotrienes that are generated by cyclooxygenase and lipoxygenase, respectively. The role of prostaglandins and leukotrienes in mediating various aspects of the inflammatory response is discussed in Chapter 13.

Antiinflammatory Effects

Administration of corticosteroids results in a complex series of changes in the actions of cells involved in inflammatory reactions. After a single dose of steroids, a net increase occurs in the number of circulating neutrophils, accompanied by a decrease in the margination, migration, and accumulation of neutrophils at sites of inflammation, which reduces the signs of acute inflammation and also interferes with the expression of delayed-type hypersensitivity skin reactions.

Corticosteroids also directly suppress the action of cells involved in the inflammatory response, inhibiting phagocytosis by neutrophils and monocytes, the production of degradative enzymes such as collagenase and plasminogen activator by neutrophils and synovial lining cells, and the production of inflammatory lymphokines and monokines such as IL-1 and tumor necrosis factor (TNF) (Table 53–2). The inhibition of these factors prevents the vasodilatation and increased vascular permeability components of the inflammatory response.

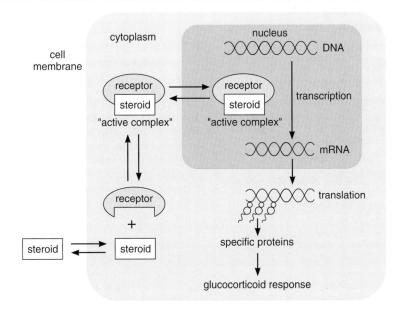

Figure 53–3. Mechanism of action of steroid hormones on a molecular level.

Table 53–2. Effects of glucocorticoids on molecules involved in inflammation.

Increased Production	Decreased Production
Lipomodulin	Collagenase
	Elastase
	Plasminogen activator
Cytokine receptors	Tumor necrosis factor
Neutral endopeptidase	Interleukin-1, IL-6, IL-8

Metabolic Effects

Like other hormones, corticosteroids affect many different tissue and organ systems. At physiologic concentrations, their various metabolic effects presumably maintain normal homeostasis, but at the high concentrations used pharmacologically (or from pathologic overproduction), an accentuation of these same metabolic effects leads to target organ dysfunction.

A summary of the metabolic effects of glucocorticoids is given in Table 53–3. In general, steroids promote catabolism. They block glucose uptake by tissues; enhance protein breakdown; and decrease new protein synthesis in muscle, skin, bone, connective tissue, fat, and lymphoid tissue. DNA synthesis and cell proliferation in fibroblasts, lymphocytes, and adipocytes are inhibited. Chronic exposure to supraphysiologic levels of corticosteroids has a type of wasting effect, that is, loss of bone, connective tissue, and muscle and gain in water and fat.

Table 53–3. Metabolic effects of glucocorticoids.

Carbohydrate metabolism
  Impairs glucose uptake and utilization by peripheral tissues
  Increases gluconeogenesis and glycogen deposition in liver

Lipid metabolism
  Stimulates lipolysis and increases free fatty acid levels, an effect countered by increased insulin release and gluconeogenesis
  Increases fat deposition in truncal and facial areas

Protein metabolism
  Inhibits synthesis and enhances breakdown of proteins in many tissues, leading to negative nitrogen balance
  Increases plasma-free amino acid levels

Nucleic acid metabolism
  Stimulates RNA synthesis in liver, inhibits RNA synthesis in other tissues
  Inhibits DNA synthesis in most tissues

Fluid and electrolyte metabolism
  May enhance sodium retention and potassium loss independent of mineralocorticoid action
  Increases glomerular filtration rate

Bone and calcium metabolism
  Decreases intestinal calcium absorption
  Decreases renal reabsorption of calcium and phosphate with resulting hypercalciuria
  Inhibits osteoblast function

Table 53–4. Side effects of glucocorticoid therapy.

Very common and should be anticipated in all patients
  Negative calcium balance leading to osteoporosis
  Increased appetite
  Centripetal obesity with muscle wasting
  Impaired wound healing
  Increased risk of infection
  Suppression of hypothalamic–pituitary–adrenal axis
  Growth arrest in children

Frequently seen
  Myopathy
  Avascular necrosis
  Hypertension
  Plethora
  Thin, fragile skin/striae/purpura
  Edema secondary to sodium and water retention
  Hyperlipidemia
  Psychiatric symptoms, particularly euphoria or depression
  Impaired glucose tolerance and diabetes
  Posterior subcapsular cataracts

Not very common, but important to recognize early
  Glaucoma
  Benign intracranial hypertension
  "Silent" intestinal perforation
  Peptic ulcer disease (often gastric)
  Hypokalemic alkalosis
  Hyperosmolar nonketotic coma
  Gastric hemorrhage

Rare
  Pancreatitis
  Hirsutism
  Panniculitis
  Secondary amenorrhea
  Impotence
  Epidural lipomatosis
  Allergy to synthetic steroids

Toxicity

The toxicities of prolonged corticosteroid therapy (listed in Table 53–4) are numerous and are the major limiting factor in the use of these agents. Susceptibility to side effects varies among patients; the reason for this is unknown. Some patients on prolonged, high-dose therapy appear to tolerate corticosteroids with few adverse effects, whereas others treated with small doses for brief intervals develop such devastating side effects as aseptic necrosis, osteoporosis, and vertebral collapse. In part, this differential sensitivity may be related to individual differences in plasma protein binding (with hypoalbuminemic patients at risk) and to variations in metabolism and clearance of synthetic steroids. Sensitivity to glucocorticoids in mice is closely linked to the H-2 histocompatibility region, and there is some evidence of analogous human leukocyte antigen (HLA) linkages in humans.

There are several useful approaches to reducing corticosteroid toxicity. One is through local application, as with topical ointments for dermatitis or administration via inhalers for asthma. Another is the use of so-called steroid-sparing drugs. These are drugs that may not have sufficient activity for use as first-line therapy but may allow a lowering of the dose of corticosteroids required to control disease activity.

ASPIRIN & OTHER NONSTEROIDAL ANTIINFLAMMATORY DRUGS

Hippocrates, Pliny, Galen, and other ancient practitioners endorsed the use of salicylate-containing extracts of willow bark for the relief of pain and the treatment of fever. The successful synthesis of acetylsalicylic acid (aspirin) at the very end of the 19th century set the stage for its subsequent large-scale production. Hundreds of different nonsteroidal antiinflammatory drugs (NSAIDs) have now been synthesized, and dozens have been introduced into clinical use. Today aspirin and NSAIDs such as ibuprofen and naproxen are among the most widely used of medications; the United States alone annually consumes 30 million pounds of aspirin. NSAIDs are used primarily for their antiinflammatory, analgesic, and antipyretic effects. In addition, low-dose daily aspirin is effective in the prevention of myocardial infarction and stroke, and increasing evidence suggests that the chronic use of aspirin and other NSAIDs reduces the risk of colorectal cancer.

Antiinflammatory Effects

The different NSAIDs have similar antiinflammatory effects in many experimental systems, suggesting that they share a similar mechanism of action (discussed in the following section). NSAIDs reduce the pain, swelling, redness, and loss of function in experimental models of inflammation as diverse as sunburn and carrageenan-induced paw edema in rats. NSAID administration reduces the rate of progressive joint destruction associated with adjuvant-induced arthritis in rats. Clinically, NSAIDs are effective in many acute and chronic inflammatory disorders, such as arthritis, tendinitis, and pericarditis, and they are analgesic, with at least some of the analgesic activities mediated by direct action in the central nervous system.

Mechanisms of Action

Aspirin and other NSAIDs at therapeutic levels inhibit the enzyme cyclooxygenase, thereby blocking the production of prostaglandins (Figure 53–4). Prostaglandins cause vasodilation and sensitize pain receptors to other inflammatory mediators such as histamine. They also are involved in central control of temperature regulation and pain sensation. The relative ability of different NSAIDs to inhibit cyclooxygenase in vitro parallels their antiinflammatory potency in vivo. Indeed, inhibition of cyclooxygenase is used as an in vitro screening test for the identification of new NSAIDs. Aspirin irreversibly inhibits cyclooxygenase by acetylating a serine residue in the active site. Inhibition by all other NSAIDs is reversible. These reversibly bind cyclooxygenase at various sites in the channel leading to the active site and sterically hinder the interaction with arachidonic acid.

There are two distinct isoforms of cyclooxygenase: COX-1 and COX-2. COX-1, a constitutive enzyme found in most tissues, is responsible for the homeostatic roles of the prostaglandins, such as protection of the gastric mucosa and platelet activation. In contrast, COX-2 is undetectable in most tissues (with the notable exceptions of the renal cortex and the central nervous system) but is rapidly induced at sites of inflammation. Macrophages, fibroblasts, and other cells express COX-2 in response to a variety of inflammatory stimuli, including cytokines such as IL-1 and TNFα. COX-2 appears to play a major role in inflammation, pain, and fever and also may participate in tissue repair after injury. In theory, selective inhibition of COX-2 should have antiinflammatory, analgesic, and antipyretic effects without toxicity due to disruption of the housekeeping functions of COX-1. Until recently, all NSAIDs available for clinical use inhibited both COX-1 and COX-2. However, two selective inhibitors of COX-2—celecoxib and rofecoxib—have now been developed and approved. Initial clinical studies indicate that celecoxib and rofecoxib reduce inflammation and pain, probably with efficacies similar to those of the nonselective NSAIDs. Whether these specific COX-2 inhibitors have less toxicity remains to be determined (see later discussion).

Inhibition of prostaglandin synthesis may not explain fully the antiinflammatory effects of NSAIDs. By blocking cyclooxygenase, NSAIDs can shunt arachidonic acid into pathways involving 5-, 12-, and 15-lipoxygenase, some of the products of which possess antiinflammatory activity. NSAIDs have been reported to inhibit cyclic adenosine monophosphate (cyclic-AMP)-dependent kinase, phospholipase C, amino acid transport across membranes, and a number of other membrane-associated events. NSAIDs inhibit a variety of neutrophil and monocyte functions, not all of which can be readily attributed to inhibition of prostaglandin production.

Toxicity

The major side effects of NSAIDs are listed in Table 53–5. Of particular importance is gastrointestinal toxicity. The mechanism is thought to involve three processes, two of which are secondary to cyclooxygenase inhibition: (1) loss of the inhibitory effects of prostaglandin E on hydrochloric acid secretion, (2) loss of the cytoprotective effect of prostaglandin E on gastric mucosa, and (3) a direct toxic effect of the NSAID, which, as an organic acid, can damage enterocytes after absorption. Certain factors place patients at higher risk for gastrointestinal complications (Table 53–6).

Between 10 and 40% of patients in controlled trials of NSAIDs stop using the drug because of upper gastrointestinal symptoms such as dyspepsia, nausea, and vomiting. NSAIDs can induce gastric and duodenal ulcers that range in severity from asymptomatic

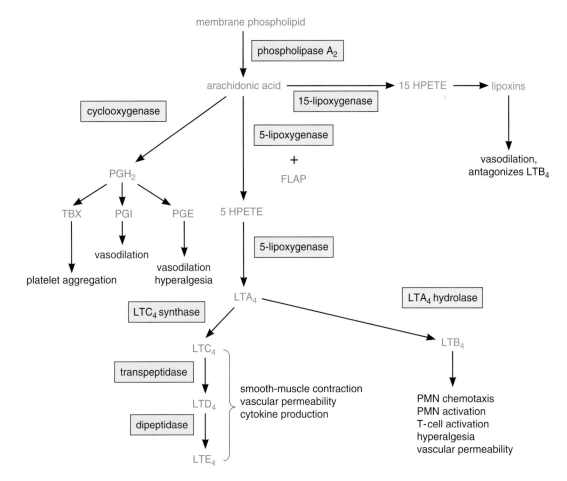

Figure 53–4. Metabolism of arachidonic acid, with contribution of metabolites to the inflammatory response. *Abbreviations:* HPETE = hydroperoxyeicotetraenoic acid; LTB = leukotriene B; FLAP = 5-lipoxygenase-activating protein; PGI prostaglandin I; TBX = thromboxane; PGH = prostaglandin H; LTC = leukotriene C; LTA = leukotriene A; PMN = polymorphonuclear neutrophil.

Table 53–5. Side effects of NSAID therapy.

Gastrointestinal
 Gastritis
 Duodenal ulcer
 Gastric ulcer

Renal
 Decreased creatinine clearance
 Acute renal failure
 Interstitial nephritis

Central nervous system
 Headache
 Confusion, memory loss, personality change, especially in
  the elderly

Toxicities not shared by all NSAIDs
 Bone marrow failure with phenylbutazone
 Rash with meclofenamate

Abbreviations: NSAIDs = nonsteroidal antiinflammatory drugs.

endoscopic findings to the cause of upper gastrointestinal bleeding and perforation. The specific COX-2 inhibitors induce several-fold fewer endoscopically detected ulcers than do the nonselective NSAIDs, but it is not yet known whether these newer drugs are associated with a reduction in clinically significant toxicity (symptomatic ulcers, bleeding ulcers, perforations). The frequency of nonulcer-related dyspepsia

Table 53–6. Characteristics associated with increased risk of upper gastrointestinal bleeding with NSAIDs.

Advanced age
History of peptic ulcer disease
Concomitant corticosteroid use
Concomitant anticoagulant use
Low functional status
Alcohol-related disease

Abbreviations: NSAIDs = nonsteroidal antiinflammatory drugs.

in patients treated with selective COX-2 inhibitors is similar to the frequency in patients on nonselective NSAIDs.

The major renal complication of NSAID use is also related to inhibition of cyclooxygenase, but the relative contributions of COX-1 and COX-2 (which also is constitutively expressed in the kidney) are under active investigation. In patients with preexisting renal disease or circulatory disease resulting in decreased renal blood flow, NSAIDs can reduce renal blood flow further and decrease the glomerular filtration rate by eliminating prostaglandin-mediated compensatory mechanisms. This becomes clinically important in some patients and can lead to renal failure, which almost always reverses on cessation of the NSAID. Renal toxicity is unusual in patients with normal renal function.

Aspirin and nonselective NSAIDs block platelet aggregation through their effects on COX-1. This antiplatelet effect can exacerbate NSAID-induced gastrointestinal bleeding but also has therapeutic uses, such as the prevention of myocardial infarction and stroke. Because the effect of aspirin on COX-1 is irreversible, aspirin is the preferred antiplatelet drug. Aspirin inhibits platelet function for the life span of the platelet, whereas the effect of the other nonselective NSAIDs is reversible. Platelets do not express COX-2, and the selective COX-2 inhibitors do not affect platelet function.

NSAIDs can precipitate severe asthma, particularly in individuals with the triad of vasomotor rhinitis, nasal polyposis, and preexisting asthma. This is not an immune-mediated response to the drug, and individuals exhibiting this form of hypersensitivity to one NSAID likely are sensitive to all NSAIDs. Loss of bronchodilating prostaglandins or local production of bronchoconstricting leukotrienes may be responsible for this idiosyncratic response to NSAIDs.

Leukotriene Antagonists

In addition to being a substrate for cyclooxygenase, arachidonic acid can be converted by 5-lipoxygenase (acting in conjunction with 5-lipoxygenase-activating protein or FLAP) to leukotriene A4, which is metabolized to either the cysteinyl leukotrienes (leukotrienes C4, D4, and E4) or to leukotriene B4 (see Figure 53–4). Because the cysteinyl leukotrienes are potent bronchoconstrictors, leukotriene antagonists have been developed for the treatment of asthma. Two classes of antileukotrienes are currently available: antagonists of the receptor (Cys-LT1) for cysteinyl leukotrienes (zafirlukast, pranlukast, and montelukast) and inhibitors of 5-lipoxygenase (zileuton). Although clinical trials have established the efficacy of these antileukotrienes in the treatment of asthma, the beneficial effect for most patients appears to be modest and less than that of inhaled corticosteroids. Certain patients, however, have marked improvement, including patients with a history of as-

pirin sensitivity. The leukotriene antagonists are generally well tolerated. A number of cases of Churg-Strauss syndrome have occurred in association with the Cys-LT1 antagonists, possibly due to the unmasking of steroid-suppressed pulmonary vasculitis when antileukotriene therapy led to tapering of corticosteroids.

COLCHICINE

Colchicine has largely been replaced in the treatment of acute gouty attacks by NSAIDs, which work quicker, are at least as efficacious, and are less toxic. It is sometimes used as an adjunctive therapy with NSAIDs in chronic or polyarticular gout and also as a prophylactic agent in low doses (0.6 mg once or twice daily) to prevent attacks.

Recently, prophylactic chronic colchicine ingestion has been found to reduce attacks of familial Mediterranean fever and to prevent the development of amyloidosis in patients with that disease. Colchicine has been reported to slow the progression of cirrhosis in patients with alcoholic liver disease.

The mechanism of action of colchicine is not completely understood. Colchicine binds to tubulin dimers, thereby preventing their polymerization to form microtubules. Microtubules are involved in many aspects of cell motion and function. The cellular target of colchicine in gout and pseudogout is the neutrophil, in which interference with microtubule formation prevents degranulation and the release of crystal-induced chemotactic factors, IL-1 and LTB_4.

DRUGS THAT SUPPRESS IMMEDIATE-HYPERSENSITIVITY REACTIONS

Cromolyn Sodium

Cromolyn sodium inhibits the release of mediators from mast cells, thereby blocking the tissue response and symptoms of IgE-mediated allergy. The precise mechanism of action of cromolyn sodium is unknown, but evidence suggests that it interferes with calcium influx through the cell membrane. It does not interfere with the binding of IgE to mast cells nor with the interaction of antigen with the IgE bound to mast cells. Rather, it suppresses the degranulation normally triggered by the cross-linking of cell surface IgE by antigen.

Cromolyn sodium is effective only prophylactically. It is poorly absorbed after oral administration and is therefore effective only when administered topically to mucous membranes. It is available as a micronized powder in a metered-dose inhaler or as a powder for inhalation in a special dispenser for asthma, as a nasal aerosolized solution for allergic rhinitis, as eye drops for allergic conjunctivitis, and as an oral preparation for use in food allergies or for systemic mastocytosis. Nedocromil sodium is chemically unrelated but therapeutically similar to cromolyn.

The toxicity of cromolyn sodium is low and relates mostly to irritation produced by the inhaled powdered drug. It has no known utility in other inflammatory diseases.

Anti-IgE Monoclonal Antibody Therapy

Efforts to block IgE-dependent events have led to the development of rhuMAb-E25, a humanized monoclonal antibody that recognizes IgE on the same site as the high-affinity Fc receptor for IgE (FcεRI). RhuMAb-E25 binds free (but not cell surface) IgE and interferes with its binding to FcεRI, thereby inhibiting allergen-dependent release of mediators from mast cells and basophils. RhuMAb-E25 remains an investigational drug, but controlled studies indicate that it has efficacy in moderate to severe allergic asthma.

Antihistamines

The two classes of antihistamines, called the H_1 and H_2 blockers, correspond to two of the three types of histamine receptors found in mammalian tissues. Only H_1 blockers are considered here because H_2 blockers do not possess noticeable antiinflammatory activity, although they are sometimes used to treat allergic diseases. The pharmacologic properties of H_1-blocking antihistamines are listed in Table 53–7.

The major therapeutic role for antihistamines is in the treatment of allergic diseases involving IgE-mediated hypersensitivity reactions. They are effective in reducing nasal and lacrimal secretions in seasonal rhinitis and conjunctivitis (hay fever). They are also effective in treating urticaria and angioedema, and they reduce pruritus associated with other dermatoses. Another major therapeutic role for antihistamines in the treatment of motion sickness and Mèniére's disease.

The principal side effects of antihistamines are sedation, dryness of mucous membranes, and constipation. Several antihistamines have been developed that lack the sedative effect, probably because of their failure to penetrate the blood-brain barrier.

A large number of drugs have antihistaminic effects. The chemical classification of these drugs and representative examples are listed in Table 53–8.

Table 53–7. Actions of histamine at H_1 receptor sites inhibited by antihistamine.

Increased capillary permeability following histamine or antigen challenge.
Smooth muscle constriction, particularly bronchial and gastrointestinal tract.
Stimulation of sensory nerve endings, leading to pruritus and sneezing.
Secretion of exocrine glands.

Table 53–8. Commonly used antihistamines (H_1 blockers).

Classic	New Generation
Alkylamines	Acrivastine[a,b]
Chlorpheniramine	
Dexchlorpheniramine	
Brompheniramine	
Triprolidine	
Ethanolamines	Ketotifen[b]
Diphenhydramine	Oxatomide[b]
Dimenhydrate	
Clemastine	
Cinarrizine[b]	
Ethylenediamines	
Tripelennamine	
Piperazines	Cetirizine[a,c]
Hydroxyzine	
Meclizine	
Phenothiazines	Mequitazine[a–c]
Promethazine	
Piperidines	Loratidine[a,c]
Cyproheptadine	Astemizole[a,c]
Azatidine	Terfenadine[a]
	Azelastine[b]

[a]Nonsedative.
[b]Not available in the United States (as of Dec., 1995).
[c]Once-a-day dosage.

Sympathomimetic Drugs

Sympathomimetic, or adrenergic, drugs mimic the effects of sympathetic nerve stimulation. They have two general mechanisms of action: (1) stimulation of adrenergic receptors and (2) increase in the release of catecholamines from sympathetic nerve endings. Some drugs have both properties.

The sympathetic nervous system is not primarily involved in the pathogenesis of allergic disease, but in certain allergic reactions—particularly anaphylactic shock and acute asthma—the vascular and visceral effects evoke a secondary sympathomimetic response to maintain homeostasis of function in the affected organs. Sympathomimetic drugs are therefore highly effective in treating many manifestations of IgE-mediated allergy.

The diverse actions of sympathomimetic amines are explained by two classes of receptors, α and β, and their subclasses, α_1, α_2, β_1, and β_2 (Table 53–9).

α_1-Adrenergic agonists cause mucosal vasoconstriction and are widely used as nasal decongestants. Examples of such drugs are phenylephrine and phenylpropanolamine. A variety of β_2-selective bronchodilators are available for treatment of asthma. These include metaproterenol, terbutaline, albuterol, pirbuterol, isoetharine, and procaterol. Epinephrine is the drug of choice for treating anaphylaxis because it has powerful α- and β-stimulating effects necessary to counteract the systemic effects of anaphylaxis.

Table 53–9. Tissue distribution and effects of different adrenergic receptors.

Receptor	Tissue Distribution	Action	Physiologic Effect
α_1	Vascular smooth muscle	Contraction	Vasoconstriction
	Radial muscle of pupil	Contraction	Dilate pupil
	Trigone sphincter muscle	Contraction	Inhibition of urination
	Pilomotor smooth muscle	Contraction	Erect hair
	Liver	Increase gluconeogenesis	Increase blood sugar
α_2	Central nervous system adrenergic receptors	Activation	Diverse
	Platelets	Aggregation	Aggregation
	Presynaptic peripheral adrenergic and cholinergic nerves	Inhibition of transmitter release	Diverse
	Some vascular smooth muscle	Contraction	Vasoconstriction
	Gastrointestinal smooth muscle	Relaxation	Decreased motility
β_1	Heart muscle	Increase cyclic-AMP[a]	Increase heart rate, force of contraction, conduction velocity
	Coronary vessel smooth muscle	Contraction	Vasoconstriction
	Fat cells	Increase cyclic-AMP	Lipolysis
β_2	Bronchial smooth muscle	Relaxation	Bronchodilation
	Liver	Increase gluconeogenesis	Increased blood sugar
	Kidney	Increased cyclic-AMP	Increased renin secretion
	Gastrointestinal smooth muscle	Relaxation	Decreased motility

Abbreviation: AMP = adenosine monophosphate.
[a]Activation of all β_1 or β_2 receptors results in increased cyclic-AMP. A more distal action is listed, if known.

Methylxanthines

The methylxanthines include caffeine and theophylline. Their principal use is as central nervous system stimulants and as bronchodilators. Theophylline is poorly soluble in water and may be administered as a salt, such as aminophylline or oxtriphylline. Theophylline and its salts are used in treatment of chronic asthma. Side effects include nervousness, insomnia, tachycardia, ventricular arrhythmias, diuresis, anorexia, nausea, vomiting, and abdominal pain. The toxicity of theophylline is related to blood levels, which are easily obtainable in most clinical laboratories.

The mechanism of action is unknown. Methylxanthines inhibit phosphodiesterase, thereby slowing the metabolism of cyclic-AMP and increasing cyclic-AMP levels. Phosphodiesterase inhibition, however, requires a much higher theophylline concentration than is clinically effective for bronchodilatation. Another potential mechanism is antagonism of adenosine. Enprofylline, however, a methylxanthine and bronchodilator, reportedly is not an adenosine antagonist.

IMMUNOMODULATORS

John Davis, Jr. MD, MPH, & David Wofsy, MD

Technologic advances have made possible the development of monoclonal antibodies (mAbs) and recombinant proteins as therapeutic agents. Moreover, improved understanding of the immune system and immune-mediated disease provides a rational basis for devising new therapeutic strategies. This section reviews the more promising of these strategies in current clinical use.

CYTOKINE INHIBITORS

Selective inhibition of particular cytokines holds considerable promise for the treatment of immune-mediated diseases ranging from asthma to multiple sclerosis. Most therapeutic efforts to block specific cytokines are still in the preclinical phase or in the early stages of clinical testing. Considerable progress, however, has been made in the development of inhibitors of TNF, a proinflammatory cytokine. The FDA recently approved two inhibitors of TNF for clinical use.

Inhibitors of Tumor Necrosis Factor

TNFα is a macrophage-derived cytokine that plays an important role in the protective inflammatory response to infection but also contributes to inflammation in rheumatoid arthritis, Crohn's disease, and other diseases. TNFβ is a T-cell-derived cytokine with similar proinflammatory properties. The two TNF receptors (p75 and p55) both bind the two forms of TNF with high affinity.

Two strategies have been pursued in an effort to block TNF. One involves a "humanized" mouse mAb (**infliximab**) that binds human TNFα (but not TNFβ) and prevents the binding of TNFα to its receptors. Infliximab is efficacious in treating Crohn's disease and has been approved for use by the FDA for the healing of fistulas in that disease. Infliximab also produces impressive improvement in the clinical manifestations of rheumatoid arthritis when used alone or in conjunction with methotrexate. Methotrexate appears to inhibit the host antibody response that can develop to the murine components of infliximab and that would otherwise compromise its long-term use.

Another therapeutic effort to block TNF led to the development of **etanercept,** a fusion protein that consists of the extracellular (ligand-binding) domain of the human TNF p75 receptor linked to the constant region of a human IgG. The p75 component of etanercept binds TNFα and TNFβ with high affinity and inhibits their interactions with endogenous TNF receptors. Etanercept has proved very effective in rheumatoid arthritis and is approved by the FDA for the treatment of that disease. Host antibody responses to this all human chimeric protein are uncommon.

Because TNF plays a crucial role in inflammation and protective immunity, the potential risk is that anti-TNF therapy may predispose patients to infection or malignancy. To date, these complications appear to be infrequent, but longer follow-up is required before it will be possible to accurately assess the magnitude of these risks.

PHARMACOLOGIC ADMINISTRATION OF CYTOKINES

There is considerable interest in the possible use of recombinant cytokines as pharmacologic agents, often with the goal of augmenting an immune response but also, in the case of antiinflammatory cytokines, of inhibiting inflammation. Some of these strategies are in early stages of development. Toxicity and limited efficacy have reduced enthusiasm for certain cytokine therapies, such as the use of IL-2 as an immune stimulant in the treatment of malignancies. Currently, the major clinical indication for cytokine therapy is with the **interferons,** a diverse but related group of cytokines with antiviral, antiproliferative, and immunomodulatory effects (see Chapter 10). Three forms have been described: interferon-α (IFNα) produced by leukocytes, interferon-β (IFNβ) produced by fibroblasts, and interferon-γ (IFNγ) produced by T cells and natural killer (NK) cells. Each of these forms of IFN has distinct biologic properties that have been exploited to create new therapies for people with viral, neoplastic, or autoimmune diseases.

IFNα has been studied extensively in the treatment of viral hepatitis. In hepatitis B, treatment with IFNα increases life expectancy and reduces the prevalence of the carrier state. In hepatitis C, IFNα shows promise, particularly in combination with other antiviral agents. Intralesional or topical administration

of IFNα has led to improvement in several viral infections, including condylomata acuminata, laryngeal papillomatosis, and herpetic keratoconjunctivitis. IFNα has also shown activity in the treatment of Kaposi's sarcoma in HIV-infected patients, but only at the expense of substantial toxicity.

IFNα has been tested as a possible treatment for a variety of neoplasms. Most patients with hairy cell leukemia respond to IFNα, although relapse is common after discontinuation of treatment. IFNα has also provided some benefit in patients with chronic myelogenous leukemia; multiple myeloma; non-Hodgkin's lymphoma; cutaneous T-cell lymphoma; and several solid tumors, including malignant melanoma, renal cell carcinoma, bladder cancer, and ovarian cancer.

IFNβ, although less well studied, also appears to be effective in the treatment of certain neoplastic conditions, particularly of the central nervous system. For example, IFNβ induces partial responses in up to 20% of patients with gliomas. Preliminary reports suggest that IFNβ may also be helpful in the treatment some autoimmune diseases, such as multiple sclerosis.

In patients with HIV infection, IFNγ has retarded progression of Kaposi's sarcoma and reduced the incidence of opportunistic infection, but it has not improved overall survival. Treatment with IFNγ improved pulmonary function in patients with idiopathic pulmonary fibrosis. The benefits of IFNγ, like the benefits of the other interferons, are achieved at the expense of side effects that reflect their biologic activities. Side effects of all of the interferons include a flu-like syndrome of fatigue, anorexia, fever, arthralgias, myalgias, and liver function abnormalities.

T-CELL-DIRECTED THERAPIES

The first therapies to use mAbs against T cells sought to deplete, or interfere with the function of, the entire T-cell population or large subpopulations of T cells. Indeed, the anti-T cell mAb OKT3, which binds the CD3 components of the antigen receptors expressed by all T cells, proved to be effective treatment for allograft rejection (Chapter 52). Such global targeting of T cells, however, has yet to produce important success in the treatment of autoimmune diseases. In the case of anti-CD4, for example, mAb therapy inhibits protective as well as pathologic immune responses. Moreover, unexpectedly prolonged depletion of CD4 T cells complicated early human trials with anti-CD4 mAbs.

Considerable current interest is focused on the development of therapeutic strategies that might achieve selective immune suppression, for example, inhibition of an autoimmune response without impairing the ability to respond to foreign pathogens. These strategies have focused on the critical cell surface interactions that occur between T cells and antigen-presenting cells (APCs) during antigen recognition. Specifically, the interaction of B7 molecules on APCs with CD28 on T cells provides an important costimulus for T-cell activation. When the costimulatory B7-CD28 interaction is disrupted in vitro, engagement of the T-cell antigen receptor induces T-cell anergy—a state of prolonged unresponsiveness— or apoptosis (see Figure 9–10). Attempts to extend this observation to in vivo systems have focused on a new strategy that takes advantage of the homology between CD28 and another T-cell surface molecule, designated CTLA-4. CTLA-4 is expressed on activated T cells and binds B7 with considerably higher avidity than does CD28. A fusion protein of the extracellular domain of CTLA-4 and the constant region of IgG1 (**CTLA4Ig**) binds B7, blocks the B7/CD28 interaction, and inhibits T-cell activation. Because in vitro blockade of B7 only induces anergy and apoptosis when concomitant stimulation of the T-cell antigen receptor occurs, CTLA4Ig may anergize or deplete in vivo only those T cells that respond to antigen at the time of administration of CTLA4Ig. The hope, therefore, is to selectively inhibit T cells recognizing autoantigens in peo-

ple with autoimmune diseases and alloantigens in transplant recipients. CTLA4Ig has been used successfully in murine models to induce tolerance to allografts and to block autoantibody production and retard autoimmune disease. Based on these observations, trials of CTLA4Ig have been initiated in humans. The first phase I trial of CTLA4Ig reported encouraging results in psoriasis. Studies of CTLA4Ig in other T-cell-mediated diseases are in progress.

A second strategy to achieve selective suppression of undesirable immune responses targets CD154 (also termed gp39 or CD40-ligand). CD154, which is expressed on activated but not on resting helper T cells, binds to CD40 on all B cells and provides a critical stimulus for B-cell proliferation, immunoglobulin production, and ultimately isotype switching (see Chapter 8). The interaction between CD40 and CD154 also promotes up-regulation of B7 expression by APC and contributes to T-cell costimulation. Anti-CD154 therapy, which disrupts the interaction of CD154 with CD40, facilitates allograft acceptance and suppresses autoimmunity in mice, and at least in certain animal models, acts in synergy with CTLA4Ig. Clinical trials of anti-CD154 therapy in human systemic lupus erythematosus are in progress.

REFERENCES

IMMUNOSUPPRESSIVE AGENTS

Crabtree GR: Generic signals and specific outcomes: Signaling through calcium, calcineurin, and NF-AT. *Cell* 1999;96:611.

Cronstein BN: The mechanisms of action of methotrexate. *Rheum Dis Clin North Am* 1997;23:739.

Davis JC, Jr et al: High dose versus low dose fludarabine in the treatment of patients with severe refractory rheumatoid arthritis. *J Rheumatol* 1998;25:1694.

Davis JC, Jr et al: A pilot study of 2-chloro-2′-deoxyadenosine in the treatment of systemic lupus erythematosus-associated glomerulonephritis. *Arthritis Rheum* 1998; 41:335.

Dooley MA, Falk RJ: Immunosuppressive therapy of lupus nephritis. *Lupus* 1997;7:630.

Ho S et al: The mechanisms of action of cyclosporin A and FK506. *Clin Immunol Immunopathol* 1996;80:S40.

Kremer JM: Methotrexate and emerging therapies. *Rheum Dis Clin North Am* 1998;24:651.

McCune WJ: Immunosuppressive drug therapy. *Curr Opin Rheumatol* 1996;8:183.

McCune WJ et al: Clinical and immunologic effects of monthly administration of intravenous cyclophosphamide in severe systemic lupus erythematosus. *N Engl J Med* 1988;318:1423.

O'Dell JR: Methotrexate use in rheumatoid arthritis. *Rheum Dis Clin North Am* 1997;23:779.

Prakash A, Jarvis B: Leflunomide: A review of its use in active rheumatoid arthritis. *Drugs* 199;58:1137.

Sievers TM et al: Mycophenolate mofetil. *Pharmacotherapy* 1997;17:155.

ANTIINFLAMMATORY AGENTS

Bause WW: Role of antihistamines in allergic disease. *Ann Allergy* 1994;72:371.

Brann DW et al: Emerging diversities in the mechanism of action of steroid hormones. *J Steroid Biochem Molec Biol* 1995;52:113.

Crofford LJ et al: Basic biology and clinical application of specific cyclooxygenase-2 inhibitors. *Arthritis Rheum* 2000;43:4.

Duval D, Freyss-Beguin M: Glucocorticoids and prostaglandin synthesis. *Prostaglandins Leukot Essent Fatty Acids* 1992;45:85.

Edwards AM: Sodium cromoglycate (Intal) as an anti-inflammatory agent for the treatment of chronic asthma. *Clin Exp Allergy* 1994;24:612.

Henderson WR: The role of leukotrienes in inflammation. *Ann Int Med* 1994;121:684.

Marcus AJ: Aspirin as prophylaxis against colorectal cancer. *N Engl J Med* 1995;333:656.

Milgrom H et al: Treatment of allergic asthma with monoclonal anti-IgE antibody. *N Engl J Med* 1999;341:1966.

Patrano C: Aspirin as an antiplatelet drug antibody. *N Engl J Med* 1994;330:1287.

Schleimer RP: An overview of glucocorticoid anti-inflammatory actions. *Eur J Clin Pharmacol* 1993:45 (suppl 1):53

Simons FER, Simons KJ: The pharmacology and use of H1 receptor-antagonist drugs antibody. *N Engl J Med* 1994;330:1663.

Ward AJ et al: Theophylline—An immunomodulatory role in asthma? *Am Rev Respir Dis* 1993;147:518.

Wenzel SE: New approaches to anti-inflammatory therapy for asthma. *Am J Med* 1998;104:287.

IMMUNOMODULATORY AGENTS

Abrams JR et al: CTLA4Ig-mediated blockade of T-cell costimulation in patients with psoriasis vulgaris. *J Clin Invest* 1999;103:1243.

Daikh DI et al: Long-term inhibition of murine lupus by brief simultaneous blockade of the B7/CD28 and CD40/gp39 costimulation pathways. *J Immunol* 1997;159:3104.

Finck BK et al: Treatment of murine lupus with CTLA4Ig. *Science* 1994;265:1225.

Maini RN et al: Therapeutic efficacy of multiple intravenous infusions of anti-tumor necrosis factor alpha monoclonal antibody combined with low-dose weekly methotrexate in rheumatoid arthritis. *Arthritis Rheum* 1998;41:1552.

McHutchison J et al: Interferon alpha-2b alone or in combination with ribavirin as initial treatment for chronic hepatitis C. *N Engl J Med* 1998;339:1485.

Reiser H, Stadescker MJ: Costimulatory B7 molecules in the pathogenesis of infectious and autoimmune diseases. *N Engl J Med* 1996;335:1369.

Targan SR et al: A short-term study of chimeric monoclonal antibody cA2 to tumor necrosis factor alpha for Crohn's disease. *N Engl J Med* 1997;337:1029.

Weinblatt ME et al: A trial of etanercept, a recombinant tumor necrosis factor receptor:Fc fusion protein, in patients with rheumatoid arthritis receiving methotrexate. *N Engl J Med* 1999;340:253.

Wong D et al: Effect of alpha-interferon treatment in patients with hepatitis B e antigen-positive chronic hepatitis B: A meta-analysis. *Ann Intern Med* 1993;119:312.

Ziesche R et al: A preliminary study of long-term treatment with interferon gamma-1b and low-dose prednisolone in patients with idiopathic pulmonary fibrosis. *N Engl J Med* 1999;341:1264.

Appendices

The CD Classification of Hematopoietic Cell Surface Markers[a]

Marker	Other Names	Cell Types/Lineages	Major Functions and Properties
CD1	T6	Cortical thymocytes, dendritic cells, B cells, intestinal epithelium	Family of nonclassical MHC class I-like proteins; specialized forms of antigen presentation
CD2	T11, sheep RBC receptor	T cells, NK cells	Binds LFA-3 (CD58); signaling
CD3	T3, Leu4	T lymphocytes	Transduces signals from T-cell receptor; T-lineage marker
CD4	T4, Leu3a	T lymphocytes, monocytes, macrophages, EBV-transformed B cells	Coreceptor for class II MHC; marker for helper T cells; signaling; receptor for human immunodeficiency virus (HIV)
CD5	T1	T lymphocytes, some B cells	Binds CD72; signaling; subset marker for B cells
CD7	Leu9	T cells, NK cells, some lymphoid and myeloid precursors	Early T-lineage marker; signaling
CD8	T8, Leu2a	T lymphocytes	Coreceptor for class I MHC; marker for cytotoxic T cells; signaling
CD10	CALLA	B-cell precursors, marrow stroma	Endopeptidase; marker for acute lymphocytic leukemia
CD11a	LFA-1 α chain	Lymphocytes, monocytes, neutrophils, NK cells	Integrin; binds ICAM-1 (CD54), ICAM-2, or ICAM-3; mediates leukocyte adhesion to other leukocytes or to endothelium
CD11b	MAC-1, CR3	NK cells, monocytes, neutrophils	Integrin; receptor for complement fragment C3bi, fibrinogen, or clotting factor X
CD11c	CR4	NK cells, monocytes, neutrophils	Integrin; receptor for complement fragment C3bi
CD14	LeuM3	Monocytes	LPS receptor
CD16	FcγRIII	Macrophages, neutrophils, NK cells	Low-affinity Fc receptor for IgG; lineage marker for NK cells
CD18	LFA-1 β chain	T and B lymphocytes, monocytes, NK cells	Integrin; binds ICAM-1 (CD54) or ICAM-2; mediates leukocyte-endothelial cell binding
CD19	B4	B lymphocytes	Signaling
CD20	B1	B lymphocytes	Signaling
CD21	CR2, B2	B lymphocytes	Receptor for complement fragment C3d, CD23, and EBV
CD22		B lymphocytes	Binds CD45RO (on T cells) or CD75 (on B cells); signaling
CD23	FcεRII	Activated B cells, macrophages, eosinophils, thymic epithelium, platelets	Low-affinity Fc receptor for IgE; ligand for CD21
CD25	IL-2R α chain, Tac	Activated T and B lymphocytes, monocytes	Low-affinity IL-2 receptor; marker for lymphocyte activation
CD28		Activated T lymphocytes (especially CD4 T cells), thymocytes	Mediates costimulation of T cells by binding B7.1 (CD80) or B7.2 (CD86) proteins on activated APCs; signaling
CD29	Integrin β1	All hematopoietic and many other cell types	Integrin; binds to extracellular matrix components
CD32	FCγRII	B lymphocytes, macrophages, neutrophils, eosinophils	Medium-affinity Fc receptor for IgG complexes; signaling

(continued)

[a] Only selected markers are listed. Certain CD designations (such as CD3) refer to heteromeric complexes of multiple polypeptide chains. Some CD proteins (such as the integrins) must associate with other proteins to mediate the functions listed here.
Abbreviations: CALLA = common acute lymphocytic leukemia antigen; LFA = leukocyte functional antigen; MAC = membrane attack complex; NK = natural killer; EBV = Epstein–Barr virus; MHC = major histocompatibility complex; ICAM = intercellular adhesion molecules; VCAM = vascular cell adhesion molecule; LPS = bacterial lipopolysaccharide; HEV = high endothelial venule; APC = antigen-presenting cell; IFN = interferon; TNF = tumor necrosis factor; IL = interleukin; MCSF = monocyte colony-stimulating factor; SCF = stem cell factor.

Marker	Other Names	Cell Types/Lineages	Major Functions and Properties
CD34		Lymph node HEV, hematopoietic stem cells, endothelium	Sialomucin; ligand for L-selectin; vascular addressin in peripheral nodes; lineage marker for hematopoietic stem cells
CD35	CR1	B lymphocytes, monocytes, neutrophils, some NK cells	Receptor for complement fragments C3b and C4b
CD38	T10	Activated lymphocytes	Unknown
CD40		B lymphocytes	Mediates T cell help by binding inducible ligand (CD40L) on surface of activated T_H cells; signaling
CD43	Leukosialin	T, B, and NK cells, monocytes	Sialomucin ligand for ICAM-1 (CD54); deficient in Wiskott-Aldrich syndrome
CD44	Hermes	T, B, and NK cells, monocytes	Hyaluronate receptor; mediates leukocyte binding to other leukocytes, to endothelium, or to extracellular matrix; signaling
CD45	Leukocyte common antigen; T200; B220 Isoforms: CD45R = 220 kd CD45RA = 205–220 kd CD45RO = 180 kd	All leukocytes	Protein tyrosine phosphatase; multiple isoforms of extracellular domain owing to alternative RNA splicing; modulates signaling; CD45RO isoform (on T cells) binds CD22 (on B cells); marker for memory (CD45RO) vs. naive (CD45RA) T cells
CD49d	VLA-4 α chain	T and B lymphocytes, monocytes	Integrin; mediates leukocyte-endothelial cell interactions by binding VCAM-1
CD54	ICAM-1	Activated lymphocytes, endothelial cells	Binds LFA-1 or CD43; receptor for rhinoviruses and for *Plasmodium falciparum*
CD55	Decay-accelerating factor	Many cell types	Degrades C3 convertase on cell surfaces; prevents complement activation
CD56	N-CAM	NK cells	NK cell adhesion; lineage marker for NK cells.
CD58	LFA-3	Activated lymphocytes, many other cells	Ligand for CD2
CD62E	E-selectin	Endothelium	Leukocyte–endothelial adhesion
CD62L	L-selectin	Leukocytes	Leukocyte–endothelial adhesion
CD62P	P-selectin	Platelets, endothelium	Leukocyte–endothelial adhesion
CD63		Neutrophils, monocytes, platelets	Activation marker for neutrophils and platelets.
CD64	FcγRI	Monocytes, macrophages	High-affinity Fc receptor for IgG
CD71	T9	Activated lymphocytes and macrophages, many proliferating cells	Transferrin receptor
CD72		B lymphocytes	Ligand for CD5
CD73	5′-Nucleotidase	Some B and T lymphocytes	Ecto-5′-nucleotidase; may regulate nucleotide uptake
CD74	Invariant chain	MHC class II-expressing cells.	Endocytic antigen presentation by MHC class II
CD79α,β	Ig-α, Ig-β	B lymphocytes	Transduces signals from B-cell antigen receptor
CD80	B7.1	B cells, dendritic cells, macrophages	APC surface ligand for T cell CD28 (help) or CTLA-4 (inhibition)
CD86	B7.2	B cells, dendritic cells, macrophages	APC surface ligand for T-cell CD28 (help) or CTLA-4 (inhibition)
CD89	FcαR	Leukocytes	Fc receptor for IgA
CD95	Fas, Apo-1	Many cell types	Induces apoptosis on binding Fas ligand (Fas-L)
CD102	ICAM-2	Endothelial cells	Binds LFA-1; leukocyte–endothelial adhesion
CD106	VCAM-1	Endothelial cells	Adhesion molecule
CD115	c-fms	Monocyte–macrophages	MCSF receptor
CD117	c-kit	Hematopoietic progenitors	SCF receptor
CD118	IFNα,βR	Many cell types	Receptor for type-1 interferons.
CD119	IFNγR	Monocyte–macrophages, B cells, endothelium	Receptor for IFNγ
CD120a,b	TNFR	Many cell types	TNF receptor types I and II
CD122	IL-2Rβ	NK cells, some B and T cells	IL-2 receptor β chain

Index

Page numbers in *italics* denote figures; those followed by "t" denote tables; those followed by "n" denote footnotes.

Abacavir, 645, 647t
ABC (ATP-binding cassette) transporters, 83
ABO blood group system, 250–251, *251,* 251t
Abortion, recurrent spontaneous, 555–556, 558–559
 in antiphospholipid syndrome, 558–559
 definition of, 558
 immunotherapy for, 559
 progesterone supplementation for, 559
ABPA. *See* Allergic bronchopulmonary aspergillosis
ACA (anticardiolipin antibodies), 448–449
Acantholysis, 504, *505*
ACE (angiotensin-converting enzyme), 187
ACE (angiotensin-converting enzyme) inhibitors, 187, 415
Acquired immune deficiency syndrome (AIDS). *See* Human immunodeficiency virus infection
Acquired immunity, 19, 61, 82
Acrodermatitis chronica atrophicans, 693
Acrosome reaction, 551
Activation-induced cell death (AICD), 70
Activation of B lymphocytes, 41–42, *42,* 46–48, *47,* 66–67, *67*
 bystander, 66
 polyclonal B-cell activators, 119
 requirements for, *48,* 48–49, 49t, 66
 T-cell help and accessory signals, 48–49, 66, 119–122, *122, 123*
Activation of endothelial cells, 25t, 26–27, 27t, 193
Activation of macrophages, 35–36
 interferon-γ and, 161
Activation of phagocytes, 68
Activation of T lymphocytes, 41–42, *42,* 46–48, *47,* 77, 136–138
 assays of, 243–245
 costimulators for, 49, 49n, 66, 122, 138, *139*
 CTLA-4 inhibition of, 139
 cytotoxic T cells, 66–67, *67*
 helper T cells, 65–66, *66*
 requirements for, *48,* 48–49, 49t
 signal transduction by T-cell receptor, 136–138, *137, 138*
Active immunization, 699–703
 adverse reactions and risk-benefit ratio for, 702
 allergic reactions to, 703
 hazards of live vaccines, 702–703
 legal liability and reporting adverse reactions to, 703, 704t
 mechanism of action of, 699–700
 previous infection and, 700
 primary and booster immunization, 700
 route of, 700
 simultaneous immunization with multiple antigens, 700–702, 709
 splenectomy and, 702
 technique of, 702

timing of, 700–702
 types of vaccines for, 79–80, 700, 701t
Acute disseminated encephalomyelitis (ADEM), 510, 516–517
 clinical features of, 517
 complications and prognosis for, 517
 differential diagnosis of, 517
 immunologic diagnosis of, 517
 immunologic features of, 516
 pathogens associated with, 516–517
 pathology of, 517
 postimmunization, 517
 treatment of, 517
Acute inflammation, 33
Acute inflammatory demyelinating polyneuropathy (AIDP), 518–519
Acute lymphoblastic leukemia (ALL), 588–591, 738
Acute myelogenous leukemia (AML), 737–738
Acute-phase response, 23–24, 24t
 cytokines in, 23, 152, 157
ADA (adenosine deaminase) deficiency, 328–330, *329*
ADCC. *See* Antibody-dependent cell-mediated cytotoxicity
Addison's disease, 316–317, 423t, 430
Addressins, vascular, 58–59, 59t
ADEM. *See* Acute disseminated encephalomyelitis
Adenohypophysitis, lymphocytic, 430
Adenosine, 195, *197*
Adenosine deaminase (ADA) deficiency, 328–330, *329*
Adhesion molecules, 8t
 on activated endothelial cells, 27, 27t
 in hematopoiesis, 6–8
 leukocyte adhesion deficiency and, 245, 337–338, *338*
 in neutrophil margination, 29, *30*
 in renal disease, 485, 485t
 in vasculitides, 451
Adjuvant(s), 73, 80
 for allergen immunotherapy, 717
 vaccines containing, 700
Adoptive T-cell therapy, for tumors, 575–576
α$_1$-Adrenergic agonists, 756
β-Adrenergic blockers, for Graves' disease, 428
β-Adrenergic bronchodilators, 363–364, 756, 757t
Adrenergic drugs, 756, 757t
Adult immunization, 709, 711t
Adult respiratory distress syndrome (ARDS), 174, 184, 546
Adult T-cell leukemia-lymphoma, 156, 569, *590,* 598–599, 653
Adverse reactions
 to drugs, 394 (*See also* Drug allergy)
 to vaccines, 702–703
Affinity maturation, 51, 126
Affinity of antigen-antibody interactions, 76
African river blindness, 686

African trypanosomiasis, 673, 679–681, *680*
Agammaglobulinemia
  malabsorption and, 304, 305
  polyarthritis and, 304
  X-linked, 117, 240, 295, 297, 302–305
Agglutination assays, 219–221, *221*
"Aggregate anaphylaxis," 374
Agranulocytosis, 435
AH_{50} assay, 232
AICD (activation-induced cell death), 70
AIDP (acute inflammatory demyelinating polyneuropathy),
    518–519
AIDS. *See* Human immunodeficiency virus infection
AIF (apoptosis-inducing factor), 15
AILD (angioimmunoblastic lymphadenopathy with
    dysproteinemia), 599
Albuterol, 363–364, 756
ALCL (anaplastic large-cell lymphoma), 600
ALG. *See* Antilymphocyte globulin
Alkylating agents, 746
ALL (acute lymphoblastic leukemia), 588–591, 738
Allelic and isotypic exclusion, 117
Allergen immunotherapy, 174, 714–717
  efficacy of, 714–715, *715*
  frequency and duration of therapy for, 714
  future strategies for, 716
    adjuvants, 717
    alternative routes of administration, 717
    modified allergens, 716–717
    peptide immunotherapy, 717
  immunologic mechanisms of, 715–716
  indications for, 714
    allergic contact dermatitis, 388
    allergic rhinitis, 358–359
    anaphylactic reaction, 376
    asthma, 364
    drug allergy, 397–398, 398, 400
  methods of, 714
  safety of, 715
Allergens
  anaphylaxis due to, 372–374
    drugs, 373, 373t
    foods, 372–373, 373t
    insect venoms, 373
    latex, 373–374
  atopic, 351–354
    animals, 354
    arthropods, 352–354
    foods, 354
    molds, 351–352, *352*
    pollens, 351, 351t, *352, 353*
  contact dermatitis due to, 387, 387t
  definition of, 349
  extracts of, 354, 354t
  hypersensitivity pneumonitis due to, 389–390, 390t
  photoallergic contact dermatitis due to, 389, 389t
  urticaria due to, 378
Allergen unit (AU), 354
Allergic asthma. *See* Asthma
Allergic bronchopulmonary aspergillosis (ABPA), 365,
    382–385, 669
  asthma and, 365, 538, 538t
  clinical diagnosis of, 384, 384t
  complications and prognosis for, 385, 385t
  in cystic fibrosis, 384
  differential diagnosis of, 384
  epidemiology of, 383
  immunologic features of, 382–383
  immunologic pathogenesis of, 383

  laboratory findings in, 383–384
  pathology of, 383
  symptoms and signs of, 383
  treatment of, 384–385
Allergic contact dermatitis, 199, 386–388, 396. *See also*
    Photoallergic contact dermatitis
  allergens associated with, 387, 387t
  clinical diagnosis of, 387
  definition of, 386
  differential diagnosis of, 387
  epidemiology of, 386
  of eyelids, 532
  immunologic diagnosis of, 387, 387t
  immunologic features of, 386
  immunologic pathogenesis of, 386
  ocular manifestations of, 532
  pathology of, 386–387
  prevention of, 388
  prognosis for, 388
  symptoms and signs of, 387
  treatment of, 388
Allergic gastroenteropathy, 349, 367–368
  complications of, 368
  definition of, 367
  differential diagnosis of, 367
  epidemiology of, 367
  immunologic features of, 367
  immunologic pathogenesis of, 367
  laboratory findings in, 367
  pathology of, 367
  prognosis for, 368
  symptoms and signs of, 367
  treatment of, 367
Allergic granulomatosis of Churg and Strauss, 455, 538
Allergic rhinitis, 19, 193, 349, 356–359
  complications of, 359
  desensitization for, 358–359
  differential diagnosis of, 357
  drug treatment of, 358
  environmental modifications for, 358
  epidemiology of, 356
  immunologic diagnosis of, 357
  immunologic features of, 356
  immunologic pathogenesis of, 357–358, *358*
  laboratory findings in, 356–357
  prognosis for, 359
  symptoms and signs of, 356
"Allergic shiners," 356
Allergy, 189. *See also* Hypersensitivity
  allergic granulomatosis and angiitis (*See* Churg-Strauss
    syndrome)
  anaphylaxis, 370–376
  asthma, 359–365
  atopic dermatitis, 365–366
  atopy and, 349
  cell-mediated hypersensitivity diseases, 386–393
    allergic contact dermatitis, 386–388, 396
    hypersensitivity pneumonitis, 389–393, 390t
    photoallergic contact dermatitis, 388–389
  chemokines and, 171
  compared with other responses, 350t
  definition of, 349
  desensitization therapy for (*See* Allergen immunotherapy)
  diagnostic testing for, 354–356
    cutaneous and intradermal testing, 354, *355,* 355t
    in vitro tests for IgE antibodies, 355, *356*
    provocation testing, 355–356
  to drugs, 394–400
  eosinophils and, 190–191

IgE-mediated, 102, 108, 191, 193, 242, 349–351
IL-4 and, 156, 350
IL-5 and, 157, 350
IL-13 and, 350
immune complex-mediated, 380–385
allergic bronchopulmonary aspergillosis, 365, 382–385
Arthus reaction, 199, 242, 380, 381t
serum sickness, 199, 201, 381–382, 381t, *382*
to latex, 373–374, 535
leukotrienes and, 194, 195
platelet-activating factor and, 195
selective IgA deficiency and, 308
T_H2 cells and, 141, 350
to transfusion, 255
urticaria and angioedema, 376–379
to vaccines, 703
Allogenic bone marrow transplantation, 738
Allograft rejection, 91. *See also* Transplantation
bone, 741
heart, 733–734
kidney, 722–725, *722–725*
liver, 728–730
pancreas, 731–732
Alloreaction, 91
Alpha-fetoprotein, 571
Alpha heavy-chain disease, 464
ALS (amyotrophic lateral sclerosis), 523
Alternative complement activation pathway, 22, *23,* 176, 179–180, 341
deficiencies in components of, 342t, 343–344
Aluminum salts, 80, 700
Alzheimer's disease, 510, 523
Amantadine, 622
Amiodarone pneumonitis, 537
AML (acute myelogenous leukemia), 737–738
Amphotericin B, 655
for blastomycosis, 660
for candidiasis, 667
for coccidioidomycosis, 664
for cryptococcosis, 668
for histoplasmosis, 665
Ampligen, 647
Amprenavir, 645, 647t
Amyloidosis, 596, 597t
Amyotrophic lateral sclerosis (ALS), 523
ANA. *See* Antinuclear antibodies
Anamnestic immune response, *69, 70*
Anaphylactic shock, 370, 371
treatment of, 375
Anaphylactoid reactions, 370, 374–375
"aggregate," 374
during anesthesia, 399
cholinergic, 374
exercise-induced, 374
idiopathic, 374–375
to ionic compounds, 374
non-IgE, 374
to polysaccharides, 374
Anaphylatoxins, 183
Anaphylaxis, 189, 202, 370–376
allergens associated with, 372–374
drugs, 373, 373t, 395
foods, 372–373, 373t
insect venoms, 373
latex, 373–374
clinical diagnosis of, 372
complications of, 376
definition of, 370
differential diagnosis of, 375

due to drug allergy, 395
general anesthetics, 399
penicillin, 398
due to passive immunization, 706
epidemiology of, 370
histamine in, 371
immunologic diagnosis of, 372, 372t
immunologic features of, 371
immunologic pathogenesis of, 349, 370–371
laboratory findings in, 371–372
lower respiratory obstruction and, 371
pathology of, 370
platelet-activating factor and, 195
prevention of, 376
prognosis for, 376
"slow-reacting substance of," 195
symptoms and signs of, 371
treatment of, 375–376
bronchial obstruction, 375
Hymenoptera insect stings, 376
laryngeal edema, 375
patient monitoring and, 375–376
shock, 375
sympathomimetic drugs, 756
urticaria, angioedema, and gastrointestinal reactions, 375
urticaria and angioedema, 371
Anaplastic large-cell lymphoma (ALCL), 600
ANCA. *See* Antineutrophil cytoplasmic antibodies
Ancylostoma duodenale, 684
Anemia
aplastic, 441–442, 737
erythrocyte production during, 2
immune hemolytic, 436–441
classification of, 437t
cold agglutinin syndromes, 439
drug-induced, 439–440, 440t
hemolytic disease of newborn, 251, 252, 257
paroxysmal cold hemoglobinuria, 440–441
serologic tests for, 436–437, 438t
warm autoimmune hemolytic anemia, 437–439
pernicious, 464–465
pure erythrocyte aplasia, 441
in rheumatoid arthritis, 407
in scleroderma, 414
in systemic lupus erythematosus, 403
Anergy, 199, 242
B-cell, 129
clinical conditions associated with, 242t
clonal, 129
definition of, 199
T-cell, 138, 759
IL-2 treatment for, 156
Anesthetics, hypersensitivity to, 399–400
Angiitis. *See* Vasculitis
Angiocentric NK/T lymphoma, 599–600
Angioedema
hereditary, 181, 378
C1 inhibitor deficiency and, 181, 345
kinins and, 187
management of, 347
urticaria and, 376–379
anaphylaxis and, 371
causes of, 378
differential diagnosis of, 378
epidemiology of, 377
immunologic diagnosis of, 377–378
immunologic features of, 376
pathogenesis of, 377
pathology of, 377

Angioedema *(continued)*
  urticaria and, *(continued)*
    symptoms and signs of, 377
    treatment of, 375, 378–379
Angiogenesis, 171
Angioimmunoblastic lymphadenopathy with dysproteinemia
    (AILD), 599
Angioimmunoblastic T-cell lymphoma, 599
Angioinvasion by fungi, 655
Angiotensin-converting enzyme (ACE), 187
Angiotensin-converting enzyme (ACE) inhibitors, 187
  for scleroderma, 415
Animal allergens, 354
Ankylosing spondylitis, 93–94, 94t, 417–418, 611
  ocular manifestations of, 528, *528*
Anthrax, 609
Antibiotics
  beta-lactam, hypersensitivity to, *398,* 398–399, *399*
  methicillin-resistant *Staphylococcus aureus,* 610
  natural, 113
  peptide, 21
  prophylaxis for bone marrow transplantation, 738
  for Reiter's syndrome, 418
  for scleroderma, 415
  for Wegener's granulomatosis, 455
Antibodies, 43. *See also* Immunoglobulin
  anticardiolipin, 448–449
  anticytoplasmic, in systemic lupus erythematosus, 405
  anti-DNA, in systemic lupus erythematosus, 404
  antiendothelial
    in renal disease, 483
    in vasculitides, 451
  antierythrocyte, in systemic lupus erythematosus, 404
  antigranulocyte, 434, 435
  antimesangial, 483
  antimitochondrial, in primary biliary cirrhosis, 472
  antineuronal, 522t
  antineutrophil cytoplasmic, 451
    in Churg-Strauss syndrome, 456
    in microscopic polyangiitis, 453
    in polyarteritis nodosa, 452
    in renal disease, 483–484, 492–493
    in ulcerative colitis, 468
    in Wegener's granulomatosis, 454–455
  antinuclear
    in antiphospholipid syndrome, 449
    in autoimmune chronic active hepatitis, 470
    in juvenile arthritis, 407
    in rheumatoid arthritis, 407
    in scleroderma, 413
    in Sjögren's syndrome, 412
    in systemic lupus erythematosus, 403–404, 404t
    testing for, 229, *230*
  antiphospholipid
    antiphospholipid syndrome, 448–449
    recurrent spontaneous abortion and, 558–559
    in stroke, 524
    in systemic lupus erythematosus, 404
  antiplasmodial, 675
  antiplatelet, 442
    in idiopathic thrombocytopenic purpura, 443, 444, 444t
    in systemic lupus erythematosus, 404–405
  antisperm, 550, 557
  antithyroid
    in Graves' disease, 427
    in Hashimoto's thyroiditis, 424–425, *425*
    in primary hypothyroidism, 428
  catalytic, 106–108
  Donath–Landsteiner, 440

  epitope recognition by, 72, 73
  in evaluation of humoral immunity, 295
  in eye disease, 527–530
  in gluten-sensitive enteropathy, 461–462
  to human serum globulins, 252–253, *253*
  laboratory methods for detection of, 215–232 *(See also*
      Laboratory tests)
  monoclonal *(See* Monoclonal antibodies)
  in myasthenia gravis, 521
  as opsonins, 68
  organ-specific, in autoimmune endocrine diseases, 422, 423t
  physicochemical basis of antigen-antibody binding, *75,*
      75–77
    cross-reactions, 76
    haptens, 76–77, *77*
    quantitative aspects, 76
  in polymyositis-dermatomyositis, 416
  precipitating, 392
  produced by active immunization, 699
  in renal disease, 481–484, 492–493
  role in tumor immunity, 572
  in scleroderma, 414
  screening for HLA antibodies, 279–280, 290t
  serum concentration of, 69
  in Sjögren's syndrome, 411, 412
  toxin neutralization by, 67–68
  viral effects on, 618t
  virus neutralization by, 68
Antibody-dependent cell-mediated cytotoxicity (ADCC), 68,
    108, 144
  in renal allograft rejection, 724
Antibody immunodeficiency. *See* B-cell immunodeficiency
    disorders
Antibody technologies, 106–108
Anticardiolipin antibodies (ACA), 448–449
Anticytoplasmic antibodies, in systemic lupus erythematosus,
    405
Antiendothelial antibodies
  in renal disease, 483
  in vasculitides, 451
Antierythrocyte antibodies, in systemic lupus erythematosus,
    404
Antifungal therapy, 655
  for blastomycosis, 660
  for candidiasis, 667
  for coccidioidomycosis, 664
  for cryptococcosis, 668
  for histoplasmosis, 665
  for paracoccidioidomycosis, 666
Anti-GBM disease. *See* Antiglomerular basement membrane
    disease
Antigen-antibody binding, 199, *200,* 215–216. *See also*
    Immune complexes
Antigen-antibody complexes. *See* Immune complexes
Antigenic determinant, 72
Antigenic shift, 707
Antigenic variation, 707
  of influenza virus, 621
Antigen-presenting cells (APCs), 38, 43–45, 63–65, 91–93
  in acute renal graft rejection, 722–724, *723–725*
  B lymphocytes, 92, 122–124, *124*
  capture, processing, and presentation of antigens by, 63–65,
      65
  definition of, 63–65
  dendritic cells, *64,* 65, 91–92
  endothelial cells, 193
  in lamina propria, 207
  macrophages, 65, *65,* 92
  professional, 65

secretion of IL-1 and TNFα by, 148–149
special forms of, 92–93
T-cell receptor binding to, 77
types of, 65
Antigens, 42, 43, *72,* 72–79
B-cell, *74,* 73–77, *75,* 239–240
binding of, 61
cancer–testes, 571
carcinoembryonic, 571
CD nomenclature system for, 2n, 234–235, 581, 761–762
cognate, 76
common acute lymphocytic leukemia, 571
definition of, 63, 72
for delayed-type hypersensitivity skin testing, 242, 242t
Duffy, 173
erythrocyte, 250–252
    ABO and H, *251,* 251–252, 251t
    Duffy, 252
    Kell, 252
    Kidd, 252
    Lewis, 251
    Rh, 251–252, 252t
    secretor, 251
flow cytometric analysis of, 235–242
H, 250–251, *251,* 251t, 611
hepatitis B, 628–629, 629t, *630*
human leukocyte, 84–87, 270–292 (*See also* Human
    leukocyte antigens)
immune response induced by, 63
immunogens, 63–65, 72–73
intracellular, 241
K, 611
laboratory methods for detection of, 215–232 (*See also*
    Laboratory tests)
in lymphocyte activation, 48–49
lymphocyte-determined membrane, 653
M, 610
mechanisms of elimination of, 67–68
    antibody-dependent cell-mediated cytotoxicity, 68
    complement activation, 68
    opsonization and phagocyte activation, 68
    toxic neutralization, 67–68
    virus neutralization, 68
multivalent, 76
myeloid, 240–241
O, 611
oncofetal, 571
onconeural, 522, 522t
oral tolerance to, *211,* 211–212
p24, 642
physicochemical basis of antigen-antibody binding, *75,* 75–77
    cross-reactions, 76
    haptens, 76–77, *77*
    quantitative aspects, 76
planted, in renal disease, 483
positive vs. negative lymphocyte selection promoted by, 70
processing and presentation of, 63–65, *65,* 82
    control of pathways for, 90
    pathways for, 82–83, 82t
sperm, 550, 557
streptococcal, 610
superantigens, T-cell receptor interactions with, 132–133, *133*
T-cell, 77–79, *78,* 82, 238–239
T-cell-independent, 119, *121*
T-cell receptor recognition of, 132
on tumors
    immunization to, 574–575
    tumor-associated, 569–571
    tumor-specific, 569–570

Antigen specificity, *62,* 62–63, 82
Antiglobulin tests, 252–253, *253,* 438t
Antiglomerular basement membrane (anti-GBM) disease, *482,*
    482–483, 491–492, 544–545
    clinical features of, *482,* 482–483, 491–492, *544,* 544–545
    differential diagnosis of, 545
    immunologic features of, 544
    immunologic pathogenesis of, 544
    pathology and immunopathology of, 492
    treatment and prognosis for, 492, 545
Antigranulocyte antibodies, 434, 435
Antihistamines, 194, 756, 756t
    for allergic rhinitis, 358
    for anaphylaxis, 375
    for urticaria, 379
Antiidiotype antiserum, 103
Antiinflammatory drugs, 750–757
    colchicine, 755
    corticosteroids, 750–752
    drugs that suppression immediate hypersensitivity reactions,
        755–757
    leukotriene antagonists, 755
    nonsteroidal antiinflammatory drugs, 753–755
Antilymphocyte globulin (ALG), 381–382
    for aplastic anemia, 442
    as graft-enhancing treatment, 719
    for transplant recipients, kidney, 721
Antimesangial antibodies, 483
Antimitochondrial antibodies, in primary biliary cirrhosis,
    472
Antineuronal antibodies, 522t
Antineutrophil cytoplasmic antibodies (ANCA)
    in renal disease, 483–484, 492–493
    in ulcerative colitis, 468
    in vasculitides, 451, 483–484
        Churg-Strauss syndrome, 456
        microscopic polyangiitis, 453
        polyarteritis nodosa, 452
        Wegener's granulomatosis, 454–455
Antinuclear antibodies (ANA)
    in antiphospholipid syndrome, 449
    in autoimmune chronic active hepatitis, 470
    in juvenile arthritis, 407
    in rheumatoid arthritis, 407
    in scleroderma, 413
    in Sjögren's syndrome, 412
    in systemic lupus erythematosus, 403–404, 404t
    testing for, 229, *230*
Antiphospholipid antibodies
    recurrent spontaneous abortion and, 558–559
    in stroke, 524
    in systemic lupus erythematosus, 404
Antiphospholipid syndrome (APS), 448–449
    immunologic features of, 448
    immunologic pathogenesis of, 448
    laboratory findings in, 449
    recurrent spontaneous abortion and, 558–559
    symptoms and signs of, 448–449
    treatment of, 449
Antiplasmodial antibodies, 675
Antiplatelet antibodies, 442
    in idiopathic thrombocytopenic purpura, 443, 444, 444t
    in systemic lupus erythematosus, 404–405
Antiretroviral therapy, 645–646
    development of, 636
    drug classes, 645, 647t
    highly active, 636, 646
    in pregnancy, 562, 640
    timing of commencement of, 646

Antiserum, 106
  antiidiotype, 103
  specific, 69
Antisperm antibodies, 550, 557
Antithymocyte globulin (ATG), 381–382
  for graft-versus-host disease, 739
  for kidney transplant recipients, 721, 724–725
Antithyroid antibodies
  in Graves' disease, 427
  in Hashimoto's thyroiditis, 424–425, *425*
  in primary hypothyroidism, 428
Antitubular basement membrane nephritis, 483, 493
Antivenins, 705t, 706
Aortitis, 456
  syphilitic, 689
APCs. *See* Antigen-presenting cells
APECED (autoimmune polyendocrinopathy-candidiasis
      ectodermal dystrophy) syndrome, 316
Aphthous ulcers, recurrent (RAU), 476–478, *477*
  etiology of, 477
  immunologic features of, 476–477
  immunologic pathogenesis of, 477–478
  treatment and prognosis for, 478
Aplastic anemia, 441–442
  antilymphocyte globulin for, 442
  bone marrow transplantation for, 442, 737
  cytokine therapy for, 436, 436t, 442
Apoptosis, 5, 14–17, *16*
  activation-induced cell death, 70
  Bcl-2 in, 15–17, 16t, 70
  of CD4 cells in HIV infection, 639
  Fas in, 15, 70
  flow cytometric analysis for, 241–242
  in immune system, 70
  mitochondrial pathways of, 15
  viral effects on, 620t
Apoptosis-inducing factor (AIF), 15
A protein, 610
APS. *See* Antiphospholipid syndrome
Arachidonic acid metabolites, 194–195, *195, 196*
ARDS (adult respiratory distress syndrome), 174, 184, 546
Arterial ischemic and infarct syndromes, 448
Arteritis. *See also* Vasculitis
  giant-cell, 456–457
  polyarteritis nodosa, 451–453
  Takayasu's, 457
Arthritis
  hypogammaglobulinemia and, 420
  juvenile, 408–411
  in Lyme disease, 693
  in polymyositis-dermatomyositis, 416
  psoriatic, 418–419
  Reiter's syndrome, 418
  rheumatoid, 406–408
  in systemic lupus erythematosus, 402, 405
  in Wegener's granulomatosis, 454
Arthropod allergens, 352–354
Arthus, Nicholas-Maurice, 380
Arthus reaction, 199, 242, 380, 381t
ASA. *See* Aspirin
Ascariasis, 685
Aspergillosis, 655, 657t, 669
  allergic bronchopulmonary, 365, 382–385, 669
  complications and prognosis for, 669
  differential diagnosis of, 669
  effect of immunologic abnormalities on course of, 661t
  epidemiology of, 669
  immunologic diagnosis of, 663t, 669
  immunologic features of, 669

  laboratory findings in, 669
  pathologic features of, 660t
  prevention of, 669
  signs and symptoms of, 669
  treatment of, 669
Aspirin (ASA), 194, 753–755. *See also* Nonsteroidal
      antiinflammatory drugs
  Alzheimer's disease risk and, 468
  bronchospasm induced by, 535
  hypersensitivity to, 400
    asthma and, 361, 362t, 375
    desensitization for, 400
  indications for, 753
  for juvenile arthritis, 410
  for Kawasaki's disease, 458
  mechanism of action of, 753
  for systemic lupus erythematosus, 405
  toxicity of, 753–755
  for uveitis associated with rheumatoid disease, 529
Assays
  agglutination, 219–221, *221*
  AH$_{50}$, 232
  antibody capture, 222, *223*
  bactericidal, 248, *248*
  Boyden chamber, 246
  CH$_{50}$, 231–232, *232*, 296–297, 341
  complement, 231, 232
  complement fixation, 217, 219t, *220*
  enzyme-linked immunoassays, 222
  enzyme-linked immunosorbent, 221–224, *222, 223*
  enzyme-linked immunospot, 245
  gene rearrangement assay for lymphocyte clonality,
      263–265
  granulocyte degranulation, 247, *247*
  hemolytic, *231*, 231–232, *232*, 232t
  hybridization, 261–262, *263, 264*
  immunoelectrophoresis, 226–227, *227*
  immunoflourescence, 228–230, *229, 230*
  immunohistochemical, 230–231
  in situ hybridization, 265, *266*
  latex agglutination, 221
  leukocyte function, 241
  lymphocyte activation, 243–245
  microparticle enzyme immunoassays, 222–224, 224t
  monocyte-macrophage, 245
  neutrophil function, 245–248
  nuclease protection, 261
  of phagocytosis, 246
  sandwich, 222, *222*
  serum protein electrophoresis, 224–226, *224–226*
  Southern blot, 262–263, *265*
  superoxide, 241, 246–247
Asthma, 349, 359–365
  adult-onset, 359, 360
  allergen bronchoprovocation testing in, 361
  allergic bronchopulmonary aspergillosis and, 365, 382–385,
      538, 538t
  aspirin sensitivity and, 361, 362t, 375, 400
  atopy and, 359
  childhood-onset, 360
  complications and prognosis for, 364–365
  definition of, 359
  differential diagnosis of, 362–363
  drug-induced, 535
    NSAIDs, 755
  eosinophilic pneumonias and, 191, 360, 538, 538t
  epidemiology of, 359
  exercise- and hyperventilation-induced, 362
  extrinsic, 359

immunologic diagnosis of, 362
immunologic features of, 359
immunologic pathogenesis of, 361–362
intrinsic, 359–360
kinins and, 187
laboratory findings in, *360*, 360–361
occupational allergens and, 362, 363t
pathology of, 361
symptoms and signs of, 360
treatment of, 363–364
   corticosteroids, 364
   cromolyn and nedocromil, 364
   desensitization, 364
   environmental control, 363
   leukotriene antagonists, 194, 364, 755
   other drugs, 364
   for status asthmaticus and respiratory failure, 364
   sympathomimetics, 363–364, 756
   xanthines, 364, 757
triggers for attacks of, 361, 362t
Ataxia-telangiectasia, 320, 324–326
complications and prognosis for, 326, *326*
differential diagnosis of, 325
immunologic diagnosis of, 325
immunologic features of, 324
immunologic pathogenesis of, 324–325
laboratory findings in, 325
symptoms and signs of, 325, *325*
treatment of, 325–326
ATG. *See* Antithymocyte globulin
Atopic dermatitis, 365–366
complications and prognosis for, 366
definition of, 365
differential diagnosis of, 366
epidemiology of, 365
immunologic diagnosis of, 365–366
immunologic features of, 365
immunologic pathogenesis of, 366
laboratory findings in, 365
pathology of, 365
symptoms and signs of, 365
treatment of, 366
Atopic keratoconjunctivitis, 527
Atopy, 189, 202, 349–369. *See also* Allergy
allergic gastroenteropathy, 367–368
allergic rhinitis, 356–359
allergies, IgE antibodies and, 349, *350*
asthma, 359–365
definition of, 349
dermatitis, 365–366
diagnostic testing for, 354–356
diseases associated with, 349, 350t
etiology of, 349–351
   autonomic imbalance, 350
   candidate genes, 349–350, 350t
   cytokines, 350–351
   environmental factors, 351
   helminthiasis, 351
etiology of, 349–351
immunologic pathogenesis of, 349
immunology of, 349
prevalence of, 349
ATP-binding cassette (ABC) transporters, 83
AU (allergen unit), 354
Autoantibodies. *See also* Antibodies
crossmatching for, 282, 290t
organ-specific, 422, 423t
Autoimmune diseases, 128–129, 141
blistering skin diseases, 495–507

autoantibody binding and, 495, *496*
bullous pemphigoid, 495–498, *497*
dermatitis herpetiformis, 501–503, *502, 503*
diagnosis of, 495
epidermolysis bullosa acquisita, 500–501
herpes gestationis, *499*, 499–500
linear IgA bullous dermatosis, 503–504
mucous membrane pemphigoid, 498–499
paraneoplastic pemphigus, 506–507
pemphigus vulgaris and pemphigus foliaceous, 504–506, *505, 506*
chemokines and, 167
chronic active hepatitis, 470–471
complement deficiencies and, 296, 343, 346–347
drug-induced, 396
endocrine, 422–432
   Addison's disease, 430
   Graves' disease, 426–428, *427*
   Hashimoto's thyroiditis, 422–425, *424, 425*
   idiopathic hypoparathyroidism, 431
   insulin-dependent diabetes mellitus, 429–430
   lymphocytic adenohypophysitis, 430
   mechanism of development of, 422, *423*
   organ-specific autoantibodies and, 422, 423t
   polyglandular syndromes, 431–432, 431t
   premature ovarian failure, 430–431
   primary hypothyroidism, 428
   transient thyroiditis syndromes, 425–426
Enterobacteriaceae and, 611
glomerulonephritis, 482–483
hematologic
   hemolytic anemias, 436–441, 437t
   neutropenia, 434
   thrombocytopenias, 442–449
inflammatory response and, 189
major histocompatibility complex alleles and, 93–94, 94t, 270
neurologic, 510–525
   acute disseminated encephalomyelitis, 516–517
   amyotrophic lateral sclerosis, 523
   chronic inflammatory neuropathies, 519
   Guillain-Barré syndrome, 518–519
   multiple sclerosis, 510–516, *512–514*
   myasthenia gravis, 519–521
   paraneoplastic syndromes, 521–523, 522t
   Rasmussen's encephalitis, 524
   stiff-person syndrome, 524
neutropenia, 434
rheumatic
   juvenile arthritis, 408–411
   polymyositis-dermatomyositis, 415–417
   rheumatoid arthritis, 406–408
   scleroderma, 413–415
   Sjögren's syndrome, 411–413
   systemic lupus erythematosus, 401–405
selective IgA deficiency and, 308
of testis and ovary, 557
type III cryoglobulins and, 219
Autoimmune polyendocrinopathy-candidiasis ectodermal dystrophy (APECED) syndrome, 316
Autologous bone marrow transplantation, 738
Autoreactive immunoglobulins, 118, 128–129
Autoreactive lymphocytes, 70, 91
Avidity model of T-cell selection, 135–136
Avidity of antigen-antibody interactions, 76n
Azathioprine, 745–746
for autoimmune chronic active hepatitis, 471
for bullous pemphigoid, 498
for microscopic polyangiitis, 454

Azathioprine, *(continued)*
  for paraneoplastic pemphigus, 507
  for pemphigus vulgaris and pemphigus foliaceous, 506
  for polyarteritis nodosa, 453
  for polymyositis-dermatomyositis, 417
  for primary biliary cirrhosis, 472
  for Reiter's syndrome, 418
  for rheumatoid arthritis, 408
  for systemic lupus erythematosus, 405
  for transplant recipients
    bone, 741
    heart, 733
    heart-lung and lung, 735
    kidney, 721
  for warm autoimmune hemolytic anemia, 439
AZT (zidovudine), 645, 647t

B7, 49, 92, 122–124, 138, *139*
  interaction with CD28, 759
  in renal allograft rejection, 723, *723*
Babesia microti, 256
Bacillus anthracis, 609
Bacillus Calmette-Guérin (BCG), 79, 615, 701t
Bacillus cereus, 609
Bacterial diseases, 607–615
  encapsulated bacteria, 607, 612–613
  immunity to, 607, 615
  intracellular bacteria, 83, 607, 614–615
  mycobacterial, 615
  serodiagnosis of, 607
  toxigenic, 607–612
Bactericidal assay, 248, *248*
Bactericidal permeability-increasing protein (BPI), 21
Bacteroides fragilis, 613
BALT (bronchus-associated lymphoid tissue), 204
Bands, *3*, 33
Bare lymphocyte syndrome, 295, 321, 322–323
  clinical features of, 322
  genetics of, 322
  immunologic features of, 322
  pathogenesis of, 322
  treatment of, 323
Basophils, 2, 192–193
  cutaneous basophil hypersensitivity, 198t, 202
  Fc receptors on, 190t, 192–193
  IgE receptors on, 349
  in inflammatory response, 192–193
  production of, *3*
  properties of, 191t
  structure of, 192, *193*
Bax, 15–17
B-cell antigen receptor (BCR), 118–119, *120, 123*
B-cell antigens, *74*, 73–77, *75*
  flow cytometric analysis of, 239–240
B-cell chronic lymphocytic leukemia (B-CLL), 591
B-cell epitopes, *74*, 73–77
  conformation and linear, 74–75, *75*
  physicochemical basis of antigen-antibody binding, *75*, 75–77
    cross-reactions, 76
    haptens, 76–77, *77*
    quantitative aspects, 76
  size and locations of, 74
B-cell immunodeficiency disorders, 240, 300t, 302–312. *See also* Combined B-cell and T-cell immunodeficiency disorders
  common variable immunodeficiency, 305–307
  immunodeficiency with hyper-IgM, 119, 240, 295, 307

immunodeficiency with thymoma, 311
immunologic evaluation for, 295, 301t, 302t
5′-nucleotidase deficiency, 311
selective deficiency of IgG subclasses, 310–311
selective IgA deficiency, 295, 307–310
selective IgM deficiency, 310
transcobalamin II deficiency, 311–312
transient hypogammaglobulinemia of infancy, 305
treatment of, 301t
X-linked agammaglobulinemia, 117, 240, 295, 297, 302–305
B-cell malignancy. *See also* Neoplasms of immune system
  CD5 B cells and, 118
  immunoglobulin gene rearrangements and, *113*, 113–114
B cells. *See* B lymphocytes
B-cell tolerance, 128–129, *129*
BCG (bacillus Calmette-Guérin), 79, 615, 701t
Bcl-2, 16t
  in apoptosis, 15–17
  in diffuse large B-cell lymphoma, 594
  in follicular lymphoma, 70, 114, 593
B-CLL (B-cell chronic lymphocytic leukemia), 591
BclXL, 16
BCR (B-cell antigen receptor), 118–119, *120*
Bee sting allergy, 372, 373, 373t, 376
  desensitization for, 714
Behçet's disease, 417
  ocular manifestations of, 532
  recurrent aphthous ulcers and, 477
Bell's palsy, 693, 696
Bence Jones proteins, 595
  in amyloidosis, 596
  in plasma cell myeloma, 595
Benign hypergammaglobulinemic purpura, 597
Beta-lactam antibiotics
  hypersensitivity to, 398–399
  structures of, *398, 399*
Bid, 16
Biliary atresia, extrahepatic, 727
Biliary cirrhosis, primary (PBC), 471–472
  clinical features of, 472
  complications and prognosis for, 472
  differential diagnosis of, 472
  epidemiology of, 471
  immunologic diagnosis of, 472
  immunologic features of, 471
  immunopathology of, *471*, 471–472
  treatment of, 472
Bilineal phenotype, 579
Biotin-dependent carboxylase deficiencies, 318
Biphenotypic cells, 580
Bird handler's disease. *See* Hypersensitivity pneumonitis
Black piedra, 656t, 661t
Blackwater fever, 674
Black widow spider bite, 705t, 706
Blastocyst, 551
Blastomycosis, 657t, 658–660
  complications and prognosis for, 660
  differential diagnosis of, 660
  effect of immunologic abnormalities on course of, 661t
  epidemiology of, 658
  immunologic diagnosis of, 660, 662t
  immunologic features of, 658
  laboratory findings in, 660
  pathologic features of, 659t
  symptoms and signs of, 658–660
  treatment of, 660
Blast transformation, 47
BLC (B-lymphocyte chemoattractant), 59, 171–172

Blistering skin diseases, 495–507
  autoantibody binding and, 495, *496*
  bullous pemphigoid, 495–498, *497*
  dermatitis herpetiformis, 501–503, *502, 503*
  diagnosis of, 495
  epidermolysis bullosa acquisita, 500–501
  herpes gestationis, *499,* 499–500
  linear IgA bullous dermatosis, 503–504
  mucous membrane pemphigoid, 498–499
  paraneoplastic pemphigus, 506–507
  pemphigus vulgaris and pemphigus foliaceous, 504–506, *505, 506*
Blood banking and immunohematology, 250–259
  blood component therapy, 258–259, 258t
  blood groups, 250
  erythrocyte antigens, 250–252, *251,* 251t, 252t
  Rh isoimmunization, 257
  transfusion reactions, 254–257, 254t
Blood-brain barrier, 510
Blood cell biology, 1–17
  cellular interactions in bone marrow, 5–8
  control of cell proliferation and survival, 13–17
  hematopoiesis, 1–5
  hematopoietic cytokines and receptors, 8–13
Blood transfusion, 250–259
  blood component therapy, 258–259, 258t
    erythrocytes, 258
    plasma products, 259
    platelets, 258–259
  blood groups, 250
  detection of antigen and antibodies to erythrocytes, 252–254
    antiglobulin tests, 252–253, *253*
    crossmatch, 254
    pretransfusion testing, 253
    type and screen, 253–254
  erythrocyte antigens and, 250–252, *251,* 251t, 252t
  hepatitis transmitted by, 632
  for kidney transplantation, 721
  reactions to, 254–257, 254t
    acute lung injury, 255
    allergic, 255
    febrile, 255
    hemolytic, 254–255
    immunologic mechanisms of, 256–257
    infection, 255–256, 255t
    posttransfusion purpura, 446
  Rh isoimmunization and, 257
  tests to detect antigen and antibodies to erythrocytes, 252–254, *253*
B-lymphocyte chemoattractant (BLC), 59, 171–172
B lymphocytes, 2, 42–43, 115–129. *See also* Lymphocytes
  activation of, 41–42, *42,* 46–48, *47,* 66–67, *67*
    bystander, 66
    polyclonal B-cell activators, 119
    requirements for, *48,* 48–49, 49t, 66
    T-cell help and accessory signals, 48–49, 66, 119–122, *122, 123*
  affinity maturation of, 51, 126
  anergic, 129
  as antigen-presenting cells, 92, 122–124, *124*
  autoreactive, 70
  CD5, 118
  chemokine receptor expression by, *169*
  development of, *3,* 40–41, *41,* 115–117, *116*
  evaluating function of, 295–296
  follicular, 206
  functions of, 43
  in HIV infection, 644

  IL-2 effects on, 156
  immature, *116,* 117
    receptor editing of, 113, 128–129
  in immune response, 63, *64, 66*–67, *67*
  immunoglobulin synthesis by, 42, *42*
  immunophenotypic stages of early differentiation of, 579t
  in lamina propria, 207
  life span of, 118
    "death by neglect," 118
  in lymph nodes, 50–51
  lymphocytotoxicity crossmatching, 281
  memory, 43, *43,* 124–125
  naive, maturation and release of, 117–118
  phenotyping of, 234–242
  plasma cells, 43, *43, 44,* 124
  role in tumor immunity, 572
  self-reactive, 128–129
  somatic hypermutation of, 126
  in spleen, 53
  subsets of, 118
  surface markers expressed on, 115–118, *116*
  tissue distribution of, 40, 41t
Bombay type, 250
Bone marrow, 1, 40
  blood cell storage pool in, 2
  cellular interactions in, 5–8
  hematopoietic stem cells in, 1–5, *3–5*
  long-term bone marrow cultures, 6–8
  lymphocyte proportions in, 41t
  microenvironments of, 6, *6–7*
  origins of cells in, 1–2, *3*
  production of lymphoid cells in, *3,* 40, *41*
  rate of blood cell production in, 2
  stromal cells of, 6–8
Bone marrow transplantation, 4, 163, 736–740
  allogenic, 738
  antibiotic prophylaxis for, 738
  autologous, 738
  complications of, 739
    graft-versus-host disease, 739, 739t
    infections, 650, 740, 740t
    venoocclusive disease of liver, 739–740
  diseases transmittable by, 737t
  donors for, 736–737
    National Marrow Donor Program, 275, 737
  history of, 736
  indications for, 737–738
    acute lymphoblastic leukemia, 738
    acute myelogenous leukemia, 737–738
    aplastic anemia, 442, 737
    bare lymphocyte syndrome, 323
    chronic myelogenous leukemia, 738
    hematologic malignancies, 587
    severe combined immunodeficiency, 321, 737
    X-linked lymphoproliferative syndrome, 331
  operative procedure for, 738–739
Bone transplantation, 740–741
  clinical recovery after, 741
  course after, 741
  immunologic rejection of, 741
  immunosuppression for, 741
  indications for, 740–741
Booster immunization, 700
Bordetella pertussis, 609–610
Borrelia, 688
Borrelia burgdorferi, 688, 692–696
Botox, 609
Botulism, 608–609, 705t
"Boutonnière" deformity, 406

"Boxcar" lesions, 228
Boyden chamber assay, 246
BPI (bactericidal permeability-increasing protein), 21
Bradykinins, *186,* 186–187, 256
BrdU (bromodeoxyuridine), 244
Breast milk
    cytomegalovirus transmission via, 649
    HIV transmission via, 562
    immunology of, 212–213
Bromodeoxyuridine (BrdU), 244
Bronchial provocation testing
    for asthma, 361
    for hypersensitivity pneumonitis, 392–393
Bronchiolitis
    obliterans, 393
    in respiratory syncytial virus, 623–625, *624*
Bronchitis
    asthmatic, 363
    chronic, 362
Bronchoalveolar lavage, 393
Bronchodilators, for asthma, 363–364, 756
Bronchus-associated lymphoid tissue (BALT), 204
Brucella, 607
Brucella abortus, 615
Brucella melitensis, 615
Brucella suis, 615
Brucellosis, 221, 615
Brugia malayi, 684–686
Bruton, Ogden, 302
Bruton agammaglobulinemia. *See* X-linked
    agammaglobulinemia
Btk gene, 117, 297, 304
Buerger's disease, 457–458
Bullous pemphigoid, 193, 495–498
    autoantibodies in, 498
    definition of, 495
    differential diagnosis of, 498
    etiology of, 495
    immunologic diagnosis of, 497–498
    immunologic features of, 495
    laboratory findings in, 496–497
    pathology of, 495–496, *497*
    prevalence of, 495
    prognosis for, 498
    signs and symptoms of, 496, *497*
    treatment of, 498
Burkitt's lymphoma, 113, *113,* 583–584, 595, 650, 651
Burns, 19
"Butterfly rash," 402
Bystander B-cell activation, 66

C1, 177, 179
C1 inhibitor, 181, 182t
    deficiency of, 181, 342t, 344–345
C1q, 177, 179
    deficiency of, 342t, 343, 346
C1q receptors, 184, 184t
C1r deficiency, 342t, 343
C1s deficiency, 342t, 343
C2, 177
    deficiency of, 342t, 343
C3, 20t, 22–23, *23,* 176, 177–179, *180,* 341
    deficiency of, 341–342, 342t, 345
C3 convertase
    alternative pathway, 180
    classical pathway, 177
C3 nephritic factor, 341–342
C3 receptors, 184–185, 184t

C4, 177
    deficiency of, 342t, 343
C4-binding protein, 181–183, 182t
    deficiency of, 342t, 345
C5 convertase, 179
C5-9, 181, *182,* 341
    deficiencies of, 342t, 344
C5a and C5b, 179, 181, 183–184, 195, 200
C8-binding protein, 185
C5a, 167
Cachectin, 151. *See also* Tumor necrosis factor α
Cachexia, 23, 151
Caffeine, 757
Calcineurin, 747
Calcium, intracellular free ions, 47
Calcium channel blockers, for scleroderma, 415
CALLA (common acute lymphocytic leukemia antigen), 571
Cancer, 578–603. *See also* Neoplasms of immune system;
        specific malignancies
    ataxia-telangiectasia and, 326, *326*
    hepatocellular, 628, 629, 631
    paraneoplastic syndromes and
        neurologic, 521–523
        pemphigus, 506–507
    p53 mutations and, 14
    polymyositis-dermatomyositis and, 416
    tumor immunology, 568–576
    type I cryoglobulins and, 218
    urticaria, angioedema and, 378
Cancer chemotherapeutic agents, 587
    adverse pulmonary effects of, 537
    neutropenia induced by, 435–436
    thrombotic thrombocytopenic purpura and, 447
Cancer–testes antigens, 571
Candidiasis, 655, 657t, 666–667
    chronic mucocutaneous, *316,* 316–317, 667
        hypoparathyroidism and, 317, 431
    complications and prognosis for, 667
    differential diagnosis of, 667
    effect of immunologic abnormalities on course of, 661t
    immunologic diagnosis of, 663t, 667
    laboratory findings in, 667
    neonatal, 666–667
    oral, *478,* 478–479
    pathologic features of, 660t
    prevention of, 667
    signs and symptoms of, 667
    species causing, 666
    treatment of, 667
Caprine arthritis-encephalitis virus, 637
Capsular polysaccharide, *612,* 612–613
    of *Bacteroides fragilis,* 613
    of *Haemophilus influenzae,* 613
    of *Klebsiella pneumoniae,* 613
    of *Neisseria* species, 613
    of *Streptococcus agalactiae,* 613
    of *Streptococcus pneumoniae,* 612
Carboxylase deficiency, biotin-dependent, 318
Carcinoembryonic antigen (CEA), 571
Carcinogens, 568–569
Cardiotrophin (CT-1), 158t
Cardiovascular system. *See also* Heart; Vasculitis
    anaphylaxis and, 371
    in systemic lupus erythematosus, 402, 403
Carpal tunnel syndrome, 407
Carrington's chronic eosinophilic pneumonia, 538, 538t, *539*
Cartilage-hair hypoplasia, 327–328, *328*
Casoni skin test, 684
Caspase-1, 150, 153t, 164

Caspase-8, 152
Caspases, 14–15
Castleman's disease, 603, 627
Catalytic antibodies, 106–108
Catheter-associated infections, 610
CCR5, 639, 641
CD1 proteins, 93
CD1d, 145
CD2, 45, 45t
CD3, 45, 45t, 66, 131, *132,* 236, *237*
CD4 cells, 45t, 46, *46 . See also* Helper T lymphocytes
  allergen desensitization and, 716
  antigen presentation to, 63, *64*
  delayed-type hypersensitivity and, 197
  depletion in HIV infection, 638–641, *643,* 643–644
    monitoring of, 646–647
  human herpesvirus 6 infection of, 654
  idiopathic CD4 lymphocytopenia, 318
  in lamina propria, 206–207
  peptide-MHC recognition by, 90
  in renal allograft rejection, 722–724, *723–725*
  thymocytes, 55, *56*
CD4 coreceptor, 133, *133*
CD5, 45t, 118
CD7, 45t
CD8 cells, 45, 45t, 46, *46 . See also* Cytotoxic T lymphocytes
  allergen desensitization and, 716
  antigen presentation to, 63
  cytotoxicity and, 45–46, 139, 141–143, 197
  intraepithelial lymphocytes, 206
  peptide-MHC recognition by, 90
  in renal allograft rejection, 722–724, *723–725*
  thymocytes, 55, *56*
CD8 coreceptor, 133
CD10, 115, *116*
CD14
  membrane, 36, *37*
  soluble, 20t, 21
CD16, 144, 317–318
CD19, 115, *116,* 236, *237*
CD21, *116,* 117
CD22, *116,* 118
CD23, *116,* 118
  Wiskott–Aldrich syndrome and, 323
CD25, 45t, 46
CD27, 154
CD27 ligand (CD70), 152t, 154
CD28, 45t, 46, 49, 138, *139*
  B7 interaction with, 759
CD29, 45t, 46
CD30, 152t, 153t, 154
CD34, 2–4, 7, 58, 240–241
CD35, *116*
CD38, 4
CD40, 49, 66, *67,* 118, 119, 151, 152t, 154
CD40 ligand (CR40L), 45t, 46, 49, 66, *67,* 119, 127, 139–140,
    152t, 153t
  anti-CD40L therapy, 759
  congenital deficiency of (*See* Hyper-IgM syndrome)
CD43, Wiskott–Aldrich syndrome and, 323
CD44, 6, 8, 8t
CD45, *116,* 122, 138, *138,* 143, 236, *238*
CD46, binding of measles virus to, 186, 625
CD48, 144
CD54, 45t
CD56, 144, 318
CD59, 182, 185t
  deficiency of, 342t, 345–346
CD69, 45t

CD73, *116,* 117
CD95, 15, 70
CD154. *See* CD40 ligand
CDC (Centers for Disease Control and Prevention), 703
CD (clusters of differentiation) antigen nomenclature system,
    2n, 234–235, 581, 761–762
CDKIs (cyclin-dependent kinase inhibitors), 14
CDKs (cyclin-dependent kinases), 13–14
CDRs (complementarity-determining regions), 103, 111
CEA (carcinoembryonic antigen), 571
Celiac disease, selective IgA deficiency and, 308
Celiac sprue. *See* Gluten-sensitive enteropathy
Cell cycle, *13,* 13–14
  DNA damage and, 14
  phases of, 13
  regulation of, 13–14
  viral effects on, 620t
Cell-mediated eye diseases, 530–533
  AIDS-related, 532–533
  Behçet's disease, 532
  contact dermatitis of eyelids, 532
  giant-cell arteritis, 532
  ocular sarcoidosis, 530–531
  phlyctenular keratoconjunctivitis, 532, *532*
  polyarteritis nodosa, 532
  sympathetic ophthalmia and Vogt-Koyanagi-Harada
    syndrome, 531–532
Cell-mediated hypersensitivity diseases, 386–393
  allergic contact dermatitis, 386–388, 396
  hypersensitivity pneumonitis, 389–393, 390t
  photoallergic contact dermatitis, 388–389
Cell-mediated immunity (CMI), 19, 43, 234
  inflammatory response, 197–199, *198,* 198t
  laboratory evaluation of, 234–248, 296, 301t, 313t
    delayed-type hypersensitivity skin testing, 242–243
    leukocyte phenotyping (flow cytometry), 234–242
    lymphocyte activation assays, 243–245
    monocyte-macrophage assays, 245
    neutrophil function assays, 245–248
Cell-mediated lympholysis test, 272
Cells
  antigen-presenting, 38, 43–45, 63, 91–93
  basophils, 191t, 192–193, *193*
  bilineal, 579
  biphenotypic, 580
  dendritic, 45, 91–92
    follicular, 50, 126–127, *127*
    interdigitating, 51, 91
  dome area, 205
  effector, 19, 42, 61, 69
  endothelial, 26–27, 27t, 193
  eosinophils, *190,* 190–191
  epithelioid, 38
  γ/δ, 143
  hematopoietic stem, 1
  Hofbauer, 552, *554*
  inflammatory, 189–193, 189t
  Ito, 682
  Kupffer, 34
  lamina propria, 204, *205,* 206–207
  Langerhans', 54, 91
  light-scattering properties in flow cytometer, 235, *235, 236*
  lineage-committed progenitors, 2, *3,* 5
  lymphocytes, 27, 27t, 40–59
    B cells, 42–43, 115–129
    T cells, 2, 43–46, 131–143
  lymphokine-activated killer, 144
  M, 205, *205*
  malignant lymphoid, 578–580

Cells *(continued)*
  mast, 191–192, 191t, *192*
  memory, 41–42, 46, 61, 124–125
  mononuclear phagocytes, 27t, 34–38
  multinucleate giant, 38
  natural killer, 2, 40, 143–145
  neutrophils, 2, 27–34, 27t
  NKT, 145–146
  "passenger," 722
  plasma, 43, *43, 44,* 124
  platelets, 193
  pre-B, *116,* 117
  pro-B, 115, *116*
  Reed-Sternberg, *600,* 600–601
  reticular, 50
  self-renewing, 1
  terminally differentiated, 1
Cell surface markers, 2–4
  CD nomenclature system for, 2n, 234–235, 581, 761–762
  determination of number and types of, 234–242
  expressed on B lymphocytes, 115–118, *116*
  expressed on dendritic cells, 65
  expressed on hematopoietic stem cells, 2–4
  expressed on natural killer cells, 144
  expressed on T lymphocytes, 45, 45t
    role in B lymphocyte activation, 48–49, 66
  flow cytometric analysis of, 236–238, *237–239*
  lymphocyte activation assays of, 243–245
Cellular assays for histocompatibility, 289–292
Cellular immunodeficiency. *See* T-cell immunodeficiency
    disorders
Centers for Disease Control and Prevention (CDC), 703
Centroblasts, 127
Centrocytes, 127
Centrocytic lymphoma, 592
Cephalosporins, *398,* 399
Cephamycins, *398*
Cercariae, 682
Cerebrovascular occlusion, 456
Cervix, uterine, 548
Cestodes, 683–684
  echinococcosis, 684
CFA (complete Freund's adjuvant), 80
CFUs (colony-forming units), 5
CGD. *See* Chronic granulomatous disease
Chagas' disease, 256
α-Chain disease, 596
γ-Chain disease, 597
μ-Chain disease, 597
Chancre, syphilitic, 688
Charcot–Leyden crystal protein, 190, 191
CH$_{50}$ assay, 231–232, *232,* 296–297, 341
Chédiak–Higashi syndrome (CHS), 295, 296, 318, 336
Chemokines, 29, 167–174
  binding to Duffy antigen, 173
  biologic activities of, 169–173
  classification of, 167, *168,* 168t
  developmental (homeostatic), 169, 171–173, 172t
    receptors for, 172t
  discovery of, 167
  functions of, 167
  in lymphocyte circulation and homing, 59
  microbial interactions with, 173
  proinflammatory, 168t, 169–171, 195, 202
  receptors for, 167–169, *168,* 168t
    as coreceptors for HIV-1, 639
    defensins as ligands for, 173
    expression by hematopoietic cells, *169*
  in renal disease, 485, 485t
  structure of, 167
  therapeutic potential of, 173–174
Chemokinesis, 246
Chemotaxis, 25t, 29, *30,* 36t, 195, 245–246
  viral effects on, 619t
Chemotherapy, 587
  adverse pulmonary effects of, 537
  neutropenia induced by, 435–436
  thrombotic thrombocytopenic purpura and, 447
Chiclero ulcer, 677
Childhood immunization schedule, 709, 710t
Chimerism
  liver transplantation and, 726
  testing for, 289
Chinese liver fluke, 681
Chitin, 655
Chlamydia, 83, 199
Chlorambucil, 746
  for bullous pemphigoid, 498
  for polyarteritis nodosa, 453
Chloroquine, for systemic lupus erythematosus, 405
Cholangitis, primary sclerosing, 472–473
Cholera, 609
Cholera vaccine, 708
Cholinergic anaphylactoid reactions, 374
Cholinergic urticaria, 378
Chromoblastomycosis, 656t
  immunologic diagnosis of, 662t
Chromosomal abnormalities
  in Burkitt's lymphoma, 113, *113,* 583–584
  evaluating immune system neoplasms for, 581–584
  in follicular lymphoma, 113–114, 584
  in L3 acute lymphoblastic leukemia, 583
Chronic granulomatous disease (CGD), 295, 334–336
  complications and prognosis for, 336
  differential diagnosis of, 335
  immunologic diagnosis of, 335
    superoxide assay, 241, 246–247, *247,* 294, 296
  immunologic features of, 334
  laboratory findings in, 334–335, *335*
  McLeod phenotype and, 252
  pathogenesis of, 334, *334*
  symptoms and signs of, 334
  treatment of, 161, 335–336
  X-linked, 334–336
Chronic inflammation, 37
Chronic inflammatory demyelinating polyradiculoneuropathy
    (CIDP), 519
Chronic lymphocytic leukemia, 118
Chronic mucocutaneous candidiasis, *316,* 316–317, 667
  hypoparathyroidism and, 317, 431
  immunologic features of, 316
  symptoms and signs of, 316–317
Chronic myelogenous leukemia (CML), 738
CHS (Chédiak–Higashi syndrome), 295, 296, 318, 336
Churg-Strauss syndrome (CSS), 455–456
  diagnosis of, 456
  immunologic features of, 455
  immunologic pathogenesis of, 455
  induced by Cys-LT1 antagonists, 755
  laboratory findings in, 456
  prognosis for, 456
  signs and symptoms of, 455–456
    allergic granulomatosis, 455, 538t, 538t
    renal disease, 492–493
  treatment of, 456
Chymase, 192
Cicatricial pemphigoid, 498–499
  ocular manifestations of, 530

Cidofovir, 650
CIDP (chronic inflammatory demyelinating polyradiculoneuropathy), 519
CIE (countercurrent immunoelectrophoresis), 216
Ciliary neurotrophic factor (CNTF), 153t, 158t
Cimetidine, 194
Cirrhosis, primary biliary, *471,* 471–472
Cladribine, 746
Class I major histocompatibility complex (MHC) proteins, 63, 66–67, 83, 84, *85, 86*
  deficiency of, 323
  recognition by inhibitory receptors on natural killer cells, 144–145
  structure of, 84, *85, 86*
  type I interferon-induced expression of, 160
Class I pathway, antigenic peptides generated by, 82t, 83
Class II major histocompatibility complex (MHC) proteins, 45t, 46, 63–65, *64,* 83, *116,* 118
  deficiency of, 295, 322–323
  interferon-γ-induced expression of, 161
  structure of, 84, *85*
Class II pathway, antigenic peptides generated by, 82–83, 82t
Class switching, heavy-chain, *125,* 125–126
Classical complement activation pathway, 22, 176–179, *178,* 341
  deficiencies in components of, 342–343, 342t
  initiation of, 177
  nonimmunologic activators of, 179
CLIP (corticotropin-like intermediate lobe peptide), *89, 90*
Clonal anergy, 129
Clonal deletion, 129
Clonality of malignant lymphoid cells, 578
Clonal restriction, 62–63, 117
Clonal selection, 62–63, 115, 118
Clonorchis sinensis, 681
Clostridium botulinum, 608–609
Clostridium perfringens, 609
Clostridium tetani, 608
Clusterin, 182t, 183
Clusters of differentiation (CD) antigen nomenclature system, 2n, 234–235, 581, 761–762
CMI. *See* Cell-mediated immunity
CML (chronic myelogenous leukemia), 738
CMV. *See* Cytomegalovirus infection
c-myc, 14, 17, 47, 113, 569, 583–584
CNTF (ciliary neurotrophic factor), 153t, 158t
Coagulation factor therapy, 259
Coagulation inhibitors, circulating, 447–448
  lupus anticoagulant, 404
Cobra venom factor, 180
Coccidioidomycosis, 657t, 660–664
  complications and prognosis for, 664
  differential diagnosis of, 664
  effect of immunologic abnormalities on course of, 661t
  epidemiology of, 662–664
  immunologic diagnosis of, 662t, 664
  immunologic features of, 660
  laboratory findings in, 664
  pathologic features of, 659t
  signs and symptoms of, 664
  treatment and prevention of, 664
Cockroaches, 353
Colchicine, 755
  for primary biliary cirrhosis, 472
Cold agglutinins, 221
Cold agglutinin syndromes, 439
Cold urticaria, 378
Collagenases, 37, 38t
Colony-forming assays, 5

Colony-forming units (CFUs), 5
Colony-stimulating factor-1 (CSF-1), 436t
Colony-stimulating factors (CSFs), *4,* 4–5, 36t, 148, 162–163
  phenotypes of knockout mice, 163t
  production during immune or inflammatory responses, 163
  receptors for, *10*
  synergism with other cytokines, 162–163
  therapeutic use of, 163, 436t
    neutropenia, 435–436
Combined B-cell and T-cell immunodeficiency disorders, 300t, 320–331
  adenosine deaminase and purine nucleoside phosphorylase deficiency, 328–330, *329*
  ataxia-telangiectasia, 324–326, *325, 326*
  combined immunodeficiency with T-cell membrane or signaling defects, 322
  complete vs. partial, 320
  evaluation for, 320
  genetic mutations and, 320
  graft-versus-host disease, *326,* 326–327, *327*
  MHC class I deficiency, 323
  MHC class II deficiency, 322–323
  Nijmegen breakage syndrome, 326
  Omenn syndrome, 323
  reticular dysgenesis, 320
  severe combined immunodeficiency, 320–321
  short-limbed dwarfism with immunodeficiency and cartilage-hair hypoplasia, 327–328, *328*
  treatment of, 301t
  Wiskott–Aldrich syndrome, 323–324, *324*
  X-linked lymphoproliferative syndrome, 330–331
Combined immunodeficiency with T-cell membrane or signaling defects, 322
Common acute lymphocytic leukemia antigen (CALLA), 571
Common cold, 19
Common variable immunodeficiency (CVID), 240, 295, 296, 305–307
  complications and prognosis for, 307
  differential diagnosis of, 307
  immunologic diagnosis of, 306–307
  immunologic features of, 305
  immunologic pathogenesis of, 305–306
  laboratory and imaging findings in, 306
  symptoms and signs of, 306
  treatment of, 307
Complement, 21–23, 175–186
  activation of, 22–23, 68, *176,* 176–181, 341
    alternative pathway, 22, *23,* 176, 179–180
    classical pathway, 22, 176–179, *178*
    mannan-binding lectin pathway, 22–23, 176, 181
  in adaptive immune response, 185–186
  C1, 177
  C2, 177
  C3, 177–179, *180*
  C4, 177
  C5-9 and membrane attack complex, 181
  complement cascade, *178*
  components of, 175t, 176
    nomenclature for, 177
  fluid-phase regulators of, 181–183, 182t
    C4-binding protein, 181–183
    C1 inhibitor, 181
    clusterin, 183
    factor H, 183
    factor I, 181–183
    factor J, 183
    protected site concept, 183
    S protein, 183
  functions of, 175

Complement, *(continued)*
  genes for, 183
  in immune complex-mediated inflammation, 200–201
  inflammation and, 183–184
  mimicry of complement proteins, 185–186
  receptors for, 31, *116,* 117, 184–185, 184t
    on eosinophils, 191
  regulatory membrane proteins of, 182t, 185
  in transfusion reactions, 256
Complementarity-determining regions (CDRs), 103, 111
Complement assays, 231, 232
Complement deficiencies, 341–347, 342t
  alternative pathway deficiencies, 343–344
  autoimmune disease and, 296, 343, 346–347
  C3 deficiency, 341–342
  classical pathway deficiencies, 342–343
  complement receptor deficiencies, 346
  control protein deficiencies, 344–346
  heterozygous vs. homozygous, 341
  laboratory evaluation for, 296–297
  management of, 347
  mannan-binding lectin pathway deficiencies, 344
  renal disease and, 485
  in systemic lupus erythematosus, 345, 346, 401, 403
  terminal component deficiencies, 344
Complement fixation assays, 217, 219t, *220*
Complete Freund's adjuvant (CFA), 80
Concanavalin A (Con A), 244, 296
Condom therapy for infertility, 558
Conjunctivitis
  allergic, 193
  vernal keratoconjunctivitis, 357
Constant region, immunoglobulin, *96, 97*
Contact dermatitis
  allergic, 199, 386–388, 396
  of eyelids, 532
  photoallergic, 388–389
Contact hypersensitivity, 243
Coral snake antivenin, 705t, 706
Cornea transplantation
  graft reactions, *533,* 533–534
    immunologic pathogenesis of, 533–534
    treatment of, 534
  HLA matching for, 292, 533, 534
Cor pulmonale, 393
Cortex of lymph node, 50
Corticosteroids, 750–752
  for Addison's disease, 430
  for allergic contact dermatitis, 388
  for allergic rhinitis, 358
  for antiglomerular basement membrane disease, 492
  antiinflammatory effects of, 751, 752t
  for asthma, 364
  for atopic dermatitis, 366
  for autoimmune chronic active hepatitis, 471
  for Behçet's disease, 417
  for bullous pemphigoid, 498
  for Churg-Strauss syndrome, 456
  for corneal graft reactions, 534
  for Crohn's disease, 468
  for epidermolysis bullosa acquisita, 501
  for giant-cell arteritis, 457
  for Henoch-Schönlein purpura, 458
  for hereditary angioedema, 347
  for herpes gestationis, 500
  for hypersensitivity pneumonitis, 393
  for idiopathic pulmonary fibrosis, 544
  for idiopathic thrombocytopenic purpura, 445
  for infertility, 558

  inhibition of IL-1 and TNFα by, 154
  for juvenile arthritis, 410
  mechanism of action of, 750–751, *751*
  metabolic effects of, 752, 752t
  for microscopic polyangiitis, 454
  for multiple sclerosis, 516
  for ocular sarcoidosis, 531
  for paraneoplastic pemphigus, 507
  for paroxysmal nocturnal hemoglobinuria, 347
  for pemphigus vulgaris and pemphigus foliaceous, 505–506
  pharmacology of, 750
  for polyarteritis nodosa, 453
  for polymyositis-dermatomyositis, 417
  for psoriatic arthritis, 419
  for pure erythrocyte aplasia, 441
  for recurrent aphthous ulcers, 478
  for relapsing panniculitis, 420
  for relapsing polychondritis, 419
  relative potency of, 750, 750t
  for rheumatoid arthritis, 408
  for scleroderma, 415
  for Sjögren's syndrome, 412
  structures of, *749,* 750
  for sympathetic ophthalmia, 532
  for systemic lupus erythematosus, 405
  for Takayasu's arteritis, 457
  toxicity of, 752, 752t
  for transplant recipients
    bone, 741
    graft-versus-host disease, 739
    heart, 733
    heart-lung and lung, 735
    kidney, 721, 724
    liver, 730
    pancreas, 732
  for uveitis associated with rheumatoid disease, 529
  for Vogt-Koyanagi-Harada syndrome, 532
  for warm autoimmune hemolytic anemia, 439
  for Wegener's granulomatosis, 455
Corticotropin-like intermediate lobe peptide (CLIP), *89, 90*
Cortisol, *749,* 750t
Cortisone, *749,* 750t
Corynebacterium diphtheriae, 609
Countercurrent immunoelectrophoresis (CIE), 216
Cowpox (vaccinia) virus, 79, 164
COX (cyclooxygenase) inhibitors, 753–755, *754*
CpG (cytosine-phosphate-guanosine) dinucleotides,
    unmethylated, 36
Cranial arteritis, 456–457
C-reactive protein, 20t, 21, 23–24
Crohn's disease, 193, 466–468
  clinical features of, 467
  complications and prognosis for, 468
  differential diagnosis of, 467–468
  epidemiology of, 466
  immunologic diagnosis of, 467
  immunologic features of, 466
  immunopathology of, 466–467, *467*
  selective IgA deficiency and, 308
  treatment of, 468
    infliximab, 757–758
Cromolyn sodium, 364, 755–756
Crossmatching, 254, 270, 280–282, 290t. *See also*
    Histocompatibility testing
  for autoantibodies, 282
  B-cell lymphocytotoxicity, 281
  flow-cytometry, 281–282, *282*
  peripheral blood lymphocyte lymphocytotoxicity, 280
  purpose of, 280

T-cell lymphocytotoxicity, 280, *281*
for transplantation, 272
heart, 291, 733
heart-lung and lung, 735
kidney, 291, 291t, 719–720
liver, 291–292, 729
pancreas, 731
Crotalid snake antivenin, 705t, 706
Crow-Fukase syndrome, 519
Cryoglobulinemia, 228, 597
Cryoglobulins, 218–219
pathologic, 597
renal disease and, 481
rheumatoid arthritis and, 407
Cryoprecipitate, 259
Cryptococcosis, 657t, 667–668
complications and prognosis for, 668
differential diagnosis of, 668
effect of immunologic abnormalities on course of, 661t
epidemiology of, 668
immunologic diagnosis of, 663t, 668
immunologic features of, 667–668
laboratory findings in, 668
pathologic features of, 659t
prevention of, 668
signs and symptoms of, 668
treatment of, 668
CSF-1 (colony-stimulating factor-1), 436t
CSFs. *See* Colony-stimulating factors
CSS. *See* Churg-Strauss syndrome
CT-1 (cardiotrophin), 158t
CTLA-4, 139, 759
tumor vaccine and, 575
CTLA4Ig, 759
CTLs. *See* Cytotoxic T lymphocytes
Cumulus oophorus, 551
Cutaneous leishmaniasis, 677–679, *678*
CVID. *See* Common variable immunodeficiency
CXCR4, 639
Cyclic neutropenia, 434
Cyclin-dependent kinase inhibitors (CDKIs), 14
Cyclin-dependent kinases (CDKs), 13–14
Cyclins, 13–14
Cyclooxygenase (COX) inhibitors, 753–755, *754*
Cyclooxygenase metabolites, 195, *195, 196*
Cyclophilin, 747
Cyclophosphamide, 746
for bone transplantation, 741
for bullous pemphigoid, 498
for kidney transplantation, 721
for microscopic polyangiitis, 454
for paraneoplastic pemphigus, 507
for pemphigus vulgaris and pemphigus foliaceous, 506
for polyarteritis nodosa, 453
for pure erythrocyte aplasia, 441
for scleroderma, 415
for systemic lupus erythematosus, 405
for warm autoimmune hemolytic anemia, 439
for Wegener's granulomatosis, 455
Cyclosporine, 747–748, *748*
for graft-versus-host disease, 739
for paraneoplastic pemphigus, 507
for pemphigus vulgaris and pemphigus foliaceous, 506
for polyarteritis nodosa, 453
for polymyositis-dermatomyositis, 417
for primary biliary cirrhosis, 472
for rheumatoid arthritis, 408
for transplant recipients
bone, 741

heart, 733
heart-lung and lung, 735
kidney, 721
liver, 730
for warm autoimmune hemolytic anemia, 439
Cysticercosis, 683
Cytochrome *c*, 15, 16
Cytogenetic analysis of immune system neoplasms, 113–114, 581–584, 586t
Burkitt's lymphoma, 113, *113,* 583–584
follicular lymphoma, 113–114, 584
L3 acute lymphoblastic leukemia, 583
Cytokines, 148–164. *See also* specific cytokines
in acute-phase response, 23, 152, 157
in allograft rejection, kidney, *723,* 723–724, *725*
antiinflammatory, 758
atopy and, 156, 157, 350–351
chemoattractant, 29, 167–174 (*See also* Chemokines)
colony-stimulating factors, 4–5, 36t, 148, 162–163, 163t
cytokine receptor families, 163, 164t
definition of, 148
functions of, 148, 164
hematopoietic, 4–5, 9–13
functions of, 8t, 9
membrane-bound, 8–9
signal transduction and receptors for, 9–13, *10, 12*
types of, 8t, 9
inhibitors of, 757–758
interferons, 159–161, *160*
interleukin-1 and tumor necrosis factor α, 148–154, 151t
interleukin-2, 154–156, *156*
interleukin-4 and interleukin-13, 156–157
interleukin-5, 157
interleukin-6 family, 157, 158t
interleukin-7, 157–158
interleukin-9, 158
interleukin-10, 158–159
interleukin-12, 159
interleukin-15, 159
interleukin-16, 159
interleukin-17, 159
interleukin-18, 159
lymphokines, 43, 148
monokines, 148
in multiple sclerosis, 511
nomenclature for, 148, 149t, 150t
paracrine and autocrine effects of, 148
phenotypes of cytokine knockout mice, 148, 153t, 155t, 163t
preeclampsia and, 564
production by recombinant DNA techniques, 148
production of, 148
assays for, 244–245
by helper T cells, 66, 140–141, 140t
by macrophages, 37, 38t
by natural killer cells, 144
by NKT cells, 145–146
by trophoblast, 552
proinflammatory, 148, 202
in renal disease, 485, 485t
role in implantation, 551
therapeutic uses of, 164, 758
HIV infection, 647
neutropenia, 435–436, 436t
transforming growth factor β, 161–162, *162*
virokines and viroreceptors, 164
Cytolysin, 142
Cytomegalovirus (CMV) infection, 649–650
in bone marrow transplant recipients, 650, 738, 740

Cytomegalovirus (CMV) infection, *(continued)*
    clinical features of, 649, 649t
    immunologic findings in, 649–650
    prevalence of, 649
    transfusion-transmitted, 255–256
    treatment and prevention of, 650, 705t
Cytosine-phosphate-guanosine (CpG) dinucleotides,
        unmethylated, 36
Cytosolic pathway, antigenic peptides generated by, 82t, 83
Cytotoxic agents, 744–746
    azathioprine, 745–746
    chlorambucil, 746
    cladribine, 746
    cyclophosphamide, 746
    fludarabine, 746
    6-mercaptopurine, 745
    methotrexate, 744–745
Cytotoxicity, 197
    antibody-dependent cell-mediated, 68, 108, 144
Cytotoxic T cell precursors (CTLp), 290
Cytotoxic T lymphocytes (CTLs), 45–46, 139, 141–143, 197
    activation of, 66–67, *67*
    assays for, 244
    functions of, 141–142
    killing by cytotoxic granules, 142, *142*
    killing by Fas ligand-Fas pathway, *142,* 142–143
    responses in HIV infection, 644
    viral effects on, 618t–619t
Cytotoxic (type II) hypersensitivity reactions, 395

DAF. *See* **Decay-accelerating factor**
DAG (diacylglycerol), 47
Dalen-Fuchs nodules, 531
Dapsone
    for bullous pemphigoid, 498
    for pemphigus vulgaris and pemphigus foliaceous, 506
DARC, 173
DCF (2′,7′-dichlorofluorescein) test, 246–247, 294, 296
ddC (zalcitabine), 645, 647t
ddI (didanosine), 645, 647y
"Death by neglect" of B lymphocytes, 118
Death domains of Fas and tumor necrosis factor receptor I,
        152
Decay-accelerating factor (DAF), 182t, 185
    deficiency of, 342t, 345–346
Decidua, 548, 551
Defensins, 20t, 21, 32
    as ligands for chemokine receptors, 173
Degranulation, 32, *32*
    assays of, 247, *247*
    extracellular, 33, *34,* 191
Delavirdine, 645, 647t
Delayed hemolytic transfusion reactions, 254–255, 254t
Delayed-type (type IV) hypersensitivity (DTH) reactions, 37,
        197–199, 386–393, 395t, 396
    allergic contact dermatitis, 386–388, 396
    in HIV infection, 644
    hypersensitivity pneumonitis, 389–393
    photoallergic contact dermatitis, 388–389
    skin testing for, 242–243, 242t, 296
        contact hypersensitivity, 243
        patch testing, 243, 387, 387t, 397
        PPD test, 242–243
Delta hepatitis, 632
Demyelinating diseases, 510–519
    acute disseminated encephalomyelitis, 516–517
    acute inflammatory demyelinating polyneuropathy, 518–519
    chronic inflammatory neuropathies, 519

molecular mimicry in, 510
    multiple sclerosis, 226, *226,* 510–516, *512–515*
Demyelinating encephalopathy, after passive immunization,
        706
Denaturing gel electrophoresis, 224, 227
Dendritic cells, 45, *64*
    as antigen-presenting cells, *64,* 65, 91–92
    blood, 91
    chemokine receptor expression by, *169,* 173
    follicular, 50, 126–127, *127*
    HIV-infected, 639
    immature, 91
    interdigitating, 51, 91
    in lamina propria, 207
    Langerhans' cells, 54, 91
    malignancies of, 602
        Langerhans' cell histiocytosis, 602
        sarcomas, 602
    maturation of, 92
    production of, *3*
        GM-CSF and, 163
    surface receptors of, 65
Dental plaque, microflora of, 474
Deoxyribonucleic acid. *See* DNA
de Quervain's thyroiditis, 425
Dermatitis. *See also* Skin conditions
    atopic, 349, 365–366
    contact, 386–389
        allergic, 199, 386–388
        of eyelids, 386–388, 532199
        photoallergic, 388–389
    herpetiformis, 501–503
        clinical features of, 501–503, *502*
        differential diagnosis of, 503
        genetics of, 501
        immunologic diagnosis of, 503, *503*
        immunologic features of, 501
        pathology of, 501
        prognosis and diseases associated with, 503
        treatment of, 503
Dermatophytosis, 656t, 661t
Dermographism, 378
Desensitization. *See* Allergen immunotherapy
Dexamethasone, *749,* 750t
Diabetes mellitus, insulin-dependent, 94t, 146, 429–430
    antigens associated with, 423t
    clinical features of, 429–430
    epidemiology of, 429
    genetics of, 429
    immunologic diagnosis of, 430
    immunologic features of, 429
    pancreas transplantation for, 730–732
    pathogenesis of, 429, 730
    pathology of, 429
    stiff-person syndrome and, 524
    treatment of, 430
Diacylglycerol (DAG), 47
Dialysis, 184
Diapedesis, 59
DIC. *See* Disseminated intravascular coagulation
2′,7′-Dichlorofluorescein (DCF) test, 246–247, 294, 296
Didanosine (ddI), 645, 647t
DiGeorge anomaly, 239, 313–316, *314*
    complications and prognosis for, 316
    differential diagnosis of, 315
    genetic factors and, 314
    immunologic diagnosis of, 315
    immunologic features of, 313
    immunologic pathogenesis of, 313–314, *314*

laboratory findings in, 315
symptoms and signs of, 314–315
treatment of, 315
Dihydrofolate reductase, 744
Dimorphic fungi, 655
Diphenylhydantoin-induced pulmonary disease, 537
Diphtheria, 609
Diphtheria antitoxin, 705t
Diphtheria toxoid, 79t, 80, 609, 610, 701t
Diphyllobothrium latum, 683
Direct antiglobulin test, 252, *253*
Disease-modifying antirheumatic drugs (DMARDs), 408
Disseminated intravascular coagulation (DIC), 152
anaphylaxis and, 371
Dissociation constant (K_d), 76
Dissociation half-life ($t_{1/2}$), 76
DMARDs (disease-modifying antirheumatic drugs), 408
DNA (deoxyribonucleic acid). *See also* Molecular genetic
techniques
amplification by polymerase chain reaction, *266, 266–267,
267,* 284
branched, 262
complementary, 260, 268
denatured, 260
flow cytometric analysis of DNA ploidy, 241
genomic arrays, 268
heteroduplex analysis, 289
hybridization assays, 261–262, *263, 264*
probes, 260–261, *262*
sequence-based typing, 284t, 287, *288*
sequence-specific oligonucleotide probing, 284–287, *286*
sequence-specific priming, 284, *285*
structure of, 260, *261*
DNA polymerases, 266
DNA vaccines, 80
for allergen immunotherapy, 717
DNA viruses, 569
Dome area cells, 205
Donath–Landsteiner antibody, 440
Donors
bone marrow, 736–737
heart, 733
heart-lung and lung, 735
kidney, 719–721
liver, 727
Dot blot hybridization, 261
Double-positive/negative T lymphocytes, 45, 55, *56,* 134
DPT vaccine, 610, 701t, 702, 709
Dracunculus medinensis, 684
Drug allergy, 394–400
acute interstitial nephritis due to, 396
acute rapid desensitization for, 397–398
autoimmune diseases due to, 396
diagnosis of, 396–397, 397t
ELISA, 397
patch testing, 397
RAST, 397
test-dose challenge, 397
drug fever due to, 396
Gell and Coombs classification of, 394–396, 395t
type II cytotoxic reactions, 395
type III immune complex-mediated reactions, 396
type I immediate reactions, 394–395
type IV delayed type reactions, 396
immunologic basis of, 394, *395*
photosensitivity reactions due to, 396
risk factors for, 394
patient-related, 394
route of administration, 394

to specific drugs, 398–400
aspirin and nonsteroidal antiinflammatory drugs, 400
beta-lactam antibiotics, *398,* 398–399, *399*
general anesthetics, 399
local anesthetics, 399–400
Drug-induced disorders
acute interstitial nephritis, 396
agranulocytosis, 435
allergic contact dermatitis, 396
allergic rhinitis, 357, 357t
anaphylactoid reactions, 374, 374t
anaphylaxis, 373, 373t, 395
antiphospholipid syndrome, 449
aplastic anemia, 442
autoimmune diseases, 396
drug fever, 396
eosinophilic pneumonias, 540, 540t
immune hemolytic anemia, 439–440, 440t
immune neutropenia, 434–435
immune thrombocytopenia, 443t, 445–446
lupus-like syndrome, 403, 537
photosensitivity, 396
respiratory diseases, 535–537, 536t, *537*
selective IgA deficiency, 309
urticaria, 378
DTF. *See* Delayed-type hypersensitivity
d4T (stavudine), 645, 647t
Duffy antigen, 173
Duffy antigens, 252
Duncan's syndrome, 295, 330–331, 650, 651
Dust mites, 352
Dwarfism, short-limbed, with immunodeficiency, 321,
327–328

EAE (experimental autoimmune encephalomyelitis), 511
EAN (experimental autoimmune neuritis), 518
EBV. *See* Epstein–Barr virus infection
Echinococcosis, 684
ECM (extracellular matrix), 6, 8
Ectocervix, 548
Eczema. *See* Atopic dermatitis
Edema, laryngeal, 375
Efavirenz, 645, 647t
Effector cells, 19, 42, 61, 69
Egg-sperm fusion, 550–551
EIAs (enzyme-linked immunoassays), 222
Eicosanoids, 194
Elastases, 37, 38t
ELC (Epstein–Barr virus-induced molecule 1 ligand
chemokine), 59, 172–173, 172t
Elderly persons, immunization of, 709, 711t
Electromyography, 416
Electrophoresis, 224–227
denaturing gel, 224, *224*
immunoelectrophoresis, 226–227, *227*
serum protein, 224–226, *224–226*
support media for, 224
zone, 224, *224–226*
Elephantiasis, 686
ELISA. *See* Enzyme-linked immunosorbent assay
ELISPOT (enzyme-linked immunospot) assay, 245
Embryonic development, 552
Emigration of neutrophils, 29, *30*
Emotional stress, urticaria and, 378
Emphysema, 362
Encapsulated bacteria, 607, 612–613
Bacteroides fragilis, 613
Haemophilus influenzae, 613

Encapsulated bacteria, *(continued)*
  immunity to, 612, *612*
  Klebsiella pneumoniae, 613
  Neisseria species, 613
  Streptococcus agalactiae, 613
  Streptococcus pneumoniae, 612
Encephalitis
  caprine arthritis-encephalitis, 637
  Japanese, 701t
  limbic, 522t, 523
  Rasmussen's, 524
  subacute sclerosing panencephalitis, 625
Encephalomyelitis
  acute disseminated, 510, 516–517
  experimental autoimmune, 511, 516
  postimmunization, 517
Endocarditis
  in antiphospholipid syndrome, 448
  verrucous, in systemic lupus erythematosus, 402
Endocervix, 548
Endocrine diseases, 422–432
  Addison's disease, 430
  idiopathic hypoparathyroidism, 431
  insulin-dependent diabetes mellitus, 429–430
  lymphocytic adenohypophysitis, 430
  mechanism of development of, 422, *423*
  organ-specific autoantibodies and, 422, 423t
  polyglandular syndromes, 431–432, 431t
  premature ovarian failure, 430–431
  thyroid diseases, 422–428
    Graves' disease, 426–428, *427*
    Hashimoto's thyroiditis, 422–425, *424, 425*
    primary hypothyroidism, 428
    transient thyroiditis syndromes, 425–426
Endocytic pathway, antigenic peptides generated by, 82–83, 82t
Endocytosis, receptor-mediated, 31
Endometrium, 548, 551
Endosalpinx, 548
Endothelial cells, 193
  activation of, 25t, 26–27, 27t, 193
  as antigen-presenting cells, 193
  in inflammatory response, 193
Endotoxin, 607–608. *See also* Lipopolysaccharide; Toxins
Enterobacteriaceae, 611
env gene, 637, 638, *638*
Environmental factors
  allergic contact dermatitis and, 387, 387t
  allergic rhinitis and, 358
  anaphylaxis and, 372–374
  asthma and, 361–363, 362t, 363t
  atopy and, 351
  carcinogens, 568–569
  fungal diseases and, 655
  hypersensitivity pneumonitis and, 389–390, 390t
  photoallergic contact dermatitis and, 389, 389t
  respiratory diseases and, 541
Enzyme-linked immunoassays (EIAs), 222
Enzyme-linked immunosorbent assay (ELISA), 221–224, 244
  antibody capture assay, 222, *223*
  biotin/avidin-enhanced, 222, *223*
  to diagnose HIV infection, 642
  for drug allergy, 397
  enzymes used for, 222
  microparticle enzyme immunoassays, 222–224, 224t
  sandwich assay, 222, *222*
  to screen for HLA antibodies, 279–280
  sensitivity of, 222
Enzyme-linked immunospot (ELISPOT) assay, 245

Enzymes
  immunodeficiency associated with deficiencies of
    adenosine deaminase and purine nucleoside
      phosphorylase, 328–330, *329*
    glucose-6-phosphate dehydrogenase, 336
    myeloperoxidase, 336
  as inflammatory mediators, 195, 197t
  restriction, 262
Eosinophilia, 190
  in allergic gastroenteropathy, 367
  in allergic rhinitis, 356–357
  in bullous pemphigoid, 496–497
  in helminth infections, 683
Eosinophilic granuloma, 602
Eosinophilic pneumonia, 537–540, 538t
  acute, 539–540
  allergic granulomatosis of Churg and Strauss, 538
  asthma and, 191, 360, 538, 538t
  chronic idiopathic (Carrington's), 538, *539*
  drug-induced, 540, 540t
  eosinophilia-myalgia syndrome, 540
  hypereosinophilic syndrome, 540
  parasite-induced, 540, 540t
  simple idiopathic pulmonary eosinophilia, 538–539
Eosinophil peroxidase, 190, 191
Eosinophils, 2, 190–191
  activation of, 191
  chemokine receptor expression by, *169*
  Fc receptors on, 190t, 191
  hypodense, 191
  IL-5 and, 157, 190–191
  in inflammatory response, 190–191
  production of, *3,* 190
  structure of, 190, *190*
Eotaxin, 171
Epidermolysis bullosa acquisita, 500–501
  clinical features of, 500–501
  differential diagnosis of, 501
  immunologic diagnosis of, 501
  immunologic features of, 500
  pathology of, 500
  prognosis for, 501
  treatment of, 501
Epinephrine
  for anaphylaxis, 375, 756
  for asthma, 363
  for urticaria and angioedema, 379
Epithelioid cells, 38
Epitopes, 72, 73
  B-cell, 73–77, *74, 75*
  T-cell, 73, *74,* 77–79, *78*
EPO. *See* Erythropoietin
Epstein–Barr virus (EBV) infection, 164, 650–653
  clinical features of, 650–651, 651t
    hairy leukoplakia, 478
    infectious mononucleosis, 650–651
    lymphoproliferative disorders, 603
    malignancies, 569, 651, 652
  drug allergy and, 394
  immunologic features of, 650–653, *652*
  laboratory diagnosis of infectious mononucleosis, 651, *651*
  mimicry of C3d by, 186
  pathogenesis of, 650
  transfusion-transmitted, 256
  treatment and prevention of, 653
Epstein–Barr virus-induced molecule 1 ligand chemokine
    (ELC), 59, 172–173, 172t
Ergosterol, 655
Erwinia, 611

Erythema, 26
Erythema migrans, 692
Erythema multiforme, 664
Erythema nodosum, 664
Erythrocyte antigens, 250–252
  ABO and H, *251,* 251–252, 251t
  Duffy, 252
  Kell, 252
  Kidd, 252
  Lewis, 251
  Rh, 251–252, 252t
  secretor, 251
Erythrocyte disorders, 436–442
  aplastic anemia, 441–442, 737
  immune hemolytic anemias, 436–441
    classification of, 437t
    cold agglutinin syndromes, 439
    drug-induced, 439–440, 440t
    hemolytic disease of newborn, 251, 252, 257
    paroxysmal cold hemoglobinuria, 440–441
    serologic tests for, 436–437, 438t
    warm autoimmune hemolytic anemia, 437–439
  paroxysmal nocturnal hemoglobinuria, 185, 346, 347, 441
  pure erythrocyte aplasia, 441
Erythrocytes
  blood groups, 250
  DARC expression on, 173
  destruction in malaria, 674
  detection of antigen and antibodies to, 252–254, 436–437
    antiglobulin tests, 252–253, *253,* 438t
    pretransfusion testing, 253
    type and screen, 253–254
  production of, 1, 2, *3*
  transfusion of, 258, 258t
Erythrocyte sedimentation rate, 24
Erythroid progenitor, 2, *3*
Erythropoietin (EPO), 5, 8t, 148, 162–163
  receptor for, 9, *10*
  therapeutic use of, 436t
Escherichia coli, 179, 611
E-selectin, 8t, 27, 27t, 29, *30*
Espundia, 677
EST (expressed sequence tag), 268
Etanercept, 408, 758
Eukaryotes, 655
Exanthem subitum, 654
Exercise-induced disorders
  "anaphylaxis," 374
  asthma, 362
Exons, 109
Exotoxins, 607. *See also* Toxins
Experimental autoimmune encephalomyelitis (EAE), 511, 516
Experimental autoimmune myasthenia gravis, 520
Experimental autoimmune neuritis (EAN), 518
Expressed sequence tag (EST), 268
Extracellular degranulation, 33, *34,* 191
Extracellular matrix (ECM), 6, 8
Extrinsic allergic alveolitis. *See* Hypersensitivity pneumonitis
Eye disorders, 527–534
  African river blindness, 686
  AIDS-associated, 532–533
  antibody-mediated, 527–530
  atopic keratoconjunctivitis, 527
  in Behçet's disease, 532
  cell-mediated, 530–533
  in cicatricial pemphigoid, 530
  in contact dermatitis, 532
  corneal graft reactions, *533,* 533–534
  in giant-cell arteritis, 532
  lens-induced uveitis, 530
  in microscopic polyangiitis, 453
  ocular sarcoidosis, 530–531
  in pemphigus vulgaris, 530
  phlyctenular keratoconjunctivitis, 532, *532*
  in polyarteritis nodosa, 452, 532
  in rheumatoid diseases, *528,* 528–529, *529*
    ankylosing spondylitis, 528, *528*
    immunologic diagnosis of, 529
    immunologic pathogenesis of, 528–529
    juvenile arthritis, 409, 528
    Reiter's syndrome, 418, 528, *529*
    relapsing polychondritis, 419
    rheumatoid arthritis, 407, 528, *528, 529*
    Sjögren's syndrome, 411, 412
    treatment of, 529
  sympathetic ophthalmia, 531–532
  in systemic lupus erythematosus, 403, 530, *530*
  in toxoplasmosis, 676
  vernal conjunctivitis, 527, *528*
  Vogt-Koyanagi-Harada syndrome, 531–532

F(ab)′2 fragment, 97
Facial palsy, in Lyme disease, 693, 696
Factor B, 180
  deficiency of, 342t, 343
Factor D, 180
  deficiency of, 342t, 343
Factor H, 182t, 183
  deficiency of, 342t, 345
Factor I, 181–183, 182t
  deficiency of, 342t, 345
Factor J, 182t, 183
Factor V, 259
Factor VIII, 259
  inhibitors of, 448
Factor XI, *186,* 186–187
Fallopian tube, 548
Farmer's lung. *See* Hypersensitivity pneumonitis
Fas, 15, 70, 152t, 154
  cytotoxic T-cell killing and, *142,* 142–143
  death domain of, 152
  phenotypes of knockout mice, 153t
Fasciola, 191
Fascioliasis, 681
Fas ligand (FasL), 15, *16,* 70, 151, 152t, 154
  phenotypes of knockout mice, 153t
Fc receptors, 31, 45t, 68, 108, 108t, *116,* 121, 126
  as accessory receptors for HIV-1, 639
  in allergic rhinitis, 367
  on inflammatory cells, 189–190, 190t
    basophils, 192–193
    eosinophils, 191
    mast cells, 192
  monoclonal antibody binding to, 241
  on myeloid cells, 241
FDCs (follicular dendritic cells), 50, 126–127, *127*
Febrile nonhemolytic transfusion reactions (FNHTRs), 255
Felty's syndrome, 333, 405, 407, 434
Fertilization, 550–551
α-Fetoprotein, 571
Fetus
  antiphospholipid syndrome and recurrent fetal loss, 448
  fertilization, implantation, and immune response to, 550–552
  hematopoiesis in, 2, *4*
  HIV infection of, 561–562
  oncofetal antigens, 571

Fever, 152
  blackwater, 674
  drug, 396
  Katayama, 683
  rheumatic, 410
  scarlet, 610
  typhoid, 614
FFP (fresh-frozen plasma), 258t, 259
Fibrin, 198
Fibrinogen, 23–24
Fibroblasts, production of IFNβ by, 160
Filariasis, 684–686
FITC (fluorescein isothiocyanate), 235
FK 506. *See* Tacrolimus
FK-binding protein-12 (FKBP12), 747, 749
Flow cytometry, 235–242
  clinical applications of, 238–242, 240t
    apoptosis, 241–242
    B-cell antigens, 239–240, 295
    DNA ploidy, 241
    intracellular antigens, 241
    leukocyte functional assays, 241
    myeloid antigens, 240–241
    T-cell antigens, 238–239
  crossmatching, 281–282, *282,* 290t
  data collection and analysis, 236–238, *237–239*
  flow cytometers for, *235,* 235–236
  fluorescence-activated cell sorters, 238, *240*
  light-scattering properties of cells, 235, *235, 236*
  sample preparation for, 236
  to screen for HLA antibodies, 280
Flt-3, 163t
Flt-3 ligand, 5, 8t
Fluconazole
  for candidiasis, 667
  for coccidioidomycosis, 664
  for cryptococcosis, 668
  for histoplasmosis, 665
Flucytosine
  for candidiasis, 667
  for cryptococcosis, 668
Fludarabine, 746
Fluid-phase regulators of complement, 181–183, 182t
  C4-binding protein, 181–183
  C1 inhibitor, 181
  clusterin, 183
  factor H, 183
  factor I, 181–183
  factor J, 183
  protected site concept, 183
  S protein, 183
Fluorescein isothiocyanate (FITC), 235
Fluorescence-activated cell sorters, 238, *240*
Fluorescence microscopy, 229
Fluorescent-treponemal antibody absorbance test (FTA-ABS),
      691, *691*
FNHTRs (febrile nonhemolytic transfusion reactions), 255
Folate antagonists, 744–745
Follicular B cells, 206
Follicular dendritic cells (FDCs), 50, 126–127, *127*
Follicular lymphoma, 70, 113–114, 584, 593
Follicular T cells, 205
Food allergens, 354, 372–373, 373t
  gluten-sensitive enteropathy and, 460–462
  villous atrophy not due to gluten sensitivity and, 462
Foreign travel, immunizations for, 709–711
Fos, 14
Foscarnet, 650
Fossa navicularis, 549
Fractalkine, 167, 168t, 171

Francisella, 221
Fresh-frozen plasma (FFP), 258t, 259
"Frustrated" phagocytosis, *34,* 247, *247*
FTA-ABS (fluorescent-treponemal antibody absorbance test),
      691, *691*
Fungal diseases, 655–671
  cutaneous, 655, 656t
  effect of immunologic abnormalities on course of, 661t
  hypersensitivity pneumonitis and, 390t
  immunity to, 655, 657t–658t
  immunologic diagnosis of, 662t–663t
  opportunistic, 655, 657t–658t, 666–671
    aspergillosis, 669
    candidiasis, 666–667
    cryptococcosis, 667–668
    mucormycosis, 669–670
    pneumocystosis, 670–671
  pathologic features of, 659t–660t
  subcutaneous, 655, 656t
  superficial, 655, 656t
  systemic, 655, 657t–658t, 658–666
    blastomycosis, 658–660
    coccidioidomycosis, 660–664
    histoplasmosis, 664–665
    paracoccidioidomycosis, 665–666
Fungi
  angioinvasion by, 655
  dimorphic, 655
  environmental sources of, 655
  mold allergens, 351–352, *352*
  structure of, 655

GAD (glutamic acid decarboxylase), 524, 730
gag gene, 637, 638, *638*
GALT (gut-associated lymphoid tissue), 204
Gamete intrafallopian transfer, 558
Gametocytes in malaria, 674
γ/δ cells, 143
Gamma-globulin fraction, 95
Ganciclovir, 650
Gas gangrene, 609
Gastrointestinal disorders, 460–469
  allergic gastroenteropathy, 349, 367–368
  anaphylaxis and, 371
  in Churg-Strauss syndrome, 456
  gluten-sensitive enteropathy, 460–462, *461*
  Helicobacter pylori-associated chronic gastritis and MALT
      lymphomas, 465
  immunoproliferative small-intestinal diseases, 464
  inflammatory bowel diseases, 465–469
    Crohn's disease, 466–468, *467*
    ulcerative colitis, *468,* 468–469
  intestinal lymphangiectasia and other protein-losing
      enteropathies, 463
  in microscopic polyangiitis, 453
  NSAID-induced, 753–755, 754t
  pernicious anemia, 464–465
  in polyarteritis nodosa, 452
  in scleroderma, 414
  in systemic lupus erythematosus, 403
  villous atrophy not due to gluten sensitivity, 462–463
  in Wegener's granulomatosis, 454
  Whipple's disease, 463
GBM. *See* Glomerular basement membrane
GBS. *See* Guillain-Barré syndrome
GCA. *See* Giant-cell arteritis
G-CSF. *See* Granulocyte colony-stimulating factor
GDP (guanosine diphosphate), 11

Gell and Coombs classification of hypersensitivity reactions, 394–396, 395t, 535
  type II cytotoxic reactions, 395
  type III immune complex-mediated reactions, 380–385, 396
  type I immediate reactions, 201–202, *202,* 394–395
  type IV delayed type reactions, 37, 197–199, 242–243, 242t, 386, 396
General anesthetics, hypersensitivity to, 399
Gene rearrangement assay for lymphocyte clonality, 263–265
Genes
  for ABO and H blood groups, 250–251
  amplification by polymerase chain reaction, *266,* 266–267, *267,* 284
  for complement proteins, 183
  for human leukocyte antigens, 84–87, *88,* 88t, *272,* 272–273
  immunoglobulin, 108–114
    supergene family, 105–106, 105t, 163, 164t
  oncogenes, 569–570
  for Rh blood group, 251–252, 252t
  T-cell receptor α and β, 131–132
  testing for mutations associated with immunodeficiency states, 297
Gene therapy, 5
Genetic factors
  atopy and, 349–350, 350t
  bare lymphocyte syndrome and, 322
  combined B-cell and T-cell immunodeficiency disorders and, 320
  complement deficiencies and, 341–347, 342t
  DiGeorge anomaly and, 314
  drug allergy and, 394
  response to immunogens and, 73
  selective IgA deficiency and, 309
Genitourinary disorders
  in polyarteritis nodosa, 452
  in Wegener's granulomatosis, 454–455
Genomic arrays, 268
Germinal center of secondary lymphoid follicle, 51, *51–53*
  B-lymphocyte chemoattractant in formation of, 172
  in humoral immune response, 126–127, *127*
Giant-cell arteritis (GCA), 456–457
  diagnosis of, 457
  immunologic features of, 456
  immunologic pathogenesis of, 456
  laboratory findings in, 456
  prognosis for, 457
  signs and symptoms of, 456
    ocular, 532
  treatment of, 457
Gingivitis, 473–476. *See also* Periodontal disease
Glands of Littré, 549
Glomerular basement membrane (GBM), 481–482
  anti-GBM disease, *482,* 482–483, 491–492, *544,* 544–545
Glomerulonephritis. *See also* Nephritis; Renal disease
  antineutrophil cytoplasmic antibodies and, 483–484
  autoimmune, 482–483
  in Churg-Strauss syndrome, 456
  complement deficiencies and, 346
  in Henoch-Schönlein purpura, 458, 491
  IgA nephropathy, 488
  in malaria, 673
  membranoproliferative, 489
  membranous, *482, 486,* 486–487
  in microscopic polyangiitis, 454
  postinfectious, 481–482, *487,* 487–488
  primary, 486–489
  secondary mediators of, 485–486
    cells, 485
    molecular mediators, 485–486, 485t
  similarity to serum sickness, 481–482

in systemic lupus erythematosus, 402, 489–491, *490,* 490t
T lymphocytes and, 484–485
in Wegener's granulomatosis, 454
α- and β-Glucans, 655
Glucocorticoids, 152, 750–752. *See also* Corticosteroids
  for allergic rhinitis, 358
  for asthma, 364
  for hereditary angioedema, 347
  for paroxysmal nocturnal hemoglobinuria, 347
Glucose-6-phosphate dehydrogenase deficiency, 336
Glutamic acid decarboxylase (GAD), 524, 730
Gluten-sensitive enteropathy (GSE), 460–462
  clinical features of, 461
  complications and prognosis for, 462
  differential diagnosis of, 462
  immunologic diagnosis of, 461–462
  immunologic features of, 460
  immunologic pathogenesis of, 461
  pathology of, 460–461, *461*
  treatment of, 462
Glycogen storage disease type 1B, 337
Glycolipid antigens, 77, 93, 145
Glycosyl phosphatidylinositol (GPI), 145, 345–346
GM-CSF. *See* Granulocyte-monocyte colony-stimulating factor
Gold salts
  for pemphigus vulgaris and pemphigus foliaceous, 506
  pneumonitis induced by, 537
Gonococcus, 613
Goodpasture's syndrome, *482,* 482–483, 491–492, 544–545
  clinical features of, *482,* 482–483, 491–492, 544–545
  differential diagnosis of, 545
  immunologic features of, 544
  immunologic pathogenesis of, 544
  pathology and immunopathology of, 492
  treatment and prognosis for, 492, 545
Good's syndrome, 311
gp39. *See* CD40 ligand
gp41, 638, 642
gp120, 638, 639
gp160, 638
GPI (glycosyl phosphatidylinositol), 145, 345–346
G-protein-coupled receptors, 169
Graft-versus-host disease (GVHD), 326–327
  acute, *326,* 326–327, 739
  in bone marrow transplant recipients, 739
  chronic, 327, 739
  clinical staging of, 739t
  diagnosis of, 327
  histocompatibility testing for prevention of, 270
  hyperacute, 327
  in immunodeficient patients, 326–327
  management of, 327
  transfusion-associated, 256–257
Gram-negative rods, 611–612
Granulocyte colony-stimulating factor (G-CSF), *4,* 8t, 162–163
  for chronic granulomatous disease, 335
  phenotypes of knockout mice, 163t
  therapeutic uses of, 163, 436t
    HIV infection, 647
    neutropenia, 435–436
Granulocyte-monocyte colony-stimulating factor (GM-CSF), *4,* 5, 8, 8t, 9
  atopy and, 350
  phenotypes of knockout mice, 163t
  receptor for, 9, 10, *10*
  therapeutic uses of, 163, 436t
    HIV infection, 647
    neutropenia, 435–436
Granulocyte-monocyte progenitor, 2, *3,* 5
Granulocytopenia, 434

Granulomas, 38, *38*
chronic granulomatous disease, 295, 334–336
in schistosomiasis, 682
syphilitic gummas, 689
Granulomatosis
allergic, of Churg and Strauss, 455, 538
bronchocentric, 545–546
lymphomatoid, 545
necrotizing sarcoid, 545
Wegener's, 454–455
Granulomatous ileitis. *See* Crohn's disease
Granzyme B, 15
Granzymes, 142
Graves' disease, 94t, 426–428
antigens associated with, 423t
clinical features of, 427
complications and prognosis for, 428
differential diagnosis of, 428
epidemiology of, 426
immunologic diagnosis of, *427*, 427–428
immunologic features of, 426
pathology of, 427
treatment of, 428
Griscelli's syndrome, 321
Group A streptococci, 610
Group B streptococci, 613
Group D streptococci, 611
GSE. *See* Gluten-sensitive enteropathy
GTPase (guanosine triphosphatase), 11
Guanosine diphosphate (GDP), 11
Guanosine triphosphatase (GTPase), 11
Guillain-Barré syndrome (GBS), 510, 518–519
clinical features of, 518
complications and prognosis for, 519
differential diagnosis of, 518
immunologic diagnosis of, 518
pathogens associated with, 518
pathology of, 518
treatment of, 518–519
Guinea worm, 684
Gumma, syphilitic, 689
Gut-associated lymphoid tissue (GALT), 204
GVHD. *See* Graft-versus-host disease

Haemophilus influenzae, **613**
Haemophilus influenzae type B vaccine, 79t, 80, 295, 613, 701t
Hageman factor, 181, *186,* 186–187, 256
Hairy cell leukemia, 594
Hairy leukoplakia, oral, 478, *478*
Hand-Schüller-Christian syndrome, 602
Hansen's disease, 615
H antigen, 250–251, *251,* 251t, 611
Haplotype, 86, 275
Haptenation, 394, *395*
Haptens, 76–77, *77*
in drug-induced immune hemolytic anemia, 440
Hashimoto's thyroiditis, 422–425
antigens associated with, 423t
clinical features of, 424
differential diagnosis of, 425
epidemiology of, 423
immunologic diagnosis of, 424–425, *425*
immunologic features of, 422
pathology of, 424, *424*
prognosis for, 425
treatment of, 425
Hassall's corpuscles, 55

HAV. *See* Hepatitis A virus infection
Hay fever. *See* Rhinitis, allergic
HBV. *See* Hepatitis B virus infection
HCV. *See* Hepatitis C virus infection
HDN (hemolytic disease of the newborn), 251, 252, 257
HDV (hepatitis delta virus) infection, 632
Heart
in antiphospholipid syndrome, 448
in Churg-Strauss syndrome, 455–456
in Kawasaki's disease, 458
in Lyme disease, 693
in polyarteritis nodosa, 452
in scleroderma, 414
in Takayasu's arteritis, 457
in Wegener's granulomatosis, 454–455
Heart-lung and lung transplantation, 734–736
allograft monitoring after, 736
complications of, 736
contraindications to, 735
donor selection for, 735
history of, 734–735
immunosuppression after, 735–736
operative procedure for, 735
organ procurement for, 735
outcome of, 736
recipient selection for, 735
idiopathic pulmonary fibrosis, 544
registry for, 735
Heart transplantation, 291, 732–734
allograft monitoring after, 733–734
chronic rejection, 734
signs of allograft dysfunction, 733–734
complications of, 734
contraindications to, 733
crossmatching for, 291, 733
donor selection for, 733
history of, 732
immunosuppression after, 733
operative procedure for, 733
organ procurement for, 733
outcome of, 734
recipient selection for, 733
registry for, 732–733
Heavy-chain diseases, 596–597
Heavy chains, immunoglobulin, 42, *96,* 96–97
class switching, *125,* 125–126
genes for, 111–112, *112*
Helicobacter pylori and MALT lymphomas, 465, 593
"Heliotrope" rash, 416
Helminthic diseases, 681–686
atopy and, 351
cestodes, 683–684
echinococcosis, 684
eosinophilic pneumonias and, 190–191, 540
nematodes, 684–686
ascariasis, 685
filariid, 685–686
trichinosis, 684–685
trematodes, 681–683
schistosomiasis, 681–683
Helper T cell precursors (HTLp), 290
Helper T lymphocytes, 45t, 46, 48–49, 139–141
activation of, 65–66, *66,* 139
allergen desensitization and, 716
cytokines secreted by, 66, 140–141, 140t
depletion in HIV infection, 638–641, *643,* 643–644
functions of, 139–140
IL-1 and TNFα actions on, 148–149
T_H1 and T_H2 cells

atopy and, 141, 350
  differentiation of, 140–141, *141*
Hemagglutination assays, 219–221, *221*
Hematologic disorders, 434–449
  erythrocyte disorders, 436–442
    aplastic anemia, 441–442, 737
    immune hemolytic anemias, 436–441, 437t
    paroxysmal nocturnal hemoglobinuria, 185, 346, 347, 441
    pure erythrocyte aplasia, 441
  in HIV infection, 645
  leukocyte disorders, 434–436, 435t
    agranulocytosis, 435
    autoimmune neutropenia, 434
    cyclic neutropenia, 434
    drug-induced immune neutropenia, 434–435
    management of neutropenia, 435–436, 436t
  platelet disorders, 442–449, 443t
    antiphospholipid syndrome, 448–449
    circulating inhibitors of coagulation, 447–448
    drug-induced immune thrombocytopenia, 445–446
    hemolytic-uremic syndrome, 447
    idiopathic thrombocytopenic purpura, 443–445
    neonatal alloimmune thrombocytopenia, 446
    posttransfusion purpura, 446
    quinine-induced immune thrombocytopenia with hemolytic-uremic syndrome, 447
    thrombotic thrombocytopenic purpura, 446–447
Hematopoiesis, 1–5
  definition of, 1
  fetal, 2
  ontogeny of, 2, *4*
  origins of cells in blood and bone marrow, 1–2, *3*
  rate of, 2, 13
  role of adhesion molecules in, 6–8, 8t
  role of cytokines in, 4–5, 8t, 9–13 (*See also* Cytokines)
Hematopoietic stem cells (HSCs), 1–5
  alternative differentiation pathways for, 1–2, *3*
  apoptosis of, 5
  expression of surface proteins on, 2–4
  fetal, 2, 4, *4*
  generation of B cells from, 115–117, *116*
  growth and differentiation of, 2–5, *4, 5*
  lymphoid, 40, *41*
  self-renewal of, 1
  storage pool of, 2
  structure of, 4
  tissue localization of, 2, *4*
  transplantation for severe combined immunodeficiency, 321
  in umbilical cord blood, 4
Hematopoietin receptor family, 9–10, *10,* 163, 164t
Hematoxylin body, 402
Hemoglobinuria
  paroxysmal cold, 440–441
  paroxysmal nocturnal, 185, 346, 347, 441
Hemolytic anemias, immune, 436–441
  classification of, 437t
  cold agglutinin syndromes, 439
  drug-induced, 439–440, 440t
  hemolytic disease of newborn, 251, 252, 257
  paroxysmal cold hemoglobinuria, 440–441
  serologic tests for, 436–437, 438t
  warm autoimmune hemolytic anemia, 437–439
Hemolytic assays, *231,* 231–232, *232,* 232t
Hemolytic disease of the newborn (HDN), 251, 252, 257
Hemolytic transfusion reactions, 254–255, 254t
Hemolytic-uremic syndrome (HUS), 447
  quinine-induced immune thrombocytopenia with, 447
  thrombotic thrombocytopenic purpura and, 447
Hemophagocytic syndromes, 603

Hemophilia, 448
Hemorrhagic Shwartzman reaction, 152
Henoch-Schönlein purpura (HSP), 458, 491
Heparin, in mast cells, 192
Hepatitis
  autoimmune chronic active, 470–471
    clinical features of, 470
    differential diagnosis of, 470–471
    immunologic diagnosis of, 470
    immunologic features of, 470
    immunopathology of, 470
    treatment of, 471
  transfusion-transmitted, 255, 255t
  transfusion-transmitted virus and, 632
Hepatitis A virus (HAV) infection, 627–628
  clinical features of, 627
  diagnosis of, 627–628
  prevention of, 628
    hepatitis A immune globulin, 628, 705t, 707
    vaccine, 79t, 628, 701t, 707
  virology of, 627
Hepatitis B virus (HBV) infection, 628–630
  chronic, 629
  clinical features of, 629
  diagnosis of, 629, 629t, *630*
  epidemiology of, 628
  hepatitis delta and, 632
  hepatocellular carcinoma and, 628, 629
  immunologic features of, 628
  immunologic pathogenesis of, 628–629
  immunologic sequelae of, 621t
  membranous glomerulonephritis and, 486
  pathology of, 628
  polyarteritis nodosa and, 452
  prevention of, 630
    hepatitis B immune globulin, 630, 705t
    postexposure prophylaxis, 630
    vaccine, 79t, 80, 630, 701t, 707
  transmission of, 628
  treatment of, 629–630
    interferon-α, 630, 758
    liver transplantation, 630, 727
  virology of, 628
    core antigen, 628
    surface antigen, 628
Hepatitis C virus (HCV) infection, 630–632
  clinical features of, 631–632
  diagnosis of, 632
  epidemiology of, 631
  hepatocellular carcinoma and, 631
  immunologic features of, 630–631
  immunologic pathogenesis of, 631
  transmission of, 631
  treatment of, 632
    interferon-α, 632, 758
    liver transplantation, 727
  virology of, 631
Hepatitis delta virus (HDV) infection, 632
Hepatitis E virus (HEV) infection, 632
Hepatitis G virus (HGV) infection, 632
Hepatobiliary disorders, 469–473
  autoimmune chronic active hepatitis, 470–471
  clinical features of, 726
  in giant-cell arteritis, 456
  hepatitis A, 627–628
  hepatitis B, 628–630
  hepatitis C, 630–632
  hepatitis D, 632
  hepatitis E, 632

Hepatobiliary disorders, *(continued)*
  hepatitis G, 632
  liver transplantation for, 291–292, 726–730
  primary biliary cirrhosis, *471,* 471–472
  primary sclerosing cholangitis, 472–473
  transfusion-transmitted hepatitis, 255, 255t, 632
  transjugular intrahepatic portasystemic shunts for, 726
  venoocclusive disease of liver after bone marrow
    transplantation, 739–740
Hepatocellular carcinoma
  hepatitis B and, 628, 629
  hepatitis C and, 631
Herd immunity, 706–707
Hereditary angioedema, 181, 378
  C1 inhibitor deficiency and, 181, 345
  kinins and, 187
  management of, 347
Herpes gestationis, 499–500
  clinical features of, 500
  definition of, 499
  differential diagnosis of, 500
  etiology of, 499
  immunologic diagnosis of, 500
  immunologic features of, 499
  pathology of, 499, *499*
  prevalence of, 499
  treatment and prognosis for, 500
Herpes saimiri virus, 164
Heteroduplex analysis, 284t, 289
Heterophile antibody test, 220–221
HEV (hepatitis E virus) infection, 632
HEVs (high endothelial venules), *58,* 58–59
Heymann's nephritis, 483
HGV (hepatitis G virus) infection, 632
HHV-8. *See* Human herpesvirus 8 infection
HHV-6 (human herpesvirus 6) infection, 653–654
High endothelial venules (HEVs), *58,* 58–59
High-molecular-weight kininogen, *186,* 186–187
Hinge region, immunoglobulin, *96, 97*
Histamine, 25t, 26, 194
  anaphylaxis and, 371
  in immediate hypersensitivity, 201–202
  in mast cells, 192, 201
  receptors for, 194, 194t
  structure of, *194*
  urticaria and, 371
Histiocytes, 35
  hemophagocytic syndromes, 602
  malignant histiocytes, 602
Histocompatibility testing, 91, 270–292
  antibody screening, 279–280
  cellular assays, 289–292, 290t, 291t
  crossmatching, 280–282
    for autoantibodies, 282
    B-cell lymphocytotoxicity, 281
    flow cytometry, 281–282, *282*
    peripheral blood lymphocytes lymphocytotoxicity, 280
    T-cell lymphocytotoxicity, 280, *281*
  HLA polymorphism and typing, *272,* 272–275, 273t, *274*
  molecular-biologic methods, 282–289, 283t, 284t
    chimerism testing, 289
    gene amplification, 284
    heteroduplex analysis, 289
    limitations of, 287–289
    restriction fragment length polymorphism, 283
    sequence-based typing, 287, *288*
    sequence-specific oligonucleotide probing, 284–287, *286*
    sequence-specific priming, 284, *285*
  serologic methods, 275–276, *276*

tissue typing by lymphocytotoxicity test, 276–279, 277t–279t
  for transplantation, 270–272, 271t, 290–292, 291t
    bone marrow, 736–737
    cornea, 292, 533, 534
    heart, 291, 733
    heart-lung and lung, 735
    kidney, 291, 291t, 719–720
    liver, 291–292, 729
    pancreas, 731
  Websites related to, 271t
Histoplasmosis, 657t, 664–665
  complications and prognosis for, 665
  differential diagnosis of, 665
  effect of immunologic abnormalities on course of, 661t
  epidemiology of, 665
  immunologic diagnosis of, 662t, 665
  immunologic features of, 664
  laboratory findings in, 665
  pathologic features of, 659t
  signs and symptoms of, 665
  treatment of, 665
HIV. *See* Human immunodeficiency virus infection
Hives. *See* Urticaria
HLAs. *See* Human leukocyte antigens
Hodgkin's disease, 154, 600–602
  clinical features of, 601
  histology of, *600,* 600–601
  immunologic diagnosis of, 601–602
  radiation therapy for, 587
  Rye classification of, 601, 601t
Homing
  of lymphocytes, 56–59, *57, 58,* 59t
  mucosal, 204, 210, *211*
Homologous restriction factor (HRF), 182t, 185
  deficiency of, 342t, 345
Hookworms, 684
H₁ receptor antagonists, 194, 756
H₂ receptor antagonists, 194, 756
HRF. *See* Homologous restriction factor
HSCs. *See* Hematopoietic stem cells
HSP (Henoch-Schönlein purpura), 458
HTLV. *See* Human T-cell lymphotrophic virus
Human herpesvirus 6 (HHV-6) infection, 653–654
Human herpesvirus 8 (HHV-8) infection, 626–627
  clinical features of, 627
  diagnosis of, 627
  immunologic features of, 626
  Kaposi's sarcoma and, 627, 641
  plasma cell myeloma and, 596, 627
  transmission of, 627
  treatment of, 627
  virology of, 626–627
    interactions with chemokine pathways, 173
Human immune globulin, 703–705, 705t
Human immunodeficiency virus (HIV) infection, 5, 636–648
  antiretroviral therapy for, 645–646
    development of, 636
    drug classes, 645, 647t
    highly active, 636, 646
    in pregnancy, 562, 640
    timing of commencement of, 646
  chemokines and, 173
  clinical features of, 641, 641t
    acute HIV mononucleosis, 641
    AIDS, 641
    blastomycosis, 658, 660
    central nervous system involvement, 640
    coccidioidomycosis, 664
    cryptococcosis, 668

fungal diseases, 655
Guillain-Barré syndrome, 518
histoplasmosis, 665
lymphomas, 603
Mycobacterium avium complex infection, 615
ocular disorders, 532–533
opportunistic infections, 641, 641t
oral disorders, 478, *478*
parasitic diseases, 673
pneumocystosis, 641, 670–671
reproductive system, 560–562
symptomatic infection, 641
tuberculosis, 615
differential diagnosis of, 645, 645t
drug allergy and, 394, 398
epidemiology of, 636, 640–641, 640t
hematologic findings in, 645
immunologic findings in, 636, 643–645
abnormal delayed-type hypersensitivity responses, 644
B-cell responses, 644
CD4 lymphocyte depletion, 638–641, *643,* 643–644
cytotoxic lymphocyte responses, 644
other abnormal responses, 645
T-cell proliferative responses, 644
immunorestorative therapy for, 156, 647–648, 758
laboratory diagnosis of, 642–643
confirmatory tests, 227, *228, 642, 642*
ELISA screening, 642
neonatal, 642–643
seroconversion, 642
latency period to onset of disease, 640–641
liver transplantation and, 727
major histocompatibility complex and, 93
monitoring patients with, 646–647
pathogenesis of, 638–640
receptors, 639
role of macrophages, 639–640, 644, 645t
viral load, 639
viral replicative cycle, 639–640, *646*
virologic set-point, 639
pediatric, 562
prevention of, 648
public education, 648
vaccines, 648, 648t, 712
transmission of, 640
blood transfusion, 255, 256
breast milk, 562
heterosexual contact, 560–561, *561,* 640
perinatal, 561–562, 640
virology of, 636–637
genomic organization, 637–638, *638*
HIV-1 and HIV-2, 637
Human leukocyte antigens (HLAs), 84–87, 270
in antiglomerular basement membrane disease, 492
in autoimmune chronic active hepatitis, 470
in Buerger's disease, 457
in dermatitis herpetiformis, 501
drug allergy and, 394
in endocrine disorders, 422, *423*
autoimmune polyglandular syndromes, 431
Graves' disease, 426
Hashimoto's thyroiditis, 423
Type I diabetes mellitus, 429
genetics of, 84–87, *88,* 88t, *272,* 272–273
in gluten-sensitive enteropathy, 460, 461
gram-negative rods and, 611
in herpes gestationis, 499
histocompatibility testing for, 270–292 (*See also*
Histocompatibility testing)

HLA-B27, 93–94
HLA sharing and recurrent pregnancy loss, 559
HLA typing, 91
inheritance of, 275
low- and high-resolution typing of, 275
in multiple sclerosis, 511, 515
in myasthenia gravis, 520
nomenclature for, 273–275, *274*
National Marrow Donor Program codes, 275
paracoccidioidomycosis and, 666
in pemphigus vulgaris, 504
placental expression of, 552
polymorphism of, 273–275, *274*
in primary biliary cirrhosis, 471
in rheumatic diseases, 529
ankylosing spondylitis, 418
Behçet's disease, 417
juvenile arthritis, 409
polymyositis-dermatomyositis, 415
psoriatic arthritis, 419
Reiter's syndrome, 418
rheumatoid arthritis, 406
systemic lupus erythematosus, 401
serologic specificities of, 273–275, 273t
Human T-cell lymphotrophic virus (HTLV) types I and II, 156, 569, 653
adult T-cell leukemia-lymphoma and, 599, 653
epidemiology of, 653
HTLV-1-associated myelopathy, 515, 653
transfusion-transmitted, 255, 255t, 256
Humidifier lung disease. *See* Hypersensitivity pneumonitis
Humoral immunity, 19, 43, 118–128, 234
B-cell antigen receptor, 118–119, *120*
B lymphocytes as antigen-presenting cells, 92, 122–124, *124*
immunoglobulin secretion, 43, 100, 124
laboratory evaluation of, 295–296
lymphoid follicles and germinal centers, 126–127, *127*
primary and secondary responses, 127–128, 128t
T-cell help and accessory signals, 119–122, *122, 123*
T-cell-independent antigens, 119, *121*
HUS. *See* Hemolytic-uremic syndrome
Hyalohyphomycosis, 658t, 661t
Hyaluronic acid, 8
Hybridization assays, 261–262, *263, 264*
Hybridoma, 106, *107*
Hydatid cysts, 683, 684
Hydralazine-induced lupus syndrome, 537
Hydroxychloroquine
for pemphigus vulgaris and pemphigus foliaceous, 506
for rheumatoid arthritis, 408
for systemic lupus erythematosus, 405
Hymenolepsis nana, 683
Hymenoptera insect stings
anaphylactic reaction to, 372, 373, 373t, 376
desensitization for, 714
Hypereosinophilic syndrome, 540
Hypergammaglobulinemia, *225*
benign hypergammaglobulinemic purpura, 597
in juvenile arthritis, 409
in scleroderma, 414
in Sjögren's syndrome, 411, 412
in visceral leishmaniasis, 679
Hyper-IgG syndrome, 337, *337*
Hyper-IgM syndrome, 119, 240, 295, 307
Hypersensitivity angiitis, 458
Hypersensitivity pneumonitis, 389–393, 390t
allergens associated with, 389–390, 390t
clinical diagnosis of, 392

Hypersensitivity pneumonitis, *(continued)*
complications of, 393
definition of, 389
differential diagnosis of, 393
epidemiology of, 389
immunologic diagnosis of, 392–393
immunologic features of, 389
laboratory findings in, 392
pathogenesis of, 391
pathology of, 390–391
prevention of, 393
prognosis for, 393
symptoms and signs of, 391–392
treatment of, 393
Hypersensitivity reactions, 189. *See also* Allergy
anaphylaxis, 189, 202, 370–376
basophils and, 193
contact, 243
cutaneous basophil (Jones-Mote), 198t, 202
cytotoxic (type II), 395–396, 395t
definition of, 349
to drugs, 394–400
after drug treatment for nematodes, 684
Gell and Coombs classification of, 394–396, 395t, 535 (*See also* specific types of reactions)
type II cytotoxic reactions, 395
type III immune complex-mediated reactions, 380–385, 396
type I immediate reactions, 201–202, *202,* 394–395
type IV delayed type reactions, 37, 197–199, 242–243, 242t, 386, 396
respiratory, 535
Hypertension
portal, 726
preeclampsia, 563–565
scleroderma and, 414, 415
systemic lupus erythematosus and, 402
Hyperthyroidism, Graves' disease, 94t, 426–428
Hypervariable regions of immunoglobulins, 103, *103*
Hyperviscosity syndrome, 227–228
Hypnozoites, 674
Hypocalcemia, DiGeorge anomaly and, 314–315
Hypogammaglobulinemia, *225,* 299
arthritis and, 420
immune globulin for, 705t
transient, of infancy, 305
Hypoparathyroidism
chronic mucocutaneous candidiasis and, 317, 431
idiopathic, 423t, 431
Hypothyroidism
chronic mucocutaneous candidiasis and, 317
in Hashimoto's thyroiditis, 424
primary, 428

IBDs. *See* **Inflammatory bowel diseases**
Ibuprofen, 7553
ICAM-1 (intercellular adhesion molecule 1), 27, 27t, 45t, 118
ICE (interleukin-1β-converting enzyme), 150
Idiopathic anaphylactoid reactions, 374–375
Idiopathic CD4 lymphocytopenia, 318
Idiopathic pulmonary fibrosis, 542–544, *543*
causes of, 542
clinical features of, 542–543
diagnosis of, 543
differential diagnosis of, 543, 544t
immunologic features of, 542
immunologic pathogenesis of, 542
treatment and prognosis for, 543–544, 758

Idiopathic thrombocytopenic purpura (ITP), 443–445
in children vs. adults, 443, 443t
clinical features of, 444
differential diagnosis of, 444–445, 444t
epidemiology of, 443
immunologic diagnosis of, 444, 444t
immunologic features of, 443
pathogenesis of, 443
platelet kinetics in, 444
treatment of, 445
Idiotype, 103
IELs (intraepithelial lymphocytes), 206, *206*
IFA (immunoflourescence assays), 228–230, *229, 230,* 495
IFN. *See* Interferon
Ig. *See* Immunoglobulin
I-κB family, 13
IL. *See* Interleukin
IMIG (intramuscular immunoglobulin), 704–705
Immediate hemolytic transfusion reactions, 254, 254t
Immediate (type I) hypersensitivity reactions, 201–202, *202,* 394–395
drugs for suppression of, 755–757
antihistamines, 756, 756t
anti-IgE monoclonal antibodies, 756
cromolyn sodium, 755–756
methylxanthines, 757
sympathomimetic drugs, 756, 757t
Immune competence evaluation, 294–297
cell-mediated immunity, 296
complement deficiencies, 296–297
humoral immunity, 295–296
indications for, 294, 294t
initial evaluation, 295
phagocyte function, 296, 301t, 333t
subsequent testing, 297
variations and limitations of, 294–295
Immune complexes, 199–200
allergies mediated by, 380–385, 396
allergic bronchopulmonary aspergillosis, 365, 382–385
Arthus reaction, 199, 242, 380, 381t
drug allergy, 396
serum sickness, 199, 201, 381–382, 381t, *382,* 396
deposition of, 199–200
formation of, 199, *200,* 215–216
in Hashimoto's thyroiditis, 424
in Henoch-Schönlein purpura, 458
inflammation mediated by, 198t, 199–201, *200*
clinical manifestations of, 201
complement activation and cellular infiltration, 200–201
laboratory tests based on antigen or antibody fixation to solid surface, 219–227
agglutination assays, 219–221, *221*
electrophoresis methods, 224–227, *224–227*
enzyme-linked immunosorbent assays, 221–224, *222, 223*
immunoprecipitation, 215, *216, 217*
laboratory tests based on formation of, 215–227
complement fixation, 217, 219t, *220*
cryoglobulins, 218–219
immunodiffusion, 216, *217, 218,* 218t
nephelometry, 216–217, *219,* 219t
prozone phenomenon, 216
in relapsing polychondritis, 419
in renal disease, 481–482
IgA nephropathy, 488
lupus nephritis, 490–491
membranoproliferative glomerulonephritis, 489
postinfectious glomerulonephritis, 488
in rheumatoid arthritis, 406

solubilization of, 346
  complement deficiencies and, 346
in systemic lupus erythematosus, 404
in vasculitides, 451
  polyarteritis nodosa, 452
Immune exclusion, 209
Immune hemolytic anemias, 436–441, 437t
  antiphospholipid syndrome and, 449
  classification of, 437t
  cold agglutinin syndromes, 439
  drug-induced, 439–440, 440t
  hemolytic disease of newborn, 251, 252, 257
  paroxysmal cold hemoglobinuria, 440–441
  serologic tests for, 436–437, 438t
  warm autoimmune hemolytic anemia, 437–439
Immune privilege, 70, 510
Immune response, 61–70, 93
  activation of B cells and cytotoxic T cells, 66–67, *67*
  activation of helper T cells, 65–66, *66*
  antigen processing and presentation, 63–65, *65*
  apoptosis, 5, 14–17, *16*
  atopy, 189, 202, 349–369
  clonal organization and dynamics of lymphocyte
        populations, 61–63, *62*
  immunogens and antigens, 63–65, 72–79
  inflammation, 24–27, 68, 189–202
  localization of, 68–69
  mechanisms of antigen elimination, 67–68
    antibody-dependent cell-mediated cytotoxicity, 68
    complement activation, 68
    opsonization and phagocyte activation, 68
    toxic neutralization, 67–68
    virus neutralization, 68
  in pregnancy, 552–555
  primary, *69,* 69–70
  programmed cell death in immune system, 70
  quantitative and kinetic aspects of, *69,* 69–70
  secondary (anamnestic), *69,* 70
  sequence of events during, 63, *64*
  specificity of, 61–63, 115
  T-cell-mediated, 63–66, *64, 65,* 139–143
  triggering of, 63
  tumor immunology, 568–576
Immunity
  acquired, 19, 61, 82
  cell-mediated, 19, 43, 197–199, *198,* 234
    laboratory methods for detection of, 234–248
  herd, 706–707
  humoral, 19, 43, 118–128, 234
  innate, 19–38, 61, 82
Immunization, 699–712. *See also* Vaccines
  active, 699–703
    adverse reactions and risk-benefit ratio for, 702
    allergic reactions to, 703
    hazards of live vaccines, 702–703
    legal liability and reporting adverse reactions to, 703, 704t
    mechanism of action of, 699–700
    previous infection and, 700
    primary and booster immunization, 700
    route of, 700
    simultaneous immunization with multiple antigens,
        700–702, 709
    splenectomy and, 702
    technique of, 702
    timing of, 700–702
    types of vaccines for, 79–80, 700, 701t
  age at, 708–709
    adults and elderly persons, 709, 711t
    children, 709, 710t

antigenic shift and antigenic variation and, 707
clinical indications for, 706
combined passive-active, 706
for foreign travel, 709–711
herd immunity and, 706–707
history of, 699, 700t
of HIV-infected persons, 644
passive, 699, 703–706
  animal sera and antitoxins for, 705
  hazards of, 706
  human immune globulin for, 703–705, 705t
  for Kawasaki syndrome, 706
  for poisonous bites, 706
  to prevent Rh isoimmunization, 705–706
postimmunization encephalomyelitis, 517
for special populations, 711
against specific diseases, 707–708
types of, 699
vaccines currently in development, 712
Immunocytoma, 592
Immunodeficiency disorders
  B-cell, 240, 302–312
  causes of, 299t
  classification of, 300t
  clinical clues to, 294
  clinical features of, 299, 300t
  combined B-cell and T-cell, 320–331
  complement deficiencies, 341–347
  fungal diseases and, 655, 661t
  hemophagocytic syndromes and, 602
  HIV infection, 636–648
  immunologic testing for, 294–297, 299, 301t
  mechanisms of, 299–300
  phagocytic dysfunction disorders, 333–339
  pulmonary manifestations of, 546
  severe combined immunodeficiency, 239, 320–321, 737
  T-cell, 239, 313–318
  treatment of, 300, 301t
Immunodiffusion, 216, *217, 218,* 218t
Immunodominance, 79, 93
Immunoelectrophoresis, 226–227, *227*
Immunoflourescence assays (IFA), 228–230, *229, 230,* 495
Immunogenicity, 72–73
Immunogens, 63–65, *64, 72,* 72–73. *See also* Antigens
  definition of, 72
  effect of adjuvants and immunomodulators on response to,
        73, 80
  genetic constitution of host animal and response to, 73
  mode of contact and response to, 73
  properties of, 72–73
  tolerance to, 73
    high-zone, 73
Immunoglobulin A (IgA), 98, 100t, 204, 207–209
  antiinflammatory properties of, 208
  biologic activities of, 102
  class switching, 209
  genes for, 207
  IgA nephropathy, 488
  linear IgA bullous dermatosis, 503–504
  in mucosal immune system, 207–209
  polymerization and interaction with secretory component, 208
  proinflammatory properties of, 208
  receptors for, on inflammatory cells, 190t
  regulation of synthesis at mucosal sites, 209–210, *210*
  resistance to proteolysis, 208
  secretory vs. circulating, 209
  selective IgA deficiency, 295, 307–310
  structure and function of, 207–208
  transport of, *208,* 208–209

Immunoglobulin barrel, 96
Immunoglobulin D (IgD), 98, 100t
  biologic activities of, 102
  receptors for, on inflammatory cells, 190t
  surface, *116*, 117
Immunoglobulin E (IgE), 98, 100t
  allergen desensitization and, 715–716
  allergy, atopy and, 102, 108, 242, 349–351, *350*
  anaphylaxis and, 349, 370–372
  biologic activities of, 102
  diseases associated with elevation of, 349, 350t
  inflammatory response mediated by, 198t, 201–202, *202*
    drugs for suppression of, 755–757
  in mucosal immune system, 209
  receptors for, 108t
    on inflammatory cells, 190t, 191, 349
  wheal-and-flare reactions, 195, 242, 354, 355t
Immunoglobulin G (IgG), 98, 100t
  allergen desensitization and, 716
  biologic activities of, 101–102
  hyper-IgG (Job's) syndrome, 337, *337*
  in mucosal immune system, 209
  receptors for, 108t
    on inflammatory cells, 190t
  subclasses of, 101, 101t, 310
    specific deficiencies of, 310–311
    specific testing for, 295
Immunoglobulin M (IgM), 98, *99*, 100t
  biologic activities of, 102
  hyper-IgM syndrome, 119, 240, 295, 307
  in mucosal immune system, 209
  selective IgM deficiency, 310
  surface, *116*, 117
Immunoglobulins, 42, 61, 95–114
  antigen-binding sites of, 97
  autoreactive, 118, 128–129
  biologic activities of, 95, 101–102
  capping of, 48
  classification of, 97–101, 98t
    allotypic forms of heavy and light chains, 100
    composition of classes and subclasses, 98–99, 100t
    heavy-chain types and subtypes, 98
    J chain and secretory component, *99*, 100–101
    light-chain types and subtypes, 97–98
  cross-linking of, 48
  enzymatic digestion products of, 97
  Fc receptors for, 108, 108t
  genes for, 108–114
    B-cell malignancy and rearrangements of, *113*, 113–114
    formation through DNA rearrangement in B cells, 108–112
    heavy-chain genes, 111–112, *112*
    light-chain genes, 109–111, *109–111*
    molecular basis of V/(D)/J rearrangement, 112–113
    natural antibiotics, 113
    supergene family, 105–106, 105t, 163, 164t
  heavy-chain class switching, *125*, 125–126
  membrane, *42*, 42–43, 99–100
  in mucosal immune system, 207–209
  normal distribution of, *310*
  opsonizing effect of, 31
  organization and diversity of, 42, 95–97, *96*
  secreted, *42*, 43, 100, 124
  three-dimensional structure of, 103–105, *104, 105*
  variable regions of, 102–103
    framework and hypervariable regions, 103, *103*
    idiotypes of, 103
    subgroups of, 103

Immunohematology, 250–259
  blood component therapy, 258–259, 258t
  blood groups, 250
  erythrocyte antigens, 250–252, *251*, 251t, 252t
  Rh isoimmunization, 257
  transfusion reactions, 254–257, 254t
Immunohistochemical assays, 230–231
Immunologic synapse, 77, *78*
Immunology, defined, 1
Immunomodulators, 73, 757–759
  cytokine inhibitors, 757–758
  inclusion in vaccines, 80
  T-cell-directed therapies, 758–759
Immunophenotypic analysis of immune system neoplasms, 580–581, 581t–583t, *584, 585,* 589t
Immunophenotypic stages of early lymphocyte differentiation, 579t
Immunophilins, 747
Immunoprecipitation, 215, *216, 217*
Immunoproliferative small-intestinal disease (IPSID), 464
Immunoreceptor tyrosine-based activation motif (ITAM), 118–119, *120*
Immunosuppressive therapy, 744–750
  for autoimmune chronic active hepatitis, 471
  for bullous pemphigoid, 498
  drugs used for, 744–750
    cyclosporine, 747–748, *748*
    cytotoxic agents, 744–746
    leflunomide, 747
    mycophenolate mofetil, 746–747
    sirolimus, 749–750
    tacrolimus, 748–749
  for Guillain-Barré syndrome, 518
  hematologic proliferations in patients receiving, 602–603
  for microscopic polyangiitis, 454
  for paraneoplastic pemphigus, 507
  for pemphigus vulgaris and pemphigus foliaceous, 506
  for polyarteritis nodosa, 453
  for polymyositis-dermatomyositis, 417
  for primary biliary cirrhosis, 472
  for psoriatic arthritis, 419
  for pure erythrocyte aplasia, 441
  for Reiter's syndrome, 418
  for rheumatoid arthritis, 408
  for scleroderma, 415
  for Sjögren's syndrome, 412
  for systemic lupus erythematosus, 405
  for transplant recipients, 719
    bone, 741
    bone marrow, 739
    heart, 733
    heart-lung and lung, 735–736
    kidney, 721, 724–725
    liver, 730
    pancreas, 732
  for Type I diabetes mellitus, 430
  for warm autoimmune hemolytic anemia, 439
  for Wegener's granulomatosis, 455
Immunotherapy
  allergen, 174, 714–717
  immunization, 699–712
  for infertility, 557–558
  peptide, 717
  for recurrent spontaneous abortion, 559
  for tumors, 574–576
Immunotoxins, 106
Implantation, 551
Inactivated vaccine, 700
Indinavir, 645, 647t

Indirect antiglobulin test, 252–254, *253*
Induration, 198
Infections
  bacterial, 607–615
  in bone marrow transplant recipients, 740, 740t
  catheter-associated, 610
  complement deficiencies and, 341, 347
  fungal, 655–671
  immunization against, 699–712
  immunodeficiency disorders and, 299
  leukocyte production during, 2
  after liver transplantation, 728
  mucosal, 204
  opportunistic
    cancer and, 574
    fungal, 655, 657t–658t
    HIV infection and, 641, 641t
  parasitic, 673–686
  polymorphonuclear neutrophil deficiency and, 245
  spirochetal, 688–696
  transfusion-transmitted, 255–256, 255t
  type II cryoglobulins and, 218
  viral, 617–634
Infectious mononucleosis, 650–651
  heterophile antibody test for, 220–221
Infertility, 555–558
  immune causes for, 557
    antisperm antibodies, 557
    autoimmune diseases of testis and ovary, 557
  immune therapies for, 557–558
    condom therapy, 558
    reproductive technologies, 558
    sperm washing, 558
Inflammation, 24–27, 68, 189–202
  acute, 33
  antiinflammatory drugs, 750–757
    colchicine, 755
    corticosteroids, 750–752
    drugs that suppression immediate hypersensitivity
        reactions, 755–757
    leukotriene antagonists, 755
    nonsteroidal antiinflammatory drugs, 753–755
  chronic, 37
  complement and, 183–184
  cytokines and, 189, 194, 202
    chemokines, 168t, 169–171, 195
    colony-stimulating factors, 163
    IL-1 and TNFα, 152
    TGFβ, 162
  dilation and increased permeability of microscopic blood
      vessels, *25,* 25–26, 26t
  granulomatous, 199
  harmful effects of, 189
  immunologically mediated, 197–202, 198t
    cell-mediated immunity, 197–199, *198*
    cutaneous basophil hypersensitivity, 202
    IgE-mediated inflammation, 201–202, *202*
    immune complex-mediated inflammation, 199–201, *200,*
        380, 381t
  mediators of, 24–25, 25t, 189, 193–196, 194t
    adenosine, 195, *197*
    arachidonic acid metabolites, 194–195, *195, 196*
    chemotactic, 195, 245–246
    definition of, 193–194
    enzymatic, 195, 197t
    histamine, 194, *194,* 194t
    platelet-activating factor, 195, *197*
    proteoglycans, 196
  signs of, 24, 68, 189

Inflammatory bowel diseases (IBDs), 465–469
  Crohn's disease, 466–468, *467*
  genetics of, 466
  immunologic mechanisms in, 466
  mouse models of, 466
  ulcerative colitis, *468,* 468–469
Inflammatory cells, 189–193, 189t
  basophils, 192–193, *193*
  endothelial cells, 26–27, 27t, 193
  eosinophils, *190,* 190–191
  Fc receptors on, 189–190, 190t
  mast cells, 191–192, 191t, *192*
  platelets, 193
Inflammatory neuropathies, 518–519
  acute inflammatory demyelinating polyneuropathy,
      518–519
  chronic, 519
Infliximab, 757–758
Influenza virus infection, 617–623
  clinical features of, 621–622
  immunologic features of, 617
  immunologic pathogenesis of, 622
  postinfectious disorders associated with, 622
  prevention of, 622–623
    vaccines, 623, 701t, 707–708
  target cells for, 621
  treatment of, 622
  virology of, 617, 621, *621*
    antigenic variation, 621
    influenza A, B, and C viruses, 621
    structural proteins, 617, 621t
Innate immunity, 19–38, 61, 82
  definition of, 19
  humoral proteins of, 19–24
    acute-phase response, 23–24, 24t
    antimicrobial enzymes and binding proteins, 20–21, 20t
    complement cascade, 21–23, *23*
    factors that recognize bacterial lipopolysaccharide, 21,
        22
    pathogen-specific macromolecules, 20, 20t
    peptide antibiotics, 21
  inflammation, 24–27
  phagocytes, 27–38
    monocyte-macrophage system, 27t, 34–38
    neutrophils, 27–34, 27t
Innocent-bystander phenomenon in drug-induced immune
      disorders
  hemolytic anemia, 439
  neutropenia, 435
  thrombocytopenia, 442
Inosine pranobex, 647
Inositol 4,5-trisphosphate (IP^3), 47
Insect allergens, 352–354
  desensitization to, 714
  Hymenoptera insects, 372, 373, 373t
In situ hybridization, 265, *266*
Insulin therapy, 430
Integrins, 6, 8t, 27, 29
  in neutrophil adhesion, 245
  in neutrophil margination, 29, *30*
Intercellular adhesion molecule 1 (ICAM-1), 27, 27t, 45t, 118
Interdigitating dendritic cells, 51, 91
Interferon-α (IFNα), 150t, 155t, 160, 758
  therapeutic uses of, 758
    malignancies, 758
    viral hepatitis, 629, 632, 758
Interferon-β (IFNβ), 150t, 155t, 160
  therapeutic uses of, 758
    multiple sclerosis, 515–516, 758

Interferon-γ (IFNγ), 36, 68, 90, 92, 150t, 155t, 161
  immunoregulatory effects of, 161
  inhibitors of, 161
  in renal allograft rejection, 723
  sources of, 145–146, 161
  therapeutic uses of, 758
    chronic granulomatous disease, 161, 335
    HIV infection, 647
    hyper-IgG syndrome, 337
Interferons (IFNs), 148, 159–161
  antiviral (type I), *160,* 160–161
  immune (type II), 161
  phenotypes of knockout mice, 155t
  receptors for, 164t
  viral effects on, 618t
Interferon-γ (IFNγ), 160
Interleukin-1β-converting enzyme (ICE), 150
Interleukin-1 (IL-1), 8t, 148–154, 149t
  actions on helper T cells, 148–149
  IL-1α and IL-1β, 150
  nonimmunologic inflammatory effects of, 152
  phenotypes of knockout mice, 153t
  production of, 150
  receptors for (IL-1RI and IL1RII), 45t, 150–151
  target cells and actions of, 151t, 153
  as therapeutic agent, 154
Interleukin-2 (IL-2), 8t, 9, *12,* 149t, 154–156
  autocrine and paracrine effects of, 66, 154
  in cytotoxic T-cell activation, 49, 67, *67*
  effects on non-T cells, 156
  functions of, 154
  helper T-cell secretion of, 66
  phenotypes of knockout mice, 155t
  receptors for, 9, 10, *10,* 45t, 66, *66,* 155, *156*
    signal transduction and, 155–156
  in renal allograft rejection, 723, *723*
  side effects of, 156
  sources of, 155
  stimulation of natural killer cells by, 144
  structure of, 154
  as therapeutic agent, 156, 436t
    HIV infection, 156, 647
    malignancies, 758
Interleukin-3 (IL-3), 8, 8t, 9, 149t, 162
  receptors for, *10,* 164t
  therapeutic use of, 436t
Interleukin-4 (IL-4), 119, 149t, 156–157
  in allergic diseases, 156
  atopy and, 350
  functions of, 157
  phenotypes of knockout mice, 155t
  receptors for, 157
  secretion by NKT cells, 145–146
Interleukin-5 (IL-5), 5, 8t, 119, 149t, 157
  atopy and, 350
  as eosinophil growth factor, 157, 190–191
  receptor for, *10*
Interleukin-6 (IL-6), 5, 8t, 23, 149t, 157, 158t
  in acute-phase response, 23, 157
  functions of, 157, 158t
  phenotypes of knockout mice, 153t
  receptors for, 45t, 157, 164t
  therapeutic use of, 436t
Interleukin-7 (IL-7), 41, 117, 149t, 157–158
  phenotypes of knockout mice, 155t
  receptor for, 157
  as therapeutic agent, 158
Interleukin-8 (IL-8), 149t, 167, 168t
  receptors for, 164t

Interleukin-9 (IL-9), 149t, 158
  receptor for, 158
Interleukin-10 (IL-10), 149t, 158–159
  immunosuppressive action of, 158
  phenotypes of knockout mice, 155t
Interleukin-11 (IL-11), 5, 149t, 157, 158t
Interleukin-12 (IL-12), 149t, 159
  for HIV infection, 647
  receptor for, 159
  use with vaccines, 80, 141
Interleukin-13 (IL-13), 149t, 156–157
  atopy and, 350
  functions of, 157
  phenotypes of knockout mice, 155t
  receptors for, 157
Interleukin-15 (IL-15), 149t, 159
Interleukin-16 (IL-16), 149t, 159
Interleukin-17 (IL-17), 149t, 159
Interleukin-18 (IL-18), 149t, 159
Interleukin-1 receptor antagonist (IL-1RA), 150
Interleukins (ILs), 36t, 148
  in hematopoiesis, *4,* 5, 9
  phenotypes of knockout mice, 153t, 155t
  properties of, 149t
  viral effects on, 619t
Interstitial fluid, 49–50
Intestinal lymphangiectasia, 463
Intestinal T-cell lymphoma, 600
Intracellular bacteria, 607, 614–615
  antigens from, 83
  Brucella species, 615
  immunity to, 614, *614*
  Legionella pneumophila, 614–615
  Listeria monocytogenes, 615
  Salmonella species, 614
Intraepithelial lymphocytes (IELs), 206, *206*
Intramuscular immunoglobulin (IMIG), 704–705
Intravenous immunoglobulin (IVIG)
  adverse reactions to, 304–305
  for common variable immunodeficiency, 307
    "aggregate anaphylaxis" due to, 374
  half-life of, 304
  human immune globulin, 703–705, 705t
  for hyper-IgG syndrome, 337
  for hyper-IgM syndrome, 307
  for idiopathic thrombocytopenic purpura, 445
  for Kawasaki's disease, 458, 706
  for neonatal alloimmune thrombocytopenia, 446
  for paraneoplastic pemphigus, 507
  passive immunization with, 703–706
  for polymyositis-dermatomyositis, 417
  preparation of, 305
  for pure erythrocyte aplasia, 441
  for severe combined immunodeficiency, 321
  for short-limbed dwarfism with immunodeficiency, 328
  for thrombocytopenic purpura, 706
  for transient hypogammaglobulinemia of infancy, 305
  for Wiskott–Aldrich syndrome, 324
  for X-linked agammaglobulinemia, 304–305
  for X-linked lymphoproliferative syndrome, 330
Introns, 109
Invariant chain, 89
In vitro fertilization, 558
IP^3 (inositol 4,5-trisphosphate), 47
IPSID (immunoproliferative small-intestinal disease), 464
Islet cell transplantation, 732
Isoetharine, 363–364, 756
Isoniazid-induced lupus syndrome, 537
Isoprinosine. *See* Inosine pranobex

Isotype switching, heavy-chain, *125,* 125–126
ITAM (immunoreceptor tyrosine-based activation motif), 118–119, *120*
Ito cells, 682
ITP. *See* Idiopathic thrombocytopenic purpura
Itraconazole
    for blastomycosis, 660
    for coccidioidomycosis, 664
    for histoplasmosis, 665
    for paracoccidioidomycosis, 666
IVIG. *See* Intravenous immunoglobulin

JAK-3 **gene, 297**
Jak/Stat signaling pathway, 11–13, *12*
Janus kinase (Jak) family, 11, *12*
Japanese encephalitis vaccine, 701t
Jarisch–Herxheimer reaction, 375, 691
J chain, *99,* 100
Job's syndrome, 337, *337*
Jones-Mote hypersensitivity, 202
Jun, 14
Juvenile arthritis, 94t, 408–411
    complications and prognosis for, 411
    differential diagnosis of, 410
    epidemiology of, 409
    growth disorders and, 410
    immunologic diagnosis of, 410
    immunologic features of, 408
    immunologic pathogenesis of, 409
    laboratory findings in, 410
    radiographic findings in, 410
    symptoms and signs of, 409–410
        ocular, 409, 528
    treatment of, 410–411

Kala-azar, 679
Kallikrein, 181
K antigens, 611
Kaposi's sarcoma, 173, 294, 478, 641
    human herpesvirus 8 and, 626–627
    ocular, 532
Kaposi's sarcoma herpesvirus. *See* Human herpesvirus 8 infection
κ-deleting element, 128
Katayama fever, 683
Kawasaki disease, 458, 706
Kell antigens, 252
Keratoconjunctivitis
    atopic, 527
    phlyctenular, 532, *532*
    sicca, 411, 412, 529
    vernal, 357, 527, *528*
Ketoconazole
    for candidiasis, 667
    for coccidioidomycosis, 664
    for paracoccidioidomycosis, 666
Keyhole limpet hemocyanin (KLH), 295
Kidd antigens, 252
Kidney disease. *See* Renal disease
Kidney transplantation, 193, 291, 291t, 719–726
    ABO testing for, 719
    blood transfusion for, 721
    cadaveric, 720
    contraindications to, 719
    crossmatching for, 720
    donor evaluation and procedures for, 720–721
    graft rejection after, 722–726
        acute, 722–725, *722–725*

        chronic, *722,* 726
    diagnosis of, 722
        hyperacute, 725–726
        pathology of, 722–726
        signs and symptoms of, 722
    HLA matching for, 291, 291t, 719–720
    immunosuppression after, 721
        corticosteroids, 721, 724
        monoclonal antibodies, 724–725
    living related and unrelated donor, 719–720
    operative procedure for, 721, *721*
    outcome of, 726
    pancreas transplantation simultaneous with, 730
    presensitization and, 720
Killed vaccine, 80, 700
Killer inhibitory receptors (KIRs), 144–145
Kinetic and quantitative aspects of immune response, *69,* 69–70
Kininogen
    high-molecular-weight, *186,* 186–187
    low-molecular-weight, 187
Kinin system, 186–187
    activation of, 187
    amplification and regulation of, 187
    functions in disease, 187
    plasma inhibitors of, 187
    proteins of, 186, *186*
KIRs (killer inhibitory receptors), 144–145
Klebsiella pneumoniae, 611, 613
KLH (keyhole limpet hemocyanin), 295
Kostmann's syndrome, 296, 333
Kupffer cells, 34

Labor and delivery, preterm, 562–563, *564*
Laboratory tests, immunologic
    to detect antigen and antibodies to erythrocytes, 252–254, 436–437
        antiglobulin tests, 252–253, *253*
        pretransfusion testing, 253
        type and screen, 253–254
    to detect antigens and antibodies, 215–232
        antigen-antibody binding, 215–227
            agglutination assays, 219–221, *221*
            complement fixation, 217, 219t, *220*
            cryoglobulins, 218–219
            electrophoresis methods, 224–227, *224–227*
            enzyme-linked immunosorbent assays, 221–224, *222, 223,* 224t
            immunodiffusion, 216, *217, 218,* 218t
            nephelometry, 218–219, *219,* 219t
            tests based on antigen or antibody fixation to solid surface, 215, 219–227
            tests based on immune complex formation, 215–227
        complement assays, 231
        hemolytic assays, 231–232
        immunohistochemical methods, 228–231
        serum viscosity, 227–228
    to detect cellular immunity, 234–248
        delayed-type hypersensitivity skin testing, 242–243
        leukocyte phenotyping (flow cytometry), 234–242
        lymphocyte activation assays, 243–245
        monocyte-macrophage assays, 245
        neutrophil function assays, 245–248
    to evaluate immune competence, 294–297
        cell-mediated immunity, 296
        complement deficiencies, 296–297
        humoral immunity, 295–296
        indications for, 294, 294t

Laboratory tests, immunologic *(continued)*
  to evaluate immune competence, *(continued)*
    initial evaluation, 295
    phagocyte function, 296
    subsequent testing, 297
    variations and limitations of, 294–295
  histocompatibility testing, 270–292, 271t
    antibody screening, 279–280
    cellular assays, 289–292, 290t, 291t
    crossmatching, 280–282, *281, 282*
    HLA polymorphism and typing, *272,* 272–275, 273t, *274*
    molecular-biologic methods, 282–289, 283t, 284t, *285, 286, 288*
    serologic methods, 275–276, *276*
    tissue typing by lymphocytotoxicity test, 276–279, 277t–279t
    for transplantation, 270–272
  for immune system neoplasms, 580–586
    cytogenetic analysis, 113–114, 581–584, 586t
    immunophenotypic analysis, 580–581, 581t–583t, *584, 585*
    molecular genetic analysis, 586
  molecular genetic techniques, 260–269
    gene rearrangement assay for lymphocyte clonality, 263–265
    genomic arrays, 268
    hybridization assays, 261–262, *263, 264*
    in situ hybridization, 265, *266*
    methods of analyzing RNA, 268
    nucleic acid probes, 260–261, *262*
    overview and prospects for, 268–269
    polymerase chain reaction, *266,* 266–267, *267*
    Southern blot, 262–263, *265*
Lacrimal gland, 529
LAD (leukocyte adhesion deficiency), 245, 295, 296, 337–338, *338*
LAK (lymphokine-activated killer) cells, 144
Lambert-Eaton myasthenic syndrome (LEMS), 521, 522t
Lamina propria cells, 204, *205,* 206–207
Lamivudine (3TC), 629, 645, 647t
Landsteiner, Karl, 250
Langerhans' cell histiocytosis (LCH), 602
Langerhans' cells, 54, 91
  HIV-infected, 639
LARC (liver and activation-regulated cytokine), 172t, 173
Large granular lymphocyte leukemia (LGLL), 597–598
Larva migrans, visceral, 540
Laryngeal edema, 375
Latent viral infections, 617
Latex agglutination assays, 221
Latex allergy, 373–374, 535
LBL. *See* Lymphoblastic lymphoma
LBP (lipopolysaccharide-binding protein), 20t, 21
LCH (Langerhans' cell histiocytosis), 602
Lectin-like receptors, 145
Lectins, 6, 48, 244, 296
Leflunomide, 408, 747
Legionella pneumophila, 614–615
Leishmania major, 141
Leishmaniasis, 673, 677–679
  cutaneous, 677–679, *678*
  transfusion-transmitted, 256
  visceral (kala-azar), 679
Leishmanin test, 678
LEMS (Lambert-Eaton myasthenic syndrome), 521, 522t
Lens-induced uveitis, 530
Lentiviruses, 636–637, 637t
Leprosy, 615
Leptospira, 688

Letterer-Siwe syndrome, 602
Leukemia, 5, 8. *See also* Neoplasms of immune system
  acute lymphoblastic, 588–591, 738
  acute myelogenous, 737–738
  adult T-cell leukemia-lymphoma, 156, 569, *590,* 598–599
  ataxia-telangiectasia and, 326, *326*
  B-cell chronic lymphocytic, 591
  bone marrow transplantation for, 737–738
  chronic lymphocytic, 118
  chronic myelogenous, 738
  hairy cell, 594
  large granular lymphocyte, *590,* 597–598
  vs. lymphoma, 580
  prolymphocytic, 591–592
  T-cell prolymphocytic, 598
  T-lymphoblastic, *590*
  T-prolymphocytic, *590*
Leukemia inhibitory factor (LIF), 153t, 157, 158t, 551
Leukocyte adhesion deficiency (LAD), 245, 295, 296, 337–338, *338*
Leukocyte chemotactic factors, 29, *30,* 36t
Leukocyte disorders, 434–436
  agranulocytosis, 435
  autoimmune neutropenia, 434
  causes of leukopenia, 434, 435t
  cyclic neutropenia, 434
  drug-induced immune neutropenia, 434–435
  management of neutropenia, 435–436, 436t
Leukocyte functional assays, 241
Leukocyte function-associated antigen 1 (LFA-1), *30,* 45t, 59, 118
Leukocytes
  chemotaxis of, 25t
  flow cytometric analysis of antigens on, 235–242
  interferons expressed by, 160
  phenotyping of, 234–242 (*See also* Flow cytometry)
  production of, 1, 2
Leukopenia, 434, 435t
  in HIV infection, 645
Leukotriene antagonists, *754,* 755
  for asthma, 194, 364, 755
Leukotrienes, 25t, 26, 194–195, *195*
  as inflammatory mediators, 195
  structures of, *196*
Lewis antigens, 251
LFA-1 (leukocyte function-associated antigen 1), *30,* 45t, 59, 118
LGLL (large granular lymphocyte leukemia), 597–598
LIF (leukemia inhibitory factor), 153t, 157, 158t, 551
Ligand(s)
  bound by surface receptors on macrophages, 35, 36t
  CD27, 152t, 154
  CD40, 45t, 46, 49, 66, *67,* 119, 127, 139–140, 152t, 153t
    anti-CD40L therapy, 759
    congenital deficiency of (*See* Hyper-IgM syndrome)
  defensins as, 173
  Epstein–Barr virus-induced molecule 1 ligand chemokine (ELC), 59, 172–173, 172t
  Fas, 15, *16,* 70, 151, 152t, 154
    phenotypes of knockout mice, 153t
  Flt-3, 5, 8t
  OX40, 152t, 209
Light chains, immunoglobulin, 42, *96,* 96–97
  genes for, 109–111, *109–111*
  surrogate, 115–117
Limbic encephalitis, 522t, 523
Lineage association of malignant lymphoid cells, 578–580, *579,* 579t
Lineage-committed progenitors, 2, *3,* 5

Linear IgA bullous dermatosis, 503–504
Lipids, 77, 93
Lipopolysaccharide-binding protein (LBP), 20t, 21
Lipopolysaccharide (LPS), 607
    disseminated intravascular coagulation and, 152
    Enterobacteriaceae and, 611
    hemorrhagic Shwartzman reaction and, 152
    IL-1 secretion in response to, 150
    in lymphocyte activation assays, 244
    recognition by humoral proteins, 21, 119
    structure of, 21, *22*
    Toll-like receptors and cellular signaling by, 36, *37*, 119
Lipoxins, 194
Lipoxygenase metabolites, 195, *195, 196*
Listeria, 83
Listeria monocytogenes, 615
Liver and activation-regulated cytokine (LARC), 172t, 173
Liver disease. *See* Hepatobiliary disorders
Liver transplantation, 726–730
    contraindications to, 727
    crossmatching for, 291–292, 729
    host tolerance to, 726
    immunosuppression after, 730
    indications for, 726–727
        autoimmune chronic active hepatitis, 471
        extrahepatic biliary atresia, 727
        hepatitis B, 630, 727
        hepatitis C, 727
        primary biliary cirrhosis, 472
        primary sclerosing cholangitis, 473
    living donor, 727
    operative procedure for, 727–728, *729*
    outcome of, 728–729
        infectious complications, 728
        primary graft nonfunction, 728
        rejection, 728–730
    support of patient waiting for, 726–727
Live vaccine, 79, 700
    hazards of, 702–703
Loa loa, 256, 684
Loboa loboi, 655
Local anesthetics, hypersensitivity to, 399–400
Löffler's syndrome, 538–539, 538t
Long-term bone marrow cultures (LTBMCs), 6–8
Lou Gehrig's disease, 523
Low-molecular-weight kininogen, 187
LPS. *See* Lipopolysaccharide
L-selectin, 8t, 29, *30,* 58, *116,* 118, 245
LTBMCs (long-term bone marrow cultures), 6–8
Lung flukes, 681
Lungs. *See also* Respiratory disease
    acute transfusion-related injury of, 255
    in adult respiratory distress syndrome, 546
    asthma, 349, 359–365
    in Churg-Strauss syndrome, 455
    drug-induced diseases of, 535–537, 536t, *537*
    hypersensitivity pneumonitis, 389–393
    idiopathic pulmonary fibrosis, 542–544, *543*
    in microscopic polyangiitis, 453
    in polyarteritis nodosa, 452
    in rheumatoid arthritis, 407
    in sarcoidosis, *541,* 541–542
    in scleroderma, 414
    in systemic lupus erythematosus, 403
    transplantation of, 734–736 (*See also* Heart-lung and lung
        transplantation)
    in Wegener's granulomatosis, 454
Lung surfactant protein A, 21
Lupus. *See* Systemic lupus erythematosus

Lupus anticoagulant, 404
Lupus nephritis, 402, 489–491
    classification of, 490t
    clinical features and course of, 489–490
    pathology and immunopathology of, *490,* 490–491
    tubulointerstitial, 493
LY-DMA (lymphocyte-determined membrane antigen), 653
Lyme disease, 410, 692–696
    clinical features of, 692–694
        acute disseminated disease, 693
        chronic disease, 693–694
        early, localized disease, 692
    diagnosis of, 695–696
    differential diagnosis of, 696
    epidemiology of, 692
    pathogenesis of, 694–695
        role of autoimmunity, 695
        spirochete persistence, 695
    prevention of, 696
        vaccine, 696, 701t, 708
    treatment and prognosis for, 696
Lymph, 49
Lymphadenopathy, 51–53
    angioimmunoblastic lymphadenopathy with dysproteinemia,
        599
    mimicking lymphoma, 603
Lymphadenopathy-associated virus. *See* Human
        immunodeficiency virus infection
Lymphangiectasia, intestinal, 463
Lymphatic circulation, 49–50, *50*
Lymphatic filariasis, 686
Lymphatic vessels, afferent and efferent, 50, *51, 57*
Lymph nodes, *50,* 50–53
    lymphocyte circulation through, 56, *57*
    lymphocyte proportions in, 41t
    structure of, 50–51, *51, 52*
Lymphoblastic lymphoma (LBL), 580, 588–591
Lymphoblasts, 47, *47*
Lymphocyte activation assays, 243–245
    activation markers, 243–244
    cytokine production, 244–245
    cytolytic T-cell responses, 244
    lymphocyte proliferation, 244
Lymphocyte-determined membrane antigen (LY-DMA), 653
Lymphocytes, 27, 27t, 40–59. *See also* B lymphocytes; T
        lymphocytes
    activation of, 41–42, *42,* 46–48, *47,* 61
        B cells, 66, *67*
        cell death induced by, 70
        cytotoxic T cells, 66–67, *67*
        helper T cells, 65–66, *66*
        requirements for, *48,* 48–49, 49t
    antigen specificity of, *62,* 62–63, 82
    apoptosis of, 70
    autoreactive, 70, 91
    B cells, 42–43, *43, 44,* 115–129
    circulation and homing of, 56–59, *57, 58,* 59t
    clonal organization and dynamics of populations of, 61–63, *62*
        gene rearrangement assay for clonality, 263–265
    definition of, 40n
    differentiation of, 2, *3*
    in immune response, 63–67, *64–67*
        decreased reactivity in pregnancy, 555
    intraepithelial, 206
    in lymphoid organs, 49–56
    memory, 41–42, 61
    naive, 41, 62
    neoplasms of, 578–603 (*See also* Neoplasms of immune
        system)

Lymphocytes, *(continued)*
number of, 40
positive vs. negative selection of, 70, 90–91
primary lymphocyte repertoire, 62
production of, *3,* 40–41, *41*
proliferation of, 42
"resting," 41
structure of, 40, *40*
T cells, 43–46, 45t, *46,* 131–143
tissue proportions of, 40, 41t
Lymphocytic adenohypophysitis, 430
Lymphocytopenia, idiopathic CD4, 318
Lymphocytosis, 295
Lymphocytotoxicity test, 276–279
B-cell crossmatching, 281
cell isolation for, 276–277
complement-dependent, 277, 290t
HLA private and public specificities, 278
peripheral blood lymphocyte crossmatching, 280
reagents for, 277–278
results of, 277, 278t
variability in, 278–279, 279t
scoring of, 277, 277t
T-cell crossmatching, 280, *281*
Lymphoid, defined, 40n
Lymphoid follicles, 50, *51, 57*
in humoral immune response, 126–127, *127*
primary vs. secondary, 50–51, *51*
splenic, 53, *53*
structures of, *52*
Lymphoid organs, 49–56
high endothelial venules in, *58,* 58–59
lymph nodes and lymphatic circulation, 49–53, *50–52*
primary, 40–41
secondary, 41
spleen, 53, *53*
tertiary, 59
thymus, 54–56, *55, 56*
tonsils, Peyer's patches, and other subepithelial organs, 53–54, *54*
Lymphokine-activated killer (LAK) cells, 144
Lymphokines, 43, 148
Lymphoma. *See also* Neoplasms of immune system
adult T-cell leukemia-lymphoma, 156, 569, *590,* 598–599
anaplastic large-cell, *590,* 600
angiocentric NK/T, 599–600
angioimmunoblastic T-cell, 599
ataxia-telangiectasia and, 326, *326*
Burkitt's and Burkitt-like, 113, *113,* 583–584, 595
classification of non-Hodgkin's lymphomas, 587–588, 588t, 589t
diffuse large B-cell, 594
follicular center, 70, 113–114, 593
HIV infection and, 603
Hodgkin's disease, *600,* 600–602, 601t
human herpesvirus 8-associated, 627
immunoblastic, 603
intestinal T-cell, 600
vs. leukemia, 580
lymphoblastic, 580, 588–591
lymphoplasmacytoid, 592
MALT, 465, 593–594
mantle cell, 592
marginal zone B-cell, 593
Mediterranean, 464
monocytoid B-cell, 594
peripheral T-cell, 599
posttransplant polymorphic, 603
small lymphocytic, 591
T-lymphoblastic, *590*

Lymphomatoid granulomatosis, 545
Lymphopenia, 295
Lymphoplasmacytoid lymphoma, 592
Lymphoplasmapheresis, for kidney transplant recipients, 721
Lymphopoiesis, 40–41
Lymphoproliferative disorders
posttransplant, 602–603
X-linked, 295
Lymphotactin, 167, 172t
Lymphotoxin α, 150t, 152t, 153t, 154
Lymphotoxin α-lymphotoxin β complex, 150t, 152t, 154
Lysosomes, 34
Lysozyme, 20, 20t, 37, 38t

mAbs. *See* **Monoclonal antibodies**
MAC. *See* Membrane attack complex
Mac-1, 29, *30*
Macrophage-derived chemokine (MDC), 172t
Macrophages, 35–38
activation of, 35–36
interferon-γ and, 161
as antigen-presenting cells, 65, *65,* 92
assays for, 245
chemokine receptor expression by, *169*
in chronic inflammation, 37
granuloma formation, 38, *38*
HIV-infected, 639–640, 644, 645t
ligands bound by surface receptors on, 35, 36t
monocyte-macrophage assays, 245
in renal disease, 485
role in tumor immunity, 573
secretory products of, 37, 38t
splenic, 53
Macropinocytosis, 83
MAGE proteins, 571
Major basic protein, 190, 191
Major determinants, 398
Major histocompatibility complex (MHC) proteins, 45, 63, 83–94. *See also* Human leukocyte antigens
allelic polymorphism of, 84–85, 88t
antigen-presenting cells, 43–45, 63–65, 91–93
assembly and presentation of peptide-MHC complexes, 87–90, *89*
class I, 63, 66–67, 83, 84, *85, 86*
deficiency of, 323
recognition by inhibitory receptors on natural killer cells, 144–145
structure of, 84, *85, 86*
type I interferon-induced expression of, 160
class II, 45t, *46,* 63–65, *64,* 83, *116,* 118
deficiency of, 295, 322–323
interferon-γ-induced expression of, 161
structure of, 84, *85*
discovery of, 84
disease and, 93–94, 94t
genes for, 85–87, *88,* 88t, *272,* 272–273
codominant expression of, 86
MHC restriction, 91
nonclassical, 86
peptide-binding sites of, 84, *87*
peptide-MHC recognition by T cells, 90–91
alloreactivity and transplant rejection, 91, 722–723, *723*
positive and negative T-cell selection, 70, 90–91
Malabsorption
agammaglobulinemia and, 304, 305
gluten-sensitive enteropathy, 460–462
of vitamin B^{12}, 464–465
Malaria, 673–675
Malassezia, 656t

Malignant histiocytosis (MH), 602
MALT (mucosa-associated lymphoid tissue), 54
MALT (mucosa-associated lymphoid tissue) lymphomas, 465,
    593–594
Mannan-binding lectin (MBL), 20–21, 20t, *23,* 181
    complement activation pathway, 22–23, 176, 181, 341
    deficiency of, 342t, 344
Mantle cell lymphoma (MCL), 592
Mantle of secondary lymphoid follicle, 51, *51, 53, 127*
MAPK (mitosis-associated protein kinase), 11
Maramyl dipeptides or tripeptides, 80
Marginal zone, splenic, 53, *53*
Marginal zone B-cell lymphoma, 593
Margination of neutrophils, 29, *30*
MASP-1 and MASP-2, 181
Mast cells, 2, 26, 191–192
    Fc receptors on, 190t, 192, 201
    IgE receptors on, 349
    in inflammatory response, 191–192
    in lamina propria, 207
    production of, *3*
    properties of, 191t
    regulators of, 192
    structure of, 191, *192*
        metachromatic granules, 191–192
Masugi nephritis, 482
Max, 14
MBL. *See* Mannan-binding lectin
M cells, 205, *205*
McLeod phenotype, 252
MCL (mantle cell lymphoma), 592
MCP (membrane cofactor protein), 182t
M-CSF. *See* Monocyte colony-stimulating factor
MDC (macrophage-derived chemokine, 172t
MDC (macrophage-derived chemokine), 172t
Measles virus infection, 625–626
    atypical, 626
    clinical features of, 625
    diagnosis of, 625–626
    immunologic features of, 625
    immunologic pathogenesis of, 626
    immunologic sequelae of, 621t
    prevention of, 626
        immune globulin, 705t
        vaccines, 79t, 626, 701t
    subacute sclerosing panencephalitis and, 625
    virology of, 186, 625
Mediterranean lymphoma, 464
Medulla of lymph node, 50, 51, *51*
Megakaryocytes, 2, *3*
MEIAs (microparticle enzyme immunoassays), 222–224, 224t
Membrane attack complex (MAC), 181, *182,* 182t
    deficiencies of, 342t, 344
Membrane cofactor protein (MCP), 182t
Membranoproliferative glomerulonephritis, 489
Membranous glomerulonephritis, 486–487
    clinical features and course of, 486
    pathology and immunopathology of, *482,* 486, *486*
    treatment of, 487
Memory cells, 41–42, 61
    B lymphocytes, 43, *43,* 124–125
    T lymphocytes, 46, 143, 242
Meningococcal vaccine, 701t
Meningococcus, 613
6-Mercaptopurine, 745
Merozoites, 674
Mesangiolysis, 483
Metabolic (respiratory) burst, 33, 36
    determination of, 246–247
Metaproterenol, 363–364, 756

Methotrexate, 744–745
    for graft-versus-host disease, 739
    for polyarteritis nodosa, 453
    for polymyositis-dermatomyositis, 417
    for Reiter's syndrome, 418
    for rheumatoid arthritis, 408
    for systemic lupus erythematosus, 405
Methylxanthines, 364, 757
MG. *See* Myasthenia gravis
MGUS (monoclonal gammopathy of undetermined
    significance), 519, 596
MHC. *See* Major histocompatibility complex proteins
MH (malignant histiocytosis), 602
Microbicidal assay, 248, *248*
Microfilariasis, transfusion-transmitted, 256
Microparticle enzyme immunoassays (MEIAs), 222–224, 224t
Microscopic polyangiitis (MPA), 453–454
    diagnosis of, 453–454
    immunologic features of, 453
    laboratory findings in, 453
    prognosis for, 454
    signs and symptoms of, 453
        renal disease, 492–493
    treatment of, 454
Minor determinants, 398
MIP-1α, 167, 171, 174
Miracidia, 682
"Missing self" hypothesis, 145
Mites, 352
Mitochondria, role in apoptosis, 15
Mitogenesis, 46
Mitogens, 48, 244, 296
    HIV infection and response to, 644
Mitosis, 13
Mitosis-associated protein kinase (MAPK), 11
Mixed lymphocyte culture (MLC) test, 272, 282, 290, 290t
MMN (multifocal motor neuropathy), 519
MMR vaccine, 702
MNS antigens, 252
Mold allergens, 351–352, *352*
Molecular genetic techniques, 260–269
    for analysis of immune system neoplasms, 586
    gene rearrangement assay for lymphocyte clonality,
        263–265
    genomic arrays, 268
    for histocompatibility testing, 282–289, 283t, 284t
        chimerism testing, 289
        gene amplification, 284
        heteroduplex analysis, 289
        limitations of, 287–289
        restriction fragment length polymorphism, 283
        sequence-based typing, 287, *288*
        sequence-specific oligonucleotide probing, 284–287, *286*
        sequence-specific priming, 284, *285*
    hybridization assays, 261–262, *263, 264*
    in situ hybridization, 265, *266*
    methods of analyzing RNA, 268
    nucleic acid probes, 260–261, *262*
    overview and prospects for, 268–269
    polymerase chain reaction, *266,* 266–267, *267*
    Southern blot, 262–263, *265*
Molecular mimicry, 510
Monobactams, *398*
Monoclonal antibodies (mAbs), 96, 106, 234
    anti-CD4, 758
        for multiple sclerosis, 516
    for antigen detection, 215, 581
    anti-IgE, 756
    binding to myeloid cell Fc receptors, 241
    in evaluation of cell-mediated immunity, 296

Monoclonal antibodies (mAbs), *(continued)*
  in evaluation of immune system neoplasms, 581
  in flow cytometry, 235–242
  for HIV infection, 648
  isotype-matched, 241
  for leukocyte phenotyping, 234
  in lymphocyte activation assays, 244, 245
  in monocyte-macrophage assays, 245
  palivizumab for respiratory syncytial virus infection, 625
  T-cell-directed, 758–759
  for transplant recipients, 719
    graft-versus-host disease, 739
    kidney, 724–725
    pancreas, 732
  for tumor therapy, 576, 587
Monoclonal gammopathy of undetermined significance
    (MGUS), 519, 596
Monoclonal lymphocytosis of uncertain significance, 591
Monocyte colony-stimulating factor (M-CSF), 8t, 148
  phenotypes of knockout mice, 163t
Monocytes, 2, *3,* 34, *35*
  assays for, 245
  chemokine receptor expression by, *169*
  Fc receptors on, 190t
Monocytoid B-cell lymphomas, 594
Monokines, 148
Mononuclear phagocytes, 27t, 34–38
  macrophages, 35–38
  monocytes, 2, *3,* 34, *35*
  neoplasms of, 602
    Langerhans' cell histiocytosis, 602
    malignant histiocytosis, 602
Monospot test, 220
Montelukast, 364, 755
Montenegro hypersensitivity skin test, 678
MPA. *See* Microscopic polyangiitis
M proteins, 610
MS. *See* Multiple sclerosis
Mucins, 6–7
Mucocutaneous candidiasis, chronic, *316,* 316–317, 667
Mucocutaneous lymph node syndrome, 458
Mucormycosis, 655, 657t, 669–670
  complications and prognosis for, 670
  differential diagnosis of, 670
  effect of immunologic abnormalities on course of, 661t
  etiologic agents for, 670
  immunologic diagnosis of, 663t, 670
  immunologic features of, 669–670
  laboratory findings in, 670
  pathologic features of, 660t
  rhinocerebral, 670
  signs and symptoms of, 670
  treatment of, 670
Mucosa-associated lymphoid tissue (MALT), 54
Mucosa-associated lymphoid tissue (MALT) lymphomas, 465,
    593–594
Mucosal immune system, 204–213
  anatomy of, 204–207
    diffuse lymphoid tissues, 204, *205, 206,* 206–207
    lymphoid aggregates, *205,* 205–206
    organized lymphoid tissues, 204
  breast milk immunology and, 212–213
  distinctive properties of, 204
  functions of, 204
  IgA in, 207–209
    regulation of synthesis at mucosal sites, 209–210, *210*
    secretory vs. circulating, 209
    structure and function of, 207–208
    transport of, *208,* 208–209

  mucosal homing, 204, 210, *211*
  oral tolerance and, *211,* 211–212
    vs. oral immunization, 212
  other immunoglobulins in, 209
  of reproductive system, 548–549, *549*
Mucous membrane pemphigoid, 498–499
  ocular manifestations of, 530
Multicystic kidney disease, *226*
Multifocal motor neuropathy (MMN), 519
Multinucleate giant cells, 38
Multiple myeloma, 95, 224, *225–227,* 228, 295, 595–596,
    627
Multiple sclerosis (MS), 226, *226,* 510–516
  clinical features of, *514,* 514–515
  complications and prognosis for, 516
  diagnosis of, 515
  differential diagnosis of, 515
  epidemiology of, 510–511
  genetics of, 511
  immunologic pathogenesis of, 511–514, *512, 513*
  pathology of, 514
  treatment of, 515–516
Mumps vaccine, 79t, 701t
Muromonab-CD3, for kidney transplant recipients, 725
Muscle relaxants, anaphylactic reactions to, 399
Musculoskeletal system
  eosinophilia-myalgia syndrome, 540
  in giant-cell arteritis, 456
  in microscopic polyangiitis, 453
  in polyarteritis nodosa, 452
  polymyositis-dermatomyositis, 415, 416
  in rheumatoid arthritis, 406–407
  in scleroderma, 414
  in systemic lupus erythematosus, 402
  in Wegener's granulomatosis, 454
Myasthenia gravis (MG), 510, 519–521
  clinical features of, 520–521
  complications and prognosis for, 521
  differential diagnosis of, 521
  epidemiology of, 520
  experimental autoimmune, 520
  genetics of, 520
  immunologic diagnosis of, 521
  immunologic features of, 519–520
  immunologic pathogenesis of, 520
  pathology of, 520, *520*
  treatment of, 521
Mycetoma, 656t
  effect of immunologic abnormalities on course of, 661t
  immunologic diagnosis of, 662t
  pathologic features of, 659t
Mycobacterium avium complex, 615
Mycobacterium bovis, 615
Mycobacterium leprae, 199, 615
Mycobacterium tuberculosis, 199, 615
  BCG vaccine against, 79, 701t
  PPD skin testing for, 242–243
Mycophenolate mofetil, 746–747
  for pemphigus vulgaris and pemphigus foliaceous, 506
  for transplant recipients, 719
    heart-lung and lung, 735
    kidney, 721
    liver, 730
    pancreas, 732
Mycoplasma pneumoniae, 221
Mycoses. *See* Fungal diseases
Mycosis fungoides, *590*
Myelodysplasia, 436
Myelo-erythroid progenitor, *3*

Myeloid cells
  definition of, 2n
  differentiation of, 2, *3, 4*
  evaluating function of, 296
  flow cytometric analysis of, 240–241
Myeloid progenitor, *3*
Myeloma proteins, 95
Myeloperoxidase, 32, 241
  deficiency of, 296, 336
Myocarditis, in systemic lupus erythematosus, 403

NADPH (reduced nicotinamide adenine dinucleotide
     phosphate) oxidase, 32
  deficiency of, 246, 296, 334
NAIT (neonatal alloimmune thrombocytopenia), 446
Naproxen, 7553
Nasal polyps, 359
National Childhood Vaccine Injury Act of 1986, 703
National Marrow Donor Program (NMDP), 275, 737
National Organ Transplant Act of 1987, 291
Natural killer (NK) cells, 2, 143–145
  cytokines produced by, 144
  deficiency of, 317–318
  development of, *3,* 40, 144
  effector functions of, 144
  IL-2 effects on, 156
  recognition of class I MHC antigens by inhibitory receptors
    on, 144–145
  role in host defense, 145
  role in tumor immunity, 572–573
  surface markers expressed by, 144
  tissue distribution of, 40, 41t, 144
  viral effects on, 618t
NBT (nitroblue tetrazolium) test, 246, 294, 296, 334, 335
Necator americanus, 684
Necrosis, 14
Necrotizing sarcoid granulomatosis, 545
Nedocromil, 364
nef gene, 638, *638*
Negative and positive selection of thymocytes, 70, 90–91,
    134–136, *135*
Neisseria gonorrhoeae, 613
Neisseria meningitidis, 613
  vaccine against, 701t
Nelfinavir, 645, 647t
Nematodes, 684–686
  ascariasis, 685
  filariid, 685–686
  trichinosis, 684–685
Neonatal alloimmune thrombocytopenia (NAIT), 446
Neoplasms of immune system, 578–603. *See also* Tumor
    immunology
  acute lymphoblastic leukemia and lymphoblastic lymphoma,
    588–591, *590*
  adult T-cell leukemia-lymphoma, 598–599
  amyloidosis and, 596, 597t
  anaplastic large-cell lymphomas, 600
  angiocentric NK/T lymphoma, 599–600
  angioimmunoblastic T-cell lymphoma, 599
  approach to diagnosis of, 580–586
    cytogenetic analysis, 581–584, 586t
    immunophenotypic analysis, 580–581, 581t–583t, *584,*
      585
    integrating data, 586
    molecular genetic analysis, 586
    morphologic examination, 580
  B-cell chronic lymphocytic leukemia and small lymphocytic
    lymphoma, 591

benign conditions mimicking or associated with, 603
benign hypergammaglobulinemic purpura, 597
Burkitt's and Burkitt-like lymphomas, 595
characteristics of malignant lymphoid cells, 578–580
  aberrant features, 580
  clonality, 578
  leukemia vs. lymphoma, 580
  lineage association, 578–580, *579,* 579t
classification of lymphomas, 587–588, 588t, 589t
clonal plasma cell disorders, 595
  plasma cell myeloma, 95, 224, *225–227,* 228, 295,
    595–596
  solitary plasmacytoma, 596
cryoglobulinemia and, 597
diffuse large B-cell lymphoma, 594
follicular center lymphomas, 593
hairy cell leukemia, 594
heavy-chain diseases and, 596–597
Hodgkin's disease, *600,* 600–602, 601t
intestinal T-cell lymphoma, 600
large granular lymphocyte leukemias, 597–598
lymphoplasmacytoid lymphoma and Waldenström's
    macroglobulinemia, 592
lymphoproliferative disorders in immunosuppressed
    patients, 602–603
MALT lymphomas, 593–594
mantle cell lymphoma, 592
marginal zone B-cell lymphomas, 593
monoclonal gammopathy of undetermined significance, 596
monocytoid B-cell lymphomas, 594
mycosis fungoides and Sézary syndrome, 598
neoplasms of mononuclear phagocytes and antigen-
    presenting cells, 602
  Langerhans' cell histiocytosis, 602
  malignant histiocytosis, 602
peripheral T-cell lymphomas, 599
prolymphocytic leukemia, 591–592
T-cell prolymphocytic leukemia, 598
therapies for, 586–587
  bone marrow transplantation, 587
  chemotherapy, 587
  monoclonal antibodies, 576, 587
  radiation therapy, 587
Nephelometry, 216–217, *219,* 219t
Nephritis. *See also* Glomerulonephritis; Renal disease
  allergic interstitial, 193
    drug-induced, 396
  Heymann's, 483
  lupus, 402, 489–491, *490,* 490t
  nephrotoxic (Masugi), 482
  Steblay, 482–483
  tubulointerstitial, 493–494
    antitubular basement membrane, 483, 493
    lupus-associated, 493
    T-lymphocyte-mediated, 484, 493–494, 494t
Nerve growth factor (NGF), 152t, 154
Neuraminidase inhibitors, 622
Neurologic disorders, 510–525
  Alzheimer's disease, 523
  amyotrophic lateral sclerosis, 523
  in Churg-Strauss syndrome, 455
  demyelinating diseases, 510–519
    acute disseminated encephalomyelitis, 516–517
    acute inflammatory demyelinating polyneuropathy,
      518–519
    chronic inflammatory neuropathies, 519
    molecular mimicry in, 510
    multiple sclerosis, 226, *226,* 510–516, *512–515*
    immunologic abnormalities in, 510, 522

Neurologic disorders, *(continued)*
  immunologic features of stroke, 524–525
  in Lyme disease, 694
  neuromuscular transmission disorders, 519–521
    Lambert-Eaton myasthenic syndrome, 521
    myasthenia gravis, 519–521, *520*
  neurosyphilis, 689, 691
  paraneoplastic syndromes, 522–523
  in polyarteritis nodosa, 452
  Rasmussen's encephalitis, 524
  in rheumatoid arthritis, 407
  stiff-person syndrome, 524
  in systemic lupus erythematosus, 403
  in Wegener's granulomatosis, 454
Neutropenia, 296, 333, 434–436
  autoimmune, 434
  cyclic, 434
  drug-induced immune, 434–435
  fungal diseases and, 655
  management of, 435–436, 436t
Neutrophil function assays, 245–248
  bacterial killing, 248, *248*
  chemotaxis, 245–246
  neutrophil adhesion, 245
  phagocytosis, 246
  respiratory burst and degranulation, *246,* 246–247, *247*
Neutrophils, 2, 27–34, 27t
  in acute inflammation, 33
  advantages and limitations of immunity based on, 33–34
  chemokine receptor expression by, *169,* 170
  disorders of function of, 248t
  Fc receptors on, 190t
  granules of, 27–28, 28t, 32
    extracellular release of contents of, 33, *34*
  margination and emigration of, 29, *30*
  oxidative microbial pathways in, 32–33, *33*
  in phagocytosis, *31,* 31–32, *32*
  production and circulation of, *3,* 28–29
  in renal disease, 485
  structure of, 27, *28*
Nevirapine, 645, 647t
Nezelof's syndrome, 321
NF-κB (nuclear factor κB) signaling pathway, *12,* 13
NGF (nerve growth factor), 152t, 154
Nickel allergy, 199
Nijmegen breakage syndrome, 326
Nikolsky's sign, 504
Nitric oxide (NO), 32–33, *33,* 35
Nitroblue tetrazolium (NBT) test, 246, 294, 296, 334, 335
Nitrofurantoin-induced lung disease, 535–537, *537*
NK cells. *See* Natural killer cells
NKp46, 144
NKT cells, 145–146
NMDP (National Marrow Donor Program), 275, 737
NNRTIs (nonnucleoside analog reverse transcriptase
    inhibitors), 645, 647t
Nomenclature
  for CD antigens, 2n, 234–235, 581, 761–762
  for complement components, 177
  for cytokines, 148, 149t, 150t
  for human leukocyte antigens, 273–275, *274*
Nonnucleoside analog reverse transcriptase inhibitors
    (NNRTIs), 645, 647t
Nonsteroidal antiinflammatory drugs (NSAIDs), 194,
    753–755
  Alzheimer's disease risk and, 468
  antiinflammatory effects of, 753
  bronchospasm induced by, 535
  for Crohn's disease, 468

  for Henoch-Schönlein purpura, 458
  hypersensitivity to, 400
  for juvenile arthritis, 410
  mechanisms of action of, 753, *754*
  for Reiter's syndrome, 418
  for relapsing polychondritis, 419
  for rheumatoid arthritis, 408
  for Sjögren's syndrome, 412
  for systemic lupus erythematosus, 405
  toxicity of, 753–755, 754t
Northern blot, 268
N regions, immunoglobulin, 111
NRTIs (nucleoside analog reverse transcriptase inhibitors),
    645, 647t
NSAIDs. *See* Nonsteroidal antiinflammatory drugs
Nuclear factor κB (NF-κB) signaling pathway, *12,* 13
Nuclease protection assay, 261
Nucleic acid probes, 260–261, *262*
Nucleoside analog reverse transcriptase inhibitors (NRTIs),
    645, 647t
5'-Nucleotidase, *116,* 117
  deficiency of, 311
NY-ESO, 571

O antigens, 611
Occupational respiratory diseases, 541
Ocular disorders. *See* Eye disorders
OKT3, 758
  for pancreas transplant recipients, 732
OKT4 epitope deficiency, 321
2'-5' Oligoadenylate (2-5A) synthetase, 160
Omenn syndrome, 321, 323
Onchocerca volvulus, 684–686
Oncofetal antigens, 571
Oncogenes, 569–570
Oncornaviruses, 637t
Oncostatin (OSM), 158t
Oophoritis, autoimmune, 557
Opportunistic infections
  cancer and, 574
  fungal, 655, 657t–658t
  HIV infection and, 641, 641t
Opsonins, 31, 36t, 68
Opsonization, 31, *32,* 68
  complement and, 175, 179
  of encapsulated bacteria, 612
  Fc receptors and, 31, 68, 108
Oral candidiasis, *478,* 478–479
Oral hairy leukoplakia, 478, *478*
Oral tolerance, *211,* 211–212
  vs. oral immunization, 212
Orchitis, autoimmune, 557
Organ-specific antibodies, in autoimmune endocrine diseases,
    422, 423t
Orodental disorders, 473–479
  AIDS-related, 478, *478*
  gingivitis and periodontitis, 473–476, *475, 476*
  juvenile periodontitis, 476
  oral candidiasis, *478,* 478–479
  recurrent aphthous ulcers, 476–478, *477*
  in Sjögren's syndrome, 411
OSM (oncostatin), 158t
Osteoprotegerin, 153t
Ostwald viscosimeter, 228
Otitis media, 359
Ouchterlony analysis, 216, *218*
Ovary, 550
  autoimmune diseases of, 557

OX40, 209
Oxidative stress
apoptosis and, 15
renal disease and, 486
OX40 ligand, 152t, 209

p21, 14
p24, 642
p53, 14, 17
p55, 757
p75, 757–758
PA. *See* Pernicious anemia
PAF (platelet-activating factor), 193, 195, *197*
Palivizumab, 625
PAN. *See* Polyarteritis nodosa
Pancreas transplantation, 730–732
complications and outcome of, 731
crossmatching for, 731
diagnosis of allograft rejection, 731–732
immunosuppression after, 732
indications for, 730
islet cell transplantation, 732
operative procedure for, 730–731, *731*
Pancreatitis, kinins and, 187
Paracoccidioidomycosis, 657t, 665–666
complications and prognosis for, 666
differential diagnosis of, 666
effect of immunologic abnormalities on course of, 661t
epidemiology of, 665–666
immunologic diagnosis of, 663t, 666
immunologic features of, 665
laboratory findings in, 666
pathologic features of, 659t
signs and symptoms of, 666
treatment of, 666
Paracortex of lymph node, 51
Paragonimiasis, 681
Paraneoplastic syndromes
neurologic, 522–523
Lambert-Eaton myasthenic syndrome, 521
pemphigus, 506–507
Parasitic diseases, 673–686
cestodes, 683–684
echinococcosis, 684
chronicity of, 673
eosinophilic pneumonias and, 540, 540t
eosinophils and, 190–191
immune responses to, 673
helminths, 681
mechanisms of evasion of, 673, *674*
protozoa, 673
nematodes, 684–686
ascariasis, 685
filariid, 685–686
trichinosis, 684–685
protozoa, 673–681
African trypanosomiasis, 679–681
leishmaniasis, 677–679
malaria, 673–675
toxoplasmosis, 675–677
transfusion-transmitted, 256
trematodes, 681–683
schistosomiasis, 681–683
Paresis, syphilitic, 689
Paroxysmal cold hemoglobinuria, 440–441
Paroxysmal nocturnal hemoglobinuria (PNH), 185, 346, 347, 441
Pars cavernosa, 549

"Passenger" cells, 722
Passive-active immunization, 706
Passive immunization, 699, 703–706
animal sera and antitoxins for, 705
hazards of, 706
human immune globulin for, 703–705, 705t
for Kawasaki syndrome, 706
for poisonous bites, 706
to prevent Rh isoimmunization, 705–706
Patch testing, 243, 387, 387t, 397
photopatch testing, 388
Pathogens, 19
bacterial, 607–615
fungal, 655–671
interactions with chemokine pathways, 173
intracellular, antigens from, 83
parasitic, 673–686
spirochetal, 688–696
viral, 617–634
Pathogen-specific macromolecules, 20, 20t
PBC. *See* Biliary cirrhosis, primary
PCP. *See Pneumocystis carinii* pneumonia
PCR (polymerase chain reaction), *266,* 266–267, *267*
Pemphigoid
bullous, 495–498, *497*
mucous membrane (cicatricial), 498–499
ocular manifestations of, 530
Pemphigus
paraneoplastic, 506–507
vulgaris and foliaceous, 504–506
clinical features of, 504–505, *505*
differential diagnosis of, 505
epidemiology of, 504
etiology of, 504
genetics of, 504
immunologic diagnosis of, 505, *506*
immunologic features of, 504
ocular manifestations of, 530
pathology of, 504, *505*
prognosis and diseases associated with, 506
treatment of, 505–506
D-Penicillamine
for primary biliary cirrhosis, 472
pulmonary disease induced by, 537
Penicillins
hypersensitivity to, 396, 398–399
desensitization for, 398, 714
metabolites of, 398, *399*
structure of, *398*
Penile urethral epithelium, 548–549
Pentamidine isethionate, 671
Peptic ulcer disease, 194
Peptide antibiotics, 21
Peptide immunotherapy, 717
Peptides, antigenic, 82–83, 82t
Peptide vaccine, 80
Peptidoglycan of bacterial cell walls, lysozyme digestion of, 20
Peptidomannans, 655
Perforin, 142
Periarteriolar lymphoid sheath, 53, *53*
Pericarditis, in systemic lupus erythematosus, 402
Periodontal disease, 339, 473–476, *476*
immunologic features of, 473–474
immunologic pathogenesis of, 474–476, *475*
juvenile, 476
microflora of dental plaque and, 474
treatment of, 476
Peripheral blood lymphocytes, 40, 41t, 49

Peripheral T-cell lymphoma (PTL), 599
Pernicious anemia (PA), 464–465
  diagnosis of, 465
  immunologic features of, 464
  immunologic pathogenesis of, 464–465
  pathology of, 465
  treatment of, 465
Pertussis, 609–610
Pertussis vaccine, 79t, 609–610, 701t, 707
Peyer's patches, 54, *54, 205,* 209–210, *211*
Phaeohyphomycosis, 658t, 661t
Phagocytes, 27–38
  activation of, 68
  dysfunction of, 300t, 333–339
    Chédiak–Higashi syndrome, 295, 296, 318, 336
    chronic granulomatous disease, 161, 241, 246–247, 252, 294, 296, 334–336
    extrinsic vs. intrinsic, 333
    glucose-6-phosphate dehydrogenase deficiency, 336
    glycogen storage disease type 1B, 337
    hyper-IgE (Job's) syndrome, 337, *337*
    infections associated with, 299, 333
    laboratory evaluation for, 296, 301t, 333t
    leukocyte adhesion defect, 245, 295, 296, 337–338, *338*
    myeloperoxidase deficiency, 296, 336
    neutropenia, 333
    periodontitis syndromes, 339
    Schwachman syndrome, 338
    specific granule deficiency, 336–337
    treatment of, 301t
    tuftsin deficiency, 338
  monocyte-macrophage system, 27t, 34–38
  neutrophils, 27–34, 27t
Phagocytosis
  assays of, 246
  macrophage, 36–37
  neutrophil, *31,* 31–32, *32*
  "frustrated," *34,* 247, *247*
Phagosomes, 31–32, *32*
PHA (phytohemagglutinin), 244, 296
Pharyngitis, streptococcal, 610
Phlyctenular keratoconjunctivitis, 532, *532*
Phorbol myristate acetate (PMA), 244
Phosphatidylserine, 15
Phospholipase C-γ1, 47
Phosphorylation, 10, 11
Photoallergic contact dermatitis, 388–389, 389t
  allergens associated with, 389, 389t
  clinical diagnosis of, 388
  clinical features of, 388
  definition of, 388
  differential diagnosis of, 388
  epidemiology of, 388
  immunologic diagnosis of, 388
  immunologic features of, 388
  immunologic pathogenesis of, 388
  pathology of, 388
  prognosis for, 389
  treatment of, 389
Photoallergic drug reactions, 396
Photopatch testing, 388
Phototoxic drug reactions, 396
Physical barriers to infection, 19
Physicochemical basis of antigen-antibody binding, *75,* 75–77
  cross-reactions, 76
  haptens, 76–77, *77*
  quantitative aspects, 76

Phytohemagglutinin (PHA), 244, 296
PIA (polysaccharide intercellular adhesin), 610
PIE (pulmonary infiltrates with eosinophilia). *See* Eosinophilic pneumonia
Pigeon breeder's disease. *See* Hypersensitivity pneumonitis
Pinocytosis, 35
Pirbuterol, 363–364, 756
Pityriasis versicolor, 656t, 661t
Pityrosporum folliculitis, 661t
PKR (RNA-dependent protein kinase), 160
Placenta
  HIV transmission across, 561–562
  as immune organ, 552
    HLA expression, 552
    Hofbauer cell, 552, *554*
    trophoblast, 552
  local immunosuppression at, 554–555
  proteins secreted by, 555
  steroid hormones secreted by, 555
Plague vaccine, 701t
Plasma cell disorders, 595
  dyscrasia, 595
  plasma cell myeloma, 95, 224, *225–227,* 228, 295, 595–596, 627
  solitary plasmacytoma, 596
Plasma cells, 43, *43, 44,* 124
  in lamina propria, 207
Plasmacytic hyperplasia, 603
Plasmapheresis
  for antiglomerular basement membrane disease, 492
  for Guillain-Barré syndrome, 518
  for paraneoplastic pemphigus, 507
  for pemphigus vulgaris and pemphigus foliaceous, 506
  for polyarteritis nodosa, 453
Plasma product transfusion, 258t, 259, 347
Plasmodium, 173, 252, 674–675
Platelet-activating factor (PAF), 193, 195, *197*
Plateletpheresis, 258
Platelets, 193
  activation of, 193
  disorders of, 442–449, 443t
    antiphospholipid syndrome, 448–449
    circulating inhibitors of coagulation, 447–448
    drug-induced immune thrombocytopenia, 445–446
    hemolytic-uremic syndrome, 447
    idiopathic thrombocytopenic purpura, 443–445
    immunologic mechanisms of platelet destruction, 442–443
    neonatal alloimmune thrombocytopenia, 446
    posttransfusion purpura, 446
    quinine-induced immune thrombocytopenia with hemolytic-uremic syndrome, 447
    thrombotic thrombocytopenic purpura, 446–447
  Fc receptors on, 190t, 193
  in inflammatory response, 193
  production of, 1, 2, *3*
  transfusion of, 258–259, 258t
    for bone marrow transplant recipients, 738
PLE (protein-losing enteropathy), 463
Pleural disease
  drug-induced, 537
  systemic lupus erythematosus and, 402
PLL (prolymphocytic leukemia), 591–592
PLT (primed lymphocyte typing), 290
PMA (phorbol myristate acetate), 244
PMNs. *See* Polymorphonuclear neutrophils
PMR (polymyalgia rheumatica), 456
Pneumococcal polysaccharide vaccine, 295, 311, 612, 701t
Pneumococcus, 612

Pneumocystis carinii pneumonia (PCP), 641, 655, 658t, 670–671
    in AIDS, 641, 670–671
    complications and prognosis for, 671
    differential diagnosis of, 671
    effect of immunologic abnormalities on course of, 661t
    immunologic diagnosis of, 671
    immunologic features of, 670
    laboratory findings in, 671
    pathologic features of, 660t
    prevention of, 671
    signs and symptoms of, 671
    treatment of, 671
Pneumonia
    eosinophilic, 537–540, 538t
    Haemophilus influenzae, 613
    Klebsiella pneumoniae, 613
    pneumococcal, 612
    Pneumocystis carinii, 641, 670–671
Pneumonitis
    amiodarone, 537
    hypersensitivity, 389–393
PNH (paroxysmal nocturnal hemoglobinuria), 185, 346, 347, 441
PNP (purine nucleoside phosphorylase) deficiency, 328–330, *329*
POEMS syndrome, 519
Poison ivy/oak, 199, 243, 386. *See also* Contact dermatitis, allergic
Pokeweed mitogen (PWM), 244
pol gene, 637, 638, *638*
Polio vaccines, 79t, 80, 634, 700, 701t, 707
Poliovirus infection, 633–634
Pollen allergens, 351, 351t, *352, 353*
    desensitization to, 714–717
Polyarteritis nodosa (PAN), 451–453
    diagnosis of, 452–453
    eye disorders in, 452, 532
    immunologic features of, 451
    immunologic pathogenesis of, 452
    laboratory findings in, 452
    localized vs. systemic, 452
    prognosis for, 453
    symptoms and signs of, 452
        ocular, 452, 532
    treatment of, 453
Polyclonal B-cell activators, 119
Polyglandular syndromes, autoimmune, 431–432, 431t
Poly(I:C), 160
Polymerase chain reaction (PCR), *266,* 266–267, *267,* 284
    reverse transcriptase, 268, 642
Polymorphic hyperplasia, 603
Polymorphisms
    human leukocyte antigens, 273–275, *274*
    restriction fragment length, 283, 284t
    single-strand conformational, 267, *267*
Polymorphonuclear neutrophils (PMNs), 27, 245. *See also* Neutrophils
    disorders of function of, 248t
    functional assays of, 245–248
        bacterial killing, 248, *248*
        chemotaxis, 245–246
        neutrophil adhesion, 245
        phagocytosis, 246
        respiratory burst and degranulation, *246,* 246–247, *247*
Polymyalgia rheumatica (PMR), 456
Polymyositis-dermatomyositis, 415–417
    classification of, 415
    complications and prognosis for, 417

    differential diagnosis of, 416–417
    immunologic diagnosis of, 416
    immunologic features of, 415
    immunologic pathogenesis of, 415
    laboratory findings in, 416
    pathology of, 415–416
    symptoms and signs of, 416
    treatment of, 417
Polymyxin B, 374
Polyneuropathy, acute inflammatory demyelinating, 518–519
Polysaccharide capsule, *612,* 612–613
    of *Bacteroides fragilis,* 613
    of *Haemophilus influenzae,* 613
    of *Klebsiella pneumoniae,* 613
    of *Neisseria* species, 613
    of *Streptococcus agalactiae,* 613
    of *Streptococcus pneumoniae,* 612
Polysaccharide intercellular adhesin (PIA), 610
Polyserositis, in systemic lupus erythematosus, 402
Portal hypertension, 726
Positive and negative selection of thymocytes, 70, 90–91, 134–136, *135*
Postcapillary venules, 26
Postinfectious glomerulonephritis, 481–482, *487,* 487–488
    clinical features and course of, 487
    pathology and immunopathology of, *487,* 487–488
    treatment of, 488
Postpartum thyroiditis, 425
Poxviruses, 164, 173
PPD (purified protein derivative) skin testing, 242–243
Pranlukast, 755
Precipitating antibodies, 392
Prednisolone, *749,* 750t
    for polyarteritis nodosa, 453
Prednisone, *749,* 750t. *See also* Corticosteroids
    for bullous pemphigoid, 498
    for graft-versus-host disease, 739
    for pure erythrocyte aplasia, 441
    for warm autoimmune hemolytic anemia, 439
Preeclampsia, 563–565
Pregnancy, 550–558
    fertilization, implantation, and immune response to fetal tissues, 550–552
        implantation, 551
        placenta as immune organ, 552, *554*
        sperm-egg fusion, 550–551
        trophoblast invasion of maternal tissues, 552, *553*
    immunity in, 552–555
        altered susceptibility to infection, 552–554
        decreased lymphocyte reactivity, 555
        immunosuppression at placenta and adjacent tissues, 554–555
        placental proteins, 555
        placental steroid hormones, 555
        proposed mechanisms of, 554
        survival of normal pregnancy, 555, *556*
    infertility, 555–558
    mother-to-infant infection transmission in
        cytomegalovirus, 649
        hepatitis B, 628
        HIV, 561–562
        syphilis, 689
        toxoplasmosis, 676
    preeclampsia, 563–565
    preterm labor and delivery, 562–563, *564*
    recurrent spontaneous abortion, 555–556, 558–559
    testing for, 221
Prekallikrein, *186,* 186–187
Prelysosomes, 89

Premature ovarian failure, 430–431
Pressure urticaria, 378
Preterm labor and delivery, 562–563, *564*
Primary active immunization, 700
Primary biliary cirrhosis (PBC), 471–472
Primary glomerulonephritis, 486–489
Primary immune response, *69,* 69–70
Primary lymphocyte repertoire, 62
Primary lymphoid organs, 40–41
Primary sclerosing cholangitis (PSC), 472–473
Primed lymphocyte typing (PLT), 290
Procainamide-induced lupus syndrome, 537
Procaspases, 15
Procaterol, 756
Progenitor cells. *See* Hematopoietic stem cells
Progesterone, for recurrent pregnancy loss, 559
Programmed cell death. *See* Apoptosis
Progressive systemic sclerosis, 146, 413–415
   complications and prognosis for, 415
   differential diagnosis of, 414
   immunologic diagnosis of, 414
   immunologic features of, 413
   immunologic pathogenesis of, 413
   laboratory findings in, 414
   pathology of, 413
   symptoms and signs of, 413–414
      gastrointestinal system, 414
      heart, 414
      joints and muscles, 414
      kidneys, 414
      lungs, 414
      onset, 413
      Sjögren's syndrome, 414
      skin, 413–414
   treatment of, 414–415
Prokaryotes, 655
Prolymphocytic leukemia (PLL), 591–592
Promastigotes of *Leishmania,* 676
Properdin, 180
   deficiency of, 342t, 343–344
Prostaglandins, 25t, 26, 194–195, *195*
   IL-1 regulation by, 150
   as inflammatory mediators, 195
   inhibition of synthesis of, 753
   prostaglandin D$_2$, 195
   structures of, *196*
Protease inhibitors, 645, 647t
Proteasomes, 83
Protected site concept, 183
Protein kinase C, 47
Protein-losing enteropathy (PLE), 463
Protein(s)
   A, 610
   bactericidal permeability-increasing, 21
   Bence Jones, 595, 596
   C4-binding, 181–183, 182t
      deficiency of, 342t, 345
   C8-binding, 185
   CD1, 93
   Charcot–Leyden crystal, 190, 191
   C-reactive, 20t, 21, 23–24
   cyclophilin, 747
   expressed on surface of hematopoietic stem cells, 2–4
   α-fetoprotein, 571
   FK-binding protein-12, 747, 749
   humoral, 19–24
   immunophilins, 747
   of influenza virus, 617, 621t
   of kinin system, 186, *186*
   lipopolysaccharide-binding, 20t, 21
   lung surfactant protein A, 21
   M, 610
   MAGE, 571
   major basic, 190, 191
   major histocompatibility complex, 45, 63, 83–94
   membrane cofactor, 182t
   myeloma, 95
   placental, 555
   S, 182t, 183
   serum amyloid protein P, 20t, 21, 23
   Stat, 11, *12*
Protein tyrosine kinases (PTKs), 10–11
   in lymphocyte activation, 46–47, *47*
Protein tyrosine phosphatase, 122
Proteoglycans, 196
Proteus, 611
Protozoal diseases, 673–681
   African trypanosomiasis, 679–681
   leishmaniasis, 677–679
   malaria, 673–675
   toxoplasmosis, 675–677
Prozone phenomenon, 216
Pruritus, 201
PSC. *See* Sclerosing cholangitis, primary
P-selectin, 8t, 27, 27t, 29, *30*
Pseudoallergic drug reactions, 399
Pseudo-Goodpasture's syndrome, 537
Pseudomonas aeruginosa, 611–612
Psoriatic arthritis, 418–419
PTKs. *See* Protein tyrosine kinases
PTL (peripheral T-cell lymphoma), 599
Pulmonary fibrosis, idiopathic, 542–544, *543*
   causes of, 542
   clinical features of, 542–543
   diagnosis of, 543
   differential diagnosis of, 543, 544t
   immunologic features of, 542
   immunologic pathogenesis of, 542
   treatment and prognosis for, 543–544, 758
Pulmonary function testing
   in asthma, 360
   in hypersensitivity pneumonitis, 392
   after lung transplantation, 736
Pulmonary infiltrates with eosinophilia (PIE). *See* Eosinophilic
      pneumonia
Pure erythrocyte aplasia, 441
Purified protein derivative (PPD) skin testing, 242–243
Purine nucleoside phosphorylase (PNP) deficiency, 328–330,
      329
Purpura
   benign hypergammaglobulinemic, 597
   Henoch-Schönlein, 458
   posttransfusion, 446
   thrombocytopenic
      idiopathic, 443–445
      intravenous immunoglobulin for, 706
      thrombotic, 446–447
Pus, 33
PWM (pokeweed mitogen), 244
Pyrogens, endogenous, 152

**Quantitative and kinetic aspects of immune response, *69,*
      69–70**
Quartan malaria, 674–675
Quinine-induced immune thrombocytopenia with hemolytic-
      uremic syndrome, 447

Rabies immune globulin, 705t
Rabies vaccine, 633, 701t, 708
Rabies virus infection, 632–633
Radiation-induced carcinogenesis, 568–569
Radiation therapy, 587
Radioallergosorbent test (RAST), 354, 355, *356,* 397
Radiographic contrast media, 374, 376
RAG-1 and RAG-2. *See* Recombination-activating genes
Ranitidine, 194
RANTES, 171, 202
Rapamycin (sirolimus), 719, 749–750
Rapid plasma reagin test, 690–691
Ras-dependent signaling pathway, 11, *12*
Rasmussen's encephalitis, 524
RAST (radioallergosorbent test), 354, 355, *356,* 397
Rattlesnake antivenin, 705t, 706
RAU. See Aphthous ulcers, recurrent
Raynaud's phenomenon, 405, 412–414, 439
Receptor editing, 113, 128–129
Receptors. *See* specific receptors
Recombination-activating genes (RAG-1 and RAG-2),
    112–113, 115, *116,* 117, 128
    Omenn syndrome and, 323
    severe combined immunodeficiency and, 321
Recombination signal sequences, *110,* 112
Red blood cells. *See* Erythrocytes
Red pulp, splenic, 53
Reduced nicotinamide adenine dinucleotide phosphate
    (NADPH) oxidase, 32
    deficiency of, 246, 296, 334
Reed–Sternberg cells, 154, *600,* 600–601
Regional enteritis. *See* Crohn's disease
Reiter's syndrome, 94t, 408, 418
    ocular manifestations of, 418, 528, *529*
Relapsing panniculitis, 419–420
Relapsing polychondritis, 419
Renal dialysis, 184
Renal disease, 481–494
    allergic interstitial nephritis, 193, 396
    in Henoch-Schönlein purpura, 458, 491
    immune mechanisms of, 481–486, 482t
        antibody-mediated, 481–484
        secondary mediators of acute inflammation, 485–486,
            485t
        T-lymphocyte-mediated, 484–485
    kidney transplantation for, 193, 291, 291t, 719–726
    NSAID-induced, 755
    primary glomerulonephritis, *486,* 486–489, *487*
    in scleroderma, 414
    in systemic lupus erythematosus, 402, 489–491, *490,* 490t,
        493
    tubulointerstitial nephritis, 493
        antitubular basement membrane nephritis, 493
        lupus-associated, 493
        T-lymphocyte-mediated, 493–494, 494t
    vasculitis-associated glomerular lesions, 491–493
        in ANCA-associated diseases, 492–493
        antiglomerular basement membrane disease, 491–492,
            544–545
        in Churg-Strauss syndrome, 456
        in microscopic polyangiitis, 453
        in polyarteritis nodosa, 452
        in Wegener's granulomatosis, 454
Repertoire broadening, 511
Reproductive system, 548–565
    fertilization, implantation, and immune response to fetal
        tissues, 550–552
        implantation, 551
        placenta as immune organ, 552, *554*
        sperm-egg fusion, 550–551
        trophoblast invasion of maternal tissues, 552, *553*
    HIV infection and, 560–562
    immunity and anatomy of, 548–550
        defenses against pathogens vs. tolerance of sperm
            "invasion," 550
        female, 548, *549*
        male, 548–549
        mucosal immunity, 549
        ovary, 550
        testis, 550
    immunity in pregnancy, 552–555
        altered susceptibility to infection, 552–554
        decreased lymphocyte reactivity, 555
        immunosuppression at placenta and adjacent tissues,
            554–555
        placental proteins, 555
        placental steroid hormones, 555
        proposed mechanisms of, 554
        survival of normal pregnancy, 555, *556*
    infertility, 555–558
    preeclampsia, 563–565
    preterm labor and delivery, 562–563, *564*
    recurrent spontaneous abortion, 555–556, 558–559
RER (rough endoplasmic reticulum), 83, 87–89
Respiratory disease, 535–546. *See also* Lungs
    adult respiratory distress syndrome, 174, 184, 546
    allergic bronchopulmonary aspergillosis, 365, 382–385
    anaphylaxis and, 371
    asthma, 349, 359–365
    diphtheria, 609
    drug-induced, 535–537, 536t
        airway involvement in, 535
        immunologic mechanisms of, 535
        lupus syndrome, 537
        mediastinal, 537
        parenchymal involvement in, 535–537, *537*
        pleural, 537
        pseudo-Goodpasture's syndrome, 537
    due to hypersensitivity responses, 535
    eosinophilic pneumonias, 537–540, 538t
    hypersensitivity pneumonitis, 389–393, 390t
    idiopathic pulmonary fibrosis, 542–544, *543*
    immunodeficiency and, 546
    influenza, 617–623
    measles, 625–626
    occupational and environmental, 541
    pertussis, 609–610
    respiratory syncytial virus infection, 623–625
    sarcoidosis, *541,* 541–542
    tuberculosis, 615
    vasculitis syndromes, 545–546, 545t
        allergic granulomatosis of Churg and Strauss, 455, 538
        bronchocentric granulomatosis, 545–546
        lymphomatoid granulomatosis, 545
        necrotizing sarcoid granulomatosis, 545
        Wegener's granulomatosis, 454
Respiratory failure
    hypersensitivity pneumonitis and, 393
    status asthmaticus and, 364
Respiratory (metabolic) burst, 33, 36
    determination of, 246–247
Respiratory syncytial virus (RSV) infection, 623–625, *624*
    clinical features of, 623
    immunologic features of, 623
    immunologic pathogenesis of, 623–624
    immunologic sequelae of, 621t
    prevention of, 624–625
        palivizumab, 625

Respiratory syncytial virus (RSV) infection, *(continued)*
  prevention of, *(continued)*
    RSV immunoglobulin, 625
    vaccines, 624–625
  treatment of, 624
  virology of, 623
"Resting" lymphocytes, 41
Restriction enzymes, 262
Restriction fragment length polymorphisms (RFLPs), 283, 284t
Restriction fragments, 262
Reticular cells, 50
  sarcomas of, 602
Reticular dysgenesis, 320
Reticulin fibers, 50
Retroviruses, 569
  classification of, 637t
  evolutional relationships among, *637*
  HIV, 636–637
  human T-cell lymphotrophic virus types I and II, 653
Reverse transcriptase, 569, 636–638, 645
Reverse transcriptase polymerase chain reaction (RT-PCR), 268, 642
rev gene, 638, *638*
RFLPs (restriction fragment length polymorphisms), 283, 284t
RFs. *See* Rheumatoid factors
Rh blood group system, 251–252, 252t
RHCE gene, 251
RHD gene, 251
Rheumatic diseases, 401–420
  autoimmune neutropenia and, 434
  Behçet's disease, 417
  juvenile arthritis, 408–411
  ocular manifestations of, *528*, 528–529, *529*
  polymyositis-dermatomyositis, 415–417
  rheumatoid arthritis, 406–408
  scleroderma, 413–415
  Sjögren's syndrome, 411–413
  spondyloarthropathies, 417–420
    ankylosing spondylitis, 417–418
    hypogammaglobulinemia and arthritis, 420
    psoriatic arthritis, 418–419
    Reiter's syndrome, 418
    relapsing panniculitis, 419–420
    relapsing polychondritis, 419
  systemic lupus erythematosus, 401–405
Rheumatic fever, 410
Rheumatoid arthritis, 406–408
  complications and prognosis for, 408
  differential diagnosis of, 408
  epidemiology of, 406
  immunologic diagnosis of, 407
  immunologic features of, 406
  immunologic pathogenesis of, 406
  kinins and, 187
  laboratory findings in, 407
  radiographic findings in, 407
  symptoms and signs of, 406–407
    articular, 406–407
    extraarticular, 407
    Felty's syndrome, 407
    ocular, 407, 528, *528*, *529*
  treatment of, 408
Rheumatoid factors (RFs), 100, 218
  eye disease and, 528–529
  in juvenile arthritis, 409, 410
  in rheumatoid arthritis, 406, 407
  in Sjögren's syndrome, 411, 412
  in systemic lupus erythematosus, 405
  in Wegener's granulomatosis, 455
Rheumatoid nodules, 407
Rh immune globulin (RhIG), 257, 705–706, 705t
Rh incompatibility, 177
Rhinitis
  allergic, 19, 193, 349, 356–359
  drug-induced, 357, 357t
  infectious, 357
  kinins and, 187
  medicamentosa, 357
  nonallergic, 357
  vernal keratoconjunctivitis, 357
Rhinosporidium seeberi, 655
Rh isoimmunization, 257
  prevention of, 705–706
Rhizopus arrhizus, 655
Rhodamine, 235
Rhoptries, 676
RhuMAb-E25, 756
Ribavirin, 632
Rickettsia, 83
Rimantadine, for influenza, 622
Ritonavir, 645, 647t
RNA-dependent protein kinase (PKR), 160
RNA (ribonucleic acid)
  methods for analysis of, 268
  probes, 260–261, *262*
RNA viruses, 569
Rotavirus vaccine, 701t, 708
Rough endoplasmic reticulum (RER), 83, 87–89
Roundworms, 684, 685
RSV. *See* Respiratory syncytial virus infection
RT-PCR (reverse transcriptase polymerase chain reaction), 268, 642
Rubella, 621t
Rubella vaccine, 79t, 701t
Rye classification of Hodgkin's disease, 601, 601t

Sabin vaccine, 79t, 80, 707
Salk HIV vaccine, 648
Salk polio vaccine, 79t, 80, 707
Salmeterol, 364
Salmonella, 179, 611
Salmonella choleraesuis, 614
Salmonella enteritidis, 614
Salmonella typhi, 614
Salt-split skin, 497
Sandwich assay, 222, *222*
Saquinavir, 645, 647t
Sarcoidosis, *541*, 541–542
  diagnosis of, 542, 542t
  differential diagnosis of, 542
  immunologic features of, 541
  immunologic pathogenesis of, 541
  ocular features of, 530–531
  pulmonary features of, 541–542
  treatment and prognosis for, 542
Sarcoma
  dendritic cell, 602
  Kaposi's, 173, 294, 478, 532, 626–627, 641
SBT (sequence-based HLA typing), 284t, 287, *288*
SC. *See* Secretory component
Scarlet fever, 610
Scavenger receptors, 36
SCF. *See* Stem cell factor
Schick test, 609
Schilling's test, 465

Schirmer's test, 412
Schistosomiasis, 191, 673, 681–683
Schistosomula, 682
Schmidt's syndrome, 431
SCID. *See* Severe combined immunodeficiency
Scleroderma. *See* Progressive systemic sclerosis
Sclerosing cholangitis, primary (PSC), 472–473
  immunologic diagnosis of, 473
  immunologic features of, 472
  immunopathogenesis of, 473
  pathology of, 473
  prognosis for, 473
  signs and symptoms of, 473
  treatment of, 473
Scorpion stings, 706
SDF-1 (stromal-derived factor 1), 171
SDS-PAGE (sodium dodecyl sulfate-polyacrylamide gel
      electrophoresis), 227
Se and *se* genes, 251
Secondary immune response, *69, 70*
Secondary lymphoid organs, 41
Secondary lymphoid tissue chemokine (SLC), 59, 172–173,
      172t
Secretor antigens, 251
Secretory component (SC), *99,* 100–101
  IgA polymerization and interaction with, *208,* 208–209
Selectins, 6–7, 8t, 27, 27t
  in neutrophil adhesion, 245
  in neutrophil margination, 29, *30*
Selective IgA deficiency, 295, 307–310
  ataxia-telangiectasia and, 325
  complications and prognosis for, 310
  differential diagnosis of, 309
  drug-induced, 309
  genetic factors and, 309
  immunologic features of, 307
  immunologic pathogenesis of, 308
  laboratory findings in, 309
  passive immunization in persons with, 706
  prevalence of, 307–308
  symptoms and signs of, 308–309
  treatment of, 309–310
Selective IgM deficiency, 310
Self-cure phenomenon, 685
Self-reactive B lymphocytes, 128–129
Self-renewing cells, 1
Sensitivity. *See* Allergy; Hypersensitivity
Sensitization, 272
Septic shock, 152
Sequence-based HLA typing (SBT), 284t, 287, *288*
Sequence-specific oligonucleotide probing (SSOP), 284–287,
      284t, *286*
Sequence-specific priming (SSP), 284, 284t, *285*
SERAX (serologic analysis of antibody responses by
      expression cloning), 570
Serologic methods, 69. *See also* Laboratory tests
  to diagnose bacterial diseases, 607
  to diagnose HIV infection, 642
  to diagnose syphilis, 690–691, *691*
  for histocompatibility testing, 275–279, *276 (See also*
      Lymphocytotoxicity test)
  serologic analysis of antibody responses by expression
      cloning, 570
Serum amyloid protein P, 20t, 21, 23
Serum protein electrophoresis (SPEP), 224–226, *224–226*
Serum sickness, 199, 201, 381–382, 396
  causes of, 381, 381t, 706
  complications and prognosis for, 382
  definition of, 381

  epidemiology of, 381
  immunologic diagnosis of, 382
  immunologic pathogenesis of, 381–382, *382*
  laboratory findings in, 382
  similarity of glomerulonephritis to, 481–482
  symptoms and signs of, 382
  treatment of, 382
Serum viscosity measurements, 227–228
Seven-transmembrane receptor family, 29
Severe combined immunodeficiency (SCID), 239, 320–321
  clinical features of, 320
  diagnosis of, 320–321
  evaluation for, 295–297
  immunologic features of, 320
  pathogenesis of, 321
  treatment of, 321
    bone marrow transplantation, 321, 737
  variants of, 321
  X-linked, 321
Sézary's syndrome, *590*
SH2 domains, 11
Sheehan's syndrome, 430
Shigella, 83, 611
Shock
  anaphylactic, 370, 371 (*See also* Anaphylaxis)
    treatment of, 375
  septic, 152
Short-limbed dwarfism with immunodeficiency, 321, 327–328
Short tandem repeats (STR) typing, 289
Shwachman syndrome, 338
Signal transduction
  cytokine receptors and, 9–13, *10*
  IL-2 receptors and, 155–156
  Jak/Stat signaling pathway, 11–13, *12*
  NF-κB signaling pathway, *12,* 13
  Ras-dependent signaling pathway, 11, *12*
  by T-cell receptor, 136–138, *137*
    CD45 and, 138, *138*
Simian immunodeficiency virus (SIV), 560, 637
Single-positive T lymphocytes, 45, *56,* 134
Single-strand conformational polymorphisms (SSCPs), 267,
      267
Sinusitis, 359
Sirolimus (rapamycin), 719, 749–750
SIV (simian immunodeficiency virus), 560, 637
Sjögren's syndrome, 94t, 411–413, 529
  complications and prognosis for, 412–413
  differential diagnosis of, 412
  immunologic diagnosis of, 412
  immunologic features of, 411
  immunologic pathogenesis of, 411
  laboratory findings in, 412
  MALT lymphomas and, 593
  pathology of, 411
  polymyositis-dermatomyositis and, 416
  progressive systemic sclerosis and, 414
  rheumatoid arthritis and, 407
  symptoms and signs of, 411–412, 412
  systemic lupus erythematosus and, 403
  treatment of, 412
Skin, 19
Skin conditions
  allergic contact dermatitis, 199, 386–388, 396
  anaphylaxis and, 371
  atopic dermatitis, 365–366
  blistering diseases, 495–507
    autoantibody binding and, 495, *496*
    bullous pemphigoid, 495–498, *497*
    dermatitis herpetiformis, 501–503, *502, 503*

Skin conditions *(continued)*
  blistering diseases, *(continued)*
    diagnosis of, 495
    epidermolysis bullosa acquisita, 500–501
    herpes gestationis, *499,* 499–500
    linear IgA bullous dermatosis, 503–504
    mucous membrane pemphigoid, 498–499
    paraneoplastic pemphigus, 506–507
    pemphigus vulgaris and pemphigus foliaceous, 504–506, *505, 506*
  in Churg-Strauss syndrome, 456
  cutaneous leishmaniasis, 677–679
  dermatophytosis, 661t
  fungal diseases, 656t
  in Lyme disease, 692, 693
  lymphocytes in, 54
  in microscopic polyangiitis, 453
  photoallergic contact dermatitis, 388–389
  in polyarteritis nodosa, 452
  polymyositis-dermatomyositis, 415–417
  in psoriatic arthritis, 418–419
  in rheumatoid arthritis, 407
  in scleroderma, 413–415
  in systemic lupus erythematosus, 402, 405
  in Takayasu's arteritis, 457
  urticaria and angioedema, 376–379
  in Wegener's granulomatosis, 454
Skin testing, 197
  for allergies, 354, *355,* 355t
  for anaphylaxis, 372, 372t
  anergy and, 199, 242, 242t
  for delayed-type hypersensitivity, 242–243, 242t, 296
  for echinococcosis, 684
  for leishmaniasis, 678
  patch testing, 243, 387, 387t, 397
    photopatch testing, 388
  severe local reactions to, 243
SLC (secondary lymphoid tissue chemokine), 59, 172–173, 172t
SLE. *See* Systemic lupus erythematosus
Sleeping sickness, 679–681, *680*
SLL (small lymphocytic lymphoma), 591
"Slow-reacting substance of anaphylaxis," 195
Small lymphocytic lymphoma (SLL), 591
Smallpox vaccine, 79, 79t, 701t
Snakebite antivenins, 705t, 706
SOCS (suppressors of cytokine signaling), 11, *12*
Sodium dodecyl sulfate-polyacrylamide gel electrophoresis (SDS-PAGE), 227
Solitary plasmacytoma, 596
Somatic hypermutation, 126
Southern, E. M., 263
Southern blot, 262–263, *265,* 586
Specific antiserum, 69
Specific granule deficiency, 336–337
SPEP (serum protein electrophoresis), 224–226, *224–226*
Sperm antigens, 550, 557
Sperm-egg fusion, 550–551
Sperm washing, 558
Spirochaetaceae, 688
Spirochetal diseases, 688–696
  Lyme disease, 692–696
  syphilis, 688–692
Spleen, 53, *53*
  lymphocyte proportions in, 41t
  onion skin lesion in systemic lupus erythematosus, 402
Splenectomy
  active immunization and, 702
  for pure erythrocyte aplasia, 441

Spondyloarthropathies, 417–420
  ankylosing spondylitis, 93–94, 94t, 417–418, 528, *528,* 611
  gram-negative rods and, 611
  hypogammaglobulinemia and arthritis, 420
  psoriatic arthritis, 418–419
  Reiter's syndrome, 418
  relapsing panniculitis, 419–420
  relapsing polychondritis, 419
Sporocysts, 682
Sporotrichosis, 656t
  effect of immunologic abnormalities on course of, 661t
  immunologic diagnosis of, 662t
  pathologic features of, 659t
Sporozoites, 674
S protein, 182t, 183
Spumiviruses, 637t
Src-family kinases, 11
SSCPs (single-strand conformational polymorphisms), 267, *267*
SSOP (sequence-specific oligonucleotide probing), 284–287, 284t, *286*
SSPE (subacute sclerosing panencephalitis), 625
SSP (sequence-specific priming), 284, 284t, *285*
Staphylococcus aureus, 132, 610
Staphylococcus epidermidis, 610
Stat proteins, 11, *12*
Status asthmaticus, 364
Stavudine (d4T), 645, 647t
Steblay nephritis, 482–483
Stem cell factor (SCF), *4, 5,* 8t, 41, 148, 162–163
  phenotypes of knockout mice, 163t
  receptor for, *10*
Stem cells. *See* Hematopoietic stem cells
Stiff-person syndrome, 524
Still's disease, 409–411
Stratum functionale, 548
Streptococcal infections, 610–611
Streptococcus agalactiae, 613
Streptococcus gordonii, 610
Streptococcus pneumoniae, 612
Streptococcus pyogenes, 610
Streptococcus sanguis, 477
Streptolysins O and S, 610
Stroke, 524–525
Stromal cells, 6–8
Stromal-derived factor 1 (SDF-1), 171
Strongyloides stercoralis, 684
STR (short tandem repeats) typing, 289
Subacute sclerosing panencephalitis (SSPE), 625
Subcapsular sinus of lymph node, 50, *51*
Subunit vaccine, 80
Sulfasalazine-induced lung disease, 537
Superantigens
  definition of, 132
  in lymphocyte activation assays, 244
  T-cell receptor interaction with, 132–133, *133*
Supergene family, immunoglobulin, 105–106, 105t, 163, 164t
Superoxide assay for chronic granulomatous disease, 241, 246–247, *247,* 294, 296
Superoxide dismutase, 192
Suppressors of cytokine signaling (SOCS), 11, *12*
"Swan neck" deformity, 407
"Swimmer's itch," 683
Switch regions, 125–126
Syk, 119, *120*
Sympathetic ophthalmia, 531–532
  clinical features of, 531
  immunologic diagnosis of, 531
  immunologic pathogenesis of, 531
  treatment of, 532

Sympathomimetic drugs, 756, 757t
  for asthma, 363–364, 756
Syncytiotrophoblast, 552
Syphilis, 688–692
  diagnosis of, 690–691, *691*
  epidemiology of, 688
  history of, 688
  latent and tertiary, 689
  pathogenesis of, 689–690
  prevention of, 692
  primary, 688
  secondary, 688–689
  transfusion-transmitted, 256
  treatment and prognosis for, 691–692
Systemic lupus erythematosus (SLE), 94t, 229, 401–405
  complications and prognosis for, 405
  differential diagnosis of, 405
  discoid, 405
  drug-induced lupus-like syndrome, 403, 537
  immunologic diagnosis of, 403–405
    anticytoplasmic antibodies, 405
    anti-DNA antibodies and immune complexes, 404
    antierythrocyte antibodies, 404
    antinuclear antibodies, 403–404, 404t
    circulating anticoagulants, antiphospholipids, and
      antiplatelet antibodies, 404–405
    complement deficiencies, 345, 346, 401, 403
    rheumatoid factors, 405
    tissue immunofluorescence, 405
  immunologic features of, 401
  immunologic pathogenesis of, 401–402
  laboratory findings in, 403
  pathology of, 402
    hematoxylin body, 402
    splenic onion skin lesion, 402
    verrucous endocarditis, 402
  symptoms and signs of, 402–403
    antiphospholipid syndrome, 449
    eyes, 403, 530, *530*
    gastrointestinal system, 403
    heart, 403
    joints and muscles, 402
    kidneys, 402, 489–491, *490,* 490t, 493
    lungs, 403
    nervous system, 403
    polyserositis, 402
    Sjögren's syndrome, 403
    skin, 402
    vascular system, 403
  treatment of, 405

Tabes dorsalis, 689
TACE (tumor necrosis factor α-converting enzyme), 151
Tachyzoites, 676
Tacrolimus, 748–749
  for transplant recipients, 719
    heart, 733
    heart-lung and lung, 735
    kidney, 721
    liver, 730
    pancreas, 732
Taenia saginata, 683
Taenia solium, 683
Tail segment, 100
Takayasu's arteritis, 405, 457
TAP-1 and TAP-2 (transporters of antigenic peptides), 83, 86,
  89, 90
Tapasin, 86, 88
Tapeworms, 683–684

TARC (thymus and activation-regulated cytokine), 172t
Tat protein, 638
TBM. *See* Tubular basement membrane
T-cell antigens, 82
  flow cytometric analysis of, 238–239
  origins of antigenic peptides, 82–83, 82t
    cytosolic pathway, 83
    endocytic pathway, 82–83
T-cell epitopes, 73, *74,* 77–79, *78*
  immunodominance and, 79, 93
  immunogenicity and, 77–79
T-cell growth factor. *See* Interleukin-2
T-cell immunodeficiency disorders, 239, 300t, 313–318. *See*
  also Combined B-cell and T-cell immunodeficiency
    disorders
  biotin-dependent carboxylase deficiencies, 318
  chronic mucocutaneous candidiasis, *316,* 316–317
  DiGeorge anomaly, 313–316, *314*
  idiopathic CD4 lymphocytopenia, 318
  immunologic evaluation for, 296, 301t, 313t
  treatment of, 301t
T-cell-independent antigens, 119, *121*
T-cell prolymphocytic leukemia (T-PLL), 598
T-cell receptor (TCR), 43–45, 61, 131–133, *132*
  αb structure and antigen recognition, 132
  α and β genes and generation of diversity, 131–132, *133*
  antigen-binding sites of, 77
  CD4 and CD8 coreceptors, 133, *133*
  epitope recognition by, 72, 73, 77
  interaction with superantigens, 132–133, *133*
  signal transduction by, 136–138, *137*
    CD45 and, 138, *138*
T cells. *See* T lymphocytes
TCR. *See* T-cell receptor
TdT (terminal deoxynucleotidyl transferase), 111, 115, *116,* 241
TECK (thymus-expressed cytokine), 54, 172, 172t
Temporal arteritis. *See* Giant-cell arteritis
Terbutaline, 364, 756
Terminal deoxynucleotidyl transferase (TdT), 111, 115, *116,* 241
Testis, 550
  autoimmune diseases of, 557
Tetanus, 608
Tetanus immune globulin, 705t
Tetanus toxoid, 79t, 80, 608, 610, 701t
Tetany, 608
Tetracycline-nicotinamide
  for bullous pemphigoid, 498
  for pemphigus vulgaris and pemphigus foliaceous, 506
TGFβ. *See* Transforming growth factor β
Theophylline, 364, 757
Third and fourth pouch/arch syndrome. *See* DiGeorge anomaly
THI (transient hypogammaglobulinemia of infancy), 305
3TC (lamivudine), 629, 645, 647t
Thrombocytopenia
  in antiphospholipid syndrome, 449
  causes of, 442
  classification of, 443t
  drug-induced, 443t, 445–446
  in HIV infection, 645
  HIV-related, 641
  immunodeficiency with eczema and (*See* Wiskott–Aldrich
    syndrome)
  neonatal alloimmune, 446
  posttransfusion purpura, 446
  quinine-induced, with hemolytic-uremic syndrome, 447
  thrombocytopenic purpura
    idiopathic, 443–445
    intravenous immunoglobulin for, 706
    thrombotic, 446–447

Thrombopoietin (TPO), 8t, 9, 162–163
  receptor for, *10*
Thrombotic thrombocytopenic purpura (TTP), 446–447
Thromboxane, 194, *196*
Thrush, 478–479
Thymocytes, 55–56, *56*
  development of, *3*, 40–41, *41*, 55–56, 133–134, *134*
  positive and negative selection of, 70, 90–91, 134–136, *135*
Thymoma, immunodeficiency with, 311
Thymus, 40–41, 54–56, *55*
  aplasia of (*See* DiGeorge anomaly)
  lymphocyte proportions in, 41t
  T lymphocytes in, 54–56, *56*
Thymus and activation-regulated cytokine (TARC), 172t
Thymus-expressed cytokine (TECK), 54, 172, 172t
Thyroid autoimmune diseases, 422–428
  Graves' disease, 426–428, *427*
  Hashimoto's thyroiditis, 422–425, *424, 425*
  primary hypothyroidism, 428
  transient thyroiditis syndromes, 425–426
TI-1 and TI-2 antigens, 119, *121*
Tinea nigra, 656t, 661t
Tinea versicolor, 656t, 661t
TIPS (transjugular intrahepatic portasystemic shunts), 726
Tissue kallikreins, 187
TLRs (Toll-like receptors), 36, *37*, 119, *121*
T lymphocytes, 2, 43–46, 131–143. *See also* Lymphocytes
  activation of, 41–42, *42*, 46–48, *47*, 77, 136–138
    assays of, 243–245
    costimulators for, 49, 49n, 66, 122, 138, *139*
    CTLA-4 inhibition of, 139
    cytokine production and, 244–245
    cytotoxic T cells, 66–67, *67*
    helper T cells, 65–66, *66*
    requirements for, *48*, 48–49, 49t
    signal transduction by T-cell receptor, 136–138, *137, 138*
  allergen desensitization and, 716
  in allograft rejection, 91
    kidney, 722–724, *723–725*
  anergic, 138, 759
    IL-2 treatment for, 156
  antigen presentation to, 63–65, *64*
  antigen specificity of, 82, 139
  autoreactive, 70, 91
  chemokine receptor expression by, *169*
  cytotoxic, 45–46, 139, 141–143
    activation of, 66–67, *67*
    assays for, 244
    functions of, 141–142
    killing by cytotoxic granules, 142, *142*
    killing by Fas ligand-Fas pathway, *142*, 142–143
    responses in HIV infection, 644
    viral effects on, 618t–619t
  development of, *3*, 40–41, *41*, 55–56, 133–134, *134*
  double-negative, 45, 55, *56*, 134
  double-positive, 45, 55, *56*
  evaluating function of, 296
  follicular, 205
  γ/δ cells, 143
  helper, 45t, 46, 48–49, 139–141
    activation of, 65–66, *66*, 139
    cytokines secreted by, 66, 140–141, 140t
    depletion in HIV infection, 638–641, *643*, 643–644
    differentiation into T$_H$1 and T$_H$2 cells, 140–141, *141*
    functions of, 139–140
    IL-1 and TNFα actions on, 148–149
  in HIV infection, 639, 643–644
  immune responses mediated by, 63–66, *64, 65*, 139–143

  immunophenotypic stages of early differentiation of, 579t
  intraepithelial, 206
  in lamina propria, 206–207
  in lymph nodes, 51
  lymphocytotoxicity crossmatching, 280, *281*
  memory, 46, 143, 242
  naive, 46, 56
  oral tolerance and, 211–212
  peptide-MHC recognition by, 90–91
    alloreactivity and transplant rejection, 91
  phenotyping of, 234–242
  positive and negative selection of, 70, 90–91, 134–136, *135*
  renal injury mediated by, 484–485
  role in tumor immunity, 571–572
  single-positive, 45, *56*, 134
  in spleen, 53
  subsets of, 45–46, 45t, 133, 139, 234
  surface molecules on, 45, 45t
    in B lymphocyte activation, 48–49, 66
  in thymus, 54–56, *56*
  tissue distribution of, 40, 41t
TNF. *See* Tumor necrosis factor
Tolerance
  B-cell, 128–129, *129*
  to immunogens, 73
  to liver transplantation, 726
  oral, *211*, 211–212
  of sperm "invasion," 550
Toll-like receptors (TLRs), 36, *37*, 119, *121*
Tonsils, 54
Toxemia of pregnancy, 563–565
Toxic shock-like syndrome, 610
Toxic shock syndrome, 132–133, 610
Toxins, 607–612
  Bacillus, 609
  Bordetella pertussis, 609–610
  Clostridium, 608–609
  Corynebacterium diphtheriae, 609
  definition of exotoxins and endotoxins, 607
  gram-negative rods, 611–612
  immunity to, 607–608, *608*
  monoclonal antibodies coupled to, 106
  neutralization of, 67–68
  Staphylococcus aureus, 610
  Streptococcus, 610–611
  TSST-1, 132
  Vibrio cholerae, 609
Toxoid vaccines, 79t, 80, 608–610
Toxoplasmosis, 83, 675–677, *676*
T-PLL (T-cell prolymphocytic leukemia), 598
TPO. *See* Thrombopoietin
TRAIL, 152t, 154
TRANCE, 152t, 153t, 154
Transcobalamin II deficiency, 311–312
Transferrin receptors, 45, 46
Transforming growth factor β (TGFβ), 14, 36t, 126, 148, 150t, 161–162
  cell sources and effects of, 161, *162*
  in IgA B-cell differentiation, 209, *210*
  inhibition of IL-1 and TNFα by, 154
  phenotypes of knockout mice, 153t
  receptors for, 161, 164t
Transfusion reactions, 254–257, 254t
  acute lung injury, 255
  allergic, 255
  febrile, 255
  hemolytic, 254–255
  immunologic mechanisms of, 256–257

infection, 255–256, 255t
in patients with selective IgA deficiency, 309–310
posttransfusion purpura, 446
Rh isoimmunization, 257
Transfusion-transmitted virus (TTV), 632
Transient hypogammaglobulinemia of infancy (THI), 305
Transient thyroiditis syndromes, 425–426
clinical features of, 425
de Quervain's thyroiditis, 425
immunologic diagnosis of, 425
immunologic features of, 425
pathology of, 425
postpartum thyroiditis, 425
prognosis for, 425
treatment of, 425
Transjugular intrahepatic portasystemic shunts (TIPS), 726
Translocations in hematologic malignancies, 113–114,
582–584, 586t
acute lymphoblastic leukemia, 591
Burkitt's lymphoma, 113, *113,* 583–584, 595
mantle cell lymphoma, 592
molecular genetic analysis of, 586
Transplantation, 719–742
bone, 740–741
bone marrow, 736–740
chimerism testing after, 289
cornea, 292, *533,* 533–534
cytokine therapy and, 436
future of, 741–742
heart, 291, 732–734
heart-lung and lung, 734–736
histocompatibility testing for, 270–272, 271t, 290–292,
291t
history of, 719
immunosuppressive therapy for, 719
kidney, 291, 291t, 719–726
liver, 291–292, 726–730
lymphoproliferative disorders after, 602–603
pancreas, 730–732
pancreatic, islet cell transplantation, 732
United Network for Organ Sharing, 291
Websites related to, 271t
Transporters of antigenic peptides (TAP-1 and TAP-2), 83, 86,
89, 90
Trematodes, 681–683
Treponema, 688
Treponema pallidum, 688
Treponema pallidum rare outer membrane proteins (TROMPs),
689–690
Triamcinolone, *749,* 750t
Trichinosis, 191, 684–685
Trichosporon beigelii, 655
Trimethoprim-sulfamethoxazole
desensitization for allergy to, 398
for pneumocystosis, 671, 738
for Wegener's granulomatosis, 455
TROMPs (*Treponema pallidum* rare outer membrane proteins),
689–690
Tropheryma whippelii, 463
Trophoblast, 552, *553*
Tropical pulmonary eosinophilia, 540
Tropical sore, 677–679
Trypanosoma cruzi, 256
Tryptase, 192, 195
TTP (thrombotic thrombocytopenic purpura), 446–447
TTV (transfusion-transmitted virus), 632
Tuberculosis, 199, 615
BCG vaccine against, 79, 701t
PPD skin testing for, 242–243

Tubular basement membrane (TBM), 482
anti-TBM disease, 483, 493
Tuftsin deficiency, 338
Tularensis, 221
Tumor immunology, 568–576
antigens on tumor cells, 569–571
common properties of tumors, 568t
development of tumors, 568–569
carcinogens, 568–569
oncogenic viruses, 569, 570
immunologic effector mechanisms potentially operative
against tumor cells, 571–573
B cells and antibody-dependent killing, 572
macrophages, 573
natural killer cells, 572–573
T cells, 571–572
immunotherapy, 574–576
adoptive T-cell therapy, 575–576
immunization to tumor antigens, 574–575
monoclonal antibodies, 576
mechanisms permitting tumor cell escape from immune
response, 573–574
Tumor necrosis factor α-converting enzyme (TACE), 151
Tumor necrosis factor α (TNFα), *12, 16,* 21, 36t, 148–149,
151–154
actions on helper T cells, 148–149
in adult respiratory distress syndrome, 546
gene for, 87, *88*
inhibitors of, 757–758
in mast cells, 192
nonimmunologic inflammatory effects of, 152
phenotypes of knockout mice, 153t
properties of, 150t
receptors for (TNFRI and TNFRII), 45t, 151–152
synthesis of, 151
target cells and actions of, 151t, 153
as therapeutic agent, 154
viral effects on, 619t
Tumor necrosis factor β (TNFβ), 87, *88,* 154
inhibitors of, 757–758
Tumor necrosis factor receptor superfamily, 152t, 154, 164t
Type I (immediate) hypersensitivity reactions, 201–202, *202,*
394–395
drugs for suppression of, 755–757
antihistamines, 756, 756t
anti-IgE monoclonal antibodies, 756
cromolyn sodium, 755–756
methylxanthines, 757
sympathomimetic drugs, 756, 757t
Type II (cytotoxic) hypersensitivity reactions, 395
Type III (immune complex-mediated) hypersensitivity
reactions, 380–385, 396
allergic bronchopulmonary aspergillosis, 365, 382–385
Arthus reaction, 199, 242, 380, 381t
drug allergy, 396
serum sickness, 199, 201, 381–382, 381t, *382,* 396
Type IV (delayed-type) hypersensitivity reactions, 37,
197–199, 242–243, 242t, 386, 396
allergic contact dermatitis, 386–388, 396
in HIV infection, 644
hypersensitivity pneumonitis, 389–393
photoallergic contact dermatitis, 388–389
skin testing for, 242–243, 242t, 296
contact hypersensitivity, 243
patch testing, 243, 387, 387t, 397
PPD test, 242–243
Typhoid fever, 614
Typhoid vaccine, 701t
Tyrosine kinase receptor family, 164t

Ufd1 gene, 314
Ulcerative colitis, 468–469
  clinical features of, 469
  complications and prognosis for, 469
  differential diagnosis of, 469
  epidemiology of, 468
  immunologic diagnosis of, 469
  immunologic features of, 468
  immunopathology of, 468–469
  selective IgA deficiency and, 308
  treatment of, 469
United Network for Organ Sharing (UNOS), 291
Ursodeoxycholic acid, 472
Urticaria
  allergic, 202, 349
  angioedema and, 376–379
    anaphylaxis and, 371
    causes of, 378
    differential diagnosis of, 378
    epidemiology of, 377
    idiopathic, 378
    immunologic diagnosis of, 377–378
    immunologic features of, 376
    pathogenesis of, 377
    pathology of, 377
    symptoms and signs of, 377
    treatment of, 375, 378–379
  cholinergic, 378
  cold, 378
  pigmentosa, 378
  pressure, 378
Uterus, 548
Uveitis, 94t
  lens-induced, 530

Vaccine Adverse Event Reporting System, 703
Vaccines, 79–80, 79t, 701t. *See also* Immunization
  adverse reactions to, 702–703, 704t
  allergic reactions to, 703
  anthrax, 609
  attenuated, 80, 700
  bacillus Calmette-Guèrin, 79, 615, 701t
  cholera, 609, 708
  currently in development, 712
  cytomegalovirus, 650
  DNA, 80
    for allergen immunotherapy, 717
  DPT, 610, 701t, 702, 709
  against encapsulated bacteria, 612
  glycoconjugate, 80
  Haemophilus influenzae type B, 79t, 80, 295, 613, 701t
  hepatitis A, 79t, 628, 701t, 707
  hepatitis B, 79t, 80, 630, 701t, 707
  HIV, 648, 648t, 712
  inactivated, 700
  inclusion of immunomodulators in, 80
  influenza, 623, 701t, 707–708
  Japanese encephalitis, 701t
  killed, 80, 700
  live, 79, 700
    hazards of, 702–703
  Lyme disease, 696, 701t, 708
  malaria, 675
  measles, 79t, 626, 701t
  meningococcal, 701t
  MMR, 702t
  mumps, 79t, 701t

  peptide, 80
  pertussis, 79t, 609–610, 701t, 707
  plague, 701t
  pneumococcal, 295, 311, 612, 701t
  polio, 79t, 80, 634, 700, 701t, 707
    Sabin, 79t, 80, 707
    Salk, 79t, 80, 707
  rabies, 633, 701t, 708
  recombinant DNA, 700
  respiratory syncytial virus, 624–625
  rotavirus, 701t, 708
  rubella, 79t, 701t
  smallpox, 79, 79t, 701t
  subunit, 80
  toxoid, 80
    diphtheria, 79t, 80, 609, 610, 701t
    tetanus, 79t, 80, 608, 610, 701t
  tumor, 574–575
  types of, 79–80, 700
  typhoid, 701t
  use of interleukin-12 with, 80, 141
  varicella, 701t, 708
  yellow fever, 701t
Vaccinia (cowpox) virus, 79, 164
Vaginal mucosa, 548
Variable number tandem repeats (VNTR) typing, 289
Variable region, immunoglobulin, *96,* 97, 102–103
  framework and hypervariable regions, 103, *103*
  idiotypes of, 103
  subgroups of, 103
Varicella vaccine, 701t, 708
Varicella-zoster immune globulin, 705t
Vascular addressins, 58–59, 59t
Vascular cell adhesion molecule 1 (VCAM-1), 6, 27, 27t, 202
Vascular leak syndrome, 156
Vasculitis, 451–458
  in Behçet's disease, 417
  Buerger's disease, 457–458
  Churg-Strauss syndrome, 455–456
  classification of, 458
  giant-cell arteritis, 456–457
  glomerular lesions associated with, 491–493
    ANCA-associated diseases, 492
    antiglomerular basement membrane disease, *482,*
      482–483, 491–492
  Henoch-Schönlein's purpura, 458
  hypersensitivity angiitis, 458
  immunologic mechanisms of, 451
    antineutrophil cytoplasmic antibodies, 451, 483–484
  Kawasaki's disease, 458
  microscopic polyangiitis, 453–454
  polyarteritis nodosa, 451–453
  in polymyositis-dermatomyositis, 416
  pulmonary, 545–546, 545t
    bronchocentric granulomatosis, 545–546
    lymphomatoid granulomatosis, 545
    necrotizing sarcoid granulomatosis, 545
  in rheumatoid arthritis, 407
  as sign of pancreatic allograft rejection, 732
  syphilitic aortitis, 689
  in systemic lupus erythematosus, 403
  Takayasu's arteritis, 457
  urticaria and, 378
  Wegener's granulomatosis, 454–455
Vasodilatation, *25,* 25–26, 25t
Vasovagal collapse, 375
VCAM-1 (vascular cell adhesion molecule 1), 6, 27, 27t, 202
V/(D)/J recombinase, 112

Venereal Disease Research Laboratory (VDRL) test, 690–691, *691*

Venous thrombosis, antiphospholipid syndrome and, 448

Venules
high endothelial, *58, 58*–59
postcapillary, 26

Vernal conjunctivitis, 357, 527, *528*

Vibrio cholerae, 609

vif gene, 638, *638*

Villous atrophy
in gluten-sensitive enteropathy, 460–462, *461*
not due to gluten sensitivity, 462–463

Vincristine, 445

Viral infections, 617–634. *See also* specific viruses
chronic, 617
clinical features of, 617
cytomegalovirus, 649–650
Epstein–Barr virus, 650–653
hepatitis, 627–632
hepatitis A, 627–628
hepatitis B, 628–630, *630*
hepatitis C, 630–632
hepatitis delta, 632
hepatitis E, 632
hepatitis G, 632
HIV, 5, 636–648
human herpesvirus 6, 653–654
human herpesvirus 8, 626–627
human T-cell lymphotrophic virus I/II, 653
immunologic sequelae of, 621t
immunopathic effects of, 617
influenza virus, 617–623, *621,* 621t
latent, 617
measles virus, 625–626
poliovirus, 633–634
rabies virus, 632–633
respiratory syncytial virus, 623–625, *624*
transfusion-transmitted virus, 632
viropathic effects of, 617

Viral load in HIV infection, 639
monitoring of, 646–647
virologic set-point, 639

Viridans streptococci, 611

Virokines, 164

Virologic set-point, in HIV infection, 639

Viroreceptors, 164

Virulence factors
bacterial, 608, *608,* 610
viral, 617

Viruses
activation of classical complement pathway by, 179
antigens from, 83
antiviral interferons, *160,* 160–161
DNA, 569
genome of, 617
interactions with chemokine pathways, 173
neutralization of, 68
oncogenic, 569, 570
retroviruses, 569
RNA, 569
strategies to evade host immune responses, 617, 618t–620t

Visceral larva migrans, 540

Visceral leishmaniasis, 679

Visna virus, 637

Vitamin B$_{12}$ malabsorption, 464–465

Vitronectin, 183

VNTR (variable number tandem repeats) typing, 289

Vogt-Koyanagi-Harada syndrome, 531–532
clinical features of, 531
immunologic diagnosis of, 531–532
immunologic pathogenesis of, 531
treatment of, 532

von Willebrand factor, 259
inhibitors against, 448
thrombotic thrombocytopenic purpura and, 447

vpr gene, 638, *638*

vpu gene, 638, *638*

Waldenström's macroglobulinemia, 224, *225,* 228, 592

Warm autoimmune hemolytic anemia, 437–439
clinical features of, 438
differential diagnosis of, 438
idiopathic vs. secondary, 438
immunologic diagnosis of, 438, 438t
immunologic features of, 437–438
prognosis for, 439
treatment of, 438–439

WAS. *See* Wiskott–Aldrich syndrome

WASP gene, 297, 323

Weber-Christian disease, 419–420

Wegener's granulomatosis, 454–455
diagnosis of, 455
immunologic features of, 454
laboratory findings in, 455
pathogenesis of, 454
prognosis for, 455
signs and symptoms of, 454–455
renal, 492–493
treatment of, 455

Western blot, 227, *228,* 642, *642*

Wheal-and-flare reactions, 195, 242, 354, 355t

Whipple's disease, 463

White blood cells. *See* Leukocytes

White piedra, 656t, 661t

White pulp, splenic, 53

Whooping cough, 609–610
vaccine against, 79t, 609–610, 701t, 707

Wiskott–Aldrich syndrome (WAS), 239, 295, 297, 320, 323–324
complications and prognosis for, 324
differential diagnosis of, 324
immunologic diagnosis of, 324
immunologic features of, 323
immunologic pathogenesis of, 323
laboratory findings in, 324
symptoms and signs of, 323–324, *324*
treatment of, 324

Wuchereria bancrofti, 256, 684–686

Xanthines, 364, 757

X-linked agammaglobulinemia (XLA), 117, 240, 295, 297, 302–305
complications and prognosis for, 305
differential diagnosis of, 304
immunologic diagnosis of, 304
immunologic features of, 302
immunologic pathogenesis of, 302
laboratory and imaging findings in, 303–304
molecular diagnosis of, 304
symptoms and signs of, 302–303, *303*
treatment of, 304–305

X-linked chronic granulomatous disease, 334–336

X-linked lymphoproliferative syndrome, 295, 330–331, 650, 651

X-linked severe combined immunodeficiency, 321

Yellow fever vaccine, 701t
Yersinia, 611

Zafirlukast, 364, 755
Zalcitabine (ddC), 645, 647t
Zanamavir, 622
ZAP-70 deficiency, 296, 297, 321

Zidovudine (AZT), 645, 647t
Zileuton, 755
Zona pellucida, 551
Zone electrophoresis, 224, *224–226*
Zone of equivalence, 215
Zoonoses, 676
Zygomycosis. *See* Mucormycosis